Textbook of Clinical Neuropsychiatry

Textbook of Clinical Neuropsychiatry

Second edition

David P Moore MD
Associate Clinical Professor, Department of Psychiatry, Associate
Clinical Professor, Department of Neurosurgery (Division of Physical
Medicine and Rehabilitation), University of Louisville School of
Medicine, Louisville, Kentucky, USA

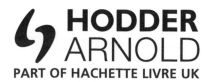

**HODDER
ARNOLD**
PART OF HACHETTE LIVRE UK

First published in Great Britain in 2001 by Arnold
This second edition published in 2008 by Hodder Arnold,
an imprint of Hodder Education, part of Hachette Livre UK,
338 Euston Road, London NW1 3BH

http://www.hoddereducation.com

British Library Cataloguing in Publication Data
A catalogue record for this book is available from the British Library

Library of Congress Cataloging-in-Publication Data
A catalog record for this book is available from the Library of Congress

ISBN-13 978 0 340 93953 6

1 2 3 4 5 6 7 8 9 10

Commissioning Editor: Philip Shaw
Project Editor: Amy Mulick
Production Controller: Karen Tate
Cover Design: Helen Townson

Typeset in 10/12 pt Minion by Charon Tec Ltd
(A Macmillan Company), Chennai, India
www.charontec.com
Printed and bound in Great Britain

Dedication

This book is dedicated to my wife, Nancy G Moore, PhD, my children, Ethan, Nathaniel, and Joshua, and to James W Jefferson, MD, for whose example and guidance I remain ever thankful. I also wish to express my gratitude to Professors Raymond Faber, Michael R Trimble and Elden Tunks, whose kind words made this second edition possible.

'*Scribere actum fidei est*'

Contents

Preface

This second edition of the *Textbook of Clinical Neuropsychiatry*, like the first, is a practical, clinically oriented text that is designed to equip readers to diagnose and treat the multitude of neuropsychiatric disorders they encounter. It is divided into three parts: Part 1 describes the diagnostic assessment of patients and details the interview, mental status examination, neurologic examination and ancillary investigations; Part 2 provides a thorough description of the various signs, symptoms and syndromes that are seen in neuropsychiatric practice; and Part 3 presents virtually all of the specific disorders seen in neuropsychiatric practice, in each instance detailing clinical features, course, etiology, differential diagnosis, and treatment.

The literature devoted to neuropsychiatric disorders is vast, encompassing, as it does, much of both neurology and psychiatry, and I have attempted to cull from this tremendous reservoir those references that are of most use to the clinician. Although the preponderance of references are from the recent past, classic authors are not neglected and readers will find references to the works of such physicians as Alzheimer, Binswanger, Bleuler, Hughlings Jackson, Kraepelin, and Kinnier Wilson. In all, over 5000 references are included, thus providing readers not only with ready access to further detail on any particular subject, but also with a window on the literature as a whole.

I am deeply indebted to the reviewers of the first edition, and to many other readers who have offered comments, critiques, and suggestions: they have enabled me to write a second edition, which, I believe, is far stronger than the first. Neuropsychiatry is a rapidly growing specialty, and it is my hope that this text will not only help solidify the field but also enable the reader to practice it successfully. As with the first edition, so too with this second one, I invite both newcomers and established practitioners to try using it in their own practices, as I think they may well find it as indispensable as I do.

David P Moore
September 2007

DIAGNOSTIC ASSESSMENT

Diagnostic assessment

1.1 DIAGNOSTIC INTERVIEW

Lord Brain (1964) noted that 'in the diagnosis of nervous diseases the history of the patient's illness is often of greater importance than the discovery of his abnormal physical signs', a sentiment echoed by Russell DeJong (1979) who asserted that 'a good clinical history often holds the key to diagnosis'.

Obtaining the history, however, as noted by DeJong (1979), 'is no simple task [and] may require greater skill and experience than are necessary to carry out a detailed examination'. The acquisition of this skill is, for most, no easy matter, requiring, above all, practice and supervision. Certain points, however, may be made regarding the setting of the interview, establishing rapport, eliciting the chief complaint, the division of the interview itself into non-directive and directive portions, concluding the interview, and the subsequent acquisition of collateral history from family or acquaintances. Even these general points, however, allow exceptions depending on the clinical situation, and the physician must be flexible and prepared to exercise initiative.

Setting

The interview should ideally be conducted in a quiet and private setting, set apart from distractions and anything that might inhibit patients as they relate the history. Importantly, that means that family and friends should be excused during the interview, as patients may feel reluctant to reveal certain facts in their presence. If the interview takes place at the bedside, the physician should be seated; standing implies that time is short, and some patients, picking up on this cue, may skip over potentially valuable parts of the history in order not to waste the physician's time. In this regard, it is also important that the physician

sets aside a sufficient amount of time to take the history, which may range from less than half an hour in uncomplicated cases related by cooperative patients to well over an hour when the history is long and complex or the patient is unable to cooperate fully. There is debate as to whether the physician should take notes during the interview: some feel it is distracting, both to the patient and the physician, whereas others recommend it in order to ensure accuracy, especially when the interview is lengthy. I agree with Victor (Victor and Ropper 2001) who feels that the practice is 'particularly recommended'. The idea is not to make a transcript but simply to jot down key points and dates, and to do so in a way that allows the physician to maintain his or her attention on what the patient is saying.

Establishing rapport

DeJong (1979) noted that 'interest, understanding, and sympathy' are essential to the successful conduct of the interview: patients who experience a sense of rapport with their physicians are more likely to be truthful and forthcoming; hence establishing rapport is of great importance.

First impressions carry great weight here: after introducing themselves, physicians should clearly relate their role in the case and then, as suggested by DeJong (1979), display 'kindness, patience, reserve, and a manner which conveys interest' throughout the interview. Provided with such a forum, most patients will, with only minor help, provide the history required to generate the appropriate differential diagnosis.

Eliciting the chief complaint

'It is well', noted Lord Brain (1964), 'to begin by asking the patient of what he complains'. The chief complaint is the epitome of the patient's illness: lacking such a focus, digressions are almost inevitable, and the history obtained may be of little diagnostic use. Thus, once introductions are out of the way the first question put by the physician should focus on what brought the patient to the hospital. Critically, as some patients may be reluctant to reveal the actual reason for their coming to the hospital, it is necessary to weigh the chief complaint offered by the patient and ask oneself whether, in fact, it sounds like a plausible reason to seek medical attention. If not, gentle probing is in order and should generally be continued until the actual chief complaint is revealed. Importantly, the physician should never accept at face value a diagnosis offered by a patient: as Bickerstaff (1980) pointed out, 'it must be made absolutely clear what the patient means by his description of his symptoms. By all means put it down in his words first, but do not be content with that . . . "Black-outs" may mean loss of consciousness, loss of vision, loss of memory, or just loss of confidence'.

Occasionally, it may not be possible to establish a chief complaint during the interview, as may occur with patients who are delirious, demented, psychotic, or simply hostile and uncooperative. In such cases, persisting overly long in the pursuit of a chief complaint may become counterproductive as patients may become resentful, and it is generally more appropriate to move on to the 'directive' portion of the interview described below, always being alert, however, to the possibility that the patient may 'slip in' the chief complaint at an unexpected moment.

The non-directive portion of the interview

Once a chief complaint has been established, the patient, as noted by Brain (1964), 'should be allowed to relate the story of his illness as far as possible without interruption, questions being put to him afterwards to expand his statements and to elicit additional information'. Some patients, once asked to expand on the chief complaint, may, with little or no prompting, provide the 'perfect' history, covering each of the following essential points:

- onset, including approximate date and mode of onset (acute, gradual, or insidious)
- presence or absence of any precipitating factors
- temporal evolution of various signs and symptoms
- presence or absence of any aggravating or alleviating factors
- treatment efforts and their results
- pertinent positives and negatives
- any history of similar experiences in the past.

Most patients will require, however, either encouragement or some gentle shepherding at various times. When patients begin to falter in their history, or seem to be leaving items out, it is appropriate to encourage them to talk by asking 'open-ended' questions such as 'Tell me more about that'. Such a method is much to be preferred over the 'question-and-answer' approach used by many. The problem with the 'question-and-answer' approach is that many patients will lose the initiative to speak, and simply await questions from the physician, which is all well and good unless, of course, the physician fails to ask the 'right' questions, in which case potentially critical aspects of the history may remain unrevealed.

Gentle shepherding may be required in cases when patients digress or take off at a tangent. One should not, of course, rudely pull the patient back to task, but rather tactfully suggest that refocusing on the illness that prompted admission might be more appropriate.

Once the essential points have been covered, it is appropriate to summarize briefly what the patient has said in order to be sure that the history, as understood by the physician, is correct. Patients should be invited to correct any misapprehensions and once the history is complete the physician should move on to the directive portion of the interview.

The directive portion of the interview

The directive portion of the interview should be introduced to the patient as a series of perhaps 'routine' questions relating to the patient's overall health. Here, one obtains information regarding the medications that the patient is taking, allergies, the past medical history, a review of systems, the family medical history and, finally, the mental status examination (discussed in Section 1.2). In this regard, two points deserve special emphasis. First, when interviewing hospitalized patients it is essential to obtain an absolutely accurate list of medicines that the patient was taking at home, prior to admission: medication changes often provide the clue to otherwise puzzling syndromes, such as delirium, which may occur during the hospital stay. Second, given the increasing importance of genetics in neuropsychiatric practice, it is essential to obtain a detailed family history regarding any neuropsychiatric illness.

During the directive portion of the interview, although a question-and-answer approach is generally appropriate the physician must always be ready to adopt a non-directive approach should the patient report a symptom or illness potentially pertinent to the chief complaint. For example, if during the review of systems the patient affirms that headaches have been present it is appropriate to stop and ask the patient to elaborate on this, with an eye towards obtaining information regarding each of the essential points described earlier.

Questions regarding alcohol/drug use and suicidal/homicidal ideation must be directly pursued if not already covered in the non-directive portion of the interview. These are, of course, delicate areas, but, if approached in a straightforward and non-judgmental way, it is remarkable how forthcoming, and indeed relieved, some patients may be at being given an opportunity to speak of them.

Concluding the interview

Once the directive portion of the interview has been completed it is appropriate to give the patient an opportunity to speak freely again. If asked whether they have anything else to add, many patients will offer important information that they may have either withheld or simply not recalled earlier. Asking patients whether they have anything they wish to ask the physician is also appropriate, as the patients' questions may reveal much about the concerns that brought them to the hospital in the first place.

Collateral history

According to Brain (1964), 'the history obtained from the patient should always be supplemented, if possible, by an account of his illness given by a relative or by someone who knows him well'. This is especially the case when patients are confused or suffer from poor memory: it is remarkable how often a collateral history will change a diagnostic impression, guide further testing or alter proposed treatments. In obtaining the collateral history, particular attention should be paid to establishing the patient's pre-morbid baseline ability to perform such routine activities of daily living as bathing, dressing, cooking, feeding, doing housework, shopping, driving or using public transportation, and paying bills. Inquiry should also be made regarding hobbies, such as playing cards or chess, or doing crossword puzzles. In cases characterized by cognitive deficits, the loss of these abilities may serve to establish the onset of the current illness.

Some have expressed concern that interviewing the family or acquaintances may violate patient confidentiality but this is simply not the case, provided that the contact knows already that the patient is in the hospital and that the physician reveals nothing about the patient while interviewing the collateral contact. No confidentiality is breached by introducing oneself as the patient's physician or by asking collateral contacts what they know about the patient.

Finally, it is also essential to review old records. This is sometimes a tedious task but, as with interviewing collateral sources, it may reveal critical information.

1.2 MENTAL STATUS EXAMINATION

The mental status examination constitutes an essential part of any neuropsychiatric evaluation and, at a minimum, should cover each of the items discussed below. Many of these may be determined during the non-directive portion of the interview; however, some, especially those concerning cognition (e.g., orientation, memory), require direct testing. As some patients may object to cognitive testing, it is important to smooth the way by indicating that these are 'routine' questions to test 'things such as memory and arithmetic', perhaps adding that 'patients who have had a stroke (or whatever illness the patient feels comfortable discussing) often have difficulties here'. Should patients remain uncooperative, it may at times be possible to infer their cognitive status indirectly; for example, during history taking, by asking the date of a recent event brought up by the patient.

As noted below, abnormalities on the mental status examination typically indicate the presence of one of the major syndromes, such as dementia (Section 5.1), delirium (Section 5.3), amnesia (Section 5.4), depression (Section 6.1), apathy (Section 6.2), mania (Section 6.3), anxiety (Section 6.5), psychosis (Section 7.1), and personality change (Section 7.2), especially the frontal lobe syndrome.

Grooming and dress

Good habits of grooming and dress may suffer in certain illnesses, sometimes with diagnostically suggestive results. Depressive patients may find that hopelessness, fatigue, and anhedonia make them give up all hope of maintaining their appearance, with the result that grooming and dress are left in a greater or lesser degree of disarray. Manic patients, overflowing with exuberance, may truly make a spectacle of themselves with decorations of make-up and garish clothing. Patients with psychosis, especially schizophrenia (Section 20.1) may be quite unkempt and at times dirty, and their clothing may be bizarre, as, for example, with multiple layers and a woollen cap, even in the summer; overall dishevellment may also be seen in frontal lobe syndrome, dementia, or delirium. Rarely, one may see evidence of neglect wherein dress and grooming suffer on only one side of the body (Section 2.1).

General description

An overall and general description of the patient's behavior is essential, and gives room for the exercise of whatever literary talents the physician may possess.

Comments should be made on the relationship of the patient to the interviewer, noting, for example, whether the patient is cooperative or uncooperative, guarded, evasive, hostile, or belligerent. The overall quality of the relationship may also be of diagnostic importance. For example, as noted by Bleuler (1924), in schizophrenia, there is often a *defect in . . . emotional rapport* (italics in original), such that 'the joy of a schizophrenic does not transport us, and his expressions of pain leave us cold'. By contrast, in mania, as noted by Kraepelin (1921), 'the patient feels the need to get out of himself, to be on more intimate terms with his surroundings', such that the physician, willingly or not, often feels engaged, in one fashion or another, with the patient; in the case of a euphoric manic it is the rare physician who can keep from smiling, and in the case of an irritable manic most physicians will find themselves becoming, at the very least, on edge.

During the interview, one may also find evidence of certain discrete personality changes. Perseveration, disinhibition, and a tendency to puerile, silly puns or jokes may suggest frontal lobe syndrome, and in epileptics one may find evidence of the interictal personality syndrome with an overall 'viscosity' or 'adhesiveness', such that patients are unable to manage changing the subject or switching tasks. Evidence of the Kluver–Bucy syndrome (Section 4.12) may also be apparent should patients repeatedly put inedible objects in their mouths or engage in indiscriminate sexual activity.

Consideration should also be given to the overall level of the patient's verbal and motor behavior, noting whether there is either psychomotor hyperactivity or retardation.

Psychomotor hyperactivity may manifest with agitation (Section 6.4) or mere restlessness, and the activity itself may or may not be purposeful. For example, hyperactivity may be quite purposeful in mania: as pointed out by Kraepelin (1899), the manic patient 'feels the need to come out of his shell [and] to have livelier relations with those around him'. By contrast, in excited catatonia (Section 3.11) behavior is typically purposeless and bizarre: Kraepelin (1899), in commenting on this difference between mania and catatonia, noted that 'the catatonic's urge to move often takes place in the smallest space, i.e. in part of the bed, whereas the manic looks everywhere for an opportunity to be active, and runs around, occupies himself with other patients, follows the doctor and gets into all kinds of mischief'.

Psychomotor retardation may range from an almost total quietude and immobility to a mere slowing of speech and behavior. Various conditions may underlie such a change. Mere exhaustion may slow patients down, but the response to rest is generally robust. Apathetic patients, lacking in motivation, may evidence little speech or behavior; depressed patients may appear similar but here one also sees a depressed mood. In akinesia (Section 3.9) there may also be a generalized slowing of all behavior; however, here one also fails to see a depressed mood. Abulia (Section 4.10) is distinguished from akinesia by the response to supervision: in contrast with patients with apathy, depression, or akinesia, the abulic patient performs at a normal rate when supervised. Delirium may be characterized by quietude and inactivity but is distinguished by the presence of confusion and deficits in memory and orientation. Catatonia of the stuporous type (Section 3.11) may be characterized by profound immobility; however, here one typically finds distinctive associated signs, such as waxy flexibility, posturing, and negativism. Finally, one should never forget hypothyroidism, wherein, as noted by Kraepelin (1899), it may take patients 'an incredibly long time to do the simplest things, to write a letter [or] to get dressed'.

Other behavioral disturbances may occur during the interview and examination, including mannerisms, stereotypies, and echopraxia. Mannerisms represent more or less bizarre transformations of speech, gesture, or other behaviors (Section 4.27). Stereotypies are a kind of perseveration wherein patients repeatedly engage in the same behaviors, to no apparent purpose (Section 4.28). Echopraxia is said to be present when patients involuntarily mimic what others, such as the examining physician, do (Section 4.29) Although each of these disturbances may be seen in schizophrenia, they are also present in other disorders such as dementia.

Mood and affect

Mood is constituted by an individual's prevailing emotional 'tone'. When this is within the broad limits of normal, one speaks of 'euthymia' or a euthymic mood; significant mood disturbances may tend toward depression, euphoria, anxiety, or irritability. Depressed mood may be characterized by 'a profound inward dejection and gloomy hopelessness' (Kraepelin 1921); in contrast, euphoria is characterized by an 'overflowing contentment' (Griesinger 1882), such patients being 'penetrated with great merriment' (Kraepelin 1921). Anxious patients are beset with apprehensions, may plead for help, and may complain of tremor and palpitations. Irritable patients are typically 'dissatisfied, intolerant [and] fault-finding' (Kraepelin 1921), often quick to react to any perceived slight or criticism.

In the case of euphoria or irritability, one should also note whether or not the mood is 'heightened', that is to say whether or not it is so abundant and at such a level that its display in strong affect is simply inevitable: for example, patients with a heightened sense of irritability may be hostile, argumentative, and uncontrollably angry, whereas other patients whose irritability is not heightened might present a picture of mere sullenness and withdrawal.

Affect has been variously defined as representing either the combination of the immediately present emotion and its accompanying expression in tone of voice, gesture, facial expression, etc. or, less commonly, as only the emotional expression itself. Although in general there is a congruence between the experienced emotion and the facial expression, disparities may arise, as in 'inappropriate affect' (Section 4.26), sensory aprosodia (Section 2.7), emotional facial palsy (Section 4.8), and 'emotional incontinence' (as seen in pseudobulbar palsy [Section 4.7]). In each of these conditions patients report a substantial difference between what they are feeling and what is 'showing' on their faces. This is perhaps most dramatic in emotional incontinence (or, as Wilson [1928] called it, 'pathological laughing and crying'), which is characterized by an uncontrollable affective display that occurs in the absence of any corresponding feeling. Thus 'incontinent' of affective display, patients may burst forth into laughter or tears upon the slightest of stimuli and be unable to control themselves despite the lack of any sense of mirth or sadness.

Given that, as with mood, affect may be depressed, euphoric, anxious, or irritable it may appear academic to distinguish between the two; however, disparities between mood and affect may arise. Mood is enduring, whereas affect is relatively changeable: in a sense, mood is to climate as affect is to weather. Thus, patients suffering from a depressed mood that has generally endured for weeks, months, or longer may at times during the day experience a normal, or near-normal affect, and in such cases if the physician depended solely on observation of the patient's affect and did not inquire of the overall enduring mood an important clinical finding might be missed.

Affect, in addition to being depressed, euphoric, anxious or irritable, may also be flattened or labile. Flattened (or 'blunted' as it is also known) affect is characterized by a lifeless and wooden facial expression, accompanied by an absence or diminution of feeling. As such, it may be distinguished from motor aprosodia (Section 2.7), wherein patients do in fact still experience feelings, although speaking in a monotone as if they had no feelings. The 'hypomimia' seen in parkinsonian conditions, such as Parkinson's disease or antipsychotic-induced parkinsonism, is distinguished in the same way: although these patients' facial movements are more or less frozen and devoid of expression they still may have strong feelings. Some investigators believe flattened affect is also present in severe depression; however, in my experience there is little difficulty in distinguishing a flattened from a depressed affect. Flattened affect is found very commonly in schizophrenia (Andreasen et al. 1979); it may also occur in some secondary psychoses (Cornelius et al. 1992) and, rarely, in dementia secondary to infarction of the mesencephalon or thalamus (Katz et al. 1987).

Labile affect is characterized by swift, and sometimes violent, changes in both felt and expressed emotion.

Disturbances of mood are seen in a large number of conditions, as discussed in the chapters on depression, mania, and anxiety. Furthermore, it must be stressed that changes in mood, and especially affect, are also very common in dementia and delirium. This is particularly important to keep in mind, given that effective treatment of delirium typically results in a normalization of affect without the need for treatment with antidepressants or other medications.

Incoherence and allied disturbances

Normally the thoughts we put into words are coherent, focused, and goal-directed: abnormalities here include incoherence, circumstantiality and tangentiality, and flight of ideas.

Incoherent speech is characterized by a disconnectedness and disorganization of words, phrases, and sentences such that what the patient says, to a greater or lesser degree, 'makes no sense'. Incoherence may be found in a number of different syndromes, and it is the presence of other signs and symptoms that alerts the clinician to which syndromal diagnosis should be pursued: cognitive deficits indicate the presence of dementia or delirium; heightened mood, pressure of speech, and hyperactivity suggest mania; and bizarre behavior, hallucinations, or delusions point to a psychosis, such as schizophrenia. In cases characterized primarily by incoherence but with few, if any, other abnormalities on the mental status examination, then a diagnosis of aphasia of the 'sensory' type should be considered (Section 2.1). There has been much ink spilt on whether it is possible to reliably distinguish the incoherence seen in schizophrenia (known as 'loosening of associations') from that seen in sensory aphasia; however, of the many articles written on this subject only two studies actually compared the speech of patients with schizophrenia with that of patients with sensory aphasia secondary to stroke (Faber et al. 1983; Gerson et al. 1977), and the results, although promising, were not definitive. In general, patients with loosening of associations spoke freely and at length and, although what they said made little sense, they had no trouble in finding words. By contrast, patients with aphasia often had at least some difficulty in finding words, and their responses to questions were typically brief. Furthermore, whereas patients with loosening of associations had little or no recognition of their incoherence, the aphasic patients often seemed at least somewhat aware of their difficulty. It has been this author's experience that these differences, although often present, are not sufficiently reliable to make the differential between loosening of associations and aphasia, and that it is much more useful to look for the presence of more or less bizarre delusions, which are typically present in any patient with loosening of associations but absent in those with aphasia.

Circumstantiality is said to be present when, perhaps in response to a question, patients take the cognitive 'long way round', traversing superfluous details and dead-ended digressions until finally getting around to the answer. In listening to such patients, the interviewer often has to suppress the urge to tell them to 'get to the point'. Tangentiality differs from circumstantiality in that the patient's thought, although coherent, takes off on a 'tangent' from the initial question, never in fact getting 'to the point'. Both of these signs are diagnostically non-specific but may be seen in the same conditions as incoherence.

Flight of ideas is, according to Kraepelin (1921), characterized by a 'sudden and abrupt jumping from one subject to another': before any given thought is fully developed, the patient's attention lights on another thought that is there to stay for only a short time before moving on yet again. This differs from incoherence in that, although incomplete, the development of the subject is coherent before the patient jumps to the next. Such a flight of ideas is classic for mania.

Other disturbances of thought or speech

Poverty of thought is characterized by a dearth of thoughts: such patients, lacking anything to say, speak very little. By contrast, patients with poverty of speech may speak much. Their speech, however, is 'empty', being filled with so many stock phrases and repetitions that little is actually 'said'. Both these disturbances may be found in schizophrenia and in certain cases of aphasia.

Thought blocking is characterized by an abrupt termination of speech, sometimes in the middle of a sentence, as if the train of thought had suddenly been 'blocked'. This is not a matter of simply running out of things to say, but rather an uncanny experience wherein thoughts suddenly stop appearing. When present to a marked degree, this experience is typically accompanied by one of the Schneiderian first rank delusions, namely 'thought withdrawal' (Section 4.31).

Pressure of speech is experienced by the patient as an 'urge to talk' that is so imperious that, as described by Kraepelin (1899), 'he cannot keep quiet for long, chatters and shouts out loud, yells, roars, bawls, whistles [and] speaks overhastily'. To be in the presence of such patients is akin to standing in front of a dam bursting with words and thoughts. Although classically seen in mania, such a disturbance may also be seen in schizophrenia, schizoaffective disorder, and, occasionally, in dementia.

Perseveration of speech (Section 4.5) is said to be present when patients either supply the same answer to successive questions or merely, and without prompting, repeat the same words or phrases over and over. This abnormality is most commonly seen in dementia or delirium. Palilalia, sometimes confused with perseveration, is characterized by an involuntary repetition of the last phrase or word of a sentence, with these repetitions occurring with increasing rapidity, but diminishing distinctness (Section 4.4).

Echolalia is characterized by an involuntary repetition by the patient of words or sentences spoken by others, and may be seen in a large number of disorders, such as dementia, aphasia, catatonia, and Tourette's syndrome.

Obsessions are distinguished from normal thoughts by the fact that they repeatedly and involuntarily come to mind despite the fact that the patient finds them unwanted and distressing.

Hallucinations

Patients are said to be hallucinated when they experience something in the absence of any corresponding actual object; such hallucinations may occur in the visual, auditory, tactile, olfactory, or gustatory sphere. Thus, a patient who 'saw' a group of people or who 'heard' people murmuring in the next room when the room was in fact empty and silent would be considered hallucinated. Hallucinated patients may or may not retain 'insight': that is to say, they may or may not recognize that their experience is not 'real'. For example, whereas one patient might say, 'I hear some people next door, but I know that it's just my imagination and they're not really there', another might be surprised to hear that the physician did not hear them also. In cases where insight is lacking, it is generally useless to disagree with patients or try and 'talk them out of it'. As Bleuler (1924) pointed out, 'it is of no avail to try to convince the patient by his own observation that there is no one in the next room talking to him; his ready reply is that the talkers just went out or that they are in the walls or that they speak through invisible apparatus'.

Certain auditory hallucinations are included among the Schneiderian first rank symptoms (Section 4.31), and should routinely be sought. They include: audible thoughts (i.e., hearing one's own thoughts 'out loud', as if they were being spoken and as if others could also hear them), hearing voices that comment on what the patients themselves are doing, and hearing voices that argue with one another.

Although classically associated with psychosis, hallucinations are just as common in delirium and dementia.

Delusions

A delusion, according to Lord Brain (1964), 'is an erroneous belief which cannot be corrected by an appeal to reason and is not shared by others of the patient's education and station'. Thus, whereas for a Russian in the middle part of the twentieth century to be convinced that the telephones were routinely 'bugged' would not, *prima facie*, be a delusion; for a Canadian of the twenty-first century to be so convinced would be suspect. Although at times it may be difficult to decide whether or not a belief is delusional, it is in most cases quite obvious: for example, the belief that a small reptilian creature sits inside one's external auditory canal and inserts thoughts is simply not plausible in any culture.

Delusions are generally categorized according to their content or theme. Thus, there are delusions of persecution, grandeur, erotic love, jealousy, sin, poverty, and reference. Delusions of reference are said to be present when patients believe that otherwise unconnected events in some way or other refer or pertain to them. Thus, patients with a delusion of persecution who believed that they were under surveillance might, upon reading a newspaper article about undercover police, hold that the article, in fact, was a kind of 'warning' or 'message' that they could not escape.

Certain delusions are also counted among the Schneiderian first rank symptoms, and these include beliefs that one is directly controlled or influenced by outside forces, that thoughts can be withdrawn, or alternatively inserted, and that thoughts are being 'broadcast' such that they can be 'picked up' and known by others.

Delusions, like hallucinations, may be seen not only in psychosis, but also in delirium or dementia.

Other disturbances of thought content

Phobias are fears that patients admit are irrational. Seen in the condition known as specific phobia (Section 20.12), they may occasionally manifest during the interview, as, for example, in claustrophobia when the patient may object to the door being closed.

Depersonalization is characterized by an uncanny sense of detachment on the patient's part from what is currently going on. Patients may complain of feeling detached, as if they weren't 'there', and, although doing things, were somehow removed and observing. As discussed in Section 4.16, this may occur not only in 'depersonalization disorder', but also in other conditions such as epilepsy.

Compulsions are characterized by irrational and overwhelming urges to do things; obsessions are thoughts that come to mind involuntarily and do so repeatedly despite patients' attempts to stop them. Discussed further in Section 4.17, these phenomena may occasionally be evident during the interview, as, for example, with a compulsion to arrange things 'just so' on the desk or bedside table or with the obsessive recurrence of a fragment of a song.

Level of consciousness

Note should be made of whether or not patients are alert. If not, attempts should be made to arouse them, ranging from calling the patient's name, to shaking the shoulder, to, if necessary, painful stimuli, such as a sternal rub. The response to these maneuvers should be noted. Terms such as 'stupor', 'torpor', or 'obtundation' are best avoided as they are used differently by different authors.

Presence or absence of confusion

Confused patients may appear to be in a daze, and some may report feeling 'fuzzy' or 'cloudy': they have difficulty ordering their own thoughts and a similar difficulty in attending to events around them. An evocative synonym for confusion is 'clouding of the sensorium'. This is a particularly important clinical finding given that the differential diagnosis between delirium and dementia rests, in large part, on its presence or absence.

Orientation

Orientation is traditionally assessed for three 'spheres' – person, place and time – and patients who can properly place themselves in each sphere are said to be 'oriented times three'. Orientation to person may be determined by asking patients for their full names; such orientation is only very rarely lost. Orientation to place is checked by asking patients to identify where they are, including the name of the city and of the building. In cases where patients hesitate to answer, perhaps because they are unsure, it is important to encourage them to take a guess. Should they misidentify the building, inquire further as to what kind of building it is. Some patients may betray a degree of concreteness here, for example, by replying 'a brick building' and, if they do, gently press further by offering some choices, for example, 'a hotel, hospital or office building', and ask them to choose one. Orientation to time is determined by asking patients the date, including the day of the week, the month, day of the month, and year. If patients

are oriented perfectly in all these three spheres then one may simply note 'oriented times three' in the chart. If they are not, it is critical to note their exact responses: simply noting 'oriented times two' fails to capture important information, including, as it does, the patient who believes it is 1948 and the patient who is off the date by only a few days.

In cases when patients are disoriented, it is appropriate to subsequently, and gently, state the correct orientation. This not only ensures that they have been told the correct orientation at least once, but also opens the door to the identification of the rare syndrome of reduplicative paramnesia (Section 4.18) (also known as 'delusional disorientation') wherein, for example, patients may correctly identify the name of the hospital but insist that the hospital is in a distant city.

Some authors also recommend checking orientation in a 'fourth' sphere, namely orientation to situation. This is typically determined during the non-directive portion of the interview, when it becomes clear whether or not patients recognize that they are ill, and in a hospital for treatment, etc. It is akin to 'insight' (discussed later in this chapter) and is probably appropriate.

Disorientation may be seen in delirium, dementia, amnesia, and psychosis.

Memory

Memory is discussed in detail in Section 5.4 and, as noted there, the most important type of memory from a clinical point of view is memory for events and facts, and it is this that is tested in the mental status examination.

Traditionally, three aspects of memory are tested: immediate, short-term, and long-term memory. Immediate recall is tested by using 'digit span'. Here, the patient is given a list of random digits, slowly, one second at a time, and then immediately asked to recall them forwards, from first to last. One starts with a list of three digits, and if the patient recalls these correctly, moves to a list four digits long, proceeding to ever longer lists until the patient either errs in recall or reaches seven digits; normal individuals can recall lists of five to seven digits in length. Once this has been accomplished, 'backward' digit recall is checked by giving a list two digits long and immediately asking the patient to recall them in reverse order. If this is done correctly one proceeds to longer lists, again until errors are made or the patient performs within the normal range of spans of three to five digits.

Short-term recall is tested by telling the patient that you will give a list of three words and that you would like him or her to memorize them because in a few minutes you will ask that they be recalled. Three unrelated words are then provided (e.g., 'rock, car, pencil') and the patient is asked to repeat them once to make sure that he or she 'has' them. Once it is clear that the patient 'has' them, wait 5 minutes and then ask the patient to recall them. Importantly, during this 5-minute interval, the interviewer should stick to neutral topics (e.g., some innocuous 'review of systems' questions) and avoid any emotionally laden subjects that might upset the patient. Normally, all three words are recalled.

Long-term memory should be checked both for personal and public events. This is often assessed informally during the non-directive portion of the interview as one ascertains whether the patient recalls what happened in the days leading up to admission, during recent holidays, or recalls where he or she worked/went to school. Recall of public events may be checked by asking about recent newsworthy events or, in a somewhat more quantitative way, by asking the patient to recall the names of the last four prime ministers or presidents.

Deficits in immediate recall are typically accompanied by confusion and generally indicate a delirium. In addition to delirium, deficits in short- and long-term memory may also be seen in dementia and amnesia. In some cases, either during testing for long-term memory or during the interview, one may find evidence of confabulation (Section 4.19), wherein the answers that patients provide are clearly false.

Abstracting ability

Abstracting ability is traditionally assessed by asking patients to interpret a proverb, such as 'Don't cry over spilled milk'. Responses to proverb testing may be 'abstract' or 'concrete', as, for example, if a patient replied, 'Well, it's already spilled.' At times, the abnormality on proverb interpretation will consist of a bizarre response instead of a concrete reply, such as 'Alien milk has no taste'. Concrete responses may be seen in delirium or dementia and typically indicate frontal lobe dysfunction. Bizarre responses suggest a psychosis, such as schizophrenia.

Calculating ability

Calculating ability is traditionally assessed with the 'serial sevens' test, wherein patients are asked to subtract seven from 100, then seven from that number, and are then asked to keep on subtracting seven until they can go no further. Fewer than one-half of normal individuals are able to do this perfectly, most making two or three errors (Smith 1962). In cases in which patients are unable to do serial sevens at all, it is appropriate to ask them to attempt simpler mathematical tasks, such as adding four plus five, or subtracting eight from 12. As discussed in Section 2.4, deficits in calculating ability may occur in a number of conditions, including dementia and delirium.

Judgment and insight

Judgment has traditionally been assessed with test questions such as 'What would you do if you smelled smoke in a theatre?'. In many instances, however, it is appropriate to pose situations more relevant to the patients' lives; thus, one might ask a police officer what should be done if a suspect refused to answer questions.

Insight, for the purposes of the mental status examination, refers not to some sophisticated appraisal of one's situation, but rather, simply, to whether or not patients recognize that they are ill or that something is wrong. This is identical to 'orientation to situation' as discussed earlier in this chapter and, if already noted, no further comment is required.

Judgment or insight may be lost in delirium, dementia, or a personality change such as frontal lobe syndrome. Insight may also be lost when anosognosia (Section 2.9) is present, as, for example, when a patient with hemiplegia is unable to recognize the deficit.

1.3 NEUROLOGIC EXAMINATION

Bleuler (1924), in his classic *Textbook of Psychiatry*, insisted that 'a *minute physical* and *especially neurological examination* must not be omitted' (italics in original) and the reader is urged to take this admonition to heart.

Over the decades, the neurologic examination has 'thinned down' somewhat and of the dozens of abnormal reflexes that used to be *de rigeur* only a few survive today. The scheme presented here constitutes a 'middle-of-the-road' approach and, although it may be found skimpy by some, others may consider it overly detailed. I plead guilty on both accounts, but urge the reader to try this approach and then to reshape it in light of future experience and wide reading. Although, in most cases, the examination may be conducted in the order suggested here, flexibility must be maintained, especially with fatigued, agitated, or uncooperative patients. Bear in mind that even with a completely uncooperative patient, much may be gathered by a simple observation of eye and facial movements, speech, movement of the extremities, gait, etc.

For most findings, further detail on, and a consideration of, the differential diagnosis of the finding may be found in the appropriate chapter, as noted below.

General appearance

In some cases, the overall appearance of the patient may immediately suggest a possible diagnosis. Examples include the moon facies of Cushing's syndrome (Haskett 1985; Spillane 1951), the puffy facial myxedema and thinning hair of hypothyroidism (Akelaitis 1936; Nickel and Frame 1958) and the massive obesity of the Bardet–Biedl and Prader–Willi syndromes (Rathmell and Burns 1938; Robinson *et al.* 1992) or the Pickwickian syndrome (Meyer *et al.* 1961).

Facial appearance, including facial dysmorphisms, may also be diagnostically suggestive (Wiedemann *et al.* 1989), as, for example, the port wine stain of Sturge–Weber syndrome, the adenoma sebaceum of tuberous sclerosis or the high forehead, large ears, and prognathism of fragile X syndrome.

Handedness

Inquire as to handedness and observe as patients handle implements such as a pen; if there is doubt, ask which hand the patient uses to throw a ball or which foot is used to kick with.

Pupils

The pupils are normally round in shape, regular in outline and centered in the iris. Their diameter should be measured and their reactions to light and to accommodation should be noted. The pupillary reaction to light is tested first by shining a penlight into one eye and observing the reaction, not only of that pupil but also in terms of the consensual reaction in the opposite pupil. After a short wait, the other eye should be tested in the same fashion. The accommodation or convergence reaction is then tested by asking the patient to focus on the examiner's finger as it is slowly moved along the midline toward a spot midway between the patient's eyes: normally, as the eyes converge, both pupils undergo constriction. A preserved reaction to accommodation in the face of an absent or sluggish reaction to light is known as an Argyll Robertson pupil and is very suggestive of neurosyphilis.

While examining the pupils, the corneal limbus should also be examined for a Kayser–Fleischer ring, as seen in Wilson's disease. This is a golden brown discoloration of the limbus, which typically begins at the 12- and 6 o'clock regions from where it gradually expands medially and laterally to eventually form a ring around the cornea.

Funduscopic examination

After examining the optic fundus for any hemorrhages or exudates, attention should be turned to the optic disk, which should be flat and sharply demarcated from the surrounding fundus. The depth of the optic cup should be noted, as should the presence or absence of venous pulsations.

Cranial nerves

CRANIAL NERVE I

The olfactory nerve is tested by first occluding one nostril and then bringing an aromatic substance, such as 'a little powdered coffee' (Brain 1964), to the patent's nostril, inquiring as to whether any odor is appreciated, and if so, what it is. In a pinch one may use a substance readily available at the bedside, such as toothpaste. There are also commercially available tests of the 'scratch and sniff' variety, which, although much more detailed, have not as yet found a place in routine clinical practice. Unilateral anosmia may occur secondary to compression of the olfactory bulb or tract by a tumor, such as a meningioma of the olfactory groove; bilateral anosmia may be seen in neurodegenerative diseases, such as Alzheimer's or Parkinson's disease (Mesholam et al. 1998), and may also be seen after head trauma, with rupture of the olfactory filaments as they pass through the cribriform plate.

CRANIAL NERVE II

The optic nerve is tested not only for acuity, but also for visual fields. Visual acuity may be informally tested by asking the patient to read text from a newspaper or, more formally, by use of a Snellen chart. If the patient has glasses or contact lenses, vision should be tested both with and without them. The visual fields may be assessed by confrontation testing: while facing each other, the physician and patient are separated by about a meter, each fixing vision on the other's nose; the physician then brings a small object (e.g., the tip of a reflex hammer) in from outside the patient's peripheral field, instructing the patient to say 'yes' as soon as it comes into view, and bringing the target in not only from either side, but also from above and below. Importantly, in cases where the patient fails to respond to an object in one hemi-field, one must consider not only the possibility of an hemianopia, but also the possibility of left visual neglect (see Neglect, p. 16).

CRANIAL NERVES III, IV, AND VI

The oculomotor, trochlear, and abducens nerves are tested by having the patient follow the physician's finger as it moves to either side and both upward and downward while the patient's head is kept stationary. Eye movements should be full and conjugate in all directions of gaze, and without nystagmus. The oculomotor nerve also innervates the upper eyelid; thus, the presence or absence of ptosis should be noted. In cases where there is limitation of voluntary up-gaze, or, more importantly, down-gaze, one should further test the patient with the 'doll's eyes' maneuver to determine if the vertical gaze palsy is either supranuclear, nuclear, or infranuclear. To perform this first lightly grasp the patient's head and then flex and extend it at the neck, watching how the eyes move. If eye movements are full then the lesion responsible for the voluntary vertical gaze palsy is supranuclear, as may be seen in disorders such as progressive supranuclear palsy.

CRANIAL NERVE V

The trigeminal nerve has both motor and sensory components. Masseter muscle strength is checked by lightly placing one's fingers on the patient's cheeks and then instructing the patient to bite down. Sensory testing, to both light touch and pin-prick, is checked in all three divisions, namely the ophthalmic, maxillary, and mandibular. The corneal reflex, which tests both the cranial nerves V and VII, may also be performed by lightly touching a wisp of cotton to the patient's cornea, after which there should be a bilateral blink.

CRANIAL NERVE VII

The facial nerve is first tested for voluntary facial movements by asking the patient to wrinkle the forehead and subsequently to show the teeth. In cases of unilateral voluntary facial paresis note must be made of which divisions of the facial nerve are involved: the upper (controlling forehead wrinkling), the lower (controlling elevation of the side of the mouth), or both. At times facial weakness may be quite subtle, manifesting perhaps only with a slight flattening of the nasolabial fold on one side.

After voluntary movements have been tested, the physician must then test for involuntary or 'mimetic' facial movements. This may be accomplished by telling a joke, or, if the physician is in less than a humorous mood, by simply observing the patient for any spontaneous smiling. Voluntary and involuntary facial movements are quite distinct neuroanatomically and thus both should be tested for (Hopf *et al.* 1992). Voluntary facial palsy affecting only the lower division indicates a lesion of the pre-central gyrus or corticobulbar fibers, whereas emotional facial palsy (Section 4.8) indicates a lesion in the supplementary motor area, temporal lobe, striatum, or pons.

CRANIAL NERVE VIII

The vestibulocochlear nerve is generally tested by gently rubbing the fingers together about 30 cm from the patient's ear and asking whether anything is heard; alternatively, one may bring a ticking watch in from a distance and ask the patient to indicate when it is first heard. If there are any abnormalities, both Weber and Rinne testing should be performed to determine whether the hearing loss is of the conduction or sensorineural type.

In the Weber test, a vibrating tuning fork is placed square on the midline of the patient's forehead and the patient is asked whether it sounds the same on both sides or is heard louder on one side than on the other. In the Rinne test, a vibrating tuning fork is placed against the styloid process and the patient is asked to indicate when the sound vanishes, at which point the tines of the tuning fork are immediately brought in close approximation to the ear and the patient is asked whether it can now be heard. With conductive hearing loss, the Weber lateralizes to the side with the hearing loss, and on Rinne testing, bone conduction (i.e., with the tuning fork against the styloid process) is louder than air conduction (i.e., with the tines of the fork vibrating in the air just outside the ear). With sensorineuronal loss, the Weber lateralizes to the 'good' side and, on

Rinne testing, air conduction is better than bone conduction bilaterally.

CRANIAL NERVES IX AND X

The glossopharyngeal and vagus nerves are tested with the gag reflex and by observation for symmetric elevation of the palate during phonation.

CRANIAL NERVE XI

The spinal accessory nerve is tested by having patients shrug their shoulders against the resistance of the physician's hand and by turning the head to one side or the other while the physician exerts contrary pressure on the jaw.

CRANIAL NERVE XII

The hypoglossal nerve is tested first by asking the patient to open the mouth and then observing the tongue, as it rests in the oropharynx, for any atrophy or fasciculations. Once this has been accomplished, the patient is asked to protrude the tongue as far as possible, noting especially whether it protrudes past the lips and also whether it deviates to one side or the other.

Sensory testing

Elementary sensory testing involves light touch, pin-prick, and vibration. Light touch may be assessed by using a wisp of cotton, or simply by a light touch with one's finger, and pin-prick sensation is tested using a disposable safety pin. Vibratory sensation is tested by touching a vibrating tuning fork to a bony structure (such as a finger joint, the lateral malleolus, or the great toe) and asking the patient whether he or she can tell if it is vibrating; if so, the tuning fork is held in place and the patient is asked to say when the vibration ceases, with the physician taking note, in a rough sort of way, of how much the tuning fork is still vibrating at that point. If there are any abnormalities in elementary sensation it is critical to determine whether or not they are bilateral. In general, it is sufficient to test sensation at both hands and both feet, reserving more detailed testing for cases in which the history suggests a more focal sensory loss.

Graphesthesia and two-point discrimination tests also constitute part of the sensory examination but these should only be used if elementary sensation is intact. Agraphesthesia is said to be present when patients, with their eyes closed, are unable to identify letters or numerals traced on their palms by a pencil or dull pin. Two-point discrimination may be tested by 'bending a paperclip to different distances between its two points . . . [starting] with the points relatively far apart . . . [then] approximated until the patient begins to make errors' (Dejong 1979). As two-point discriminatory ability varies on different parts of the body (from 2 to 4 mm at the fingertips to 20–30 mm on the dorsum of the hand), what is most important here is to compare both sides to look for a difference.

Agraphesthesia and diminished two-point discrimination suggest a lesion in the parietal cortex; elementary sensory loss, especially to pin-prick, is also seen with parietal cortex lesions but in addition may occur with lesions of the thalamus, brainstem, cord, or of the peripheral nerves.

Cerebellar testing

In addition to observing the patient's gait for ataxia, as discussed below, cerebellar testing also involves finger-to-nose and heel-to-knee-to-shin testing, testing for rapid alternating movements and observing for dysarthria.

In the finger-to-nose test, patients are instructed to keep their eyes open, extend the arm with the index finger outstretched, and then to touch the nose with the index finger. In the heel-to-knee-to-shin test, patients, while seated or recumbent, are asked to bring the heel into contact with the opposite knee and then to run that heel down the shin below the knee. In both tests one observes for evidence of dysmetria (as, for example, when the nose is missed in the finger-to-nose test) and for intention tremor, wherein, for example, there is an oscillation of the finger and hand as it approaches the target (in this case the nose, with this tremor worsening as the finger is brought progressively closer to the nose).

Rapid alternating movements also assess cerebellar function. Here, while seated, patients are asked to pronate the hand and gently slap an underlying surface (e.g., a tabletop or the patient's own thigh) and then supinate the same hand and again gently slap the underlying surface. Once they have the hang of it, patients are then asked to repeat these movements as quickly and carefully as possible. Decomposition of this movement, known as dysdiadochokinesia, if present, is generally readily apparent on this test.

Dysarthria may also represent cerebellar dysfunction and may be casually assessed by simply listening carefully to the patient's spontaneous speech, noting any evidence of slurring. In doubtful cases one may ask the patient to repeat a test phrase, such as 'Methodist Episcopal' or 'Third Riding Artillery Brigade' (DeJong 1979). Importantly, dysarthria may also be seen with lesions of the motor cortex or associated subcortical structures.

Station, gait, and the Romberg test

Station is assessed by asking patients to stand with their feet normally spaced, and observing for any sway or loss of balance. At this point, if station is adequate, one should perform the Romberg test by telling patients that you will ask them to put their feet close together, as if 'at attention', and then to close their eyes, reassuring them that you will have your hands close by and that you will not let them fall.

If they are comfortable with these instructions then the test can be carried out, observing the patients for perhaps half a minute to see whether or not any swaying develops once the eyes are closed. A 'positive' Romberg test indicates a loss of position sense, as may be seen with a peripheral neuropathy or damage to the posterior columns.

Gait is tested by asking the patient to walk a straight line down a hall, then walking 'heel to toe' in a tandem walk, and, finally, if these are done adequately, by asking the patient to walk 'on the outside of your feet, like a "cowboy"'.

An ataxic gait, seen in cerebellar disorders, is wide based and staggering: steps are irregular in length, the feet are often raised high and brought down with force, and the overall course is zigzagging. In a 'magnetic' gait, as seen in hydrocephalus or bilateral frontal lesions, the feet seem stuck to the floor as if magnetized or glued to it. In a steppage gait, seen in peripheral neuropathies, the normal dorsiflexion of the feet with walking is lost and patients raise their feet high to avoid tripping on their toes. In a spastic gait, seen with hemiplegic patients, the affected lower extremity is rigid in extension and the foot is plantar flexed: with each step, the leg is circumducted around and the front of the foot is often scraped along the floor. In very mild cases of hemiplegia, the gait, to casual inspection, may not be abnormal; however, when patients walk 'on the outside' of their feet, one often sees dystonic posturing of the upper extremity on the involved side. Parkinsonian gait is described in Abnormal movements, p. 14.

Strength

Strength may, according to Brain (1964), be graded as follows: 0, no contraction; 1+, a flicker or trace of movement; 2+, active movement providing that gravity is eliminated; 3+, active movement against gravity; 4+, active movement against some resistance; and 5+, full strength. In the process of assessing muscular strength one should also observe for any atrophy, fasciculations, or myotonia. Myotonia is sometimes apparent in a handshake, as patients may have trouble relaxing their grip, and may also be assessed by using a reflex hammer to lightly tap a muscle belly, such as at the thenar eminence, and watching for distinctive myotonic dimpling.

Common patterns of weakness include monoparesis, if only one limb is involved, hemiparesis if both limbs on one side are weak, paraparesis if both lower extremities are weak, and quadriparesis (or, alternatively, tetraparesis), if all four extremities are weakened. In cases when strength = 0 then one speaks not of paresis but of paralysis, and uses the terms monoplegia, hemiplegia, paraplegia, or quadriplegia. When weakness is present, note should be made whether the proximal or distal portions of the limb are primarily involved; in cases of hemiparesis in which both limbs are not equally affected, the limb that is more affected should be noted.

Drift

A positive pronator drift test may be the first evidence of hemiparesis. This test, according to DeJong (1979), is accomplished by asking patients (with their eyes closed) to fully extend their upper extremities, palms up, and then maintain that position: a positive test consists of 'slow pronation of the wrist, slight flexion of the elbow and fingers, and a downward and lateral drift of the hand'.

Rigidity

Rigidity should, at a minimum, be assessed at the elbows, wrists, and knees by passive flexion and extension at the joint, with close attention to the appearance of spastic, lead pipe, or cogwheel rigidity. Spastic rigidity, seen with upper motor neuron lesions, is most noticeable on attempted extension of the upper extremity at the elbow and attempted flexion of the lower extremity at the knee. Furthermore, in spasticity, one may see the 'clasp knife' phenomenon. Here, on attempted rapid extension of the upper extremity at the elbow, an initial period of minimal resistance is quickly followed by a 'catch' of increased resistance, which, in turn, is eventually followed by a loosening, with the whole experience reminiscent of what it feels like to open the blade on clasp knife. Lead pipe rigidity, seen in parkinsonism, is, in contrast with spastic rigidity, characterized by a more or less constant degree of rigidity throughout the entire range of motion, much as if one were manipulating a thick piece of solder. Cogwheel rigidity, also seen in parkinsonism, may accompany lead pipe rigidity or occur independently. This is best appreciated by gently holding the patient's elbow in the cup of your hand while pressing down on the patient's biceps tendon with your thumb. Once the arm is thus supported, with your other hand gradually extend the arm. When cogwheeling is present, a 'ratcheting' motion will be appreciated with your thumb, much as if there were a 'cogwheel' inside the joint.

After testing for these forms of rigidity, one should then test for gegenhalten at the elbow by repeatedly extending and flexing the arm, feeling carefully for any increasing rigidity. Evidence for this generally indicates frontal lobe damage.

Abnormal movements

Tremor (Section 3.1) is generally of one of three types: rest, postural, or intention. Rest tremor is most noticeable when the extremity is at rest, as for example when the patient is seated with the hands resting in the lap. Postural tremor becomes evident when a posture is maintained, as, for example, when the arms are held straight out in front with the fingers extended and spread. Intention tremor (as described in Cerebellar testing, p. 13) appears when the

patient carries out an intended action, as, for example, touching the index finger to the nose. Other forms are also possible, for example, Holmes' tremor, which has both postural and intention elements. Tremor is further characterized in terms of amplitude (from fine to coarse) and frequency (ranging from slow [3–5 cps] to medium [6–10 cps] to rapid [11–20 cycles per second, cps]).

Myoclonus (Section 3.2) consists of 'a shock-like muscular contraction' (Brain 1964) and may be focal, segmental, or generalized, occurring either spontaneously in response to some sudden stimulus (e.g., a loud noise) or as 'intention' or 'action' myoclonus that appears upon intentional movement. This is an especially valuable sign and the physician should remain alert to its occurrence throughout the interview and examination.

Motor tics (Section 3.3) are sudden involuntary movements that, importantly, resemble purposeful movements, such as shoulder shrugs, facial grimaces, or head jerks. Unlike myoclonus, tics involve 'a number of muscles in their normal synergic relationships' (Brain 1964).

Chorea (Section 3.4), according to Brain (1964), is characterized by 'quasi-purposive, jerky, irregular, and non-repetitive' movements that are very brief in duration, generally erupting randomly on different parts of the body.

Athetosis (Section 3.5) 'consists of slow, writhing movements' (Brain 1964) that are generally most evident in the distal portions of a limb; they are persistent and seem to flow into one another in a serpentine fashion.

Ballismus (Section 3.6), which is generally unilateral, consists of 'wild flaillike, writhing, twisting or rolling movements that may be intense and may lead to exhaustion' (DeJong 1979). In severe cases the flinging movements of the extremity may actually throw the patient off the chair or bed.

Dystonia (Section 3.7), in contrast with ballismus, consists of slow and sustained movements that variously twist or contort the involved body part. It may be focal (e.g., moving the head to one side or 'cramping' the hand), segmental (e.g., spreading to an adjacent body part, as with the head turning and the shoulder elevating), or generalized (e.g., in severe cases, creating a human 'pretzel').

Parkinsonism (Section 3.8), when fully developed, stamps patients with a distinctive clinical picture. A flexion posture is evident, with the patient being stooped over with the arms and legs held in flexion, and a rhythmic 'pill-rolling' rest tremor of the hands may be seen, especially with the hands resting on the lap. The face is often 'masked' and expressionless, and bradykinesia is evident in the slowness with which all movements are executed. Gait is shuffling and one may also see festination wherein the patient seems to hurry 'with small steps in a bent attitude, as if trying to catch up [with] his center of gravity' (Brain 1964).

Akathisia (Section 3.10) is typified by an inability to keep still. If standing, patients may rock back and forth or 'march in place' and, if seated, there may be a restless fidgeting, with crossing and uncrossing of the arms or legs. In severe cases, the compulsion to move is irresistible, and patients may constantly pace back and forth. Characteristically, the restlessness is worse when lying down or seated, and most patients find some relief upon standing or moving about.

Catatonia (Section 3.11) of the stuporous type (Barnes *et al.* 1986) is characterized by varying degrees of immobility, mutism, and a remarkable phenomenon known as waxy flexibility (or catalepsy), wherein, as noted by Kraepelin (1899), the limbs, after being passively placed in any position, 'retain this position until they receive another impetus or until they follow the law of gravity as a result of extreme muscular fatigue'.

Asterixis (Section 3.12) (Leavitt and Tyler 1964) is tested for by having patients hold their upper limbs in full extension, with the hands being held in hyperextension: asterixis, if present, appears as a precipitous loss of muscle tone, such that the hands 'flap' down. When present, this may appear immediately and recur frequently, or may be delayed for up to half a minute.

Heightened startle response (Section 3.14) (Saenz-Lope *et al.* 1984) is often precipitated by a sudden loud noise and may go beyond being simply excessively 'jumpy'; some patients may actually be thrown to the ground during the startle.

Deep tendon reflexes

At a minimum, the following deep tendon reflexes should be tested: biceps jerk, triceps jerk, supinator jerk, knee jerk, and ankle jerk (Brain 1964). The results may, according to DeJong (1979), be graded as 0 for absent, + for present but diminished, ++ for normal, +++ for increased, and ++++ for markedly hyperactive. Hyperactive deep tendon reflexes may also be accompanied by ankle clonus. Testing for clonus is accomplished by placing your hand under the ball of the patient's foot and then briskly dorsiflexing the foot. When clonus is present, the foot will then briskly and spontaneously undergo plantar flexion. Keeping a light upward pressure on the ball of the foot may precipitate repetitive clonic jerking, and in some cases this may be self-perpetuating or 'sustained'.

In those cases in which patients remain so tense that their reflexes cannot be elicited, several maneuvers may render the examination possible (Bickerstaff 1980): for the upper limbs, the patient should clench his teeth tightly or while one arm is being examined he should clench the fist of the other. For the lower limbs these measures can still be used but the well-tried method of Jendressak is more reliable; the patient interlocks the flexed fingers of the two hands and pulls one against the other at the moment the reflex is stimulated.

Babinski sign

The Babinski sign, considered by DeJong (1979) as 'the most important sign in clinical neurology', may be elicited by lightly dragging a blunt object across the sole of the patient's foot: beginning at the heel, proceeding along the lateral aspect of the sole and then turning medially to cross under the ball of the foot. One then observes for the 'plantar response' of the toes, noting whether it is 'flexor' or 'extensor'. The normal response is 'flexor', wherein the toes undergo flexion. An 'extensor' response is considered abnormal and constitutes the Babinski sign, which, when fully present, consists of dorsiflexion of the great toe and fanning of the rest. The presence of the Babinski sign is a reliable indicator of damage to the corticospinal tract.

Primitive reflexes

Certain reflexes present in infancy or early childhood normally disappear. When these reappear in adult years they are known as 'primitive reflexes' (Section 4.6) and may indicate frontal lobe disease.

The palmomental reflex is tested for by repeatedly and rapidly dragging an object, such as the tip of a reflex hammer, across the thenar eminence: when the reflex is present, one sees 'a wrinkling of the skin of the chin and slight retraction and sometimes elevation of the angle of the mouth' (DeJong 1979).

The snout reflex is said to be present when gentle tapping or pressure just above the patient's upper lip, in the midline, is followed by a puckering or protrusion of the lips; in advanced cases, the reflex may be elicited by merely 'sweeping a tongue blade briskly across the upper lip' (DeJong 1979).

The grasp reflex may be elicited by laying one's finger across the patient's palm such that it may be readily dragged out between the patient's thumb and index finger. If the reflex is present, the patient's fingers will grasp the physician's finger as it is slowly dragged across the palm (Walshe and Robertson 1933).

The grope reflex may be elicited by simply lightly touching the patient's hand with one's finger: when present, the patient's hand will automatically make groping movements until the physician's finger is found and grasped (Seyffarth and Denny-Brown 1948).

Aphasia and mutism

Aphasia represents a disturbance in the comprehension and/or production of spoken language. Testing involves listening to the patient's spontaneous speech, giving simple spoken commands, and determining whether the patient understands them, and asking the patient to repeat a test phrase, such as 'No ifs, ands, or buts'.

As discussed in detail in Section 2.1, there are three basic forms of aphasia: motor (also known as expressive or Broca's), sensory (also known as receptive or Wernicke's), and global. In motor aphasia, patients are able to follow commands, although their speech, despite being coherent, is effortful, sparse, and often 'telegraphic', (i.e., lacking in prepositions and conjunctions). In sensory aphasia, in contrast, patients have a greater or lesser degree of difficulty in following oral commands, especially complex ones; furthermore, speech is quite fluent, even voluble, rather than being effortful: however, there is a greater or lesser degree of incoherence such that what the patient says makes 'no sense'. Finally, the global type of aphasia represents a combination of these two: patients have trouble following commands, speech is effortful and sparse, and what the patient says is more or less incoherent.

Each of these three types may also occur as a 'transcortical' variant, and this is said to be present when patients are able to repeat a test phrase accurately and without effort. Other variants, less common, are also possible and these are discussed Section 2.1.

Mutism (Section 4.1) is said to be present when there is no speech.

Alexia and agraphia

Alexia (Section 2.2) and agraphia (Section 2.3) represent, respectively, difficulties in reading and writing, and although often seen in combination with aphasia, may also appear in pure form. Testing is accomplished simply by asking the patient to read something, perhaps a headline, and then to write something, such as an address.

Aprosodia

Aprosodia (Section 2.7) represents a disturbance in the production or comprehension of the 'emotional' and melodic aspects of speech (Ross 1981). Thus, the patient's own speech may be monotone, lacking all prosodic elements, or the patient may have difficulty in appreciating the emotional tone of another's voice. A lack of prosody in the patient's own speech is generally apparent as the history is related; testing for the patient's ability to 'comprehend' prosody may require that patients close their eyes and then listen as the physician repeats the same neutral phrase repeatedly but with different intonations (e.g., happy, angry, or sad), asking each time what the tone was.

Aprosodia must be distinguished from flattened affect and parkinsonian hypomimia, and this differential was discussed above previously in this chapter under Mood and affect.

Apraxia

Apraxia may be ideational/ideomotor, constructional, or dressing.

Ideational and *ideomotor apraxia* (DeJong 1979; Heilman 1973) are tested by first asking the patient to mime using a common implement, such as a comb or a pair of scissors, and then, if the patient has any difficulty in performing the mime, by providing the implement and asking the patient to make use of it. In ideational apraxia, both miming and actual use are defective, whereas with ideomotor apraxia the patient, although unable to mime, has no trouble correctly employing the actual implement.

Constructional apraxia is tested for by asking the patient to draw a simple figure, such as a 'stick person', or to copy a geometric design (DeJong 1979) such as a cube.

Dressing apraxia is casually assessed by observing the patient put on clothing: when present, patients may put their arms in the wrong sleeve or perhaps attempt to put their shirt on backwards (Hecaen *et al.* 1956).

Agnosias

Agnosia, as discussed in Section 2.9 exists in various forms: for example, visual agnosia, tactile agnosia, and anosognosia. In each form, despite the fact that relevant elementary sensory abilities are intact there is an inability to recognize things.

Visual agnosia, or the inability to recognize an object by sight, is tested by pointing to a common object, such as a comb, and asking patients not only to name it, but also to describe its use.

Tactile agnosia represents an inability to recognize an object by touch: with the eyes closed, the patient is given a common object, such as a key, and asked both to identify it and to describe its use.

Anosognosia is said to be present when patients fail to recognize a deficit, such as hemiparesis, or grossly minimize it, for example, by characterizing a severely hemiparetic limb as simply 'stiff'.

Other agnosias, also described in Section 2.9, which are generally not routinely tested for, include color agnosia, prosopagnosia (the inability to recognize faces), auditory agnosia (the inability to recognize common sounds), topographagnosia (a loss of a sense of direction), simultanagnosia (an inability to visually 'grasp' the whole of a scene to see all of its parts simultaneously), and asomatagnosia (a denial of the 'ownership' of a body part, as may be seen in some cases of hemiparesis).

Neglect

Neglect, discussed in Section 2.10, is characterized by an involuntary failure to attend to or notice phenomena on one side or the other; this may be either visual or motor.

Visual neglect is tested by seating the patient squarely in front of a table, with the patient's trunk kept parallel to the edge of the table (Beschin *et al.* 1997). First, draw a line horizontally across a piece of paper, at least 15 cm long (Tegner and Levander 1991) and then place the paper directly in front of, and square to, the patient. The patient is then asked to bisect the line. Next, draw numerous short marks in a random fashion on a piece of paper, placing the paper squarely in front of the patient and asking the patient to mark or cancel out all the lines. Finally, position a blank piece of paper in front of the patient with the instruction to draw a clock face on it, with all the numbers, from one to twelve, on the drawing. These constitute, respectively, the line bisection, line cancellation, and clock-drawing tests, and visual neglect is said to be present if the line is bisected off the midline, a significant percentage of the random lines on one side are not cancelled out, or the numerals on the clock face are bunched to one side.

Motor neglect is tested by asking the patient to perform a task that requires the use of both upper extremities, such as fastening a button: when motor neglect is present, the patient 'underutilizes' the 'neglected' side and attempts to perform the task primarily with one hand, despite the fact that with strong urging normal bilateral manual coordination is possible (Laplane and Degos 1983).

Extinction

Extinction, also discussed in Section 2.10, is considered a subtype of neglect, and, like neglect, may be either visual or tactile (Valler *et al.* 1994).

Visual extinction may be tested immediately after performing confrontation testing of the visual fields. While retaining the same position with respect to the patient, the physician holds both hands outstretched laterally to the edge of the peripheral fields and then simultaneously wiggles both index fingers, asking the patient to point to the finger/fingers that are moving. When visual extinction is present, the patient notes the motion of only one finger.

Tactile extinction may be tested during routine sensory testing. While the patient's eyes are closed, the physician instructs the patient to report which hand or hands are being touched – touching first one hand, then the other and then both simultaneously. When tactile extinction is present, only one hand will be reported as touched during simultaneous stimulation.

1.4 NEUROIMAGING

Computed tomography (CT) and magnetic resonance imaging (MRI) have revolutionized neuroimaging. Before the advent of CT in 1972, physicians were limited to skull radiographs, radionuclide scanning, and pneumoencephalography, none of which retains any use for imaging the brain today.

For both CT and MRI, imaging is accomplished on a voxel-by-voxel basis. A voxel (from *volume element*) is a specific three-dimensional volume of tissue, each voxel subsequently being represented on the scan by a pixel (from *picture element*). Early-generation scanners allowed for only a limited number of voxels; consequently, tissue resolution was poor and the corresponding scan created by the pixels was fuzzy and relatively unedifying. However, technical progress has allowed for a much higher number of voxels and pixels with the result that, especially in the case of MRI, the scans are breathtakingly accurate representations of the intracranial contents.

The technology of CT scanning is similar to that utilized in traditional radiography and is thus conceptually easily grasped by most physicians. MR scanning, however, relies on a fundamentally different technology, which, for most, requires some getting used to.

This chapter will briefly discuss CT and MRI, and then consider their relative merits for clinical neuroimaging.

CT scanning

CT scanning, developed by Hounsfield (1972), is based upon determining the attenuation of an X-ray beam by any given voxel of tissue. The degree of attenuation is expressed in Hounsfield units (Phelps *et al.* 1975): by convention, these range from -1000 (for air) to $+1000$ (for bone), tissues of biologic interest being assigned intermediate values, for example, 0 for water, ~30 for white matter, ~35 for gray matter, ~75 for freshly clotted blood, and ~150–200 for calcified gray matter. A gray scale is then created to represent the various attenuation coefficients, very low-attenuation (or 'hypodense') areas such as air in the sinuses appearing black, and very high-attenuation (or 'hyperdense') tissues, such as blood, bone, or other areas of heavy calcification, appearing more or less white.

CT scanning is most reliable for supratentorial structures: the posterior fossa is particularly likely to be obscured by various artifacts (Mostrum and Ytterbergh 1986).

Enhancement is accomplished by the intravenous injection of an iodinated contrast material, which, as it has a high attenuation coefficient, makes the tissue into which it extravasates appear more dense.

Angiography may also be accomplished with CT scanning; however, this requires a large injection of contrast material.

MR scanning

The physics underlying MRI are complex (Edelman and Warach 1993; Pykett 1982; Pykett *et al.* 1982), so what follows is a very simplified, and very brief, general overview. To begin, consider hydrogen atoms, their nuclei composed of but one proton. Each proton spins at a very fast rate, thus creating a magnetic field and, as it were, becoming a very small magnet itself. These proton 'magnets' are normally arrayed in random directions, but if a very strong external magnetic field is applied, they will all align themselves parallel to the external magnetic field. In such a situation, if a radio pulse of appropriate frequency is fired at the protons, they will absorb this energy, with the result that they begin to spin with an eccentric axis, no longer in parallel alignment to the external magnetic field. Over a variable period of time, however, the protons fall back into line, in so doing releasing the energy absorbed from the earlier radio pulse. The speed with which the protons undergo realignment is determined by various factors, including the availability of nearby tissues that may absorb energy and the presence of any surrounding magnetic inhomogeneities or tissues that, of themselves, have magnetic properties. The released energy may be measured and constitutes the 'signal' of the voxel in question.

Routine MRI imaging includes T1, T2, and FLAIR (fluid-attenuated inversion recovery) sequences and, whenever one is interested in documenting old bleeds, a gradient echo (or T2*) sequence should also be ordered. The appearance of various tissues and abnormalities differs on each of these sequences. On T1-weighted images, cerebrospinal fluid (CSF) appears black, gray matter is medium-gray in appearance, white matter is light-gray, and both edema and gliosis are dark. On T2-weighted images, CSF appears bright, gray matter is medium-gray, white matter is dark-gray, and both edema and gliosis are light-colored. On FLAIR sequences, CSF is quite dark, gray matter is light-gray and white matter somewhat lighter, and edema and gliosis are quite bright. Overall, T1-weighted scans provide the sharpest delineation of structures, but are less sensitive to pathology. T2-weighted and FLAIR scans provide less clear delineation of structures, but are far more sensitive to pathology and, of these two, FLAIR is the most sensitive. Gradient echo scanning is reserved for situations wherein one suspects that the patient has had, in the distant past, intracerebral hemorrhage. In this situation, blood has degraded to hemosiderin, and T2*-weighted scanning is exquisitely sensitive for this, displaying an area of greatly reduced signal intensity.

The enhancement of MRI is accomplished by the injection of a paramagnetic substance such as gadolinium and is best appreciated on T1-weighted scans (Berry et al. 1986; Brant-Zawadzki et al. 1986): on such images, as illustrated in Figure 1.1, the tissues into which the gadolinium has

extravasated have a much higher signal intensity and appear much brighter.

Consideration should also be given to ordering diffusion-weighted images (DWIs) (Schaeffer et al. 2000). DWI is exquisitely sensitive to cytotoxic edema (Warach et al. 1995) (somewhat less so to vasogenic edema), and, as discussed below, has become an essential tool in the diagnosis of cerebral infarction (Fisher and Albers 1999; Neumann-Haefelin et al. 2000). In cases in which there is uncertainty as to whether the increased signal intensity on a diffusion-weighted image represents cytotoxic edema or vasogenic edema, an 'apparent diffusion coefficient' (ADC) map should be ordered: on ADC mapping, areas of cytotoxic edema appear very dark, whereas areas of vasogenic edema have an increased signal intensity.

Angiography may also be performed with MRI. Such magnetic resonance angiography (MRA) may be performed either with 'time of flight (TOF) imaging' or via 'phase contrast imaging': of the two, the TOF technique produces more informative images.

Clinical indications

As with any diagnostic test, the decision to request either CT or MRI should be guided by one's diagnostic suspicions. Furthermore, it is critical to provide the radiologist with a brief summary of the history and findings, along with one's presumptive diagnosis, so that the best imaging parameters may be selected.

MRI is preferable to CT in most clinical situations (Armstrong and Keevil 1991; Bradley et al. 1984; Haughton et al. 1986), with the exception of suspected intracranial calcification (Holland et al. 1985). However, MRI should not be utilized whenever the patient harbors a metallic object that might undergo any potentially dangerous movement during the application of the external magnetic field. Examples include: aneurysmal clips, depth electrodes, intracranial bullets or shrapnel, some CSF shunts, some cochlear implants, cardiac pacemakers, transcutaneous electrical nerve stimulation (TENS) units, some prosthetic valves, some arterial stents, various orthopedic devices, some penile implants, wire sutures, and, importantly, any metallic object in the eye. This last contraindication deserves special attention as some patients may not be aware of the presence of a metallic ocular foreign body (e.g., a lathe operator struck in the eye with a minute sliver of metal decades earlier): if any doubt exists, plain films of the orbits should be acquired first. Metallic objects that may be removed include hearing aids, dentures, TENS units, insulin pumps, and some intrauterine devices.

Some common indications (such as suspected cerebral infarction) for CT or MRI are discussed as follows.

CEREBRAL INFARCTION

Cerebral infarction demonstrates a definite evolution of pathologic stages, progressing from cytotoxic edema to

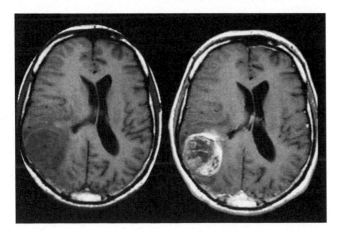

Figure 1.1   Both of these T1-weighted magnetic resonance (MR) scans are of the same patient with a high-grade glioma in the right hemisphere; on the left, the tumor appears as an area of decreased signal intensity but, with enhancement, as seen in the scan on the right, the tumor displays increased signal intensity and 'lights up'. (Reproduced from Gillespie and Jackson 2000.)

vasogenic edema and finally to necrosis, with varying degrees of cavitation.

On CT scanning (Bories *et al.* 1985; Johnson 1994) there is loss of definition of the gray-white boundary within the first 6 hours, and over the next 18 hours an area of slight radiolucency develops in the appropriate vascular territory. After 24 hours, this area becomes better defined and, with the development of vasogenic edema, a mass effect on surrounding structures develops, peaking at from 3–5 days. Edema gradually resolves over 2–4 weeks, and eventually a fairly circumscribed area of radiolucency appears, corresponding to the residual encephalomalacia. Contrast enhancement generally appears after 3 days, and resolves in a matter of weeks.

MRI with diffusion-weighted imaging (DWI) is exquisitely sensitive to the cytotoxic edema of infarction, revealing an increased signal intensity within the first few hours, and indeed, in some cases within minutes (Yoneda *et al.* 1999). T2-weighted and FLAIR images will reveal increased signal intensity in the area of infarction within 6 hours and this tends to persist. Gadolinium enhancement becomes apparent within a matter of days, and resolves in from 1 to 2 months.

Although CT scanning is typically utilized first in cases of suspected cerebral infarction, this is primarily due to its ease of use and availability, and to its efficacy in the detection of intracerebral hemorrhage. It is not because CT is superior to MRI in the detection of acute infarction; indeed, there is no question that MRI is by far superior to CT in this regard (Fiebach *et al.* 2001; Gonzalez *et al.* 1999; Lansberg *et al.* 2000).

INTRACEREBRAL HEMORRHAGE

On CT scanning (Dolinskas *et al.* 1977) intracerebral hemorrhage is immediately apparent as an area of increased radiodensity. Over the following weeks this gradually resolves to an area of isodensity and, eventually, after months, an area of radiolucency appears.

With MR scanning the evolution of the image is more complex (Gomori *et al.* 1985; Patel *et al.* 1996). During the 'hyperacute' phase, when the hemoglobin in the red blood cells is, for the most part, still in its oxyhemoglobin form, there may be little definitive change on MR scanning. It was initially felt that this hyperacute phase lasted several hours; however, recent studies have indicated that intracellular hemoglobin may begin to degrade to deoxyhemoglobin early on, within these first few hours. In the following acute phase, spanning the next few days, there is unequivocal degeneration of intracellular oxyhemoglobin into deoxyhemoglobin, and the bleed now appears as an area of decreased signal intensity on T2-weighted scans. During the early subacute phase, which lasts roughly from day three to day seven, the intracellular deoxyhemoglobin further degrades into methemoglobin and the lesion at this point appears as an area of increased signal intensity on T1-weighted scans, with persisting decreased signal intensity on the T2-weighted scan. The late subacute phase ensues and lasts for months; during this phase red blood cells rupture and methemoglobin is released into the extracellular space, creating increased signal intensity on both T1- and T2-weighted scans. Finally, during the chronic stage, there is degradation of methemoglobin and chronic deposition of hemosiderin, with low signal intensity on both T1 and T2 scans and a virtual black hole on gradient echo scans.

Although, as in the case of suspected ischemic infarction, CT is routinely used initially in suspected intracerebral hemorrhage, this again appears to be more a matter of availability, given that MRI performed within the first few hours appears just as sensitive (Kidwell *et al.* 2004; Schellinger *et al.* 1999). Furthermore, in evaluating patients months after suspected intracerebral hemorrhage there is no question that MRI, utilizing gradient echo sequences, is far more sensitive than CT (Wardlaw *et al.* 2003).

SUBARACHNOID HEMORRHAGE

Subarachnoid hemorrhage is routinely detected by CT scanning as an area of hyperdensity corresponding to the free blood within the subarachnoid space (van der Wee *et al.* 1995; van Gijn and van Dongen 1982). As in the case with suspected ischemic infarction or intracerebral hemorrhage, CT is generally used first in possible subarachnoid hemorrhage; however, MRI, using FLAIR sequence, may be just as accurate (Wiesmann *et al.* 2002).

LACUNAR INFARCTIONS

Chronic lacunar infarctions, often missed on CT scanning, appear on MR scanning as areas of decreased signal intensity on T1-weighted scans and increased signal intensity on T2-weighted scans (Brown *et al.* 1988). As with large cortical infarcts, DWI may reveal acute lacunar infarcts (Singer *et al.* 1998) and is especially helpful in indicating which lacunae are 'fresh' (Oliveira-Filho *et al.* 2000); indeed, DWI may demonstrate the occurrence of lacunar infarctions despite the absence of any history of a clinical event (Choi *et al.* 2000). Importantly, lacunae must be distinguished from prominent Virchow–Robin spaces (Heier *et al.* 1989; Jungreis *et al.* 1988), which, unlike lacunae, tend to be bilaterally symmetric and quite regular in shape.

BINSWANGER'S DISEASE

Binswanger's disease, also known as subcortical arteriosclerotic leukoencephalopathy, is characterized by irregular, patchy and often confluent areas of more or less complete demyelinization in the centrum semiovale and periventricular white matter. Although these patchy lesions may, in some cases, be seen on CT scans as ill-defined areas of hypodensity, they are much better appreciated on MR scanning as areas of decreased signal intensity on T1-weighted scans and, most especially, as areas of increased signal intensity on T2-weighted scans (Kinkel *et al.* 1985). These patchy lesions must be distinguished from certain normal variants (Fazekas *et al.* 1991), such as bilaterally symmetric and smoothly contoured periventricular 'caps' and 'rims', and what are known as unidentified bright objects (UBOs): scattered punctate foci of increased signal intensity on T2-weighted images.

INTRACRANIAL CALCIFICATION

Intracranial calcification, as may be seen in Fahr's syndrome, tuberous sclerosis, or Sturge–Weber syndrome, is better demonstrated on CT scanning, on which it is evident as an area of hyperdensity, than on MR scanning, where it may be difficult to detect (Holland *et al.* 1985; Wasenko *et al.* 1990).

TUMORS

Tumors are, overall, better demonstrated by MR than CT scanning (Armstrong and Keevil 1991; Bradley *et al.* 1984; Brant-Zawadzki *et al.* 1984). With both CT and MR scanning, enhancement increases sensitivity (Sze *et al.* 1990) and, in the case of gliomas, the degree of enhancement may serve as a guide to the malignancy of the tumor, with increased enhancement indicating greater malignancy with both CT (Tchang *et al.* 1977) and MR (Dean *et al.* 1990; Graif and Steiner 1986) scanning. In the case of meningiomas, the administration of contrast is especially important (Vassilouthis and Ambrose 1979; Zimmerman *et al.* 1985): on unenhanced CT scanning, the tumor, although often hyperdense, may be isodense, and on MR scanning there is often no change at all in signal intensity on either T1- or T2-weighted scans. With contrast, however, almost all meningiomas will enhance on both CT and MR scanning.

TRAUMATIC BRAIN INJURY

Although CT is generally the first technique used in patients with traumatic brain injury and is often the only one, it is clear that MRI is far superior in the detection of contusions, and, especially, diffuse axonal injury (Jenkins *et al.* 1986; Kelly *et al.* 1988; Mittl *et al.* 1994; Orrison *et al.* 1994; Zimmerman *et al.* 1986).

MULTIPLE SCLEROSIS

Multiple sclerosis is characterized by plaques of demyelinization that may be either active (with evidence of definite inflammation) or chronic and inactive. CT scanning (Hershey *et al.* 1979; Mushlin *et al.* 1993) demonstrates plaques as areas of hypodensity, and active plaques may be identified by contrast enhancement. MR scanning is far more sensitive than CT scanning, even when CT scanning is carried out using double contrast (Mushlin *et al.* 1993; Young *et al.* 1981).

On MR scanning (Katz *et al.* 1993; Nesbit *et al.* 1991; Ormerod *et al.* 1987), inactive plaques appear as areas of decreased signal intensity on T1-weighted scans and increased signal intensity on T2-weighted scans; active plaques demonstrate gadolinium enhancement. Serial MR scanning (Grossman *et al.* 1988; Guttmann *et al.* 1995; Thompson *et al.* 1992) may be used to follow the progress of the disease and may indeed reveal clinically 'silent' lesions. Furthermore, recently activated plaques may be detected by gadolinium enhancement before there is any clinical evidence of their presence (Kermode *et al.* 1990; Miller *et al.* 1988). MRI has revolutionized the diagnosis of multiple sclerosis and no evaluation of a patient suspected of harboring this dreaded disease is complete without it.

MESIAL TEMPORAL SCLEROSIS

Mesial temporal sclerosis, the most common cause of complex partial seizures, is better detected by MRI than CT (Franceschi *et al.* 1989). On MR scanning, mesial temporal sclerosis is apparent with atrophy (best seen on T1-weighted scans) and, on T2-weighted scans, increased signal intensity in the same area: importantly, these changes are generally best seen on coronal images (Berkovic *et al.* 1991).

NEURONAL MIGRATION DISORDERS

Neuronal migration disorders are a common cause of simple or complex partial seizures and of grand mal seizures of focal onset. For the most part, they manifest as subependymal nodular heterotopias, either laminar or band heterotopias in the white matter itself, or areas of cortical dysplasia or microdysgenesis. Although CT scanning may detect subependymal heterotopias (especially if they are calcified) MR scanning is superior, picking up not only these lesions, but also band and laminar heterotopias (Altman *et al.* 1988; Barkovich and Kjos 1992; Huttenlocher *et al.* 1994), as illustrated in Figure 1.2.

AIDS DEMENTIA

AIDS dementia has imaging characteristics similar to those described for Binswanger's disease and is better imaged with MRI than CT (Chrysikopoulos *et al.* 1990). Furthermore, MRI is also more sensitive than CT for AIDS-related illnesses such as toxoplasmosis (Porter and Sande 1992) and progressive multifocal leukoencephalopathy (Guilleux *et al.* 1986; Krup *et al.* 1985).

HERPES SIMPLEX VIRAL ENCEPHALITIS

Herpes simplex viral encephalitis, the most common cause of sporadic encephalitis (and a very important diagnosis given its amenability to treatment) is far better imaged by MRI than CT (Gasecki and Steg 1991); indeed, CT scanning may be normal during the critical first few days (Greenberg *et al.* 1981). Herpes simplex encephalitis usually affects first the mesial temporal structures, producing an increased signal intensity on T2-weighted scanning (Tien *et al.* 1993).

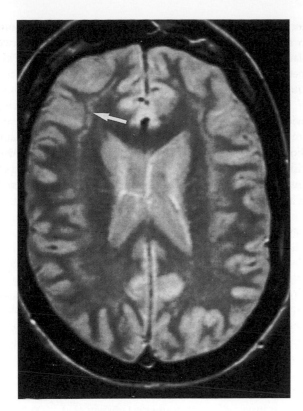

Figure 1.2 A T1-weighted magnetic resonance imaging scan demonstrates a laminar band heterotopia, as indicated by the arrow, in exquisite detail. (Reproduced from Hopkins *et al.* 1995.)

PITUITARY ADENOMA

Pituitary macroadenomas may be seen on both CT and MR scanning; microadenomas, however, are generally seen only with MR scanning (Levy and Lightman 1994), which, in the case of prolactinomas, may be used to monitor the results of treatment with bromocriptine (Pojunas *et al.* 1986).

1.5 ELECTROENCEPHALOGRAPHY

The existence of cerebral electrical activity was demonstrated in animals in 1875 by an English physician, Richard Caton (1875), and the first human electroencephalogram (EEG) was reported by Hans Berger in 1929 (Berger 1929). By the middle of the twentieth century, the EEG had become very important in the diagnosis of such intracranial lesions as tumors but, with the advent of CT and MRI the indications for electroencephalography have changed, and most EEGs are currently obtained in the course of the diagnosis or management of seizures or epilepsy and in the evaluation of delirium. This chapter discusses EEG instrumentation, the normal EEG, various EEG abnormalities, activation procedures (e.g., hyperventilation), normal variants, and the various artifacts that may mimic pathologic abnormalities.

As with any other diagnostic test, electroencephalography must be properly performed to yield the most useful data (Epstein *et al.* 2006a). In particular, the awake EEG should include at least 20 minutes of artifact-free recording, followed, when appropriate, by the activating procedures of hyperventilation, photic stimulation, and sleep, which should itself last an additional 20 minutes.

In contrast with CT and MR scanning, there is nothing 'intuitively' obvious about an EEG tracing: anyone familiar with neuroanatomy can almost immediately grasp an MR scan. Looking at an EEG tracing is, however, like looking at an electrocardiogram (ECG); without a considerable amount of preparation on the part of the physician, the EEG tracing is no more informative about the state of the brain than the ECG is about the heart. Consequently, this section on EEG is relatively longer than that on neuroimaging, as well as more detailed.

Instrumentation

Electrodes are attached to the scalp and are connected via wires to the EEG machine. Pairing of these wires, and the electrodes from which they stem, allows one to construct numerous different channels. In older, analog machines, this pairing is performed utilizing 'selector switches': however, in the now standard digital machines, an analog-to-digital-converter allows for the creation of channels at the touch of a keyboard. Within the EEG machine itself, one finds amplifiers and filters that respectively amplify the very weak electrical signals arising from the cortex and filter out as much as possible electrical activity that arises from either extracerebral sources or from the brain, and which is of little clinical interest.

The amplified and filtered electrical impulse of each channel is then used, in analog machines, to cause a deflection of the appropriate pen over a continuously moving sheet of paper, thus creating the actual tracing (EEG). With digital machines, there are, of course, no pens or paper tracings; however, this terminology has stayed with us. In a standard recording, the sheet moves at a constant rate of 30 mm/s, and the sensitivity of the pen is set such that an impulse of 50 μV causes a deflection of 7 mm.

The specific arrangement of electrodes on the scalp is known as an array, and the international 10–20 system described by Jasper (1958) remains a world-wide standard (Epstein *et al.* 2006b). In this system, imaginary lines are drawn on the head between specific landmarks (e.g., the nasion and inion) and the electrodes are placed along them at certain fractional intervals, i.e., either 10 percent or 20 percent of the total length of the imaginary line. These electrodes are designated with letters that refer to their location, and with numbers that indicate whether they are on the left side of the head, the right side or in the sagittal midline; thus, F_p = frontopolar, F = frontal, T = temporal, O = occipital, C = central, P = parietal, and A = auricular; odd numbers indicate the left side of the head, even numbers the right side, and zero ('z') the sagittal midline. Figure 1.3 demonstrates these placements, and Table 1.1 provides the full name for each electrode. Note, however,

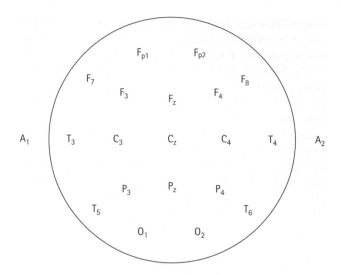

Figure 1.3   Electroencephalography (EEG) electrode placement according to the international 10–20 system (see text for details).

Table 1.1   Electrode names in the 10–20 system

Name	Position
F_{p1}, F_{p2}	Prefrontal
F_7, F_8	Anterior temporal
T_3, T_4	Mid-temporal
T_5, T_6	Posterior temporal
O_1, O_2	Occipital
F_3, F_4	Frontal
C_3, C_4	Central
P_3, P_4	Parietal
A_1, A_2	Auricular
F_z	Frontal midline
C_z	Central vertex
P_z	Parietal midline

that clarification is needed regarding electrodes F7 and F8; although, logically, one might expect these to be called 'frontal', they are commonly referred to instead as 'anterior temporal' leads as, for the most part, they reflect activity arising from the anterior portion of the temporal lobes.

This international 10–20 system may be extended and modified by adding more electrodes (Chatrian *et al.* 1985; Epstein *et al.* 2006b), and this may be resorted to in order to improve localization or to increase spatial resolution and allow for better computed EEG analysis. Supplemental leads may also be added to better detect and localize foci in the temporal lobe. 'True' anterior temporal leads (to be distinguished from the admittedly misnamed F7 and F8 electrodes) are placed by drawing a line between the external auditory canal and the lateral canthus, and placing the electrode anterior to the external auditory canal one-third of the way forward along, and 1 cm above, this line (Homan *et al* 1988; Silverman 1960). Nasopharyngeal leads, as the name suggests, are inserted into the nostril in order to sample the medial aspect of the temporal lobe (MacLean 1949). Sphenoidal leads are invasive, requiring a trochar to place them through the masseter muscle and up posterior to the zygomatic arch: these also attempt to sample the medial aspect of the temporal lobe (Risinger *et al.* 1989).

There is a debate over which one or combination of supplemental leads is most appropriate for detecting temporal lobe foci. The addition of anterior temporal leads provides more sensitivity than a routine 10–20 array, and it appears that anterior temporal leads are either of roughly equivalent (Sperling and Engel 1985) or superior sensitivity (Sadler and Goodwin 1989) to nasopharyngeal leads. It is not clear how anterior temporal leads compare in sensitivity to sphenoidal leads: some studies find them equivalent (Homan *et al.* 1988; Sadler and Goodwin 1989); however, others find sphenoidal leads superior (Sperling *et al.* 1986). Whenever temporal lobe foci are sought, at the very least 'true' anterior leads should be ordered with other supplemental leads held in reserve.

As noted earlier, the electroencephalography machine allows electrodes to be paired in various ways, and the pattern of such pairings is known as a montage. Three standard montages are recommended: a referential montage and two bipolar montages, namely a longitudinal bipolar montage and a transverse bipolar montage (Epstein *et al.* 2006c).

In a referential montage, each scalp electrode is paired with the same 'reference' electrode, usually the ipsilateral ear, producing channels such as F_7-A_1, T_3-A_1, and T_5-A_1. The scalp electrode is commonly referred to as the 'active' electrode, in contrast with the reference electrode, which is termed 'indifferent'. However, this terminology is not accurate because the ear electrode in fact picks up electrical activity arising from the temporal lobe and is thus only 'relatively' indifferent. In some instances, other electrodes, or combinations of electrodes, will be used instead of one ear: thus, the reference electrode may be found on the angle of the mandible or an 'average reference electrode' may be produced by averaging the electrical activity of a large number of scalp electrodes (Goldman 1950).

In a bipolar montage, scalp electrodes are paired in two directions – longitudinal and transverse. In a longitudinal bipolar montage, the pairings proceed ipsilaterally, from anterior to posterior, producing 'chains' of channels, such as $F_{p1}-F_3$, F_3-C_3, C_3-P_3, and P_3-O_1. In a transverse bipolar montage, the chain proceeds across the scalp, from left to right, for example F_7-F_3, F_3-F_z, F_z-F_4, F_4-F_8. It is appropriate to note here that in the chains of a bipolar montage one individual electrode may serve as the second electrode in one channel and the first electrode of the next; for example, in the chain noted above, containing channels $F_{p1}-F_3$, F_3-C_3, C_3-P_3, and P_3-O_1, note that electrode F_3 serves as the second electrode for the first channel ($F_{p1}-F_3$) and the first electrode for the next channel (F_3-C_3). As will be noted later in the discussion of interictal epileptiform abnormalities, the commonality of one electrode to two successive channels in a bipolar montage allows for a localization of epileptic foci.

Normal EEG

The electrical activity recorded by the EEG arises from the apical dendrites of cortical pyramidal neurons (Humphrey 1968; Purpura and Grundfest 1956). Although the electrical activity associated with an action potential is too brief to be recorded on an EEG (i.e., lasting less than 1 ms), activity derived from both inhibitory and excitatory postsynaptic potentials lasts much longer (from 15 to 200 ms) and it is this activity that is reflected in the EEG (Humphrey 1968). The electrical activity arising from one neuron is obviously too weak to affect the surface electrodes, so it is upon the summed activity of numerous neurons that the EEG depends. Furthermore, it must be borne in mind that abnormal electrical activity occurring deep below the cortex may not 'reach' the scalp electrodes (Cooper et al. 1965) and thus certain deep lesions, such as lacunar infarcts, may not cause any abnormality on the EEG although have profound clinical consequences (MacDonnell et al. 1988).

Electroencephalographic activity may or may not be rhythmic and it appears that rhythmicity occurs secondary to the activity of the thalamus, which acts like a pacemaker or 'conductor', exerting rhythmic control over the cortical 'orchestra', and bringing large groups of neurons into synchrony (Dempsey and Morrison 1942; Steriade et al. 1990). This dependence of cortical neurons upon the thalamus for rhythmic firing was demonstrated by experiments in which the destruction of the thalamus abolished rhythmic cortical activity (Jasper 1949).

The EEG consists of various waves that may differ in terms of morphology, amplitude, and duration. Thus, in terms of morphology, an individual wave may be monophasic, diphasic, triphasic, or polyphasic, depending on how many times the 'baseline' is crossed by the wave in question. Amplitude is measured in microvolts from the crest to the trough of the wave: customarily, amplitudes under 20 μV are considered low, those between 20 and 50 μV, medium, and those over 50 μV, high (some electroencephalographers will, however, rather than using this absolute scale, consider the amplitude of a given wave relative to the overall amplitude of background activity: thus, if the background activity were generally of 60 μV, a 30-μV wave, using this relative scale, might be considered low). It is therefore critical that the electroencephalographer specifies whether an absolute or a relative scale is being used when reporting amplitude. The duration of the wave is measured in milliseconds: waves lasting less than 70 ms are referred to as 'spikes' and those lasting from 70 to 200 ms as 'sharp waves'; those lasting for over 200 ms are spoken of either as 'slow waves' or simply 'waves'.

Waves may be isolated or recurrent. If recurrent, their frequency is reported in cycles per second (Hz): by convention, frequencies less than 4 Hz are termed 'delta', those from 4 to under 8 Hz 'theta', those from 8 to 13 Hz 'alpha', and those over 13 Hz as 'beta' waves. Some electroencephalographers also use the terms 'slow' and 'fast', 'slow' referring to both delta and theta activity (i.e., anything under 8 Hz) and 'fast' referring to any activity in the beta range (i.e., over 13 Hz). Recurrent activity may also be rhythmic and regular in occurrence, or arrhythmic and irregular.

The EEG will normally have a recognizable background activity that is more or less persistent and similar throughout the recording. Upon this background, one may at times see isolated events that, for one reason or another, stand out from the background, such events being referred to as 'transients'. Transients may, in turn, consist either of an isolated spike or wave, or a 'complex' of two or more of these. Complexes themselves are further described in terms of whether they are isolated or recurrent, and if recurrent, whether they recur irregularly or regularly. 'Spindles' comprise a specific type of transient complex, consisting of a group of rhythmic waves that gradually increase in amplitude, and then just as gradually decrease.

The normal adult awake EEG, as seen during relaxed wakefulness with the eyes closed, contains an alpha rhythm and a beta rhythm. These two terms must not be used loosely: for example, although much EEG activity may occur in the alpha *frequency*, the activity must fulfill certain other criteria to qualify as an alpha *rhythm*. In a minority of individuals, a *mu rhythm* may also be seen.

The *alpha rhythm* consists of more or less regular sinusoidal activity, ranging in amplitude from 20 to 60 μV (averaging about 50), occurring in the alpha range and most prominent posteriorly. The alpha rhythm is generally 'blocked' by eye opening, being replaced by lower amplitude, and faster/irregular activity. Although the frequency of the alpha rhythm is the same on each side, the actual waves themselves are generally out of phase. Further, there is also generally an amplitude difference between the two sides, with the left side alpha being of lower amplitude than the right. Generally, this amplitude differential is no more than 20 percent; however, the range of normal here is wide, with some normal individuals having differentials up to 50 percent. The alpha rhythm is best seen in a state of relaxed wakefulness with the eyes closed. In a small minority of cases, variants of the alpha rhythm may occur (Goodwin 1947), wherein the frequency of the sinusoidal activity is either in the 4- to 5-Hz range ('slow' alpha variant) or 16- to 20-Hz range ('fast' alpha variant). These variants represent 'harmonics' of the more typical alpha rhythm.

The *beta rhythm* consists of bilateral beta activity of an amplitude of 30 μV or less, seen best anteriorly, which is blocked unilaterally by contralateral tactile stimulation, movement, or merely an intention to move. Although the waves are generally out of phase, the frequency is bilaterally symmetric. An amplitude variance of up to 35 percent from side to side is considered normal. Beta activity is often increased by sedatives such as benzodiazepines and barbiturates (Brown and Penry 1973; Frost et al. 1973; Greenblatt et al. 1989).

The *mu rhythm* represents another normal type of EEG activity, one that is not seen as routinely as the alpha or beta rhythms and is present in only about 10 percent of normal adults. The mu rhythm consists of theta or alpha activity (ranging from 7 to 11 Hz) that appears as long transients ('trains') lasting at least several seconds and appearing in the centroparietal region. Although these occur bilaterally, the trains are often not synchronous, with one side having a train and then losing it, and then a train appearing a little later on the opposite side. The mu rhythm is generally 50 μV or less in amplitude. The mu rhythm, like the beta rhythm, may also be unilaterally blocked by contralateral phenomena (Chatrian 1964; Chatrian *et al.* 1959) including movement (Chatrian *et al.* 1959), intention to move (Klass and Bickford 1957) and tactile stimuli (Magnus 1954).

Each of these three normal rhythms may represent a kind of 'idling' of the underlying cerebral cortex. This hypothesis, poetic as it might be, gains support from the various blocking maneuvers. For example, if the alpha rhythm represents an idling occipital cortex one would expect it to be blocked when the occipital cortex is brought into gear by visual stimuli.

The normal adult sleep EEG demonstrates both REM (rapid eye movement) and non-REM (NREM: non-rapid eye movement) sleep. REM sleep is, as the name suggests, characterized by rapid, saccadic, conjugate eye movements and is typically associated with dreaming. NREM sleep is generally not associated with dreaming, and during such sleep, the eyes are either still, or slowly roving about. NREM sleep may further be divided into four stages: I, II, III, and IV, with each of these stages having a distinctive electroencephalographic signature (Erwin *et al.* 1984; Rechtschaffen and Kales 1968). In order to identify the various stages one must be familiar with several different transient events: vertex sharp transients, K complexes, sleep spindles, and positive occipital sharp transients (POSTs).

Vertex sharp transients (also known as 'V waves') are intermittently occurring, bilaterally symmetric sharp waves of high amplitude (rarely more than 250 μV) seen most prominently at the vertex. K complexes are very similar to vertex sharp transients, differing only in that they generally consist of a diphasic slow wave. Sleep spindles are transients lasting from half a second to several seconds, consisting of rhythmic activity in the 11- to 14-Hz range, which, as with all spindles, demonstrates a gradual increase and decrease in amplitude, with a maximum of generally less than 50 μV. These sleep spindles occur simultaneously on both sides and, although maximal centrally, are widespread. POSTs (Vignaendra *et al.* 1974) consist of sharp waves of positive polarity seen posteriorly in the occipital regions. They are monophasic and generally of no more than 50 μV in amplitude; although they are seen bilaterally, they are not synchronous. Furthermore, they are not rhythmic and can be seen at irregular intervals of anywhere from several to one per second.

With these various transients in mind, the four sleep stages may now be defined. The onset of stage I is marked by 'alpha dropout', with slowing of the background rhythm into the delta–theta range (2–7 Hz); soon thereafter vertex sharp transients appear. Stage II is characterized by a persistence of the slowing and the vertex sharp transients, but with the appearance of K complexes, sleep spindles and POSTs. Stage III is characterized by further slowing (20–50 percent of the background activity being in the delta range), an absence of vertex sharp transients, a fading out of K complexes and sleep spindles, but a persistence of POSTs. Stage IV is identified by gross slowing (more than 50 percent delta activity), an absence of vertex sharp transients and K complexes, and only rare sleep spindles and POSTs.

The entire night's sleep typically occurs in cycles, each cycle lasting from 80 to 120 minutes. The first cycle begins as the patient drifts into stage I, progressing down through stages II and III to stage IV and thence back up through stages III and II to stage I, from which REM sleep emerges. The end of REM sleep signals the end of the first cycle and the beginning of the next. During one night's sleep, subjects normally pass through three to five of these cycles, and with each successive cycle, the amount of time spent in stage IV sleep decreases.

EEG abnormalities

The various EEG abnormalities discussed here include decreased amplitude, slowing (either focal or generalized), interictal ('epileptiform') and ictal abnormalities, periodic complexes, triphasic waves, and the burst-suppression pattern.

DECREASED AMPLITUDE

Low-amplitude EEG activity may result either from an alteration in the media between the cortex and the recording electrode or from decreased electrogenesis by the cortex (Aird and Shimuzu 1970). For example, both grease and an abnormally thick skull (e.g., in Paget's disease) act as insulators, and fluid collections, such as subgaleal, epidural, or subdural hematomas, act as 'shunts' that divert the electrical field away from the overlying electrode. Cortical electrogenesis may be reduced either because of actual destruction, as in Alzheimer's disease or tumors, or decreased neuronal activity, as in metabolic deliria or post-ictal states. Decreased amplitude may be either generalized or focal.

Generalized low-amplitude EEGs of from 20 to 10 μV may be seen in 5–10 percent of normal adults; an amplitude of less than 10 μV is rare in normal subjects. When the general amplitude is reduced to below 20 μV, it is helpful to be able to compare the current record with past ones, or to make serial recordings in order to determine whether the low amplitude is stable or worsening. It is also critical to ensure that the recording is made during relaxed wakefulness: tense or anxious patients, or those engaging in some more or less demanding mental activity, will have low-amplitude recordings. A generalized decrease in amplitude may be seen in conditions characterized by widespread cortical neuronal loss (e.g., Alzheimer's disease,

Huntington's disease [Scott *et al.* 1972], Creutzfeldt–Jakob disease [Burger *et al.* 1972], post-anoxic encephalopathy, or AIDS dementia [Harden *et al.* 1993]) or widespread neuronal dysfunction (e.g., metabolic deliria such as hepatic or uremic encephalopathy, or other conditions such as hypothyroidism, hypothermia, uncomplicated alcohol withdrawal [Walker *et al.* 1956] or post-ictally after a grand mal seizure).

Focal low-amplitude EEGs may be seen in conditions that cause a unilateral increase in the media (e.g. subdural hematoma [Lusins *et al.* 1976]) and either unilateral neuronal destruction (e.g., infarction or tumor [Aird and Shimuzu 1970]) or dysfunction (e.g., transient ischemic attacks, migraine, and post-ictally after a partial seizure [Kaibara and Blume 1988]).

In evaluating amplitude asymmetries of the alpha rhythm, one must not forget that the left side normally has an amplitude of up to 50 percent less than the right; it is thus only when the alpha rhythm on the left is at least 50 percent less than that on the right that one can declare with certainty that an abnormality is present. The beta rhythm is generally bilaterally symmetric, but even here an amplitude asymmetry is not unusual in normal individuals; thus, for the beta rhythm, any asymmetry must be more than 35 percent before it can be declared outside the normal range.

A unilateral reduction in amplitude of the beta rhythm indicates a frontal lesion. In general, a unilateral reduction of the alpha rhythm suggests a lesion of the underlying occipital cortex, but in the case of the alpha rhythm an amplitude reduction may also be seen with distant lesions in the frontal or parietal cortices or the ipsilateral thalamus.

Amplitude asymmetry may occasionally be spurious, as for example with 'breach' rhythms. Here, in conditions where the skull has been breached, for example with a burr hole or fracture (regardless of how much scar tissue has formed), an excessive amplitude is seen on the side with the breach, making the normal amplitude activity on the other side appear low by comparison (Cobb *et al.* 1979).

SLOWING

Slowing on the EEG may be either focal or generalized.

Focal slowing

Focal slowing may consist of either theta or delta activity, and is seen in a variety of focal conditions, including infarcts and tumors (Daly and Thomas 1958; Gastaut *et al.* 1979; Gilmore and Brenner 1981), subdural hematoma (Lusins *et al.* 1976), post-ictally after a focal onset seizure (Gilmore and Brenner 1981), after some migraine headaches (Hockaday and Whitty 1969), and early in herpes simplex encephalitis (Upton and Gumpert 1970).

Generalized slowing

Generalized slowing appears in the theta or delta range and may be either bilaterally asynchronous or synchronous. Asynchronous generalized slowing is most commonly seen

in metabolic or toxic delirium (Pro and Wells 1977; Romano and Engel 1944). Metabolic deliria accompanied by generalized asynchronous slowing include hepatic encephalopathy and uremic encephalopathy, and the deliria occurring secondary to hyperglycemia, hypoglycemia, hypernatremia, hyponatremia, hypercalcemia, or hypocalcemia. Toxic deliria associated with similar slowing include those due to phenytoin (Roseman 1961), valproate (Adams *et al.* 1978), and either carbamazepine or phenobarbital (Schmidt 1982). Generalized slowing may also be seen during alcohol intoxication (Walker *et al.* 1956) and in Wernicke's encephalopathy. Interestingly, however, the delirium of delirium tremens, rather than slowing, is accompanied by an increase of beta activity (Kennard *et al.* 1945; Schear 1985). The delirium seen with bacterial meningitis or viral encephalitis is also marked by generalized slowing. Various dementing disorders may also be accompanied by generalized asynchronous slowing, including Alzheimer's disease (Deisenhammer and Jellinger 1974; Johannesson *et al.* 1977), Binswanger's disease (Caplan and Schoene 1978), Parkinson's disease (Neufeld *et al.* 1988), diffuse Lewy body disease (Briel *et al.* 1999), progressive supranuclear palsy (Su and Goldensohn 1973), normal pressure hydrocephalus (Wood *et al.* 1974), vitamin B12 deficiency (Walson *et al.* 1954), post-anoxic encephalopathy (Hockaday *et al.* 1965), AIDS dementia (Harden *et al.* 1993), and Creutzfeldt–Jakob disease (Burger *et al.* 1972) (including the new-variant type [Zeidler *et al.* 1997]).

A mild degree of generalized asynchronous slowing may also be seen as a normal variant in a small minority of subjects; furthermore, occasional scattered theta transients are not at all abnormal in normal subjects over the age of 60 years (Kooi *et al.* 1964). Generalized slowing also, of course, occurs with sleep, and thus slowing in a drowsy patient who is slipping in and out of sleep is of little significance.

Synchronous bilaterally generalized slowing typically occurs episodically, and in such cases is termed IRDA (intermittent rhythmic delta activity). In most adults, IRDA is predominantly frontal, and is termed FIRDA (frontal intermittent rhythmic delta activity) (Zurek *et al.* 1985), whereas in children IRDA is generally occipital and referred to as OIRDA (Watemberg *et al.* 2007). Although FIRDA was classically associated with deep midline lesions (Daly *et al.* 1953), it has now become clear that FIRDA is most commonly seen in metabolic and toxic deliria (Schaull *et al.* 1981), especially in patients with pre-existing ischemic lesions (Watemberg *et al.* 2002); FIRDA has also been reported in association with diffuse Lewy body disease (Calzetti *et al.* 2002), Creutzfeldt–Jakob disease (Wieser *et al.* 2004), and in association with high-dosage antipsychotics (Koshino *et al.* 1993). There is one other, relatively rare, type of IRDA which is restricted to the temporal areas: this TIRDA, rather than being seen in delirium, most commonly occurs in patients with complex partial seizures (Normand *et al.* 1995), especially, as might be expected, in those with foci in the temporal lobes (Di Gennaro *et al.* 2003).

INTERICTAL AND ICTAL EEG ABNORMALITIES

In patients with seizures or epilepsy, abnormalities seen between seizures are termed 'interictal', whereas those seen during a seizure are designated as 'ictal'.

Interictal activity

Interictal activity consists of what are known as epileptiform discharges. These interictal epileptiform discharges (IEDs) are paroxysmal transients that 'shoot' out from the background rhythm (Pedley 1980). These paroxysmal transients may consist of isolated spikes or sharp waves or may appear as complexes, such as spike-and-sharp wave, spike-and-slow wave, sharp-and-slow wave, polyspikes, or polyspike-and-wave discharges. Although epileptiform activity may be seen in a very small percentage of subjects who have never had a seizure (Ajmone-Marsan and Zivin 1970; Gibbs et al. 1943; Gregory et al. 1993; Zivin and Ajmone-Marsan 1968), and may also occur as a side-effect of certain medications (e.g., lithium [Helmchen and Kanowski 1971], clozapine [Malow et al. 1994], meperidine [Kaiko et al. 1983]), and in patients with autism (Kim et al. 2006) or developmental dysphasia (Picard et al. 1998), they are typically present only in patients with a history of seizures. Importantly, however, although most epileptic patients will have interictal epileptiform abnormalities (Goodin and Aminoff 1984), the absence of such a finding on the first EEG does not rule out a diagnosis of epilepsy, as it may take up to four or more EEGs before an IED is 'caught' (Salinsky et al. 1987). Furthermore, in evaluating a patient who has had a seizure, it is important to obtain the EEG within the first 24 hours, as EEGs obtained later than this are less likely to reveal IEDs (King et al. 1998). It must be borne in mind, however, that in a very small minority of patients with unquestionable epilepsy routine EEGs will simply not display IEDs (Ajmone-Marsan and Zivin 1970; Martins da Silva et al. 1984; Morris et al. 1988).

Interictal epileptiform activity may be generalized, focal, or multifocal:

Generalized bisynchronous IEDs indicate the presence of one of the idiopathic generalized epilepsies, such as petit mal epilepsy (either childhood or juvenile onset), juvenile myoclonic epilepsy, or epilepsy with any tonic–clonic seizures. In petit mal epilepsy, one sees the classic, roughly 3-Hz generalized and bisynchronous spike and dome discharges (Dalby 1969); in the other forms, the IEDs may be spike-and-wave, polyspike or polyspike-and-wave in character (Betting et al. 2006) (importantly, in this latter group a minority of patients displayed atypical findings, including focal discharges).

Focal epileptiform activity strongly suggests an underlying focal epileptogenic lesion (e.g., a tumor, scar, or area of cortical dysplasia), whereas multifocal epileptiform activity, as might be expected, suggests widespread and multiple lesions (e.g., subsequent to severe traumatic brain injury). The task of localizing focal epileptiform activity is facilitated by having in mind a spatial image of the electrical

activity itself. Most paroxysmal electrical discharges are 'surface negative' (Matsuo and Knott 1977), i.e., their electrical potential is negative with regard to the normal baseline. Furthermore, most of these discharges cover a fairly wide area: although the discharge may be 'seen' under only one electrode, this is quite rare and in the vast majority of cases it covers a wider area, subtending two or more adjacent electrodes. The electrical activity itself may be visualized as a landscape, which may in turn contain various topographic features: gently rolling electrical hills and valleys represent the normal EEG background, whereas deep chasms can be likened to epileptiform discharges plunging down from the background. With this image in mind, one can understand the changes produced on either a referential or bipolar montage.

To take an example, consider an epileptiform discharge producing an electrical 'chasm' on the left hemisphere that is large enough to subtend electrodes F_3, C_3, and P_3, as illustrated in Figure 1.4. Keep in mind also that, in this example, the 'walls' of the chasm, rather than going straight up and down, instead gently slope down to the greatest electrical depth. Thus, proceeding from F_{p1} to F_3 the depth falls, from F_3 to C_3 it continues to fall to its nadir, from C_3 to P_3 it rises, and from P_3 to O_1 it continues to rise back to the surface. Assume, for the purpose of this example, that the gently rolling landscape exists at an electrical potential of $-25\,\mu V$, and that this is what electrodes F_{p1}, O_1, and A_1 'see'. Furthermore, assume also that electrode F_3, being over the gently downsloping wall of the chasm, sees a potential of $-50\,\mu V$, and that electrode C_3, being over the nadir of the chasm, sees a potential of $-100\,\mu V$. Electrode P_3, being over the following wall of the chasm, sees $-50\,\mu V$, and electrode O1 encompasses the normal landscape of $-25\,\mu V$. Depending on whether a referential or bipolar montage is used, the EEG recording of this same landscape will look quite different.

As noted earlier, in a referential recording each scalp, or active electrode, is paired with the same reference electrode, in this example the ipsilateral ear; thus, in this example, as

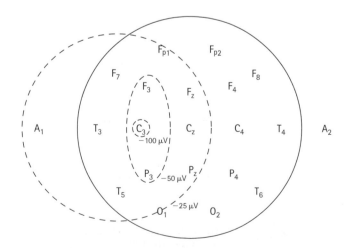

Figure 1.4 Surface-negative epileptiform discharge, of greatest extent at electrode C_3 (see text for details).

illustrated in Figure 1.5, there are five channels to consider: $F_{p1}-A_1$, F_3-A_1, C_3-A_1, P_3-A_1, and O_1-A_1. Channel $F_{p1}-A_1$, with both electrodes 'seeing' the same potential, would register no difference; channel F_3-A_1 would see a difference of $25\,\mu V$ (i.e., looking up from a depth of -50 to the surface, which is at -25); channel C_3-A_1 would see a difference of $75\,\mu V$ (looking up from a depth of -100 to the surface at -25); channel P_3-A_1 a difference of $25\,\mu V$ (looking up from -50 to -25), and the last channel, O_1-A_1, with both electrodes seeing $-25\,\mu V$, would register 0. As seen in Figure 1.4, the greatest pen deflection is seen in the channel containing the electrode, in this example C_3, which lies over the deepest part of the electrical chasm. Thus, with referential recordings, it is the channel showing the greatest amplitude that serves to localize the focus of the electrical paroxysm.

It may be noted that the pen deflections in channels F_3-A_1, C_3-A_1, and P_3-A_1 are all positive, and this is according to the convention (Knott 1985) that whenever, in going from the first to second lead of any channel, one is

'looking' up, the pen goes up, but if one is 'looking' down the pen likewise goes down.

The situation with bipolar recordings is quite different: here, it is not amplitude that is important but a phenomenon known as phase reversal (Knott 1985; Lesser 1985). Take the same example of an electrical paroxysm as used above, but this time cover it, as illustrated in Figure 1.6, with a longitudinal chain of electrodes, starting at F_{p1} and including, sequentially, F_3, C_3, P_3, and O_1. Then construct the following channels: $F_{p1}-F_3$, F_3-C_3, C_3-P_3, and, finally, P_3-O_1. Now consider what each channel will record. For channel $F_{p1}-F_3$, one looks down from F_{p1} at -25 to F_3 at -50, for a difference of $-25\,\mu V$. For the next channel, F_3-C_3, one continues to look down into the electrical chasm, now looking down from -50 to -100, for a difference of $-50\,\mu V$. At the next channel, C_3-P_3, however, something very different happens; here, standing at the nadir of the chasm at -100, one is looking 'up' to -50, for a difference of $+50\,\mu V$. Similarly, for the next channel, P_3-O_1, one continues to look up, but here from -50 to -25, for a difference of $+25\,\mu V$.

Figure 1.6 shows the various pen tracings seen for each channel. As may be noted, both channels $F_{p1}-F_3$ and

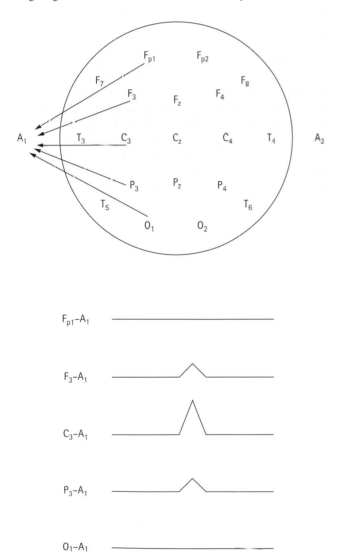

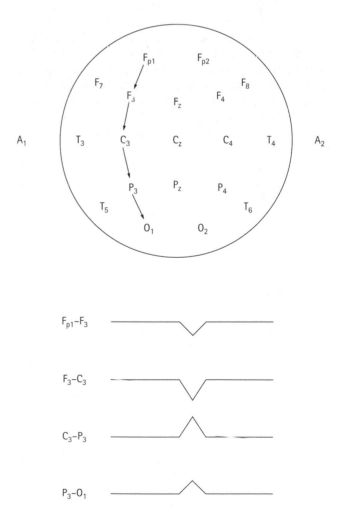

Figure 1.5 Referential recording of the epileptiform discharge shown in Figure 1.4 (see text for details).

Figure 1.6 Bipolar recording of the epileptiform discharge shown in Figure 1.4 (see text for details).

F_3-C_3 show a downward or negative pen deflection. What happens next, however, is most critical: the next two channels, C_3-P_3 and P_3-O_1, both show an upward or positive deflection. It is apparent here that there has been a phase reversal as one goes from channel F_3-C_3 to channel C_3-P_3. This indicates that, in going from channel F_3-C_3 to channel C_3-P_3, one has 'crossed' over the depth of the electrical chasm; furthermore, as the electrode that both these channels have in common is C_3, it is now clear that the depth of the chasm lies under that electrode; that is to say phase reversal is seen at electrode C_3.

In some cases, focal epileptiform activity will not exhibit phase reversal with a bipolar montage. Specifically, when the focus is either proximal to the start of the chain or distal to its end, phase reversal is not possible. For example, consider a longitudinal chain linking F_{p1}, F_3, C_3, P_3, and O_1, and then imagine that the focus is located anterior to F_{p1}. In this case, all the pen deflections will be positive. Conversely, if the focus were distal to O_1, all the pen deflections would be negative.

Ictal activity

Ictal discharges consist of rhythmic activity that, unlike interictal epileptiform discharges, is sustained, at the very least, for a matter of seconds, with most ictal discharges lasting minutes. These ictal discharges may be either generalized at the onset or display a focal onset.

Ictal discharges that are generalized from the onset are typically seen in the idiopathic generalized epilepsies: myoclonic seizures are typically accompanied by polyspike or polyspike-and-wave sustained discharges, and petit mal seizures by sustained spike-and-dome discharges very similar to those seen interictally (Browne et al. 1974).

Ictal discharges that are focal at the onset may remain so for the duration of the seizure, and in most of these cases, clinically one sees a simple partial seizure of one sort or the other. In cases when there is spread to a more or less focal area contralaterally a complex partial seizure is often seen, and in those cases when the generalization involves the entire cortex, a grand mal seizure is the typical accompaniment. Although in some cases in which there was some preceding interictal epileptiform activity the ictal discharges may resemble the interictal ones, in most cases ictal discharges are morphologically different (Blume et al. 1984; Geiger and Horner 1978). In general, the ictal activity is rhythmic and may occur at any frequency, from delta to beta; rarely, instead of primarily a change in frequency, one may see a change in amplitude, namely an 'electrodecremental' pattern in which the seizure is accompanied only by a paroxysmal loss of amplitude.

Remarkably, in the case of partial seizures, the surface EEG may remain normal, even in the face of indisputable seizures. In the case of simple partial seizures (Cockerell et al. 1996; Devinsky et al. 1989; Seshia and McLachlan 2005) this is seen in the majority; however, with complex partial seizures it is noted in only a very small percentage (Lieb et al. 1976).

PERIODIC COMPLEXES

Periodic complexes generally consist of one or more sharp waves combined with one or more slow waves that recur on a regular basis, at intervals ranging from 1 to 15 seconds, often on a background of generalized slowing. Although they may begin with a focal predominance, they fairly soon become generalized and synchronous, often with a frontal prominence. Such periodic complexes are often associated with myoclonus and are classically seen in such disorders as subacute sclerosing panencephalitis (Cobb 1966; Cobb and Hill 1950) and Creutzfeldt–Jakob disease (Aguglia et al. 1987; Burger et al. 1972; Chiofalo et al. 1980; Levy et al. 1986; Steinhoff et al. 1996). Importantly, although almost all patients with Creutzfeldt–Jakob disease eventually develop periodic complexes (Browne et al. 1986) (generally within the first 3 months [Levy et al. 1986]), these may be absent (Bortone et al. 1994; Zochodne et al. 1988), and this appears to be particularly the case with new-variant Creutzfeldt–Jakob disease (Will et al. 1996). Periodic complexes have also been noted in various other conditions, including herpes simplex viral encephalitis (Upton and Gumpert 1970), post-anoxic encephalopathy (Hockaday et al. 1965), Alzheimer's disease and diffuse Lewy body disease (Doran and Larner 2004; Tschampa et al. 2001), and baclofen intoxication (Hormes et al. 1988).

Triphasic waves constitute a specific kind of periodic complex. These are slow waves that, as the name indicates, possess a triphasic morphology. They typically occur in a generalized, bilaterally synchronous fashion, often with a frontal predominance, either singly, in an isolated fashion, or in longer bursts. Although they are classically associated with hepatic encephalopathy (Karnatze and Bickford 1984; Summerskill et al. 1956), they may be seen in other types of metabolic delirium (Fisch and Klass 1988) such as that of uremia, hypercalcemia, hypoglycemia, hypernatremia, or hyponatremia, and have also been noted in a toxic delirium secondary to lithium (Kaplan and Birbeck 2006).

Periodic lateralized epileptiform discharges (PLEDS) constitute another specific form of periodic complex. These consist of lateralized epileptiform discharges (either spikes or sharp waves) that occur with a fairly regular periodicity, varying from once every half a second to every 5 seconds (Chatrian et al. 1964; Markand and Daly 1971). As described in two large studies (Garcia-Morales et al. 2002; Gurer et al. 2004), in most cases PLEDS are associated with lesions affecting the cortex. Although subcortical white matter lesions may also be responsible, this is far less common; the most common lesions are infarctions, followed by tumors, abscesses, and subdural hematomas. Other conditions include Creutzfeldt–Jakob disease, herpes simplex encephalitis, and post-anoxic encephalopathy and, rarely, alcohol withdrawal (Chu 1980). In most cases, PLEDS occur during the acute onset of these underlying lesions and then gradually remit; in a small minority of cases, however, they may persist chronically. Clinically, most patients will also have seizures (Baykan et al. 2000); importantly, however, with rare exceptions (Singh *et al.* 2005), the PLEDS themselves do not constitute ictal discharges, but, from an electroencephalographic point of view, constitute innocent bystanders.

Bilateral independent periodic lateralized epileptiform discharges (BIPLEDS) constitute a variant of PLEDS, with, as the name suggests, the appearance of these lateralized epileptiform discharges first on one side, then the other. This pattern may be seen in herpes simplex encephalitis or anoxic encephalopathy (de la Paz and Brenner 1981), and with bilateral infarctions of the frontal (Nicolai *et al.* 2001), or temporal lobes (Fushimi *et al.* 2003).

BURST-SUPPRESSION

The burst-suppression pattern is characterized by bursts of generalized, bilaterally symmetric and synchronous delta activity, lasting in the order of 1–3 seconds and occurring every 3–10 seconds, in between which the background activity is suppressed to a very low amplitude or, at a normal sensitivity, to a flat line. This pattern is seen in states of severe cortical dysfunction, for example subacute sclerosing panencephalitis (Markand and Panzi 1975), viral encephalitis, or post-anoxic coma (Hockaday *et al.* 1965). Although it is typically bilateral, it may occasionally be seen unilaterally, as for example after a very large infarction.

Activation procedures

Hyperventilation, photic stimulation, and sleep are all considered to be activation procedures in that they may activate certain abnormalities that would otherwise not be apparent on the routine EEG. In patients suspected of having reflex seizures, exposing the patient to the putative epileptogenic stimulus may also be considered in order to activate the focus.

HYPERVENTILATION

Hyperventilation is normally followed by a build-up of generalized, bilaterally symmetric and synchronous high-amplitude slow waves, maximal frontally in adults (Goldberg and Strauss 1959). Abnormalities that may occur include asymmetric or focal slowing and epileptiform abnormalities. Asymmetric or focal slowing has the same significance as spontaneous slowing, as discussed previously in this chapter. Epileptiform abnormalities are very common in the case of petit mal seizures, with most of these patients showing typical 3-Hz spike-and-dome epileptiform changes (Dalby 1969); indeed, in these patients hyperventilation is a more sensitive diagnostic procedure than is a 6-hour recording (Adams and Lueders 1981). In the case of complex partial seizures, however, only a small minority of cases will display activation (Adams and Lueders 1981; Gabor and Ajmone-Marsan 1969; Miley and Forster 1977; Morgan and Scott 1970). In addition to IEDs, seizures may also be induced by hyperventilation but this is very uncommon

(Holmes *et al.* 2004), except in patients with treatment-resistant focal seizures, in whom it occurred in one-quarter of all patients (Guaranha *et al.* 2005).

Hyperventilation is generally contraindicated in patients with sickle cell disease (Protass 1978) or those with significant cerebrovascular or cardiovascular disease.

PHOTIC STIMULATION

Photic stimulation is accomplished by positioning a stroboscopic light about 30 cm from the patient's face, the eyes being either open or closed. The light is then flashed at various frequencies (e.g., 3, 5, 10, 13, 15, 17, 20, and 25 Hz), each frequency being allotted about 10 seconds. In about two-thirds of normal adults this stroboscopic illumination will produce the photic driving response, wherein bilaterally symmetric and synchronous waves appear at a frequency equal to either the stroboscopic frequency or some harmonic of it (Hughes 1960). Normally, although the photic driving is maximal occipitally, it may extend to the parietal or temporal area. Maximal photic driving is generally seen when the strobe frequency is close to the patient's normal alpha rhythm and, as with the alpha rhythm, the amplitude of the photic driving response is often lower on the left side. With very high-frequency stroboscopic activity the resultant wave forms may resemble spikes. Abnormalities seen with photic driving include unexpected amplitude asymmetries, photomyoclonic responses, and photoparoxysmal responses. Amplitude asymmetries wherein the left side has an amplitude of less than 50 percent that of the right, or wherein the right side has an amplitude less than that of the left, indicate a definite abnormality. The photomyoclonic response (Meier-Ewert and Broughton 1976) consists of a myoclonic twitching of the eyelids and, in severe cases, myoclonus of the head and neck; it may be seen in a very small minority of normal individuals (Kooi *et al.* 1960) and more commonly in those withdrawing from alcohol or sedative hypnotics (Fisch *et al.* 1989; Gastaut *et al.* 1958). The photoparoxysmal response consists of epileptiform changes (Bickford *et al.* 1952) and is most common in those with petit mal or one of the other idiopathic generalized epilepsies (Stevens 1962; Wolf and Gooses 1986). A minority of patients with the photoparoxysmal response will experience a seizure during the photic stimulation (Seddigh *et al.* 1999).

SLEEP

Sleep may activate epileptiform activity (Sammaritano *et al.* 1991); indeed, IEDs are seen only during sleep in up to one-third of patients with complex partial seizures (Niedermeyer and Rocca 1972). The sleep portion of the recording should last at least 20 minutes and include both stages I and II of sleep. In some cases, patients will simply drift off to sleep on their own at the end of the awake recording session, whereas in others the administration of chloral hydrate will be required. Some authors recommend sleep deprivation not only to ensure that the patient falls asleep during the recording, but also in the belief that sleep deprivation *per se* is activating: this is a controversial notion, supported by some (Ellingson *et al.* 1984; Leach *et al.* 2006; Mattson *et al.* 1965), but not all, studies (Pratt *et al.* 1968; Veldhuizen *et al.* 1983). In interpreting a sleep EEG it is important to distinguish epileptiform activity from normally occurring POSTs and vertex sharp waves. In addition to revealing epileptiform abnormalities, sleep recordings may, at times, reveal other abnormalities, for example the early onset of REM sleep as may be seen in narcolepsy or in alcohol or anxiolytic withdrawal (Kales *et al.* 1974).

REFLEX ACTIVATION

In cases of definite or suspected 'reflex' epilepsy, it may be appropriate, as discussed in Section 7.3 to expose the patient to the triggering event itself. Thus, in 'musicogenic' epilepsy, the appropriate tune may be played, and in 'reading' epilepsy, the appropriate passage read, etc. Consideration must, of course, be given to the risk of inducing a seizure during the recording.

Normal variants

Normal variants may resemble epileptiform changes (e.g., small sharp spikes [SSS]) or pathologic slow waves (e.g., subclinical rhythmic EEG discharges of adults [SREDA]).

SSS, also known as benign epileptiform transients of sleep (BETS), are, as the name suggests, low-amplitude, very sharp spikes (i.e., less than 50 μV in amplitude and less than 50 ms in duration) that are seen intermittently during drowsiness in both temporal areas, either intermittently or in a bilaterally synchronous fashion (Klass and Westmoreland 1985; White *et al.* 1977).

Phantom spike-and-wave (also known as 6-cps spike-and-wave) (Klass and Westmoreland 1985; Thomas and Klass 1968) is characterized by brief trains of rhythmic 6-Hz activity that are generalized, bilaterally symmetric, and synchronous, generally lasting no longer than a second or two. The name comes from the fact that the rhythmic activity is composed of a peculiar spike-and-wave complex wherein the spike is of such relatively low amplitude and brevity that, next to the much more prominent wave, it, like the 'Phantom', is rarely seen.

'Occipital spikes of blind persons', an aptly named electrographic syndrome, may be seen in patients with congenital or acquired blindness and is characterized by intermittent spikes confined to the occipital area.

SREDA (O'Brien *et al.* 1998; Westmoreland and Klass 1981) is characterized by lengthy trains of rhythmic theta or, less commonly, delta activity, seen best in the centroparietal areas. The trains themselves are often of abrupt onset and may be preceded by some sharp waves. They

generally last about a minute and are most commonly seen with hyperventilation in the elderly.

Rhythmic mid-temporal discharges (Gibbs *et al.* 1963; Klass and Westmoreland 1985), also known as rhythmic theta bursts of drowsiness, consist of lengthy trains of rhythmic theta activity that occur in both temporal areas, either synchronously or independently. The trains themselves often last about 10 seconds but they may endure for as long as a minute. This variant was once referred to as the psychomotor variant but this terminology has been abandoned as there is no connection between rhythmic mid-temporal discharges and complex partial seizures.

Ctenoids, also known as '14- and 6-cps positive bursts' (Klass and Westmoreland 1985; Lombroso *et al.* 1966) consist of brief trains, lasting half a second to one second, of 6- or 14-Hz rhythmic waves that occur in the temporal regions either independently or in a bilaterally synchronous fashion. They are best seen during stages I and II of sleep, and the waves themselves have a distinctive arciform morphology.

Wicket spikes (Klass and Westmoreland 1985; Reiher and Lebel 1977) consist of brief trains of rhythmic activity at a frequency of 6–11 Hz, which are most prominent in the temporal regions where they may appear independently or in a bilaterally synchronous fashion. Like ctenoids, the waves themselves have an arciform morphology. In some cases, rather than trains, wicket spikes may occur in an isolated fashion: such isolated wicket spikes may be distinguished from IEDs by the absence of a following slow wave (Krauss *et al.* 2005).

Lambda waves (Barlow and Ciganek 1969; Evans 1953; Green 1957; Scott *et al.* 1967) are isolated, bilaterally synchronous occipital waves that occur just after saccadic eye movements made by patients as they scan a detailed scene or picture. The waves themselves are of 20–50 μV in amplitude and 200–300 ms in duration; they have a characteristic triangular or sawtooth-shaped morphology. These may be eliminated by having the patient stare at a blank sheet of paper, and this technique should be utilized and noted by the EEG technologist.

Artifacts

Artifacts may be grouped according to the EEG activity that they most closely resemble, including interictal epileptiform discharges, slow waves, or decreased amplitude. There is also a 60-cps artifact, which is usually readily identified as it does not resemble any naturally occurring EEG activity.

RESEMBLING INTERICTAL EPILEPTIFORM DISCHARGES

Drip artifact (Linnenger *et al.* 1981) reflects the electrical disturbance occurring each time a drip occurs in an intravenous line. It may appear so similar to an epileptiform discharge that its correct identification may depend on the EEG technician noting on the record when the drips occur.

Electrode pop reflects, as it were, a sudden 'spark' at an individual electrode, often occurring secondary to some impurity. Although it strongly resembles an epileptiform spike the fact that it is restricted to one electrode betrays its artifactual nature, as true epileptiform spikes are almost always seen at more than one electrode.

Electrocardiography (ECG) artifact represents cardiac electrical activity picked up by the EEG. In the case of a regular cardiac rhythm, its artifactual nature is immediately obvious as epileptiform spikes simply do not occur with such monotonous regularity. When irregularly occurring premature ventricular contractions are present, however, the distinction may be more difficult and indeed may depend on simultaneously recording the ECG.

Muscle artifact reflects electrical activity arising from the contraction of the scalp musculature and may appear in any one of three ways: as isolated irregularly appearing 'blips', or as 'blips' superimposed on a 'muddy' black line, the blips occurring either arrhythmically or rhythmically. The key to the identification of muscle 'blips' is their extreme brevity.

RESEMBLING SLOW WAVES

Eye movements may induce artifacts (Peters 1967). In the case of vertical movements, the artifact is seen in the frontopolar leads and, if horizontal, in the anterior temporal leads. Heuristically, the eye may be considered to be a 'battery', the cornea being positive and the retina negative; thus, whichever electrode the eye 'looks' toward becomes more positive, and whichever one the eyes 'look' away from becomes, conversely, more negative. Consider, for example, the results with a longitudinal bipolar montage when the patient engages in horizontal eye movement looking to the left: F_7 becomes more positive relative to T_3, and thus, in the channel F_7-T_3 the pen deflection is downwards; conversely, F_8 becomes more negative relative to T_4, and thus, in channel F_8-T_4, the pen deflection is up. Next, consider the situation with vertical eye movements, as occurs during a blink (Matsuo et al. 1975), recalling that when a blink occurs, the eyes, in Bell's phenomenon, undergo upward rotation. In this case, both frontopolar electrodes, F_{p1} and F_{p2}, become positive relative to their immediate neighbors, F_3 and F_4, and thus channels $F_{p1}-F_3$ and $F_{p2}-F_4$ both show a negative deflection. Eye movement artifacts, whether horizontal or vertical, are suggested by their bilateral synchrony. In the case of horizontal movements, a further indication is the fact that the resulting pen deflections on either side are in opposite directions. In the case of vertical eye movements occurring with blinking, the occurrence of eyelid flutter may make identification a little more difficult because the resulting artifact will appear similar to a bifrontal slow wave focus.

Movement artifact occurs when the electrodes are actually moved, as most commonly occurs when the occipital electrodes (pressed between the patient's head and the underlying pillow) are slightly dislodged by the minimal head movements that occur either with respiration or, when present, tremor. The regularity of the resulting artifact, the identity of its frequency with the respiratory rate or the tremor frequency, and its restriction to the occipital leads all highlight its true nature.

Glossokinetic artifact occurs with tongue movement. The tip of the tongue is negative, and its up and down movement may produce slow waves in the frontal or temporal areas. Asking the patient to say 'la la la' during the recording allows for ready identification of this artifact.

Pulse artifact occurs in situations when an electrode is accidentally placed over a relatively large scalp artery, which, with every passing pulse, slightly moves the electrode resting on it. The fact that the resulting artifact occurs at a regular rate, identical to the cardiac rate, suggests its true identity: in doubtful cases, a simultaneous ECG will reveal that the pulse artifact follows, after a slight delay, every QRS complex, the delay reflecting the time required for the pulse to travel from the heart to the scalp.

Perspiration on the scalp, as may occur if the patient is febrile or anxious, both alters the resistance of the overlying electrodes and allows for some slight slippage between the electrodes and the scalp: the resulting artifact consists of very slow waves (e.g., 0.5 Hz) of very high amplitude, which occur in a generalized, bilateral, but asynchronous fashion.

RESEMBLING DECREASED AMPLITUDE

Increased electrode resistance may lead to what appears to be decreased amplitude at one electrode. Its restriction, however, to but one electrode betrays its artifactual nature as pathologic conditions capable of causing decreased amplitude are rarely so restricted in location that they will be reflected at only one electrode position.

Defective calibration of one channel may result in a decreased deflection of that channel's pen. Its isolation to one pen suggests the correct diagnosis; furthermore, the fact that the same pen continues to show decreased deflection with changing montages confirms the diagnosis.

SIXTY CYCLE PER SECOND ARTIFACT

A 60-Hz artifact occurs secondary to interference from a nearby alternating current source, typically appearing on the EEG as a thick 'muddy' line. If there is any doubt as to the source of such a 'muddy' line, lowering the paper speed to 15 mm/s will confirm the diagnosis by allowing the resolution of the line into orderly 60-Hz deflections.

1.6 LUMBAR PUNCTURE

In the not-too-distant past, lumbar puncture was a standard procedure and it was the rare neuropsychiatric patient admitted to hospital who escaped this procedure. Although the need for this test has dropped dramatically with the advent of modern neuroimaging using CT and MRI, there are still certain clinical situations, as discussed below, in which it is vital. This section will discuss the indications and contraindications for lumbar puncture, its technique and complications, and the various tests, both standard and otherwise, that may be ordered.

Indications and contraindications

Lumbar puncture is indicated in cases of encephalitis or meningitis, and in those uncommon cases wherein sub-arachnoid hemorrhage is strongly suspected although the CT scan is negative. Lumbar puncture is also indicated when the following disorders are suspected: neurosyphilis, multiple sclerosis, Creutzfeldt–Jakob disease, certain cases of vasculitis, and benign intracranial hypertension.

Lumbar puncture is contraindicated when there is infection of any of the tissues near the site of the proposed puncture. Conditions that present a risk of bleeding during the puncture also constitute contraindications, and these include thrombocytopenia (with platelet counts below 50 000) and treatment with either heparin or warfarin. In cases when puncture must be performed, consideration may be given to use of platelet transfusion, protamine, or vitamin K. Evidence of increased intracranial pressure is often considered a contraindication, but this holds only where there is a risk of herniation, whether subfalcine, uncal, transtentorial, or cerebellar. Thus, the presence of mass lesions and acute infarctions generally argue against lumbar puncture. However, there are some cases of raised intracranial pressure wherein the risk of herniation is low, as for example in benign intracranial hypertension and some cases of subarachnoid hemorrhage; in these instances lumbar puncture may be safely performed and indeed may be carried out therapeutically. As a rule, imaging with either CT or MRI should be performed in every patient before lumbar puncture: the only exception here would be when bacterial meningitis is strongly suspected and delay could prove fatal.

Technique (Roos 2003)

The patient is placed in the left lateral decubitus position on a firm surface, with his or her back brought up to the edge of the bed or gurney. Pillows are placed under the head and neck as well as between the legs, and the back is kept strictly vertical by assuring that the right shoulder and hip are directly above the left shoulder and hip, respectively. The patient is then helped into a fetal position by flexing the head and legs, thus opening the spaces between the spinous processes. In adults, the needle should generally be inserted in the L3–L4 interspace, a spot which may be found by palpating the superior iliac crests and then drawing an imaginary line between them: the appropriate interspace generally lies just below this line. After palpating

the appropriate area, the target may be marked by indenting the skin with a fingernail. The area is then prepped with betadine and alcohol, and sterile drapes are placed. Most physicians will then infiltrate the superficial tissues with half a cubic centimeter of a local anesthetic; however, some, on the theory that this puncture causes as much pain as the actual lumbar puncture, will forgo it. In order to reduce the risk of a post-lumbar puncture headache (Evans et al. 2000), a 20- or 22-gauge needle should be used (higher gauge needles, up to 26 gauge, are even safer in this regard [Tourtellotte et al. 1972], but given their small size the flow of CSF may be quite sluggish), and the bevel of the needle should be parallel to the longitudinal axis of the patient, as this angle allows for separation, rather than laceration, of dural fibers. Atraumatic needles are even less prone to cause headache (Lavi et al. 2006; Strupp et al. 2001) but they are more difficult to use. The needle itself should be held perpendicular to the patient's back and angled slightly cephalad, generally toward the patient's umbilicus (with due regard for sagging umbilici in obese patients). The needle is then gently inserted: at a depth of from 4 to 5 cm, there is often a palpable 'give' as the dura is pierced, followed by a less obvious 'pop' when the arachnoid is punctured. Once these landmark events have transpired, the stylet should be slowly removed (rapid removal may suck a nerve rootlet into the lumen) and one should watch to see if any fluid emerges. 'Dry taps' generally indicate improper placement and, if the patient is tolerating the procedure, the stylet should be replaced, the needle gently withdrawn, and another attempt made. As fluid emerges, the patient may be allowed to relax and to slightly extend the legs. In cases when an opening pressure is desired, a manometer is attached to the needle and the pressure of water read (in centimeters). Given that compression of the abdomen may elevate the pressure, it is necessary for obese patients to relax their legs sufficiently to release any pressure on the abdomen before reading the pressure. In any case, the CSF is then collected into three containers and these are then promptly sealed. When sufficient fluid has been obtained, the stylet is replaced, the needle is withdrawn, and firm pressure is applied to the puncture site, followed by the application of an adhesive plaster. The patient may then be allowed to be up ad lib; bed rest at this point does not decrease the risk of a post-lumbar puncture headache (Dieterich and Brandt 1985).

Recently, it has become common to perform lumbar puncture under fluoroscopic guidance, with the procedure itself performed by a radiologist.

Complications

The most common complication of a lumbar puncture is headache and this may occur in about one-quarter of all cases. The headache occurs typically a day or two after the puncture, and may last from days to a couple of weeks: it is generalized and may be either steady or throbbing in character, and is worse when sitting or standing and generally relieved by recumbancy. Treatment involves bed rest and analgesics; caffeine sodium benzoate, in a dose of 500 mg i.v., may also be used and is typically dramatically effective (Choi *et al.* 1996). If these fail, and the headache is severe, a 'blood patch' may be placed by injecting about 10 cubic centimeters (cm^3) of the patient's blood on to the puncture site: this procedure, however, should not be routine for it may cause a radiculopathy in up to one-third of all cases. The mechanism underlying the headache involves leakage of fluid through the dural hole, which allows the brain to 'sag', thus stretching pain-sensitive structures. This sagging may also stretch cranial nerves, resulting in tinnitus, deafness, or diplopia; rarely, these cranial nerve palsies may occur in the absence of headache.

Other complications include backache, subarachnoid bleeding, radiculopathy, and, as noted above, herniation.

Standard measurements

A number of determinations are considered standard and should be requested in all cases. These include the appearance of the fluid, cell count and differential, total protein, glucose, stain and appropriate culture, and tests for syphilis. Measurement of the opening pressure was once standard but is now rarely required.

APPEARANCE

Normal CSF is crystal clear. A 'ground glass' appearance may occur in the presence of 200 or more red blood cells (RBCs), whereas red counts over 1000 may impart a pinkish cast to the fluid. A hazy fluid may occur in the presence of 200 or more white cells, and larger white counts may make the fluid cloudy in appearance.

Xanthochromia, or a yellowish discoloration, may occur in any situation when the total protein is over 150 mg/dL. Such a discoloration may also occur in jaundice (serum bilirubin >6 mg/dL), cases of carotenemia and in patients treated with rifampin. Another very important cause of xanthochromia is hemolysis (as may be seen eight or more hours after a subarachnoid hemorrhage), wherein lysed red cells leak hemoglobin breakdown products, such as bilirubin, into the CSF.

Frankly bloody CSF may occur either in cases of subarachnoid hemorrhage or after a traumatic, or 'bloody', tap. Traumatic taps occur in about 10 percent of lumbar punctures and, rather than reflecting poor technique, they generally result from the accidental nicking of a vein in the epidural plexus. These two possibilities may be differentiated by the 'three-tube test', wherein one simply watches for any change in appearance between the first, second, and third tubes collected. In subarachnoid hemorrhage, the fluid in the third tube is as bloody as that in the first, whereas in a traumatic tap there is substantial clearing of the fluid by the third tube. These two conditions may also be distinguished by centrifuging the first tube, and inspecting the supernatant. In traumatic taps the supernatant is clear, whereas in subarachnoid hemorrhage the presence of hemolyzed red cells creates xanthochromia. Importantly, however, xanthochromia may be absent early on, for, as noted above, hemolysis generally takes at least 8 hours to occur.

CELL COUNT AND DIFFERENTIAL

Normal CSF is free of red cells but may contain up to five white cells, either lymphocytic or mononuclear. Red cells may be seen in subarachnoid hemorrhage and cases of either contusion or intracerebral/intraventricular hemorrhage.

A pleocytosis, i.e., increased number of white cells, is seen in a large number of conditions. Note that a polymorphonuclear predominance generally indicates a bacterial infection: although viral, fungal, or tubercular infections may initially display a polymorphonuclear predominance a lymphocytic one is far more common, especially after the infection has passed the acute stage.

When the CSF is frankly bloody, as in subarachnoid hemorrhage or with a traumatic tap, the CSF white blood count (WBC) is of course elevated by white cells derived directly from the systemic circulation. As a rule of thumb, one may correct for this by subtracting one white cell from the total CSF count for every 1000 red cells.

Total protein

Most of the protein in the CSF consists of albumin; other constituents include gamma-globulins, other globulins (alpha and beta) and prealbumin. The total protein in normal CSF ranges from 15 to 45 mg/dL.

When the fluid is grossly bloody, the total protein is corrected by subtracting about 1 mg for each 1000 RBCs.

Glucose

Normally, CSF glucose runs anywhere from 50 to 65 percent of serum glucose and hence normal CSF values range from 45 to 80 mg/dL. In all cases, the serum glucose should be measured, however, given that 2–4 hours are required for equilibration between serum and CSF, the timing of the blood draw varies according to the fed state of the patient: when the patient is fasting, the blood draw may be just before the puncture; when the patient has eaten, however, the blood draw should be 2–4 hours before the scheduled puncture.

Elevated CSF glucose is of no concern. Reductions in CSF glucose may occur with hypoglycemia, in bacterial or fungal meningitides, or other inflammatory disorders.

Stains and cultures

The CSF should always be Gram-stained and, whenever tuberculosis is suspected, an acid-fast stain should also be requested. An 'India ink prep' is traditional when cryptococcal infection is suspected; however, the availability of polymerase chain reaction (PCR) assays has made this almost superfluous. Appropriate cultures should also be requested, whether bacterial, tubercular, or fungal.

Tests for syphilis

It is good practice to always request a CSF-VDRL test with titer. Furthermore, in cases where the clinical picture is consistent with neurosyphilis but the CSF-VDRL is negative it is entirely appropriate to obtain a CSF-FTA, given that the CSF-FTA is a far more sensitive test than the CSF-VDRL (Davis and Schmitt 1989; Timmermans and Carr 2004).

Opening pressure

Measurement of the opening pressure, although once considered standard, is rarely required in modern practice: one exception consists of cases of suspected benign intracranial hypertension. The normal opening pressure ranges from 6 to 20 cm of water; values of below 5 cm may be seen with systemic dehydration, subarachnoid block, or following a prior lumbar puncture. Elevations of over 20 cm are seen in cases of benign intracranial hypertension, meningitis, cerebral venous occlusion, and with mass lesions, hemorrhages, or acute infarctions.

Other determinations

Other determinations are requested depending on one's diagnostic suspicions, and may include PCR assay and testing for various antibodies and antigens: in these regards, consultation with an infectious disease specialist, if not already in the works, is always appropriate, given the rapid advances made in these fields. Other tests to consider include the immunoglobulin G (IgG) index, oligoclonal bands, myelin basic protein and the 14-3-3 protein.

Polymerase chain reaction assay represents a rapid, sensitive, and specific means for detecting various infections. Viruses detected include herpes simplex, varicella zoster, Epstein-Barr, JC virus, HIV, and cytomegalovirus (CMV) (Steiner et al. 2005). Furthermore, almost all bacteria may also be identified (Poppert et al. 2005). Fungal and tubercular infections may also be detected.

Antibodies to arboviruses, rabies virus, *Borrelia burgdorferi* and *Coccidioides immitis* may be tested for, as may antigens specific for *Cryptococcus* and *Histoplasma*, and these should be ordered in the appropriate clinical setting.

The IgG index provides a reliable measure of increased production of IgG within the CNS. Elevations of total IgG itself may represent a false-positive, given that the immunoglobulin level in the CSF reflects not only intrathecal synthesis of globulin, but also transfer of globulins from the systemic circulation. Consequently, it is necessary to correct the CSF level by obtaining what is known as the 'IgG index'. The IgG index = (IgG[CSF]/IgG[serum])/ (albumin[CSF]/albumin[serum]). IgG index values above 0.65 indicate intrathecal synthesis. To calculate this, of course, one must also obtain blood for a serum protein electrophoresis, and this should be done just before the lumbar puncture.

Oligoclonal bands, that is to say anywhere from three to five bands seen on electrophoresis, are seen in a number of conditions, including multiple sclerosis, lupus, Behçet's syndrome, neurosarcoidosis, and infections, whether viral, bacterial, or fungal.

Myelin basic protein is found in diseases characterized by myelin breakdown, such as multiple sclerosis. An increased myelin basic protein, however, is certainly not specific for multiple sclerosis, being found in various other conditions, such as encephalitis, lupus, vasculitidies, and recent infarction.

The 14-3-3 protein should be tested for in suspected cases of Creutzfeldt–Jakob disease. Although this is very sensitive for Creutzfeldt–Jakob disease, false-positives have been noted in large number of conditions such as encephalitis, recent infarction, multiple sclerosis, Hashimoto's encephalopathy, paraneoplastic limbic encephalitis, astrocytoma, and even degenerative disorders such as Alzheimer's disease, diffuse Lewy body disease, and amyotrophic lateral sclerosis (Lemstra et al. 2000; Martinez-Yelamos et al. 2001; Van Everbroeck et al. 2005).

REFERENCES

Adams DJ, Lueders H. Hyperventilation and 6-hour EEG recording in evaluation of absence seizures. *Neurology* 1981; **31**:1175–7.

Adams DJ, Lueders H, Pippinger CH. Sodium valproate in the treatment of intractable seizure disorders: a clinical and electroencephalographic study. *Neurology* 1978; **28**:152–7.

Aguglia U, Farnarier G, Tinuper P et al. Subacute spongiform encephalopathy with periodic paroxysmal activities: clinical evaluation and serial EEG findings in 20 cases. *Clin Electroencephalogr* 1987; **18**:147–58.

Aird RB, Shimizu M. Neuropathological correlates of low-voltage EEG foci. *Arch Neurol* 1970; **22**:75–80.

Ajmone-Marsan C, Zivin LS. Factors related to the occurrence of typical paroxysmal abnormalities in the EEG records of epileptic patients. *Epilepsia* 1970; **11**:361–81.

Akelaitis AJE. Psychiatric aspects of myxedema. *J Nerv Ment Dis* 1936; **83**:22–36.

Altman NR, Purser RK, Rost MJD. Tuberous sclerosis: characteristics at CT and MR imaging. *Radiology* 1988; **167**:523–32.

Andreasen NC. Affective flattening and criteria for schizophrenia. *Am J Psychiatry* 1979; **136**:944–7.

Armstrong P, Keevil SF. Magnetic resonance imaging. 2. Clinical uses. *BMJ* 1991; **303**:105–9.

Barkovich AJ, Kjos BO. Gray matter heterotopias: MR characteristics and correlation with developmental and neurologic manifestations. *Radiology* 1992; **182**:493–9.

Barlow JS, Ciganek L. Lambda responses in relation to visual evoked responses in man. *Electroencephalogr Clin Neurophysiol* 1969; **26**:183–92.

Barnes MP, Saunders M, Walls TJ et al. The syndrome of Karl Ludwig Kahlbaum. *J Neurol Neurosurg Psychiatry* 1986; **49**:991–6.

Baykan B, Kinay D, Gokyigit A *et al.* Periodic lateralized epileptiform discharges: association with siezures. *Seizure* 2000; **9**:402–6.

Berger H. Uber das clektrenkephalogramm des menschen. *Archiv Psychiat Nervenkr* 1929; **87**:527–70.

Berkovic SF, Andermann F, Olivier A *et al.* Hippocampal sclerosis in temporal lobe epilepsy demonstrated by magnetic resonance imaging. *Ann Neurol* 1991; **29**:175–82.

Berry I, Brant-Zawadzki M, Osaki L *et al.* Gd-DTPA in clinical MR of the brain. 2. Extra-axial lesions and normal structures. *AJR* 1986; **147**:1231–5.

Beschin N, Cubelli R, Della Sala S *et al.* Left of what? The role of egocentric coordinates in neglect. *J Neurol Neurosurg Psychiatry* 1997; **63**:483–9.

Betting LE, Mory SB, Lopes-Cendes I *et al.* EEG features in idiopathic generalized epilepsy: clues to diagnosis. *Epilepsia* 2006; **47**:523–8.

Bickerstaff ER. *Neurological examination in clinical practice*, 4th edn. Oxford: Blackwell Scientific, 1980.

Bickford RG, Sem-Jacobsen CW, White PT *et al.* Some observations on the mechanism of photic and photo-Metrazol activation. *Electroencephalogr Clin Neuropshysiol* 1952; **4**:275–82.

Bleuler E. *Textbook of psychiatry*, translated by Brill AA. New York: Macmillan, 1924. Reissued by Arno Press, New York, 1976.

Blume WT, Young GB, Lemieux JF. EEG morphology of partial epileptic seizures. *Electroencephalogr Clin Neurophysiol* 1984; **57**:295–302.

Bories J, Derhy S, Chiras J. CT in hemispheric ischemic attacks. *Neuroradiology* 1985; **27**:468–83.

Bortone E, Bettoni L, Giorgi C *et al.* Reliability of EEG in the diagnosis of Creutzfeldt–Jakob disease. *Electroencephalogr Clin Neurophysiol* 1994; **90**:323–30.

Bradley WG, Waluch W, Yadley RA *et al.* Comparison of CT and MR in 400 patients with suspected disease of the brain and cervical spinal cord. *Radiology* 1984; **152**:695–702.

Brain W. *Clinical neurology*, 2nd edn. London: Oxford University Press, 1964.

Brant-Zawadzki M, Badami JP, Mills CM *et al.* Primary intracerebral tumor imaging: a comparison of magnetic resonance and CT. *Radiology* 1984; **150**:435–40.

Brant-Zawadzki M, Berry I, Osaki L *et al.* Gd-DTPA in clinical MR of the brain. 1. Intraaxial lesions. *AJR* 1986; **147**:1223–30.

Briel RC, McKeith IG, Barber WA *et al.* EEG findings in dementia with Lewy bodies and Alzheimer's disease. *J Neurol Neurosurg Psychiatry* 1999; **66**:401–3.

Brown JJ, Hesselink JR, Rothrock JF. MR and CT of lacunar infarcts. *Am J Neuroradiol* 1988; **9**:477–82.

Browne P, Cathala F, Castaigne P *et al.* Creutzfeldt–Jakob disease: clinical analysis of a consecutive series of 230 neuropathologically verified cases. *Ann Neurol* 1986; **20**:597–602.

Browne TR, Penry JK. Benzodiazepines in the treatment of epilepsy. *Epilepsia* 1973; **14**:277–310.

Browne TR, Penry JK, Porter RJ *et al.* Responsiveness before, during and after spike-wave paroxysms. *Neurology* 1974; **24**:659–65.

Burger LJ, Rowan AJ, Goldensohn ES. Creutzfeldt–Jakob disease. An electroencephalographic study. *Arch Neurol* 1972; **26**:428–33.

Calzetti S, Bortone E, Negrotti A *et al.* Frontal intermittent rhythmic delay activity (FIRDA) in patients with dementia with Lewy bodies: a diagnostic tool? *Neurol Sci* 2002; **23**(suppl. 2):S65–6.

Caplan LR, Schoene WL. Clinical features of subcortical arteriosclerotic encephalopathy (Binswanger disease). *Neurology* 1978; **28**:1206–15.

Caton R. The electrical currents of the brain. *BMJ* 1875; **2**:278.

Chatrian GE. Characteristics of unusual EEG patterns: incidence, significance. *Electroencephalogr Clin Neurophysiol* 1964; **17**:471–2.

Chatrian GE, Petersen MC, Lazarte JE. The blocking of the rolandic wicket rhythm and some central changes related to movement. *Electroencephalogr Clin Neurophysiol* 1959; **11**:497–510.

Chatrian GE, Shaw CM, Leffman H. The significance of periodic lateralized epileptiform discharges in EEG: an electrographic, clinical and pathological study. *Electroencephalogr Clin Neurophysiol* 1964; **17**:177–93.

Chatrian GE, Lettich F, Nelson PL. Ten percent electrode system for topographic studies of spontaneous and evoked EEG activities. *Am J EEG Technol* 1985; **25**:83–92.

Chiofalo N, Fuentes A, Galvez S. Serial EEG findings in 27 cases of Cretuzfeldt–Jakob disease. *Arch Neurol* 1980; **37**:143–5.

Choi A, Laurito CE, Cunningham FE. Pharmacologic management of postdural puncture headache. *Ann Pharmacother* 1996; **30**:831–9.

Choi SH, Na DL, Chung CS *et al.* Diffusion-weighted MRI in vascular dementia. *Neurology* 2000; **54**:83–9.

Chrysikopoulos HS, Press GA, Grafe MR *et al.* Encephalitis caused by human immunodeficiency virus: CT and MR imaging manifestations with clinical and pathological confirmation. *Radiology* 1990; **175**:185–91.

Chu NS. Periodic lateralized epileptiform discharges with preexisting focal brain lesions: role of alcohol withdrawal and anoxic encephalopathy. *Arch Neurol* 1980; **37**:551–4.

Cobb WA. The periodic events of subacute sclerosing panencephalitis. *Electroencephalogr Clin Neurophysiol* 1966; **21**:278–94.

Cobb WA, Hill D. Electroencephalogram in subacute progressive encephalitis. *Brain* 1950; **73**:392–404.

Cobb WA, Guiloff RJ, Cast J. Breach rhythm: the EEG related to skull defects. *Electroencephalogr Clin Neurophsyiol* 1979; **47**:251–71.

Cockerell OC, Rothwell J, Thomson PD *et al.* Clinical and physiological features of epilepsia partialis continua. Cases ascertained in the UK. *Brain* 1996; **119**:393–407.

Cooper R, Winter AL, Crown JJ *et al.* Comparison of subcortical, cortical and scalp activity using indwelling electrodes in man. *Electroencephalogr Clin Neurophysiol* 1965; **18**:217–28.

Cornelius JR, Day NL, Fabrega H *et al.* Characterizing organic delusional syndrome. *Arch Gen Psychiatry* 1991; **48**:997–9.

Dalby MA. Epilepsy and three per second spike and wave rhythms. A clinical electroencephalographic and prognostic evaluation of 346 patients. *Acta Neurol Scand* 1969; **45**(suppl. 40):1–180.

Daly DD, Thomas JE. Sequential alterations in the electroencephalograms of patients with brain tumors. *Electroencephalogr Clin Neurophysiol* 1958; **10**:395–404.

Daly DD, Whelan JL, Bickford RG *et al.* The electroencephalogram in cases of tumor of the posterior fossa and third ventricle. *Electroencephalogr Clin Neurophysiol* 1953; **5**:203–16.

Davis LE, Schmitt JW. Clinical significance of cerebrospinal fluid tests for neurosyphilis. *Ann Neurol* 1989; **25**:50–5.

Dean BL, Drayer BP, Bird CR. Gliomas: classification with MR imaging. *Radiology* 1990; **174**:411–15.

Deisenhammer E, Jelinger K. EEG in senile dementia. *Electroencephalogr Clin Neurophysiol* 1974; **36**:91–3.

DeJong RN. *The neurologic examination*, 4th edn. New York:Harper & Row, 1979.

Dempsey EW, Morrison RS. The production of rhythmically recurrent cortical potentials after localized thalamic stimulation. *Am J Physiol* 1942; **135**:293–300.

Devinsky O, Sato S, Kufta CV *et al.* Electroencephalographic studies of simple partial seizures with subdural electrode recordings. *Neurology* 1989; **39**:527–33.

Dieterich M, Brandt T. Is obligatory bedrest after lumbar puncture obsolete? *Eur Arch Psychiatr Neurol Sci* 1985; **235**:71–5.

Di Gennaro G, Quarato PP, Onorati P *et al.* Localizing significance of temporal intermittent rhythmic delta activity (TIRDA) in drug-resistant focal epilepsy. *Clin Neurophysiol* 2003; **114**:70–8.

Dolinskas C, Bilaniuk LT, Zimmerman RA *et al.* Computed tomography of intracerebral hematomas. I. Transmission CT observations of hematoma resolution. *AJR* 1977; **129**:681–8.

Doran M, Larner AJ. EEG findings in dementia with Lewy bodies causing diagnostic confusion with sporadic Creutzfeldt–Jakob disease. *Eur J Neurol* 2004; **11**:838–41.

Edelman RR, Warach S. Magnetic resonance imaging. *N Engl J Med* 1993; **328**:708–16.

Ellingson RJ, Wilken K, Bennet DR. Efficacy of sleep deprivation as an activation procedure in epilepsy patients. *J Clin Neurophysiol* 1984; **2**:83–101.

Epstein CM, Bej MD, Foldvary-Schaefer N *et al.* American Clinical Neurophysiology Society. Guideline 1: Minimum technical requirements for performing clinical electroencephalography. *J Clin Neurophysiol* 2006a; **23**:86–91.

Epstein CM, Bej MD, Foldvary-Schaefer N *et al.* American Clinical Neurophysiology Society. Guideline 5: Guideline for standard electrode position nomenclature. *J Clin Neurophysiol* 2006b; **23**:107–10.

Epstein CM, Bej MD, Foldvary-Schaefer N *et al.* American Clinical Neurophysiology Society. Guideline 6: A proposal for standard montages to be used in clinical EEG. *J Clin Neurophysiol* 2006c; **23**:111–17.

Erwin CW, Somerville ER, Radtke RA. A review of electroencephalographic features of normal sleep. *Clin Neurophysiol* 1984; **1**:253–74.

Evans CC. Spontaneous excitation of the visual cortex and association areas – lambda waves. *Electroencephalogr Clin Neurophysiol* 1953; **5**:69–74.

Evans RW, Armon C, Frohman EM *et al.* Assessment: Prevention of post-lumbar puncture headaches. *Neurology* 2000; **55**:909–14.

Faber R, Abrams R, Taylor MA *et al.* Comparison of schizophrenic patients with formal thought disorder and neurologically impaired patients with aphasia. *Am J Psychiatry* 1983; **140**:1348–51.

Fazekas F, Schmidt R, Offenbacher H *et al.* Prevalence of white matter and periventricular magnetic resonance hyperintensities in asymptomatic volunteers. *J Neuroimag* 1991; **1**:27–9.

Fiebach J, Jansen O, Schellinger P *et al.* Comparison of CT with diffusion-weighted RMI in patients with hyperacute stroke. *Neuroradiology* 2001; **43**:628–32.

Fisch BJ, Klass DW. The diagnostic specificity of triphasic wave patterns. *Electroencephalogr Clin Neurophysiol* 1988; **70**:1–8.

Fisch BJ, Hauser WA, Brust JCM *et al.* The EEG response to diffuse and patterned photic stimulation during acute untreated alcohol withdrawal. *Neurology* 1989; **39**:434–6.

Fisher M, Albers GW. Applications of diffusion-perfusion magnetic resonance imaging in acute ischemic stroke. *Neurology* 1999; **52**:1750–6.

Franceschi M, Triulzi F, Ferini-Strambi L *et al.* Focal cerebral lesions found by magnetic resonance imaging in cryptogenic nonrefractory temporal lobe epilepsy patients. *Epilepsia* 1989; **30**:540–6.

Frost JD, Carrie JRG, Borda RP *et al.* The effects of Dalmane (flurazepam hydrochloride) on human EEG characteristics. *Electroencephalogr Clin Neurophysiol* 1973; **34**:171–5.

Fushimi M, Matsubichi N, Sekine A *et al.* Benign bilateral independent periodic lateralized epileptoform discharges. *Acta Neurol Scand* 2003; **108**:55–9.

Gabor AJ, Ajmone-Marsan C. Co-existence of focal and bilateral diffuse epileptiform discharges in epileptics. *Epilepsia* 1969; **10**:453–72.

Garcia-Morales I, Garcia MT, Galan-Davila L *et al.* Periodic lateralized epileptiform discharges: etiology, clinical aspects, seizures, and evolution in 130 patients. *J Clin Neurophysiol* 2002; **19**:172–7.

Gasecki AP, Steg RE. Correlation of early MRI with CT scan, EEG and CSF: analyses in a case of biopsy-proven herpes simplex encephalitis. *Eur Neurol* 1991; **31**:372–5.

Gastaut H, Trevisan C, Naquet R. Diagnostic value of electroencephalographic abnormalities provoked by intermittent photic stimulation. *Electroencephalogr Clin Neurophysiol* 1958; **10**:194–5.

Gastaut JL, Michael B, Hassan S *et al.* Electroencephalography in brain edema (127 cases of tumor investigated by cranial computerized tomography). *Clin Neurophysiol* 1979; **46**:239–55.

Geiger LR, Horner RN. EEG pattern at the time of focal seizure onset. *Arch Neurol* 1978; **35**:276–86.

Gerson SN, Benson F, Frazier SH. Diagnosis: schizophrenia versus posterior aphasia. *Am J Psychiatry* 1977; **134**:966–9.

Gibbs FA, Gibbs EL, Lennox WG. Electroencephalographic classification of epileptic patients and control subjects. *Arch Neurol Psychiatry* 1943; **50**:111–28.

Gibbs FA, Rich CL, Gibbs EL. Psychomotor variant type of seizure discharge. *Neurology* 1963; **13**:991–8.

van Gijn J, van Dongen KJ. The time course of aneurysmal hemorrhage on computed tomograms. *Neuroradiology* 1982; **23**:153–6.

Gillespie J, Jackson A. *MRI and CT of the brain.* London: Arnold, 2000.

Gilmore PC, Brenner RP. Correlation of EEG, computerized tomography, and clinical findings: a study of 100 patients with focal delta activity. *Arch Neurol* 1981; **38**:371–2.

Goldberg HH, Strauss H. Distribution of slow activity induced by hyperventilation. *Electroencephalogr Clin Neurophysiol* 1959; **11**:615.

Goldman D. The clinical use of the 'average' reference electrode in monopolar recording. *Electroencephalogr Clin Neurophysiol* 1950; **2**:209–12.

Gomori M, Grossman RI, Goldberg HI *et al.* High field magnetic resonance imaging of intracranial hematomas. *Radiology* 1985; **157**:87–93.

Gonzalez RG, Schaefer PW, Buonanno FS *et al.* Diffusion-weighted MR imaging: accuracy in patients imaged within 6 hours of stroke symptom onset. *Radiology* 1999; **210**:155–62.

Goodin DS, Aminoff MJ. Does the interictal EEG have a role in the diagnosis of epilepsy? *Lancet* 1984; **1**:837–9.

Goodwin JE. Significance of alpha variants and their relationship to epileptiform syndrome. *Am J Psychiatry* 1947; **104**:369–79.

Graif M, Steiner RE. Contrast-enhanced magnetic resonance imaging of the central nervous system: a clinical review. *Br J Psychiatry* 1986; **59**:865–73.

Green J. Some observations on lambda waves and peripheral stimulation. *Electroencephalogr Clin Neurophysiol* 1957; **9**:691–704.

Greenberg SB, Taber L, Septimus E *et al.* CT in brain biopsy-proven herpes simplex encephalitis. Early normal results. *Arch Neurol* 1981; **38**:58–9.

Greenblatt DJ, Ehrenberg BL, Gunderman J *et al.* Pharmacokinetic and electroencephalographic study of intravenous diazepam, midazolam, and placebo. *Clin Pharmacol Ther* 1989; **45**:356–65.

Gregory RP, Oates T, Merry RTG. EEG epileptiform abnormalities in candidates for aircrew training. *Electroencephalogr Clin Neurophysiol* 1993; **86**:75–7.

Griesinger W. *Mental pathology and therapeutics.* New York: William Wood, 1882.

Grossman RI, Braffman BH, Brorson JR *et al.* Multiple sclerosis: serial study of gadolinium-enhanced MR imaging. *Radiology* 1988; **169**:117–22.

Guaranha MSB, Garzon E, Buchpiguel CA *et al.* Hyperventilation revisited: physiolgical effects and efficacy on focal seizure activation in the era of video-EEG monitoring. *Epilepsia* 2005; **46**:69–7.

Guilleux M-H, Steiner RE, Young IR. MR imaging in progressive multifocal leukoencephalopathy. *Am J Neuroradiol* 1986; **7**:1033–5.

Gurer G, Yemisci M, Saygi S *et al.* Structural lesions in periodic lateralized epileptiform discharges (PLEDS). *Clin EEG Neurosci* 2004; **35**:88–93.

Guttmann CRG, Abn SS, Hsu L *et al.* Evolution of multiple sclerosis lesions on serial MRI. *Am J Neuroradiol* 1995; **16**:1481–91.

Harden CL, Daras M, Tuchman AJ *et al.* Low amplitude EEGs in demented AIDS patients. *Electroencephalogr Clin Neurophysiol* 1993; **87**:54–6.

Haskett RF. Diagnostic categorization of psychiatric disturbance in Cushing's syndrome. *Am J Psychiatry* 1985; **142**:911–16.

Haughton VM, Rimm AA, Sobocinski KA *et al.* A blinded clinical comparison of MR imaging and CT in neuroradiology. *Radiology* 1986; **160**:751–5.

Hecaen H, Penfield W, Bertrand C *et al.* The syndrome of apractagnosia due to lesions of the minor cerebral hemisphere. *Arch Neurol Psychiatry* 1956; **75**:400–34.

Heier LA, Bauer CJ, Schwartz J *et al.* Large Virchow–Robin spaces: MR–clinical correlation. *Am J Neuroradiol* 1989; **10**:929–36.

Heilman KM. Ideational apraxia – a re-definition. *Brain* 1973; **96**:861–4.

Helmchen H, Kanowski S. EEG changes under lithium treatment. *Electroencephalogr Clin Neurophysiol* 1971; **30**:269.

Hershey LA, Gado MH, Trotter JL. Computerized tomography in the diagnostic evaluation of multiple sclerosis. *Ann Neurol* 1979; **5**:32–9.

Hockaday JM, Whitty CW. Factors determining the electroencephalogram in migraine: a study of 560 patients, according to clinical type of migraine. *Brain* 1969; **92**:769–88.

Hockaday JM, Potts F, Epstein E *et al.* Electroencephalographic changes in acute cerebral anoxia from cardiac or respiratory arrest. *Electroencephalogr Clin Neurophysiol* 1965; **18**:575–86.

Holland BA, Kucharcyzk W, Brant Zawadzki M *et al.* MR imaging of calcified intracranial lesions. *Radiology* 1985; **157**:353–6.

Holmes MD, Dewaraja AS, Vanhatalo S. Does hyperventilation elicit epileptic seizures? *Epilepsia* 2004; **45**:618–20.

Homan RW, Jones MC, Rawat S. Anterior temporal electrodes in complex partial seizures. *Electroencephalogr Clin Neurophysiol* 1988; **70**:105–9.

Hopf HC, Muller-Forell W, Hopf NJ. Localization of emotional and volitional facial paresis. *Neurology* 1992; **42**:1918–23.

Hopkins A, Shorvon S, Cascino G. *Epilepsy*, 2nd edn. London: Arnold, 1995.

Hounsfield GN. Computerized transverse axial scanning (tomography). I. Description of the system. *Br J Psychiatry* 1972; **46**:1016–22.

Hormes JT, Benarroch EE, Rodriguez M *et al.* Periodic sharp waves in baclofen-induced encephalopathy. *Arch Neurol* 1988; **45**:814–15.

Hughes JR. Usefulness of photic stimulation in routine clinical electroencephalography. *Neurology* 1960; **10**:777–82.

Humphrey DR. Re-analysis of the antidromic cortical response: II. On the contribution of all discharges and PSPs to the evoked potential. *Electroencephalogr Clin Neurophysiol* 1968; **25**:421–42.

Huttenlocher PR, Taravath S, Mojjahedi S. Periventricular heterotopia and epilepsy. *Neurology* 1994; **44**:51–5.

Jasper H. Diffuse projection systems: the integrative action of the thalamic reticular system. *Electroencephalogr Clin Neurophysiol* 1949; **1**:405–20.

Jasper HH. The ten-twenty electrode system of the International Federation. *Electroencephalogr Clin Neurophysiol* 1958; **10**:371-3.

Jenkins A, Teasdale G, Hadley MD *et al.* Brain lesions detected by magnetic resonance imaging in mild and severe head injuries. *Lancet* 1986; **2**:445-6.

Johannesson G, Brun A, Gustafson I *et al.* EEG in presenile dementia related to cerebral blood flow and autopsy findings. *Acta Neurol Scand* 1977; **56**:89-103.

Johnson MH. CT evaluation of the earliest signs of stroke. *Radiologist* 1994; **1**:189-99.

Jungreis CA, Kanal E, Hirsch W *et al.* Normal perivascular spaces mimicking lacunar infarction: MR imaging. *Radiology* 1988; **169**:101-4.

Kaibara M, Blume WT. The postictal electroencephalogram. *Electroencephalogr Clin Neurophysiol* 1988; **70**:99-104.

Kaiko RF, Foley KM, Grabisnki PY *et al.* Central nervous system excitatory effects of meperidine in cancer patients. *Ann Neurol* 1983; **13**:180-5.

Kales A, Bixler EO, Tan TL *et al.* Chronic hypnotic drug use. Ineffectiveness, drug-withdrawal insomnia and dependence. *JAMA* 1974; **227**:513-17.

Kaplan PW, Birbeck G. Lithium-induced confusional states: nonconvulsive status epilepticus or triphasic encephalopathy? *Epilepsia* 2006; **47**:2071-7.

Karnatze DS, Bickford RG. Triphasic waves: a reassessment of their clinical significance. *Electroencephalogr Clin Neurophysiol* 1984; **57**:193-8.

Katz DI, Alexander MP, Mandell AM. Dementia following strokes in the mesencephalon and diencephalons. *Arch Neurol* 1987; **44**:1127-33.

Katz DI, Taubenberger JK, Cannella B *et al.* Correlation between magnetic resonance imaging findings and lesion development in chronic, active multiple sclerosis. *Ann Neurol* 1993; **5**:661-9.

Kelly AB, Zimmerman RD, Snow RB *et al.* Head trauma: comparison of MR and CT-experience in 100 patients. *Am J Neuroradiol* 1988; **9**:699-708.

Kennard MA, Beuding E, Wortis SB. Some biochemical and electroencephalographic changes in delirium tremens. *Q J Stud Alcohol* 1945; **6**:4-14.

Kermode AG, Thompson AJ, Tofts P *et al.* Breakdown of the blood-brain barrier precedes symptoms and other magnetic resonance imaging signs of new lesions in multiple sclerosis. *Brain* 1990; **113**:1477-89.

Kidwell CS, Chalela JA, Saver JL *et al.* Comparison of MRI and CT for detection of acute intracerebral hemorrhage. *JAMA* 2004; **292**:1823-30.

Kim HL, Donnelly JH, Tonay AE *et al.* Absence of seizures despite high prevalence of epileptiform EEG abnormalities in children with autism monitored in a tertiary care center. *Epilepsia* 2006; **47**:394-8.

King MA, Newton MR, Jackson GD *et al.* Epileptology of the first seizure presentation: a clinical, EEG and MRI study of 300 consecutive patients. *Lancet* 1998; **352**:1007-11.

Kinkel W, Jacobs L, Polachini I *et al.* Subcortical arteriosclerotic encephalopathy (Binswanger's disease): computed tomographic, nuclear magnetic resonance, and clinical correlation. *Arch Neurol* 1985; **42**:951-9.

Klass DW, Bickford RG. Observations on the rolandic arceau rhythm. *Electroencephalogr Clin Neurophysiol* 1957; **9**:570.

Klass DW, Westmoreland BF. Nonepileptogenic epileptiform electroencephalographic activity. *Ann Neurol* 1985; **18**:627-35.

Knott JR. Further thoughts on polarity, montages and localization. *J Clin Neurophysiol* 1985; **2**:63-75.

Kooi KA, Thomas MH, Mortensen FN. Photoconvulsive and photomyoclonic responses in adults. An appraisal of their clinical significance. *Neurology* 1960; **10**:113-40.

Kooi KA, Guvener AM, Tupper CJ *et al.* Electroencephalographic pattern of the temporal regions in normal adults. *Neurology* 1964; **14**:1029-35.

Koshino Y, Murata I, Murata T *et al.* Frontal intermittent rhythmic delta activity in schizophrenic patients receiving antipsychotic drugs. *Clin Electroenphalogr* 1993; **24**:13-18.

Kraepelin E. *Manic-depressive insanity and paranoia*, translated by Barclay RM. Edinburgh: E&S Livingstone, 1921. Republished by Arno Press, New York, 1976.

Kraepelin E. *Psychiatry. A textbook for students and physicians*, 1899, translated by Metoui H, Ayed S. Canton, MA: Science History Publications, 1990.

Krauss GL, Abdallah A, Lesser R *et al.* Clinical and EEG features of patients with EEG wicket rhythm misdiagnosed with epilepsy. *Neurology* 2005; **64**:1879-83.

Krup LB, Lipton RB, Swerlow ML *et al.* Progressive multifocal leukoencephalopathy: clinical and radiographic features. *Ann Neurol* 1985; **17**:344-9.

Lansberg MG, Albers GW, Beaulieu G *et al.* Comparison of diffusion-weighted MR and CT in acute stroke. *Neurology* 2000; **54**:1557-61.

Laplane D, Degos JD. Motor neglect. *J Neurol Neurosurg Psychiatry* 1983; **46**:152-8.

Lavi R, Yernitzky D, Rowe JM *et al.* Atraumatic Whitacre needle for diagnostic lumbar puncture: a randomized trial. *Neurology* 2006; **67**:1492-4.

Leach JP, Stephen LJ, Salveta C *et al.* Which electroencephalography (EEG) for epilepsy? The relative usefulness of different EEG protocols in patients with possible epilepsy. *J Neurol Neurosurg Psychiatry* 2006; **77**:1040-2.

Leavitt S, Tyler H. Studies in asterixis. *Arch Neurol* 1964; **10**:360-8.

Lemstra AW, van Meegen MT, Vreyling JP *et al.* 14-3-3 testing in diagnosing Creutzfeldt-Jakob disease. A prospective study in 112 patients. *Neurology* 2000; **55**:514-16.

Lesser RP, Luders H, Dinner DS *et al.* An introduction to the basic concepts of polarity and localization. *J Clin Neurophysiol* 1985; **2**:45-61.

Levy A, Lightman SS. Diagnosis and management of pituitary tumors. *BMJ* 1994; **308**:1087-91.

Levy SR, Chiappa KH, Burke CJ *et al.* Early evolution and incidence of electroencephalographic abnormalities in Creutzfeldt-Jakob disease. *J Clin Neurophysiol* 1986; **3**:1-21.

Lieb JP, Walsh GO, Babb TL *et al.* A comparison of EEF seizure patterns recorded with surface and depth electrodes in patients with temporal lobe epilepsy. *Epilepsia* 1976; **17**:137-60.

Linnenger AW, Volow MR, Gianturco DT. Intravenous infusion artifact. *EEG Technol* 1981; **21**:167–73.

Lombroso CT, Schwartz IH, Clark DM *et al*. Ctenoids in healthy youths: Controlled study of 14- and 6-per second positive spiking. *Neurology* 1966; **16**:1152–8.

Lusins J, Jaffe R, Bender MB. Unoperated subdural hematoma: long-term follow-up study by brain scan and electroencephalography. *J Neurosurg* 1976; **44**:601–7.

MacDonnell RAL, Donnan GA, Baldin PF *et al*. The electroencephalogram in acute ischemic stroke. *Arch Neurol* 1988; **45**:520–4.

MacLean PD. A nasopharyngeal lead. *Electroencephalogr Clin Neurophysiol* 1949; **1**:110–12.

Magnus O. The cerebral alpha-rhythm ('rhythme en arceau'). *Electroencephalogr Clin Neurophysiol* 1954; **6**:349–50.

Malow BA, Reese KB, Sato S *et al*. Abnormalities during clozapine treatment. *Electroencephalogr Clin Neurophysiol* 1994; **91**:205–11.

Markand ON, Daly DD. Pseudo-periodic lateralized paroxysmal discharges in electroencephalogram. *Neurology* 1971; **21**:975–81.

Markand ON, Panzi JG. The electroencephalogram in subacute sclerosing panencephalitis. *Arch Neurol* 1975; **32**:719–26.

Martinez-Yelamos A, Saiz A, Sanchez-Valle R *et al*. 14-3-3 protein in the CSF as prognostic marker in early multiple sclerosis. *Neurology* 2001; **57**:722–4.

Martins da Silva A, Aarts JH, Binne CD *et al*. The circadian distribution of interictal epileptiform EEG activity. *Electroencephalogr Clin Neurophysiol* 1984; **58**:1–13.

Matsuo F, Knott JR. Focal positive spikes in electroencephalography. *Electroencephalogr Clin Neurophysiol* 1977; **42**:15–25.

Matsuo F, Peters JF, Reilly EL. Electrical phenomena associated with movements of the eyelid. *Electroencephalogr Clin Neurophysiol* 1975; **38**:507–11.

Mattson RH, Pratt KL, Calverley JR. Electroencephalograms of epileptics following sleep deprivation. *Arch Neurol* 1965; **13**:310–15.

Meier-Ewart R, Broughton RJ. Photomyoclonic response of epileptic and nonepileptic subjects during wakefulness, sleep, and arousal. *Electroencephalogr Clin Neurophysiol* 1976; **23**:301–4.

Mesolham RI, Moberg PJ, Mahr RN *et al*. Olfaction in neurodegenerative disease: a meta-analysis of olfactory functioning in Alzheimer's and Parkinson's diseases. *Arch Neurol* 1998; **55**:84–90.

Meyer JS, Gotham J, Tazaki Y *et al*. Cardiorespiratory syndrome of extreme obesity with papilledema. *Neurology* 1961; **11**:950–8.

Miley CM, Forster FM. Activation of complex partial seizures by hyperventilation. *Arch Neurol* 1977; **34**:371–3.

Miller DH, Rudge P, Johnson G *et al*. Serial gadolinium enhanced magnetic resonance imaging in multiple sclerosis. *Brain* 1988; **111**:927–39.

Mittl RL, Grossman RI, Hieble JF *et al*. Prevalence of MR evidence of diffuse axonal injury in patients with mild head injury and normal CT findings. *Am J Neuroradiol* 1994; **15**:1583–9.

Morgan MH, Scott DF. EEG activation in epilepsies other than petit mal. *Epilepsia* 1970; **11**:255–61.

Morris HH, Dinner DS, Luders H *et al*. Supplementary motor seizures: clinical and electroencephalographic findings. *Neurology* 1988; **38**:1075–82.

Mostrum V, Ytterbergh C. Artifacts in computed tomography of the posterior fossa: a comparative phantom study. *J Comput Assist Tomogr* 1986; **10**:560–6.

Mushlin AI, Detsky AS, Phelps CE *et al*. The accuracy of magnetic resonance imaging in patients with suspected multiple sclerosis. *JAMA* 1993; **269**:3146–51.

Nesbit GM, Forbes GS, Scheithauer BW *et al*. Multiple sclerosis: histopathologic and MR and/or CT correlation in 37 cases at biopsy and three cases at autopsy. *Radiology* 1991; **180**:467–74.

Neufeld MY, Inzelberg R, Korczyn AD. EEG in demented and non-demented parkinsonian patients. *Acta Neurol Scand* 1988; **78**:1–5.

Neumann-Haefelin T, Moseley ME, Albers GW. New magnetic resonance imagining methods for cerebrovascular disease: emerging clinical applications. *Ann Neurol* 2000; **47**:559–70.

Nickel SN, Frame B. Neurologic manifestations of myxedema. *Neurology* 1958; **8**:511–17.

Nicolai J, van Putten MJ, Tavy DL. BIPLEDS in a kinetic mutism caused by bilateral anterior cerebral artery infarction. *Clin Neurophysiol* 2001; **112**:1726–8.

Niedermeyer E, Rocca V. The diagnostic significance of sleep electroencephalograms in temporal lobe epilepsy: a comparison of scalp and depth tracings. *Eur Neurol* 1972; **7**:119–29.

Normand MM, Wszolek ZK, Klass DW. Temporal intermittent rhythmic delta activity in electroencephalograms. *J Clin Neurophysiol* 1995; **12**:280–4.

O'Brien TJ, Sharbrough FW, Westmoreland BF *et al*. Subclinical rhythmic electrographic discharges of adults (SREDA) revisited: a study using digital EEG analysis. *J Clin Neurophysiol* 1998; **15**:493–501.

Oliveira-Filho J, Ay H, Schaeffer PW *et al*. Diffusion-weighted magnetic resonance imaging identifies the 'clinically relevant' small-penetrator infarcts. *Arch Neurol* 2000; **57**:1009–14.

Ormerod IEC, Miller DH, McDonald WI *et al*. The role of NMR imaging in the assessment of multiple sclerosis and isolated neurological lesions. *Brain* 1987; **110**:1579–616.

Orrison WW, Gentry RL, Simac GK *et al*. Blinded comparison of cranial CT and MR in closed head injury evaluation. *Am J Neuroradiol* 1994; **15**:351–6.

Patel MR, Edelman RR, Warach S. Detection of hyperacute primary intraparenchymal hemorrhage by magnetic resonance imaging. *Stroke* 1996; **27**:2321–4.

de la Paz D, Brenner RP. Bilateral independent periodic lateralized epileptiform discharges: clinical significance. *Arch Neurol* 1981; **38**:713–15.

Pedley TA. Interictal epileptiform discharges: discriminating characteristics and clinical correlations. *Am J EEG Technol* 1980; **20**:101–19.

Peters JF. Surface electrical fields generated by eye movements. *Am J EEG Technol* 1967; **7**:27–40.

Phelps ME, Hoffman EJ, Ter-Pogossian MM. Attenuation coefficients of various body tissues, fluids and lesions at photon energies of 18 keV to 136 keV. *Radiology* 1975; **117**:537–83.

Picard A, Cheliout Hearaut F, Bouskraoui M *et al.* Sleep EEG and developmental dysphasia. *Dev Med Child Neurol* 1998; **40**:595–9.

Pojunas KW, Daniels DL, Williams AL *et al.* MR imaging of prolactin-secreting microadenomas. *Am J Neuroradiol* 1986; **7**:209–13.

Poppert S, Essig A, Stoehr B *et al.* Rapid diagnosis of bacterial meningitis by real-time PCR and fluorescence in situ hybridization. *J Clin Microbiol* 2005; **43**:3390–7.

Porter SB, Sande MA. Toxoplasmosis of the central nervous system. *N Engl J Med* 1992; **327**:1643–8.

Pratt KL, Mattson RH, Weikers NJ *et al.* EEG activation of epileptics following sleep deprivation: a prospective study of 114 cases. *Electroencephalogr Clin Neurophysiol* 1968; **24**:11–15.

Pro JD, Wells CE. The use of the electroencephalogram in the diagnosis of delirium. *Dis Nerv Syst* 1977; 38:804–8.

Protass L. Hyperventilation in sickle cell disease. *Arch Int Med* 1978; **138**:29.

Purpura DP, Grundfest H. Nature of dendritic potentials and synaptic mechanism in cerebral cortex of cat. *J Neurophysiol* 1956; **19**:573–95.

Pykett IL. NMR imaging in medicine. *Sci Am* 1982; **246**:78–88.

Pykett SL, Newhouse JH, Buonanno BS *et al.* Principles of nuclear magnetic imaging. *Radiology* 1982; **143**:157–68.

Rathmell TK, Burns MA. The Laurence–Moon–Biedl syndrome occurring in a brother and a sister. *Arch Neurol Psychiatry* 1938; **39**:1033–42.

Rechtschaffen A, Kales A. *A manual of standardized terminology, technique and scoring system for sleep stages of human subjects.* Washington DC: US Government Printing Office, 1968.

Reiher J, Lebel M. Wicket spikes: clinical correlates of a previously undescribed EEG pattern. *Can J Neurol Sci* 1977; **4**:39–47.

Risinger MW, Engel J, Van Ness PC *et al.* Ictal localization of temporal lobe seizures with scalp sphenoidal recordings. *Neurology* 1989; **39**:1288–93.

Robinson WP, Bottani A, Yagang X. Molecular, cytogenetic, and clinical investigations of Prader–Willi syndrome patients. *Am J Hum Genet* 1992; **49**:1219–34.

Romano J, Engel GL. Delirium, I: electroencephalographic data. *Arch Neurol Psychiatry* 1944; **51**:356–77.

Roseman E. Dilantin toxicity: a clinical and electroencephalographic study. *Neurology* 1961; **11**:912–21.

Roos KL. Lumbar puncture. *Semin Neurol* 2003; **23**:105–14.

Ross ED. The aprosdias: functional–anatomic organization of the affective components of language in the right hemisphere. *Arch Neurol* 1981; **38**:561–9.

Sadler RM, Goodwin J. Multiple electrodes for detecting spikes in partial complex seizures. *Can J Neurol Sci* 1989; **16**:326–9.

Saenz-Lope E, Herranz-Tanarro FJ, Masdeu JC *et al.* Hyperekplexia: a syndrome of pathological startle responses. *Ann Neurol* 1984; **15**:36–41.

Salinsky M, Kanter R, Dashieff RM. Effectiveness of multiple EEGs in supporting the diagnosis of epilepsy: an operational curve. *Epilepsia* 1987; **28**:331–4.

Sammaritano J, Gigli GL, Gotman J. Interictal spiking during wakefulness and sleep and the localization of foci in temporal lobe epilepsy. *Neurology* 1991; **41**:290–7.

Schaeffer PW, Grant PE, Gonzalez RG. Diffusion-weighted MR imaging of the brain. *Radiology* 2000; **217**:331–45.

Schaul N, Lueders H, Sachdev K. Generalized bilaterally synchronous bursts of slow waves in the EEG. *Arch Neurol* 1981; **38**:690–2.

Schear HE. The EEG pattern in delirium tremens. *Clin Electroencephalog* 1985; **16**:30–2.

Schellinger PD, Jansn O, Fiebach JB *et al.* A standardized MRI stroke protocol: comparison with CT in hyperacute intracerebral hemorrhage. *Stroke* 1999; **30**:765–8.

Schmidt D. The influence of antiepileptic drugs on the electroencephalogram: a review of controlled clinical studies. *Electroencephalogr Clin Neurophysiol* 1982 (suppl.); **36**: 453–66.

Scott DF, Groetheysen UC, Bickford RG. Lambda responses in the human electroencephalogram. *Neurology* 1967; **17**:770–8.

Scott DF, Heathfield KWG, Toone B *et al.* The EEG in Huntington's disease: a clinical and neuropathological study. *J Neurol Neurosurg Psychiatry* 1972; **35**:97–102.

Seddigh S, Thomke F, Vogt Th. Complex partial seizures provoked by photic stimulation. *J Neurol Neurosurg Psychiatry* 1999; **66**:801–2.

Seshia SS. McLachlan RS. Aura continua. *Epilepsia* 2005; **46**:454–5.

Seyffarth H, Denny-Brown D. The grasp reflex and the instinctive grasp reaction. *Brain* 1948; **71**:109–83.

Singh G, Wright MA, Sander JW *et al.* Periodic lateralized epileptiform discharges (PLEDS) as the sole electrographic correlate of a complex partial seizure. *Epileptic Disord* 2005; **7**:37–41.

Silverman D. The anterior temporal electrode and the ten-twenty system. *Electroencephalogr Clin Neurophysiol* 1960; **12**:735–7.

Singer MB, Chong J, Lu D *et al.* Diffusion-weighted MRI in acute subcortical infarction. *Stroke* 1998; **29**:133–6.

Smith A. The serial sevens subtraction test. *Arch Neurol* 1962; **17**:78–80.

Sperling MR, Engel J. Electroencephalographic recordings from the temporal lobe: a comparison of ear, anterior temporal and nasopharyngeal electrodes. *Ann Neurol* 1985; **17**:510–13.

Sperling MR, Mednius JR, Engel J. Mesial temporal spikes: a simultaneous comparison of sphenoidal, nasopharyngeal and ear electrodes. *Epilepsia* 1986; **27**:81–6.

Spillane JD. Nervous and mental disorders in Cushing's syndrome. *Brain* 1951; **74**:72–94.

Steiner L, Budka H, Chaudhuri A *et al.* Viral encephalitis: a review of diagnostic methods and guidelines for management. *Eur J Neurol* 2005; **12**:331–43.

Steinhoff BJ, Racker S, Herrendorf G *et al.* Accuracy and reliability of periodic sharp wave complexes in Creutzfeldt–Jakob disease. *Arch Neurol* 1996; **53**:162–6.

Steriade M, Gloor P, Llinas RD et al. Basic mechanisms of cerebral rhythmical activities. Electroencephalogr Clin Neurophysiol 1990; 76:481–508.

Stevens JR. Central and peripheral factors in epileptic discharge: clinical studies. Arch Neurol 1962; 7:330–8.

Strupp M, Schueler O, Straube A et al. 'Atraumatic' Sprotte needle reduces the incidence of post-lumbar puncture headaches. Neurology 2001; 57:2310–12.

Su P, Goldensohn ES. Progressive supranuclear palsy: electroencephalographic studies. Arch Neurol 1973; 29:183–6.

Summerskill WHJ, Davidson EA, Sherlock S et al. The neuropsychiatric syndrome associated with hepatic cirrhosis and extensive portal circulation. Q J Med 1956; 25:245.

Sze G, Milano E, Johnson C et al. Detection of brain metastases: comparison of contrast-enhanced MR with unenhanced MR and enhanced CT. Am J Neuroradiol 1990; 11:785–91.

Tchang S, Scotti G, Terbrugge K et al. Computed tomography as a possible aid to histological grading of supratentorial tumors. J Neurosurg 1977; 46:735–9.

Tegner R, Levander M. The influence of stimulus properties on visual neglect. J Neurol Neurosurg Psychiatry 1991; 54:882–7.

Thomas JE, Klass DW. Six-per-second spike-and-wave pattern in the electroencephalogram: a reappraisal of its clinical significance. Neurology 1968; 18:587–93.

Thompson AJ, Miller D, Youl B et al. Serial gadolinium-enhanced MRI in relapsing/remitting multiple sclerosis of varying disease duration. Neurology 1992; 42:60–3.

Tien RD, Felsberg GJ, Osumi AK. Herpes virus infection of the CNS: MR findings. AJR 1993; 161:283–9.

Timmermans M, Carr J. Neurosyphilis in the modern era. J Neurol Neurosurg Psychiatry 2004; 75:1727–30.

Tourtellotte WW, Henderson WG, Tucker RP et al. A randomized, double-blind clinical trial of post-lumbar puncture headache in normal individuals. Headache 1972; 12:73–8.

Tschampa HJ, Neumnn M, Zerr I et al. Patients with Alzheimer's disease and dementia with Lewy bodies mistaken for Creutzfeldt–Jakob disease. J Neurol Neurosurg Psychiatry 2001; 71:33–9.

Upton A, Gumpert J. Electroencephalography in diagnosis of herpes simplex encephalitis. Lancet 1970; 1:650–2.

Valler G, Rusconi ML, Bignamimi L et al. Anatomical correlates of visual and tactile extinction in humans: a clinical CT scan study. J Neurol Neurosurg Psychiatry 1994; 57:464–70.

Van Everbroeck BRJ, Boons J, Cras P. 14-3-3 Isoform detection distinguishes sporadic Creutzfeldt–Jakob disease from other dementias. J Neurol Neurosurg Psychiatry 2005; 76:100–2.

Vassilouthis J, Ambrose J. Computerized tomography scanning appearances of intracranial meningiomas: an attempt to predict the histological features. J Neurosurg 1979; 50:320–7.

Veldhuizen R, Binnie CD, Beintema DJ. The effect of sleep deprivation on the EEG in epilepsy. Electroencephalogr Clin Neurophysiol 1983; 55:505–12.

Victor M, Ropper AH. Principles of neurology, 7th edn. New York: McGraw Hill, 2001.

Vignaendra V, Mathews RL, Chatrian GE. Positive occipital sharp transients of sleep: relationships to nocturnal sleep cycle in man. Electroencephalogr Clin Neurophysiol 1974; 37:239–46.

Walker A, Pescor FT, Fraser HF et al. Electroencephalographic changes associated with chronic alcohol intoxication and the alcohol abstinence syndrome. Am J Psychiatry 1956; 113:106–14.

Walshe FMR, Robertson EG. Observations upon the form and nature of the 'grasping' movements and 'tonic innervation' seen in certain cases of lesions of the frontal lobe. Brain 1933; 56:40–70.

Walson JM, Kiloh LG, Osselton JW et al. The electroencephalogram in pernicious anemia and subacute combined degeneration of the spinal cord. Electroencephalogr Clin Neurophysiol 1954; 6:45–64.

Warach S, Gaa J, Stewart B et al. Acute human stroke studied by whole echo-planar diffusion-weighted imaging. Ann Neurol 1995; 37:231–44.

Wardlaw JM, Keir SL, Dennis MS. The impact of delays in computed tomography of the brain on the accuracy of diagnosis and subsequent management in patients with minor stroke. J Neurol Neurosurg Psychiatry 2003; 74:77–81.

Wasenko JJ, Rosenbloom SA, Duchesneau PM et al. The Sturge–Weber syndrome: comparison of MR and CT characteristics. Am J Neuroradiol 1990; 11:131–4.

Watemberg N, Alehan F, Dabby R et al. Clinical and radiologic correlates of frontal intermittent rhythmic delta activity. J Clin Neurophysiol 2002; 19:535–9.

Watemberg N, Linder I, Dabby R et al. Clinical correlates of occipital intermittent rhythmic delta activity (OIRDA) in children. Epilepsia 2007; 48:330–4.

van der Wee N, Rinkel GJ, Hasan D et al. Detection of subarachnoid hemorrhage on early CT: is lumbar puncture still needed after a negative scan? J Neurol Neurosurg Psychiatry 1995; 58:357–9.

Westmoreland BF, Klass DW. A distinctive rhythmic EEG discharge of adults. Electroencephalogr Clin Neurophysiol 1981; 51:186–91.

White JC, Langston JW, Pedley TA. Benign epileptiform transients of sleep: clarification of the small sharp spike controversy. Neurology 1977; 17:1061–8.

Wiedemann H-R, Kunze J, Grosse F-R et al. An atlas of clinical syndromes, 3rd edn. St Louis, MO: Mosby-Wolfe, 1989.

Wieser HG, Schwarz U, Blatter T et al. Serial EEG findings in sporadic and iatrogenic Creutzfeldt-Jakob disease. Clin Neurophysiol 2004; 115:2467–78.

Wiesmann M, Mayer TE, Yousry I et al. Detection of hyperacute subarachnoid hemorrhage of the brain by using magnetic resonance imaging. J Neurosurg 2002; 96:684–9.

Will RG, Ironside JW, Zeidler M et al. A new variant of Creutzfeldt–Jakob disease in the UK. Lancet 1996; 347:921–5.

Wilson SA. Modern problems in neurology. London: Edward Arnold, 1928.

Wolf P, Gooses R. Relation of photosensitivity to epileptic syndromes. J Neurol Neurosurg Psychiatry 1986; 49:1386–91.

Wood JW, Bartlet D, James AE et al. Normal pressure hydrocephalus: diagnosis and patient selection for shunt surgery. Neurology 1974; 24:517–26.

Yoneda Y, Tokui K, Hanihara T *et al.* Diffusion-weighted magnetic resonance imaging: detection of ischemic injury 39 minutes after onset in a stroke patient. *Ann Neurol* 1999; **45**:794–7.

Young IR, Hall AS, Pallis CA *et al.* Nuclear magnetic resonance imaging of the brain in multiple sclerosis. *Lancet* 1981; **2**:1063–6.

Zeidler M, Stewart GE, Barraclough CR *et al.* New variant Creutzfeldt–Jakob disease: neurological features and diagnostic tests. *Lancet* 1997; **35**:903–7.

Zimmerman RD, Fleming CA, Saint-Louis LA *et al.* Magnetic resonance imaging of meningiomas. *Am J Neuroradiol* 1985; **6**:149–57.

Zimmerman RD, Bilaniuk LT, Hackney DB *et al.* Head injury: early results of comparing CT and high-field MR. *Am J Neuroradiol* 1986; **7**:757–64.

Zivin L, Ajmone-Marsan C. Incidence and prognostic significance of 'epileptiform' activity in the EEG of non-epileptic subjects. *Brain* 1968; **91**:751–79.

Zochodne DW, Young GB, McLachlan RS *et al.* Creutzfeldt–Jakob disease without periodic sharp wave complexes: a clinical, electroencephalographic and pathologic study. *Neurology* 1988; **38**:1056–60.

Zurek R, Schiemann-Delgado J, Froescher W *et al.* Frontal intermittent rhythmical delta activity and anterior bradyarrythmia. *Clin Electroencephalogr* 1985; **16**:1–10.

PART II

SIGNS, SYMPTOMS, AND SYNDROMES

2

'Cortical' signs and symptoms

2.1 APHASIA

Aphasia is a fascinating clinical phenomenon, as it represents a disruption of that most human of all characteristics, namely language. The classification of the various types of aphasia has a long and contentious history: although the approach offered here is currently dominant, further research may require a more or less substantial revision.

Clinical features

Aphasia is characterized by impairments in one or more aspects of spoken language. Assessment begins with observation of the patient's spontaneous speech, with particular attention to fluency, comprehension, and coherence and also to the presence of what is known as paraphasia – a peculiar kind of misuse of words. Following this, one tests specifically for any improvement of speech with repetition and for the patient's ability to name objects.

Fluency, or its absence, is immediately apparent. Fluent speech occurs at a normal, or perhaps even increased rate: phrases and sentences are present, and there is a normal complement of prepositions, conjunctions, adjectives, and adverbs. Non-fluent speech, by contrast, is effortful, slowed, and 'telegraphic'. Given that many readers have perhaps never seen a telegraph, some words are in order regarding this descriptive term. The cost of a telegraph was apportioned according to its length, and hence efforts were made by telegraphers to omit as may words as possible while maintaining the sense of the original message. Consequently, telegraphs often lacked prepositions, conjunctions, adverbs, and adjectives. Non-fluent aphasias share this characteristic and, as this was first described in the age of telegraphs, the term 'telegraphic' was applied.

Comprehension, or its lack, becomes apparent during interaction with the patient. For example, during the neurologic examination it may appear that the patient has trouble understanding certain commands as, for example, when one instructs the patient to take the index finger and touch the nose. If one suspects a perhaps more subtle deficit in comprehension, it is appropriate to present a more complex command, for example, 'Now I want you to touch your right knee with your left hand'.

Coherence, or, again, its lack, becomes apparent during conversation with the patient. In this regard, it is critical to engage the patient in prolonged conversation, and to avoid a 'yes–no' format that denies the patient the opportunity to speak at length: all too often, physicians come away from a brief 'yes–no' interview without any sense of how incoherent their patient actually is. Incoherent speech is characterized by the presence of such disconnectedness and disorganization of words, phrases, and sentences that what the patient says 'makes no sense'.

Paraphasias represent a specific distortion in word usage, and come in one of two forms: phonemic (also known as literal) paraphasia, and semantic (also known as verbal) paraphasia. In phonemic paraphasia, a letter or syllable is replaced or added thus producing an incorrect word: for example, rather than saying 'put it on the table', the patient with a phonemic paraphasia may say 'put it on the stable'. In semantic paraphasia, by contrast, an entire word is substituted: for example, rather than saying "the book is on the table", the patient with a semantic paraphasia may say 'the book is on the mirror'.

Repetition may have a remarkable effect in some cases of aphasia. As in some cases speech improves with repetition, tell the aphasic patient that you are going to ask him to repeat something and then provide the patient with a test phrase, such as 'this is a hospital'. If the patient repeats this correctly and without hesitation then give a more complex phrase, for example 'to get out of the hospital, take the elevator to the first floor and then turn right'.

Finally, the ability to name things may be tested by pointing to an object in the room, such as a lamp, or perhaps by holding up a pencil and asking the patient to name it. If the patient does so correctly then proceed to parts of the object in question, such as the lampshade, light bulb, etc. If the patient has difficulty then provide cues, such as 'it's something that provides light' or 'it begins with the letter L'. If cues are not helpful, tell the patient the name of the object and ask whether or not that is the correct name.

After making all these determinations, it is generally possible to classify the patient's aphasia into one of the following types (all described in detail below): motor, transcortical motor, sensory, transcortical sensory, global, transcortical mixed, conduction, pure word deafness, and anomic. Importantly, however, it must be borne in mind that this classificatory scheme is but an approximation: clinical reality often overflows the nosologic boundaries we erect and atypical cases are not at all uncommon (Brown and Simonson 1957). One must also be prepared for surprises: for example, in bilingual patients one may see a different aphasia for each language: in one case of a native Spanish speaker who had Hebrew as a second language, there was a motor aphasia for Spanish and a sensory one for Hebrew (Silverberg and Gordon 1979).

Each of the various types of aphasia is described further below, with comments on its localizing value. Before proceeding, however, a word is in order regarding aphasia's lateralizing value. Roughly 90 percent of the general population is right-handed and in 99 percent of these individuals the left hemisphere is dominant for language. Among left-handers, the majority also exhibit language dominance in the left hemisphere (Goodglass and Quadfasel 1954; Humphrey and Zangwill 1952), and among the remainder some form of mixed dominance is generally present. Consequently, and especially in right-handers, the presence of aphasia lateralizes the lesion to the left hemisphere. However, exceptions to this rule in right-handers have been noted, and such cases are referred to as 'crossed aphasia' (Bakar et al. 1996; Brown and Wilson 1973; Holmes and Sadoff 1966). Crossed aphasia has been noted for motor aphasia (Hindson et al. 1984; Trojanowski et al. 1980), transcortical motor aphasia (Ghika-Schmid and Bogousslavsky 2000), sensory aphasia (Alexander et al. 1989; Henderson 1983; Sweet et al. 1984), global aphasia (Assal et al. 1981), and mixed transcortical aphasia (Cappa et al. 1993).

MOTOR APHASIA

Motor aphasia, also known as Broca's aphasia or expressive aphasia, is characterized by non-fluent, effortful speech that is laconic, often circumlocutory, and telegraphic. Comprehension is preserved and although one may miss hearing the expected prepositions, conjunctions, and the like, coherence is generally preserved and, paraphasias, if present, are rare. Repetition does not improve speech; naming, although effortful, is generally preserved.

Motor aphasia can be a very frustrating experience and patients tend to become irritable or depressed (Benson 1973). Asking about the patient's experience can be edifying. Try, for example, saying to the patient 'Some patients who have trouble speaking do so because they're not clear what they want to say, whereas others know exactly what they want to say but can't get the words out. Is that the kind of trouble you're having? Do you know what you want to say but can't get it out?' Patients with motor aphasia often nod their heads vigorously, relieved that the physician understands their plight. Interestingly, emotionally laden speech, such as cursing, may be relatively unaffected, and some patients may evidence a remarkably preserved ability to sing (Yamadori et al. 1977).

In most cases, the responsible lesion is seen to involve the posterior portion of the inferior frontal gyrus (Mohr et al. 1978; Naeser and Hayward 1978; Tonkonogy and Goodglass 1981). Given that most lesions extend beyond the inferior frontal gyrus, it is very common to find associated deficits, such as a right-sided hemiparesis: indeed, although noted (Henderson 1985; Masdeu and O'Hara 1983), it is very uncommon to find an isolated motor aphasia without any accompanying deficits.

Motor aphasia has also been noted with a thalamic lesion (Megens et al. 1992) and with infarction of the putamen and adjacent anterior limb of the internal capsule (Naeser et al. 1982).

TRANSCORTICAL MOTOR APHASIA

Transcortical motor aphasia is essentially identical to motor aphasia, with the exception that repetition is preserved. Transcortical motor aphasia is most often seen with lesions of the medial aspect of the left frontal lobe, as may occur with infarctions in the area of distribution of the anterior cerebral artery (Alexander and Schmitt 1980; Bogousslavsky and Regli 1990; Freedman et al. 1984; Racy et al. 1979; Rubens 1975). A syndrome similar to transcortical motor aphasia may also occur with lesions of the putamen or thalamus (Alexander and LoVerme 1980; Ghika-Schmid and Bogousslavsky 2000; McFarling et al. 1982).

SENSORY APHASIA

Sensory aphasia, also known as Wernicke's aphasia or receptive aphasia, is characterized by fluent speech that is more or less incoherent and contaminated by frequent paraphasias; such patients also have difficulty comprehending commands, especially complex ones. In its most severe form, one sees what as known as 'jargon aphasia', or speech that is almost totally incomprehensible.

In some cases, patients may appear relatively unconcerned, despite a severe deficit. In other cases, patients may become agitated and suspicious, and some may develop delusions of persecution (Benson 1973, Singer et al. 1989).

Sensory aphasia may be seen with lesions involving the temporoparietal area (Naeser and Hayward 1978), especially Wernicke's area on the posterior surface of the superior temporal gyrus (Selnes *et al.* 1985); it may also be seen with lesions of the white matter subjacent to Wernicke's area (Naeser and Hayward 1978) and lesions affecting the putamen and adjacent posterior limb of the internal capsule (Naeser *et al.* 1982).

TRANSCORTICAL SENSORY APHASIA

Transcortical sensory aphasia resembles sensory aphasia, except that repetition is intact. Transcortical sensory aphasia may be seen with lesions of the parietotemporal area that spare Wernicke's area (Selnes *et al.* 1985), or with lesions of the left thalamus, principally the dorsomedial nucleus (Bogousslavsky *et al.* 1988a; Tuszynski and Petito 1988).

GLOBAL APHASIA

Global aphasia is characterized by a combination of speech that is effortful and sparse with an inability to follow complex commands. Coherence is diminished; however, this is often difficult to assess, given that many patients are reduced to single words or over-learned stock phrases. Repetition does not improve their speech.

Global aphasia is most commonly seen with very large lesions involving the frontal, parietal, and temporal cortices (Bogousslavsky 1988; Naeser and Hayward 1978) and, as such, is typically accompanied by a hemiparesis. Exceptions to this rule do occur, however, and global aphasia secondary to cortical lesions may occur without hemiparesis when there are two distinct lesions – one in the frontal, and one in the temporoparietal cortex; such a scenario has been noted with multiple embolic infarctions (Hanlon *et al.* 1996; Tranel *et al.* 1987; Van Horn and Hawes 1982). Global aphasia has also been noted with a lesion of the thalamus (Kumar *et al.* 1996) and of the putamen and adjacent anterior and posterior limbs of the internal capsule (Naeser *et al.* 1982).

TRANSCORTICAL MIXED APHASIA

This aphasia, which could also just as well be called 'transcortical global aphasia', is essentially identical to global aphasia except for the fact that speech improves with repetition.

Transcortical mixed aphasia may be seen with lesions that, in one way or other, 'isolate' the posterior portion of the superior temporal gyrus and adjacent angular gyrus from the rest of the cortex, and has been reported with watershed infarction (Bogousslavsky *et al.* 1988b) and infarction of the medial aspects of the left frontal and parietal cortices (Ross 1980).

CONDUCTION APHASIA

In conduction aphasia speech is fluent, but there is a degree of incoherence and paraphasias are present. In striking contrast with sensory aphasia, however, comprehension is preserved. Furthermore, and remarkably so in light of the preserved comprehension, patients are unable to repeat complex sentences.

Conduction aphasia is classically associated with damage to the arcuate fasciculus (Benson *et al.* 1973; Damasio and Damasio 1980; Tanabe *et al.* 1987) but has also been noted with infarction of the caudate nucleus (Godefroy *et al.* 1994).

PURE WORD DEAFNESS

Pure word deafness is a remarkable syndrome characterized by an isolated inability to comprehend spoken words and to repeat phrases. Spontaneous speech is both fluent and coherent, and there are no paraphasias. One patient commented, 'Voice comes but no words . . . There is no trouble at all with the sound. Sounds come. I can hear, but I cannot understand it' (Hemphill and Stengel 1940). Another patient, although able to recognize non-speech sounds such as telephone rings or automobile horns, could not understand spoken words: he commented, 'I can hear you talking but I can't translate it' (Kanshepolsky *et al.* 1973).

Pure word deafness has been noted with bilateral damage to the superior temporal gyrus (Coslett *et al.* 1984; Kanshepolsky *et al.* 1973) and with bilateral damage to the inferior colliculi (Meyer *et al.* 1996; Pan *et al.* 2004).

Transcortical pure word deafness, wherein patients, although unable to understand the spoken word are yet able to repeat it, may or may not occur in pure form: a possible case was noted with a lesion of the left angular gyrus (Heilman *et al.* 1981).

ANOMIC APHASIA

Anomic aphasia is characterized by a more or less isolated inability to correctly name objects. Speech, although overall fluent and coherent, is marked by circumlocutions and a tendency to use indefinite nouns, such as 'it' or 'thing' when the correct word fails to come to mind. Comprehension is preserved.

Although cueing is not effective, if the examiner provides the correct name, the patient generally recognizes it.

Although isolated anomic aphasia does not have strong localizing value, pathology in the temporal lobe may be suspected, especially as seen in frontotemporal dementia. Anomic aphasia may also occur in the course of a delirium and as a side-effect of certain medications, such as topiramate (Mula *et al.* 2003) and both tricyclic (Schatzberg *et al.* 1978) and monoamine oxidase inhibitor (Goldstein and Goldberg 1986) antidepressants.

ATYPICAL APHASIA

Atypical aphasias are not uncommon and simply do not fit into the categories noted above. They are particularly associated with subcortical lesions (Ciemens 1970; Damasio *et al.* 1982a).

Etiology

As noted above, the various different types of aphasia, although generally lateralizing to the left hemisphere, localize, according to the type present, to multiple different areas of the cortex and, less commonly, subcortical structures. Determining the nature of the underlying lesion is facilitated by attending to the mode of onset of the aphasia, whether acute or gradual, and whether or not it is occurring in a more or less isolated fashion or in the context of another syndrome, notably either dementia or delirium.

Aphasia of acute onset, in most cases, represents a stroke, either ischemic or hemorrhagic. In this situation, it is not uncommon for the patient to initially present with mutism: over time, as perilesional edema subsides, the mutism resolves, leaving one of the classic aphasias in its wake (Pedersen *et al.* 1995). Rarely, a similar onset may be seen secondary to an emerging plaque in multiple sclerosis (Achiron *et al.* 1992; Devere *et al.* 2000; Lacour *et al.* 2004; Olmos-Lau *et al.* 1977). Aphasia of paroxysmal onset may occur on an ictal basis, representing either a simple partial or a complex partial seizure. In the case of simple partial seizures, aphasia may be the sole symptom (Hamilton and Mathews 1979; Labar *et al.* 1992) or may be accompanied by some twitching of the right side of the face (Williamson *et al.* 1985); when aphasia occurs as part of a complex partial seizure (Devinsky *et al.* 1994; Knight and Cooper 1986) one also finds other typical symptoms, such as confusion or automatisms. Post-ictal states may also be characterized by aphasia, and this strongly suggests that the seizure focus is in the left hemisphere (Gabr *et al.* 1989; Privitera *et al.* 1991).

Aphasia of gradual onset may occur secondary to an appropriately situated tumor or abscess and has also been noted in progressive multifocal leukoencephalopathy (Astrom *et al.* 1958; Krupp *et al.* 1985): all of these conditions are readily identified on MR scanning. Such gradual onsets may also occur in a condition known as primary progressive aphasia (PPA). PPA represents the effects of a focal onset of various neurodegenerative disorders (Josephs *et al.* 2006; Knibb *et al.* 2006), including Alzheimer's disease (Clark *et al.* 2003; Galton *et al.* 2000; Green *et al.* 1990; Greene *et al.* 1996), frontotemporal dementia (Mesulam *et al.* 2007; Turner *et al.* 1996), Pick's disease (Graff-Radford *et al.* 1990; Karbe *et al.* 1993; Kertesz *et al.* 1994; Wechsler *et al.* 1982), corticobasal ganglionic degeneration (Geda *et al.* 2007; Ikeda *et al.* 1996), and progressive supranuclear palsy (Knibb *et al.* 2006); the syndrome has also been reported secondary to Creutzfeldt–Jakob disease (Mandell *et al.* 1989). Clinically, most patients present with a motor or anomic aphasia or, less commonly, a sensory aphasia (Clark *et al.* 2003; Mendez and Zander 1991). Over a long period of time, and as the aphasia gradually worsens, a dementia eventually appears, thus betraying the nature of the underlying process (Le Rhun *et al.* 2005).

Aphasia may also appear in the context of a pre-existing dementia, and this may occur in each of the disorders, noted above, that may also cause the syndrome of primary progressive aphasia. In passing, it may be noted that, with the exception of frontotemporal dementia, it is rare that these neurodegenerative disorders present with an isolated aphasia. Aphasia is also common in the midst of a delirium, and here one typically finds elements of either a sensory or an anomic aphasia.

In children, aphasia may also be seen as part of the Landau–Kleffner syndrome (Hirsch *et al.* 1990; Mantovani and Landau 1980; Paquier *et al.* 1992) and the syndrome of developmental dysphasia: in developmental dysphasia both motor (Sato and Dreifuss 1973) and sensory (Bartak *et al.* 1975; Cohen *et al.* 1989; Paul *et al.* 1983) types have been described.

Differential diagnosis

Motor aphasia must be distinguished from dysarthria. Dysarthric, or slurred, speech, may appear somewhat effortful, but there are no word finding pauses or circumlocutions and, if one listens carefully one finds a normal complement of prepositions, adjectives, etc.

Sensory aphasia must be distinguished from other causes of incoherence, notably the loosening of associations seen in schizophrenia and the rambling and variably incoherent speech seen in delirium and advanced cases of dementia. This differential is relatively easy if one pays attention to the clinical context and associated symptoms.

Loosening of associations, in contrast with sensory aphasia (Faber *et al.* 1983; Gerson *et al.* 1977), is generally associated with more voluble speech; furthermore, patients with loosening of associations are also less concerned about their incoherence than are patients with sensory aphasia: indeed, patients with loosening often are absolutely unconcerned in this regard. Although these points may be helpful in distinguishing loosening from sensory aphasia, they represent differences in degree only and may not be that helpful clinically. In my experience it is far more useful to attend to the presence of associated symptoms, such as bizarre behavior, auditory hallucinations, and bizarre delusions, which are almost universally present in cases of schizophrenia associated with loosening of associations and, by contrast, are absent in cases of sensory aphasia: as noted above, delusions or persecution may be present in patients with sensory aphasia but bizarre delusions are absent.

Rambling and more or less incoherent speech is typical of delirium and advanced cases of dementia, and some might argue that the difference between this and sensory aphasia is moot and go on to simply say that this finding, in fact, represents a sensory aphasia. From a clinical point of view, however, the important point is not to resolve this debate but rather to note whether in patients with rambling and incoherent speech there are associated cognitive deficits, such as disorientation, confusion, short-term memory loss, etc. If these are present, then one pursues the differential as noted in Section 5.1 (dementia) and Section 5.3 (delirium).

Pure word deafness must be distinguished from deafness, and this may be accomplished by attending to the patient's reaction to sounds other than speech. Patients with pure word deafness, although unable to comprehend spoken words, nevertheless are able to respond appropriately to other sounds, such as the ringing of a telephone of the sound of a car horn (Coslett *et al.* 1984; Kanshepolsky *et al.* 1973). Deaf patients, in contrast, fail to respond to these non-speech sounds (Bahls *et al.* 1988; Le Gros Clark and Russel 1938).

Isolated alexia (Section 2.2) or agraphia (Section 2.3) must also be differentiated from aphasia, and this is readily accomplished if one keeps in mind that aphasia is primarily a disturbance in spoken language: although disturbances in written language typically accompany the disturbed speech they do not appear in isolation, that is to say in the presence of intact speech, as they do in alexia or agraphia.

Treatment

In addition to treatment, if possible, of the underlying condition, speech therapy and, controversially, drug treatment may be considered.

Speech therapy is generally reserved for cases of aphasia secondary to stroke or other more or less static lesions; its effectiveness in cases of aphasia secondary to disorders which, in the natural course of events tends to progress (e.g., tumors, neurodegenerative disorders), is not clear.

Drug therapy has been attempted with bromocriptine, donepezil, and amphetamine, with inconclusive results. Bromocriptine has been studied in the treatment of motor aphasia secondary to stroke in four double-blind studies, with one positive result (Bragoni *et al.* 2000) and three negative ones (Ashtary *et al.* 2006; Gupta *et al.* 1995; Sabe *et al.* 1995). In one double-blind study of patients with chronic aphasia of various different types, donepezil was superior to placebo on some measures (Bertheir *et al.* 2006). Dextroamphetamine, in one double-blind study (Walker-Batson *et al.* 2001), showed some short-term benefit in a group of patients with various aphasia types secondary to stroke but this benefit was not maintained to a statistically significant degree over the long haul. Given these inconclusive results, prudence may dictate abstaining from drug treatment pending further studies.

2.2 ALEXIA

As noted in the immediately preceding chapter, alexia (the inability to read) may be seen in conjunction with aphasia;

this chapter, however, is concerned with alexia occurring in an isolated fashion, that is to say in patients who, although still able to understand the spoken word and to speak fluently and coherently, are yet unable to comprehend the written word.

Clinical features

Alexia may or may not be accompanied by agraphia, or the inability to write: cases of alexia without agraphia are also referred to as 'pure' alexia or 'pure word blindness'.

The experience of alexia is quite remarkable. One patient with alexia without agraphia (Cohen *et al.* 1976), an English teacher, in describing her situation, commented: 'I can write and I can see, but I can't read.' She went on to note that 'it was as if the writing were in a foreign language.' She attempted to cope with the deficit during class by memorizing what she had written on the blackboard and the strategy would work, unless, of course, the memory faded – turning back to the blackboard, she then found herself unable to read what she'd written just minutes earlier.

Remarkably, in alexia without agraphia, some patients, although unable to read words, are still able to read individual letters, and this preserved ability enables patients with pure alexia to circumvent their deficit by utilizing a 'letter-by-letter' reading strategy. Here, patients read each letter out loud, and in hearing the letters, they reconstruct the word, which is then understood (Stommel *et al.* 1991; Warrington and Langdon 1994).

In cases of alexia without agraphia, one often, but not always, finds a right hemianopia. In cases of alexia with agraphia, one also typically sees elements of the Gerstmann's syndrome, such as finger agnosia, right–left disorientation and acalculia.

Etiology

A brief review of the visual pathways may be helpful in understanding the mechanisms involved in alexia. To begin, recall that fibers of the optic tract terminate in the lateral geniculate body of the thalamus. From the lateral geniculate body, the geniculocalcarine tract arises and proceeds to the calcarine cortex, located on the medial aspect of the ipsilateral occipital cortex. Fibers from the left calcarine cortex proceed directly anteriorly toward the left angular gyrus, whereas fibers from the right calcarine cortex must first pass forward, and then cross in the splenium of the corpus callosum, after which they proceed laterally to an eventual juncture with the fibers that originated in the left calcarine cortex. These conjoined fibers then proceed anteriorly, to terminate finally in the left angular gyrus.

It appears that the left angular gyrus subserves both reading and writing. Hence, lesions of the gyrus itself cause the syndrome of alexia with agraphia. Lesions, however, which spare the angular gyrus but which deprive it of visual afferents from both hemispheres cause 'pure' alexia, i.e., alexia without agraphia.

This deprivation of the angular gyrus of visual afferents from both hemispheres may occur via a number of different mechanisms. First, and most commonly, one finds a lesion in the splenium of the corpus callosum (which severs afferents from the right occipital cortex) in combination with a lesion of the medial aspect of the left occipital cortex (which destroys afferents from the left occipital cortex) (Ajax et al. 1977; Damasio and Damasio 1983). This first mechanism occurs most commonly secondary to an infarction in the area of distribution of the left posterior cerebral artery, which nourishes both the splenium and the medial aspect of the left occipital cortex. Second, there may be a combination of a lesion affecting the left lateral geniculate body (thus depriving visual afferents from the left hemisphere) and one affecting the splenium (thus severing afferents from the right hemisphere) (Stommel et al. 1991). Third, just subjacent to the angular gyrus there may be a lesion located in the white matter, which destroys the conjoined fibers from both occipital lobes (Greenblatt 1976).

As noted earlier, cases of alexia without agraphia may be accompanied by a right hemianopia, and this occurs with either the first or second mechanisms just described. In cases occurring via the third mechanism, however, the visual fields remain unaffected.

As in the case of spoken language, so too for written language the left hemisphere is dominant in almost all right-handers and in most left-handers also. Exceptions, however, do occur. For example, cases of 'crossed' alexia have been noted in which right-handed patients suffered alexia due to right hemisphere lesions (Fincham et al. 1975; Henderson et al. 1985). Furthermore, there is also a case report of a left-handed patient who developed alexia due to a right hemisphere lesion (Pillon et al. 1987).

Most cases of alexia occur on the basis of stroke, as a result of an ischemic infarction or, less commonly, an intracerebral hemorrhage. Other possible lesions include appropriately situated tumors (Turgman et al. 1979; Vincent et al. 1977) or plaques of multiple sclerosis (Day et al. 1987; Dogulu et al. 1996; Mao-Draayer and Panitch 2004).

Differential diagnosis

Aphasia is distinguished by an inability to understand the spoken word.

Neglect may include a kind of alexia (often referred to as 'hemialexia') wherein patients fail to attend to the left part of a word and thus misread it (Kinsbourne and Warrington 1962). For example, a patient with left neglect might, upon being presented with the written word 'birdhouse', read 'house'.

Dementing disorders, such as Alzheimer's disease (Arsland et al. 1993), may cause alexia but this is seen in the context of other cognitive deficits, such as disorientation, short-term memory loss, etc.

The term 'alexia', by convention, refers to cases of an acquired inability to read in those who had once mastered this skill. In cases characterized by an inability, despite adequate intelligence and educational opportunity, to acquire this skill, one speaks of 'developmental dyslexia' (discussed in Section 9.17).

Treatment

Speech therapy may also be considered in addition to treatment, where possible, of the underlying lesion.

2.3 AGRAPHIA

Agraphia, or the inability to write, may be seen, as discussed in Section 2.1, in conjunction with aphasia; this chapter, however, is concerned with agraphia occurring in an isolated fashion, that is to say in patients who, despite being unable to write, are able to both speak and understand the spoken word without significant difficulty.

Clinical features

Agraphia may occur in one of two fashions, either in a 'pure' form, or as part of Gerstmann's syndrome, where one also finds finger agnosia, right–left disorientation and acalculia.

Etiology

As might be expected, agraphia typically appears secondary to lesions in the left hemisphere. Most cases occur secondary to lesions affecting the parietotemporal cortex (Rosati and De Bastiani 1979), including either the supramarginal or angular gyri (Roeltgen and Heilman 1984); cases have also been reported secondary to lesions in or near 'Exner's area' (in the posterior portion of the middle frontal gyrus) (Anderson et al. 1990; Tohgi et al 1995) or in the dorsomedial nucleus of the thalamus (Ohno et al. 2000).

Agraphia may also be confined to the left hand in right-handed patients as part of a disconnection syndrome occurring secondary to a lesion of the corpus callosum (Yamadori et al. 1980)

Agraphia typically occurs as part of a stroke syndrome, secondary to either ischemic infarction or intracerebral hemorrhage.

Differential diagnosis

Poor handwriting, as may be seen with tremor, dystonia, paresis or parkinsonian micrographia, is readily apparent, provided one simply observes the patient's attempt at writing.

Apraxia may lead to disturbed handwriting; however, associated features typically suggest the correct diagnosis. In ideational apraxia, one also sees difficulty in employing other 'tools', thus patients, in addition to difficulty in utilizing a pen or pencil, will also have difficulty in handling a comb, scissors, etc. In constructional apraxia, there will be additional difficulties in copying geometric figures, drawing stick figures, etc.

Delirium and dementia may be accompanied by agraphia, but the correct syndromal diagnosis is immediately suggested by associated cognitive deficits, such as confusion, disorientation, short-term memory loss, etc.

Agraphia may also occur on a developmental basis and in these cases, it is referred to by convention as dysgraphia. Developmental dysgraphia, discussed in Section 9.18, is distinguished from acquired agraphia in that in developmental cases, writing skills, despite adequate intelligence and educational opportunity, were simply never acquired, whereas in acquired agraphia, these skills were acquired, only to be lost.

Treatment

Speech therapy should be considered in addition to treatment, if possible, of the underlying lesion.

2.4 ACALCULIA

Acalculia, that is to say an acquired inability to do arithmetic, may be seen as part of Gerstmann's syndrome, wherein it is accompanied by finger agnosia, right–left disorientation and agraphia, or it may occur in an isolated fashion, and it is this isolated acalculia that is dealt with here.

Clinical features

Acalculia may become obvious to patients when they find themselves unable to make change or balance their checkbooks or may only become apparent during the mental status examination. Typically, on the mental status examination, the patient's ability to do simple, one- or two-digit addition and subtraction is tested and, if these are done well, the patient is then asked to perform 'serial 7s'. In this venerable test, the patient is asked to subtract 7 from 100, then to subtract 7 from that number and to keep on subtracting sevens until he or she can go no further: making more than two or three errors is considered abnormal (Smith 1962). If there is a clinical suspicion of acalculia and these tests are done well, it is appropriate to then test the patient's ability to do multiplication and division, as in some cases the various computational processes may be differentially affected (Lampl *et al.* 1994).

Etiology

Isolated acalculia has been noted with lesions of the left parietal cortex (Lampl *et al.* 1994; Takayama *et al.* 1994), especially the angular gyrus (Benson and Weir 1972; Bernal *et al.* 2003), the posterior inferior frontal cortex (Tohgi *et al.* 1995), striatum (Corbett *et al.* 1986), or anterior thalamus (Mendez *et al.* 2003). In almost all cases, acalculia occurs as part of a stroke syndrome.

Differential diagnosis

Dementia or delirium is typically accompanied by acalculia; however, here the associated cognitive deficits, such as confusion, disorientation, short-term memory loss, etc., suggest the correct syndromal diagnosis.

Aphasia is also typically accompanied by acalculia.

Perseveration, as may be seen with frontal lesions, may pantomime acalculia. For example, perseveration in the 'serial 7s' test may lead to the following responses: '93, 83, 73, 63 . . .'.

In cases where patients are able to perform calculations 'in their head', but are unable to do so on paper, suspicion should be aroused for neglect or apraxia. In neglect, patients may misread written numbers (e.g., reading '48' for '1948') and in apraxia they may be unable to properly order written numbers on the page.

Acalculia occurring on a developmental basis (as discussed in Section 9.19) is distinguished from acquired acalculia in that in developmental cases patients are unable to acquire mathematical skills despite adequate intelligence and educational opportunity, whereas in acquired cases this ability was developed only to be subsequently lost.

Treatment

In addition, if possible, to treatment of the underlying lesion, speech therapy may be considered. Hand-held calculators, of course, should also be utilized.

2.5 GERSTMANN'S SYNDROME

In 1924, Josef Gerstmann described a remarkable syndrome characterized by the tetrad of finger agnosia, right–left disorientation, agraphia, and acalculia. Although there has been controversy in the past regarding whether this occurs in 'pure' form or not, the case reports cited below indicate that, although rare, the pure syndrome does in fact occur.

Clinical features

In later papers in English, Gerstmann (1940, 1942, 1957) further described the syndrome. He noted that in finger agnosia the patient cannot name the fingers either of his/her or the examiner's hand, and that this deficit is usually more pronounced with regard to the index, middle, and ring fingers. Right–left disorientation may become apparent when patients are instructed, say, to touch their right knee with their left hand: patients with this sign may use the incorrect hand or may touch the ipsilateral knee. Agraphia and acalculia are tested for by having the patient write a brief paragraph and then asking him or her to perform progressively more difficult calculations.

As noted by Gerstmann (1940), it is not uncommon to see an associated right hemianopia and a degree of alexia.

Etiology

Classically, Gerstmann's syndrome, as pointed out by Gerstmann himself (1940), localizes to the angular gyrus (Gold *et al.* 1995). The syndrome has also been noted with lesions of the white matter subjacent to the angular gyrus (Mayer *et al.* 1999), and with lesions involving both the angular and supramarginal gyri (Roeltgen *et al.* 1983; Tucha *et al.* 1997). Although most cases are due to infarction, Gerstmann's syndrome has also been noted with tumors (Tucha *et al.* 1997), systemic lupus erythematosus (Jung *et al.* 2001), trauma (Mazzoni *et al.* 1990), and subdural hematoma (Maeshima *et al.* 1998). Although left-sided lesions are by far the most common cause, Gerstmann's syndrome has been noted with a right-hemisphere lesion (Moore *et al.* 1991).

Note that Gerstmann's syndrome may also occur on a developmental basis (Benson and Geschwind 1970; PeBenito 1987; Suresh and Sebastian 2000).

Differential diagnosis

The various elements of the tetrad may occur in patients with dementia or delirium; however, here the associated cognitive deficits, such as confusion, disorientation and short-term memory loss, will suggest the correct syndromal diagnosis.

Certain neurodegenerative disorders, such as Alzheimer's disease, may, albeit rarely, present in a 'focal' fashion, with the syndrome of 'posterior cortical atrophy', which, in addition to elements of Gerstmann's syndrome, also includes Balint's syndrome, aphasia, apraxia, and neglect (Renner *et al.* 2004; Tang-Wei *et al.* 2004).

Treatment

Consideration may be given to a course of speech therapy in addition to treatment, if possible, of the underlying lesion.

2.6 HYPERGRAPHIA

Hypergraphia, as defined by Mungas (Hermann *et al.* 1988), is characterized by a tendency to excessive writing that goes beyond any social, occupational, or educational requirements. The text produced is for the most part coherent, and, rather than consisting of the mere perseverative reproduction of phrases, words or letters, displays a more or less complete working-up of various related themes.

Clinical features

In evaluating a patient's written production for evidence of hypergraphia, attention must be paid to the pre-morbid level of written output. Thus, for a patient who premorbidly wrote very little, the appearance of a tendency to write several pages a day would be clinically significant. Particular attention must also be made to the presence or absence of perseveration: hypergraphic productions tend to read like letters, articles or chapters, in that there are more or less clear themes, which again are more or less fully elaborated in a more or less coherent fashion.

Etiology

Hypergraphia may be seen in the interictal personality syndrome, mania, and in schizophrenia.

The interictal personality syndrome (see Section 7.2), seen in patients with chronic epilepsy typically includes hypergraphia (Hermann *et al.* 1988; Okamura *et al.* 1993; Waxman and Geschwind 1974, 1975) and is suggested by the history of chronic epilepsy and the appearance of other aspects of the syndrome, such as deep and persistent affect, verbosity, a pre-occupation with religious, ethical or philosophical concerns, hyposexuality, and irritability.

Mania may be characterized by hypergraphia, wherein it represents the written equivalent of pressured speech. Kraepelin (1976) noted that manics may produce an 'astonishing' number of documents, all from 'the pleasure in writing'. The presence of other typical symptoms, such as increased energy, pressured speech, a decreased need for sleep, etc. indicate the correct diagnosis.

Schizophrenia may also lead to hypergraphia and Kraepelin (1971) commented on the 'very numerous and monotonous' documents that may appear, all marked by neologisms, delusional thoughts, and a degree of incoherence.

Differential diagnosis

Hypergraphia must be distinguished from an appropriate increase in written output and from mere perseverative writing. Increased written output is normal in professional authors and others whose personal or professional lives require writing. With perseveration, when it appears in written form, the written output itself consists of the same phrase, word, or even letter written repeatedly again and again, sometimes filling page after page. Here, there is no theme evident and no elaborative working-up of ideas. This kind of graphic perseveration has been referred to as 'automatic writing behavior' and has been noted with a right hemispheric tumor (Imamura *et al.* 1992), right hemisphere stroke (due to either infarction in the area of distribution of the right middle cerebral artery or to putaminal hemorrhage) (Evyapan and Kumral 2001), and in dementia characterized in part by a frontal lobe syndrome (Frisoni *et al.* 1993; van Pugt *et al.* 1996).

Treatment

Treatment is directed at the underlying condition.

2.7 APROSODIA

Prosody refers to the affective or emotional aspects of speech, which are conveyed by the inflection, rhythm, and tone with which patients speak (Monrad-Krohn 1947a,b); aprosodia, in turn, represents a defect either in speaking with normal prosody or in comprehending the prosody with which others speak. In a sense, as will become apparent below, aprosodia is to the right hemisphere as aphasia is to the left hemisphere. The scheme presented here follows closely that presented by Ross (Gorelick and Ross 1987; Ross 1981).

Aprosodia, although not as obvious as aphasia, may have profound effects on a patient's life. In many aspects of life, it is not so much *what* we say that counts, as it is *how* we say it, and it is this aspect that is impaired in aprosodia.

Clinical features

In assessing patients for aprosodia, attention is paid to the following aspects of speech: the presence or absence of a monotonous voice; the ability of the patient to comprehend what another is feeling by simply hearing the intonation in the other's voice; the presence or absence of a 'mismatch' between what the patient says he is feeling and the prosody with which he speaks; and, finally, for any improvement in prosodic deficits by repetition.

Monotony is said to be present when the patient's speech is devoid of inflection or changes in tone – stripped, as it were, of emotional valence. When there is doubt about this, it may be appropriate, at some point during the interview, to ask an emotionally charged question and then to listen carefully to see whether the patient's response remains monotonous. If it does, then it is critical to ask the patient what he is feeling during the response. Furthermore, one may simply ask the patient if he has had any trouble in expressing himself by his tone of voice. Formal testing may be accomplished by providing a neutral phrase, such as 'I am going to the movies', and asking the patient to speak that phrase on three successive occasions with three different intonations, namely happy, angry, and sad.

Comprehension on the patient's part of the prosody with which others speak may be difficult to assess during the interview, as most physicians have been trained to keep a studied neutrality in their tone of voice. Consequently, it is necessary to ask the patient if he has had any difficulty in understanding what others are feeling. When there is doubt, one may also ask friends or family members of the patient whether the patient seems to have had any trouble understanding what they are feeling. In some cases, others may report that the only way to get across to the patient what they are feeling is to state it explicitly, rather than relying on tone of voice. Formal testing may be accomplished by telling the patient that you are going to say something (e.g., as above, 'I am going to the movies') with different tones of voice (e.g., happy, angry, or sad) and that you want him to report what tone you are using. In performing this test, one must stand behind the patient in order to prevent the patient from seeing your facial expressions or gestures.

A 'mismatch' between what the patient is feeling and the prosody with which he speaks as he describes his feeling may become apparent during the interview. For example, after the patient has described a traumatic experience, one may ask 'how are you feeling now?'. If the patient says 'I'm feeling very sad,' yet there is a lilt to his voice then a mismatch is present. Or conversely, after the patient has described a gratifying experience, one may again ask how he is feeling. If he says 'Great, just great' yet his tone of voice is somber and lugubrious then again one has demonstrated that a 'mismatch' is present. Importantly, a monotonous tone does not indicate a 'mismatch': to say that a mismatch is present, there must be a dissonance between what the patient says he is feeling and the tone with which he reports that feeling.

Repetition is tested by telling the patient that you are going to say something with different tones of voice, and that you want him to repeat what you said with the exact tone in which you said it. One may then proceed with the neutral phrase 'I am going to the movies', said first with a happy tone, then a sad one and finally an angry one.

It should be noted that in aprosodia there is also often an accompanying change in gesture and facial expression. For example, if monotony is present, one may see an absence of gesturing and a lack of facial expression. This association is not invariable, however, and in many cases gesture and expression will remain intact in the face of a significant disturbance of prosody.

After the above assessment, it is generally possible to categorize the patient's aprosodia into one of the following categories: motor, transcortical motor, sensory, transcortical sensory, global, transcortical mixed, conduction, and pure affective deafness. Each is discussed below, with comments on its localizing value. Before proceeding, however, it is appropriate to note, as indicated earlier, that in almost all cases, aprosodia indicates a right hemisphere lesion. Cases of 'crossed' aprosodia, in which right-handed patients developed aprosodia secondary to a lesion in the left hemisphere, although reported (Darby 1993; Ross *et al.* 1989), are rare.

MOTOR APROSODIA

In motor aprosodia, speech is monotonous, but comprehension is intact and there is no 'mismatch'; repetition does not relieve the monotonous tone. The presence of motor aprosodia may be quite disconcerting to patients. One of Ross and Mesulam's (1979) patients complained that she had great difficulty in disciplining her children because when she said to them that she was angry they didn't respond, because she didn't sound angry. She eventually came up with a way to circumvent her motor aprosodia by adding a parenthetical statement, such as 'God damnit, I mean it' or 'I am angry and I mean it,' afterward, thereby getting across what she was feeling. Of note, however, in this case, 'even the parenthetical statement was voiced in a complete monotone'.

Motor aprosodia most commonly occurs secondary to lesions in the posterior frontal operculum (Gorelick and Ross 1987; Ross 1981; Ross and Mesulam 1979); cases have also been reported with lesions in the internal capsule (Ross *et al.* 1981) and basal ganglia (Speedie *et al.* 1993).

TRANSCORTICAL MOTOR APROSODIA

Transcortical motor aprosodia is essentially identical to motor aprosodia except that the monotonous tone of voice disappears with repetition. A case was reported secondary to a lesion in the anterior limb of the internal capsule (Ross 1981).

SENSORY APROSODIA

In sensory aprosodia there is a normal range of intonation in the patient's spontaneous speech. Comprehension, however, is impaired, and one finds mismatches; repetition is also impaired in that when patients repeat the neutral phrase, the intonation of their speech will not be the same as that of the examiner.

Sensory aprosodia has been noted with lesions affecting the temporoparietal cortex (Darby 1993; Gorelick and Ross 1987; Ross 1981); a case has also been reported secondary to a lesion of the thalamus and adjacent posterior limb of the internal capsule (Wolfe and Ross 1987).

TRANSCORTICAL SENSORY APROSODIA

This aprosodia is similar to sensory aprosodia with the exception that repetition is performed well, with the patient accurately mimicking the examiner's tone of voice. Cases have been described secondary to a lesion of the anterior temporal cortex (Ross 1981), and the striatum and adjacent posterior limb of the internal capsule (Gorelick and Ross 1987).

GLOBAL APROSODIA

In global aprosodia, speech is monotonous and comprehension of other's prosody is poor; repetition does not improve the patient's prosodoic output. Global aprosodia has been noted with lesions affecting both the frontal operculum and the posterior temporal cortex (Darby 1993; Ross 1981).

TRANSCORTICAL MIXED APROSODIA

Transcortical mixed aprosodia, which might just as well be called transcortical global aprosodia, is essentially identical to global aprosodia with the exception that the patient's prosody improves with repetition. A case has been reported with a lesion involving the frontoparietal cortex (Ross 1981).

CONDUCTION APROSODIA

In conduction aprosodia spontaneous speech shows a normal range of intonation, and comprehension is intact. Remarkably, however, there is a 'mismatch' between the patient's statement as to how he is feeling and the tone with which that statement is made. Furthermore, and remarkably so in light of the preserved comprehension of prosody, patients are unable to repeat sentences with the prosody spoken by the examiner. Conduction aprosody appears to be very rare; a case was reported with a lesion involving the temporoparietal cortex (Gorelick and Ross 1987).

PURE AFFECTIVE DEAFNESS

In this condition, spontaneous speech shows a normal range of intonation and there is no mismatch present. Despite these preserved abilities; however, patients are unable to comprehend the prosody with which others speak. Remarkably, however, patients are able to mimic the examiner's intonation upon repetition testing.

Cases of pure affective deafness have been reported with lesions affecting the posterior frontal and immediately subjacent temporal operculum (Gorelick and Ross 1987; Ross 1981) and also with a large lesion affecting the occipitoparietal cortex (Gorelick and Ross 1987).

Etiology

Almost all reported cases of aprosodia have occurred as part of a stroke syndrome, secondary to either ischemic infarction or, much less commonly, intracerebral hemorrhage. A case has also been reported of a gradually progressive motor aprosodia secondary to a progressive focal atrophy of the right frontal lobe (Ghacibeh and Heilman 2003). Further, there is also a report of motor aprosodia occurring paroxysmally as a simple partial seizure (Bautista and Ciampetti 2003).

Various forms of aprosodia may also be seen in dementia, as for example Alzheimer's disease (Perez-Trullen and Modrego Pardo 1996); however, here associated cognitive deficits, such as disorientation and short-term memory loss, will suggest the correct syndromal diagnosis.

Differential diagnosis

Motor aprosodia must be distinguished from flattened affect and hypophonia. Flattened affect is typically accompanied by a monotone voice; however, here there is also a 'flattening' of the patient's feelings: patients with flattened affect typically report having no feelings and this is in contrast with motor aprosodia wherein patients, although speaking in a monotone, still have feelings, sometimes quite strong ones. Hypophonia, as seen in parkinsonism, is a speech deficit characterized by whispering and low volume, which stands in contrast with the normal volume seen in motor aprosodia.

Sensory aprosodia must be distinguished from emotional incontinence and from inappropriate affect. Emotional incontinence, as discussed in Section 4.7, is characterized by episodes of involuntary laughing or crying (accompanied by, respectively, a mirthful or sad tone of voice) during which the patient has no feelings, except, perhaps, a sense of consternation at being unable to control the emotional display. This, superficially, is similar to the 'mismatch' seen in sensory aprosodia; however, on closer inspection there are differences. First, there is, in fact, no actual 'mismatch' in the sense of a patient feeling one thing and displaying a discordant tone of voice as he reports that feeling, for in emotional incontinence patients often are emotionally neutral during the episode. Second, in contrast with aprosodia, which in almost all cases is constant and more or less chronic, emotional incontinence occurs in discrete episodes, in between which there is a congruence between what the patient feels and the tone with which that feeling is reported.

Inappropriate affect is very similar to sensory aprosodia, in that in both these signs there is a mismatch between what the patient feels and the tone of voice in which that feeling is expressed. Differentiating between the two requires attention to comprehension of prosody, which is present in patients with inappropriate affect, and absent in those with sensory aprosodia.

Finally, aphasia must be clearly distinguished from aprosodia. Aphasia represents a disturbance in *what* is said, aprosodia a disturbance in *how* it is said. Consider, for example, two patients who are both grief-stricken over a recent loss. The first one, having a motor aphasia (Broca's aphasia), although restricted to simply repeating the word 'sad . . . sad . . . sad' over and over again, might yet say it so lugubriously that the listener has no doubt about the depth of the patient's grief. By contrast, the second patient, with a motor aprosodia, although able to say the words 'I've never felt so sad in my entire life', would say them in such a monotone that the listener might well doubt whether the patient was, in fact, really feeling any sadness.

Treatment

Speech therapy may be helpful in addition to treatment, if possible, of the underlying condition.

2.8 APRAXIA

Apraxia is said to be present when, despite preserved strength, sensation, and coordination, patients are unable to carry out purposeful activities. In the literature, there are a large number of different kinds of apraxia described; in this chapter, four of these are considered: ideomotor, ideational, constructional, and dressing.

Clinical features

Each of the four kinds of apraxia is described below.

IDEOMOTOR AND IDEATIONAL APRAXIA

Ideomotor and ideational apraxia both have to do with the use of tools, considered in a broad sense, such as combs, knives and forks, and scissors. Bedside testing is readily accomplished using either some plastic knives/forks from the hospital cafeteria or a plastic blunt-ended pair of scissors carried discreetly in the pocket of one's white coat. Begin first by asking the patient to pantomime the use of a knife and fork, or perhaps a pair of scissors, and observe the performance. In some cases, the evidence for apraxia is obvious, as patients appear perplexed and are unable to make any appropriate movements. In other cases, there may be some doubt, as for example when patients use a body part as the tool itself. An example of this might be when, in attempting to pantomime using scissors to cut an imaginary piece of paper, the patient moves the index and middle fingers as if they were the blades of the scissors, rather than making a repetitive, squeezing kind of motion with the hand, as one does when the scissors are actually present. Some authorities consider this an example of apraxia; however, in this author's experience normal individuals are as likely to use their fingers as scissors as not. If the patient does display significant difficulty in mimicking the use of a tool, the next step is to provide the tool and ask the patient to use it; in this case, one pulls out the scissors and offers them, along with a piece of paper, and observes the response. In some cases, patients are able to pick up the tool and use it with little or no difficulty. In others, however, the perplexity persists: patients may pick up the scissors by the wrong end, turn them upside down, or otherwise hold them in a useless position. Cases wherein patients are unable to pantomime use of a tool but then go on to use the actual tool without difficulty are considered examples of ideomotor apraxia; cases wherein the difficulty with mimicking is followed by a significant difficulty in actually using the tool are considered examples of ideational apraxia.

Ideomotor apraxia rarely, if ever, constitutes a chief complaint, given that, in the normal course of events, most individuals simply do not engage in pantomime. Ideational apraxia, however, may bring patients to clinical attention as, for example, when patients who are unable to use a knife and fork begin to eat with their hands, or those who are unable to utilize a toothbrush develop severe bad breath.

CONSTRUCTIONAL APRAXIA

Constructional apraxia is said to be present when patients are unable to copy figures or to spontaneously draw them, and bedside testing is performed with pencil and paper. First, draw some simple geometric forms, such as a triangle, and ask the patient to copy them. Next, ask the patient to draw a daisy, a house, and a stick figure. In assessing the results, one is obviously not judging artistic merit, but rather, attention is focused on any disorganization of the drawn figure.

DRESSING APRAXIA

In dressing apraxia there is, as the name implies, a significant difficulty in getting dressed, which cannot be accounted for by weakness, fatigue, or clumsiness. One patient, described by Hecaen et al. (1956) 'mentioned spontaneously that he had had a great deal of trouble in dressing and that he must frequently be helped by his wife. "I get puzzled in dressing. I get my clothes mixed." He said he put his arms in the wrong sleeve of his shirt or he put the back of his shirt in front'.

Etiology

IDEOMOTOR AND IDEATIONAL APRAXIA

Both ideomotor and ideational apraxia may occur in a more or less isolated fashion, or they may be found in the context of a larger syndrome such as delirium or dementia.

When occurring in an isolated fashion, the onset may be either acute or gradual. Acute onsets almost always occur as part of a stroke syndrome. In these cases, ideomotor apraxia may be seen with lesions in the left hemisphere, of either the parietal cortex (Heilman 1973), lentiform nucleus (Agostoni et al. 1983), or thalamus (Agostoni et al. 1983; Nadeau et al. 1994). Ideational apraxia, similarly, is also seen with left hemisphere lesions, including the parietal cortex (De Renzi et al. 1988), lentiform nucleus (De Renzi et al. 1986), and thalamus (De Renzi et al. 1986; Warren et al. 2000). Gradual onsets may occur with mass lesions, such as tumors, in the same locations; more commonly, however, gradual onsets are seen in certain neurodegenerative

diseases. Of the neurodegenerative diseases that can present with ideomotor or ideational apraxia, corticobasal ganglionic degeneration is the most important, and in such cases one typically finds an associated asymmetric parkinsonism (Riley et al. 1990; Rinne et al. 1994). Other neurodegenerative disorders that may present with these apraxias include Alzheimer's disease (Ross et al. 1996) and Pick's disease (Fukui et al. 1996). In all of these neurodegenerative disorders the gradually progressive apraxia is eventually joined by a dementia.

Isolated ideomotor (Kazui ad Sawada 1993) or ideational (Watson and Heilman 1983) apraxia may also occur as part of a disconnection syndrome, wherein the apraxia is confined to the left upper extremity. In these cases, a lesion of the corpus callosum, by severing fibers running from the left parietal cortex to the right parietal cortex, deprives the right parietal cortex of 'guidance' and hence purposeful movements of the left arm cannot be made.

Ideomotor and ideational apraxia are very commonly found in delirium and advanced dementia and in these cases constitute but one of a large number of cortical deficits accompanying the associated cognitive changes, such as confusion, short-term memory loss, disorientation, etc.

CONSTRUCTIONAL APRAXIA

Constructional apraxia is seen with lesions, generally infarctions, of the right parietal cortex (Piercy et al. 1960); rarely constructional apraxia may be seen with a right thalamic lesion (Motomura et al. 1986). Rarely, a disconnection constructional apraxia may occur wherein, again because of a callosal lesion, drawing with the right hand is severely impaired, whereas drawing with the left hand is relatively good by contrast (Giroud and Dumas 1995).

DRESSING APRAXIA

Dressing apraxia may be seen with lesions, again generally ischemic infarctions, of the right parietal cortex (Brain 1941; Hacean et al. 1956).

Differential diagnosis

Sensory aphasia, given the overall difficulty with comprehension, may make it very difficult to test for ideomotor, ideational, or constructional apraxia.

Visual agnosia may complicate testing for ideational apraxia, in that patients may simply not recognize the tool that you are asking them to use. Consequently, if patients do display apparent ideational apraxia, it is necessary to ask them to name the offered tool and if they have difficulty with that one should go on to ask them to describe what the tool is used for in order to rule out mere anomia. Anomic patients may not be able to say the name of the tool, but can describe its use; agnosic patients, by contrast, will neither be able to name it nor describe its use.

Neglect of the left side, as may be seen with right parietal lesions, may simulate constructional apraxia to a degree. In neglect, however, the deficient drawing is present only on the left side of the figure, whereas the right side of the figure is drawn more or less normally; in contrast, in constructional apraxia both the left and right halves of the figure are poorly drawn. Left neglect may also simulate dressing apraxia, as patients may leave the left side of their dressing unattended to, with the left shirt sleeve dangling or the left shoe untied. Here, however, as with the differential with constructional apraxia, the clue to the diagnosis of neglect is the presence of adequate dressing on the right side of the body.

Treatment

Speech and occupational therapy should be considered in addition to treatment, if possible, of the underlying cause.

2.9 AGNOSIAS

Agnosia is a condition characterized by a failure, despite adequate sensation, to recognize phenomena. There are a number of different kinds of agnosia and these may be grouped as described below.

Certain agnosias are distinguished by the sensory modality affected. Thus, in visual agnosia, there is a failure to recognize an object by sight, in tactile agnosia, by touch, and in auditory agnosia by the sound made by the object. Other agnosias are characterized by a specific kind of feature that cannot be recognized: in prosopognosia there is difficulty in recognizing faces, in topographagnosia landmarks go unrecognized and patients get lost, and in color agnosia patients cannot recognize various colors. Two other agnosias are marked by an inability to recognize certain facts: in anosognosia, patients fail to recognize certain signs and symptoms, as for example hemiparesis; in asomatognosia patients fail to recognize that a body part, for example a hemiparetic arm, belongs to them. Finally, there is a form of agnosia, namely simultanagnosia, wherein patients fail to simultaneously recognize all the objects in their view, as if one or more of them had actually disappeared. Each of these agnosias is now discussed in turn.

Visual agnosia

Visual agnosia, or the inability to recognize and name objects by sight, is a rare disorder.

CLINICAL FEATURES

In visual agnosia, patients, despite adequate visual acuity, are unable to recognize familiar objects by sight alone. Thus, if shown a pair of scissors, they will be unable to name it and they will be unable to say what it is used for. Interestingly, however, if they are given the object and allowed to handle it, they are able to recognize it by touch.

Visual agnosia may be broken down into two subtypes: apperceptive and associative. The clinical differentiation of these subtypes is based on the patient's ability, after being shown the object in question, to either draw it or pick it out from a photograph or drawing of a group of different objects (one of which is the object in question). In apperceptive visual agnosia patients can neither make a drawing of the object nor can they pick it out of a group of objects. In associative visual agnosia, however, patients are able to perform these tasks.

At a phenomenological level, it seems that when apperceptive subtype patients are shown an object they do not experience an image of it and, lacking such an image, have no subsequent recognition and, of course, no ability to make a drawing. In associative visual agnosia, however, an image does occur, as evidenced by patient's ability to make a drawing of the object or to pick it out of a group of objects. Despite the presence of an image, however, there is an inability to make a connection between that image and the concept of that object, and thus a failure to recognize it, name it, or say what it is used for.

Of note, visual agnosia is typically more severe for small objects, such as a pair of scissors, than it is for large objects, such as chairs or desks, which patients are generally able to recognize and name. Furthermore, the presence of a larger object may, by providing a context, allow a patient to recognize a smaller object, which, if seen in isolation, he or she would be unable to name. For example, if shown a pair of scissors on a desk-top, the patient might be able to name it, whereas if shown the scissors in isolation, perhaps by placing them on the bed sheet, the patient would be unable to do so.

ETIOLOGY

Apperceptive visual agnosia has been noted with bilateral infarction of the occipital lobes, which spare the striate cortex but involve the secondary visual cortices; the adjacent temporal lobes are often also involved but only in their more posterior extent (Benson and Greenburg 1969; Ferreira *et al.* 1998; Shelton *et al.* 1994).

Associative visual agnosia may occur secondary to bilateral infarction of the medial occipitotemporal cortex and subcortical white matter, especially involving the lingual, fusiform, and parahippocampal gyri (Albert *et al.* 1979). Cases have also been reported secondary to a left unilateral occipitotemporal infarct coupled with infarction of the splenium of the corpus callosum (Feinberg *et al.* 1994). This latter mechanism represents a kind of 'disconnection' syndrome wherein, although the right occipital lobe is untouched, the lesion of the splenium disconnects it from the left hemisphere.

Theoretically, it appears reasonable to say that in the apperceptive subtype the destruction of the secondary visual cortex prevents, as it were, the 'working-up' of the raw visual experience into a coherent image. In the associative subtype, sparing of the secondary visual cortices allows for the development of an image, but destruction of the more anterior occipitotemporal cortex renders impossible an association between the image and the concepts that the patient has regarding various objects.

DIFFERENTIAL DIAGNOSIS

Motor aphasia, when at all severe, is distinguished by the effortful speech. In milder cases, characterized primarily by a word-finding difficulty, the distinction is based on the patient's ability to 'circumlocute' and say what the object is used for: in Broca's aphasia, patients, when shown a pair of scissors, although unable to say the word 'scissors', yet are able to say it is used for cutting, whereas in visual agnosia patients are unable to describe the use of the object.

Anomic aphasia may be distinguished by the patient's response to being allowed to handle the object. The anomic patient, upon handling the pair of scissors, will still remain unable to come up with the name, whereas the agnosic patient will recognize and name the object.

TREATMENT

Speech/language and occupational therapy may be effective, especially with regard to helping patients develop compensatory strategies.

Tactile agnosia

Tactile agnosia is characterized by an inability to recognize objects by touching and handling them, despite normal light touch, pin-prick, vibratory and two-point discriminatory sensation, and despite an ability to describe the shape of the object in question (Platz 1996).

CLINICAL FEATURES

After making sure that the patient's eyes are kept closed, place a common object, such as a key, in the patient's hand and ask the patient to identify it by touch alone. If the patient has any difficulty in doing so, ask for a description of the object. In cases of tactile agnosia, although the patient can describe the object's shape (e.g., as having a serrated edge), there is an inability to name it or to describe its function. At this point, ask the patient to take a look at the object and name it: in tactile agnosia, the patient will be able to name it immediately by sight.

Importantly, because tactile agnosia may occur unilaterally in either hand it is necessary to test both hands, using a different object each time; furthermore, it is also necessary to tell the patient to use only one hand at a time and not to palpate the object with both hands.

ETIOLOGY

Tactile agnosia generally occurs secondary to a lesion in the inferior parietal cortex (Caselli 1993), on either the right (Platz 1996) or the left (Reed et al. 1996).

DIFFERENTIAL DIAGNOSIS

Astereognosia is similar clinically to tactile agnosia in that patients are unable to recognize objects by touch alone; the difference lies in the fact that patients with astereognosia are unable to describe the shape of the object, whereas patients with tactile agnosia can.

Anomic aphasia may also appear similar to tactile agnosia in that anomic patients also are unable to name an object by touching it. In contrast with tactile agnosia, however, patients with anomic aphasia are unable to name the object although they can describe its use (e.g., 'it's for opening a lock').

TREATMENT

Except in the visually impaired, treatment is rarely required.

Auditory agnosia

Auditory agnosia, or, more explicitly, environmental auditory agnosia, is a very rare condition characterized by an inability to recognize such environmental sounds as the ringing of a telephone or the honking of a horn, despite normal hearing and a normal ability to understand the spoken word (Vignolo 1982).

CLINICAL FEATURES

Auditory agnosia may come to attention when patients fail to answer the phone or perhaps, with potentially disastrous consequences, fail to respond to the honking of a car horn. Bedside testing may be accomplished by standing behind the patient and ringing a bell or perhaps snapping your fingers, and then asking the patient what he heard. In environmental auditory agnosia, patients will acknowledge hearing something but they will be unable to say what it was.

ETIOLOGY

Auditory agnosia has been reported with an infarction of the posterior portion of the right temporal lobe (Fujii et al. 1990); it has also been noted to evolve out of a syndrome of cortical deafness secondary to lesions affecting the auditory radiations of the retrolenticular portion of the internal capsule bilaterally (Taniwaki et al. 2000).

DIFFERENTIAL DIAGNOSIS

Deafness is readily distinguished in that here there is no response to any sound. Pure word deafness, as discussed in

Section 2.1, is a form of aphasia in which patients are unable to comprehend the meaning of the word, although they are able to recognize environmental sounds and the spoken word as a word.

TREATMENT

Speech/language therapy may enable the patient to develop compensatory strategies.

Prosopagnosia

The term prosopagnosia is derived from the Greek word for face, '*prosopon*', and refers to a remarkable condition in which patients are unable to recognize others by looking at their faces (Sergent and Poncet 1990).

CLINICAL FEATURES

Patients with prosopagnosia, although able to recognize faces as faces, and indeed able to describe accurately the facial features of others, are yet unable to identify the other person (Tranel *et al.* 1988). Remarkably, these patients, although unable to identify others by their facial features, may be able to identify them by other features, such as their voice, dress, or characteristic gait (Damasio *et al.* 1982b).

Some examples may help to clarify this remarkable condition. In one case, the patient, a party to a lawsuit, had come to identify his own lawyer by the setting in which the two of them generally met, namely the lawyer's office; all went well until trial, when the patient, unable to recognize people in the courtroom, went up to the opposing counsel and began to discuss confidential details of the case 'with disastrous consequences' (Pevzner *et al.* 1962). In another case, a patient had come to rely on his wife's clothing as a means of identifying her: at a party, he found himself unable to recall what she had put on and although she walked right by him he failed to recognize her (Hecaen and Angelergues 1962). In a similar vein, another patient 'failed to recognize a physician who had just examined him after the doctor had substituted his suit jacket for his white coat' (Hecaen and Angelergues 1962). Finally, and most remarkably, some patients are not able to recognize themselves when they look in the mirror (Damasio *et al.* 1980).

As might be expected, such patients, in addition to being unable to recognize old acquaintances by their facial features, are also unable to utilize facial features to recognize new acquaintances (Malone *et al.* 1982).

ETIOLOGY

Prosopagnosia generally occurs secondary to bilateral lesions of the inferior occipitotemporal area (Cohn *et al.* 1986; Damasio *et al.* 1980, 1982b; Meadows 1974b; Pevzner *et al.* 1962); rarely prosopagnosia may occur secondary to a unilateral occipitotemporal lesion on the right

(Cohen *et al.* 1994; Landis *et al.* 1986, 1988; Rosler *et al.* 1997; Wada and Yamamoto 2001). In all these cases, the prosopagnosia occurred as part of a stroke syndrome, generally secondary to ischemic infarction.

Prosopagnosia has also been noted secondary to resection of the posterior portion of the right temporal lobe (Mesad *et al.* 2003) and after a right hemispherectomy (Sergent and Villemure 1989). There are also rare reports of progressive prosopagnosia occurring secondary to progressive atrophy of the right temporal lobe (Evans *et al.* 1995; Joubert *et al.* 2003).

Interestingly, prosopagnosia may also occur on a paroxysmal basis as a simple partial seizure: in one case, a patient with left occipitotemporal scarring had seizures characterized by a sense of 'flickering lights' followed by a brief episode of prosopagnosia (Agnetti *et al.* 1978).

Finally, there are also rare reports of prosopagnosia occurring on a developmental basis (Kress and Daum 2003).

DIFFERENTIAL DIAGNOSIS

Anomic aphasia may render patients incapable of coming up with the name of another person; in such cases, however, in contrast with prosopagnosia, there is no difficulty in recognizing the other person or in specifying the relationship that exists between the patient and the other person.

TREATMENT

Speech/language and occupational therapy may assist the patient in developing compensatory strategies.

Topographagnosia

At the outset, it should be noted that there is some debate regarding the definition of topographagnosia and, consequently, the reader, in perusing journal articles, should pay particular attention to the definition peculiar to the authors of the article. In this text, topographagnosia refers to a condition in which patients, despite adequate memory and vision, are unable to find their way in surroundings that had not previously caused any difficulty. This group of patients may be further subdivided into two types, namely one wherein the difficulty lies in an inability to recognize familiar landmarks (termed here 'landmark agnosia') and another wherein, despite a preserved ability to recognize landmarks, there is an inability to utilize these landmarks in deciding which way to proceed (herein referred to as 'topographical disorientation').

CLINICAL FEATURES

Finding one's way depends both on recognizing landmarks and on knowing which way to proceed upon encountering those landmarks. Thus, if one's accustomed route home from the office involves walking down Main Street to the Bank and then turning right, then in order to successfully navigate this route one must first recognize the Bank as the landmark and then, second, know that at this landmark one must turn right.

In landmark agnosia, difficulty arises at the level of recognizing the Bank as a landmark. Although the patient may recognize the building, and even describe it, it is not recognized as a landmark and hence the patient is as likely to walk past it as to turn.

In topographic disorientation, the situation is a little different. Here, the patient does recognize the Bank as a landmark, but, having lost a 'sense of direction', the patient is unable to figure out whether to turn to the right or left, or simply proceed onward. Some examples may flesh this out. In one case, a patient 'had sudden difficulty finding her way out of a subway station she had used daily for years. She had no difficulty recognizing the surrounding buildings, but she was unable to find her way to work or to her own home despite multiple attempts' (Alsaadi et al. 2000). In another case, the patient: '. . . suddenly lost his way home, where he was going on foot. The buildings in front of him were familiar to him, so he could recognize them right away. However, he did not know which direction his home was from there. Relying on cues from buildings, surrounding scenery and signs, but taking several wrong turns along the way, he eventually arrived in front of his own home, and knew immediately that it was in fact his own home' (Takahashi et al. 1997).

ETIOLOGY

Landmark agnosia has been reported with infarction involving the medial occipitotemporal area (primarily the fusiform and lingual gyri, with some involvement of the parahippocampal gyrus), either unilaterally on the right or bilaterally (Aguirre and D'Esposito 1999). An example was also reported as a sequela to herpes simplex encephalitis wherein there was damage to both temporal lobes, with the right side being much more severely involved (McCarthy et al. 1996).

Topographical disorientation has also been reported with infarction of the bilateral fusiform, lingual, and parahippocampal gyri (Alsaadi et al. 2000), and also with infarction of the right parahippocampal gyrus (Habib and Sirigu 1987; Luzzi et al. 2000). Interestingly, cases have also been reported secondary to infarction of the splenium (Alsaadi et al. 2000) or right retrosplenial cortex (Takahashi et al. 1997).

Further, there are also case reports of topographagnosia occurring on a transient basis, with episodes lasting from 5 to 30 minutes (Stracciari et al. 1994). During these episodes, apart from the topographagnosia, patients are otherwise normal and recovery is complete. Most patients were women in their middle or later years and, although the etiology is unknown, it is speculated to be similar to that of transient global amnesia.

DIFFERENTIAL DIAGNOSIS

Patients with amnesia may lose their way in unfamiliar surroundings. The basis for this, however, lies in an inability to commit to memory features of the new environment, and this stands in contrast with topographagnosia wherein memory is intact. Furthermore, patients with amnesia typically have no trouble finding their way in environments that they have travelled in before, provided, of course, that any retrograde amnesia has not obscured their recall.

Patients with dementia or delirium often lose their way and although this may be on the basis of memory loss (or, in the case of delirium, confusion), it can also occur in patients with relatively preserved memory, and in these cases it is perhaps appropriate to consider the topographagnosia as but one indicator of widespread cortical damage or dysfunction. The existence of other cognitive deficits, however, indicates the correct syndromal diagnosis.

TREATMENT

Speech/language and occupational therapy may assist the patient in developing compensatory strategies.

Color agnosia

CLINICAL FEATURES

In color agnosia, patients, despite normal color vision, are unable to recognize and name the color of objects (Kinsbourne and Warrington 1964; Meadows 1974a).

DIFFERENTIAL DIAGNOSIS

Color agnosia must be distinguished from acquired *color blindness* or, as it is also known, central achromatopsia (Damasio et al. 1980), this distinction being readily accomplished with Ishihara plates. Whereas patients with achromatopsia are unable to read the plates, patients with color agnosia are. The patient with achromatopsia exists in a world of grays; by contrast, the patient with color agnosia, although able to discern hues, cannot name them.

ETIOLOGY

Color agnosia may occur with lesions of the splenium and the medial portion of the left occipital cortex, and is often seen in association with alexia without agraphia (Geschwind and Fusillo 1966).

TREATMENT

Occupational therapy may assist in devising compensatory strategies.

Anosognosia

Anosognosia, a term coined by Babinski in 1914, is characterized by a failure to recognize neuropsychiatric deficits. Although hemiparesis is the deficit most commonly involved (and indeed anosognosia for hemiparesis is very common in the first few months after stroke [Hier 1983a,b]), other deficits, as noted below, may also go unrecognized.

CLINICAL FEATURES

The severity of the anosognosia may range from a mere tendency to minimize the extent of the deficit to a strong denial that any deficit at all exists (Baier and Karnath 2005). Upon questioning patients with anosognosia for hemiparesis, some patients may admit there is something wrong but then go on to say that the paretic limb is only 'a bit stiff', or perhaps suffers from some 'heaviness' (Cutting 1978; Roth 1949); in other cases, 'the patient behaves as though he knew nothing about his hemiplegia, as though it had not existed, as though his paralyzed limbs were normal' (Gerstmann 1942). Even more remarkably, in some cases the patient may insist that the paralyzed limb, although motionless, is in fact moving (Feinberg et al. 2000).

Other deficits that may go unrecognized include hemianopia, cortical blindness, chorea, and cognitive or behavioral deficits.

Anosognosia for hemianopia after stroke was noted in over one-half of patients in one study (Celesia et al. 1997), a fact that emphasizes the absolute necessity of meticulous visual field testing.

Anosognosia for cortical blindness, known as Anton's syndrome, represents a most remarkable clinical phenomenon (Bergman 1957; Redlich and Dorsey 1945; Symonds and MacKenzie 1957). Patients, although blind, may insist that their vision is perhaps only slightly impaired, that the light is too dim, or they may flatly insist that there is nothing wrong with their vision at all; attempting to walk, they predictably bump into things, trip, and fall.

Abnormal movements may also go unrecognized, and this is particularly the case with chorea in Huntington's disease (Snowden et al. 1998), wherein patients often stoutly maintain that there is absolutely nothing wrong.

Cognitive and behavioral deficits may also be denied by patients with dementia, who may insist on keeping their own checkbooks or driving with disastrous results.

ETIOLOGY

Anosognosia for hemiparesis is most typically seen as part of a stroke syndrome with infarction in the area of distribution of the superior division of the middle cerebral artery involving both the parietal and frontal lobes. Although the vast majority of cases involve infarction of the right hemisphere with left hemiparesis (Cutting 1978; Roth 1949), cases have been reported of anosognosia for right hemiparesis; furthermore, it is speculated that the relative rarity of reports of anosognosia for right hemiparesis may actually be due to an associated sensory aphasia, which makes testing for anosognosia very difficult (Weinstein et al. 1969). Anosognosia for hemiparesis may also be seen with infarction or hemorrhage of the following areas: right posterior limb of the internal capsule and adjacent lenticular nucleus (House and Hodges 1988), right thalamus (Liebson 2000; Motomura et al. 1986), and the pons, on either the right or the left side (Bakchine et al. 1997; Evyapan and Kumral 1999).

Anosognosia for hemianopia has been noted with unilateral infarction in the area of distribution of the posterior cerebral artery (Celesia et al. 1997) and Anton's syndrome, with bilateral infarctions in the area of distribution of the posterior cerebral arteries.

Anognosia for chorea, as noted above, has been noted in Huntington's disease.

Cognitive and behavioral deficits are often denied in patients with Alzheimer's disease (Kashiwa et al. 2005; Starkstein et al. 1997), frontotemporal dementia (Eslinger et al. 2005), and traumatic brain injury (Sbordone et al. 1998; Flashman and McCallister 2002).

DIFFERENTIAL DIAGNOSIS

In all cases, anosognosia must be differentiated from emotionally motivated denial. This distinction must not be based on the vehemence with which patients deny any disability, as some patients with anosognosia may be quite insistent in their assertion that nothing is wrong; rather it should be based on the patient's response to a display of sympathy from others. Whereas patients with anosognosia are unmoved by sympathy, patients 'in denial' will often break down and tearfully discuss the fears aroused by their disabilities.

Anosognosia for cognitive deficits may be mimicked by a frontal lobe syndrome, wherein disinhibition and jocularity prevent patients from acting on any recognition they might have of their deficits.

TREATMENT

Patients should be seen in rehabilitation therapies and, pending resolution of the anosognosia, protective measures may be required.

Asomatognosia

In asomatognosia, patients with left hemiparesis fail to experience the hemiparetic extremity as belonging to them.

CLINICAL FEATURES

In some cases, patients, in addition to denying that the paretic arm is theirs, may go on to say that in fact the arm belongs to someone else, perhaps a family member (Brock and Merwarth 1957; Feinberg et al. 1990). This can lead to a rather bizarre interview: in one case (Sandifer 1946), a female patient with a left hemiplegia, when her paretic left hand was held up in front of her, indicated that it was not hers but belonged to the physician. When the physician attempted to correct her by pointing out that the hand in question had her wedding ring on it, the patient responded, 'That's my ring, you've got my ring, Doctor.'

In doubtful cases, it may be helpful to lift up the paretic left arm, bring it over into the right hemispace and ask the patient whose arm it is (Feinberg et al. 1990).

ETIOLOGY

Most cases are due to infarction involving the right parietal cortex in the area of the supramarginal gyrus (Feinberg et al. 1990); cases have also been reported secondary to infarction involving the right striatum and adjacent internal capsule (Healton et al. 1982) and to hemorrhage in the right thalamus (Liebson 2000; Motomura et al. 1986). Rarely, asomatognosia may constitute the sole symptomatology of a simple partial seizure, wherein the seizure focus was in the right parietal lobe (So and Schauble 2004).

DIFFERENTIAL DIAGNOSIS

In the alien hand syndrome, although patients experience the left arm as being under the control of some 'alien' entity, they still acknowledge that the arm is theirs; furthermore, in the alien hand syndrome the left arm is quite active, whereas in asomatognosia the arm is paretic.

TREATMENT

Rehabilitation therapies may be helpful.

Simultanagnosia

Simultanagnosia, first described by Wolpert in 1924, is a remarkable syndrome in which patients, despite normal visual acuity, intermittently fail to see all parts of their environment simultaneously, with certain objects literally falling out of view, as if they had become temporarily invisible.

CLINICAL FEATURES

Simultanagnosia may present clinically either because objects 'disappear' or, conversely, 'appear'. In one case (Coslett and Saffran 1991), a patient, while walking through the apartment she had lived in for 25 years, 'fell over her dining room table' because she didn't see it as she crossed the room. The same patient reported the converse experience while watching a movie. In the movie, a character was having a heated argument, and the patient, while watching the movie, 'noted to her surprise and consternation that the character she had been watching was suddenly sent reeling across the room, apparently as a consequence of a punch thrown by a character she had never seen'.

Bedside testing may be accomplished either by asking patients to describe everything they see in their room, or by showing them a picture or photograph of a complex scene, and asking, again, for them to describe every object that they see.

ETIOLOGY

Simultanagnosia has been noted with infarction of the right temporo-occipital area (Cohen et al. 1994; Coslett and Saffran 1991), and with bilateral infarction of the posterior occipitoparietal area (Rizzo and Hurtig 1987; Rizzo and Robin 1990). Cases have also been reported secondary to progressive neurodegenerative conditions in the syndrome of posterior cortical atrophy (Tang-Wei et al. 2004).

Simultanagnosia may also occur as part of Balint's syndrome (Section 4.14) and, given this, all patients with simultanagnosia should be tested for optic ataxia and optic apraxia.

DIFFERENTIAL DIAGNOSIS

Hemianopia and visual neglect are experienced to only one side in contrast with simultanagnosia, wherein objects may be 'lost' from any point of the visual field.

TREATMENT

Speech/language and occupational therapy may enable patients to develop compensatory strategies.

2.10 NEGLECT

In this aptly named syndrome, patients, in one fashion or another, neglect or fail to attend to phenomena on one side, usually the left. Neglect may either be visual or motor: in visual neglect (also known as spatial neglect), as might be expected, objects are not attended to in one of the hemifields; in motor neglect, there is an 'underutilization' of the limbs on one side, as if, in a sense, the patient 'neglects' to use them.

Clinical features

Both forms of neglect are considered in turn, beginning with visual neglect. Importantly, the physician must test for both visual and motor neglect before concluding that neglect, per se, is, or is not, present. This is the case because visual and motor neglect may occur independently of each other (Laplane and Degos 1983).

VISUAL NEGLECT

Visual neglect may come to clinical attention in a variety of ways. Patients may fail to comb their hair, shave, or put on make-up on the neglected side, and food on the neglected side of a dinner plate may go uneaten. In talking with a group, patients may fail to speak with those on the neglected side, and, if patients are looking for something, the may fail to find it if it is on the neglected side, even if it is in plain view. In one case (Cherington 1974) left neglect ruined a patient's chess game: although chess pieces on the right side of the board were moved as always, those on the left, neglected, remained in position, and were easy prey for his opponent. In another case (Frantz 1950), a patient, while driving, began to run into things (such as pedestrians) on the left. Importantly, as in all cases of visual neglect, these collisions did not occur because of a hemianopia: the patient had full visual fields but simply did not attend to things to his left.

Interestingly, visual neglect may also extend to *imagined* scenes. In one study, for example, patients with neglect were instructed to imagine that they were standing on one side of a famous plaza and then describe what they saw: as might be expected, in their description of the imagined scene, they failed to speak of things on the plaza that were located on the left of the imagined scene (Bisiach and Luzzatti 1978).

Bedside testing for visual neglect may be accomplished with three 'paper and pencil' tests: line bisection, line cancellation, and clock drawing. In order to obtain reliable results for these tests, the patient must be seated squarely in front of a table, the trunk parallel to the edge of the table and the piece of paper placed directly in front of the patient, such that the midline of the paper is continuous with the patient's midline. Although patients may move their head in any direction, and look in any direction, this relative position of the paper and the patient's trunk must be maintained. The reason why the position of the patient's trunk is so important in these three tests is that if the trunk is angled toward the neglected side the portion of the visual field subject to neglect will shrink, to the point at which the tests may become falsely negative (Beschin *et al.* 1997; Karnath and Hartje 1993).

In the line bisection test a single line is drawn lengthwise on the piece of paper, with the middle of the line resting at the midline of the piece of paper. The patient is then asked to make a mark directly on the middle of the line. When left neglect is present, the mark made by the patient will be to the right of the true midline. Importantly, the line should be of the order of 10 cm or longer because if the line is substantially shorter than this, there may be a 'crossover' effect, whereby the patient with left neglect will place the mark not to the right but to the left of the true midline (Anderson 1997; Tegner and Levander 1991).

In the line cancellation test (Albert 1973) the examiner places a large number of short, straight lines randomly on the surface of the piece of paper, the different lines being oriented at various and random angles, and then asks the patient to simply mark off each line. In a positive test, the proportion of lines marked off to the left of the midline will be substantially less than the proportion marked off to the right.

In the clock-drawing test, the patient is asked to draw a large circle on the paper and then to put in all 12 numbers, as on a clockface. In a positive test, the numbers will be more or less 'bunched up' on the right side. In a similar test, patients are asked to draw a daisy; in a positive test, the petals of the daisy will end up being bunched on the right-hand side. Importantly, patients should be asked to simply 'draw a daisy' and not given instructions to 'arrange' the petals around a circle, because when patients are given such an instruction, the neglect may 'vanish' as the petals are arranged, one by one, evenly around the circle (Ishiai *et al.* 1997).

Importantly, each one of these tests must be performed before concluding that the bedside examination is negative, as some patients with neglect may 'pass' one, but not another (Azouvi *et al.* 2002; Binder *et al.* 1992; Ishiai *et al.* 1993).

Another bedside test for visual neglect involves testing for what is known as visual extinction. To test for visual extinction, establish first, with confrontation testing, that the visual fields are full. Stand directly in front of the patient, perhaps an arm's length away, and spread your arms to the sides such that your hands end up level with the patient's eyes and perhaps 30 cm in front of the patient. Next, ask the patient to stare at your nose and to point to the finger that wiggles, all the while continuing to look straight at your nose. To perform the test, wiggle one index finger at a time: if the patient points to each finger when it wiggles, then, at least on this confrontation testing, the fields are full. At this point, while maintaining the same position, wiggle both fingers simultaneously: with a positive test, the movement on the neglected side is 'extinguished' and the patient points only to the movement on the unaffected side.

MOTOR NEGLECT

Motor neglect (Laplane and Degos 1983; Triggs *et al.* 1994) may come to clinical attention in a peculiarity of gait: on the affected side, there may be reduced arm swing, and the leg, generally being underutilized and 'left behind', is seen to be 'dragged' along to keep up with the leg on the unaffected side. When patients are in a wheelchair, the arm on the affected side may dangle down from the shoulder and be dragged along passively on the floor as the wheelchair is pushed forward; for patients in bed, the affected leg may be 'left behind', still stretched out on the bed, as the patient swings the leg on the unaffected side over the edge of the bed while attempting to rise. A more subtle form of motor neglect may occur as patients neglect to chew on the neglected side, with food consequently dribbling out (Andre *et al.* 2000).

Bedside testing for motor neglect may be accomplished by asking patients to clap their hands or fasten a button: when motor neglect is present, the arm on the neglected side will either not participate in the task or do so only minimally. Importantly, this is not the result of a lack of strength or coordination: with strong urging, patients are generally able to bring the affected arm into play such that there is more or less full bimanual cooperation in the task at hand.

Etiology

As indicated earlier, left neglect, due to a lesion in the right hemisphere, is clinically far more prominent than right neglect. Although right neglect certainly does occur, it is less common, less severe, and, in the case of stroke, less enduring (Beis *et al.* 2004; Stone *et al.* 1991).

Although neglect may occur secondary to both cortical and to subcortical lesions, in the great majority of cases, it is a lesion of the cortex that is responsible (Vallar and Perani 1986; Vallar *et al.* 1994). Cortical lesions capable of causing neglect may be found in the frontal lobe (primarily in the posterior portion of the inferior frontal gyrus [Daffner *et al.* 1990; Husain and Kennad 1996; Heilman and Valenstein 1972; Maeshima *et al.* 1994; Stein and Volpe 1983]), the parietal lobe (Bender 1945; Cherington 1974; Critchley 1949; Frantz 1950) (primarily in the inferior parietal lobule [Mort *et al.* 2003; Vallar and Perani 1986]), and in the temporal lobe (primarily the medial aspect of the parahippocampal gyrus [Mort *et al.* 2003]). Subcortical structures implicated include the caudate nucleus (Caplan *et al.* 1990; Kumral *et al.* 1999), the putamen (Hier *et al.* 1977), and the thalamus (Kumral *et al.* 1995; Motomura *et al.* 1986; Watson *et al.* 1981). Rarely, neglect has been noted with a lesion of the posterior limb of the internal capsule (Bogousslavsky *et al.* 1988c; Ferro and Kertesz 1984) and with a combined lesion of the medial aspect of the occipital lobe and the splenium (Chung Park *et al.* 2005).

Although neglect is most commonly seen as part of a stroke syndrome, it may also occur with other focal lesions (such as tumors) and may also be seen as but one sign in a dementing disorder such as Alzheimer's disease.

Differential diagnosis

Visual neglect must be distinguished from hemianopia and constructional apraxia. Hemianopic patients, of course, will fail to attend to objects in the hemianopic field, given that they simply do not see them. Confrontational testing for visual fields, done with sufficient vigor, however, reveals full fields in patients with neglect. In constructional apraxia, drawing a clock face or daisy may be very difficult; however, here one sees a random pattern of errors, rather than a 'bunching up' on the unneglected side.

Motor neglect must be distinguished from hemiparesis, and this distinction is made, as indicated earlier, on the basis of the response to vigorous encouragement. Patients with neglect eventually respond to vigorous direction, whereas patients with hemiparesis simply cannot.

Treatment

Various rehabilitation techniques are helpful for visual neglect, including prism adaptation (Frassinetti *et al.* 2002; Keane *et al.* 2006), neck muscle vibration (Schindler *et al.* 2002), and visual scanning training.

REFERENCES

Achiron A, Ziv I, Djaldetti R *et al.* Aphasia in multiple sclerosis: clinical and radiologic correlation. *Neurology* 1992; **42**:2195–7.

Agnetti V, Carreras M, Pinna L *et al.* Ictal prosopagnosia and epileptogenic damage of the dominant hemisphere. *Cortex* 1978; **14**:50–7.

Agostoni E, Coletti A, Orlando G *et al.* Apraxia in deep cerebral lesions. *J Neurol Neurosurg Psychiatry* 1983; **46**:804–8.

Aguirre GK, D'Esposito M. Topographical disorientation: a synthesis and txonomy. *Brain* 1999;**122**:1613–28.

Ajax ET, Schenkenberg T, Kosteljanetz M. Alexia without agraphia and the inferior splenium. *Neurology* 1977; **27**:685–8.

Albert ML. A simple test of visual neglect. *Neurology* 1973; **23**:658–64.

Albert ML, Soffer D, Silverberg R *et al.* The anatomic basis of visual agnosia. *Neurology* 1979; **29**:876–9.

Alexander MP, LoVerme SR. Aphasia after left hemispheric intracerebral hemorrhage. *Neurology* 1980; **30**:1193–202.

Alexander MP, Schmitt MA. The aphasia syndrome of stroke in the left anterior cerebral artery territory. *Arch Neurol* 1980; **37**:97–100.

Alexander MP, Fischette MR, Fischer RS. Crossed aphasias can be mirror image anomalous: case reports, review and hypothesis. *Brain* 1989; **112**:953–73.

Alsaadi T, Binder JR, Lazar RM *et al.* Pure topographic disorientation: a distinctive syndrome with varied localization. *Neurology* 2000; **54**:1864–6.

Anderson B. Pieces of the true crossover effect in neglect. *Neurology* 1997; **49**:809–12.

Anderson SW, Damasio AR, Damasio H. Troubled letters but not numbers. Domain specific cognitive impairments following focal damage in the frontal cortex. *Brain* 1990; **113**: 749–66.

Andre JM, Beis JM, Morin N *et al.* Buccal hemineglect. *Arch Neurol* 2000; **57**:1734–41.

Arsland D, Larsen JP, Hoien T. Alexia in dementia of the Alzheimer's type. *Acta Neurol Scand* 1993; **88**: 434–9.

Ashtary F, Janghorbani M, Chitsaz A *et al.* A randomized, double-blind trial of bromocriptine efficacy in nonfluent aphasia after stroke. *Neurology* 2006; **66**: 914–16.

Assal G, Perentes E, Deruaz J-P. Crossed aphasia in a right-handed patient. *Arch Neurol* 1981; **38**: 455–8.

Astrom K-E, Mancall EL, Richardson EP. Progressive multifocal leukoencephalopathy: a hitherto unrecognized complication of chronic lymphatic leukaemia and Hodgkin's disease. *Brain* 1958; **81**:93–111.

Azouvi P, Samuel C, Louis-Dreyfus A *et al*. Sensitivity of clinical and behavioral tests of spatial neglect after right hemisphere stroke. *J Neurol Neurosurg Psychiatry* 2002; **73**:160–6.

Babinski J. Contribution a l'etude des troubles mentaux dans l'hemiplegie organique cerebrale (anosognosie). *Rev Neurol* 1914; **27**:845–7.

Bahls FH, Chatrian GE, Mesher RA *et al*. A case of persistent cortical deafness: clinical, neurophysiologic, and neuropathologic observations. *Neurology* 1988; **38**:1490–3.

Baier B, Karnath H-O. Incidence and diagnosis of anosognosia for hemiplegia. *J Neurol Neurosurg Psychiatry* 2005; **76**:358–61.

Bakar M, Kirshner HS, Wertz RT. Crossed aphasia: functional brain imaging with PET or SPECT. *Arch Neurol* 1996; **53**:1026–32.

Bakchine S, Ctassaro I, Seilhan D. Anosognosia for hemiplegia after a brainstem haematoma: a pathological case. *J Neurol Neurosurg Psychiatry* 1997; **63**:686–7.

Bartak L, Rutter M, Cox A. A comparative study of infantile autism and specific developmental receptive language disorders. I. The children. *Br J Psychiatry* 1975; **126**:127–45.

Bautista RE, Ciampetti MZ. Expressive aprosody and amusia as a manifestation of right hemisphere seizures. *Epilepsia* 2003;**44**:466–7.

Beis JM, Keller C, Morin N *et al*. Right spatial neglect after left hemisphere stroke: qualitative and quantitative study. *Neurology* 2004; **63**:1600–5.

Bender MB. Extinction and precipitation of cutaneous sensations. *Arch Neurol Psychiatry* 1945; **54**:1–9.

Benson DF. Psychiatric effects of dysphasia. *Br J Psychiatry* 1973; **123**:555–66.

Benson DF, Geschwind N. Developmental Gerstmann syndrome. *Neurology* 1970; **20**:293–8.

Benson DF, Greenberg JP. Visual form agnosia. A specific defect in visual discrimination. *Arch Neurol* 1969; **20**:82–9.

Benson DF, Wier WF. Acalculia: acquired anarithmetria. *Cortex* 1972; **8**:465–72.

Benson DF, Sheremata WA, Bouchard R *et al*. Conduction aphasia: a clinicopathological study. *Arch Neurol* 1973; **28**:339–46.

Bergman PS. Cerebral blindness. *Arch Neurol Psychiatry* 1957; **78**:568–84.

Bernal B, Ardila A, Altman NR. Acalculia: an fMRI study with implications with respect to brain plasticity. *Int J Neurosci* 2003; **113**:1505–23.

Berthier MI, Green C, Higueras C *et al*. A randomized, placebo-controlled study of donepezil in poststroke aphasia. *Neurology* 2006; **67**:1687–9.

Beschin N, Cubelli R, Della Sala S *et al*. Left of what? The role of egocentric coordinates in neglect. *J Neurol Neurosurg Psychiatry* 1997; **63**:483–9.

Binder J, Marshall R, Lazar R *et al*. Distinct syndromes of hemineglect. *Arch Neurol* 1992; **49**:1187–94.

Bisiach E, Luzzatti C. Unilateral neglect of representational space. *Cortex* 1978; **14**:129–33.

Bogousslavsky J. Global aphasia without other lateralizing signs. *Arch Neurol* 1988; **45**:143.

Bogousslavsky J, Regli F. Anterior cerebral artery territory infarction in the Lausanne stroke registry: clinical and etiologic considerations. *Arch Neurol* 1990; **47**:144–50.

Bogousslavsky J, Regli F, Uske A. Thalamic infarcts: clinical syndromes, etiology, and prognosis. *Neurology* 1988a; **38**:837–48.

Bogousslavsky J, Regli F, Assal G. Acute transcortical mixed aphasia: a carotid occlusion syndrome with pia and watershed infarcts. *Brain* 1988b; **111**:631–41.

Bogousslavsky J, Miklossy J, Regli F *et al*. Subcortical neglect: neuropsychological, SPECT, and neuropathological correlations with anterior choroidal artery territory infarction. *Ann Neurol* 1988c; **23**:448–52.

Bragoni M, Altieri M, Di Piero V *et al*. Bromocriptine and speech therapy in non-fluent chronic aphasia after stroke. *Neurol Sci* 2000;**21**:19–22.

Brain WR. Visual disorientation with special reference to lesions of the right cerebral hemisphere. *Brain* 1941; **64**:244–72.

Brock S, Merwarth HR. The illusory awareness of body parts in cerebral disease. *Arch Neurol Psychiatry* 1957; **77**: 366–75.

Brown JR, Simonson J. A clinical study of 100 aphasic patients: observations on lateralization and localization of lesions. *Neurology* 1957; **7**:777–83.

Brown JW, Wilson FR. Crossed aphasia in a dextral: a case report. *Neurology* 1973; **23**:907–11.

Caplan LR, Schmahmann JD, Kase CS *et al*. Caudate infarcts. *Arch Neurol* 1990; **47**:133–43.

Cappa SF, Perani D, Bressi S *et al*. Crossed aphasia: PET follow up study of two cases. *J Neurol Neurosurg Psychiatry* 1993; **56**:665–71.

Caselli RJ. Ventrolateral and dorsomedial somatosensory association cortex damage produces distinct somesthetic syndromes in humans. *Neurology* 1993; **43**:762–71.

Celesia G, Brigell MG, Vaphiades MS. Hemianopic anosognosia. *Neurology* 1997; **49**:88–97.

Cherington MS. Single case study: visual neglect in a chess player. *J Nerv Ment Dis* 1974; **159**:145–7.

Chung Park K, Jeong Y, Hwa Lee B *et al*. Left hemispatial visual neglect associated with a combined right occipital and splenial lesion: another disconnection syndrome. *Neurocase* 2005; **11**: 310–18.

Ciemens VA. Localized thalamic hemorrhage: a case of aphasia. *Neurology* 1970; **20**:776–82.

Clark DG, Mendez MF, Farag E *et al*. Clinicopathologic case report: progressive aphasia in a 77-year-old man. *J Neuropsychiatr Clin Neurosci* 2003; **15**:231–8.

Cohen DN, Salanga VD, Hully W *et al*. Alexia without agraphia. *Neurology* 1976; **26**:455–9.

Cohen L, Gray F, Meyrignal C *et al*. Selective deficity of visual size perception: two cases of hemimicropsia. *J Neurol Neurosurg Psychiatry* 1994; **57**:73–8.

Cohen M, Campbell R, Yaghmai F. Neuropathological abnormalities in developmental dysphasia. *Ann Neurol* 1989; 25:567–70.

Cohn R, Neumann MA, Wood DH. Prosopagnosia: a clinicopathological study. *Ann Neurol* 1986; 20:177–82.

Corbett AJ, McCosker EA, Davidson OR. Acalculia following a dominant-hemisphere subcortical infarct. *Arch Neurol* 1986; 43:964–6.

Coslett HB, Saffran E. Simultanagnosia: to see but not two see. *Brain* 1991; 114:1523–45.

Coslett HB, Brashear HR, Heilman KM. Pure word deafness after bilateral primary auditory cortex infarcts. *Neurology* 1984; 34:347–52.

Critchley M. Phenomenon of tactile inattention with special reference to parietal lesions. *Brain* 1949; 72:538–61.

Cutting J. Study of anosognosia. *J Neurol Neurosurg Psychiatry* 1978; 41:548–55.

Daffner KR, Ahern GL, Weintraub S et al. Dissociated neglect behavior following sequential stroke in the right hemisphere. *Ann Neurol* 1990; 28:97–101.

Damasio AR, Damasio H. The anatomic basis of pure alexia. *Neurology* 1983; 33:73–83.

Damasio AR, Yamada T, Damasio H et al. Central achromatopsia: behavioral, anatomic and physiologic aspects. *Neurology* 1980; 30:1064–71.

Damasio AR, Damasio H, Rizzo M et al. Aphasia with nonhemorrhagic lesion in the basal ganglia and internal capsule. *Ann Neurol* 1982a; 39:15–20.

Damasio AR, Damasio H, Van Hoesen GW. Prosopagnosia: anatomic basis and behavioral mechanisms. *Neurology* 1982b; 32:331–41.

Damasio H, Damasio AR. The anatomical basis of conduction aphasia. *Brain* 1980; 30:337–50.

Darby DG. Sensory aprosodia: a clinical clue to lesions of the inferior division of the right middle cerebral artery? *Neurology* 1993; 43:567–72.

Day JT, Fisher AG, Mastaglia FL. Alexia with agraphia in multiple sclerosis. *J Neurol Sci* 1987; 78:343–8.

De Renzi E, Lucchelli F. Ideational apraxia. *Brain* 1988; 111:1173–85.

De Renzi E, Faglioni P, Scarpa M et al. Limb apraxia in patients with damage confined to the left basal ganglia or thalamus. *J Neurol Neurosurg Psychiatry* 1986; 49:1030–8.

Devere TD, Trotter JL, Cross AH. Acute aphasia in multiple sclerosis. *Arch Neurol* 2000; 57:1207–9.

Devinsky O, Kelley K, Yacubia EMT et al. Postictal behavior. *Arch Neurol* 1994; 51:254–9.

Dogulu CF, Kansu T, Karabudak R. Alexia without agraphia in multiple sclerosis. *J Neurol Neurosurg Psychiatry* 1996; 61:528.

Eslinger PJ, Dennis K, Moore P et al. Metacognitive deficits in frontotemporal dementia. *J Neurol Neurosurg Psychiatry* 2005; 76:1630–5.

Evans JJ, Heggs AJ, Antoun N et al. Progressive prosopagnosia associated with selective right temporal lobe atrophy: a new syndrome? *Brain* 1995; 118:1–13.

Evyapan D, Kumral D. Pontine anosognosia for hemiplegia. *Neurology* 1999; 53:647–9.

Evyapan D, Kumral E. Visuospatial stimulus-bound automatic writing behavior: a right hemisphere stroke syndrome. *Neurology* 2001; 56:245–7.

Faber R, Abrams R, Taylor MA et al. Comparison of schizophrenic patients with formal thought disorder and neurologically impaired patients with aphasia. *Am J Psychiatry* 1983; 140:1348–51.

Feinberg TE, Haber LD, Leeds NE. Verbal asomatognosia. *Neurology* 1990; 40:1391–4.

Feinberg TE, Schindler RJ, Ochoa E et al. Associative visual agnosia and alexia without prosopagnosia. *Cortex* 1994; 30:395–411.

Feinberg TE, Roane DM, Ali J. Illusory limb movements in anosognosia for hemiplegia. *J Neurol Neurosurg Psychiatry* 2000; 68:511–13.

Ferreira CT, Ceccaldi M, Giusiano B et al. Separate visual pathways for perception of actions and objects: evidence from a case of apperceptive agnosia. *J Neurol Neurosurg Psychiatry* 1998; 65:382–5.

Ferro JM, Kertesz A. Posterior internal capsule infarction associated with neglect. *Arch Neurol* 1984; 41:422–4.

Fincham RW, Nibelink DW, Aschenbrenner CA. Alexia with left homonymous hemianopia without agraphia. *Neurology* 1975; 25:1164–8.

Flashman LA, McCallister TW. Lack of awareness and its impact in traumatic brain injury. *Neurorehabilitation* 2002; 17:285–96.

Frantz KE. Amnesia for left limbs and loss of interest and alteration in left fields of vision. *J Nerv Ment Dis* 1950; 112:240–4.

Frassinetti F, Angeli V, Meneghello F et al. Long-lasting amelioration of visuospatial neglect by prism adaptation. *Brain* 2002; 125:608–23.

Freedman M, Alexander MP, Naeser MA. Anatomic basis of transcortical motor aphasia. *Neurology* 1984; 34:409–17.

Frisoni GB, Scuatti A, Biancetti A et al. Hypergraphi and brain damage. *J Neurol Neurosurg Psychiatry* 1993; 56:576–7.

Fuji T, Fukatsu R, Watabe S et al. Auditory sound agnosia without aphasia following a right temporal lesion. *Cortex* 1990; 26:263–8.

Fukui T, Sugita K, Kawamura M et al. Primary progressive apraxia in Pick's disease: a clinicopathologic report. *Neurology* 1996; 47:467–73.

Gabr M, Luders H, Dinner D et al. Speech manifestations in lateralizaton of temporal lobe seizures. *Ann Neurol* 1989; 25:82–7.

Galton CJ, Patterson K, Xuereb JH et al. Atypical and typical presentations of Alzheimer's disease: a clinical, neuro-psychological, neuroimaging and pathological study. *Brain* 2000; 123:484–98.

Gerson SN, Benson DF, Frazier SH. Diagnosis: schizophrenia versus posterior aphasia. *Am J Psychiatry* 1977; 134:966–9.

Gerstmann J. Fingeragnosie: eine umschriebene storung der orientierung am eigenen korper. *Wein Klin Wschr* 1924; 37:1010–12.

Gerstmann J. Syndrome of finger agnosia, disorientation for right and left, agraphia and acalculia. *Arch Neurol Psychiatry* 1940; 44:398–408.

Gerstmann J. Problem of misperception of disease and of impaired body territories with organic lesions: relation to body scheme and its disorders. *Arch Neurol Psychiatry* 1942; **48**:890–913.

Gerstmann J. Some notes on the Gerstmann syndrome. *Neurology* 1957; **7**:866–9.

Geschwind N. Disconnexion syndromes in animals and man. *Brain* 1965; **88**:585–644.

Geschwind N, Fusillo M. Color-naming defects in association with alexia. *Arch Neurol* 1966; **15**:137–46.

Ghacibeh GA, Heilman KM. Progressive affective aprosodia and prosoplegia. *Neurology* 2003; **60**: 1192–4.

Ghika-Schmid F, Bogousslavsky J. The acute behavioral syndrome of anterior thalamic infarction: a propsective study. *Ann Neurol* 2000; **48**:220–7.

Giroud M, Dumas R. Clinical and topographical range of callosal infarction: a clinical and radiological correlation study. *J Neurol Neurosurg Psychiatry* 1995; **59**:238–42.

Godefroy O, Rousseaux M, Pruvo JP *et al.* Neuropsychological changes related to unilateral lenticulostriate infarcts. *J Neurol Neurosurg Psychiatry* 1994; **57**:480–5.

Gold M, Adair JC, Jacobs DH *et al.* Right-left confusion in Gerstmann's syndrome: a model of body centered spatial orientation. *Cortex* 1995; **31**:267–83.

Goldstein DM, Goldberg RL. Monoamine oxidase inhibition-induced speech blockage. *J Clin Psychiatry* 1986; **47**:604.

Goodglass H, Quadfasel FA. Language laterality in left-handed aphasics. *Brain* 1954; **77**:521–48.

Gorelick PB, Ross ED. The aprosodias: further functional–anatomical evidence for the organization of affective language in the right hemisphere. *J Neurol Neurosurg Psychiatry* 1987; **50**:553–60.

Graff-Radford NR, Damasio AR, Hyman BT *et al.* Progressive aphasia in a patient with Pick's disease: a neuropsychological, radiologic and anatomic study. *Neurology* 1990; **40**:620–6.

Green J, Morris JC, Sandson J *et al.* Progressive aphasia: a precursor of global dementia? *Neurology* 1990; **40**:423–9.

Greenblatt SH. Subangular alexia without agraphia or hemianopia. *Brain Lang* 1976; **3**:229–45.

Greene JDW, Patterson K, Xuereb J *et al.* Alzheimer disease and nonfluent progressive aphasia. *Arch Neurol* 1996; **53**: 1072–8.

Gupta MR, Micoch AG, Scolaro C *et al.* Bromocriptine treatment of nonfluent aphasia. *Neurology* 1995; **45**:2170–3.

Habib M, Sirigu A. Pure topographical disorientation: a definition and anatomical basis. *Cortex* 1987; **23**:73–85.

Hamilton NG, Mathews T. Aphasia: the sole manifestation of focal status epilepticus. *Neurology* 1979; **29**:745–8.

Hanlon RE, Lux WE, Dromerick AW. Global aphasia without hemiparesis: language profiles and lesion distribution. *J Neurol Neurosurg Psychiatry* 1996; **66**:365–9.

Hecaen H, Angelergues R. Agnosia for faces (prosopagnosia). *Arch Neurol* 1962; **7**:92–100.

Hecaen H, Penfield W, Bertrand C *et al.* The syndrome of apractagnosia due to lesions of the minor cerebral hemisphere. *Arch Neurol Psychiatry* 1956; **75**:400–34.

Healton EB, Navarro C, Bressman S *et al.* Subcortical neglect. *Neurology* 1982; **32**:776–8.

Heilman KM. Ideational apraxia – a re-definition. *Brain* 1973; **96**:861–4.

Heilman KM, Valenstein E. Frontal lobe neglect in man. *Neurology* 1972; **22**:660–4.

Heilman KM, Rothi L, McFarling D *et al.* Transcortical sensory aphasia with relatively spared spontaneous speech and naming. *Arch Neurol* 1981; **38**:236–9.

Hemphill RE, Stengel E. A study on pure word deafness. *J Neurol Neurosurg Psychiatry* 1940; **3**:251–62.

Henderson VW. Speech fluency in crossed aphasia. *Brain* 1983; **106**:837–57.

Henderson VW. Lesion localization in Broca's aphasia. Implications from Broca's aphasia without hemiparesis. *Arch Neurol* 1985; **42**:1210–12.

Henderson VW, Friedman RB, Teng EL *et al.* Left hemisphere pathways in reading: inferences from pure alexia without hemianopia. *Neurology* 1985; **35**:962–8.

Hermann BP, Whitman S, Wyler AR *et al.* The neurological, psychosocial and demographic correlates of hypergraphia in patients with epilepsy. *J Neurol Neurosurg Psychiatry* 198; **51**:203–8.

Hier DB, Davis KR, Richardson EP *et al.* Hypertensive putaminal hemorrhage. *Ann Neurol* 1977; **2**:152–9.

Hier DB, Mondlock J, Caplan LR. Behavioral abnormalities after right hemisphere stroke. *Neurology* 1983a; **33**:337–44.

Hier DB, Mondlock J, Caplan LR. Recovery of behavioral abnormalities after right hemisphere stroke. *Neurology* 1983b; **33**:345–50.

Hindson DA, Westmoreland DE, Carroll WA *et al.* Persistent Broca's aphasia after right cerebral infarction in a right-hander. *Neurology* 1984; **34**:387–9.

Hirsch E, Marescaux C, Maquet P *et al.* Landau-Kleffner syndrome: a clinical and EEG study of five cases. *Epilepsia* 1990; **31**:756–67.

Holmes JE, Sadoff RL. Aphasia due to a right hemisphere tumor in a right-handed man. *Neurology* 1966; **16**:392–7.

House A, Hodges J. Persistent denial of hardship after infarction of the right basal ganglia: a case study. *J Neurol Neurosurg Psychiatry* 1988; **51**:112–15.

Humphrey ME, Zangwill OL. Dysphasia in left-handed patients with unilateral brain lesions. *J Neurol Neurosurg Psychiatry* 1952; **15**:184–93.

Husain M, Kennard C. Visual neglect associated with frontal lobe infarction. *J Neurol* 1996; **243**:652–7.

Ikeda K, Akiyama H, Iritani S *et al.* Corticobasal degeneration with primary progressive aphasia and accentuated cortical lesion in superior temporal gyrus: case report and review. *Acta Neuropathol* 1996; **92**: 534–9.

Imamura T, Yamadori A, Tsuburaya K. Hypergraphia associated with a brain tumor of the right cerebral hemisphere. *J Neurol Neurosurg Psychiatry* 1992; **54**:25–7.

Ishiai S, Sugishita M, Ichikawa T *et al.* Clock-drawing test and unilateral spatial neglect. *Neurology* 1993; **43**: 106–10.

Ishiai S, Seki K, Koyama Y *et al.* Disappearance of unilateral spatial neglect following a simple instruction. *J Neurol Neurosurg Psychiatry* 1997; **63**:23–7.

Josephs KA, Duffy JR, Strand EA et al. Clinicopathological and imaging correlates of progressive aphasia and apraxia of speech. Brain 2006; 129:1385–98.

Joubert S, Felician O, Barbeau E et al. Impaired configurational processing in a case of progressive prosopagnosia associated with predominant right temporal lobe atrophy. Brain 2003; 126:2537–50.

Jung RE, Yeo RA, Sibbit WL et al. Gerstmann syndrome in systemic lupus erythematosus: neuropsychological, neuroimaging and spectroscopic findings. Neurocase 2001; 7:515–21.

Kanshepolsky J, Kelley JJ, Waggener JD. A cortical auditory disorder: clinical, audiologic and pathologic aspects. Neurology 1973; 23:699–705.

Karbe H, Kertesz A, Polk M. Profiles of language impairment in primary progressive aphasia. Arch Neurol 1993; 50:192–201.

Karnath HO, Hartje W. Decrease of contralateral neglect by neck muscle vibration and spatial orientation of trunk midline. Brain 1993; 116:383–96.

Kashiwa Y, Kitabayashi Y, Narumoto J et al. Anosognosia in Alzheimer's disease: association with patient characteristics, psychiatric symptoms and cognitive deficits. Psychiatry Clin Neurosci 2005; 59:697–704.

Kazui S, Sawasa T. Callosal apraxia without agraphia. Ann Neurol 1993; 33:401–3.

Keane S, Turner C, Sherrington C et al. Use of fresnel prism glasses to treat stroke patients with hemispatial neglect. Arch Phys Med Rehabil 2006; 87:1668–72.

Kertesz A, Hudson L, Mackenzie IRA et al. The pathology and nosology of primary progressive aphasia. Neurology 1994; 44:2065–72.

Kinsbourne M, Warrington EK. A variety of reading disability associated with right hemisphere lesions. J Neurol Neurosurg Psychiatry 1962; 25:339–44.

Kinsbourne M, Warrington EK. Observations on color agnosia. J Neurol Neurosurg Psychiatry 1964; 27:296–9.

Knibb J, Xuereb JH, Patterson K et al. Clinical and pathological characterization of progressive aphasia. Ann Neurol 2006; 59:156–65.

Knight RT, Cooper J. Status epilepticus manifesting as reversible Wernicke's aphasia. Epilepsia 1986; 27:301–4.

Kraepelin E. Dementia praecox and paraphrenia. Huntington, NY: Robert E. Krieger, 1971.

Kraepelin E. Manic-depressive insanity and paranoia. NY: Arno Press, 1976.

Kress T, Dau M. Developmental prosopagnoia: a review. Behav Neurol 2003; 14:109–21.

Krupp LB, Lipton RB, Swerdlow ML et al. Progressive multifocal leukoencephalopathy: clinical and radiologic features. Ann Neurol 1985; 17:344–9.

Kumar R, Masih AK, Pardo J. Globl aphasia due to thalamic hemorrhage: a case report and review of the literature. Arch Phys Med Rehabil 1996; 77:1312–15.

Kumral E, Kocaer T, Ertubey NO et al. Thalamic hemorrhage: a prospective study of 100 patients. Stroke 1995; 26:964–70.

Kumral E, Evyapan D, Balkir N. Acute caudate vascular lesions. Stroke 1999; 30:100–8.

Labar DR, Solomon GE, Wells CR. Aphasia as the sole manifestation of simple partial status epilepticus. Epilepsia 1992; 33:84–7.

LacourA, de Seze J, Revenco E et al. Acute aphasia in multiple sclerosis. Neurology 2004; 62:974–7.

Lampl Y, Eshel Y, Gilad R et al. Selective acalculia with sparing of the subtraction process in a patient with left parietotemporal hemorrhage. Neurology 1994; 44:1759–61.

Landis T, Cummings JL, Benson DF et al. Loss of topographic familiarity: an environmental agnosia. Arch Neurol 1986; 43:132–6.

Landis T, Regard M, Bliestle A et al. Prosopagnosia and agnosia for noncanonical views. Brain 1988; 111:1287–97.

Laplane D, Degos JD. Motor neglect. J Neurol Neurosurg Psychiatry 1983; 46:152–8.

Leibson E. Anosognosia and mania associated with right thalamic haemorrhage. J Neurol Neurosurg Psychiatry 2000; 68:107–8.

Le Gros Clark WE, Russell WR. Cortical deafness without aphasia. Brain 1938; 61:375–83.

Le Rhun E, Richard F, Pasquier F. Natural histoy of primary progressive aphasia. Neurology 2005; 65:887–91.

Luzzi S, Pucci E, Di Bella P et al. Topographical disorientation consequent to amnesia of spatial location in a patient with right parahippocampal damage. Cortex 2000; 36:427–34.

Maeshima S, Funahashi K, Ogura M et al. Unilateral spatial neglect due to right frontal lobe hematoma. J Neurol Neurosurg Psychiatry 1994; 57:89–93.

Maeshima S, Okumura Y, Nakai K et al. Gerstmann's syndrome associated with chronic subdural haematoma: a case report. Brain Inj 1998; 12:697–701.

Malone DR, Morris HH, Kay MC et al. Prosopagnosia: a double dissociation between the recognition of familiar and unfamiliar faces. J Neurol Neurosurg Psychiatry 1982; 45:820–2.

Mandell AM, Alexander MP, Carpenter S. Creutzfeldt–Jakob disease presenting as isolated aphasia. Neurology 1989; 39:55–8.

Mantovani JF, Landau WM. Acquired aphasia with convulsive disorder: course and prognosis. Neurology 1980; 30:524–9.

Mao-Draayer Y, Panitch H. Alexia without agraphia in multiple sclerosis: case report with magnetic resonance imaging localization. Mult Scler 2004; 10:705–7.

Masdeu JC, O'Hara RJ. Motor aphasia unaccompanied by faciobrachial weakness. Neurology 1983; 33:519–21.

Mayer E, Martory M-D, Pegna AJ et al. A pure case of Gerstmann's syndrome with a subangular lesion. Brain 1999; 122:1107–20.

Mazzoni M, Pardossi L, Cantini R et al. Gerstmann syndrome: a case report. Cortex 1990; 26:459–67.

McCarthy RA, Evans JJ, Hodges JR. Topographic amnesia: spatial memory disorder, perceptual dysfuncton, or category specific semantic memory impairment? J Neurol Neurosurg Psychiatry 1996; 60:318–25.

McFarling D, Rothi LJ, Heilman KM. Transcortical aphasia from ischemic infarcts of the thalamus: a report of two cases. J Neurol Neurosurg Psychiatry 1982; 45:107–12.

Meadows JC. Disturbed perception of colours associated with localized cerebral lesions. Brain 1974a; 97:615–32.

Meadows JC. The anatomical basis of prosopagnosia. *J Neurol Neurosurg Psychiatry* 1974b; **37**:489–501.

Megens J, van Loon J, Goffin J *et al.* Subcortical aphasia from a thalamic abscess. *J Neurol Neurosurg Psychiatry* 1992; **55**:319–22.

Mendez MF, Zander BA. Dementia presenting with aphasia: clinical characteristics. *J Neurol Neurosurg Psychiatry* 1991; **54**:542–5.

Mendez MF, Papasian NC, Lim GT. Thalamic acalculia. *J Neuropsychiatry Clin Neurosci* 2003; **15**:115–16.

Mesad S, Laff R, Devinsky O. Transient postoperative prosopagnosia. *Epilepsy Behav* 2003; **4**:567–70.

Mesulam M, Johnson N, Kreftt TA *et al.* Progranuin mutations in primary progressive aphasia. The PPA1 and PPA3 families. *Arch Neurol* 2007; **64**:43–7.

Meyer B, Kral T, Zentner J. Pure word deafness after resection of a tectal plate glioma with preservation of wave V of brain stem auditory evoked potentials. *J Neurol Neurosurg Psychiatry* 1996; **61**:423–4.

Mohr JP, Pessin MP, Finkelstein S *et al.* Broca aphasia: pathologic and clinical. *Neurology* 1978; **28**:311–24.

Monrad-Krohn GH. Dysprosody or altered 'melody of language'. *Brain* 1947a; **70**:405–15.

Monrad-Krohn GH. The prosodic quality of speech and its disorders. *Acta Psychiatr Neurol Scand* 1947b; **22**:255–69.

Moore MR, Saver JL, Johnson KA *et al.* Right parietal stroke with Gerstmann's syndrome. Appearance on computed tomograph, magnetic resonance imaging, and single-photon emission computed tomography. *Arch Neurol* 1991; **48**:432–5.

Mort DJ, Malhorta P, Mannan SK *et al.* The anatomy of visual neglect. *Brain* 2003; **126**:1986–97.

Motomura N, Yamadori A, Mori E *et al.* Unilateral spatial neglect due to hemorrhage in the thalamic region. *Acta Neurol Scand* 1986; **74**:190–4.

Mula M, Trimble MR, Thompson P *et al.* Topiramate and word-finding difficulties in patients with epilepsy. *Neurology* 2003; **60**:1104–7.

Nadeau SE, Reltgen DP, Sevush S *et al.* Apraxia due to a pathologically documented thalamic infarction. *Neurology* 1994; **44**:2133–7.

Naeser MA, Hayward RW. Lesion localization in aphasia with cranial computed tomography and the Boston diagnostic aphasia exam. *Neurology* 1978; **28**:545–51.

Naeser MA, Alexander MP, Helm-Estabrooks N *et al.* Aphasia with predominantly subcortical lesion sites: description of three capsular/putaminal aphasia syndromes. *Arch Neurol* 1982; **39**:2–14.

Ohno T, Bando M, Nagura H *et al.* Apraxic agraphia due to thalamic infarction. *Neurology* 2000; **54**:2336–9.

Okamura T, Fukai M, Yamadori A *et al.* A clinical study of hypergraphia in epilepsy. *J Neurol Neurosurg Psychiatry* 1993; **56**:556–9.

Olmos-Lau N, Ginsberg MD, Geller JB. Aphasia in multiple sclerosis. *Neurology* 1977; **27**:623–6.

Orton ST. 'Word blindness' in school children. *Arch Neurol Psychiatry* 1925; **14**:581–615.

Pan C-L, Kuo M-F, Hsieh S-T. Audiory agnosia caused by a tectal germinoma. *Neurology* 2004; **63**:2387–9.

Paquier PF, Van Dongen HR, Loonen CB. The Landau–Kleffner syndrome or 'acquired aphasia with convulsive disorder': long-term follow-up of six children and a review of the recent literature. *Arch Neurol* 1992; **49**:354–9.

Paul R, Cohen DJ, Caparulo BK. A longitudinal study of patients with severe developmental disorders of language learning. *J Am Acad Child Adolesc Psychiatry* 1983; **22**:525–34.

PeBenito R. Developmental Gerstmann syndrome: case report and review of the literature. *J Dev Behav Pediatr* 1987; **8**:229–32.

Pedersen PM, Jorgensen HS, Nakayama H *et al.* Aphasia in acute stroke: incidence, determinants, and recovery. *Ann Neurol* 1995; **38**:659–66.

Perez-Trullen JM, Modrego Pardo PJ. Comparative study of aprosody in Alzheimer's disease and in multi-infarct dementia. *Dementia* 1996; **7**:59–62.

Pevzner S, Bornstein B, Loewenthal M. Prosopagnosia. *J Neurol Neurosurg Psychiatry* 1962; **25**:336–8.

Piercy M, Hecaen H, de Ajuriaguerra J. Constructional apraxia with unilateral cerebral lesions – left and right sided cases compared. *Brain* 1960; **83**:225–42.

Pillon B, Bakchine S, Lhermitte F. Alexia without agraphia in a left-handed patient with a right occipital lesion. *Arch Neurol* 1987; **44**:1257–62.

Platz T. Tactile agnosia: causistic evidence and theoretical remarks on modality-specific meaning representations and sensorimotor integration. *Brain* 1996; **119**:1565–74.

Privitera MD, Morris GL, Gilliam F. Postictal language assessment and lateralization of complex partial seizures. *Ann Neurol* 1991; **30**:391–3.

Racy A, Jannotta FS, Lehner LH. Aphasia resulting from occlusion of the left anterior cerebral artery: report of a case with an old infarct in the left rolandic region. *Arch Neurol* 1979; **36**:221–4.

Redlich FC, Dorsey JF. Denial of blindness by patients with cerebral disease. *Arch Neurol Psychiatry* 1945; **53**:407–17.

Reed CL, Caselli RJ, Farah MJ. Tactile agnosia: underlying impairment and implications for normal tactile object recognition. *Brain* 1996; **119**:875–88.

Renner JA, Burns JM, Hou CE *et al.* Progressive posterior cortical dysfunction. A clinicopathologic series. *Neurology* 2004; **63**:1175–80.

Riley DE, Lang AE, Lewis A *et al.* Cortical-basal ganglionic degneration. *Neurology* 1990; **40**:1203–12.

Rizzo M, Hurtig R. Looking but not seeing: attention, perception, and eye movements in simultanagnosia. *Neurology* 1987; **37**:1642–8.

Rizzo M, Robin DA. Simultanagnosia: a defect of sustained attention yields insight on visual information processing. *Neurology* 1990; **40**:447–55.

Rinne JO, Lee MS, Thompson PD *et al.* Corticobasal degeneration: a clinical study of 36 cases. *Brain* 1994; **117**:1183–96.

Roeltgen DP, Helman KM. Lexical agraphia. Further support for the two-system hypothesis of linguistic agraphia. *Brain* 1984; **107**:811–27.

Roeltgen DP, Sevush S, Heilman KM. Pure Gerstmann's syndrome form a focal lesion. *Arch Neurol* 1983; **40**:46–67.

Rosati G, De Bastiani P. Pure agraphia: a discrete form of aphasia. *J Neurol Neurosurg Psychiatry* 1979; **42**:266–9.

Rosler A, Lanquillon S, Dippel O *et al.* Impairment of facial recognition in patients with right cerebral infarcts quantified by computer aided 'morphing'. *J Neurol Neurosurg Psychiatry* 1997; **62**:261–4.

Ross ED. Left medial parietal lobe and receptive language functions: mixed transcortical aphasia after left anterior cerebral artery infarction. *Neurology* 1980; **30**:144–51.

Ross ED. The aprosodias: functional–anatomic organization of the affective components of language in the right hemisphere. *Arch Neurol* 1981; **38**:561–9.

Ross ED, Mesulam M-M. Dominant language functions of the right hemisphere: prosody and emotional gesturing. *Arch Neurol* 1979; **36**:144–8.

Ross ED, Harney JH, deLacoste-Utamsing C *et al.* How the brain interprets affective and propositional language into a unified behavioral function: hypothesis based on clinicoanatomic evidence. *Arch Neurol* 1981; **38**:745–8.

Ross ED, Anderson B, Morgan-Fisher A. Crossed aprosodia in strongly dextral patients. *Arch Neurol* 1989; **46**:206–9.

Ross SJM, Graham N, Stuart-Green L *et al.* Progressive biparietal atrophy: an atypical presentation of Alzheimer's disease. *J Neurol Neurosurg Psychiatry* 1996; **61**:388–95.

Roth N. Disorders of body image caused by lesions of the right parietal lobe. *Brain* 1949; **72**:89–111.

Rubens AB. Aphasia with infarction in the territory of the anterior cerebral artery. *Cortex* 1975; **11**:239–50.

Rumsey JM, Donohue BC, Brady DR *et al.* A magnetic resonance imaging study of planum temporale asymmetry in men with developmental dyslexia. *Arch Neurol* 1997; **54**:1481–4.

Sabe L, Salvarezza F, Garcia Cuerva A *et al.* A randomized, double-blind, placebo-controlled study of bromocriptine in nonfluent aphasia. *Neurology* 1995; **45**:2272–4.

Sandifer PH. Anosognosia and disorders of body scheme. *Brain* 1946; **68**:122–37.

Sato S, Dreifuss FE. Electroencephalographic findings in a patient with developmental expressive aphasia. *Neurology* 1973; **23**:181–5.

Sbordone RJ, Seranian GD, Ruff RM. Are the subjective complaints of traumatically brain injured patients reliable? *Brain Inj* 1998; **12**:505–15.

Schatzberg AF, Cole JO, Blumer DP. Speech blockage: a tricyclic side effect. *Am J Psychiatry* 1978; **135**:600–1.

Schindler I, Kerkhoff G, Karnath H-O *et al.* Neck vibration induces lasting recovery in spatial neglect. *J Neurol Neurosurg Psychiatry* 2002;**73**:412–19.

Selnes OA, Knopman DS, Miccum N *et al.* The central role of Wernicke's area in sentence repetition. *Ann Neurol* 1985; **17**:549–57.

Sergent J, Poncet M. From covert to overt recognition of faces in prosopagnosia. *Brain* 1990; **113**:989.

Sergent J, Villemure JG. Prosopagnosia in a right hemispherectomized patient. *Brain* 1989; **112**:975–95.

Shelton PA, Bowers D, Duara D *et al.* Apperceptive visual agnosia: a case study. *Brain Cogn* 1994; **25**:1–23.

Silverberg R, Gordon HW. Differential aphasia in two bilingual individuals. *Neurology* 1979; **29**:51–5.

Singer S, Cummings JL, Benson DF. Delusions and mood disorders in patients with chronic aphasia. *J Neuropsychiatry Clin Neurosci* 1989; **1**:40–5.

Smith A. The serial sevens subtraction test. *Arch Neurol* 1962; **17**:78–80.

Snowden JS, Craufurd D, Griffiths HL *et al.* Awareness of involuntary movements in Huntington disease. *Arch Neurol* 1998; **55**:801–5.

So EL, Schauble BS. Ictal asomatognosia as a cause of epileptic falls. Simultaneous video EMG, and invasive EEG. *Neurology* 2004; **63**:2153–4.

Speedie LJ, Wertman E, Ta'ir J *et al.* Disruption of automatic speech following a right basal ganglia lesion. *Neurology* 1993; **43**:1768–74.

Starkstein SE, Chemerinski E, Sabe L *et al.* Prospective longitudinal study of depression and anosognosia in Alzheimer's disease. *Br J Psychiatry* 1997; **171**:47–52.

Stein S, Volpe BT. Classical 'parietal' neglect syndrome after subcortical right frontal lobe infarction. *Neurology* 1983; **33**:797–9.

Stommel EW, Friedman RJ, Reeves AG. Alexia without agraphia associated with spleniogeniculate infarction. *Neurology* 1991; **41**:587–8.

Stone SP, Wilson B, Wroot A *et al.* The assessment of visuo-spatial neglect after acute stroke. *J Neurol Neurosurg Psychiatry* 1991; **54**:345–50.

Stracciari A, Lorusso S, Pazzaglia P. Transient topographical amnesia. *J Neurol Neurosurg Psychiatry* 1994; **57**:1423–5.

Suresh PA, Sebastian S. Developmental Gerstmann's syndrome: a distinct clinical entity of learning disabilities. *Pediatr Neurol* 2000; **22**:267–78.

Sweet EWS, Panis W, Levine DN. Crossed Wernicke's aphasia. *Neurology* 1984; **34**:475–9.

Symonds C, MacKenzie I. Bilateral loss of vision from cerebral infarction. *Brain* 1957; **80**:415–55.

Takahashi N, Kawamura M, Shiota J *et al.* Pure topographic disorientation due to right retrosplenial lesion. *Neurology* 1997; **49**:464–9.

Takayama Y, Sugishita M, Akiguchi I *et al.* Isolated acalculia due to left parietal lesion. *Arch Neurol* 1994; **51**:286–91.

Tanabe H, Sawada T, Inoue N *et al.* Conduction aphasia and arcuate fasciculus. *Acta Neurol Scand* 1987; **76**:422–7.

Tang-Wei DF, Graff-Radford NR, Boeve BF *et al.* Clinical, genetic, and neuropathlogic characteristics of posterior cortical atrophy. *Neurology* 2004; **63**:1168–74.

Taniwaki T, Tagawa K, Sato F *et al.* Auditory agnosia restricted to environmental sounds following cortical deafness and generalized auditory agnosia. *Clin Neurol Neurosurg* 2000; **102**:156–62.

Tegner R, Levander M. The influence of stimulus properties on visual neglect. *J Neurol Neurosurg Psychiatry* 1991; **54**:882–7.

Toghi H, Saitoh K, Takahashi S *et al*. Agraphia and acalculalia after a left prefrontal (F1, F2) infarction. *J Neurol Neurosurg Psychiatry* 1995; **58**:629–32.

Tonkonogy J, Goodglass H. Language function, foot of the third frontal gyrus, and rolandic operculum. *Arch Neurol* 1981; **38**:486–90.

Tranel D, Biller J, Damasio H *et al*. Global aphasia without hemiparesis. *Arch Neurol* 1987; **44**:304–8.

Tranel D, Damasio AR, Damasio H. Intact recognition of facial expression, gender, and age in patients with impaired recognition of face identity. *Neurology* 1988; **38**:690–6.

Triggs WJ, Gold M, Gerstle G *et al*. Motor neglect associated with a discrete parietal lesion. *Neurology* 1994; **44**:1164–6.

Trojanowski JQ, Green RC, Levine DN. Crossed aphasia in a dextral: a clinicopathological study. *Neurology* 1980; **30**:709–13.

Tucha O, Steup A, Smely C *et al*. Toe agnosia in Gerstmann syndrome. *J Neurol Neurosurg Psychiatry* 1997; **63**:399–403.

Turner RS, Kenyon LC, Trojanowski JQ *et al*. Clinical, neuroimaging, and pathologic features of progressive nonfluent aphasia. *Ann Neurol* 1996; **39**:166–73.

Turgman J, Goldhammer Y, Braham J. Alexia, without agraphia, due to brain tumor: a reversible syndrome. *Ann Neurol* 1979; **6**:265–8.

Tuszynski MH, Petito CK. Ischemic thalamic aphasia with pathologic confirmation. *Neurology* 1988; **38**:800–2.

Vallar G, Perani D. The anatomy of unilateral neglect after right-hemisphere stroke lesions. A clinical/CT-scan correlation study in man. *Neuropsychologia* 1986; **24**:609–22.

Vallar G, Rusconi ML, Bignamini L *et al*. Anatomical correlates of visual and tactile extinction in humans: a clinical CT scan study. *J Neurol Neurosurg Psychiatry* 1994; **57**:464–70.

Van Horn G, Hawes A. Global aphasia without hemiparesis: a sign of embolic encephalopathy. *Neurology* 1982; **32**:403.

van Pugt P, Kees L, Cras P. Increased writing activity in neurological conditions: a review and clincial study. *J Neurol Neurosurg Psychiatry* 1996; **61**:510–14.

Vignolo LA. Auditory agnosia. *Phil Trans R Soc Lond Biol Sci* 1982; **298**:49–57.

Vincent FM, Sadowsky CH, Saunders RL *et al*. Alexia without agraphia, hemianopia or color-naming defect: a disconnection syndrome. *Neurology* 1977; **27**:689–91.

Wada Y, Yamamoto T. Selective impairment of facial recognition due to a haematoma restricted to the right fusiform and lateral occipital region. *J Neurol Neurosurg Psychiatry* 2001; **71**:254–7.

Walker-Batson D, Curtis S, Natarajan R *et al*. A double-blind, placebo-controlled study of the use of amphetamine in the treatment of aphasia. *Stroke* 2001; **32**:2093–8.

Warren JD, Thompson PD. Diencephalic amnesia and apraxia after left thalamic infection. *J Neurol Neurosurg Psychiatry* 2000; **68**:248.

Warrington EK, Langdon D. Spelling dyslexia: a deficit in the visual word-form. *J Neurol Neurosurg Psychiatry* 1994; **57**:211–16.

Watson RT, Heilman KM. Callosal apraxia. *Brain* 1983; **106**:391–403.

Watson RT, Valenstein E, Heilman KM. Thalamic neglect. Possible role of the medial thalamus and nucleus reticularis in behavior. *Arch Neurol* 1981; **38**:501–6.

Waxman SG, Geschwind N. Hypergraphia in temporal lobe epilepsy. *Neurology* 1974; **24**:629–36.

Waxman SG, Geschwind N. The interictal behavior syndrome of temporal lobe epilepsy. *Arch Gen Psychiatry* 1975; **32**: 1580–6.

Wechsler AF, Verity A, Rosenschein S *et al*. Pick's disease: a clinical, computed tomographic, and histologic study with Golgi impregnation observations. *Arch Neurol* 1982; **39**:287–90.

Weinstein EA, Cole M, Mitchell MS *et al*. Anosognosia and aphasia. *Arch Neurol* 1969; **10**:376–86.

Williamson PD, Spencer DD, Spencer SS *et al*. Episodic aphasia and epileptic focus in the nondominant hemisphere: relieved by section of the corpus callosum. *Neurology* 1985; **35**:1069–71.

Wolfe GI, Ross ED. Sensory aprosodia with left hemiparesis from subcortical infarction: right hemisphere analogue of sensory-type aphasia with right hemiparesis? *Arch Neurol* 1987; **44**:668–71.

Wolpert I. Die simultanagnosie-storung der gasamtauffassung. *Z Ges Neurol Psychiatr* 1924; **93**:397–415.

Yamadori A, Osumi Y, Masuhara S *et al*. Preservation of singing in Broca's aphasia. *J Neurol Neurosurg Psychiatry* 1977; **40**:221–4.

Yamadori A, Osumi Y, Ikeda H *et al*. Left unilateral agraphia and tactile anomia: disturbances seen after occlusion of the anterior cerebral artery. *Arch Neurol* 1980; **37**: 88–91.

Abnormal movements

3

3.1 TREMOR

Tremor is a more or less rhythmic oscillatory movement, most commonly seen in the upper extremities, which occurs secondary to the rapidly alternating contraction of agonist then antagonist muscles.

Clinical features

From a clinical point of view, it is most useful to distinguish three different types of tremor, namely postural, rest, and intention; other types (e.g., Holmes' tremor) also occur and are discussed later in this chapter, but are far less common.

Postural tremor is most apparent when the patient maintains a posture, as for example by extending the arms straight forward, with the fingers outstretched and slightly spread apart. This tremor typically occurs at a frequency of from 6 to 10 Hz, and ranges in amplitude from a fine tremor (which may be almost unnoticeable to casual inspection) to a coarse tremor (which may effectively preclude even the simplest of activities, such as bringing a cup of water to the lips). Some authors also refer to this tremor as an 'action' tremor, in that it occurs when the patient takes an 'action', for example by extending the arms. Not all authors are in agreement with this term, however, and it is not used further here.

Rest tremor, as the name indicates, is seen when the involved extremity is at rest as, for example, when, with the patient seated, the hands are resting in the lap. This tremor occurs at a frequency of from 3 to 5 Hz and is typically 'pill-rolling' in character, in that the oscillatory activity of the thumb, sweeping back and forth in proximity to the ventral surface of the fingers, resembles the movements one would make if one were rolling a pill back and forth in one's hand.

Intention tremor comes to light during finger-to-nose testing. To perform this, ask the patient to extend the upper extremity, with the index finger extended out, and then to bring the index finger in to touch the nose. Normally, the movement is smooth throughout; when intention tremor is present, however, an oscillatory movement develops as the index finger closes in on the target. Some authors refer to this as a 'kinetic' tremor, indicating that it appears with movement; however, this term has not gained currency and the term 'intention' is used in this text.

Other tremors, far less common, include 'task-specific' tremors, orthostatic tremor, 'rabbit' tremor, Holmes' tremor, and 'wing-beating' tremor.

'Task-specific' tremors resemble postural tremors; however, they only appear when the patient is engaged in a specific activity, such as writing, throwing darts, etc.

Orthostatic tremor (Heilman 1984), as the name suggests, occurs when patients stand up. This is a rapid tremor of the lower extremities, which patients often describe as a sense of quivering, which may cause a sense of unsteadiness or even cause patients to fall. As this tremor may be invisible, it is necessary to palpate the inner aspects of the patient's thighs immediately after the patient stands up to assess its presence.

'Rabbit' tremor is a rest tremor confined to the jaw and presents an appearance similar to that of a rabbit chewing.

Holmes' tremor, named after Gordon Holmes who first described it in 1904, is a slow frequency tremor (at a rate of from 2 to 4 Hz) of the upper, and occasionally lower, extremity, with rest, intentional, and postural components. The appearance of this tremor with sustained posture may be quite remarkable, with a rolling, sinuous motion of the upper arm and a 'flapping' motion of the hand. In the past this tremor has been referred to as a 'rubal' or 'midbrain' tremor, however these terms are discouraged, given that, as discussed below, this tremor may occur in the absence of involvement of the nucleus ruber or of any part of the midbrain.

'Wing-beating' tremor involves the upper extremities, which are flexed at the elbows: the tremor itself is primarily proximal and results in an oscillation of the upper extremities that appears similar to the motions a bird makes as it flaps its wings.

Etiology

The various etiologies of each of the types of tremor discussed above are summarized in Table 3.1, and discussed below.

POSTURAL TREMOR

One of the most common causes of isolated postural tremor is drug toxicity, and of the various responsible mediations listed in Table 3.1 the tricyclic antidepressants

(Kronfol *et al.* 1983), lithium (Gelenberg and Jefferson 1995; Vestergaard *et al.* 1988), and valproic acid (Hyman *et al.* 1979) are especially important.

Alcohol withdrawal is so commonly associated with tremor that this condition is commonly referred to as 'the shakes'. This is probably one of the most commonly missed diagnoses, primarily either because the patient denies excessive use of alcohol or because the physician simply does not inquire. The same 'missed diagnosis' may occur with tremor due to benzodiazepine or other sedative-hypnotic withdrawal.

Metabolic and endocrinologic conditions are also common causes. Hypoglycemia should be suspected when tremor occurs in diabetics or post-prandially. Hyperthyroidism should be suspected when the tremor is accompanied by diaphoresis, heat intolerance, proptosis, etc. Pheochromocytoma-induced tremor is rare, and is suggested by associated paroxysms of hypertension.

Delirium may be accompanied by tremor, and in such cases the tremor is often coarse and quite prominent (Jankovic and Fahn 1980). Delirium tremens (Latin for 'trembling delirium') is, of course, the first consideration.

Table 3.1 Causes of tremor

Postural tremor
Medication-induced
Caffeine
Sympathomimetics (e.g., pseudoephedrine)
Amphetamine
Theophylline
Antidepressants (tricyclics, SSRIs, venlafaxine)
Lithium
Valproic acid
Antipsychotics
Amiodarone

Alcohol and sedative hypnotic withdrawal (Sections 21.5 and 21.6)

Metabolic and endocrinologic
Hypoglycemia
Hyperthyroidism (Section 16.3)
Pheochromocytoma

Associated with delirium
Delirium tremens (Section 21.5)
Neuroleptic malignant syndrome (Section 22.1)
Serotonin syndrome (Section 22.5)
Other encephalopathies (uremic [Section 13.18], hepatic [Section 13.19], etc.)

Associated with anxiety or depression
Generalized anxiety disorder (Section 20.16)
Depression (Section 20.6)
Anxiety attacks (Section 6.5)

Other causes
Essential tremor (Section 8.32)
Multiple sclerosis (Section 17.1)

Peripheral neuropathies
Mercury intoxication (Section 13.12)
Tertiary neurosyphilis (Section 14.15)

Rest tremor
Parkinsonian conditions (e.g., Parkinson's disease, diffuse Lewy body disease [Section 3.8])
Antipsychotic medications

Intention tremor
Disease of the cerebellar cortex, dentate nucleus or outflow tracts

Toxicity
Alcohol intoxication
Sedative hypnotic intoxication
Lithium intoxication

Other types of tremor
Task-specific tremors
Primary writing tremor

Orthostatic tremor
Idiopathic orthostatic tremor
Secondary orthostatic tremor (e.g., head trauma, hydrocephalus, pontine lesions)

Rabbit tremor
Rabbit syndrome (Section 22.4)

Holmes' tremor
Lesions of the dentate nucleus or its outflow tracts, the thalamus or the pons

Wing-beating tremor
Wilson's disease (Section 8.16)

SSRI, selective serotonin reuptake inhibitor.

The serotonin syndrome should be suspected whenever a delirium with tremor follows initiation of treatment with a combination or serotoninergic agents, and the neuroleptic malignant syndrome whenever the syndrome is preceded by initiating treatment with an antipsychotic or by decreasing or discontinuing a dopaminergic agent. Other 'metabolic encephalopathies' may also be accompanied by tremor, including hepatic and uremic encephalopathy.

Anxiety or 'agitated' depression may be characterized by persistent tremor, and anxiety attacks may also be accompanied by tremor, as may be seen in panic disorder.

Of the other causes of postural tremor, among the late- to middle-aged and elderly, essential tremor is perhaps the most common. Multiple sclerosis, in addition to the more commonly associated intention tremor, may also cause postural tremor. Certain peripheral neuropathies, such as chronic inflammatory demyelinating peripheral neuropathy (CIDP) and Charcot–Marie–Tooth disease, may also cause postural tremor but this is rare. Other rare causes include mercury intoxication and tertiary neurosyphilis (general paresis of the insane [GPI]).

REST TREMOR

Rest tremor is a cardinal sign of parkinsonism, and of the multiple causes of parkinsonism discussed in Section 3.8 (under Parkinsonism), Parkinson's disease, diffuse Lewy body disease and multiple system atrophy, along with treatment with first-generation antipsychotics, stand out as the most common.

INTENTION TREMOR

Intention tremor is most commonly due to disease of the cerebellar cortex, the dentate nucleus or the outflow tracts of the dentate nucleus. Consideration should be given to degenerative conditions (e.g., alcoholic cerebellar degeneration of one of the spinocerebellar ataxias [Section 8.17]), multiple sclerosis (Section 17.1), and, especially in young adults, Wilson's disease (Section 8.16). Severe intoxication with alcohol or sedative hypnotics (e.g., benzodiazepines) is also typified by intention tremor, and this may also constitute one of the disabling sequelae of lithium intoxication.

OTHER TYPES

Task-specific tremors are inherited conditions and appear to be associated with the more common task-specific dystonias, such as 'writer's cramp' (Bain *et al.* 1995; Klawans *et al.* 1982a; Soland *et al.* 1996a).

Orthostatic tremor, as noted, may occur on either an idiopathic basis or secondary to other causes, such as head trauma, hydrocephalus or, rarely, lesions of the pons (Benito-Leon *et al.* 1997).

The rabbit syndrome (discussed further in Section 22.4) occurs as a side-effect of antipsychotics.

Holmes' tremor, as pointed out by Holmes himself (1904), localizes the lesion to the dentate nucleus or its

outflow tracts, and has been specifically reported with lesions of the dentate nucleus (Krauss *et al.* 1995), superior cerebellar peduncle (Krack *et al.* 1994; Krauss *et al.* 1995), dorsal midbrain tegmentum (Krauss *et al.* 1995), the red nucleus and adjacent structures (Holmes 1904; Remy *et al.* 1995), the posterior thalamus (Krauss *et al.* 1992; Miwa *et al.* 1996; Tan *et al.* 2001), and the pontine tegmentum (Miyagi *et al.* 1999; Shepherd *et al.* 1997).

Wing-beating tremor, although classic for Wilson's disease, is among the presenting signs of this disease in only a small minority of cases (Starosta-Rubinstein *et al.* 1987); this tremor, rarely, has also been reported with thalamic infarction (Ghika *et al.* 1994).

Differential diagnosis

A postural tremor often occurs in normal individuals and in these cases is referred to as a 'physiologic tremor'. Normally, this physiologic tremor is so fine that it is invisible to the naked eye. However, with fatigue, or during systemic illnesses, it may become apparent.

Myoclonus is distinguished from postural tremor in that rather than being characterized by an oscillatory motion it consists of a 'jerk' followed by a relaxation phase. In tremor there is alternating contraction of agonist and antagonist musculature, whereas in myoclonus there is only contraction of one group. Rhythmicity may also help distinguish these two: tremor is always more or less rhythmic whereas myoclonus, although at times rhythmic, is most often intermittent.

Asterixis may appear when the arms are outstretched, especially if the hands are somewhat dorsiflexed during this maneuver, and thus may be confused with postural tremor. The differential rests, as with myoclonus, on the absence of oscillation. In asterixis, there is a sudden relaxation, such that the hands 'drop'; this is then followed by a slower, voluntary resumption of the dorsiflexed position.

Clonic movements, as may occur during a simple partial motor seizure, may simulate postural tremor; however, here, again, there is no oscillation, but rather a rhythmic contraction of one muscle group followed by a relaxation. Furthermore, and in contrast with postural tremor that is almost always bilateral, simple partial motor seizures are almost always unilateral.

'Dystonic tremor' refers to a jerking motion of a dystonic limb. Although the term has currency, this is not a true tremor but more of an intermittent jerk that typically disappears when the patient relaxes and gives way to the developing dystonic spasm.

Simulated tremor, as may occur in conversion disorder, malingering or factitious illness, is suggested when the tremor changes markedly in frequency or amplitude, and especially when this occurs with distraction. Weighting the involved limbs may also be diagnostically useful: in simulated tremor, rather than a reduction of amplitude, one often sees an increase (Deuschl *et al.* 1998).

Treatment

In the case of medication-associated tremor, dose reduction is often sufficient; when this is not practical, for example in lithium treatment, consideration may be given to symptomatic treatment with propranolol (Lapierre 1976). Treatment is otherwise directed at the underlying cause, and most of these are discussed in the respective chapters. For primary writing tremor, consideration may be given to propranolol or primidone (Bain *et al.* 1995), botulinum injections (Singer *et al.* 2005), or the use of a writing device (Espay *et al.* 2005a). Orthostatic tremor may respond to clonazepam or gabapentin (Onofrj *et al.* 1998; Rodrigues *et al.* 2006), and Holmes' tremor may respond to carbidopa/levodopa (Remy *et al.* 1995; Samie *et al.* 1990; Tan *et al.* 2001; Velez *et al.* 2002), clonazepam (Jacob and Pratap Chand 1998), trihexyphenidyl (Krack *et al.* 1994), or levetiracetam (Striano *et al.* 2007).

3.2 MYOCLONUS

Myoclonus is an important diagnostic sign, and, in addition to close observation during the interview and examination, patients should be questioned as to whether or not they have had any jerking motions. In patients with delirium the presence of myoclonus immediately suggests the serotonin syndrome or Hashimoto's encephalopathy; in patients with dementia its presence immediately raises the possibility of Creutzfeldt–Jakob disease.

Clinical description

Myoclonus consists of sudden rapid muscular jerks, followed by a slower relaxation phase. These myoclonic jerks may be focal, multifocal, or generalized, and they vary in amplitude from being almost imperceptible to a gross movement that can, in severe cases, throw an arm up or knock a patient off balance. Although occasionally rhythmic myoclonus may be seen, myoclonic jerks, in most cases, occur at irregular intervals with a frequency varying from only several per day up to multiple occurrences every minute. Although in most cases myoclonus occurs spontaneously, at times one may see stimulus-sensitive myoclonus to either a sudden touch or a loud noise; furthermore, in some cases myoclonus only occurs with 'action', as for example when the patient extends the arms.

Etiology

In attempting to determine the cause of myoclonus, it is useful to consider first whether the patient has a delirium or a dementia, or has epilepsy. If the cause is still unclear then one should consider the possibility of medication toxicity and, if the diagnosis remains obscure, a number of other miscellaneous causes may be considered. Each of these diagnostic possibilities is listed in Table 3.2 and discussed further below.

In patients with delirium, the presence of myoclonus strongly suggests the serotonin syndrome and a diligent search should be made for recent use of a combination of serotoninergic drugs. Hashimoto's encephalopathy should also be considered, especially in cases with ataxia or seizures, and anti-thyroid antibodies should be tested for. Metabolic deliria associated with myoclonus include uremic encephalopathy and hyperosmolar non-ketotic hyperglycemia, and these will be revealed on a chemistry profile. Encephalopathic pellagra should be considered in alcoholics with delirium, especially when there is also an associated, albeit mild, parkinsonism. Baclofen withdrawal delirium, as may occur when chronic, high-dose baclofen is abruptly discontinued, or when a baclofen pump malfunctions, is characterized, in addition to delirium, by myoclonus and fever, and in many respects, including treatment response, resembles the serotonin syndrome. Myoclonus may play a minor role in the overall clinical picture of an arbovirus encephalitis or an episode of complex partial status epilepticus. Bismuth intoxication is rare but myoclonus plays a prominent role in its symptomatology. Other intoxications that may be characterized by myoclonus include those with leaded gasoline, bromide, or mercury.

In patients with dementia, myoclonus immediately suggests Creutzfeldt–Jakob disease; consideration should also be given to post-anoxic encephalopathy. Subacute sclerosing panencephalitis, in either children or adults, is rare but is classically associated with myoclonus. A large number of other disorders capable of causing dementia may also be associated with myoclonus (see Table 3.2); however, in these the myoclonus plays only a very minor role in the overall clinical picture.

Certain epilepsies are characterized by myoclonus, and in patients with grand mal or petit mal seizures the presence of myoclonus should suggest the diagnosis of juvenile myoclonic epilepsy or one of the progressive myoclonic epilepsies, such as Unverricht–Lundborg disease, myoclonic epilepsy with ragged red fibers, or Lafora body disease. In adults, the very rare Kufs' disease should also be considered.

Medications that are capable of causing myoclonus are listed in Table 3.2 and of these the anti-epileptic drugs gabapentin and lamotrigine stand out, as do the opioids meperidine and hydromorphone. With regard to the opioids, in some cases myoclonus may appear early on in treatment; however, in others it is only after prolonged treatment that the myoclonus appears; in these cases it is suspected that the myoclonus is occurring due to the accumulation of toxic metabolites and not secondary to the parent compound (Mercadante 1998). This same late evolution has also been noted with fluoxetine, with which years of treatment may pass before myoclonus appears. Although little need be said regarding the other medications, some words are in order regarding tardive myoclonus. Tardive myoclonus is a rare variant of tardive dyskinesia and, like all the tardive

Table 3.2 Causes of myoclonus

Associated with delirium
Serotonin syndrome (Feighner et al. 1990; Sternbach 1991)
Hashimoto's encephalopathy (Castillo et al. 2006; Ghika-Schmid et al. 1996)
Uremic encephalopathy (Mahoney and Arieff 1982)
Hyperosmolar non-ketotic hyperglycemia (Morres and Dire 1989)
Encephalopathic pellagra (Serdaru et al. 1988)
Baclofen withdrawal (Meythaler et al. 2003)
Arbovirus encephalitis (Kleinschmidt-DeMasters et al. 2004)
Encephalitis lethargica (Blunt et al. 1997; Walsh 1920)
Complex partial status epilepticus (Kaplan 1996)
Bismuth intoxication (Supino-Viterbo et al. 1977)
Leaded gasoline intoxication (Goldings and Stewart 1982)
Bromide intoxication (Obeso et al. 1986)
Mercury intoxication (Roullet et al. 1994)

Associated with dementing disorders
Creutzfeldt–Jakob disease (Brown et al. 1986)
Post-anoxic encephalopathy (Werharhan et al. 1997)
Subacute sclerosing panencephalitis (both child [Dawson 1934] and adult [Prashanth et al. 2006] onset)
Diffuse Lewy body disease (Louis et al. 1997)
Corticobasal ganglionic degeneration (Rinne et al. 1994)
Multiple system atrophy (both striatonigral [Wenning et al. 1995] and olivopontocerebellar variants [Rodriguez et al. 1994])
Progressive supranuclear palsy (Collins et al. 1995)
Huntington's disease (both adult [Salt et al. 2006] and juvenile [Siesling et al. 1997] onset)
Alzheimer's disease (Benesch et al. 1993; Chen et al. 1991)
Dentatorubropallidoluysian atrophy (Becher et al. 1997)
Acquired immune deficiency syndrome (AIDS) dementia (Maher et al. 1997; Navin et al. 1986)
Dialysis dementia (Chokroverty et al. 1976; Garrett et al. 1988; Lederman and Henry 1978)

Epilepsies
Juvenile myoclonic epilepsy (Jain et al. 1998; Panayiotopoulos et al. 1994; Pedersen and Petersen 1998)

Unverricht–Lundborg disease (Koskiniemi et al. 1974; Magaudda et al. 2006)
Myoclonic epilepsy with ragged red fibers (Berkovic et al. 1989)
Lafora body disease (Yokoi et al. 1968)
Kufs' disease (Berkovic et al. 1988; Nijssen et al. 2002)

Medications
Gabapentin (Zhang et al. 2005)
Lamotrigine (Crespel et al. 2005)
Meperidine (Kaiko et al. 1983)
Hydromorphone (Hofmann et al. 2006)
SSRIs (Barucha and Sethi 1996)
Tricyclic antidepressants (Casas et al. 1987; DeCastro 1985; Garvey and Tollefson 1987; Lippmann et al. 1977)
Trazodone (Garvey and Tollefson 1987; Patel et al. 1988)
Lithium (Caviness and Evidente 2003)
Buspirone (Ritchie et al. 1988)
Clozapine (Bak et al. 1995; Barak et al. 1996)
Levodopa (Klawans et al. 1975)
Amantadine (Matsunaga et al. 2001)
Trimethoprim/sulfamethoxazole (Dib et al. 2004)
Tardive myoclonus (Abad and Ovsiew 1993; Little and Jankovic 1987; Wojick et al. 1991)

Miscellaneous causes
Lance–Adams syndrome of post-anoxic action myoclonus (Lance and Adams 1963)
Infarction of the frontoparietal cortex (Sutton and Meyere 1974) or thalamus (Kim 2001; Lehericy et al. 2001)
Spinal cord lesions (De La Sayette et al. 1996; Hoehn and Cherrington 1977; Keswani et al. 2002)
Paraneoplastic myoclonus (Bataller et al. 2001)
Whipple's disease (Louis et al. 1996)
Celiac disease (Tison et al. 1989)
Myoclonus dystonia ('essential myoclonus' [Mahloudji and Pikielny 1967])

SSRI selective serotonin reuptake inhibitor.

dyskinesia subtypes, occurs only after long exposure to antipsychotics; although tardive myoclonus may appear in isolation, it is often accompanied by tardive dystonia.

Regarding the miscellaneous causes of myoclonus, several comments are in order. As noted earlier, myoclonus is characteristic of post-anoxic dementia; however, an episode of anoxia may be followed by myoclonus alone and in such cases the term 'Lance–Adams syndrome' is used, in honor of Lance and Adams who first described it in 1963. Lesions, for example infarction of the frontoparietal cortex or the thalamus, may cause myoclonus and months or longer may elapse between the infarct and the appearance of the abnormal movement. Lesions of the spinal cord, such as infarction, myelitis or trauma, may cause myoclonus, which may be either focal, reflecting the segment involved, or generalized: this generalized form, often referred to as propriospinal

myoclonus, typically affects the trunk and extremities. Paraneoplastic myoclonus reflects autoimmune involvement of the brainstem and is often accompanied by opsoclonus (Digre 1986). Rare causes of myoclonus include Whipple's disease and celiac disease. Finally, myoclonus may also occur on an inherited basis, namely as the syndrome of myoclonus–dystonia (Asmus et al. 2002; Doheny et al. 2002; Foncke et al. 2006; Grimes et al. 2002; Schule et al. 2004). This syndrome, also known as 'essential myoclonus', is inherited on an autosomal dominant basis with incomplete penetrance. Onset is in childhood or adolescence, and, in addition to myoclonus there may also be cervical or task-specific dystonia (e.g., writer's cramp). Of interest, there appears to be an association between myoclonus–dystonia and obsessive–compulsive disorder and alcoholism (Hess et al. 2007; Saunders-Pullman et al. 2002).

Differential diagnosis

Asterixis is distinguished from myoclonus in that, rather than consisting of a jerking motion, it is characterized by a sudden drop, or abrupt relaxation; furthermore, rather than occurring spontaneously, it appears only when the outstretched hands are held in dorsiflexion. Some authors consider asterixis to be a kind of myoclonus, namely 'negative' myoclonus, in that it consists of a sudden loss of muscle tonus rather than an active contraction. Given, however, that the etiologies of asterixis and myoclonus are not identical, it may be prudent, from a clinical point of view, to keep the two separate.

Tremor is distinguished from myoclonus by its continuous nature. In tremor, there is an ongoing and alternating contraction of agonist and antagonist muscles, producing a persistent, oscillatory motion. By contrast, in myoclonus there is a distinct relaxation phase following each jerk: following the contraction of the agonist musculature, rather than an immediately following contraction of the antagonist muscle, there is merely a relaxation of the agonist musculature.

Tics are characterized by premonitory urges and by their temporary suppressibility by voluntary effort, features which are not seen in myoclonus. Furthermore, although some tics are quite simple in nature, and thus may appear similar to myoclonic jerks, they may also be complex, resembling fragments of voluntary activity, a feature that, again, is not seen in myoclonus.

Choreic movements may be difficult to distinguish from myoclonic jerks. One helpful feature is the tendency of chorea to appear and disappear on different parts of the body with lightning-like fluidity; myoclonus is rarely so mercurial. Furthermore, in some cases choreic movements may be complex and, like some tics, may resemble voluntary behaviors, thus distinguishing themselves from myoclonic jerks, which are always simple in nature.

Hypnic jerks, also known as 'sleep starts', are myoclonic jerks that occur during the transition from wakefulness to stage I sleep; they are considered a normal variant.

There is also a condition known as palatal myoclonus (Lapresle 1986); however, the name itself may be a misnomer. In this condition there is a very rapid and rhythmic movement of the palate, which may be appreciated by the patient as a kind of clicking. The movement itself is more of a tremor than anything else and hence the name of this condition might better be 'palatal tremor'.

Treatment

Treatment is aimed, whenever possible, at the underlying cause, and this is discussed in the respective chapters. If symptomatic treatment is required, consideration may be given to clonazepam, levetiracetam, or valproic acid (Van Zandijcke 2003).

3.3 MOTOR TICS

Motor tics, although classically associated with Tourette's syndrome, may also occur as a side-effect to various medications or in various other disorders (e.g., Sydenham's chorea).

Clinical features

Motor tics are sudden, rapid movements that, to varying degrees, resemble purposeful actions. They range from such simple tics as brow-wrinkling, facial grimacing, head-shaking, or shoulder-shrugging to more complex activities such as gesturing or rising from a chair. In most cases, the actual tics are preceded by a 'premonitory urge' that rises in intensity until it is finally relieved by the tic's appearance. Although some patients are able to suppress the tic for a time, considerable effort is required to do so: Kinnier Wilson (Wilson 1928) noted that 'the strain in holding back is as great as the relief in letting go', and reported that one of his patients, in describing the experience, said that 'you can't help it any more than you can sneezing'.

Although in some cases there may be 'focal' tics, with the same tic recurring uninterruptedly over time, tics are 'multifocal' in most instances, with different tics occurring at different locations.

Etiology

Table 3.3 lists the various causes of motor tics. The most common cause of tics, by far, is Tourette's syndrome or a variant of Tourette's, known as chronic motor tic disorder. As noted in Section 8.25, the onset of Tourette's and chronic motor tic disorder is usually in childhood; however, it must also be borne in mind that Tourette's can go into remission, only to recur in later life; hence, in cases of adult-onset tics it is critical to inquire as to a history of childhood tics (Chouinard and Ford 2000; Klawans and Barr 1985).

Tics may also occur as a side-effect to medications, albeit rarely, and if Tourette's appears to be an unlikely cause then the patient's medication history should be scrutinized for any of the stimulants, anti-epileptics, antidepressants, or antipsychotics listed in Table 3.3, keeping in mind that in some cases a long period of time may elapse between initiation of treatment with an offending medication and the emergence of tics. As noted in Table 3.3, tics may also occur after chronic treatment with antipsychotics, as a subtype of tardive dyskinesia.

Tics may occur during the long-term course of various choreiform disorders, such as Sydenham's chorea, Huntington's disease, and choreoacanthocytosis; indeed, in the case of choreoacanthocytosis eventually over one-half of patients will develop tics. Furthermore, albeit rarely, these choreiform disorders may actually present with tics, as has been noted in Sydenham's chorea (Kerbeshian *et al.* 1990), Huntington's disease (Angelini *et al.* 1998), and choreoacanthocytosis (Feinberg *et al.* 1991).

Of the other causes of tics, consideration is given to autism, and to a history of carbon monoxide poisoning, traumatic brain injury, or encephalitis. Rare causes include pantothenate kinase-associated neurodegeneration, infarction of the basal ganglia, Behçet's syndrome and peripheral injury. In the case of tics that are secondary to peripheral injury (e.g., trauma to the neck followed by a tic of the head), the tics are persistently focal, occurring only in proximity to the site of the injury. Finally, in cases of adult-onset tics for which no cause may be determined, consideration may be given to the possibility of an auto-immune attack on the basal ganglia.

Table 3.3 Causes of motor tics

Tourette's syndrome (Cardoso et al. 1996; Lees et al. 1984)

Medications
Cocaine (Cardoso and Jankovic 1993; Pascual-Leone and Dhuna 1990)
Methylphenidate (Denckla *et al.* 1976)
Pemoline (Bachman 1981; Mitchell and Mathews 1980)
Atomoxetine (Ledbetter 2005)
Lamotrigine (Lombroso *et al.* 1999; Sotero de Menezes *et al.* 2000)
Carbamazepine (Robertson *et al.* 1993)
Phenobarbital (Burd *et al.* 1986)
Escitalopram (Altindag *et al.* 2005)
Sertraline (Altindag *et al.* 2005)
Clomipramine (Moshe *et al.* 1994)
Fluoxetine (Eisenhauer and Jermain 1993)
Haloperidol (Gualtieri and Patterson 1986)
Thioridazine (Gualtieri and Patterson 1986)
Clozapine (Lindenmeyer *et al.* 1995)
Tardive tics (Bharucha and Sethi 1995; Stahl 1980)

Choreiform disorders
Sydenham's chorea (Cardoso *et al.* 1997; Creak and Guttmann 1935)
Huntington's disease (Jankovic and Ashizawa 1995)
Choreoacanthocytosis (Hardie *et al.* 1991)

Other causes
Autism (Ringman and Jankovic 2000)
Carbon monoxide poisoning (Ko *et al.* 2004)
Traumatic brain injury (Krauss and Jankovic 1997)
Post-encephalitis (herpes zoster [Northam and Singer 1991], varicella-zoster [Dale *et al.* 2003])
Pantothenate kinase-associated neurodegeneration (Scarano *et al.* 2002)
Infarction of the basal ganglia (Kwak and Jankovic 2002)
Behçet's syndrome (Budman and Sarcevic 2002)
With peripheral injury (Factor and Moltho 1997)
Autoimmune conditions (Edwards *et al.* 2004)

Differential diagnosis

Tics must be distinguished from myoclonus, chorea, hemifacial spasm, tic douloureux, and stereotypies. One differential feature which distinguishes tics from each of these differential possibilities is the premonitory urge, which is classic for a tic, but absent in all these other conditions.

Myoclonus may resemble a simple tic but, in addition to lacking a premonitory urge, myoclonic jerks, unlike tics, are not suppressible by voluntary effort.

Choreiform movements may be either simple in nature or somewhat complex, resembling purposeful acts, and thus may be difficult to distinguish from tics. As in the case of myoclonus, however, choreiform movements are neither associated with a premonitory urge nor are they suppressible. Furthermore, whereas at times tics may be repetitive, choreiform movements rarely are; rather they appear and reappear on different parts of the body, typically with lightning-like rapidity.

Hemifacial spasm, again, lacks a premonitory urge and is non-suppressible. Furthermore, it is repetitive, involves only musculature innervated by the facial nerve, and is confined, as the name suggests, to one side of the face.

Tic douloureux is primarily a condition of painful spasms of the face, immediately distinguishing it from tics, which are not painful. Furthermore, the 'tic' of tic douloureaux is more of a wince after the spasm of pain than a true, autonomous motor tic.

Stereotypies, as with all these differential possibilities, lack premonitory urges; furthermore, they are readily suppressible and, in contrast with tics, patients find no difficulty in keeping the stereotypy suppressed.

Treatment

Treatment is directed at the underlying cause. When this is ineffective or not possible, consideration may be given to the use of low-dose second-generation antipsychotics.

3.4 CHOREA

Choreiform movements, classically seen in Huntington's disease, may also occur as a side-effect to various medications or as part of a host of other disorders.

Clinical features

Choreic movements consist of brief jerks, of greater or lesser complexity, which appear and disappear on different parts of the body with an amazing fluidity and rapidity, often flitting like summer lightning; they may first appear on the face, then the arm, or perhaps the leg, then again showing up in the hand. Although they are purposeless, some patients may attempt to disguise a choreiform movement by merging it into a purposeful one; thus, a choreic jerk of the arm up to the head may be melded into a purposeful movement of the hand across the top of the head, as if the movement, all along, had been meant to smooth back the hair. Gait is often disturbed in chorea, and may become lurching: when severely affected the gait has a 'dancing and prancing' quality to it; and it is from this that the term 'chorea' (Latin for 'the dance') is derived.

Etiology

The various causes of chorea are listed in Table 3.4. These causes are divided into several groups: those secondary to

medications or intoxicants (e.g., as seen in tardive dyskinesia or with oral contraceptives); those of gradual onset in late adolescence or adult years (of which Huntington's disease is the most important); those of childhood or early adolescent onset, such as Sydenham's chorea; and, finally, a miscellaneous group, of which stroke is probably the most important.

Of medications capable of causing chorea, perhaps the most important group is the antipsychotics, which, after chronic use, can cause tardive dyskinesia, which, in turn, classically presents with chorea. Of note, and in contrast with most other causes of chorea, the chorea seen in tardive dyskinesia, although it can be generalized, tends to remain

Table 3.4   Causes of chorea

Secondary to medications or intoxicants
Tardive dyskinesia (Sachdev 2000)
Oral contraceptives (Gamboa *et al.* 1971; Green 1980; Nausieda *et al.* 1979)
Phenytoin (Kooiker and Sumi 1974; Nausieda *et al.* 1978)
Valproic acid (Lancman *et al.* 1994)
Gabapentin (Buetefisch *et al.* 1996; Chudnow *et al.* 1997)
Phenobarbital intoxication (Lightman 1978)
Lamotrigine (Zesiewicz *et al.* 2006)
Cocaine (Daras *et al.* 1994)
Amphetamine (Lundh and Tunving 1981)
Methylphenidate (Extein 1978; Weiner *et al.* 1978)
Pemoline (Sallee *et al.* 1989)
Levodopa (Mones *et al.* 1971)
Baclofen (both during treatment [Crystal 1990] and upon discontinuation [Kirubakaren *et al.* 1984])
Lithium intoxication (Podskalny and Factor 1996)
Neuroleptic malignant syndrome (Rosebush and Stewart 1989)
Fluoxetine (Bharucha and Sethi 1996)
Paroxetine (Fox *et al.* 1997)
Trazodone (McNeill 2006)
Trihexyphenidyl (Nomoto *et al.* 1987)
Alpha-interferon (Moulignier *et al.* 2002)
Cimetidine (Kushner 1982)
Leaded gasoline intoxication (Goldings and Stewart 1982)

With gradual onset in late adolescence or adult years
Huntington's disease (Heathfield 1967)
Huntington disease-like syndrome 1 and 2 (Stevanin *et al.* 2003)
Choreoacanthocytosis (Critchley *et al.* 1968; Hardie *et al.* 1991; Sakai *et al.* 1981)
McLeod syndrome (Danek *et al.* 2001; Jung *et al.* 2001)
Dentatorubropallidoluysian atrophy (Becher *et al.* 1997; Warner *et al.* 1994, 1995)
Fahr's syndrome (Manyam *et al.* 2001)
Acquired hepatocerebral degeneration (Finlayson and Superville 1981; Victor *et al.* 1965)
Wilson's disease (Steinberg and Sternlieb 1984)
Schizophrenia (Owens *et al.* 1982)
Senile chorea (Bourgeois *et al.* 1980; Delwaide and Desseilles 1977; Klawans and Barr 1981; Varga *et al.* 1982)

With onset in childhood or early adolescence
Sydenham's chorea (Bland and Jones 1952; Cardoso *et al.* 1997; Nausieda *et al.* 1980a)
Cerebral palsy (Rosenbloom 1994)
Lesch–Nyhan syndrome (Jankovic *et al.* 1988; Lesch and Nyhan 1964; Nyhan 1972)
Pantothenate kinase-associated neurodegeneration (Dooling *et al.* 1974)
Ataxia telangiectasia (Woods and Taylor 1992)
Benign hereditary chorea (Behan and Bone 1977; Fernandez *et al.* 2001)

Miscellaneous causes
Stroke (infarction of basal ganglia [Chung *et al.* 2004] or thalamus [Lera *et al.* 2000])
Acquired immune deficiency syndrome (AIDS) (Gallo *et al.* 1996; Pardo *et al.* 1998; Piccolo *et al.* 1999)
Anti-phospholipid syndrome (Cervera *et al.* 1997; Sunden-Cullberg *et al.* 1998; Paus *et al.* 2001)
Systemic lupus erythematosus (Donaldson and Espiner 1971; Fermaglich *et al.* 1973)
Chorea gravidarum (Wilson and Preece 1932a,b)
Paraneoplastic syndrome (Croteau *et al.* 2001; Heckmann *et al.* 1997; Kinirons *et al.* 2003; Vernino *et al.* 2002)
Hyperosmolar non-ketotic hyperglycemia (Chang *et al.* 1996)
Hypernatremia (Speracio *et al.* 1976)
Hyperthyroidism (Fidler *et al.* 1971; Van Uitert and Russakoff 1979)
Post-hypoglycemic (Hefter *et al.* 1993; Lai *et al.* 2004)
Delayed post-anoxic encephalopathy (Davous *et al.* 1986; Hori *et al.* 1991; Schwartz *et al.* 1985)
'Post pump' chorea (Medlock *et al.* 1993)
B12 deficiency (Pachetti *et al.* 2002)
Polycythemia vera (Gautier-Smith and Prankard 1967)
New-variant Creutzfeldt–Jakob disease (McKee and Talbot 2003)
Mercury intoxication (Snyder 1972)
Cervical cord compression (Tan *et al.* 2002)
Paroxysmal dystonic choreoathetosis (Demirkiran and Jankovic 1995)
Paroxysmal chorea with hyperthyroidism (Fishbeck and Layzer 1979)

somewhat localized to the face. Oral contraceptives may cause chorea, and this is more likely to occur in females with a history of Sydenham's chorea or with either systemic lupus erythematosus or the anti-phospholipid syndrome. Of the anti-epileptic drugs capable of causing chorea, phenytoin is most commonly involved, with the others only rarely being at fault. Of the stimulants implicated in chorea, cocaine is prominent, and chorea in these cases is often referred to as 'crack dancing'. Of note, after repeated intoxication with either cocaine (Daras et al. 1994) or amphetamines (Lundh and Tunving 1981), the chorea, rather than subsiding with abstinence, may persist. Levodopa-induced chorea may occur as either a 'peak dose' side-effect or, less commonly, may be seen as the blood level rises and as it falls, with an interval 'clear' of chorea during peak blood levels. Baclofen, as noted in Table 3.4, may cause chorea not only during treatment, but also with discontinuation of chronic treatment. Lithium may cause chorea but this is only with lithium intoxication at high blood levels: although in most cases the chorea clears as the blood level falls, in some cases it may persist for months (Zorumski and Bakris 1983). The neuroleptic malignant syndrome is a rare disorder seen with an abrupt diminution of dopaminergic tone, due either to treatment with a dopamine blocker, such as an antipsychotic, or to discontinuation of a dopaminergic agent, such as levodopa: in addition to chorea, one also sees delirium, diaphoresis, fever, tachycardia, and rigidity. Regarding the other medications in Table 3.4 little need be said, except that chorea represents a very rare side-effect to them.

Of the choreas with gradual onset in late adolescence or early adult years, Huntington's disease is the most common cause: most patients fall ill in their thirties with the gradual onset of a progressively worsening chorea that is eventually joined by a dementia; this is an autosomal dominant condition and sporadic cases are very rare. There are other neurodegenerative disorders that present in a more or less similar fashion to Huntington's disease, and these must be considered in the differential diagnosis. Two of them are so similar, clinically, to Huntington's that they go by the name 'Huntington disease-like syndrome', types 1 and 2: the differential here often rests solely on genetic testing. Other disorders that come into the differential often have distinguishing clincial features. Thus, both choreoacanthocytosis and the X-linked McLeod syndrome are associated with elevated creatinine kinase (CK) levels and acanthocytosis; choreoacanthocytosis may also cause tics, dystonia, and, classically, mutilative lip biting. Dentatorubropallidoluysian atrophy, another Huntington 'look-alike', is suggested by the presence of ataxia. Fahr's syndrome may present with chorea but this is usually accompanied by other abnormal movements, such as dystonia or parkinsonism, and computed tomography (CT) scanning will immediately reveal calcification of the basal ganglia. Acquired hepatocerebral degeneration, seen only in patients with longstanding hepatic disease and a history of recurrent episodes of hepatic encephalopathy, in addition to chorea, may also cause tremor and ataxia. Wilson's disease, rarely, may present with chorea; however, other abnormal movements (e.g., dystonia, tremor) are far more common (Starosta-Rubinstein et al. 1987): nevertheless, given the tragic nature of missing the diagnosis of this treatable disease, it should remain prominent on the differential. Schizophrenia may cause chorea but this is usually quite mild and is far overshadowed, clinically, by the classic psychotic symptoms. Finally, in cases of late onset 'pure' chorea, without associated features, consideration should be given to a diagnosis of 'senile chorea'.

Of the childhood- or early adolescent-onset choreas, Sydenham's chorea is by far the most common. Although it is often accompanied by other evidence of rheumatic fever, such as carditis or polyarthritis, the onset of the chorea may at times be delayed for so long that the other signs of rheumatic fever have already gone into remission, leaving a case of 'pure' Sydenham's chorea. The chorea is of subacute onset, over weeks, and, although typically generalized, is often most prominent in the face and upper extremities. In a small minority there may be only hemichorea. Although Sydenham's chorea may in some patients present solely with chorea, there are in the majority other neuropsychiatric features, most notably obsessions and compulsions (Swedo et al. 1993). In Sydenham's chorea, the chorea, in almost all cases, eventually undergoes spontaneous remission, generally within 5–9 months. The other causes listed in Table 3.4, however, are chronic. Cerebral palsy, of the 'extrapyramidal' type, may cause chorea and its appearance may be delayed for several years after birth. The Lesch–Nyhan syndrome is immediately suggested by the classic mutilative lip biting, which usually become apparent as soon as the child gets teeth. Pantothenate kinase-associated neurodegeneration may cause chorea; however, this is usually accompanied by dystonia. Ataxia telangiectasia may also cause chorea but this is usually preceded by ataxia. Finally, in cases of chronic childhood-onset chorea when other disorders are unlikely, one may consider the diagnosis of benign hereditary chorea.

Of the miscellaneous causes of chorea, stroke and acquired immune deficiency syndrome (AIDS) are among the most common in a general hospital setting (Piccolo et al. 1999). Infarction of the basal ganglia or thalamus may cause either a hemichorea or, less commonly, generalized chorea, and in many cases the onset of the chorea may be delayed for months (Kim 2001a). In AIDS patients chorea may occur secondary either to opportunistic infections or as part of an HIV encephalopathy. Chorea may also occur on an autoimmune basis, either as part of the anti-phospholipid syndrome or systemic lupus erythematosus. Chorea gravidarum (Latin for 'chorea of pregnant women') should obviously be suspected when chorea occurs during pregnancy, and in most of these cases the patient will have either the anti-phospholipid syndrome or systemic lupus erythematosus, or will have a history of Sydenham's chorea. Patients with a paraneoplastic syndrome may also present with chorea but this is soon joined by other elements of a paraneoplastic syndrome, such as delirium, seizures, ataxia, and peripheral neuropathy. Metabolic causes of chorea include hyperosmolar non-ketotic hyperglycemia and, very rarely, hypernatremia, and both of these are readily diagnosed by a chemical survey. Hyperthyroidism may cause a persistent chorea, and the diagnosis is suggested by the associated tremor, diaphoresis, and heat intolerance. Chorea may also occur as a sequela to hypoxic coma or as part of a delayed post-anoxic encephalopathy, and, in children, may follow cardiac surgery, the so-called 'post pump' chorea. Of the other etiologies of persistent chorea listed in Table 3.4, little more need be said except that they only very rarely cause choreiform movements. Finally, note should be made of episodic, paroxysmal chorea. This may occur as part of paroxysmal dystonic choreoathetosis, wherein it is typically accompanied by dystonia (discussed further in Section 3.7), and may also, albeit very rarely, occur as part of hyperthyroidism.

Differential diagnosis

Choreiform movements must be distinguished from myoclonus, tics, athetosis, and from the abnormal oromandibular movements seen in edentulous patients.

Myoclonic jerks are always simple in nature, and hence when choreic jerks are complex, as they sometimes may be, the differential is straightforward. Simple choreic jerks, however, may be more difficult to distinguish from myoclonic jerks. One clue is the 'mercurial' nature of chorea, with jerks appearing and disappearing, fluidly, from one part of the body to another: myoclonic jerks rarely display such lightning-like changes.

Tics, like choreic movements, may be either simple or complex, and thus complexity cannot be used to differentiate them from choreic movements. Tics, however, like myclonus, rarely display the mercurial transience of choreic movements. Furthermore, tics are associated with a premonitory urge and are, at least partially, suppressible; these features are not characteristic of chorea.

Athetotic movements are longer lasting and more sustained in character than are choreic ones; furthermore, rather than being jerky they are 'slow and writhing in character', as pointed out by Kinnier Wilson (Wilson 1955).

Edentulous patients may display oromandibular movements reminiscent of chorea; however, in this condition there are no abnormal movements elsewhere on the body and the tongue is not involved (Koller 1983).

Treatment

Treatment is directed at the underlying condition, as discussed in the respective chapters. In many cases this involves symptomatic treatment with an antipsychotic, and in this regard one of the second-generation antipsychotics, for example risperidone, may be considered.

3.5 ATHETOSIS

Athetosis, a term coined by Hammond in 1871, is derived from the Greek word *athetos*, and means 'without fixed position'.

Clinical features

Athetosis is characterized by purposeless, slow, continuously writhing movements that tend to flow, one into the other, in an unceasing, serpentine pattern. They may be unilateral or bilateral, and are typically seen in the extremities; more often the upper than the lower extremity, and more often on the distal portions of the involved extremity. The movements, when seen in the hand, may mimic, in a grotesque fashion, the movements of the fingers made when playing the piano or, in some cases, may remind the observer of the hand movements made by Balinese dancers.

Etiology

The various causes of athetosis are listed in Table 3.5.

Cerebral palsy of the 'dyskinetic' type, due generally to either hypoxia or, in the past, kernicterus, may leave patients with bilateral or 'double' athetosis.

Infarction of the lenticular nucleus or thalamus may cause athetosis, and in some cases the emergence of this abnormal movement may be delayed for weeks or months after the stroke (Dooling and Adams 1975; Kim 2001a).

Severe proprioceptive sensory loss, as may be seen with infarction of the parietal cortex or thalamus, or with lesions of the cervical cord or dorsal root ganglia, may also be followed by athetosis. In the literature this is often referred to as 'pseudoathetosis'; however, given that clinically these cases are essentially indistinguishable from

Table 3.5 Causes of athetosis

Cerebral palsy ('double athetosis') (Rosenbloom 1994)

Infarction of the basal ganglia or thalamus (Carpenter 1950; Papez *et al.* 1938; Spiller 1920)

Associated with proprioceptive sensory loss due to infarction of the parietal cortex of thalamus or to lesions of the cervical cord or dorsal root ganglia (Ghika and Bogousslavsky 1997; Sharp *et al.* 1994)

Miscellaneous causes
Acquired hepatocerebral degeneration (Finlayson and Superville 1981)
Fahr's syndrome (Manyam *et al.* 2001)
Pantothenate kinase-associated neurodegeneration (Rozdilsky *et al.* 1968)
Medication side-effect (tiagabine [Tombini *et al.* 2006], donepezil [Tanaka *et al.* 2003])
Post-mercury intoxication (Snyder 1972)
Post-cyanide intoxication (Rosenow *et al.* 1995)

those seen with infarction of the lenticular nuclei, this distinction may not be useful.

Of the miscellaneous causes of athetosis, consideration may be given to acquired hepatocerebral degeneration, Fahr's syndrome and pantothenate kinase-associated neurodegeneration; however, in each of these conditions other features often dominate the clinical picture: in acquired hepatocerebral degeneration, chorea, tremor, and dystonia may be seen; in Fahr's syndrome, parkinsonism and calcification of the basal ganglia on CT scanning; and, in pantothenate kinase-associated neurodegeneration, dystonia. There are also single case reports of athetosis occurring as a side-effect to either tiagabine or donepezil. Finally, athetosis may occur as a sequela to intoxication with either mercury or cyanide.

Differential diagnosis

Choreiform movements, as noted in the preceding chapter, tend to be jerky and to appear and reappear on different parts of the body; in contrast, athetotic movements are writhing in character, sustained, and generally remain localized to a particular limb.

Dystonic movements are relatively fixed in character, and lack the writhing quality of athetosis.

Treatment

Botulinum toxin has been utilized in the treatment of double athetosis seen in cerebral palsy (Gooch and Sandell 1996); in cases of athetosis secondary to stroke, deep brain stimulation has been utilized (Katayama *et al.* 2003). It is not at all clear whether pharmacologic treatment with antipsychotics or other agents might be beneficial.

3.6 BALLISM

Ballism, or ballismus, comes originally from the Greek word *ballismos*, which means a jumping movement; it is also related to the Latin *ballista*, which refers to an ancient military machine, similar to a catapult, used for throwing large stones.

Clinical features

Ballistic movements involve the extremities: most commonly both the upper and lower extremities are involved on one side, producing hemiballism; occasionally one may see monoballism (with involvement of only one extremity) or biballism (with bilateral, generalized involvement). The proximal musculature is preferentially involved and the movements are wild and flinging in nature, sometimes to a degree that may throw patients off balance.

Etiology

The various causes of ballism are noted in Table 3.6.

Stroke, whether due to ischemic infarction or, less commonly, intracerebral hemorrhage, is the most common cause of ballism (Vidakovic *et al.* 1994). Although the subthalamic nucleus is most commonly involved, damage to related structures, such as the striatum, thalamus or, very rarely, the substantia nigra, may also cause ballism. In most cases, a hemiballism occurs, and, as might be expected, in most of these cases, the lesion is found in the contralateral hemisphere. However, exceptions to this lateralizing rule do occur and ipsilateral hemiballism has been noted with lesions of the subthalamic nucleus (Crozier *et al.* 1996; Moersch and Kernohan 1939) or the striatum (Borgohain *et al.* 1995).

Other focal lesions may also cause hemiballism, and this has been noted in the subthalamic nucleus for both metastatic tumors and multiple sclerosis plaques.

Of the miscellaneous causes of ballism, the most important from a clinical point of view is non-ketotic hyperosmolar hyperglycemia, as may be seen in elderly diabetics. This syndrome may present with either generalized or hemiballism; of note, in cases of hemiballism, T1-weighted MR scanning may reveal hyperintensity of the contralateral striatum. In all cases, the ballism resolves with restoration of euglycemia; however, it may take days or weeks for full recovery to occur. Rarely, both systemic lupus erythematosus and Sydenham's chorea may cause ballism, presumably on the basis of an autoimmune attack on the subthalamic nucleus. Traumatic brain injury is another rare cause and,

Table 3.6   Causes of ballism

Stroke (infarction or intracerebral hemorrhage)
Subthalamic nucleus (Carpenter 1955; Martin and Alcock 1934; Melamed *et al.* 1978; Pfeil 1952; Whittier 1947)
Striatum (Defebvre *et al.* 1990; Kase *et al.* 1981; Schwarz and Barrows 1960; Srinivas *et al.* 1987)
Thalamus (Antin *et al.* 1867; Dewey and Jankovic 1989; Kulisevsky *et al.* 1993)
Substantia nigra (Caparros-Lefebvre *et al.* 1994)

Other focal lesions
Tumors (Glass *et al.* 1984)
Multiple sclerosis (Riley and Lang 1988; Waubant *et al.* 1997)

Miscellaneous causes
Non-ketotic hyperglycemia (Chu *et al.* 2002; Lee *et al.* 1999; Lin and Chang 1994; Lin *et al.* 2001)
Systemic lupus erythematosus (Dewey and Jankovic 1989; Vidakovic *et al.* 1994)
Sydenham's chorea (Konagaya and Konagaya 1992)
Traumatic brain injury with damage to the subthalamic nucleus (Vakis *et al.* 2006)
Hyperthyroidism (Ristic *et al.* 2004)
Medications (phenytoin [Opida *et al.* 1978], oral contraceptives [Driesen and Wolters 1986], bupropion [de Graaf *et al.* 2003])

in the case in question, there was damage, as might be expected, to the subthalamic nucleus. Hyperthyroidism may also cause ballism, albeit rarely, and there are isolated case reports of ballism occurring as a side-effect to phenytoin, oral contraceptives, and bupropion.

Differential diagnosis

The hallmark of ballism is its wild, flinging nature, and it is this characteristic that distinguishes it from other abnormal movements, such as dystonia, athetosis and chorea. Dystonic movements are fixed and more or less immobile; although in athetosis there is some motility, it is slow and writhing in character. Choreic jerks, when severe, may approach the flinging character of ballistic movements but choreic jerks appear and reappear on different parts of the body in contrast with the consistent presence of ballism on one or more limbs.

Treatment

Of the various symptomatic treatments for ballism, by far the best established agents are the antipsychotics; among these haloperidol (Davis 1976; Klawans et al. 1976a) has the longest track record. Other first-generation agents to consider include perphenazine (Johnson and Fahn 1977) and chlorpromazine (Klawans et al. 1976a). Of second-generation antipsychotics, risperidone (Evidente et al. 1999), olanzapine (Mukand et al. 2005), and clozapine (Stojanovic et al. 1997) have also been used. Regardless of which agent is chosen, it is appropriate to start with a low dose (e.g., 1–2 mg of haloperidol or 0.25–0.5 mg of risperidone) and to gradually titrate the dose upward. Periodic attempts should be made to taper and, if possible, discontinue antipsychotics over the following months.

Other pharmacologic agents to consider include sertraline (Okun et al. 2001), topiramate (Gatto et al. 2004), and divalproex (Chandra et al. 1982; Lenton et al. 1981) (although not all reports are favorable for divalproex [Lang 1985]). In severe treatment-resistant cases, consideration may be given to pallidotomy (Yamada et al. 2004), deep brain stimulation of the thalamus (Tsubokawa et al. 1995), or intrathecal baclofen (Francisco 2006).

3.7 DYSTONIA

Dystonia, a term coined by Oppenhiem in 1911, refers to a more or less sustained contortion of one or more body parts.

Clinical features

Dystonic movements may arise either spontaneously or when a patient begins a voluntary movement. The contortion arises from the simultaneous contraction of both agonist and antagonist muscles, and persists for variable periods of time. Some common varieties deserve to be mentioned. Dystonia of the cervical muscles may rotate or twist the head in one direction or the other (torticollis), pull it over to one side (laterocollis), or forward (anterocollis), or backward (retrocollis). Dystonic contraction of the oromandibular musculature may cause a forced yawning type of movement, and when the orbicularis oculi muscles undergo dystonic contracture blepharospasm occurs. The extraocular musculature may be involved, creating what is known as an 'oculogyric crisis', with tonic conjugate gaze deviation, generally superiorly and laterally. When the upper extremity is involved, the arm may be twisted, and in the hand the thumb may be adducted with the fingers hyperextended. Lower extremity involvement is typified by inversion and plantar flexion of the foot. The axial musculature may also be involved resulting in variable contortions of the trunk. Finally, there are also cases where dystonia occurs only with specific movements. As noted earlier, in some cases dystonia may be precipitated by movement, and this may occur with non-specific movements, such as turning the head, or lifting an arm. There are, however, dystonias wherein only very specific activities, such as writing or typing, precipitate the dystonia.

Dystonias are often described with reference to the number and contiguity of body parts involved. Thus, in focal dystonia, only one body part is involved (e.g., the upper extremity alone), whereas in segmental dystonia, two adjacent parts are affected (e.g., the neck and upper extremity): 'hemidystonia' is a term reserved for a specific segmental dystonia wherein the upper and lower extremity are both involved. In multifocal dystonia, two or more non-adjacent parts are affected; in generalized dystonia, bilateral involvement is seen.

In some cases, patients may be able to relieve a dystonia by utilizing what is known as a 'sensory trick', or geste antagoniste. For example, by simply placing a hand gently on the cheek a patient with torticollis may abort the twisting motion of the neck musculature, and a patient with a generalized dystonia precipitated by walking may find relief by walking backward.

Etiology

The various causes of dystonia are listed in Table 3.7, in which they are divided into several groups. The first group, known as the primary dystonias, is composed of 'pure' dystonias that occur either idiopathically or on an inherited basis. The next group, known as the 'dystonia plus' syndromes, is also characterized by inherited disorders; however, here the dystonia is accompanied by other abnormal movements, such as parkinsonism or myoclonus. Following this are the secondary dystonias. This is a heterogeneous group, including medication-induced dystonias (e.g., antipsychotics), those occurring as part of a neurodegenerative disorder, those occurring secondary to focal lesions

Table 3.7 Causes of dystonia

Primary dystonias

Primary torsion dystonia (Johnson *et al.* 1962; Marsden and Harrison 1974; Schmidt *et al.* 2006)

Idiopathic cervical dystonia (Chan *et al.* 1991; Jankovic *et al.* 1991; Sorensen and Hamby 1966)

Meige's syndrome (Defazio *et al.* 1999; Tolosa 1981)

Breughel's syndrome (Gilbert 1996)

Spasmodic dysphonia (Brin *et al.* 1998)

Axial dystonia (Bhatia *et al.* 1997b)

Task-specific dystonia (Cohen and Hallett 1988; Sheehy and Marsden 1982)

'Dystonia plus' syndromes

Dopa-responsive dystonia (Harwood *et al.* 1994; Nygaard and Duvoisin 1986; Nygaard *et al.* 1990; Sawle *et al.* 1991; Tassin *et al.* 2000)

Myoclonus dystonia (Asmus *et al.* 2002; Doheny *et al.* 2002; Grimes *et al.* 2002; Schule *et al.* 2004)

Rapid-onset dystonia parkinsonism (Zaremba *et al.* 2004)

Lubag (Evidente *et al.* 2002)

Secondary dystonias

Medication-induced

Antipsychotics

Tardive dystonia (a variant of tardive dyskinesia)

Levodopa (Cubo *et al.* 2001; Kidron and Melamed 1987; Melamed 1979; Nausieda *et al.* 1980b)

Bupropion (Detweiller and Harpold 2002)

Fluoxetine (Dominguez-Moran *et al.* 2001)

Sertraline (Walker 2002)

Buspirone (LeWitt *et al.* 1993)

Carbamazepine (Stryjer *et al.* 2002)

Gabapentin (Pina and Modrego 2005, Reeves *et al.* 1996)

Tiagabine (Wolanczyk and Grabowska-Grzyb 2001)

Valproic acid (Oh *et al.* 2004)

Cocaine withdrawal (Choy-Kwong and Lipton 1989)

MDMA ('Ecstasy') (Priori *et al.* 1995)

Lamivudine (Song *et al.* 2005)

Alpha-interferon (Atasoy *et al.* 2004)

Flunarazine (Koukoulis *et al.* 1997)

Cimetidine (Romisher *et al.* 1987)

Neurodegenerative disorders

Wilson's disease (Svetel *et al.* 2001; Walshe and Yealand 1992)

Lesch–Nyhan syndrome (Jankovic *et al.* 1988)

Pantothenate kinase-associated neurodegeneration (Hayflick *et al.* 2003; Swaiman 1991)

Corticobasal-ganglionic degeneration (Litvan *et al.* 1997b; Riley *et al.* 1990; Rinne *et al.* 1994, Vanek and Jankovic 2001)

Progressive supranuclear palsy (Barclay and Lang 1997)

Multiple system atrophy (Boesch *et al.* 2002)

Fahr's syndrome (Manyam *et al.* 2001)

Dentatorubropallidoluysian atrophy (Warner *et al.* 1995)

Neuroacanthocytosis (Hardie *et al.* 1991)

Huntington's disease (Louis *et al.* 2000)

Spinocerebellar ataxia (Nandagopal and Moorthy 2004)

Focal lesions

Infarction or hemorrhage of the basal ganglia, thalamus, or parietal cortex

Mass lesions of the basal ganglia, frontal lobe, or cerebellum

Miscellaneous causes

Traumatic brain injury (Burke *et al.* 1980; Lee *et al.* 1994; Munchau *et al.* 2000)

Post-anoxic (Bhatt *et al.* 1993)

Central pontine myelinolysis (Maraganore *et al.* 1992; Yoshida *et al.* 2000)

Cyanide intoxication (Rosenow *et al.* 1995; Valenzuela *et al.* 1992)

Methanol intoxication (Quartarone *et al.* 2000)

Manganese intoxication (Lu *et al.* 1994)

Post-encephalitic (encephalitis lethargica [Alpers and Patten 1927], Japanese encephalitis [Kalita and Misra 2000, Murgod *et al.* 2001])

Acquired immune deficiency syndrome (AIDS) (Factor *et al.* 2003)

Creutzfeldt–Jakob disease (Hellmann and Melamed 2002)

Tourette's syndrome (Stone and Jankovic 1991)

Cerebral palsy (Saint Hilaire *et al.* 1991)

Cervical cord lesion (Cammarota *et al.* 1995)

Thoracic outlet syndrome (Quartarone *et al.* 1998)

Peripheral trauma (Schott 1985; O'Riordan and Hutchinson 2004)

Esophageal reflux ('Sandifer syndrome' [Shahnawaz *et al.* 2001])

Paroxysmal dystonias

Non-kinesigenic paroxysmal dystonic choreoathetosis

Kinesigenic paroxysmal dystonic choreoathetosis

Exercise-induced paroxysmal dystonic choreoathetosis

Nocturnal paroxysmal dystonia

Ictal dystonia (Kuba *et al.* 2003; Newton *et al.* 1992)

Miscellaneous causes (multiple sclerosis [Waubant *et al.* 2001, Zenzola *et al.* 2001], Fahr's syndrome [Volonte *et al.* 2001], traumatic brain injury and infarction of the basal ganglia [Demerkirian and Jankovic 1995])

(e.g., infarctions of the basal ganglia), and those occurring secondary to a large number of miscellaneous causes. Finally, there is a group of paroxysmal dystonias, characterized clinically by dystonia occurring only in discrete, brief episodes. In general clinical practice, dystonia is most commonly caused by one of the primary dystonias.

Of the primary dytonias, the classic example is primary torsion dystonia, or 'dystonia musculorum deformans' as it was originally named by Oppenheim (1911). This typically has an onset in childhood or adolescence, presenting with a focal dystonia, often of the lower extemity, and gradual progression to generalized involvement. The other primary dystonias generally have an onset in adult years and typically remain more or less focal. Idiopathic cervical dystonia, as the name clearly suggests, manifests with a cervical dystonia; Meige's syndrome is characterized by blepharospasm, Breughel's syndrome by oromandibular dystonia, and spasmodic dysphonia, again as the name suggests, by dysphonia. Rarely, only the trunk may be involved, creating the syndrome of axial dystonia. As noted above, some dystonias occur only with specific activities, and these are known as the 'task-specific dystonias': examples include writer's, typist's, and musician's cramp.

In considering the 'dystonia plus' syndromes, by far the most important disorder to keep in mind is dopa-responsive dystonia. This disorder has an onset in childhood with dystonia of the lower extremity, and thus figures in the differential diagnosis of primary torsion dystonia. The reason why it should always be considered is because, in contrast with primary torsion dystonia, it is eminently treatable, often responding dramatically to low-dose levodopa. The other 'dystonia plus' syndromes are rare. Myoclonus–dystonia (discussed also in Section 3.2) has an onset in childhood or adolescence and is characterized by myoclonus and dystonia, often a cervical or a task-specific dystonia. Rapid-onset dystonia–parkinsonism presents in adult years acutely with a combination of dystonia and parkinsonism, with symptoms escalating over days or weeks and then stabilizing. Lubag (also known as X-linked dystonia–parkinsonism) is an X-linked disorder seen only in Filipino men, presenting first with dystonia but eventually joined by parkinsonism.

In considering the secondary dystonias, each subgroup will be treated in turn, beginning with medication-induced dystonias.

Of the medications capable of causing dystonia, by far the most common are the first-generation antipsychotics, such as haloperidol and fluphenazine (Keepers *et al.* 1983; Swett 1975). These usually occur within a matter of days of either starting the medication or substantially increasing the dose (Ayd 1961; Keepers *et al.* 1983), and are most likely to occur in young males (Boyer *et al.* 1987). Focal dystonias, including oculogyric crisis, torticollis, and involvement of the upper limb are most common; in some cases, segmental spread may occur and, rarely, an acute antipsychotic-induced dystonia may become generalized. Lingual dystonia may also occur, and patients may become dysarthric and complain of a 'thick tongue'; very rarely, laryngeal dystonia with respiratory embarrassment may occur (Christodoulou and Kalaitzi 2005; Flaherty and Lahmeyer 1978). Interestingly, in patients with schizophrenia, antipsychotic-induced dystonias may be accompanied by a transient increase of psychotic symptoms (Chiu 1989; Thornton and McKenna 1994). Although first-generation antipsychotics are most commonly at fault, dystonia has been noted, albeit rarely, with second-generation agents such as olanzapine (Alevizos *et al.* 2003) and aripiprazole (Desarkar *et al.* 2006); there are also case reports of dystonia occurring upon discontinuation of clozapine (Ahmed *et al.* 1998; Mendhekar

and Duggal 2006). Furthermore, it must be borne in mind that other dopamine blockers, such as metoclopramide, may also cause dystonia (Chistodoulou and Kalaitzi 2005). In patients who are treated chronically with antipsychotics, tardive dystonia, a variant of tardive dyskinesia, may also occur: this generally presents with a focal dystonia affecting the neck or face, which may undergo segmental spread and, rarely, become generalized (Burke *et al.* 1982; Kiriakakis *et al.* 1998; Wojick *et al.* 1991; Yassa *et al.* 1986), in which case it may be disabling (Yadalam *et al.* 1990). Interestingly, should mania occur, a pre-existing tardive dystonia may undergo substantial improvement (Kiriakakis *et al.* 1998; Yazici *et al.* 1991). As with acute dystonias, tardive dystonia may also rarely be seen with second-generation agents such as olanzapine, although it is more common with first-generation agents (Gunal *et al.* 2001).

The most common offender of the other medications that are capable of causing dystonia is levodopa, as utilized in the treatment of Parkinson's disease: in such cases dystonia may appear either as a peak-dose dyskinesia or, more commonly, as an end-of-dose 'wearing off' phenomenon. The remaining medicines listed in Table 3.7 only rarely cause dystonia: most references are limited to single case reports.

Turning now to the neurodegenerative disorders capable of causing dystonia, the most important disorder to keep in mind is Wilson's disease, given that, unlike all the other disorders in this group, it is treatable. The onset of Wilson's disease occurs between childhood and early adult years and, in a minority of cases, it may present with dystonia (Starosta-Rubinstein *et al.* 1987): the dystonia may consist of torticollis, dystonia of the upper or lower extremity, an oculogyric crisis (Lee *et al.* 1999), or a facial dystonia of the oromandibular type, which may leave the patient with a fixed, vacuous, wide-mouthed smile. Other symptoms and signs, including personality change, gait abnormalities and tremor, eventually accrue. Given that treatment is available, testing for copper and ceruloplasmin levels should be performed if there is any suspicion of Wilson's disease. The occurrence of progressive dystonia in early childhood should suggest the Lesch–Nyhan syndrome, especially when accompanied by mutilative lip biting. Pantothenate kinase-associated neurodegeneration presents in childhood or adolescence with progressive dystonia, usually of the upper extremity, eventually joined by other abnormal movements (such as chorea or tremor) and then by a dementia (Dooling *et al.* 1974). The other neurodegenerative disorders listed in Table 3.7 all have an onset in adult or later years, and, in addition to dystonia, typically are characterized by other abnormal movements. Thus, corticobasal ganglionic degeneration, progressive supranuclear palsy, multiple system atrophy, and Fahr's syndrome are characterized, in addition to dystonia, by parkinsonism, and dentatorubropallidoluysian atrophy, neuracanthocytosis and Huntington's disease are marked by chorea. In the case of Huntington's disease, although dystonia generally appears only in far-advanced disease, there are rare cases of Huntington's disease in which the presentation was with dystonia. Finally, there are rare case reports of spinocerebellar ataxia presenting, not with the expected ataxia, but with dystonia.

Of focal lesions capable of causing dystonia, by far the most common are infarctions of either the basal ganglia (Krystkowiak *et al.* 1998; Russo 1983) or thalamus (Lehericy *et al.* 2001): of note, in these cases, it may take weeks, months, or, rarely, years, before the dystonia appears (Lehericy *et al.* 1996). There are also rare reports of cortical infarction causing dystonia, as for example of the parietal cortex (Burguera *et al.* 2001). Mass lesions may also cause dystonia, as has been reported for tumors of the basal ganglia (Martinez-Cage and Marsden 1984), frontal lobe (Soland *et al.* 1996b), and cerebellum (Alarcon *et al.* 2001; Krauss *et al.* 1997).

Of the miscellaneous secondary causes of dystonia, traumatic brain injury is perhaps the most common, and in such cases lesions of the basal ganglia are seen. Dystonia may also appear in a post-anoxic encephalopathy, and there are also case reports of dystonia occurring after central pontine myelinolysis, wherein 'extrapontine' myelinolysis, involving the basal ganglia, also occurred. Other clear-cut precipitating events, rarely associated with dystonia, include intoxication with cyanide, methanol, or manganese. Encephalitis may have dystonia as a sequela, and this has been noted after encephalitis lethargica and Japanese encephalitis. AIDS may be characterized by dystonia, and this has been noted in cases of AIDS that are complicated by progressive multifocal encephalopathy and toxoplasmosis. In one case report Creutzfeldt–Jakob disease was noted to present with dystonia. Tourette's syndrome, in addition to tics, may also, albeit rarely, cause dystonia, and cerebral palsy may also be characterized by dystonia. Remarkably, there are also reports of dystonia occurring with cervical cord lesions and with lesions outside the central nervous system, such as the thoracic outlet syndrome or with peripheral trauma: in cases of peripheral trauma, dystonia may also accompany reflex sympathetic dystrophy (van Hilten *et al.* 2001). Finally, dystonia may also occur in association with gastroesophageal reflux disease, in which case one speaks of the 'Sandifer's syndrome': although this is generally reported only in children, adult cases have also been noted.

The last group in Table 3.7 contains the paroxysmal dystonias, which may be divided into primary and secondary forms (Demerkiran and Jankovic 1995). The primary forms are divided into three types, depending on whether the dystonia occurs spontaneously or with precipitants: spontaneously occurring dystonias are referred to as 'paroxysmal non-kinesigenic dystonic choreathetosis'; those precipitated immediately by some movement, as 'paroxysmal kinesigenic dystonic choreoathetosis'; and those occurring only after relatively prolonged exercise, as 'exercise-induced paroxysmal dystonic choreoathetosis'. Each of these primary paroxysmal dystonias has an onset in childhood or adolescence, and in all cases the attacks last generally in the order of minutes, rarely extending to hours; during the attacks most patients will have dystonia, generally a hemisdystonia or a generalized dystonia, which may be accompanied by chorea. Although sporadic cases do occur, most are familial, following a pattern consistent with autosomal dominant inheritance. Further, specific, details for each type follow below.

In paroxysmal non-kinesigenic dystonic choreoathetosis (Bressman *et al.* 1988; Demirkiran and Jankovic 1995; Fink *et al.* 1997; Jarman *et al.* 1997, 2000; Lance 1977; Matsuo *et al.* 1999; Mount and Reback 1940; Richards and Barnett 1968; Rosen 1964) attacks are more likely when patients are fatigued or have been indulging in alcohol, caffeine, or nicotine. A locus has been identified on chromosome 2, and there appears to be considerable genetic heterogeneity (Bruno *et al.* 2007; Chen *et al.* 2005, Spacey *et al.* 2006).

Paroxysmal kinesigenic dystonic choreoathetosis (Bruno *et al.* 2004; Demirkiran and Jankovic 1995; Kertesz 1967; Lance 1977; Stevens 1966) is suggested by the history of attacks occurring immediately upon some movement, such as walking, running or, in some cases, simply standing up. Another distinguishing feature of this type is the fact that treatment with an anti-epileptic drug (AED) such as carbamazepine reliably prevents attacks, often at a low dose (Wein *et al.* 1996). In this disorder, a locus has been identified on chromosome 16; however, as for non-kinesigenic cases, there is also considerable genetic heterogeneity (Valente *et al.* 2000).

In exercise-induced paroxysmal dystonic choreoathetosis (Bhatia *et al.* 1997a; Munchau *et al.* 2000) attacks occur only after fairly prolonged exercise, such as walking or cycling, and they subside fairly soon with rest. A genetic locus has not as yet been identified.

The secondary paroxysmal dystonias include the syndrome of nocturnal paroxysmal dystonia, ictal dystonia, and a miscellaneous group.

Nocturnal paroxysmal dystonia is characterized by brief attacks of dystonia that arise from non-REM sleep and are associated with partial awakening. There are probably distinct subtypes in this syndrome, with some cases representing a parasomnia (Lee *et al.* 1985) and others representing seizures (Lugaresi and Cirignotta 1981; Lugaresi *et al.* 1986; Provini *et al.* 1999; Tinuper *et al.* 1990): in the latter subtype the response to an AED, such as carbamazepine, is usually good.

Ictal dystonia may also be seen during otherwise typical complex partial seizures, and in such cases the dystonia fairly reliably lateralizes the epileptic focus to the contralateral hemisphere.

Finally, the miscellaneous group includes multiple sclerosis (with plaques in the thalamus or posterior limb of the internal capsule), Fahr's syndrome, and traumatic brain injury or infarction of the basal ganglia.

Differential diagnosis

Athetosis is somewhat similar to dystonia, in that in both abnormal movements contortion is present; the difference between the two lies in the degree of mobility seen. In dystonia, the contortion gradually assumes a final form, and then remains fairly fixed; by contrast, in athetosis, the contortion constantly changes, in a writhing, almost serpentine, fashion.

Treatment

For most of the causes listed in Table 3.7, treatment is discussed in the respective chapter for the disorder in question. In the case of antipsychotic-induced dystonia, emergent treatment may be accomplished with diphenhydramine, given intramuscularly or intravenously in a dose of 25–50 mg, or benztropine, given intramuscularly in a dose of 2 mg; if needed, oral benztropine, in a similar dose, may be given on a preventive basis. For other causes where treatment is not well established, consideration may be given to empirical trials of benztropine, clonazepam, baclofen or AEDs, such as carbamazepine; botulinum toxin may be considered, and, as a last resort, deep brain stimulation of the globus pallidus is an option.

3.8 PARKINSONISM

Parkinsonism is a syndrome of multiple different etiologies: although Parkinson's disease is the most common cause of parkinsonism, it must always be kept in mind that it is but one of many possible causes, and the physician must dutifully consider the other causes before deciding that a patient with parkinsonism has Parkinson's disease.

Clinical features

Fully developed, classic parkinsonism is, once recognized, almost unforgettable. Patients stand in a flexion posture, bent at the waist and neck, and with the arms held forward in flexion and the knees somewhat bent. A rhythmic pill-rolling rest tremor is seen, most notably in the hands. When patients attempt to do anything, bradykinesia is apparent, with almost all movements initiated and carried out slowly. The gait is shuffling and patients typically take small steps; at times the phenomenon of 'festination' is seen, wherein, with ongoing ambulation, patients begin to lean forward and take ever smaller, but ever faster steps, almost as if they were trying to catch up with their forward-leaning center of gravity. Some patients may also display another gait abnormality known as 'freezing' (Giladi et al. 1992): here, patients become unable to initiate ambulation, as if they were 'frozen'. This curious phenomenon typically occurs at a threshold of some sort, for example a doorway or the start of a hallway.

Other motor abnormalities are evident on examination, and include rigidity, postural instability, and micrographia. Rigidity is evident in the limbs, and is present with both passive extension and flexion. This rigidity may be 'lead pipe' in character, in that it is of the same severity throughout the full range of motion, or there may be what is known as 'cogwheel' rigidity. Cogwheeling is perhaps most easily appreciated at the elbow by supporting the elbow in the palm of one's hand, placing the thumb over the biceps tendon and then, with the other hand, alternately slowly extending and flexing the forearm: when cogwheeling is present, a peculiar 'ratcheting' sensation is appreciated in the thumb over the biceps tendon, as if the extension of the forearm were proceeding one 'cog' at a time. Postural instability may be suggested by a history of falls, and may be detected using the 'pull test': to perform this test, stand several feet behind the patient and, after warning the patient what is to come, place your hands on the patient's shoulders and gently, but briskly, pull back. Normal individuals will quickly make a compensatory step back and catch their balance; those with parkinsonism, however, will fail to make compensatory movements and begin to tumble backward (in this regard, if the patient is large, it is appropriate to position yourself with your back to a wall in order to prevent a double fall). Micrographia is manifest by handwriting that becomes small and scratchy: in some cases, multiple samples of the patient's handwriting collected over months and years may provide 'graphic' evidence of a progression of the syndrome.

Other abnormalities that may be seen in classic parkinsonism include hypomimia, hypophonia, palilalia, and bradyphrenia. Hypomimia (also known as 'masked facies') is an abnormality of facial expression wherein the muscles of facial expression seem frozen and there is little blinking: Kinnier Wilson (Wilson 1955) described it as a 'starched' expression. In hypophonia, the voice becomes low, soft, and monotone; in severe cases it is reduced to an unintelligible mumbling. Palilalia is said to be present when the patient involuntarily repeats the last word of a phrase or sentence with ever increasing rapidity and ever increasing indistinctness. Bradyphrenia is the cognitive analog of bradykinesia and is characterized by a slowness of thought.

Of all of these signs and symptoms, the 'cardinal' ones for diagnosis are tremor, bradykinesia, rigidity, and postural instability.

Etiology

The various causes of parkinsonism are listed in Table 3.8, where they are divided into several groups. In the first group are neurodegenerative disorders, each of which causes a parkinsonism of gradual onset and progression: this group, as a whole, is by far the most common cause of parkinsonism, and of the disorders in this group, Parkinson's disease is the most frequent. The next group consists of parkinsonism secondary to medications and in almost all of these cases the parkinsonism is of relatively acute onset: of all of these medications the antipsychotics, by far, are the most common offenders. Next considered are cases secondary

Table 3.8   Causes of parkinsonism

Neurodegenerative disorders
Parkinson's disease (Hughes *et al.*, 1993; Martin *et al.* 1973)
Diffuse Lewy body disease (Byrne *et al.* 1989; Hely *et al.* 1996)
Multiple system atrophy (Watanabe *et al.* 2002; Wenning
   et al. 1995)
Progressive supranuclear palsy (Collins *et al.* 1995; Litvan *et al.*
   1996; Maher and Lees 1986; Nath *et al.* 2003)
Corticobasal ganglionic degeneration (Litvan *et al.* 1997b; Rinne
   et al. 1994)
Frontotemporal dementia with parkinsonism linked to chromosome
   17 (Boeve *et al.* 2005; Yasuda *et al.* 2005)
Dentatorubropallidoluysian atrophy (Warner *et al.* 1995)
Neuroacanthocytosis (Hardie *et al.* 1991)
Wilson's disease (Starosta-Rubinstein *et al.* 1987)
Fahr's syndrome (Klawans *et al.* 1976b; Tambyah *et al.* 1993)
Alzheimer's disease (Clark *et al.* 1997; Goodman 1953; Scarmeas
   et al. 2004)
Hallervorden–Spatz disease (Alberca *et al.* 1987; Jankovic *et al.* 1985)
Juvenile-onset Huntington's disease (Bird and Paulson 1971;
   Campbell *et al.* 1961; Siesling *et al.* 1997)
Kufs' disease (Nijssen *et al.* 2002)
Lubag (Evidente *et al.* 2002)
Spinocerebellar ataxia (Furtado *et al.* 2002; Shan *et al.* 2001)
Rapid onset dystonia parkinsonism (Brashear *et al.* 1996, 1997, 2007;
   Kabacki *et al.* 2005; Kramer *et al.* 1999; Pittock *et al.* 2000)
Hereditary mental depression and parkinsonism (Perry *et al.* 1975;
   Tsuboi *et al.* 2002)
Guamian amyotrophic lateral sclerosis–parkinsonism complex
   (Garruto *et al.* 1981; Hirano *et al.* 1967; Malamud *et al.* 1961)

Secondary to medications
Antipsychotics (Hardie and Lees 1988)
Metoclopramide (Indo *et al.* 1982; Sethi *et al.* 1989)
Prochlorperazine (Edelstein and Knight 1987)
Neuroleptic malignant syndrome (Rosebush and Stewart 1989;
   Velamoor *et al.* 1994)
Valproic acid (Armon *et al.* 1996; Easterford *et al.* 2004; Iijima
   et al. 2002)
Alpha-methyldopa (Strang 1966)
Lithium (Holroyd and Smith 1995)
Selective serotonin reuptake inhibitors (SSRIs) (e.g., fluoxetine [Ernst
   and Steur 1993], paroxetine [Jimenez-Jimenez *et al.* 1994])
Phenelzine (Teusink *et al.* 1984)
Calcium channel blockers (e.g., cinnarizine, flunarazine, amlodipine
   [Marti-Masso and Poza 1998; Sempere *et al.* 1995])

Amiodarone (Werner and Olanow 1989)
Disulfiram (de Mari *et al.* 1993; Laplane *et al.* 1992)
Budesonide (Prodan *et al.* 2006)
Cytosine arabinoside (Luque *et al.* 1987)
Kava extract (Meseguer *et al.* 2002)

Secondary to toxins and substances of abuse
Alcohol withdrawal (Carlen *et al.* 1981)
Methanol (Guggenheim *et al.* 1971; McLean *et al.* 1980;
   Verslegers *et al.* 1988)
MPTP (Ballard *et al.* 1985; Tetrud *et al.* 1989)
Inhalant abuse (Uitti *et al.* 1994)
Manganese (Abd El Naby and Hassanein 1965; Huang *et al.*
   1989)
Cyanide poisoning (Uitti *et al.* 1985)
Diquat (Sechi *et al.* 1992)
Organophosphates (Bhatt *et al.* 1999)

Secondary to other precipitating events
Dementia pugilistica (Harvey and Davis 1974; Martland
   1928)
Post-anoxic encephalopathy (Bhatt *et al.* 1993; Bucher *et al.*
   1996; Goto *et al.* 1997)
Carbon monoxide poisoning (Choi 1983; Grinker 1926;
   Klawans *et al.* 1982b)
Encephalitis lethargica (Duvoisin and Yahr 1965; Rail *et al.*
   1981)
Arbovirus encephalitis (e.g., western equine [Mulder *et al.*
   1951; Schultz *et al.* 1977], Japanese [Pradhan *et al.* 1999])

Miscellaneous causes
Stroke (see text for references)
'Arteriosclerotic parkinsonism' (Murrow *et al.* 1990)
Acquired hepatocerebral degeneration (Burkhard *et al.* 2003)
Hepatic encephalopathy (Federico and Zochodne 2001)
'Encephalopathic' pellagra (Serdaru *et al.* 1988)
Central pontine myelinolysis (Dickoff *et al.* 1988; Tomita
   et al. 1997)
Multiple sclerosis (Federlein *et al.* 1997)
Hydrocephalus (Racette *et al.* 2004)
Systemic lupus erythematosus (Dennis *et al.* 1992)
Sjögren's syndrome (Walker *et al.* 1999)
Acquired immune deficiency syndrome (AIDS) (Hersh *et al.*
   2001)
Neurosyphilis (Sandyk 1983)
Hypoparathyroidism (Stuerenburg *et al.* 1996)

MPTP, methylphenyltetrahydropyridine.

to toxins and substances of abuse, such as methanol. Following this, there is a group of cases secondary to other, more or less obvious, precipitating events, such as repeated head trauma, or anoxia. Finally, there is a group of miscellaneous causes, prominent among which are stroke and the controversial entity known as 'vascular parkinsonism'.

Among the neurodegenerative disorders, Parkinson's disease, in addition to being the most common, is also the

most likely to cause 'classic' parkinsonism as described above. Onset is typically with tremor, with or without rigidity, or less commonly with rigidity alone; symptoms generally appear unilaterally, typically in one of the upper extremities, and over time spread occurs in a gradual fashion to involve the contralateral extremity and, eventually, all four extremities. The classic picture may also be more or less faithfully imitated by diffuse Lewy body disease and multiple system atrophy; however, certain features may enable a clinical differentiation of these two disorders from Parkinson's disease. Diffuse Lewy body disease, as noted in Section 8.6, may present with relatively 'pure' parkinsonism; however, in almost all cases, one also sees, within a year of such a presentation, the development of a dementia which is marked by confusion and visual hallucinations: although patients with Parkinson's disease may also become demented, this usually does not occur until after many years have passed (Biggins et al. 1992; Marder et al. 1995; Mayeux et al. 1992). Multiple system atrophy (of the 'striatonigral' variant) may likewise cause a fairly pure parkinsonism; however, here one generally also sees evidence of degeneration of either the cerebellum or brainstem nuclei (Colosimo et al. 1995; Litvan et al. 1997a; Wenning et al. 1994, 1999), with the development of either ataxia and/or autonomic failure with postural dizziness, syncope, erectile dysfunction, or urinary retention/incontinence.

The next three neurodegenerative disorders in the list, namely progressive supranuclear palsy, corticobasal ganglionic degeneration and frontotemporal dementia, are less likely to cause a classic parkinsonism and are more likely to have clearly distinctive characteristics. Progressive supranuclear palsy tends to present with frequent, unexplained falls, and the ensuing parkinsonism is generally symmetric in onset and marked by rigidity rather than tremor; furthermore, the patient's posture, rather than one of flexion, is usually quite erect, with the neck often held in a rigid dystonic extension (Litvan et al. 1996; Steele 1972); finally, and most importantly, within several years one typically sees a supranuclear ophthalmoplegia, especially for downward gaze. Corticobasal ganglionic degeneration typically presents with bradykinesia and a markedly asymmetric parkinsonism of an upper limb, marked by a dystonic rigidity; tremor is unusual and, moreover, one typically finds cortical sensory loss and apraxia. One of the frontotemporal dementias (frontotemporal dementia and parkinsonism linked to chromosome 17) presents not only with parkinsonism, but also with a personality change of the frontal lobe type, with such symptoms as disinhibition, puerile humor, perseveration, etc.

The remaining neurodegenerative disorders in the list are far less common than those just discussed, and most also have distinctive features. Both dentatorubropallidoluysian atrophy and choreoacanthocytosis cause chorea. Wilson's disease may cause a parkinsonian rigidity but this is generally accompanied by dysarthria or dystonia. In Fahr's syndrome, although parkinsonism may be seen in an isolated fashion, it is typically accompanied by other signs, such as ataxia (Nyland and Skre 1977) or intention tremor (Mathews 1957), and neuroimaging will reveal calcification of the basal ganglia. Alzheimer's disease may be complicated by a mild parkinsonism, but this occurs only many years after the typical dementia is well established. Adolescent-onset parkinsonism may occur with pantothenate kinase-associated neurodegeneration or in the Westphal variant of Huntington's disease, but in both cases other signs are typically also present, such as dystonia in pantothenate kinase-associated neurodegeneration and either dystonia or chorea in the Huntington's disease. Kufs' disease, a very rare disorder, may cause parkinsonism, but this is typically preceded by myoclonus and seizures. Lubag (also known as X-linked dystonia parkinsonism) is an X-linked disorder seen only in Filipino men, which typically presents with dystonia, followed by parkinsonism. Spinocerebellar ataxia type 2 may present with a combination of ataxia and parkinsonism or, very rarely, with parkinsonism alone. Rapid-onset dystonia–parkinsonism has a remarkable onset in adult years characterized by the appearance, over days or weeks, of a combination of parkinsonism and dystonia that subsequently settles into a stable chronicity. Hereditary mental depression and parkinsonism is a rare familial disorder that presents in midlife with depression, and which is joined, in a matter of years, by a gradually progressive parkinsonism and, eventually, hypoventilation. Guamian amyotrophic lateral sclerosis–parkinsonism complex is a rare disorder occurring exclusively in residents of Guam, parts of Japan, and some other Pacific islands.

Turning now to the group of medications capable of causing parkinsonism, the most frequent offenders by far are the antipsychotics. Among the antipsychotics, although first-generation agents (e.g., haloperidol or fluphenazine) are most likely to cause this side-effect, parkinsonism has also been caused by second-generation agents, such as risperidone or olanzapine (Carlson et al. 2003). Although in the vast majority of cases the parkinsonism gradually subsides after the discontinuation of treatment, in a small minority, primarily in the elderly, it may persist indefinitely (Bocola et al. 1996). Other dopamine blockers, such as metoclopramide or prochlorperazine may also cause parkinsonism, a fact often not appreciated by many physicians. When parkinsonism occurs in patients treated with dopamine blockers, the neuroleptic malignant syndrome, although rare, must also be considered: this syndrome typically presents with a delirium, followed shortly by parkinsonism and other symptoms such as coarse tremor, fever, tachycardia, labile hypertension, and diaphoresis. Although the vast majority of cases of the neuroleptic malignant syndrome are caused by treatment with antipsychotics (including clozapine [Miller et al. 1991]), cases have also occurred secondary to the withdrawal of dopaminergic agents such as amantadine (Cunningham et al. 1991; Harsch 1987) and levodopa (Sechi et al. 1984; Toru et al. 1981). Valproic acid may also cause parkinsonism, and, uniquely among medications capable of causing this side-effect, the parkinsonism here may be of delayed onset, after from 6 months to 4 years (Ristic et al. 2006), thus obscuring the causal role of the drug. The other medications listed in Table 3.8 only rarely cause parkinsonism.

The next group to consider are toxins and substances of abuse and the first to consider here is alcohol, wherein parkinsonism occurs not as a complication of alcohol intoxication but rather appears during the course of alcohol withdrawal in a small minority of cases. In evaluating chronic alcoholics who have parkinsonism, one should also consider the possibility that the patient, unable to obtain alcohol, may have used methanol: severe cases of methanol intoxication may be complicated by putaminal necrosis with parkinsonism. The next substance to consider is methylphenyltetrahydropyridine (MPTP): this is a contaminant of illicitly prepared meperidine (Langston *et al.* 1983), and addicts who injected the contaminated meperidine developed a parkinsonism of rapid onset. A final example of substances of abuse capable of causing parkinsonism are the inhalants, wherein, rarely, intoxication may be complicated by a parkinsonism that then persists. With regard to toxins *per se*, the classic offender is manganese. Manganese exposure may occur in manganese mines, steel mills, battery factories, or via drinking contaminated well water and may be followed, after a variable latent interval, by a gradually progressive parkinsonism. The parkinsonism itself is characterized primarily by rigidity and bradykinesia; tremor may be present but is only rarely of the pill-rolling type. Certain additional features may also be present, including dystonia and what is known as a 'cock-walk'. Dystonic rigidity may be found in the neck or in the face, creating a vacuous, rigid grin (Charles 1927). The cock-walk, which may be seen in up to one-third of patients (Abd El Naby and Hassanein 1965) stems from a dystonic rigidity of the feet, such that patients walk on their metatarsophalangeal joints (as if in high heels [Huang *et al.* 1997]), at times looking for all the world like they are imitating the walk of a rooster. Interestingly, manganese-induced parkinsonism may progress long after exposure has ceased (Huang *et al.* 1993). Another toxin to consider is cyanide, wherein exposure typically occurs after a suicidal overdose with potassium cyanide: in these cases, parkinsonism may ensue after a latent interval spanning from weeks (Rosenberg *et al.* 1989) to 1 year (Carella *et al.* 1988); in some cases, dystonia or athetosis may also be present (Rosenow *et al.* 1995). Finally, parkinsonism has also been reported secondary to exposure to the herbicide diquat and to organophosphate pesticides.

Other, more or less obvious, precipitating events include repeated head trauma, anoxia, carbon monoxide poisoning, and encephalitis. Repeated head trauma, as may occur in boxers, may be followed, after a latent interval of 5–40 years, by the gradual evolution of a condition known as 'dementia pugilistica', comprising parkinsonism, dysarthria, ataxia, and dementia. Anoxic coma may, in those who survive, be followed weeks to months later by parkinsonism characterized primarily by rigidity and bradykinesia. Carbon monoxide poisoning may also be followed by parkinsonism, generally after a latent interval of from days to weeks. Of the encephalitides associated with parkinsonism, the classic example is encephalitis lethargica, wherein parkinsonism occurred after a latent interval of 1–20 years, and was often accompanied by oculogyric crises and blepharospasm: importantly, although there have been no further epidemics of encephalitis lethargica since 1928, sporadic cases still occur (Howard and Lees 1987). Arboviral encephalitides associated with parkinsonism include western equine encephalitis, wherein parkinsonism may appear after a latent interval of from a week to several months, and Japanese encephalitis, wherein parkinsonism may appear not only as a delayed sequela but also as part of the acute encephalitic syndrome.

The final group to consider is the miscellaneous one, and of the disorders in this group, stroke may be considered first. Infarctions of the basal ganglia or of the midbrain (affecting the substantia nigra), rarely, have been noted to cause a contralateral hemiparkinsonism (Boecker *et al.* 1996; Fenelon and Houeto 1997; Kulisevsky *et al.* 1995). With multiple lacunar infarctions of the basal ganglia, one may also see vascular parkinsonism. This is a perhaps controversial entity, as some authors doubt its existence. There are, however, convincing reports of classic parkinsonism occurring in this setting (Bruetsch and Williams 1954; Keschner and Sloane 1931; Tolosa and Santamaria 1984; Zijlmans *et al.* 1995). In most cases, however, rather than a classic picture, the parkinsonism here is characterized primarily by rigidity and bradykinesia: tremor is usually absent, and evidence of damage to the corticospinal tracts (e.g., spasticity and hyper-reflexia) and corticobulbar tracts (pseudobulbar palsy) is generally present.

Liver disease may also, albeit rarely, be associated with parkinsonism. Acquired hepatocerebral degeneration, seen in patients with cirrhosis, typically causes a complex movement disorder, with postural tremor, athetosis, dystonia, ataxia, and, in a substantial minority, parkinsonism with prominent rigidity and bradykinesia. Acute hepatic encephalopathy, with elevated ammonia levels, may also cause parkinsonism, but this is relatively rare.

Niacin deficiency causes pellagra, and this may occur in two forms. When the deficiency develops slowly, 'classic' pellagra develops, with dementia, diarrhea and a rash on sun-exposed areas; when, however, the deficiency develops suddenly, 'encephalopathic' pellagra occurs, with delirium and parkinsonism, marked primarily by rigidity. This acute onset 'encephalopathic' pellagra is not accompanied by a rash (Ishii and Nishihara 1981) and, typically, is seen only in chronic alcoholics in developed countries.

Central pontine myelinolysis may be complicated by parkinsonism; however, as might be expected, this is not secondary to myelinolysis in the pons but to the 'extrapontine' myelinolysis that may also occur in this syndrome wherein the striatum is involved. Multiple sclerosis, rarely, may cause parkinsonism, in one case due to a midbrain plaque involving the subsantia nigra. The remaining disorders in Table 3.8 are each very rare causes of parkinsonism.

Differential diagnosis

A fully developed, classic parkinsonism is distinctive and very difficult to confuse with other movement disorders. Difficulty, however, may arise when only fragments of the syndrome are present, as may be the case early on in the evolution of the syndrome. Thus, care must be taken to distinguish the rest tremor of parkinsonism from a postural tremor, as may be seen, say, in essential tremor. Care must also be taken to distinguish the shuffling gait of parkinsonism from the 'magnetic' gait seen in patients with hydrocephalus, wherein the feet seem stuck or magnetized to the floor. Further, in patients who present primarily with rigidity a careful distinction must be made with dystonia: parkinsonian rigidity, as noted earlier, is typically accompanied by the phenomenon of cogwheeling, something not seen in dystonia; furthermore, the rigidity of parkinsonism does not contort the limb, hand or foot, in contrast with dystonia, for which such contortions are the rule.

Treatment

Most of the disorders listed in Table 3.8 are discussed in their respective chapters, and, as pointed out in those chapters, symptomatic treatment, if required, is generally similar to that utilized in Parkinson's disease, involving use of levodopa, direct-acting dopaminergic agents or perhaps anticholinergics. Of note, levodopa is almost always effective in Parkinson's disease, and thus if a patient with parkinsonism fails to respond to levodopa then it is unlikely that the parkinsonism in question is occurring on the basis of Parkinson's disease. In the case of parkinsonism secondary to medications, discontinuation of the offending drug is generally in order; however, in some cases, in particular where antipsychotics are involved, this may not be possible: here, treatment with the anticholinergic benztropine is generally effective.

3.9 AKINESIA

The term 'akinesia' is, essentially, synonymous with 'bradykinesia', but is preferentially used when this phenomenon is 'pure' and unaccompanied by other signs or symptoms, in particular when it appears in the absence of parkinsonism.

Clinical features

In motor akinesia, both the initiation and execution of actions are slowed, as if the patient were encased in molasses. All activities may be affected, including talking, walking, or getting dressed. In cognitive (or, as it is sometimes called, 'psychic') akinesia, thoughts are likewise slow to appear and the 'stream' of thought is quite sluggish: some patients may complain of feeling like a 'zombie'.

Etiology

The causes of akinesia are listed in Table 3.9. Of all of these, by far the most common cause is treatment with a

Table 3.9 Causes of akinesia

Antipsychotic medications (Rifkin et al. 1975; Van Putten and May 1978)
Stroke (infarction or hemorrhage of the caudate nucleus) (Kumral et al. 1999)
Post-anoxic (Feve et al. 1993)
Neurodegenerative disorders
Progressive supranuclear palsy (Matsuo et al. 1991)
Pantothenate kinase-associated neurodegeneration (Molinuevo et al. 2003)

first-generation antipsychotic, in which case the akinesia generally develops slowly, over days or weeks, following initiation of treatment or a substantial dose increase. Pure akinesia may also occur with infarction or hemorrhage of the caudate nucleus and has been noted as a rare sequela to anoxic coma, wherein patients suffered necrosis of the globus pallidus. Finally, pure akinesia has rarely occurred as a 'forme fruste' of both progressive supranuclear palsy and of pantothenate kinase-associated neurodegeneration, without any of the symptoms typical of these disorders, such as parkinsonism or dystonia.

Differential diagnosis

The most important differential consideration is the syndrome of parkinsonism, and in evaluating patients with akinesia a careful search must be made for symptoms such as a flexion posture, tremor, shuffling gait, rigidity, or postural instability: the presence of any of these in an akinetic patient indicates parkinsonism, and the differential should then proceed as outlined in Section 3.8.

Other syndromes to consider include akinetic mutism, abulia, depression, and hypothyroidism. In akinetic mutism, there is essentially a total failure to initiate any activity, whereas with akinesia, in contrast, activity does occur, albeit after a delay. In abulia, there is also a failure to initiate activity; however, here, if patients are closely supervised, activity, once initiated, proceeds at a normal rate, in contrast with akinesia, wherein the execution of activity remains slow. Depression, when marked by psychomotor retardation, may present a picture quite similar to akinesia; however, here one sees other symptoms, such as depressed mood, fatigue, insomnia, etc., symptoms that are absent in akinesia. Finally, hypothyroidism, when severe, may cause a slowing of both activity and thought, thus mimicking akinesia; here, however, one sees other typical symptoms and signs, such as cold sensitivity, constipation, hoarseness, hair loss, puffiness, and bradycardia.

Treatment

Akinesia secondary to antipsychotics typically responds to treatment with the anticholinergic benztropine in doses of from 1 to 3 mg daily. The treatment of akinesia occurring from other causes is not well worked out; consideration might be given to a trial of benztropine or, should that fail, levodopa.

3.10 AKATHISIA

Akathisia, a term coined by Ladislav Haskovec in 1901 (Hascovec 1901), is derived from the Greek, and means, literally, 'an inability to sit still'. This is a very important syndrome to recognize, given that it may be disabling and that it is, in general, eminently treatable.

Clinical features

As described by multiple authors (Ayd 1961; Braude *et al.* 1983; Gibb and Lees 1986; Halstead *et al.* 1994; Sachdev and Kruk 1994), akathisia is characterized by a sense of restlessness and an inability to keep still; there is a dysphoric feeling of having to move, and, in most cases, this 'compulsion' to move is translated into action in various ways. If seated, patients shift restlessly from one position to another and may tap their feet or repeatedly cross and uncross their legs or arms. If standing, patients may rock back and forth, shifting their weight alternatively from one foot to another, or may actually 'march in place'. Restless pacing may occur as patients give way to the irresistible impulsion to move about. In almost all cases, this restless urge to pace or move about is worse when seated, and worst when lying down, most patients obtaining at least some relief by standing up. Coupled with this motoric restlessness, many patients also experience a 'cognitive' or 'psychic' akathisia manifest by restless thoughts: thoughts come too fast, are crowded and may shoot about the mind 'like ping-pong balls'. In some cases, this buzzing jumble of thoughts defies expression in speech and patients may become mute.

Although mild akathisia may be tolerable to some patients, more extreme forms may become unbearable, resulting in suicide attempts (Drake and Ehrlich 1985; Rothschild and Locke 1991) or assaultive behavior (Siris 1985).

The appearance of akathisia may also exacerbate symptoms of other illnesses. For example, when antipsychotics are given to patients with Tourette's syndrome to ameliorate tics, the subsequent appearance of an akathisia may lead to an exacerbation of the tics themselves (Weiden and Bruin 1987). Furthermore, patients with schizophrenia who develop an akathisia may experience a dramatic exacerbation of their psychotic symptoms (Van Putten 1975; Van Putten *et al.* 1974). Importantly, patients with schizophrenia who experience an akathisia-mediated exacerbation of their illness may neither appear restless nor complain of restlessness if questioned (Weiden and Bruin 1987): in one of the author's patients with schizophrenia, an akathisia manifested with muteness and withdrawal,

Table 3.10 Causes of akathisia

Medications:
Antipsychotics (including both acute akathisia [Van Putten *et al.* 1984] and tardive akathisia [Dufresene and Wagner 1988; Hershon *et al.* 1972; Lang 1994])
Droperidol (Foster *et al.* 1996)
Prochlorperazine (Fleishman *et al.* 1994)
Metoclopramide (Fleishman *et al.* 1994; Jungmann and Schofflang 1982)
Selective serotonin reuptake inhibitors (SSRIs) (e.g., fluoxetine [Lipinski *et al.* 1989], paroxetine [Baldassano *et al.* 1996])
Diltiazam (Jacobs 1983)
Interferon-alpha (Horikawa *et al.* 1999)

Parkinson's disease (Comella and Goetz 1994; Lang and Johnson 1987)

Basal ganglia lesions (Stuppaeck *et al.* 1995)

and it was only after treatment with propranolol that the patient was able to describe the akathetic 'chaos of thoughts' that had besieged her.

Akathisia often goes undiagnosed, especially if it is mild (Fleishman *et al.* 1994). Consequently, whenever antipsychotics, other dopamine blockers, or selective serotonin reuptake inhibitors (SSRIs) are prescribed it is important to subsequently enquire after any motoric or cognitive restlessness.

Etiology

Of the various causes of akathisia listed in Table 3.10, by far the most common are medications: among these medications, antipsychotics are the major offenders. Akathisia secondary to antipsychotics may occur either acutely or, as tardive akathisia, after chronic treatment. Acute antipsychotic-induced akathisia, although most commonly seen with first-generation antipsychotics, such as haloperidol, has, albeit rarely, also been noted with second-generation agents, such as olanzapine (Jauss *et al.* 1998) and quetiapine (Catalano *et al.* 2005). Typically, symptoms appear some 5–6 days after initiating treatment or substantially increasing the dose (Sachdev and Kruk 1994): exceptions to this rule, however, do occur, with some cases arising in the first day and others being delayed for up to a month (Van Putten *et al.* 1984). Tardive akathisia, a variant of tardive dyskinesia, is symptomatically similar to acute akathisia (Burke *et al.* 1989) and appears gradually, generally only after a year or more of treatment with an antipsychotic; tardive akathisia has also been noted after chronic treatment with metoclopramide (Shearer *et al.* 1984).

In all likelihood, akathisia induced by antipsychotics is secondary to dopamine blockade and, as might be expected, other dopamine blockers may also cause this syndrome, including droperidol, prochlorperazine, and metoclopramide. The SSRIs have also been associated with akathisia, and in this situation the underlying mechanism may involve decreased activity of mesencephalic ventral tegmental dopaminergic neurons secondary to serotoninergically mediated inhibition. The other two medications in Table 3.10, namely diltiazem and alpha-interferon, have only rarely been associated with akathisia.

Parkinson's disease may cause akathisia, and here the diagnosis may be elusive given that the typical motor restlessness may be obscured by bradykinesia. Consequently, patients must be questioned closely regarding both any 'inner' sense of restlessness and any evidence of cognitive akathisia.

Finally, akathisia has been reported secondary to bilateral necrosis of the basal ganglia after carbon monoxide intoxication.

Differential diagnosis

The restless legs syndrome may be confused with akathisia as there is in both cases motor restlessness and a tendency to pace the floor. Patients with the restless legs syndrome, however, generally experience parasthesiae in the legs and find some relief in rubbing their feet, characteristics not seen in akathisia; conversely, patients with akathisia often 'march in place', a sign not seen in the restless legs syndrome (Walters et al. 1991).

Agitation (as may be seen in disorders such as schizophrenia, 'agitated' depression, mania, dementia, delirium, and traumatic brain injury) is typically accompanied by restlessness, and in cases when patients with one of these disorders are treated with an antipsychotic or an SSRI, as is very often the case, the differential question can become quite acute. A common scenario involves a patient with agitation who is given an antipsychotic, initially improves, then, days later, becomes more agitated, and the question here is whether the increasing agitation is due to the underlying disorder or to an antipsychotic-induced akathisia. In some of these cases, the appearance of a tendency to 'march in place' or of complaints of a worsening of symptoms upon being seated or lying down, may suggest the correct diagnosis, but when these clues are absent the differential may not be possible on clinical grounds and a 'diagnosis by treatment response' may be in order. As noted below, akathisia responds well to treatment with various agents, and a prompt clinical improvement after initiation of, say, propranolol, would strongly suggest that the correct diagnosis is akathisia.

As noted above, patients with schizophrenia may experience an exacerbation of their psychotic symptoms due to akathisia, and when this occurs, as it may at times, without any motor restlessness, the only clue to the diagnosis may be that the exacerbation of the psychotic symptoms occurred days after the initiation of an antipsychotic or a substantial dose increase. Should the diagnosis here be missed, a 'vicious cycle' may ensue: believing that the increase in psychotic symptoms was secondary to the underlying schizophrenia, the physician may increase the dose of the antipsychotic, thus causing a worsening of the akathisia, and a worsening of the psychosis. Whenever there is doubt here, a 'diagnosis by treatment response', as just described above, is probably in order.

A similar scenario may also occur in patients with depression who are treated with an SSRI. Here, and again days or a week or more after beginning the SSRI, the patient may complain of an increase in suicidal ideation, or, in some cases, may experience suicidal ideation de novo. In such cases, the concurrent appearance of any restlessness, whether motoric or cognitive, should prompt an attempt at 'diagnosis by treatment response'.

Treatment

With regard to medication-induced akathisia, consideration may be given to either discontinuing the offending medication or substantially reducing the dose (Braude et al. 1983). When this is impractical or when the clinical situation demands immediate relief, any one of a large number of medications may be considered. Propranolol remains the standard, and is generally effective in total daily doses of 20–80 mg (Adler et al. 1985, 1986, 1993; Lipinski et al. 1984); provided that the drug is well tolerated, and only partial relief has been obtained, higher doses may be utilized. Mirtazapine, in a dose of 15 mg, appears similar to propranolol (Poyurovsky et al. 2006). Benztropine, in doses of from 1 to 3 mg may be utilized (Adler et al. 1993; DiMascio et al. 1976) but anticholinergic side-effects make this less attractive. Cyproheptadine, in a dose of 8 mg b.i.d. is also effective (Fischel et al. 2001), but sedation may prove a limiting factor. Clonazepam, in doses of 0.5–2.5 mg/day, is another alternative (Kutcher et al. 1989). Vitamin B6 is also effective; however, the doses required are high, ranging from 600 to 1200 mg/day (Lerner et al. 2004) and at these doses toxicity may ensue, with the development of a sensory neuropathy (Parry and Bredesen 1985).

The treatment of tardive akathisia is discussed in Section 22.2.

The treatment of akathisia secondary to Parkinson's disease is not well worked out; consideration may be given to propranolol (Adler et al. 1991) or one of the other agents mentioned above.

3.11 CATATONIA

The term catatonia was coined by the German psychiatrist Karl Kahlbaum in 1874, who described it in patients with schizophrenia. Since then, however, it has become quite apparent that schizophrenia, although one of the more common causes of catatonia, constitutes but one of the many etiologies of this syndrome.

Clinical features

Catatonia, as described by Kraepelin in 1899 (Kraepelin 1990) and Bleuler (1924), occurs in one of two forms: stuporous (or retarded) catatonia and excited catatonia (Morrison 1973). The stuporous form is the most common, and will be described first.

STUPOROUS CATATONIA

The cardinal signs of stuporous catatonia are immobility, waxy flexibility (also known as cataplexy or *cerea flexibalitas*) and mutism. Associated symptoms include posturing, 'echo' phenomena (i.e. echolalia and echopraxia), negativism, and automatic obedience.

Immobility in catatonic stupor may persist for hours, days, or longer, with little or no change in the patient's position. Some may simply lie in bed, their legs rigidly extended and adducted; others may almost curl up into a ball, resting on the floor, a chair or the bed. The eyes may be open or closed; if the eyes are open, patients often stare fixedly ahead. Patients may not move even to relieve themselves and may become foul with urine or feces. Some may not even swallow, allowing saliva or food to dribble from their mouths; indeed, if food is placed in the mouth, there is a risk of aspiration, which may be fatal (Bort 1976). Importantly, although patients appear to lack conscious activity, most remain alert, and some, upon recovery, may evidence an astonishingly accurate recall of events that occurred during the stupor. Interestingly, a patient's immobility may occasionally undergo a sudden lysis: for example, if a ball is gently thrown to an immobile patient, the patient may suddenly loosen up and catch the ball.

Waxy flexibility derives its name from the fact that, upon passive movement of the limbs, the examiner encounters a rigidity similar to what one would expect upon bending a waxen object, such as a softened candle. In most cases, in addition to this waxy flexibility, one also finds that the patient's limbs tend to stay in whatever position the examiner places them, no matter how uncomfortable and regardless of whether or not the examiner instructs the patient to maintain the position of the limb. Bleuler (1924) recommended a bedside test for waxy flexibility that involved taking 'the patient's pulse and, as if inadvertently, "holding" his arm high and extended. Then, after taking the pulse rate, I release the arm.' The test was considered to be positive when the patient's arm remained suspended in essentially the same position. Another bedside test involves checking for the presence of a 'psychological pillow'. Here, when the patient is lying supine in bed with the head resting on a pillow, the head is lifted slightly and the pillow removed. In a positive test, the patient's head remains in essentially the same position, as if the pillow were still present.

Mutism in catatonic stupor ranges from partial to complete. Those with only partial mutism may mumble or whisper incomprehensible words or phrases.

Posturing is said to occur when patients automatically and spontaneously assume more or less bizarre postures, which are then maintained. The arms may be spread in a cruciform position, or the head thrown back in full extension; some may huddle into balls or stand, stork-like, on one leg.

Echo phenomena, as noted, consist of either echolalia, wherein the patient automatically, and without prompting, repeats back what the examiner said, or echopraxia, wherein, again without prompting, the patient automatically mimics the examiner's movements, gestures, or posture.

Negativism does not represent mere contrariness, stubbornness or passive aggressiveness, for in each of these phenomena, patients have not lost control and may be able to cooperate in situations that, to them, appear to be to their advantage. In contrast, negativism presents as a mulish, almost instinctual tendency to resist, which may be either passive, wherein the patient, in response to a command, simply does nothing, or active, wherein the patient does the opposite of what is requested. Negativistic patients may refuse to come to an interview, take a bath, change their clothes, take medicines, or even eat food placed in front of them. In extreme cases, negativism may extend to the patient's own urges, leading, for example, to extreme constipation with fecal impaction. Patients with active negativism may get up from a table when food is placed on it or may back out of a doorway if asked to walk through it. Typically, there is no 'reasoning' with negativistic patients, as they generally remain mute and inaccessible.

Automatic obedience represents, in a sense, the converse of negativism, in that these patients automatically do what is expected of them, without question or hesitation, regardless of whether the consequences are absurd or harmful. This is far from mere agreeableness as patients often seem to behave in a robotic or automaton-like manner.

EXCITED CATATONIA

Excited catatonia is characterized by bizarre, frenzied, and purposeless hyperactivity. Uninvolved with others, almost sealed off in their own world, patients may gesticulate, march in place or loudly declaim; verbigeration (rapid, bizarre, and senseless speech) may also occur.

In rare instances, excited catatonia may undergo a progression into a condition known as Stauder's lethal catatonia. Here there is an escalation in the hyperactivity, followed by fever, tachycardia, hypotension, and leukocytosis, and in some cases death (Castillo *et al.* 1989; Mann *et al.* 1986). The recognition of this syndrome is critical, for even when the patient is *in extremis* (with temperatures as high as 41°C [106°F]), treatment with electroconvulsive therapy may result in recovery (Aronson and Thompson 1950).

Etiology

The various causes of stuporous catatonia and of excited catatonia are listed in Table 3.11.

Table 3.11 Causes of catatonia

Stuporous catatonia

Schizophrenia (Johnson 1984; Morrison 1973)

Depressive episode of either major depressive disorder or
bipolar disorder (Barnes *et al.* 1986)

Manic episode of bipolar disorder (Abrams and Taylor 1976;
Taylor and Abrams 1977)

Periodic catatonia (Gjessing 1974)

Medications
  Antipsychotics (Weinberger and Wyatt 1978)
  Disulfiram (Reisberg 1978; Weddington *et al.* 1980)
  Ciprofloxacin (Akhtar and Ahmad 1993)
  Azithromycin (Plana *et al.* 2006)
  Levetiracetam (Chouinard *et al.* 2006)
  Benzodiazepine withdrawal (Rosebush and Mazurek 1996)

Epileptic conditions
  Complex partial seizures (Engel *et al.* 1978; Gomez *et al.*
    1982; Lim *et al.* 1986; Shah and Kaplan 1980)
  Post-ictal psychosis (Logsdail and Toone 1988)
  Interictal psychosis (Kristensen and Sindrup 1979; Slater
    and Beard 1963)
  Psychosis of forced normalization (Pakainis *et al.* 1987)

Viral encephalitis
  Herpes simplex encephalitis (Raskin and Frank 1974)
  Encephalitis lethargica (Bond 1920; Kirby and Davis 1921)

Miscellaneous conditions
  Stroke (Saver *et al.* 1993)
  Vitamin B12 deficiency (Berry *et al.* 2003)
  Wilson's disease (Davis and Borde 1993)
  Systemic lupus erythematosus (Lanham *et al.* 1985; Mac
    and Pardo 1983)
  Limbic encephalitis (Tandon *et al.* 1988)
  Hepatic encephalopathy (Jaffe 1967)
  Lyme disease (Pfister *et al.* 1993)
  Subacute sclerosing panencephalitis (Koehler and Jakumeit
    1976)
  Tay–Sachs disease (Rosebush *et al.* 1995)
  Thrombotic thrombocytopenic purpura (Read 1983)

Excited catatonia

Schizophrenia (Morrison 1973)

Viral encephalitis (Penn *et al.* 1972)

STUPOROUS CATATONIA

The overwhelming majority of cases of stuporous catatonia occur in the course of schizophrenia, a manic episode of bipolar disorder, or a depressive episode of either major depressive disorder or bipolar disorder; in the case of depression, catatonia is more likely to occur in elderly patients (Starkstein *et al.* 1996). These diagnoses are made primarily on the basis of the clinical context within which the catatonia occurs. In the case of schizophrenia one finds a preceding

psychosis, in mania, a preceding syndrome of stages I and II of mania, and in a depressive episode, a preceding typical depressive syndrome. It must be emphasized that obtaining a history from family or others is indispensable in making these diagnoses. Periodic catatonia may also be mentioned here; this is a very rare condition characterized, as the name suggests, by recurrent episodes of catatonia; recent research suggests a genetic basis (Stober *et al.* 2002).

Of the medications that are capable of causing stuporous catatonia, by far the most common offenders are the antipsychotics, especially high-potency first-generation agents, such as haloperidol, used in high dosage (e.g., over 20 mg) (Gelenberg and Mandel 1977). Disulfiram must also be kept in mind, as the diagnosis may be obscured by the fact that disulfiram-induced catatonia may not appear for months after the disulfiram has been administered. Catatonia secondary to ciprofloxacin, azithromycin, and levetiracetam are very rare events. Although benzodiazepine treatment *per se* does not cause catatonia, this syndrome may occur in a very small minority of patients going through benzodiazepine withdrawal.

Epileptic conditions capable of causing stuporous catatonia include complex partial seizures, post-ictal psychosis, interictal psychosis, and the rare psychosis of forced normalization.

Complex partial seizures, in addition to the typical confusion, may manifest with catatonia. The diagnosis is suggested immediately by the paroxysmal onset of the disturbance, and, in most cases, by its relatively brief duration. It must be borne in mind, however, that some cases of complex partial status epilepticus with catatonia may persist for days or even longer.

Post-ictal psychosis is generally seen only after a flurry of grand mal or complex partial seizures, and may rarely present with catatonia. Typically, there is a lucid interval, lasting for days, between the last seizure and the onset of the psychosis, and the psychosis itself generally persists for days to months before spontaneously remitting.

Interictal psychosis is a chronic condition that evolves gradually only after many years of uncontrolled epilepsy and which may, rarely, present with catatonia.

The psychosis of forced normalization is a very rare disorder occurring in patients with uncontrolled epilepsy, which has been brought under control with aggressive treatment with AEDs, with the clinical improvement being accompanied by a 'forced normalization' of the electroencephalogram (EEG). Once again, and rarely, this may present with catatonia. The diagnosis is suggested by the seemingly paradoxical onset of a psychosis after the seizures have been stopped; further support for the diagnosis comes by comparing an EEG that has been carried out during the psychosis with one performed before aggressive anti-epileptic treatment and finding the 'normalization'.

Viral encephalitis may present with stuporous catatonia (Barnes *et al.* 1986; Kim and Perlstein 1970; Misra and Hay 1971; Wilson 1976), with the diagnosis being suggested by fever and headache, and this has been noted with herpes simplex viral encephalitis and encephalitis lethargica (although there have been no further epidemic cases of encephalitis lethargica since 1928, sporadic cases still occur; the most recent case with catatonia was reported in 2000 [Shill and Stacy 2000]).

The miscellaneous causes of stuporous catatonia are quite heterogeneous. Regarding catatonia occurring in stroke, a case of 'hemicatatonia' was noted with infarction of the parietal cortex. Furthermore, in about 2 percent of acute stroke patients waxy flexibility was found ipsilateral to the infarcted hemisphere, with a hemiparesis contralaterally (Saposnik *et al.* 1999): it must be noted that in these cases, the only catatonic symptom found was waxy flexibility, and that had to be specifically sought after. The other causes listed in Table 3.11 only very rarely cause catatonia.

EXCITED CATATONIA

Excited catatonia is seen virtually exclusively in schizophrenia; I could find only one convincing case due to another cause, namely in a patient with eastern equine encephalitis (see Table 3.11).

With regard to schizophrenia, it must be kept in mind that, over long periods of time, patients may have alternating episodes of either stuporous or excited catatonia.

Differential diagnosis

The differential diagnosis of the stuporous and excited forms of catatonia are quite different, and thus each is treated separately.

STUPOROUS CATATONIA

Stuporous catatonia must be distinguished from stupor of other causes, akinetic mutism, abulia, and the neuroleptic malignant syndrome.

Stupor of other cause is generally associated with a decreased level of consciousness, in contrast with the alertness seen in catatonia. Furthermore, in stupor eye movements may be roving, in contrast with the preservation of saccadic eye movements in catatonia.

Akinetic mutism, being characterized by immobility and mutism in an alert patient, is clearly quite similar to catatonia, and the clinical distinction may rest on the demonstration of waxy flexibility or associated catatonic symptoms, such as posturing, echo phenomena or negativism – symptoms not seen in akinetic mutism.

Abulia, may, at first glance, appear similar to catatonia, in that abulic patients, lacking any motivation or initiative, may be immobile. The diagnosis is readily apparent upon merely urging the patient to act: the abulic patient will comply, and continue to comply, with instructions (provided that supervision is ongoing), whereas with the catatonic patient there will be no response.

The neuroleptic malignant syndrome may be included in the differential when patients are treated with antipsychotics.

Rigidity is present, and may be either lead pipe or cogwheeling in character: when lead-pipe rigidity is present, the picture may resemble catatonia; however, the rigidity seen in the neuroleptic malignant syndrome is not accompanied by a tendency for the limbs to maintain whatever position they were placed in. Other symptoms, typical of the neuroleptic malignant syndrome, but not seen in uncomplicated catatonia, may also appear and aid in the differential: these include confusion, fever, and autonomic instability.

EXCITED CATATONIA

Excited catatonia must be distinguished from mania and from simple agitation.

Mania, during stages I and II, is marked by hyperactivity, however here the activity is purposeful and not bizarre. Furthermore, in stages I and II of mania one also finds symptoms such as heightened mood and pressure of speech, which are absent in excited catatonia. In some cases of stage III mania, however, the hyperactivity may fragment and lose purpose, and in these cases the differential may rest on obtaining a history of the preceding, typical, stages I and II.

Agitation typically is not characterized by bizarreness, which is always seen in excited catatonia.

Treatment

In cases of stuporous catatonia in which treatment of the underlying cause is ineffective or for which emergent treatment is required, consideration may be given to either lorazepam or electroconvulsive therapy (ECT). Most cases of stuporous catatonia will show prompt, albeit temporary, improvement, with parenteral lorazepam (e.g., 2 mg i.v.) (Bush *et al.* 1996; Rosebush *et al.* 1990; Salam *et al.* 1987); more lasting improvement may follow a course of ECT (Bush *et al.* 1996; Malur *et al.* 2001). Pending improvement, a careful watch must be maintained for dehydration, deep venous thrombosis with pulmonary embolism, and aspiration pneumonia.

Excited catatonia, as noted above, is seen almost exclusively in schizophrenia, and treatment proceeds as outlined in Section 20.1.

3.12 ASTERIXIS

Asterixis, first described by Adams and Foley in 1953, is a very important diagnostic sign as, in most cases, it indicates a metabolic encephalopathy due to hepatic, renal, or respiratory failure.

Clinical features

Asterixis represents a precipitous loss of muscle tone (Adams and Foley 1949; Leavitt and Tyler 1964) and is typically tested for by asking patients to hold their arms straight to the front with the hands hyperextended at the wrist as far back as possible, and holding that position for at least 30 seconds. When asterixis is present, there will be arrhythmically occurring 'flaps' of the hands down, followed, after a brief, but distinct, moment, by recovery back to the hyperextended position; although in most cases both hands will 'flap' down simultaneously, occasionally asterixis will be strictly unilateral, a finding with, as discussed below, considerable diagnostic significance. In cases where patients are unable to hold their arms forward, an alternative approach to eliciting asterixis involves having the patient rest the arms prone on the bed and then asking him or her to hyperextend the hands off the bed, again holding that position for at least 30 seconds.

Etiology

As noted in Table 3.12, asterixis may be seen in the course of a metabolic encephalopathy, such as hepatic encephalopathy, as a side-effect to various medications, and during the course of stroke due either to infarction or hemorrhage. From a diagnostic point of view it is critical to keep in mind whether the asterixis is bilateral or unilateral. Asterixis occurring in the course of a metabolic encephalopathy or as a side-effect is always bilateral; asterixis occurring as part of

Table 3.12 Causes of asterixis

Metabolic encephalopathy
Hepatic encephalopathy (Adams and Foley 1949, 1953; Read *et al.* 1961)
Uremic encephalopathy (Mahoney and Arieff 1982; Raskin and Fishman 1976; Tyler 1965)
Respiratory failure (Austen *et al.* 1957; Bacchus 1958)

Medication side-effect
Phenytoin (Chi *et al.* 2000; Murphy and Goldstein 1974)
Carbamazepine (Rittmannsberger and Lebihuber 1992)
Gabapentin (Babiy *et al.* 2005)
Pregabalin (Heckmann *et al.* 2005)
Valproate (Bodensteiner *et al.* 1981)
Lithium (Stewart and Williams 2000)
Levodopa (Glantz *et al.* 1982)
Clozapine (Rittsmannberger 1996)
Trimethoprim/sulfamethoxazole (Dib *et al.* 2004)
Ifosfamide (Meyer *et al.* 2002)
Metrizamide (Bertoni *et al.* 1981)

Infarction or hemorrhage
Cortex
Basal ganglia
Internal capsule
Thalamus
Midbrain
Pons
Cerebellum

a stroke syndrome, although occasionally bilateral, is, in the vast majority of cases, unilateral. Thus, if a patient has unilateral asterixis, the presumption must be that it is occurring secondary to infarction or hemorrhage in one of the areas described below.

Of the metabolic encephalopathies, hepatic encephalopathy is so commonly associated with asterixis that, for a time, the term 'liver flap' was used as a synonym for asterixis. Uremic encephalopathy is almost always associated with asterixis; in cases of respiratory failure, however, it may be less common.

Of the medications capable of causing asterixis as a side-effect, the AEDs and lithium are the most frequent offenders, with the other agents only uncommonly being implicated. Metrizamide myelography may be followed by a delirium accompanied by asterixis.

Infarction or hemorrhage of the cortex (most commonly the frontal cortex), basal ganglia, internal capsule, thalamus, midbrain, pons, and cerebellum may each cause asterixis, which, as noted above, is generally unilateral, and, with the exception of cerebellar lesions, is contralateral to the lesion (Degos *et al.* 1979; Kim *et al.* 2001b; Rio *et al.* 1995; Stell *et al.* 1994; Tatu *et al.* 2000). Notably, of all these areas, it is the thalamus that is most commonly involved.

Differential diagnosis

Myoclonus is distinguished by the fact that it represents not an abrupt loss of tone with a 'flap' down but rather an abrupt gain of tone with a resultant 'jerk'. Tremor is distinguished by the presence of a more or less rhythmic oscillatory movement secondary to alternating contraction of agonist and antagonist musculature.

Treatment

Treatment is directed at the underlying condition; symptomatic treatment is not required.

3.13 MIRROR MOVEMENTS

Mirror movements are normal in early childhood and may persist into adult years; they may also be seen in certain disorders, for example stroke with hemiparesis.

Clinical features

Mirror movements are typically seen in the hands, and may in some cases involve the arm. They may be elicited by asking patients to perform a fine motor task with one hand, for example sequential finger–thumb apposition. As the patient performs the maneuver, simply observe the other hand for the mirrored movement. With hemiparetic patients, a simpler strategy involves telling the patient you are going to test grip strength in one hand at a time. Then place the second and third fingers of each of your hands into the patient's hands and ask the patient to grip with only one hand. Mirror gripping may then be appreciated in the other hand. Interestingly, such mirroring in hemiparetic patients is most commonly seen in the unaffected hand (Nelles et al. 1998).

Etiology

Mirror movements, as noted, are normal in young children, and may persist into adult years; in some cases a familial tendency is noted (Rasmussen 1993). Mirror movements may also be seen in Kallmann's syndrome (Krams et al. 1999), the Klippel–Feil syndrome, Parkinson's disease (Espay et al. 2005b) and, most notably, in stroke patients with hemiparesis (Nelles et al. 1998).

Differential diagnosis

There is no other sign or symptom that mimics mirror movements.

Treatment

Treatment is rarely required; anecdotally, motor retraining has been successful (Cincotta et al. 2003).

3.14 PATHOLOGIC STARTLE

Although a startle response is a normal human reaction, in some cases it may, in one fashion or another, be exaggerated, in which case it is appropriate to speak of 'pathologic startle'.

Clinical features

The startle response is a brief, but sudden and violent, reaction to an unexpected stimulus, such as a loud noise or a bright light; in severe cases, a mere touch, as a tap on the shoulder, may be sufficient. During the startle response, the eyes blink, the face contorts in a grimace, there is flexion of the neck and trunk, and flexion and abduction of the arms; in severe cases, patients may be thrown off balance and fall.

Etiology

The various causes of pathologic startle are listed in Table 3.13; in pursuing this differential, the first step is to ascertain whether or not in between the episodes of pathologic startle there is a persistent state of autonomic

Table 3.13   Causes of pathologic startle

Post-traumatic stress disorder
Generalized anxiety disorder
Alcohol or sedative hypnotic withdrawal

Sympathomimetics
Hyperekplexia (Brown et al. 1991; Saenz-Lope et al. 1984; Tijssen et al. 2002)
Brainstem lesions (see text)
Post-anoxic encephalopathy (Brown et al. 1991)
Traumatic brain injury (Brown et al. 1991)
Creutzfeldt–Jakob disease (Hansen et al. 1998)
'Jumping Frenchmen of Maine' (Saint-Hilaire et al. 1986)
Latah (Bartholomew 1994)
Myriachit (Stevens 1965)

hyperactivity, with anxiety and a greater or lesser degree of tremulousness, as this persistent state is characteristic of the most common causes of pathologic startle, namely post-traumatic stress disorder, generalized anxiety disorder, alcohol or sedative-hypnotic withdrawal, and various sympathomimetics, such as caffeine (Howard and Ford 1992).

The other conditions listed in Table 3.13 generally do not leave the patient with persistent autonomic symptoms. Hyperekplexia is an inherited disorder, generally following an autosomal dominant pattern, which, in the 'major' form, has an onset in early infancy, and in the 'minor' form, in childhood. Brainstem lesions may also cause pathologic startle, and this has been noted with pontine lesions, such as infarction (Kimber and Thompson 1997) or a plaque of multiple sclerosis (Ruprecht et al. 2002), or with upper medullary lesions, such as demyelinization (Della Marca et al. 2007); compression of either the pons (Gambardella et al. 1999) or medulla (Salvi et al. 2000) by an ectatic artery may also be at fault. Post-anoxic encephalopathy, traumatic brain injury, and Creutzfeldt–Jakob disease may all be associated with startle, and the diagnosis is suggested by the associated cognitive deficits.

Finally, there are several 'culture-bound' syndromes wherein individuals who are normally shy, may, in response to an unexpected and 'startling' stimulus, engage in remarkable behavior characterized not only by pathologic startle, but also by other distinctive behaviors, such as cursing, swearing and, at times, echolalia. These are generally considered voluntary behaviors and have been noted, famously, among French–Canadian lumberjacks of the nineteenth century (the 'Jumping Frenchmen of Maine'), and in residents of Malaysia (where it is referred to as 'latah') and Siberia (where it has been termed 'myriachit').

Differential diagnosis

A startle reaction is a normal human response, and can be elicited in most individuals by a stimulus such as an unexpected gunshot; pathologic startle should be considered present only when the startle response is severe, frequent, and provoked by relatively minor stimuli.

Startle epilepsy (Aguglia *et al* 1984; Gimenez-Roldan and Martin 1980; Manford *et al.* 1996; Saenz-Lope *et al.* 1984) may be confused with pathologic startle. Startle epilepsy represents a form of reflex epilepsy, wherein a startling stimulus is followed first by a startle response and then by a tonic seizure. The differential is fairly easy if the patient is observed, and on two counts: first, in the tonic seizure, one sees, not flexion, but extension; second, there is loss of consciousness during the tonic seizure.

Treatment

Treatment is directed at the underlying cause; when this is ineffective, clonazepam may be utilized.

REFERENCES

Abad V, Ovsiew F. Treatment of persistent myoclonic tardive dystonia with verapamil. *Br J Psychiatry* 1993; **162**:554 6.

Abd El Naby S, Hassanein M. Neuropsychiatric manifestations of chronic manganism. *J Neurol Neurosurg Psychiatry* 1965; **28**:282–5.

Abrams R, Taylor MA. Catatonia. A prospective clinical study. *Arch Gen Psychiatry* 1976; **33**:579–81.

Adams RD, Foley J. The neurological changes in the more common types of liver disease. *Trans Am Neurol Assoc* 1949; **74**:217–19.

Adams RD, Foley JM. The neurological disorder associated with liver disease. *Assoc Res Nerv Ment Dis Proc* 1953; **32**:198–237.

Adler LA, Angrist B, Peselow E *et al.* Efficacy of propranolol in neuroleptic-induced akathisia. *J Clin Psychopharmacol* 1985; **5**:164–6.

Adler LA, Angrist B, Peselow E *et al.* Controlled assessment of propranolol in the treatment of neuroleptic-induced akathisia. *Br J Psychiatry* 1986; **149**:42–5.

Adler LA, Angrist B, Weinreb H *et al.* Studies on the time course and efficacy of beta-blockers in neuroleptic-induced akathisia and the akathisia of idiopathic Parkinson's disease. *Psychopharmacol Bull* 1991; **27**:107–11.

Adler LA, Peselow E, Rosenthal M *et al.* A controlled comparison of the effects of propranolol, benztropine and placebo on akathisia: an interim analysis. *Psychopharmacol Bull* 1993; **29**:283–6.

Aguglia U, Tinuper P, Gastaut H. Startle-induced epileptic seizures. *Epilepsia* 1984; **25**:712–20.

Ahmed S, Chengappa KN, Naidu VR *et al.* Clozapine-withdrawal-emergent dystonias and dykinesias: a case series. *J Clin Psychiatry* 1998; **59**:472–7.

Akhtar S, Ahmad H. Ciprofloxacin-induced catatonia. *J Clin Psychiatry* 1993; **54**:115–16.

Alarcon F, Tolosa E, Munoz E. Focal limb dystonia in a patient with a cerebellar mass. *Arch Neurol* 2001; **58**:1125–7.

Alberca RA, Chinchon I, Vadillo J *et al.* Late onset parkinsonian syndrome in Hallervorden–Spatz Disease. *J Neurol Neurosurg Psychiatry* 1987; **50**:1665–8.

Alevizos B, Papageorgiou C, Christodoulou GN. Acute dystonia caused by a low dosage of olanzapine. *J Neuropsychiatr Clin Neurosci* 2003; **15**:241.

Alpers BJ, Patten CA. Paroxysmal spasm of the eyelids as a postencephalitic manifestation. *Arch Neurol Psychiatry* 1927; **18**:427–32.

Altindag A, Yanik M, Asoglu M. The emergence of tics during escitalopram and sertraline treatment. *Int Clin Psychopharmacol* 2005; **20**:177–8.

Angelini L, Sgro V, Erba A *et al.* Tourettism as clinical presentation of Huntington's disease with onset in childhood. *Ital J Neurol Sci* 1988; **19**:383–5.

Antin SP, Prockop LD, Cohen SM. Transient hemiballism. *Neurology* 1967; **17**:1068–72.

Armon C, Shin C, Miller P *et al.* Reversible parkinsonism and cognitive impairment with chronic valproate use. *Neurology* 1996; **47**:626–35.

Aronson MJ, Thompson SV. Complications of acute catatonic excitement. *Am J Psychiatry* 1950; **107**:216–20.

Asmus F, Zimprich A, Tezenas du Montcel S *et al.* Myoclonus-dystonia syndrome: epsilon-sarcoglycan mutations and phenotype. *Ann Neurol* 2002; **52**:489–92.

Atasoy N, Ustundag Y, Konuk N *et al.* Acute dystonia during pegylated interferon alpha therapy in a case with chronic hepatitis B infection. *Clin Neuropharmacol* 2004; **27**:105–7.

Austen FK, Carmichael MW, Adams RD. Neurologic manifestations of chronic pulmonary insufficiency. *N Engl J Med* 1957; **257**:579 90.

Ayd FJ. A survey of drug-induced extrapyramidal reactions. *J Am Med Assoc* 1961; **175**:1054–60.

Babiy M, Stubblefield MD, Herklotz M *et al.* Asterixis related to gabapentin as a cause of falls. *Am J Phys Med Rehabil* 2005; **84**:136–40.

Bacchus M. Encephalopathy and pulmonary disease. *Arch Int Med* 1958; **102**:194–8.

Bachman DS. Pemoline-induced Tourette's disorder: a case report. *Am J Psychiatry* 1981; **138**:1116–17.

Bain PG, Findley LJ, Britton TC *et al.* Primary writing tremor. *Brain* 1995; **118**:1461–72.

Bak TH, Bauer M, Schaub RT *et al.* Myoclonus in patients treated with clozapine: a case series. *J Clin Psychiatry* 1995; **56**:418–22.

Baldassano CF, Truman CJ, Nierenberg A *et al.* Akathisia: a review and case report following paroxetine treatment. *Compr Psychiatry* 1996; **37**:122–4.

Ballard PA Tetrud JW, Langston JW. Permanent human parkinsonism due to 1-methyl-4-phenyl-1,2,3,6-tetrahydropyridine (MPTP): seven cases. *Neurology* 1985; **35**:949–56.

Barak Y, Levine J, Weisz R. Clozapine-induced myoclonus: two case reports. *J Clin Psychopharmacol* 1996; **16**:339–40.

Barclay CL, Lang AE. Dystonia in progressive supranuclear palsy. *J Neurol Neurosurg Psychiatry* 1997; **62**:352–6.

Barnes MP, Saunders M, Walls TJ et al. The syndrome of Karl
Ludwig Kahlbaum. J Neurol Neurosurg Psychiatry 1986;
49:991–6.

Bartholomew RE. Disease, disorder or deception? Latah as
habit in a Malay extended family. J Nerv Ment Dis 1994;
182:331–8.

Barucha KJ, Sethi DD. Complex movement disorders induced by
fluoxetine. Mov Disord 1996; 11:324–6.

Bataller L, Graus F, Salz A et al. Clinical outcome in adult-onset
idiopathic or paraneoplastic opsoclonus-myoclonus. Brain
2001; 124:437–43.

Becher MW, Rubinsztein DC, Leggo J et al. Dentatorubral and
pallidoluysian atrophy (DRPLA): clinical and neuropathological
findings in genetically confirmed North American and
European pedigrees. Mov Disord 1997; 12:519–30.

Behan PO, Bone I. Hereditary chorea without dementia. J Neurol
Neurosurg Psychiatry 1977; 40:687–91.

Benesch CG, McDaniel KD, Coc C et al. End-stage Alzheimer's
disease: Glasgow coma scale and neurologic examination.
Arch Neurol 1993; 50:1309–15.

Benito-Leon J, Rodriguez J, Orti-Pareja M et al. Symptomatic
orthostatic tremor in pontine lesions. Neurology 1997;
49:1439–41.

Berkovic SF, Carpenter S, Andermann F et al. Kufs' disease: a
critical reappraisal. Brain 1988; 111:27–62.

Berkovic SF, Carpeneter S, Evans A et al. Myoclonus epilepsy and
ragged-red fibers (MERRF). Brain 1989; 112:1231–60.

Berry N, Sagar R, Tripathi BM. Catatonia and other psychiatric
symptoms with vitamin B12 deficiency. Acta Psychiatr Scand
2003; 108:156–9.

Bertoni JM, Schwartzman RJ, Van Horn G et al. Asterixis and
encephalopathy following metrizamide myelography:
investigations into possible mechanisms and review of the
literature. Ann Neurol 1981; 9:366–70.

Bharucha KJ, Sethi KD. Tardive Tourettism after exposure to
neuroleptic therapy. Mov Disord 1995; 10:791–3.

Bharucha KJ, Sethi KD. Complex movement disorders induced by
fluoxetine. Mov Disord 1996; 11:324–6.

Bhatia KP, Soland VL, Bhatt MH. Paroxysmal exercize-induced
dystonia: eight new sporadic cases and a review of the
literature. Mov Disord 1997a; 12:1007–12.

Bhatia KP, Quinn NP, Marsden CD. Clinical features and natural
history of axial predominant adult onset primary dystonia.
J Neurol Neurosurg Psychiatry 1997b; 63:788–91.

Bhatt MH, Obeso JA, Marsden CD. Time course of postanoxic
akinetic-rigid and dystonic syndromes. Neurology 1993;
43:314–17.

Bhatt MH, Elias MA, Mankodi AK. Acute and reversible
parkinsonism due to organophosphate pesticide intoxication.
Five cases. Neurology 1999; 52:1467–71.

Biggins CA, Boyd JL, Harrop FM et al. A controlled, longitudinal
study of dementia in Parkinson's disease. J Neurol Neurosurg
Psychiatry 1992; 55:566–71.

Bird MT, Paulson JW. The rigid form of Huntington's chorea.
Neurology 1971; 21:271–6.

Bland EF, Jones TD. The natural history of rheumatic fever: a 20
year perspective. Ann Int Med 1952; 37:1006–26.

Bleuler E. Textbook of psychiatry, 1924, translated by Brill AA.
New York: Arno Press, 1976.

Blunt SB, Lane RJ, Turjanski N et al. Clinical features and
management of two cases of encephalitis lethargica. Mov
Disord 1997; 12:354–9.

Bocola V, Fabbrini G, Sollecito A et al. Neuroleptic induced
parkinsonism: MRI findings in relation to clinical course after
withdrawal of neuroleptic drugs. J Neurol Neurosurg
Psychiatry 1996; 60:213–16.

Bodensteiner JB, Morris HH, Golden GS. Asterixis associated with
sodium valproate. Neurology 1981; 31:194–5.

Boecker H, Weindl A, Leenders K et al. Secondary parkinsonism
due to focal substantia nigra lesions: a PET study with
[18F]FDG and [18F]flourodopa. Acta Neurol Scand 1996;
93:387–92.

Boesch SM, Wenning GK, Ransmayr G et al. Dystonia in multiple
system atrophy. J Neurol Neurosurg Psychiatry 2002;
73:300–3.

Boeve BF, Tremont-Lukats IW, Waclawik AJ et al. Longitudinal
characteristics of two siblings with frontotemporal dementia
and parkinsonism linked to chromosome 17 associated with
the S305N tau mutation. Brain 2005; 128:752–72.

Bond ED. Epidemic encephalitis and katatonic symptoms. Am J
Insanity 1920; 76:261–4.

Borgohain R, Singh AK, Thadani R et al. Hemiballismus due to
an ipsilateral striatal hemorrhage: an unusual localization.
J Neurol Sci 1995; 130:22–4.

Bort RF. Catatonia, gastric hyperacidity, and fatal aspiration: a
preventable syndrome. Am J Psychiatry 1976; 133:446–7.

Bourgeois M, Bouilh P, Tignol J et al. Brief communication:
spontaneous dyskinesias vs. neuroleptic-induced dyskinesias in
270 elderly subjects. J Nerv Ment Dis 1980; 168:177–8.

Boyer WF, Bakalar NH, Lake CR. Anticholinergic prophylaxis of
acute haloperidol-induced dystonic reactions. J Clin
Psychopharmacol 1987; 7:164–6.

Brashear A, Farlow MR, Butler I et al. Variable phenotype of
rapid-onset dystonia–parkinsonism. Mov Disord 1996;
11:151–6.

Brashear A, DeLeon D, Bressman SB et al. Rapid-onset
dystonia–parkinsonism in a second family. Neurology 1997;
48:1066–9.

Brashear A, Dubyns WB, de Carvhalo Aguiar P et al. The
phenotypic spectrum of rapid onset dystonia-parkinsonism
(RDP) and mutations in the ATP1A3 gene. Brain 2007;
130:828–35.

Braude WM, Barnes TRE, Gore SM. Clinical characteristics of
akathisia: a systematic investigation of acute psychiatric
in-patient admissions. Br J Psychiatry 1983; 143:139–50.

Bressman SB, Fahn S, Burke RE. Paroxysmal non-kinesigenic
dystonia. Adv Neurol 1988; 50:403–13.

Brin MF, Blitzer A, Stewart C. Laryngeal dystonia (spasmodic
dysphonia): observations of 901 patients and treatment with
botulinum toxin. Adv Neurol 1998; 78:237–52.

Brown P, Cathala F, Castaigne P et al. Creutzfeldt–Jakob disease:
clinical analysis of a consecutive series of 230
neuropathologically verified cases. Ann Neurol 1986;
20:597–602.

Brown P, Rothwell JC, Thompson PD *et al*. The hyperekplexias and their relationship to the normal startle reflex. *Brain* 1991; **114**:1903–28.

Bruetsch WL, Williams CL. Arteriosclerotic muscular rigidity with special reference to gait disturbances. *Am J Psychiatry* 1954; **111**:332–6.

Bruno MK, Hallett M, Gwinn-Hardy K *et al*. Clinical evaluation of idiopathic paroxysmal kinesigenic dyskinesia. New diagnostic criteria. *Neurology* 2004; **63**:2280–7.

Bruno MK, Lee H-Y, Auberger GWJ *et al*. Genotype–phenotype correlation of paroxysmal non-kinesigenic dyskinesia. *Neurology* 2007; **68**:1782–9.

Bucher SF, Seelos KC, Dodel RC *et al*. Pallidal lesions: structural and functional magnetic resonance imaging. *Arch Neurol* 1996; **53**:682–6.

Budman C, Sarcevic A. An unusual case of motor and vocal tics with obsessive-compulsive symptoms in a young adult with Behcet's syndrome. *CNS Spectr* 2002; **7**:878–81.

Buetefisch CM, Gutierrez A, Gutmann L. Choreoathetotic movements: a possible side-effect of gabapentin. *Neurology* 1996; **46**:851–2.

Burd L, Kerbeshian J, Fisher W *et al*. Anticonvulsant medications: an iatrogenic cause of tic disorders. *Can J Psychiatry* 1986; **31**:419–23.

Burguera JA, Bataller L, Valero C. Action hand dystonia after cortical parietal infarction. *Mov Disord* 2001; **16**:1183–5.

Burke RE, Fahn S, Gold AP. Delayed-onset dystonia in patients with 'static' encephalopathy. *J Neurol Neurosurg Psychiatry* 1980; **43**:789.

Burke RE, Fahn S, Jankovic J *et al*. Tardive dystonia: late-onset and persistent dystonia caused by antipsychotic drugs. *Neurology* 1982; **32**:1335–46.

Burke RE, Kang UJ, Jankovic J *et al*. Tardive akathisia: an analysis of clinical features and response to open therapeutic trials. *Mov Disord* 1989; **4**:147–75.

Burkhard PR, Delavelle J, Du Pasquier R *et al*. Chronic parkinsonism associated with cirrhosis: a distinct subset of acquired hepatocerebral degeneration. *Arch Neurol* 2003; **60**:521–8.

Bush G, Fink M, Pertrides G *et al*. Catatonia. II. Treatment with lorazepam and electroconvulsive therapy. *Arch Psychiatr Scand* 1996; **9**:137–43.

Byrne EJ, Lennox G, Lowe J *et al*. Diffuse Lewy body disease: clinical features in 15 cases. *J Neurol Neurosurg Psychiatry* 1989; **52**:709–17.

Cammarota A, Gershank OS, Garcia S *et al*. Cervical dystonia due to spinal cord ependymoma: involvement of cervical cord segments in the pathogenesis of dystonia. *Mov Disord* 1995; **10**:500–3.

Campbell AMG, Corner B, Norman RM *et al*. The rigid form of Huntington's disease. *J Neurol Neurosurg Psychiatry* 1961; **24**:71–7.

Caparros-Lefebvre D, Deleume JF, Bradai N *et al*. Ballism caused by bilateral infarction in the substantia nigra. *Mov Disord* 1994; **9**:108.

Cardoso F, Jankovic J. Cocaine-related movement disorders. *Mov Disord* 1993; **8**:175–8.

Cardoso F, Veado CCM, de Oliveira JT. A Brazilian cohort of patients with Tourette's syndrome. *J Neurol Neurosurg Psychiatry* 1996; **60**:209–12.

Cardoso F, Eduardo C, Silva AP *et al*. Chorea in fifty consecutive patients with rheumatic fever. *Mov Disord* 1997; **12**:701–3.

Carella F, Grassi MP, Savoiardo M *et al*. Dystonic-parkinsonian syndrome after cyanide poisoning: clinical and MRI findings. *J Neurol Neurosurg Psychiatry* 1988; **51**:1345–8.

Carlen PL, Lee MA, Jacob M *et al*. Parkinsonism provoked by alcoholism. *Ann Neurol* 1981; **9**:84–6.

Carlson CD, Cavazzoni PA, Berg PH *et al*. An integrated analysis of acute treatment-emergent extrapyramidal syndrome in patients with schizophrenia during olanzapine clinical trials: comparisons with placebo, haloperidol, risperidone or clozapine. *J Clin Psychiatry* 2003; **64**:898–906.

Carpenter MB. Ballism associated with partial destruction of the subthalamic nucleus of Luys. *Neurology* 1955; **5**:479–89.

Carpenter MR. Athetosis and the basal ganglia. *Arch Neurol* 1950; **63**:895–901.

Casas M, Garcia-Ribera C, Alvarez E *et al*. Myoclonic movements as a side-effect of treatment with therapeutic doses of clomipramine. *Int J Psychopharmacol* 1987; **2**:333–6.

Castillo E, Rubin RT, Holsboer-Trachsler E. Clinical differentiation between lethal catatonia and neuroleptic malignant syndrome. *Am J Psychiatry* 1989; **146**:324–8.

Castillo P, Woodruff B, Caselli R *et al*. Steroid-responsive encephalopathy associated with autoimmune thyroiditis. *Arch Neurol* 2006; **63**:197–202.

Catalano G, Grace JW, Catalano MC *et al*. Acute akathisia associated with quetiapine use. *Psychosomatics* 2005; **46**:291–301.

Caviness JN, Evidente VG. Cortical myoclonus during lithium exposure. *Arch Neurol* 2003; **60**:401–4.

Cervera R, Asherson RA, Font J *et al*. Chorea in the antiphospholipid syndrome. Clinical, radiologic, and immunologic characteristics of 50 patients from our clinics and the recent literature. *Medicine* 1997; **76**:203–12.

Chan DB, Lang MF, Fahn S. Idiopathic cervical dystonia. *Mov Disord* 1991; **6**:119–26.

Chandra V, Wharton S, Spunt AL. Amelioration of hemiballismus with sodium valproate. *Ann Neurol* 1982; **12**:407.

Chang M-H, Li J-Y, Lee S-R *et al*. Non-ketotic hyperglycaemic chorea: a SPECT study. *J Neurol Neurosurg Psychiatry* 1996; **60**:428–30.

Charles JR. Manganese toxaemia, with special reference to the effects of liver feeding. *Brain* 1927; **50**:30–43.

Chen D-H, Matsushita M, Rainier S *et al*. Presence of alanine-to-valine substitutions in myofibrillogenesis regulator 1 in paroxysmal nonkinesigenic dyskinesia. *Arch Neurol* 2005; **62**:597–600.

Chen J-Y, Stern Y, Sano M *et al*. Cumulative risks of developing extrapyramidal signs, psychosis, or myoclonus in the course of Alzheimer's disease. *Arch Neurol* 1991; **48**:1141–3.

Chi WM, Chua kS, Kong KH. Phenytoin-induced asterixis – uncommon or underdiagnosed? *Brain Inj* 2000; **14**:847–50.

Chiu LPW. Transient recurrence of auditory hallucinations during acute dystonia. *Br J Psychiatry* 1989; **155**:110–13.

Choi IS. Delayed neurologic sequelae in carbon monoxide intoxication. *Arch Neurol* 1983; **40**:433–5.

Chokroverty S, Bruetman ME, Berger V *et al.* Progressive dialytic encephalopathy. *J Neurol Neurosurg Psychiatry* 1976; **39**:411–19.

Chouinard MJ, Nguyen DK, Clement JF *et al.* Catatonia induced by levertiracetam. *Epilepsy Behav* 2006; **8**:303–7.

Chouinard S, Ford B. Adult onset tic disorders. *J Neurol Neurosurg Psychiatry* 2000; **68**:738–43.

Choy-Kwong M, Lipton RB. Dystonia related to cocaine withdrawal: a case report and pathogenic hypothesis. *Neurology* 1989; **39**:996–7.

Christodoulou C, Kalaitzi C. Antipsychotic drug-induced acute laryngeal dystonia: two case reports and a mini review. *J Psychopharmacol* 2005; **19**:307–11.

Chu K, Kang DW, Kim DE *et al.* Diffusion-weighted and gradient echo magnetic resonance findings of hemichorea-hemiballismus associated with diabetic hyperglycemia: a hyperviscosity syndome? *Arch Neurol* 2002; **59**:448–52.

Chudnow RS, Dewey RB, Lawson CR. Choreoathetosis as a side-effect of gabapentin therapy in severely neurologically impaired patients. *Arch Neurol* 1997; **54**:910–12.

Chung SJ, Im JH, Lee MC *et al.* Hemichorea after stroke: clinical-radiological correlation. *J Neurol* 2004; **251**:725–9.

Cincotta M, Borgheresi A, Balzini L *et al.* Separate ipsilateral and contralateral corticospinal projections in congenital mirror movements: neurophysiological evidence and significance for motor rehabilitation. *Mov Disord* 2003; **18**:1294–1300.

Clark CM, Ewbank D, Lerner A *et al.* The relationship between extrapyramidal signs and cognitive performance in patients with Alzheimer's disease enrolled in the CERAD study. *Neurology* 1997; **49**:70–5.

Cohen LG, Hallett M. Hand cramps: clinical features and electromyographic patterns in a focal dystonia. *Neurology* 1988; **38**:1005–12.

Collins SJ, Ahlskog JE, Parisi JE *et al.* Progressive supranuclear palsy: neuropathologically based diagnostic clinical criteria. *J Neurol Neurosurg Psychiatry* 1995; **58**:167–73.

Colosimo C, Albanese A, Hughes AJ *et al.* Some specific clinical features differentiate multiple system atrophy (striatonigral variety) from Parkinson's disease. *Arch Neurol* 1995; **52**:294–8.

Comella CL, Goetz CG. Akathisia in Parkinson's disease. *Mov Disord* 1994; **9**:545–9.

Creak M, Guttmann E. Chorea, tic, compulsive utterances. *J Ment Sci* 1935; **81**:834–9.

Crespel A, Genton P, Berrandame M *et al.* Lamotrigine associated with exacerbation or de novo myoclonus in idiopathic generalized epilepsies. *Neurology* 2005; **65**:762–4.

Critchley EMR, Clark DB, Wikler A. Acanthocytosis and neurological disorder without abetalipoproteinemia. *Arch Neurol* 1968; **18**:134–40.

Croteau D, Owainati A, Dalmau J *et al.* Response to cancer therapy in a patient with a paraneoplastic choreiform disorder. *Neurology* 2001; **57**:719–22.

Crozier S, Lehericy S, Verstichel P *et al.* Transient hemiballism/hemichorea due to ipsilateral subthalamic nucleus infarction. *Neurology* 1996; **46**:267–8.

Crystal HA. Baclofen therapy may be associated with chorea in Alzheimer's disease. *Ann Neurol* 1990; **28**:839.

Crystal HA, Dixon DW, Lizardi JE *et al.* Antemortem diagnosis of diffuse Lewy body disease. *Neurology* 1990; **40**:1523–8.

Cubo E, Gracies JM, Benabou R *et al.* Early morning off-medication dyskinesias, dystonia, and choreic subtypes. *Arch Neurol* 2001; **58**:1379–82.

Cunningham MA, Darby DG, Donnan GA. Controlled-release delivery of L-dopa associated with nonfatal hyperthermia, rigidity and autonomic dysfunction. *Neurology* 1991; **41**:942–3.

Dale RC, Church AJ, Heyman I. Striatal encephalitis after varicella zoster infection complicated by Tourettism. *Mov Disord* 2003; **18**:1554–6.

Danek A, Tison F, Rubio J *et al.* The chorea of McLeod syndrome. *Mov Disord* 2001; **16**:882–9.

Daniel SE, de Bruin VMS, Lees AJ. The clinical and pathological specturm of Steele–Richardson–Olszewski syndrome (progressive supranuclear palsy): a reappraisal. *Brain* 1995; **118**:759–70.

Daras M, Koppel BS, Atos-Radzion E. Cocaine-induced choreoathetoid movements ('crack dancing'). *Neurology* 1994; **44**:751–2.

Davis EJB, Borde M. Wilson's disease and catatonia. *Br J Psychiatry* 1993; **162**:256–9.

Davis JM. Response of hemiballismus to haloperidol. *JAMA* 1976; **235**:281–2.

Davous P, Rondot P, Marion MH *et al.* Severe chorea after acute carbon monoxide poisoning. *J Neurol Neurosurg Psychiatry* 1986; **49**:206–8.

Dawson JR. Cellular inclusions in cerebral lesions of epidemic encephalitis. *Arch Neurol Psychiatry* 1934; **31**:685–700.

DeCastro RM. Antidepressants and myoclonus: case report. *J Clin Psychiatry* 1985; **46**:284–7.

Defazio G, Berardelli A, Abruzzese G *et al.* Risk factors for spread of blepharospasm: a multicentre investigation of the Italian movement disorders study group. *J Neurol Neurosurg Psychiatry* 1999; **67**:613–19.

Defebvre L, Destee A, Cassim F *et al.* Transient hemiballism and striatal infarct. *Stroke* 1990; **21**:967–8.

Degos J-D, Verroust J, Bouchareine A *et al.* Asterixis in focal brain lesion. *Arch Neurol* 1979; **36**:705–7.

De La Sayettte V, Schaeffer S, Querel C *et al.* Lyme neuroborreliosis presenting with propriospinal myoclonus. *J Neurol Neurosurg Psychiatry* 1996; **64**:420.

Della Marca G, Retuccia D, Mariotti P *et al.* Pathologic startle following brainstem lesion. *Neurology* 2007; **68**:47.

Delwaide PJ, Desseilles M. Spontaneous buccolingualfacial dyskinesia in the elderly. *Acta Neurol Scand* 1977; **56**:256–62.

Demirkiran M, Jankovic J. Paroxysmal dyskinesias: clinical features and classification. *Ann Neurol* 1995; **38**:571–9.

Denckla MB, Bemporad JR, MacKay MC. Tics following methylphenidate administration: a report of 20 cases. *JAMA* 1976; **235**:1349–51.

Dennis MS, Byrne EJ, Hopkinson EN *et al.* Neuropsychiatric systemic lupus erythematosis in elderly people: a case series. *J Neurol Neurosurg Psychiatry* 1992; **55**:1157–61.

Desarkar P, Thakur A, Sinha V. Aripiprazole-induced acute dystonia. *Am J Psychiatry* 2006; **163**:1112–13.

Deshmukh DK, Joshi VS, Agarwal MR. Rabbit syndrome – a rare complication of long-term neuroleptic medication. *Br J Psychiatry* 1990; **157**:293.

Detweiller MB, Harpold GJ. Bupropion-induced acute dystonia. *Ann Pharmacother* 2002; **36**:251–4.

Deuschl G, Koester B, Luecking CH *et al.* Diagnostic and pathophysiological aspects of psychogenic tremor. *Movement Disord* 1998; **13**:294–302.

Dewey RB, Jankovic J. Hemiballism–hemichorea. Clinical and pharmacologic findings in 21 patients. *Arch Neurol* 1989; **46**:862–7.

Dib E, Bernstein S, Benesch C. Multifocal myoclonus induced by trimethoprim-sulfamethoxazole in a patient with nocardia infection. *N Engl J Med* 2004; **350**:88–9.

Dickoff DJ, Raps M, Yahr MD. Striatal syndrome following hyponatremia and its rapid correction: a manifestation of extrapontine myelinolysis confirmed by magnetic resonance imaging. *Arch Neurol* 1988; **45**:112–14.

Digre KB. Opsoclonus in adults – report of three cases and review of the literature. *Arch Neurol* 1986; **43**:1165–75.

DiMascio A, Bernardo DL, Greenblatt DJ *et al.* A controlled trial of amantadine in drug-induced extrapyramidal disorders. *Arch Gen Psychiatry* 1976; **33**:599–602.

Doheny DO, Brin MF, Morrison CE *et al.* Phenotypic features of myoclonus-dystonia in three kindreds. *Neurology* 2002; **59**:1187–94.

Dominguez-Moran JA, Callejo JM, Fernandex-Ruiz LC *et al.* Acute paroxysmal dystonia induced by fluoxetine. *Mov Disord* 2001; **16**:767–9.

Donaldson IM, Espiner EA. Disseminated lupus erythematosus presenting as chorea gravidarum. *Arch Neurol* 1971; **25**:240–4.

Dooling EC, Adams RD. Pathologic anatomy or posthemiplegic athetosis. *Brain* 1975; **98**:29–48.

Dooling EC, Schoene WC, Richardson EP. Halervorden–Spatz syndrome. *Arch Neurol* 1974; **30**:70–83.

Drake RE, Ehrlich J. Suicide attempts associated with akathisia. *Am J Psychiatry* 1985; **142**:499–501.

Driesen JJ, Wolters EC. Bilateral ballism induced by oral contraceptives *J Neurol* 1986; **233**:379.

Dufresne RL, Wagner RL. Antipsychotic-withdrawal akathisia versus antipsychotic-induced akathisia: further evidence for the existence of tardive akathisia. *J Clin Psychiatry* 1988; **49**:435–8.

Duvoisin RC, Yahr MD. Encephalitis and parkinsonism. *Arch Neurol* 1965; **12**:227–39.

Easterford K, Clugh P, Kellett M *et al.* Reversible parkinsonism with normal beta-CIT-SPECT in patients exposed to sodium valproate. *Neurology* 2004; **62**:1435–7.

Edelstein H, Knight RT. Severe parkinsonism in two AIDS patients taking prochlorperazine. *Lancet* 1987; **2**:341–2.

Edwards MJ, Dale RC, Church AJ *et al.* Adult-onset tic disorders, motor stereotypies, and behavioral disturbance associated with antibasal ganglia antibodies. *Mov Disord* 2004; **19**:1190–6.

Eisenhauer G, Jermain DM. Fluoxetine and tics in an adolescent. *Ann Pharmacother* 1993; **27**:725–6.

Engel J, Ludwig BI, Fetell M. Prolonged partial complex status epilepticus: EEG and behavioral observations. *Neurology* 1978; **28**:863–9.

Ernst NH, Steur J. Increase of parkinsonian disability after fluoxetine medication. *Neurology* 1993; **43**:211–13.

Espay AJ, Hung SW, Sanger TD *et al.* A writing device improves writing in primary writing tremor. *Neurology* 2005a; **64**:1648–50.

Espay AJ, Li JY, Johnston L *et al.* Mirror movements in parkinsonism: evaluation of a new clinical sign. *J Neurol Neurosurg Psychiatry* 2005b; **76**:1355–8.

Evidente VG, Gwinn-Hardy K, Caviness JN *et al.* Risperidone is effective in severe hemichorea/hemiballismus. *Mov Disord* 1999; **14**:377–9.

Evidente VG, Advincula J, Esteban R *et al.* Phenomenology of 'Lubag' or X-linked dystonia-parkinsonism. *Mov Disord* 2002; **17**:1271–7.

Extein I. Methylphenidate-induced choreoathetosis. *Am J Psychiatry* 1978; **135**:252–3.

Factor SA, Moltho ES. Adult-onset tics associated with peripheral injury. *Mov Disord* 1997; **12**:1052–5.

Factor SA, Troche-Panetto M, Weaver SA. Dystonia in AIDS: report of four cases *Mov Disord* 2003; **18**:1492–8.

Federico P, Zochodne DW. Reversible parkinsonism and hyperammonemia associated with portal vein thrombosis. *Acta Neurol Scand* 2001; **103**:198–200.

Federlein J, Postert Th, Allgeier A *et al.* Remitting parkinsonism as a symptom of multiple sclerosis and the associated magnetic resonance imaging findings. *Mov Disorders* 1997; **12**:1090–1. 1994; **241**:537–42.

Feighner JP, Boyer WF, Tyler DL *et al.* Adverse consequences of fluoxetine–MAOI combination therapy. *J Clin Psychiatry* 1990; **51**:222–5.

Feinberg TE, Cianci CD, Morrow JS *et al.* Diagnostic tests for choreoacanthocytosis. *Neurology* 1991; **41**:1000–6.

Fenelon G, Houeto J-L. Unilateral parkinsonism following a large infarct in the territory of the lenticulostriate arteries. *Mov Disorders* 1997; **12**:1086–90.

Fermaglich J, Streib E, Auth T. Chorea associated with systemic lupus erythematosus. *Arch Neurol* 1973; **28**:276–7.

Fernanadez M, Raskind W, Matsushita M *et al.* Hereditary benign chorea: clinical and genetic features of a distinct disease. *Neurology* 2001; **57**:106–10.

Feve AP, Fenelon G, Wallays C *et al.* Axial motor disturbances after hypoxic lesions of the globus pallidus. *Mov Disord* 1993; **8**:321–6.

Fidler SM, O'Rourke RA, Buchsbaum HW. Choreoathetosis as a manifestation of thyrotoxicosis. *Neurology* 1971; **21**:55–7.

Fink JK, Hedera P, Mathay JG *et al.* Paroxysmal dystonic choreoathetosis linked to chromosome 2q: clinical analysis and proposed pathophysiology. *Neurology* 1997; **49**:177–83.

Finlayson MH, Superville B. Distribution of cerebral lesions in acquired hepatocerebral degeneration. *Brain* 1981; **104**:79–95.

Fischel T, Hermesh H, Aizenberg D et al. Cyproheptadine versus propranolol for the treatment of acute neuroleptic-induced akathisia: a comparative double-blind study. J Clin Psychopharmacol 2001; 21:612–15.

Fishbeck KH, Layzer RB. Paroxysmal choreoathetosis associated with thyrotoxicosis. Ann Neurol 1979; 6:453–4.

Flaherty JA, Lahmeyer HW. Larnyngeal–pharyngeal dystonia as a possible cause of asphyxia with haloperidol treatment. Am J Psychiatry 1978; 135:1414–15.

Fleishman SB, Lavin MR, Sattler M et al. Antiemetic-induced akathisia in cancer patients receiving chemotherapy. Am J Psychiatry 1994; 151:763–5.

Foncke EMJ, Gerrits MLF, van Ruissen F et al. Distal myoclonus and later onset in a large Dutch family with myoclonus-dystonia. Neurology 2006; 67:1677–80.

Foster PN, Stickle BR, Laurence AS. Akathisia following low-dose droperidol for antiemesis in day-case patients. Anaesthesia 1996; 51:491–4.

Fox GC, Ebeid S, Vincenti G. Paroxetine-induced chorea. Br J Psychiatry 1997; 170:193–4.

Francisco GE. Successful treatment of posttraumatic hemiballismus with intrathecal baclofen therapy. Am J Phys Med Rehabil 2006; 85:779–82.

Friedman A, Sienkiewicz J. Psychotic complications of long-term levodopa treatment of Parkinson's disease. Acta Neurol Scand 1991; 84:111–13.

Furtado S, Ferrer M, Tsuboi Y et al. SCA-2 presenting as parkinsonism in an Alberta family. Clinical, genetic and PET findings. Neurology 2002; 59:1625–7.

Gallo BV, Shulman LM, Weiner WJ et al. HIV encephalitis presenting with severe generalized chorea. Neurol 1996; 46:1163–5.

Gambardella A, Valentino P, Annesi G et al. Hyperekplexia in a patient with a brainstem vascular anomaly. Acta Neurol Scand 1999; 99:255–9.

Gamboa ET, Issacs G, Harter DH. Chorea associated with oral contraceptive therapy. Arch Neurol 1971; 25:112–14.

Garrett PJ, Mulcahey D, Carmody M et al. Aluminium encephalopathy: clinical and immunologic features. Q J Med 1988; 69:775–83.

Garruto RM, Gajdusek DC, Chen KM. Amyotrophic lateral sclerosis and parkinsonism-dementia among Filipino immigrants to Guam. Ann Neurol 1981; 10:341–50.

Garvey MJ, Tollefson GD. Occurrence of myoclonus in patients treated with cyclic antidepressants. Arch Gen Psychiatry 1987; 44:269–72.

Gatto EM, Uribe Roca C, Raina G et al. Vascular hemichorea/hemiballism and topiramate. Mov Disord 2004; 19:836–8.

Gaultieri CT, Patterson DR. Neuroleptic-induced tics in two hyperactive children. Am J Psychiatry 1986; 143:1176–7.

Gautier-Smith PC, Prankerd TAJ. Polycythemia vera and chorea. Acta Neurol Scand 1967; 43:357–64.

Gelenberg AJ, Jefferson JW. Lithium tremor. J Clin Psychiatry 1995; 56:283–7.

Gelenberg AJ, Mandel MR. Catatonic reactions to high-potency neuroleptic drugs. Arch Gen Psychiatry 1977; 34:947–50.

Ghika J, Bogousslavsky J. Spinal pseudoathetosis: a rare, forgotten syndrome, with a review of old and recent descriptions. Neurology 1997; 49:432–7.

Ghika J, Bogousslavsky J, Henderson J et al. The 'jerky dystonic unsteady hand': a delayed motor syndrome in posterior thalamic infarctions. J Neurol 1994; 241:537–42.

Ghika-Schmid F, Ghika J, Regli F et al. Hashimoto's myoclonic encephalopathy: an underdiagnosed treatable condition? Mov Disord 1996; 11:555–67.

Gibb WRG, Lees AJ. The clinical phenomenon of akathisia. J Neurol Neurosurg Psychiatry 1986; 49:861–6.

Giladi N, McMahon D, Przedborski S et al. Motor blocks in Parkinson's disease. Neurology 1992; 42:333–9.

Gilbert GJ. Brueghel syndrome: its distinction from Meige syndrome. Neurology 1996; 46:1767–9.

Gimenez-Roldan S, Martin M. Startle epilepsy complicating Down syndrome during adulthood. Ann Neurol 1980; 7:78–80.

Gjessing LR. A review of periodic catatonia. Biol Psychiatry 1974; 8:23–45.

Glantz R, Weiner WJ, Goetz CG et al. Drug-induced asterixis in Parkinson's disease. Neurology 1982; 32:553–5.

Glass JP, Jankovic J, Borit A. Hemiballism and metastatic brain tumor. Neurology 1984; 34:204–7.

Goldings AS, Stewart RM. Organic lead encephalopathy: behavioral change and movement disorder following gasoline inhalation. J Clin Psychiatry 1982; 43:70–2.

Gomez EA, Comstock BS, Rosario A. Organic versus functional etiology in catatonia: case report. J Clin Psychiatry 1982; 43:200–1.

Gooch JL, Sandell TV. Botulinum toxin for spasticity and athetosis in children with cerebral palsy. Arch Phys Med Rehabil 1996; 77:508–11.

Goodman L. Alzheimer's disease: a clinico-pathologic analysis of twenty-three cases with a theory on pathogenesis. J Nerv Ment Dis 1953; 118:97–130.

Goto S, Kunitoku N, Suyama N et al. Posteroventral pallidotomy in a patient with parkinsonism caused by hypoxic encephalopathy. Neurology 1997; 49:707–10.

de Graaf L, Admiraal R, van Puijenbroeck EP. Ballism associated with bupropion use. Ann Pharmacother 2003; 37:302–3.

Graham JM, Grunewald RA, Sagar HJ. Hallucinosis in idiopathic Parkinson's disease. J Neurol Neurosurg Psychiatry 1997; 63:434–40.

Green PM. Chorea induced by oral contraceptives. Neurology 1980; 30:1131–2.

Grimes DA, Han F, Lang AE et al. A novel focus for inherited myoclonus-dystonia on 18p11. Neurology 2002; 59:1183–6.

Grinker RR. Parkinsonism following carbon monoxide poisoning. J Nerv Ment Dis 1926; 64:18–28.

Guggenheim MA, Couch JR, Weinberg W. Motor dysfunction as a permanent complication of methanol ingestion: presentation of a case with a beneficial response to levodopa treatment. Arch Neurol 1971; 24:550–4.

Gunal DI, Onultan O, Afsar N et al. Tardive dystonia associated with olanzapine therapy. Neurol Sci 2001; 22:331–2.

Gwinn-hardy K, Chen JY, Liu H-C *et al*. Spinocerebellar ataxia type 2 with parkinsonism in ethnic Chinese. *Neurology* 2000; **55**:800–5.

Halstead SM, Barnes TRE, Speller JC. Akathisia: prevalence and associated dysphoria in an in-patient population with chronic schizophrenia. *Br J Psychiatry* 1994; **164**:177–83.

Hammond WA. *A treatise on diseases of the nervous system*. New York: Appleton-Century Crofts, 1871.

Hansen HC, Zschocke S, Sturenbur HJ *et al*. Clinical changes and EEG patterns preceding the onset of periodic sharp wave complexes in Creutzfeldt–Jakob disease. *Acta Neurol Scand* 1998; **97**:99–106.

Hansotia P, Cleeland CS, Chun RWM. Juvenile Huntington's chorea. *Neurology* 1968; **18**:217–24.

Hardie RJ, Lees AJ. Neuroleptic-induced Parkinson's syndrome: clinical features and results of treatment with levodopa. *J Neurol Neurosurg Psychiatry* 1988; **51**:850–4.

Hardie RJ, Pullon HWH, Harding AE *et al*. Neuroacanthocytosis: a clinical, haematological and pathological study of 19 cases. *Brain* 1991; **114**:13–49.

Harsch HH. Neurologyoleptic malignant syndrome: physiological and laboratory findings in a series of nine cases. *J Clin Psychiatry* 1987; **48**:328–33.

Harvey PKP, Davis JN. Traumatic encephalopathy in a young boxer. *Lancet* 1974; **2**:928–9.

Harwood G, Hierons R, Fletcher NA *et al*. Lessons from a remarkable family with dopa-responsive dystonia. *J Neurol Neurosurg Psychiatry* 1994; **57**:460–3.

Haskovec L. L'akathisie. *Rev Neurol* 1901; **9**:1107–9.

Hayflick SJ, Westaway SK, Levinson B *et al*. Genetic, clinical, and radiographic delineation of Hallervorden–Spatz syndrome. *N Engl J Med* 2003; **348**:33–40.

Heathfield KWG. Huntington's chorea. *Brain* 1967; **90**:203–32.

Heckman JG, Lang CJG, Druschky D *et al*. Chorea resulting from paraneoplastic encephalitis. *Mov Disord* 1997; **12**:464–6.

Heckmann JG, Ulrich H, Dutsch M *et al*. Pregabalin-associated asterixis. *Am J Phys Med Rehabil* 2005; **84**:724.

Hefter H, Mayer P, Benecke R. Persistent chorea after recurrent hypoglycemia. A case report. *Eur Neurol* 1993; **33**:244–7.

Heilman KH. Orthostatic tremor. *Arch Neurol* 1984; **41**:880–1.

Hellman MA, Melamed E. Focal dystonia as the presenting sign in Creutzfeldt–Jakob disease. *Mov Disord* 2002; **17**:1097–8.

Hely MA, Reid WGJ, Halliday GM *et al*. Diffuse Lewy body disease: clinical features in nine cases without coexistent Alzheimer's disease. *J Neurol Neurosurg Psychiatry* 1996; **60**:531–8.

Hersh BP, Rajendran PR, Battinelli D. Parkinsonism as the presenting feature of HIV infection: improvement on HAART. *Neurology* 2001; **56**:278–9.

Hershon HI, Kennedy PF, McGuire RJ. Persistence of extrapyramidal disorders and psychiatric relapse after withdrawal of long-term phenothiazine therapy. *Br J Psychiatry* 1972; **120**:41–50.

Hess CW, Raymond D, de Carbalho Aguiar P *et al*. Myoclonus-dystonia, obsessive-compulsive disorder, and alcohol dependence in SGCE mutation carriers. *Neurology* 2007; **68**:522–4.

Hirano A, Arumugasamy N, Zimmerman HM. Amyotrophic lateral sclerosis: a comparison of Guam and classical cases. *Arch Neurol* 1967; **16**:357–63.

Hoehn MM, Cherington M. Spinal myoclonus. *Neurology* 1977; **27**:942.

Hofmann A, Tangri N, Lafontaine A-L *et al*. Myoclonus as an acute complication of low-dose hydromorphone in multiple system atrophy. *J Neurol Neurosurg Psychiatry* 2006; **77**:994–5.

Holmes G. On certain tremors in organic cerebral lesions. *Brain* 1904; **27**:327–75.

Holroyd S, Smith D. Disabling parkinsonism due to lithium: a case report. *J Geriatr Psychiatry Neurol* 1995; **8**:118–19.

Hori A, Hirose G, Kataoka S *et al*. Delayed postanoxic encephalopathy after strangulation: serial neuroradiological and neurochemical studies. *Arch Neurol* 1991; **48**:871–4.

Horikawa N, Yamazaki T, Sagawa M *et al*. A case of akathisia during interferon-alpha therapy for chronic hepatitis type C. *Gen Hosp Psychiatry* 1999; **21**:134–5.

Howard R, Ford R. From the jumping Frenchmen of Maine to post-traumatic stress disorder: the startle response in neuropsychiatry. *Psychol Med* 1992; **22**:695–707.

Howard RS, Lees AJ. Encephalitis lethargica: a report of four recent cases. *Brain* 1987; **110**:19–33.

Huang C-C, Chu N-S, Lu C-S *et al*. Chronic manganese intoxication. *Arch Neurol* 1989; **46**:1104–6.

Huang C-C, Lu C-S, Chu N-S *et al*. Progression after chronic manganese exposure. *Neurology* 1993; **43**:1479–83.

Huang C-C, Chu N-S, Lu C-S *et al*. Cock gait in manganese intoxication. *Mov Disorders* 1997; **12**:807–8.

Hughes AJ, Daniel SE, Blankson S *et al*. A clinicopathologic study of 100 cases of Parkinson's disease. *Arch Neurol* 1993; **50**:140–8.

Hyman NM, Dennis PD, Sinclair KG. Tremor due to sodium valproate. *Neurology* 1979; **29**:1172–80.

Iijima M. Valproate-induced parkinsonism in a demented elderly patient. *J Clin Psychiatry* 2002; **63**:75.

Indo T, Ando K. Metoclopramide-induced parkinsonism. Clinical characteristics of ten cases. *Arch Neurol* 1982; **39**; 494–6.

Ishii N, Nishihara Y. Pellagra among chronic alcoholics: clinical and pathological study of 20 necropsy cases. *J Neurol Neurosurg Psychiatry* 1981; **44**:209–15.

Jacob PC, Pratap Chand R. Post-traumatic rubral tremor responsive to clonazepam. *Mov Disord* 1998; **13**:977–8.

Jacobs MB. Diltiazem and akathisia. *Ann Intern Med* 1983; **99**:794–5.

Jaffe N. Catatonia and hepatic dysfunction. *Dis Nerv Syst* 1967; **28**:606–8.

Jain S, Padma MV, Puri A *et al*. Juvenile myoclonic epilepsy: disease expression among Indian families. *Acta Neurol Scand* 1998; **97**:1–7.

Jankovic J, Ashizawa T. Tourettism associated with Huntington's disease. *Mov Disord* 1995; **10**:103–5.

Jankovic J, Fahn S. Physiologic and pathologic tremors. *Ann Int Med* 1980; **93**:460–5.

Jankovic J, Kirkpatrick JB, Blomquist KA *et al*. Late-onset Hallervorden–Spatz disease presenting as familial parkinsonism. *Neurology* 1985; **35**:227–34.

Jankovic J, Caskey TC, Stout T et al. Lesch–Nyhan syndrome: a study of motor behavior and cerebrospinal fluid neurotransmitters. Ann Neurol 1988; 23:466–9.

Jankovic J, Leder S, Warner D et al. Cervical dystonia: clinical findings and associated movement disorders. Neurology 1991; 41:1088–91.

Jarman PR, Davis MB, Hodgson SV et al. Paroxysmal dystonic choreoathetosis: genetic linkage studies in a British family. Brain 1997; 120:2125–30.

Jarman PR, Bhatia KP, Davie C et al. Paroxysmal dystonic choreoathetosis: clinical features and investigation of pathophysiology in a large family. Mov Disord 2000; 15:648–57.

Jauss M, Schroder J, Pantel J et al. Severe akathisia during olanzapine treatment of acute schizophrenia. Pharmacopsychiatry 1998; 31:146–8.

Jimenez-Jimenez FJ, Tejeiro J, Martinez-Junquera G et al. Parkinsonism exacerbated by paroxetine. Neurology 1994; 44:2406.

Johnson J. Stupor: review of 25 cases. Acta Psychiatr Scand 1984; 70:370–7.

Johnson WG, Fahn S. Treatment of vascular hemiballism and hemichorea. Neurology 1977; 27:634–6.

Johnson WG, Schwartz G, Barbeau A. Studies of dystonia musculorum deformans. Arch Neurol 1962; 7:301–13.

Jung HH, Hergersberg M, Kneifel S et al. McLeod syndrome: a novel mutation, predominant psychiatric manifestations, and distinct striatal imaging findings. Ann Neurol 2001; 49:384–92.

Jungmann E, Schoffling C. Akathisia and metoclopramide. Lancet 1982; 2:221.

Kabacki K, Isbruch K, Schilling K et al. Genetic heterogeneity in rapid onset dystonia-parkinsonism: description of a new family. J Neurol Neurosurg Psychiatry 2005; 76:860–2.

Kahlbaum K. Die Katatonie oder das Spanungsirresein. Berlin, Hirsch, 1874.

Kaiko RF, Foley KM, Grabinski PY et al. Central nervous system excitatory effects of meperidine in cancer patients. Ann Neurol 1983; 13: 180–5.

Kalita J, Misra UK. Markedly severe dystonia in Japanese encephalitis. Mov Disord 2000; 15:1168–72.

Kane J, Rifkin A, Quitkin F et al. Extrapyramidal side-effects with lithium treatment. Am J Psychiatry 1978; 135:851–3.

Kaplan PW. Nonconvulsive status epilepticus in the emergency room. Epilepsia 1996; 37:643–50.

Karp BI, Laureno R. Pontine and extrapontine myelinolysis: a neurologic disorder following rapid correction of hyponatremia. Medicine 1993; 72:359–73.

Kase CS, Maulsby GO, deJuan E et al. Hemichorea–hemiballism and lacunar infarction in the basal ganglia. Neurology 1981; 31:452–5.

Katayama Y, Yamamoto T, Kobayshi K et al. Deep brain and motor cortex stimulation for post-stroke movement disorders and post-stroke pain. Acta Neurochir 2003; 87:121–3.

Keepers GA, Clappison VJ, Casey DE. Initial anticholinergic prophylaxis for neuroleptic-induced extrapyramidal syndromes. Arch Gen Psychiatry 1983; 40:1113–17.

Kelwala S, Pomara N, Stanley M et al. Lithium-associated accentuation of extrapyramidal symptoms in individuals with Alzheimer's disease. J Clin Psychiatry 1984; 45:342–4.

Kerbeshian J, Burd L, Pettit R. A possible post-streptococcal movement disorder with chorea and tics. Dev Med Child Neurol 1990; 32:642–4.

Kertesz A. Paroxysmal kinesigenic choreoathetosis: an entity within the paroxysmal choreoathetosis syndrome. Description of 10 cases, including 1 autopsied. Neurology 1967; 17:680–90.

Keschner M, Sloane P. Encephalitic, idiopathic and arteriosclerotic parkinsonism: a clinicopathologic study. Arch Neurol Psychiatry 1931; 25:1011–41.

Keswani SC, Kossoff EH, Krauss GL et al. Amelioration of spinal myoclonus with levetiracetam. J Neurol Neurosurg Psychiatry 2002; 73:456–9.

Kidron D, Melamed E. Forms of dystonia in patients with Parkinson's disease. Neurology 1987; 37:1009–11.

Kim CH, Perlstein MA. Encephalitis with catatonic schizophrenic symptoms. Ill Med J 1970; 138:503–7.

Kim JS. Delayed onset mixed involuntary movements after thalamic stroke. Clinical, radiological and pathophysiological findings. Brain 2001a; 124:299–309.

Kim JS. Asterixis after unilateral stroke: Lesion localization of 30 patients. Neurology 2001b; 56:533–6.

Kimber TE, Thompson PD. Symptomatic hyperekplexia occurring as a result of pontine infarction. Mov Disord 1997; 12:815–16.

Kinirons P, Fulton A, Keoghan M et al. Paraneoplastic limbic encephalitis (PLE) and chorea associated with CRMP-5 neuronal antibody. Neurology 2003; 61:1623–4.

Kirby GH, Davis TK. Psychiatric aspects of epidemic encephalitis. Arch Neurol Psychiatry 1921; 5:491–51.

Kiriakakis V, Bhatia K, Quinn NP et al. The natural history of tardive dystonia: a long-term follow-up study of 107 cases. Brain 1998; 121:2053–66.

Kirubakaren V, Mayfield D, Rengachary S. Dyskinesia and psychosis in a patient following baclofen withdrawal. Am J Psychiatry 1984; 141:692–3.

Klatka LA, Louis ED, Schiffer RB. Psychiatric features in diffuse Lewy body disease: a clinicopathologic study using Alzheimer's disease and Parkinson's disease comparison groups. Neurology 1996; 47:1148–52.

Klawans HL, Barr A. Prevalence of spontaneous lingual-facial-buccal dyskinesias in the elderly. Neurology 1981; 31:558–9.

Klawans HL, Barr A. Recurrence of childhood multiple tic in late adult life. Arch Neurol 1985; 42:1079–80.

Klawans HL, Goetz CG, Bergen D. Levodopa-induced myoclonus. Arch Neurol 1975; 32:331–4.

Klawans HL, Moses H, Nausieda PA et al. Treatment and prognosis of hemiballism. N Engl J Med 1976a; 295:1348–50.

Klawans HL, Lipton M, Simon L. Calcification of the basal ganglia as a cause of levodopa-resistant parkinsonism. Neurology 1976b; 26:221–5.

Klawans HL, Glantz R, Tanner CM et al. Primary writing tremor: a selective action tremor. Neurology 1982a; 32:203–6.

Klawans HL, Stein RW, Tanner CM et al. A pure parkinsonian syndrome following acute carbon monoxide intoxication. Arch Neurol 1982b; 39:302–4.

Kleinschmidt-DeMasters BK, Marder BA, Levi ME et al. Naturally acquired West Nile virus encephalomyelitis in transplant recipients: clinical, laboratory, diagnostic and neuropathological features. Arch Neurol 2004; 61:1210–20.

Ko SB, Ahn TB, Kim JR et al. A case of adult-onset tic disorder following carbon monoxide intoxication. Can J Neurol Sci 2004; 31:268–70.

Koehler J, Jakumeit U. Subacute sclerosing panencephalitis presenting as Leonhard's speech-prompt catatonia. Br J Psychiatry 1976; 129:29–31.

Koller WC. Edentulous orodyskinesia. Neurology 1983; 13:97–9.

Koller WC, Cochran JW, Klawans HL. Calcification of the basal ganglia: computerized tomography and clinical correlation. Neurology 1979; 29:328–33.

Konagaya M, Konagaya Y. MRI in hemiballism due to Sydenham's chorea. J Neurol Neurosurg Psychiatry 1992; 55:238–9.

Kooiker JC, Sumi SM. Movement disorder as a manifestation of diphenylhydantoin intoxication. Neurology 1974; 24:68–71.

Koskiniemi M, Donner M, Majuri H et al. Progressive myoclonus epilepsy: a clinical and histopathological study. Acta Neurol Scand 1974; 50:307–32.

Koukoulis A, Herrerd JS, Gomez-Alonso J. Blepharospasm induced by flunarazine. J Neurol Neurosurg Psychiatry 1997; 63:412–13.

Krack P. Deuschl G, Kapa M et al. Delayed onset of 'rubral tremor' 23 years after brainstem trauma. Mov Disord 1994; 9:240–2.

Kraepelin E. Psychiatry. A textbook for students and physicians, 6th edn, 1899, translated by Metoui H, Ayed S. Canton, MA: Science History Publications, 1990.

Kramer PL, Mineta M, Klein C et al. Rapid-onset dystonia-parkinsonism: linkage to chromosome 19q13. Ann Neurol 1999; 46:176–82.

Krams M, Quinton R, Ashburner J et al. Kallmann's syndrome: mirror movements associated with bilateral corticospinal tract hypertrophy. Neurology 1999; 52:816–22.

Krauss JK, Jankovic J. Tics secondary to craniocerebral trauma. Mov Disord 1997; 12:776–82.

Krauss JK, Nobbe F, Wakhloo AK et al. Movement disorders in astrocytomas of the basal ganglia and the thalamus. J Neurol Neurosurg Psychiatry 1992; 55:1162–7.

Krauss JK, Wakhloo AK, Nobbe F et al. MR pathological correlations of severe posttraumatic tremor. Neurol Res 1995; 17:409–16.

Krauss JK, Seeger W, Jankovic J. Cervical dystonia with tumors of the posterior fossa. Mov Disord 1997; 12:443–7.

Kristensen O, Sindrup EH. Psychomotor epilepsy and psychosis. III. Social and psychological correlates. Acta Neurol Scand 1979; 59:1–9.

Kronfol Z, Greden JF, Zis AP. Imipramine-induced tremor: effects of a beta-adrenergic blocking agent. J Clin Psychiatry 1983; 44:225–6.

Krystkowiak P, Martinat P, Defebvre L et al. Dystonia after striatopallidal and thalamic stroke: clinicoradiological correlations and pathophysiological mechanism. J Neurol Neurosurg Pyschiatry 1998; 65:703–8.

Kuba R, Rektor I, Brazdil M. Ictal limb dystonia in temporal lobe epilepsy: an invasive video-EEG finding. Eur J Neurol 2003; 10:641–9.

Kulisevsky J, Berthier ML, Pujol J. Hemiballismus and secondary mania following right thalamic infarction. Neurology 1993; 43:1422–4.

Kulisevsky J, Asuncion A, Berthier ML. Bipolar disorder and unilateral parkinsonism after a brainstem infarction. Mov Disord 1995; 10:799–802.

Kumral E, Evyapan D, Balkir K. Acute caudate vascular lesions. Stroke 1999; 30:100–8.

Kushner MJ. Chorea and cimetidine. Ann Intern Med 1982; 96:126.

Kutcher SP, Williamson P, MacKenzie S et al. Successful clonazepam treatment of neuroleptic-induced akathisia in older adolescents and young adults. J Clin Psychopharmacol 1989; 9:403–6.

Kwak CH, Jankovic J. Tourettism and dystonia after subcortical stroke. Mov Disord 2002; 17:821–5.

Lai SL, Tseng YL, Hsu MC et al. Magnetic resonance imaging and single-photon emission computed tomography changes in hypoglycemia-induced chorea. Mov Disord 2004; 19:475–8.

Lance JW. Familial paroxysmal dystonic choreoathetosis and its differentiation from related syndromes. Ann Neurol 1977; 2:285–93.

Lance JW, Adams RD. The syndrome of intention or action myoclonus as a sequel to hypoxic encephalopathy. Brain 1963; 86:111–36.

Lancman ME, Asconape MJ, Penry JK. Choreiform movements associated with the use of valproate. Arch Neurol 1994; 51:702–4.

Lang AE. Persistent hemiballismus with lesions outside the subthalamic nucleus. Can J Neurol Sci 1985; 12:125–8.

Lang AE. Withdrawal akathisia: case reports and a proposed classification of chronic akathisia. Mov Disord 1994; 9:188–92.

Lang AE, Johnson K. Akathisia in idiopathic Parkinson's disease. Neurology 1987; 37:477–81.

Langston JW, Ballard P, Tetrud JW et al. Chronic parkinsonism in humans due to a product of meperidine-analog synthesis. Science 1983; 249:979–80.

Lanham JG, Brown MM, Hughes GRV. Cerebral systemic lupus erythematosus presenting with catatonia. Postgrad Med J 1985; 61:329–30.

Lapierre YD. Control of lithium tremor with propranolol. Can Med Assoc J 1976; 114:619–20.

Laplane D, Attal N, Sauron B et al. Lesions of basal ganglia due to disulfiram neurotoxicity. J Neurol Neurosurg Psychiatry 1992; 55:925–9.

Lapresle J. Palatal myoclonus. Adv Neurol 1986; 43:265–73.

Leavitt S, Tyler H. Studies in asterixis. Arch Neurol 1964; 10:360–8.

Ledbetter M. Atomoxetine associated with onset of a motor tic. J Child Adolesc Psychopharmacol 2005; 15:331–3.

Lederman RJ, Henry CE. Progressive dialysis encephalopathy. Ann Neurol 1978; 4:199–204.

Lee B-C, Hwang S-H, Chang GY. Hemiballismus–hemichorea in older diabetic women: a clinical syndrome with MRI correlation. *Neurology* 1999; **52**:646–8.

Lee BI, Lesser RP, Pippenger CE *et al.* Familial paroxysmal hypnogenic dystonia. *Neurology* 1985; **35**:1357–60.

Lee MS, Rinne JO, Ceballos-Baumann A *et al.* Dystonia after head trauma. *Neurology* 1994; **44**:1374–8.

Lee MS, Kim YD, Lyoo CH. Oculogyric crises as an initial manifestation of Wilson's disease. *Neurology* 1999; **52**:1714–15.

Lees AJ, Robertson M, Trimble MR *et al.* A clinical study of Gilles de la Tourette syndrome in the United Kingdom. *J Neurol Neurosurg Psychiatry* 1984; **47**:1–8.

Lehericy S, Vidailhet M, Dormont D *et al.* Striatopallidal and thalamic dystonia: a magnetic resonance imaging anatamoclinical study. *Arch Neurol* 1996; **53**:241–50.

Lehericy S, Grand S, Pollak P *et al.* Clinical characteristics and topography of lesions in movement disorders due to thalamic lesions. *Neurology* 2001; **57**:1055–66.

Lenton RJ, Cofti M, Smith RG. Hemiballismus treated with sodium valproate. *BMJ* 1981; **283**:17–18.

Lera G, Scipioni O, Garcia S *et al.* A combined pattern of movement disorders resulting from posterolateral thalamic lesions of a vascular nature: a syndrome with clinico-radiologic correlation. *Mov Disord* 2000; **15**:120–6.

Lerner V, Bergman J, Statsensko N *et al.* Vitamin B6 treatment in acute neuroleptic-induced akathisia: a randomized, double-blind, placebo-controlled study. *J Clin Psychiatry* 2004; **65**:1550–4.

Lesch M, Nyhan WL. A familial disorder of uric acid metabolism and central nervous system function. *Am J Med* 1964; **36**:561–70.

Lewis I, Johnson IM. Chorea: an unusual manifestation of cerebral metastases. *Neurology* 1968; **18**:948–52.

LeWitt PA, Walters A, Hening W *et al.* Persistent movement disorders induced by buspirone. *Mov Disord* 1993; **8**:331–4.

Lightman SL. Phenobarbital dyskinesia. *Postgrad Med J* 1978; **54**:114–15.

Lim J, Yagnik P, Schrader P *et al.* Ictal catatonia as a manifestation of nonconvulsive status epilepticus. *J Neurol Neurosurg Psychiatry* 1986; **49**:833–6.

Lin J-J, Chang M-K. Hemiballism–hemichorea and non-ketotic hyperglycemia. *J Neurol Neurosurg Psychiatry* 1994; **57**:748–50.

Lin J-J, Lin GY, Shih C *et al.* Presentation of striatal hyperintensity on T1-weighted MRI in patients with hemiballism-hemichorea caused by non-ketotic hyperglycemia: report of seven new cases and a review of the literature. *J Neurol* 2001; **248**:750–5.

Lindenmeyer J-P, Da Silva D, Buendia A *et al.* Tic-like syndrome after treatment with clozapine. *Am J Psychiatry* 1995; **152**:649.

Lipinski JF, Zubenko GS, Cohen BM *et al.* Propranolol in the treatment of neuroleptic induced akathisia. *Am J Psychiatry* 1984; **141**:412–15.

Lipinski JF, Mallya A, Zimmerman P *et al.* Fluoxetine-induced akathisia: clinical and theoretical implications. *J Clin Psychiatry* 1989; **50**:339–42.

Lippmann S, Moskovitz R, O'Tuama L. Tricyclic-induced myoclonus. *Am J Psychiatry* 1977; **134**:90–1.

Little JT, Jankovic J. Tardive myoclonus: a case report. *Mov Disord* 1987; **2**:307–11.

Litvan I, Mangone CA, McKee A *et al.* Natural history of progressive supranuclear palsy (Steele–Richardson–Olszewski syndrome) and clinical predictors of survival: a clinicopathologic study. *J Neurol Neurosurg Psychiatry* 1996; **61**:615–20.

Litvan I, Goetz CG, Jankovic J *et al.* What is the accuracy of the clinical diagnosis of multiple system atrophy? A clinicopathologic study. *Arch Neurol* 1997a; **54**:937–44.

Litvan I, Agid Y, Goetz C *et al.* Accuracy of the clinical diagnosis of corticobasal degeneration: a clinicopathologic study. *Neurology* 1997b; **48**:119–25.

Logsdail SJ, Toone BK. Postictal psychoses: a clinical and phenomenological description. *Br J Psychiatry* 1988; **152**:246–52.

Lombroso CT. Lamotrigene-induced tourettism. *Neurology* 1999; **52**:1191–4.

Louis ED, Lynch T, Kaufmann P *et al.* Diagnostic guidelines in central nervous system Whipple's disease. *Ann Neurol* 1996; **40**:561–8.

Louis ED, Klatka LA, Liu Y *et al.* Comparison of extrapyramidal features in 31 pathologically confirmed cases of diffuse Lewy body disease and 34 pathologically confirmed cases of Parkinson's disease. *Neurology* 1997; **48**:376–80.

Louis ED, Anderson KE, Moskowitz C *et al.* Dystonia-predominant adult-onset Huntington disease: association between motor phenotype and age of onset in adults. *Arch Neurol* 2000; **57**:1326–30.

Lu CS, Huang CC, Chu NS *et al.* Levodopa failure in chronic manganism. *Neurology* 1994; **44**:1600–2.

Lugaresi E, Cirignotta F. Hypnogenic paroxysmal dystonia: epileptic seizure or a new syndrome? *Sleep* 1981; **4**:129–38.

Lugaresi E, Cirignotta F, Montagna P. Nocturnal paroxysmal dystonia. *J Neurol Neurosurg Psychiatry* 1986; **49**:375–80.

Lundh H, Tunving K. An extrapyramidal choreiform syndrome caused by amphetamine addiction. *J Neurol Neurosurg Psychiatry* 1981; **44**:728–30.

Luque FA, Selhorst JB, Petruska P. Parkinsonism induced by high-dose cystosine arabinoside. *Mov Disord* 1987; **2**:219–22.

Mac DS, Pardo MP. Systemic lupus erythematosus and catatonia: a case report. *J Clin Psychiatry* 1983; **44**:155–6.

Magaudda A, Ferlazzo E, Nguyen V-H *et al.* Unverricht–Lundborg disease: a condition with self-limited progression: long-term follow-up of 20 patients. *Epilepsia* 2006; **47**:860–6.

Maher ER, Lees AJ. The clinical features and natural history of Steele–Richardson–Olszewski syndrome (progressive supranuclear palsy). *Neurology* 1986; **36**:1005–8.

Maher J, Choudri S, Halliday W *et al.* AIDS dementia complex with generalized myoclonus. *Mov Disord* 1997; **12**:593–7.

Mahloudji M, Pikielny R. Hereditary essential myoclonus. *Brain* 1967; **90**:669–74.

Mahoney CA, Arieff AI. Uremic encephalopathies: clinical, biochemical, and experimental features. *Am J Kidney Dis* 1982; **2**:324–36.

Malamud N, Hirano A, Kurland LT. Pathoanatomic changes in amyotrophic lateral sclerosis on Guam. *Neurology* 1961; **5**:401–14.

Malur C, Pasol E, Francis A. ECT for prolonged catatonia. *J ECT* 2001; **17**:55–9.

Manford MR, Fish DR, Shorvon SD. Startle provoked epileptic seizures: features in 19 patients. *J Neurol Neurosurg Psychiatry* 1996; **61**: 151–6.

Mann SC, Caroff SN, Bleir HR et al. Lethal catatonia. *Am J Psychiatry* 1986; **143**:1374–81.

Manyam BV, Walters AS, Naria KR. Bilateral striatopallidodentate calcinosis: clinical characteristics of patients seen in a registry. *Mov Disord* 2001; **16**:258–64.

Maraganore DM, Folger WN, Swanson JW et al. Movement disorders as sequelae of central pontine myelinolysis: report of three cases. *Mov Disord* 1992; **7**:142–8.

Marder K, Ming-Xin T, Cote L et al. The frequency and associated risk factors for dementia in patients with Parkinson's disease. *Arch Neurol* 1995; **52**:695–701.

de Mari M, De Blasi R, Lamberti P et al. Unilateral pallidal lesion after acute disulfiram intoxication: a clinical and magnetic resonance imaging study. *Mov Disorders* 1993; **8**:247–9.

Marsden CD, Harrison MJG. Idiopathic torsion dystonia (dystonia musculorum deformans): a review of forty-two patients. *Brain* 1974; **97**:793–810.

Marti-Masso JF, Poza JJ. Cinnarizine-induced parkinsonism: ten years later. *Mov Disord* 1998; **13**:453–6.

Martin JP, Alcock NS. Hemichorea associated with a lesion of the corpus luysii. *Brain* 1934; **57**:504–16.

Martin WE, Loewenson RB, Resch JA et al. Parkinson's disease: clinical analysis of 100 patients. *Neurology* 1973; **23**: 783–90.

Martinez-Cage JM, Marsden CD. Hemi-dystonia secondary to localized basal ganglia tumors. *J Neurol Neurosurg Psychiatry* 1984; **47**:704–9.

Martland HS. Punch drunk. *J Am Med Assoc* 1928; **91**:1103–7.

Mathews WB. Familial calcification of the basal ganglia with response to parathormone. *J Neurol Neurosurg Psychiatry* 1957; **20**:172–7.

Matsunaga K, Uozumi T, Qingrui L et al. Amantadine-induced cortical myoclonus. *Neurology* 2001; **56**:279–80.

Matsuo H, Takashima H, Kishikawa M et al. Pure akinesia: an atyical manifestation of progressive supranuclear palsy. *J Neurol Neurosurg Psychiatry* 1991; **54**:397–400.

Matsuo H, Kamakura K, Saito M et al. Familial paroxysmal dystonic choreoathetosis. Clinical findings in a large Japanese family and genetic linkage to chromosome 2q. *Arch Neurol* 1999; **56**:721–6.

Mayeux R, Denaro J, Hemenegildo N et al. A population-based investigation of Parkinson's disease with and without dementia: relationship to age and gender. *Arch Neurol* 1992; **49**:492–7.

McKee D, Talbot P. Chorea as a presenting feature of variant Creutzfeldt–Jakob disease. *Mov Disord* 2003; **18**:837–8.

McLean DR, Jacobs H, Mielke BW. Methanol poisoning: a clinical and pathological study. *Ann Neurol* 1980; **8**:161–7.

McNeill A. Chorea induced by low-dose tranzodone. *Eur Neurol* 2006; **55**:101–12.

Medlock MD, Cruse RS, Winek SJ et al. A 10-year experience with postpartum chorea. *Ann Neurol* 1993; **34**:820–6.

Melamed E. Early-morning dystonia, a late effect of long-term levodopa therapy in Parkinson's disease. *Arch Neurol* 1979; **36**:308–10.

Melamed E, Korn-Lubetzk I, Reches A et al. Hemiballismus: detection of focal hemorrhage in subthalamic nucleus by CT scan. *Ann Neurol* 1978; **4**:582.

Mendhekar DN, Duggal HS. Isolated oculogyric crisis on clozapine discontinuation. *J Neuropsychiatry Clin Neurosci* 2006; **18**:424–5.

Menza MA, Cocchiola J, Golbe LI. Psychiatric symptoms in progressive supranuclear palsy. *Psychosomatics* 1995; **36**:550–4.

Mercadante S. Pathophysiology and treatment of opioid-related myoclonus in cancer patients. *Pain* 1998; **74**:5–9.

Meseguer E, Taboada R, Sanchez V et al. Life-threatening parkinsonism induced by Kava-Kava. *Mov Disord* 2002; **17**:195–6.

Meyer T, Ludolph AC, Munch C. Ifosfamide encephalopathy presenting with asterixis. *J Neuol Sci* 2002; **15**:85–8.

Meythaler JM, Roper JF, Brunner RC. Cyproheptadine for intrathecal baclofen withdrawal. *Arch Phys Med Rehabil* 2003; **84**:638–42.

Miller DD, Sharafuddin MJA, Kathol RG. A case of clozapine-induced neuroleptic malignant syndrome. *J Clin Psychiatry* 1991; **52**:99–101.

Misra PC, Hay GG. Encephalitis presenting as acute schizophrenia. *Br Med J* 1971; **1**:532–3.

Mitchell E, Mathews KL. Gilles de la Tourette's disorder associated with pemoline. *Am J Psychiatry* 1980; **137**:1618–19.

Miwa H, Harori K, Kondo T et al. Thalamic tremor: case reports and implications of the tremor-generating mechanism. *Neurology* 1996; **46**:75–9.

Miyagi Y, Shima F, Ishido K et al. Posteroventral pallidotomy for midbrain tremor after a pontine hemorrhage. Case report. *J Neurosurg* 1999; **91**:885–8.

Moersch FP, Kernohan JW. Hemiballismus: a clinicopathologic study. *Arch Neurol Psychiatry* 1939; **41**:365–72.

Molinuevo JL, Marti MJ, Blesa R et al. Pure akinesia: an unusual phenotype of Hallervorden–Spatz syndrome. *Mov Disord* 2003; **18**:1351–3.

Mones RJ, Elizan TS, Siegel GJ. Analysis of L-dopa induced dyskinesias in 51 patients with parkinsonism. *J Neurol Neurosurg Psychiatry* 1971; **34**:668–73.

Morres CA, Dire DJ. Movement disorders as a manifestation of nonketotic hyperglycemia. *J Emerg Med* 1989; **7**:359–64.

Morrison JR. Catatonia. Retarded and excited types. *Arch Gen Psychiatry* 1973; **28**:515–16.

Moshe K, Iulian I, Seth K et al. Clomipramine-induced tourettism in obsessive-compulsive disorder: clinical and theoretical implications. *Clin Neuropharmacol* 1994; **17**:338–43.

Moulignier A, Allo S, Zittoun R et al. Recombinant interferon-alpha-induced chorea and frontal subcortical dementia. Neurology 2002; 58:328–30.

Mount LA, Reback S. Familial paroxysmal choreoathetosis: preliminary report of an hitherto undescribed clinical syndrome. Arch Neurol Psychiatry 1940; 44:841–7.

Mukand JA, Fitzsimmons C, Wennemer HK et al. Olanzapine for the treatment of hemiballismus: a case report. Arch Phys Med Rehabil 2005; 86:587–90.

Mulder DW, Parrott M, Thaler M. Sequelae of western equine encephalitis. Neurology 1951; 1:318–27.

Munchau A, Mathen D, Cox T et al. Unilateral lesions of the globus pallidus: report of four patients presenting with focal or segmental dystonia. J Neurol Neurosurg Psychiatry 2000; 69:494–8.

Murgod UA, Muthane UB, Ravi V et al. Persistent motor disorders following Japanese encephalitis. Neurology 2002; 57:2313–15.

Murphy MJ, Goldsein MN. Diphenylhydantoin-induced asterixis. A clinical study. JAMA 1974; 29:538–40.

Murrow RW, Schweiger GD, Kepes JJ et al. Parkinsonism due to a basal ganglia lacunar state: clinicopathologic correlation. Neurology 1990; 40:897–900.

Nandagopal R, Moorthy SG. Dramatic levodopa responsiveness of dystonia in a sporadic case of spinocerebellar ataxia type 3. Postgrad Med J 2004; 80:363–5.

Nath U, Ben-Shlomo Y, Thomson RG et al. Clinical features and natural history of progressive supranuclear palsy. Neurology 2003; 60:910–16.

Nausieda PA, Koller WC, Klawans HL et al. Phenytoin and choreic movements. N Engl J Med 1978; 298:1093–4.

Nausieda PA, Koller WC, Weiner WJ et al. Chorea induced by oral contraceptives. Neurology 1979; 29:1605–9.

Nausieda PA, Grossman BJ, Koller WC et al. Sydenham chorea: an update. Neurology 1980a; 30:331–4.

Nausieda PA, Weiner WJ, Klawans HL. Dystonic foot response of parkinsonism. Arch Neurol 1980b; 37:132–6.

Navin B, Jordan B, Price R. The AIDS-dementia complex. I. Clinical features. Ann Neurol 1986; 19:517–24.

Nelles G, Cramer SC, Schaechter JD et al. Quantitative assessment of mirror movements after stroke. Stoke 1998; 29:1182–7.

Newton MR, Berkovic SF, Austin MC et al. Dystonia, clinical lateralization, and regional blood flow changes in temporal lobe seizures. Neurology 1992; 42:371–7.

Nijssen PC, Brusse E, Leyton AC et al. Autosomal dominant adult neuronal ceroid lipofuscinosis: parkinsonism due to both striatal and nigral dysfunction. Mov Disord 2002; 17:482–7.

Nomoto M, Thompson PD, Sheehy MP et al. Anticholinergic-induced chorea in the treatment of focal dystonia. Mov Disord 1987; 2:53–6.

Northam RS, Singer HS. Postencephalitic acquired Tourette-like syndrome in a child. Neurology 1991; 41:592–3.

Nygaard TG, Duvoisin RC. Hereditary dystonia–parkinsonism syndrome of juvenile onset. Neurology 1986; 36:1424–8.

Nygaard TG, Trugman JM, de Yebenes JG et al. Dopa-responsive dystonia: the spectrum of clinical manifestations in a large North American family. Neurology 1990; 40:66–9.

Nyhan WL. Clinical features of the Lesch–Nyhan syndrome. Arch Int Med 1972; 130:186–92.

Nyland H, Skre H. Cerebral calcinosis with late onset encephalopathy: unusual type of pseudo-pseudohypoparathyroidism. Acta Neurol Scand 1977; 56:309–25.

Obeso JA, Viteri C, Martinez Lage JM et al. Toxic myoclonus. Adv Neurol 1986; 43:225–30.

Oh J, Park KD, Cho HJ et al. Spasmodic dysphonia induced by valproic acid. Epilepsia 2004; 45:880–1.

Okun MS, Riestra RA, Nadeau SE. Treatment of ballism and pseudobulbar affect with sertraline. Arch Neurol 2001; 58:1682–4.

Oppenheim H. Uber eine eigenartige krampfkrankheit des kindlichen und jugendlichen alters (dysbasia lordotica progressiva, dystonia musculorum deformans). Neurol Centrabla 1911; 30:1090–107.

Onofrj M, Thomas A, Paci C et al. Gabapentin in orthostatic tremor: results of a double-blind crossover with placebo in four patients. Neurology 1998; 51:880–2.

Opida CL, Korthals JK, Somasunderam M. Bilateral ballismus in phenytoin intoxication. Ann Neurol 1978; 3:186.

Owens DGC, Johnstone EC, Frith CD. Spontaneous involuntary disorders of movement: their prevalence, severity, and distribution in chronic schizophrenics with and without treatment with neuroleptics. Arch Gen Psychiatry 1982; 39:452–61.

Pacchetti C, Cristina S, Nappi G. Reversible chorea and focal dystonia in vitamin B12 deficiency. N Engl J Med 2002; 347:295.

Pakainis A, Drake MA, John K et al. Forced normalization: acute psychosis after seizure control in seven patients. Arch Neurol 1987; 44:289–92.

Panayiotopoulos CP, Obeid T, Tahan AR. Juvenile myoclonic epilepsy: a 5-year prospective study. Epilepsia 1994; 35:285–96.

Pantano P, Di Cesare S, Ricci M et al. Hemichorea after a striatal ischemic lesion: evidence of thalamic disinhibition using single-photon emission computed tomography: a case report. Mov Disord 1996; 11:445–7.

Papez JW, Hertzman J, Rundles RW. Athetosis and pallidal deficiency. Arch Neurol Psychiatry 1938; 40:789–9.

Pardo J, Marcos A, Bhathal H et al. Chorea as a form of presentation of human immunodeficiency virus-associated dementia complex. Neurology 1998; 50:568–9.

Parry GJ, Bredesen DE. Sensory neuropathy with low-dose pyridoxine. Neurology 1985; 35:1466–8.

Pascual-Leone A, Dhuna A. Cocaine-associated multifocal tics. Neurology 1990; 40:999–1000.

Patel HC, Bruza D, Yerogani V. Myoclonus with trazodone. J Clin Psychopharmacol 1988; 8:152.

Paus S, Potzach B, Risse JH et al. Chorea and antiphospholipid antibodies: treatment with methotrexate. Neurology 2001; 56:137–8.

Pedersen SB, Petersen KA. Juvenile myoclonic epilepsy: clinical and EEG features. Acta Neurol Scand 1998; 97:160–3.

Penn H, Racy J, Lapham L et al. Catatonic behavior, viral encephalopathy, and death. Arch Gen Psychiatry 1972; 27:758–61.

Perry TL, Bratty PJA, Hansen S et al. Hereditary mental depression and parkinsonism with taurine deficiency. Arch Neurol 1975; 32:108–13.

Pfeil ET. Hemiballismus: hemichorea. J Nerv Ment Dis 1952; 116:36–47.

Pfister H-W, Preac-Mursic V, Wilske B et al. Catatonic syndrome in acute severe encephalitis due to Borrelia burgdorferi infection. Neurology 1993; 43:433–5.

Piccolo I, Causarano R, Sterzi R et al. Chorea in patients with AIDS. Acta Neurol Scand 1999; 100:332–6.

Pina MA, Modrego PJ. Dystonia induced by gabapentin. Ann Pharmacother 2005; 39:380–2.

Pittock SJ, Joyce C, O'Keane V et al. Rapid-onset dystonia-parkinsonism. A clinical and genetic analysis of a new kindred. Neurology 2000; 55:991–5.

Plana MT, Blanch J, Romero S et al. Toxic catatonia secondary to azithromycin. J Clin Psychiatry 2006; 67:492–3.

Podskalny GD, Factor SA. Chorea caused by lithium intoxication. A case report and literature review. Mov Disord 1996; 11:733–7.

Poyurovsky M, Pashinian A, Weizman R et al. Low-dose mirtazapine: a new option in the treatment of antipsychotic-induced akathisia. A randomized, double-blind, placebo- and propranolol-controlled trial. Biol Psychiatry 2006; 59:1071–7.

Pradhan S, Pandey N, Shashank S et al. Parkinsonism due to predominant involvement of substantia nigra in Japanese encephalitis. Neurology 1999; 53:1781–6.

Prashanth LK, Taly AB, Ravi V et al. Adult subacute sclerosing panencephalitis: clinical profile of 39 patients from a tertiary care center. J Neurol Neurosurg Psychiatry 2006; 77:630–3.

Priori A, Bertolasi L, Berardelli A et al. Acute dystonic reaction to Ecstasy. Mov Disord 1995; 10:353.

Prodan CI, Monnot M, Ross ED et al. Reversible dementia with parkinsonian features associated with budesonide use. Neurology 2006; 67:723.

Provini F, Plazzi G, Tinuper P et al. Nocturnal frontal lobe epilepsy. A clinical and polygraphic overview of 100 consecutive cases. Brain 1999; 122:1017–31.

Quartarone A, Girlanda P, Risitano G et al. Focal hand dystonia in a patient with thoracic outlet syndrome. J Neurol Neurosurg Psychiatry 1998; 65: 272–4.

Quartarone A, Girlanda P, Vita G et al. Oromandibular dystonia in a patient with bilateral putaminal necrosis after methanol poisoning: an electrophysiological study. Eur Neurol 2000; 44:127–8.

Racette BA, Esper GJ, Antenor J et al. Pathophysiology of parkinsonism due to hydrocephalus. J Neurol Neurosurg Psychiatry 2004; 75:1617–19.

Rail D, Scholtz C, Swash M. Post-encephalitic parkinsonism: current experience. J Neurol Neurosurg Psychiatry 1981; 44:670–6.

Raskin DE, Frank SW. Herpes encephalitis with catatonic stupor. Arch Gen Psychiatry 1974; 31:544–6.

Raskin NH, Fishman RA. Neurologic disorders in renal failure. N Engl J Med 1976; 294:143–8, 204–10.

Rasmussen P. Persistent mirror movements: a clinical study of 17 children, adolescents and young adults. Dev Med Child Neurol 1993; 35:699–707.

Read AE, Laidlaw J, Sherlock S. Neuropsychiatric complications of portocaval anastamosis. Lancet 1961; 1:961–4.

Read SL. Catatonia in thrombotic thrombocytopenic purpura. J Clin Psychiatry 1983; 44:343–4.

Reeves AL, So EL, Sharbrough FW et al. Movement disorders associated with the use of gabapentin. Epilepsia 1996; 37:988–90.

Reisberg B. Catatonia associated with disulfiram therapy. J Nerv Ment Dis 1978; 166:607–9.

Remy P, de Recondo A, Defer G et al. Peduncular 'rubral' tremor and dopaminergic innervation: a PET study. Neurology 1995; 45:472–7.

Richards RN, Barnett HJ. Paroxysmal dystonic choreoathetosis. A family study and review of the literature. Neurology 1968; 18:461–9.

Rifkin AR, Quitkin F, Klein DF. Akinesia: a poorly recognized drug-induced extrapyramidal behavioral disorder. Arch Gen Psychiatry 1975; 32:672–4.

Riley D, Lang AE. Hemiballism in multiple sclerosis. Mov Disord 1988; 3:88–94.

Riley DE, Lange AE, Lewis A et al. Cortical-basal ganglionic degeneration. Neurology 1990; 40:1203–12.

Ringman JM, Jankovic J. Occurrence of tics in Asperger's syndrome and autistic disorder. J Child Neurol 2000; 15:394–400.

Rinne JO, Lee MS, Thompson PD et al. Corticobasal degeneration: a clinical study of 36 cases. Brain 1994; 117:1183–96.

Rio J, Montalban J, Pujadas F et al. Asterixis associated with anatomic cerebral lesions: a study of 45 cases. Acta Neurol Scand 1995; 91:377–81.

Ristic AJ, Svetel M, Dragasevic N et al. Bilateral chorea-ballism associated with hyperthyroidism. Mov Disord 2004; 19:982–3.

Ristic AJ, Vojvodic N, Jankovic S et al. The frequency of reversible parkinsonism and cognitive decline associated with valproate treatment: a study of 364 patients with different types of epilepsy. Epilepsia 2006; 47:2183–5.

Ritchie EC, Bridenbaugh RH, Jabbari B et al. Acute generalized myoclonus following buspirone administration. J Clin Psychiatry 1988; 49:242–3.

Rittsmannberger H. Asterixis induced by psychotropic drug treatment. Clin Neuropharmacol 1996; 19:349–55.

Rittsmannberger H, Lebihuber F. Asterixis induced by carbamazepine therapy. Biol Psychiatry 1992; 32:364–8.

Robertson PL, Garofalo EA, Silverstein FS et al. Carbamazepine-induced tics. Epilepsia 1993; 34:965–8.

Rodrigues JP, Edwards DJ, Walters SE et al. Blinded placebo crossover study of gabapentin in primary orthostatic tremor. Mov Disord 2006; 21:900–5.

Rodriguez ME, Artieda J, Zubieta JL et al. Reflex myoclonus in olivopontocerebellar atrophy. J Neurol Neurosurg Psychiatry 1994; 57:316–19.

Romisher S, Feller R, Dougherty J et al. Tagamet-induced acute dystonia. Ann Emerg Med 1987; 16:1162–4.

Rosebush PI, Mazurek MF. Catatonia after benzodiazepine withdrawal. *J Clin Psychopharmacol* 1996; **16**:315–19.

Rosebush P, Stewart T. A prospective analysis of 24 episodes of neuroleptic malignant syndrome. *Am J Psychiatry* 1989; **146**:717–25.

Rosebush PI, Hildebrand AM, Furlong BG et al. Catatonic syndrome in a general hospital psychiatric population: frequency, clinical presentation, and response to lorazepam. *J Clin Psychiatry* 1990; **51**:347–53.

Rosebush PI, MacQueen GM, Clarke JTR et al. Late-onset Tay–Sachs disease presenting as catatonic schizophrenia: diagnostic and treatment issues. *J Clin Psychiatry* 1995; **56**:347–53.

Rosen JA. Paroxysmal choreoathetosis. *Arch Neurol* 1964; **11**:385–7.

Rosenberg NL, Myers JA, Martin WRW. Cyanide-induced parkinsonism: clinical, MRI and 6–flurodopa PET studies. *Neurology* 1989; **39**:142–4.

Rosenbloom L. Dyskinetic cerebral palsy and birth asphyxia. *Dev Med Child Neurol* 1994; **36**:285–9.

Rosenow F, Herholz K, Lanfermann H et al. Neurological sequelae of cyanide intoxication – the patterns of clinical, magnetic resonance imaging, and positron emission tomography findings. *Ann Neurol* 1995; **38**:825–8.

Rothschild AJ, Locke CA. Reexposure to fluoxetine after serious suicide attempts by three patients: the role of akathisia. *J Clin Psychiatry* 1991; **52**:491–3.

Roullet E, Nizou R, Jedynak P et al. Intention and action myoclonus disclosing occupational mercury poisoning. *Rev Neurol* 1984; **140**:55–8.

Rozdilsky B, Cummings JN, Huston AF. Hallervorden–Spatz disease: late infantile and adult types, report of two cases. *Acta Neuropathol* 1968; **10**:1–16.

Ruprecht K, Warmuthmetz M, Waespe W et al. Symptomatic hyperekplexia in a patient with multiple sclerosis. *Neurology* 2002; **58**:503–4.

Russo LS. Focal dystonia and lacunar infarction of the basal ganglia: a case report. *Arch Neurol* 1983; **40**:61–2.

Sachdev P, Kruk J. Clinical characteristics and predisposing factors in acute drug-induced akathisia. *Arch Gen Psychiatry* 1994; **51**:963–74.

Sachdev PS. The current status of tardive dyskinesia. *Aust N Z J Psychiatry* 2000; **34**:355–69.

Saenz-Lope E, Herranz FJ, Masdeu JC. Startle epilepsy: a clinical study. *Ann Neurol* 1984; **16**:78–81.

Sahananthan GL, Geshon S. Imipramine withdrawal: an akathisia-like syndrome. *Am J Psychiatry* 1973; **130**:1286–7.

Saint-Hilaire M-H, Saint-Hilaire J-M, Granger L. Jumping Frenchmen of Maine. *Neurology* 1986; **36**:1269–71.

Saint-Hilaire M-H, Burke RE, Bressman SB et al. Delayed onset dystonia due to perinatal or early childhood asphyxia. *Neurology* 1991; **41**:216–22.

Sakai T, Mawatari S, Hiroshi I et al. Choreoacanthocytosis: clues to clinical diagnosis. *Arch Neurol* 1981; **38**:335–8.

Salam SA, Pillai AK, Beresford TP. Lorazepam for psychogenic catatonia. *Am J Psychiatry* 1987; **144**:1082–3.

Sallee FR, Stiller RL, Perel JM et al. Pemoline-induced abnormal involuntary movements. *J Clin Psychopharmacol* 1989; **9**:125–9.

Salt C, Lauter T, Kraus PH et al. Dose-dependent improvement of myoclonic hyperkinesia due to valproic acid in eight Huntington's disease patients: a case series. *BMC Neurol* 2006; **6**:11.

Salvi F, Mascalchi M, Bortolotti C et al. Hypertension, hyperekplexia, and pyramidal paresis due to vascular compression of the medulla. *Neurology* 2000; **55**:1381–4.

Samie MR, Selhorst JB, Koller WC. Post-traumatic midbrain tremor. *Neurology* 1990; **40**:62–6.

Sandyk R. Parkinsonism secondary to neurosyphilis. A case report. *S Afr Med J* 1983; **63**:665–6.

Saposnik G, Bueri JA, Rey RC et al. Catalepsy after stroke. *Neurology* 1999; **53**:1132–5.

Saunders-Pullman R, Shriberg J, Heiman G et al. Myoclonus dystonia. Possible association with obsessive-compulsive disorder and alcohol dependence. *Neurology* 2002; **58**:242–5.

Saver JL, Greenstein P, Ronthal M et al. Asymmetric catalepsy after right hemisphere stroke. *Mov Disord* 1993; **8**:69–73.

Sawle GV, Leenders KL, Brooks DJ et al. Dopa-responsive dystonia: [18F]dopa positron emission tomography. *Ann Neurol* 1991; **30**:24–30.

Scarano V, Pellechia MT, Filia A et al. Hallervorden–Spatz syndrome resembling a typical Tourette syndrome. *Mov Disord* 2002; **17**:618–20.

Scarmeas N, Hadjieorgiou GM, Papadimitrou A et al. Motor signs during the course of Alzheimer's disease. *Neurology* 2004; **63**:975–82.

Schmidt A, Jabusch H-C, Altenmuller E et al. Dominantly transmitted focal dystonia in a family of patients with musician's cramp. *Neurology* 2006; **67**:691–3.

Schott GD. The relationship of peripheral trauma and pain to dystonia. *J Neurol Neurosurg Psychiatry* 1985; **48**:698–701.

Schule B, Kock N, Svetl M et al. Genetic heterogeneity in ten families with myoclonus-dystonia. *J Neurol Neurosurg Psychiatry* 2004; **75**:1181–5.

Schultz DR, Barthal JS, Garrett C. Western equine encephalitis with rapid onset parkinsonism. *Neurology* 1977; **27**:1095–6.

Schwartz A, Hennerici M, Wegener OH. Delayed choreoathetosis following acute carbon monoxide poisoning. *Neurology* 1985; **35**:98–9.

Schwarz GA, Barrows LJ. Hemiballism without involvement of Luy's body. *Arch Neurol* 1960; **2**:420–34.

Sechi GP, Tanda F, Mutani R. Fatal hyperpyrexia after withdrawal of levodopa. *Neurology* 1984; **34**:249–51.

Sechi GP, Agnetti V, Piredda M et al. Acute and persistent parkinsonism after use of diquat. *Neurology* 1992; **42**:261–2.

Sempere AP, Duarte J, Cabezas C et al. Parkinsonism induced by amlopidine. *Mov Disord* 1995; **10**:115–16.

Serdaru M, Hausser-Hauw C, Laplane D et al. The clinical spectrum of alcoholic pellagra encephalopathy. *Brain* 1988; **111**:829–42.

Sethi KD, Patel B, Meador KJ. Metoclopramide-induced parkinsonism. *South Med J* 1989; **82**:1581–2.

Sethi KD, Patel BP. Inconsistent response to divalproex sodium in hemichorea/hemiballism. *Neurology* 1990; **40**:1630–1.

Shah P, Kaplan SL. Catatonic symptoms in a child with epilepsy. *Am J Psychiatry* 1980; **137**:738–9.

Shahnawaz M, van der Westhuizen LR, Gledhill RF. Episodic cervical dystonia associated with gastro-oesophageal reflux. A case of adult-onset Sandifer syndrome. *Clin Neurol Neurosurg* 2001; **103**:212–15.

Shan D-E, Soong B-W, Sun C-M et al. Spinocerebellar ataxia type 2 presenting as familial levodopa-responsive parkinsonism. *Ann Neurol* 2001; **50**:812–15.

Sharp FR, Rando TA, Greenberg SA et al. Pseudochoreoathetosis: movements associated with loss of proprioception. *Arch Neurol* 1994; **51**:1103–9.

Shearer PM, Bownes IT, Curran P. Tardive akathisia and agitated depression during metoclopramide therapy. *Acta Psychiatr Scand* 1984; **70**:428–31.

Sheehy MP, Marsden CD. Writer's cramp – a focal dystonia. *Brain* 1982; **105**:461–80.

Shepherd GMG, Tauboll E, Bakke SJ et al. Midbrain tremor and hypertrophic olivary degeneration after pontine hemorrhage. *Mov Disord* 1997; **12**:432–7.

Shill HA, Stacy MA. Malignant catatonia secondary to sporadic encephalitis lethargica. *J Neurol Neurosurg Psychiatry* 2000; **69**:402–3.

Siesling S, Vegter-Van der Vlis M, Roos RAC. Juvenile Huntington's disease in the Netherlands. *Pediatr Neurol* 1997; **17**:34–43.

Singer C, Papapetropoulos S, Spielholz NI. Primary writing tremor: report of a case successfully treated with botulinum toxin A injections and discussion of the underlying mechanism. *Mov Disord* 2005; **20**:1387–8.

Siris SG. Three cases of akathisia and 'acting out'. *J Clin Psychiatry* 1985; **46**:395–7.

Slater E, Beard SW. The schizophrenia-like psychoses of epilepsy. I. Psychiatric aspects. *Br J Psychiatry* 1963; **109**:95–112.

Snyder RD. The involuntary movements of chronic mercury poisoning. *Arch Neurol* 1972; **26**:379–81.

Soland V, Bhatia KP, Volonte MA et al. Focal task-specific tremors. *Mov Disord* 1996a; **11**:665–70.

Soland V, Evoy F, Rivest J. Cervical dystonia due to a frontal meningioma. *Mov Disord* 1996b; **11**:336–7.

Song X, Hu Z, Zhang H. Acute dystonia induced by lamivudine. *Clin Neuropharmacol* 2005; **28**:193–4.

Sorensen BF, Hamby WB. Spasmodic torticollis: results in 71 surgically treated patients. *Neurology* 1966; **16**:867–78.

Sotero de Menezes MA, Rho JM, Murphy P et al. Lamotrigine-induced tic disorder: report of five pediatric cases. *Epilepsia* 2000; **41**:862–7.

Spacey SD, Adams PJ, Lam PCP et al. Genetic heterogeneity in paroxysmal nonkinesiogenic dyskinesia. *Neurology* 2006; **66**:1585–90.

Speracio RR, Anziska B, Schutta HS. Hypernatremia and chorea. A report of two cases. *Neurology* 1976; **26**:46–50.

Spiller WG. Acquired double athetosis (dystonia lenticularis). *Arch Neurol Psychiatry* 1920; **4**:370–86.

Spitz MC, Jankovic J, Killian JM. Familial tic disorder, parkinsonism, motor neuron disease and acanthocytosis: a new syndrome. *Neurology* 1985; **35**:366–70.

Srinivas K, Rao VM, Subbulakshmi N et al. Hemiballism after striatal hemorrhage. *Neurology* 1987; **37**:1428–9.

Stahl SM. Tardive Tourette syndrome in an autistic patient after long-term neuroleptic administration. *Am J Psychiatry* 1980; **137**:1267–9.

Starkstein SE, Petracca G, Teson A et al. Catatonia in depression: prevalence, clinical correlates, and validation of a scale. *J Neurol Neurosurg Psychiatry* 1996; **60**:326–32.

Starosta-Rubinstein S, Young AB, Kluin K et al. Clinical assessment of 31 patients with Wilson's disease: correlations with structural changes on magnetic resonance imaging. *Arch Neurol* 1987; **44**:365–70.

Steele JC. Progressive supranuclear palsy. *Brain* 1972; **95**:693–704.

Steinberg IN, Sternlieb I. *Wilson's disease*. Philadelphia: WB Saunders, 1984.

Stell R, Davis S, Carroll WM. Unilateral asterixis due to a lesion of the ventrolateral thalamus. *J Neurol Neurosurg Psychiatry* 1994; **57**:116.

Sternbach H. The serotonin syndrome. *Am J Psychiatry* 1991; **148**:705–13.

Stevanin G, Fujigasaki H, Lebre A-S et al. Huntington's disease-like phenotype due to trinucleotide repeat expansion in the *TBP* and *JPH3* genes. *Brain* 2003; **126**:1599–603.

Stevens H. 'Jumping Frenchmen of Maine'. Myriachit. *Arch Neurol* 1965; **12**:311–14.

Stevens H. Paroxysmal choreo-athetosis. *Arch Neurol* 1966; **14**.415–20.

Stewart JT, Williams LS. A case of lithium-induced asterixis. *J Am Ger Soc* 2000; **48**:457.

Stober G, Seelow, D, Ruschendork et al. Periodic catatonia: confirmation of linkage to chromosome 15 and further evidence for genetic homogeneity. *Hum Genet* 2002; **111**:523–30.

Stojanovic M, Sternic N, Kostic VS. Cloazapine in hemiballismus: report of two cases. *Clin Neuropharmacol* 1997; **20**:171–4.

Stone LA, Jankovic J. The coexistence of tics and dystonia. *Arch Neurol* 1991; **48**:862–5.

Strang RR. Parkinsonism occurring during methyldopa therapy. *Can Med Assoc J* 1966; **95**:928–9.

Striano P, Elefante A, Coppola A et al. Dramatic response to levetiracetam in post-ischemic Holmes' tremor. *J Neurol Neurosurg Psychiatry* 2007; **78**:438–9.

Stryjer R, Strous RD, Bar F et al. Segmental dystonia as the sole manifestation of carbamazepine toxicity. *Gen Hosp Psychiatry* 2002; **42**:114–15.

Stuerenburg HJ, Hansen HC, Thie A et al. Reversible dementia in idiopathic hypoparathyroidism associated with normocalcemia. *Neurology* 1996; **47**:474–6.

Stuppaeck CH, Miller CH, Ehrmann H et al. Akathisia induced by necrosis of the basal ganglia after carbon monoxide intoxication. *Mov Disord* 1995; **10**:229–31.

Sunden-Cullberg J, Tedroff J, Aquilonius SM. Reversible chorea in primary antiphospholipid syndrome. *Mov Disord* 1998; **13**:147–9.

Supino-Viterbo V, Sicard C, Risvegliato M *et al.* Toxic encephalopathy due to ingestion of bismuth salts: clinical and EEG studies of 45 patients. *J Neurol Neurosurg Psychiatry* 1977; **40**:748–52.

Sutton GG, Meyere RF. Focal reflex myoclonus. *J Neurol Neurosurg Psychiatry* 1974; **37**:207–17.

Svetel M, Kozic D, Stefanova E *et al.* Dystonia in Wilson's disease. *Mov Disord* 2001; **16**:719–23.

Swaiman KK. Hallervorden–Spatz syndrome and brain iron metabolism. *Arch Neurol* 1991; **48**:1285–93.

Swedo SE, Leonard HL, Schapiro NB *et al.* Sydenham's chorea: physical and psychological symptoms of St Vitus dance. *Pediatrics* 1993; **91**:706–13.

Swett C. Drug-induced dystonia. *Am J Psychiatry* 1975; **132**:532–4.

Tabaton M, Mancardi G, Loeb C. Generalized chorea due to bilateral small, deep cerebral infarcts. *Neurology* 1985; **35**:588–9.

Tambyah PA, Ong BKC, Lee KO. Reversible parkinsonism and asymptomatic hypocalcemia with basal ganglia calcification 26 years after thyroid surgery. *Am J Med* 1993; **94**:444–5.

Tan EK, Lo YL, Chan LL *et al.* Cervical disc prolapse with cord compression presenting with choreoathetosis and dystonia. *Neurology* 2002; **58**:661–2.

Tan H, Turali G, Ay H *et al.* Rubral tremor after thalamic infarction in childhood. *Pediatr Neurol* 2001; **25**:409–12.

Tanaka M, Yokode M, Kita T *et al.* Donepezil and athetosis in an elderly patient with Alzheimer's disease. *J Am Geriatr Soc* 2003; **51**:889–90.

Tandon R, Walden M, Falcon S. Catatonia as a manifestation of paraneoplastic encephalopathy. *J Clin Psychiatry* 1988; **49**:121–2.

Tassin J, Durr A, Bonnet A-M *et al.* Levodopa-responsive dystonia: GTP cyclohydrolase I or parkin mutation? *Brain* 2000; **123**:1112–21.

Tatu L, Moulin T, Martin V *et al.* Unilateral pure thalamic asterixis: clinical, electromyographic, and topographic patterns. *Neurology* 2000; **54**:2339–42.

Taylor MA, Abrams R. Catatonia: prevalence and importance in the manic phase of manic-depressive illness. *Arch Gen Psychiatry* 1977; **34**:1223–5.

Tetrud JW, Langston JW, Garbe PL *et al.* Mild parkinsonism in persons exposed to 1-methyl-4-phenyl-1,2,3,6-tetrahydropyridine (MPTP). *Neurology* 1989; **39**:1483–7.

Teusink JP, Alexopoulos GS, Shamoian CA. Parkinsonism side-effects induced by a monoamine oxidase inhibitor. *Am J Psychiatry* 1984; **141**:118–19.

Thornton A, McKenna PJ. Acute dystonic reactions complicated by psychotic phenomena. *Br J Psychiatry* 1994; **164**:115–18.

Tijssen MA, Vergouwe MN, van Dijk JG *et al.* Major and minor forms of hereditary hyperekplexia. *Mov Disord* 2002; **17**:826–30.

Tinuper P, Cerullo A, Cirignotta F *et al.* Nocturnal paroxysmal dystonia with short-lasting attacks: three cases with evidence for an epileptic frontal lobe origin of seizures. *Epilepsia* 1990; **31**:549–56.

Tison F, Arne P, Henry P. Myoclonus and adult coeliac disease. *J Neurol* 1989; **236**:307–8.

Tolosa ES. Clinical features of Meige's disease (idiopathic orofacial dystonia): a report of 17 cases. *Arch Neurol* 1981; **38**:147–51.

Tolosa ES, Santamaria J. Parkinsonism and basal ganglia infarcts. *Neurology* 1984; **34**:1516–18.

Tombini M Pacifici L, Passarelli F *et al.* Transient athetosis induced by tiagabine. *Epilepsia* 2006; **47**:799–800.

Tomita I, Satoh H, Satoh A *et al.* Extrapontine myelinolysis presenting with parkinsonism as a sequel of rapid correction of hyponatremia. *J Neurol Neurosurg Psychiatry* 1997; **62**:422–3.

Toru M, Matsuda O, Makiguchi K *et al.* Single case study: neuroleptic malignant syndrome-like state following a withdrawal of antiparkinsonian drugs. *J Nerv Ment Dis* 1981; **169**:324–7.

Trautner RJ, Cummings JL, Read SL *et al.* Idiopathic basal ganglia calcification and organic mood disorders. *Am J Psychiatry* 1988; **145**:350–3.

Tsuboi Y, Wxzolek ZK, Kusuhara T *et al.* Japanese family with parkinsonism, depression, weight loss, and cortical hypoventilation. *Neurology* 2002; **58**:1025–30.

Tsubokawa T, Katayama Y, Yamamoto T. Control of persistent hemiballismus by chronic thalamic stimulation. Report of two cases. *J Neurosurg* 1995; **82**:501–5.

Tyler HR. Neurological complications of dialysis, transplantation and other forms of treatment in chronic uremia. *Neurology* 1965; **15**:1081–8.

Uitti RJ, Rajput AH, Ashenhurst EM *et al.* Cyanide-induced parkinsonism: a clinicopathologic report. *Neurology* 1985; **35**:921–5.

Uitti RJ, Snow BJ, Shinotoh H *et al.* Parkinsonism induced by solvent abuse. *Ann Neurol* 1994; **35**:616–19.

Vakis A, Krasoudakis A, Koutendakis D. Transient post-traumatic hemiballism. Report of a case. *J Neurosurg Sci* 2006; **50**:21–3.

Valente EM, Spacey SD, Wali GM *et al.* A second paroxysmal kinesigenic choreoathetosis locus (*EKD2*) mapping on 16q13–q22 indicates a family of genes which give rise to paroxysmal disorders on human chromosome 16. *Brain* 2000; **123**:2040–5.

Valenzuela R, Court J, Godoy J. Delayed cyanide induced dystonia. *J Neurol Neurosurg Psychiatry* 1992; **55**:198–9.

van Hilten JJ, van de Beek WJ, Vein AA *et al.* Clinical aspects of multifocal or generalized tonic dystonia in reflex sympathetic dystrophy. *Neurology* 2001; **56**:1762–5.

Vanek Z, Jankovic J. Dystonia in corticobasal degeneration. *Mov Disord* 2001; **16**:252–7.

Van Putten T. The many faces of akathisia. *Compr Psychiatry* 1975; **16**:43–7.

Van Putten T, May PRA. 'Akinetic depression' in schizophrenia. *Arch Gen Psychiatry* 1978; **35**:1101–7.

Van Putten T, Mutalipassi LR, Malkin MD. Phenothiazine-induced decompensation. *Arch Gen Psychiatry* 1974; **30**:102–5.

Van Putten T, May PRA, Marder SR. Akathisia with haloperidol and thiothixene. *Arch Gen Psychiatry* 1984; **41**:1036–9.

Van Uitert RL, Russakoff LM. Hyperthyroid chorea mimicking psychiatric disease. *Am J Psychiatry* 1979; **136**:1208–10.

Van Zandjke M. Treatment of myoclonus. *Acta Neurol Belg* 2003; **103**:66–70.

Varga E, Sugerman AA, Varga V *et al*. Prevalence of spontaneous oral dyskinesia in the elderly. *Am J Psychiatry* 1982; **139**:329–31.

Velamoor VR, Norman RMG, Caroff SN *et al*. Progression of symptoms in neuroleptic malignant syndrome. *J Nerv Ment Dis* 1994; **182**:168–73.

Velez M, Cosentino C, Torres L. Levodopa-responsive rubral (Holmes') tremor. *Mov Disorder* 2002; **17**:741–2.

Verino S, Tuite P, Adler CH *et al*. Paraneoplastic chorea associated with CRMP-5 neuronal antibody and lung carcinoma. *Ann Neurol* 2002; **51**:625–30.

Verslegers W, Van den Kerchove M, Crols R *et al*. Methanol intoxication. Parkinsonism and decreased met-enkephalin levels due to putaminal necrosis. *Acta Neurol Belg* 1988; **88**:163–71.

Vestergaard P, Poulstrup I, Schou M. Prospective studies on a lithium cohort. 3. Tremor, weight gain, diarrhea, psychological complaints. *Acta Psychiatr Scand* 1988; **78**:434–41.

Victor M, Adams RD, Cole M. The acquired 'non-Wilsonian' type of chronic hepatocerebral degeneration. *Medicine* 1965; **44**:345–96.

Vidakovic A, Dragasevic N, Kostic VS. Hemiballism: report of 25 cases. *J Neurol Neurosurg Psychiatry* 1994; **57**:945–9.

Volonte MA, Perani D, Ianzi R *et al*. Regression of ventral striatum hypometabolism after calcium calcitrol therapy in paroxysmal kinesigenic chorcoathetosis due to idiopathic primary hypoparathyroidism. *J Neurol Neurosurg Psychiatry* 2001; **71**:691–5.

Walker L. Setrarline-induced akathisia and dystonia misinterpreted as a panic attack. *Psychiatr Serv* 2002; **53**:1477–8.

Walker RH, Spiera H, Brin MF *et al*. Parkinsonism associated with Sjogren's syndrome: three cases and a review of the literature. *Mov Disord* 1999; **14**:262–8.

Walsh F. On the symptom complexes of lethargic encephalitis with special reference to the involuntary muscular contractions. *Brain* 1920; **43**:197–219.

Walshe JM, Yealland M. Wilson's disease: the problem of delayed diagnosis. *J Neurol Neurosurg Psychiatry* 1992; **55**:692–6.

Walters AS, Hening W, Rubinstein M *et al*. A clinical and polysomnographic comparison of neuroleptic-induced akathisia and the idiopathic restless legs syndrome. *Sleep* 1991; **14**:339–45.

Warner TT, Lennox GG, Janota I *et al*. Autosomal-dominant dentatorubropallidoluysian atrophy. *Mov Disord* 1994; **9**:289–96.

Warner TT, Williams LD, Walker RWH *et al*. A clinical and molecular genetic study of dentatorubropallidoluysian atrophy in four European families. *Ann Neurol* 1995; **37**:452–9.

Watanabe H, Saito Y, Terao S *et al*. Progression and prognosis in multiple system atrophy. An analysis of 230 Japanese patients. *Brain* 2002; **125**:1070–83.

Waubant E, Simonetta-Moreau M, Clanet M *et al*. Left arm monoballism as a relapse in multiple sclerosis. *Mov Disord* 1997; **12**:1091–2.

Waubant E, Alize P, Tourbah A *et al*. Paroxysmal dystonia (tonic spasm) in multiple sclerosis. *Neurology* 2001; **57**:2320–1.

Weddington WW, Marks RC, Verghese JP. Disulfiram encephalopathy as a cause of the catatonic syndrome. *Am J Psychiatry* 1980; **137**:1217–19.

Weiden P, Bruin R. Worsening of Tourette's disorder due to neuroleptic-induced akathisia. *Am J Psychiatry* 1987; **144**:504–5.

Wein T, Andermann F, Silver K *et al*. Exquisite sensitivity of paroxysmal kinesigenic choreoathetosis to carbamazepine. *Neurology* 1996; **47**:1104–5.

Weinberger DR, Wyatt RJ. Catatonic stupor and neuroleptic drugs. *JAMA* 1978; **239**:1846.

Weiner WJ, Nausieda PA, Klawans HL. Methylphenidate-induced chorea: case report and pharmacologic implications. *Neurology* 1978; **28**:1041–4.

Wenning GK, Ben-Shlomo Y, Magalhaes M *et al*. Clinical features and natural history of multiple system atrophy: an analysis of 100 cases. *Brain* 1994; **117**:835–45.

Wenning GK, Ben-Shlomo Y, Magalhaes M *et al*. Clinicopathological study of 35 cases of multiple system atrophy. *J Neurol Neurosurg Psychiatry* 1995; **58**:160–6.

Wenning GK, Scherfler C, Granata R *et al*. Time course of symptomatic orthostatic hypotension in patients with postmortem confirmed parkinsonian syndromes: a clinicopathological study. *J Neurol Neurosurg Psychiatry* 1999; **67**:620–3.

Werhahan KJ, Brown P, Thompson PD *et al*. The clinical features and prognosis of chronic posthypoxic myoclonus. *Mov Disord* 1997; **12**:216–20.

Werner EG, Olanow CW. Parkinsonism and amiodarone therapy. *Ann Neurol* 1989; **25**:630–2.

Whittier JR. Ballism and subthalmic nucleus (nucleus hypothalamicus; corpus Luysi). Review of the literature and study of thirty cases. *Arch Neurol Psychiatry* 1947; **58**:672–92.

Wilson LG. Viral encephalopathy mimicking functional psychosis. *Am J Psychiatry* 1976; **133**:165–70.

Wilson P, Preece M. Chorea gravidarum. *Arch Int Med* 1932a; **49**:471–533.

Wilson P, Preece M. Chorea gravidarum. *Arch Int Med* 1932b; **49**:671–97.

Wilson SAK. *Modern problems in neurology*. London: Edward Arnold, 1928.

Wilson SAK. *Neurology*, 2nd edn. London: Butterworth, 1955.

Wojick JD, Falk WE, Fink JS *et al*. A review of 32 cases of tardive dystonia. *Am J Psychiatry* 1991; **148**:1055–9.

Wolanczyk T, Grabowski-Grzyb A. Transient dystonias in three patients treated with tiagabine. *Epilepsia* 2001; **42**:944–6.

Woods C, Taylor A. Ataxia telangiectasia in the British Isles: the clinical and laboratory features of 70 affected individuals. *Q J Med* 1992; **82**:169–79.

Yadalam KG, Korn ML, Simpson GM. Tardive dystonia: four case histories. *J Clin Psychiatry* 1990; **51**:17–20.

Yamada K, Haraa M, Goto S. Response of postapoplectic hemichorea/hemiballism to GPI pallidotomy: progressive improvement resulting in complete relief. *Mov Disord* 2004; **19**:1111–14.

Yassa R, Nair V, Dimitry A. Prevalence of tardive dystonia. *Acta Psychiatr Scand* 1986; **73**:629–33.

Yasuda M, Nakamura Y, Kaamata T *et al.* Phenotypic heterogeneity within a new family with the *MAPT* P301S mutation. *Ann Neurol* 2005; **58**:920–8.

Yazici O, Kantemir E, Tastaban Y *et al.* Spontaneous improvement of tardive dystonia during mania. *Br J Psychiatry* 1991; **158**:847–50.

Yokoi S, Austin J, Witmer F *et al.* Studies in myoclonus epilepsy (Lafora body form). *Arch Neurol* 1968; **19**:15–33.

Yoshida Y, Akanuma J, Tochikubo S *et al.* Slowly progressive dystonia following central pontine and extrapontine myelinolysis. *Intern Med* 2000; **39**:956–60.

Zaremba J, Mierzewska H, Lysiak Z *et al.* Rapid-onset dystonia-parkinsonism: a fourth family consistent with linkage to chromosome 19q13. *Mov Disord* 2004; **19**:1506–10.

Zenzola A, De Mari M, De Blasi R *et al.* Paroxysmal dystonia with thalamic lesion in multiple sclerosis. *Neurol Sci* 2001; **22**:391–4.

Zesiewicz TA, Sullivan KL, Hauser RA. Chorea induced by lamotrigine. *J Child Neurol* 2006; **21**:357.

Zhang C, Glenn DG, Bell WL *et al.* Gabapentin-induced myolonus in end-stage renal disease. *Epilepsia* 2005; **46**:156–8.

Zijlmans JCM, Thijssen HOM, Vogels OJM *et al.* MRI in patients with suspected vascular parkinsonism. *Neurology* 1995; **45**:2183–8.

Zorumski CF, Bakris GL. Choreoathetosis associated with lithium: case report and literature review. *Am J Psychiatry* 1983; **140**:1621–2.

4

Other signs and symptoms

4.1 MUTISM

The term mutism is derived from the Latin *mutus*, meaning 'inability to speak'.

Clinical features

Mute patients, as noted, do not speak; although in some cases patients may make some noises such as grunts, there is no verbalization.

Etiology

As noted in Table 4.1, mutism may appear in several different clinical settings. Perhaps the most common one in neuropsychiatric practice is the acute onset of mutism during a stroke. Mutism may also appear gradually in far-advanced neurodegenerative disorders, such as frontotemporal dementia, and is a prominent feature of several other syndromes, including akinetic mutism, catatonia, and severe cases of psychomotorically retarded depression. Finally, there is a miscellaneous group of causes including intrinsic laryngeal pathology, medications, and, in children, cerebellar surgery.

Stroke, when characterized by aphasia or aphemia, may cause acute mutism. Motor aphasia and transcortical motor aphasia may both, initially, present with mutism: over time, the mutism resolves, leaving the patient with the typical aphasic syndrome, as discussed in detail in Section 2.1. Thus, after resolution of the mutism, the patient with motor aphasia will be left with non-fluent speech but intact comprehension, and the patient with transcortical motor aphasia will be similar but will show improvement of speech with repetition.

Aphemia is an uncommon stroke syndrome characterized by mutism but, in contrast with the aphasias, there is a preserved ability to write; furthermore, as the mutism resolves, patients are left, not with an aphasia, but with a hoarse dysarthria. Aphemia, in most cases, is accompanied by a right hemiparesis and occurs secondary to a small lesion in the posterior aspect of the left inferior frontal gyrus or the immediately subjacent white matter.

Neurodegenerative disorders capable of causing dementia may also cause a mutism of gradual onset: in this situation, however, the mutism generally occurs only at the 'tail end' of a long dementing process. Such an evolution has been noted in frontotemporal dementia and Alzheimer's disease. Some neurodegenerative disorders may also present with aphasia, in the syndrome known as 'primary progressive

Table 4.1 Causes of mutism

Stroke
As presentation of certain aphasias
    Motor aphasia (David and Bone 1984; Masdeu and O'Hara
      1983)
    Transcortical motor aphasia (Alexander and Schmitt 1980;
      Bogousslavsky and Regli 1990)
Aphemia (Schiff *et al.* 1983)

Neurodegenerative disorders
Frontotemporal dementia (Neary *et al.* 1993; Snowden *et al.*
  1992)
Alzheimer's disease (Mayeux *et al.* 1985)
Primary progressive aphasia (Gorno-Tempini *et al.* 2006)

Other syndromes characterized by mutism
Catatonia (Kraepelin 1990)
Depression (Benegal *et al.* 1992)
Akinetic mutism (Cairns *et al.* 1941)

Miscellaneous causes of mutism
Intrinsic laryngeal pathology
Medications
    Tacrolimus (Wijdicks *et al.* 1994)
    Cyclosporine (Valldeoriola *et al.* 1996)
Cerebellar surgery (Catsman-Berrevoets *et al.* 1999; Van Dongen
  et al. 1994)

aphasia', which, over time, may evolve into mutism; this is discussed further in Section 2.1.

Other syndromes characterized by mutism include catatonia, severe depression, and akinetic mutism, and in all three of these the mutism is accompanied by immobility. Several features allow these syndromes to be differentiated one from another. Catatonia is typically accompanied by the very distinctive finding of waxy flexibility, a sign absent in the other two syndromes. Depression of the psychomotorically retarded type, when severe, may be accompanied by mutism; however, in these cases one finds a history of a preceding more typical depressive syndrome, with depressed mood, anergia, anhedonia, and disturbances of appetite and sleep. When a patient with mutism and immobility lacks any of these findings then the diagnosis of akinetic mutism should be seriously considered.

Of the miscellaneous causes of mutism, intrinsic laryngeal pathology (e.g., laryngitis, laryngeal tumors) is the most common, and in these cases the mutism is preceded by hoarseness. Medications capable of inducing mutism include tacrolimus and cyclosporine. Finally, in children who have undergone cerebellar surgery a syndrome of mutism may occur, either immediately postoperatively or within a few days.

Differential diagnosis

Aphasia, dysarthria, and hypophonia are all distinguished by the obvious fact that patients with these disorders do, in fact, speak. Although the speech may be effortful, as in aphasia, slurred, as in dysarthria, or low and monotone, as in hypophonia, it is still there.

Selective, or, as it was once called, *elective*, mutism is a condition seen in shy and withdrawn children who, although capable of speech with family members, become 'selectively' mute when with strangers or in school (Dummit *et al.* 1997; Elson *et al.* 1965; Steinhausen and Juzi 1996; Wergeland 1979).

Conversion muteness and malingered muteness typically occur as isolated findings, a feature that distinguishes them from mutism occurring secondary to the causes noted under 'etiology', wherein the mutism is accompanied by distinctive findings on history or examination.

Treatment

Treatment is directed at the underlying disorder; speech therapy may be attempted in cases of mutism secondary to stroke.

4.2 AKINETIC MUTISM

The name of this syndrome captures its most distinctive features, namely immobility and mutism.

Clinical features

For the most part, patients are mute and immobile, and, although at first glance they appear to be in a stupor, closer observation reveals lively conjugate eye movements as patients track objects in the room, such as physicians and nurses. In some cases, the mutism and akinesia may persist through all adversities, but in others, patients may respond to an especially adverse stimulus with a feeble motion of a limb or perhaps by uttering a word. Food may be eaten if placed in the mouth but patients do not seek it, and urine and feces may be passed in the bed. Importantly, there is no rigidity, especially no waxy flexibility, and no negativism.

Some examples may serve to flesh out this definition. The first is taken from Cairns' original description of akinetic mutism (Cairns *et al.* 1941):

> In the fully developed state he makes no sound and lies inert, except that his eyes regard the observer steadily or follow the movement of objects, and they may be diverted by sound. Despite his steady gaze, which seems to give promise of speech, the patient is quite mute, or he answers only in whispered monosyllables. Oft-repeated commands may be carried out in a feeble, slow, and incomplete manner, but usually there are no movements of a voluntary character: no restless movements, struggling or evidence of negativism. Emotional movement is almost in abeyance. A painful stimulus produces reflex withdrawal of the

limb and, if the stimulus is maintained, slow, feeble, voluntary movements of the limbs may occur in an attempt to remove the source of the stimulation, but usually without tears, noise, or other manifestations of pain or displeasure. The patient swallows readily but has to be fed. Food seen may be recognized as such, but there is evidently little appreciation of its taste and other characteristics: objects normally chewed or sucked may be swallowed whole. There is total incontinence of urine and feces.

Cairns' cases, occurring with third-ventricular tumors, were generally of gradual or subacute onset. Another case (Nielsen 1951), secondary to infarction of the cingulate gyri, bears detailed reporting given the remarkable abruptness of its onset. The patient was a 46-year-old woman who:

> was ironing when she suddenly stopped on the spot, complained of a severe headache, but remained standing. Her son put her to bed, where she lay motionless, without even speaking. She stared at the ceiling and did not ask for anything, not even for a drink. After 9 days she was hospitalized and on the ward she continued akinetic and mute. Under strong stimulation she did say, 'It hurts,' and 'Water,' but that was all. She was obviously conscious and took note of her environment but lay day after day motionless, not deigning to call for bed pan or food.

Etiology

Akinetic mutism has been noted with intraventricular masses of the third ventricle, which compressed the surrounding diencephalon (Cairns *et al.* 1941), following surgical damage to the hypothalamus (Ross and Stewart 1981), in obstructive hydrocephalus (Messert *et al.* 1966), and with infarction of the anterior cingulate gyri (Barris and Schuman 1953; Faris 1969; Freemon 1971; Nielsen 1951). Akinetic mutism has also been seen as a side-effect of cyclosporine (Bird *et al.* 1990) and in a patient treated with total body irradiation and amphotericin B (Devinsky *et al.* 1987).

Differential diagnosis

Akinetic mutism must be distinguished from other conditions capable of causing immobility and mutism, including catatonia, depression, the persistent vegetative state, the locked-in syndrome, and stupor.

Catatonia is distinguished by the presence of waxy flexibility, a sign not seen in akinetic mutism. Depression, when severe and characterized by psychomotor retardation, may resemble akinetic mutism; however, in this instance history will reveal a typical depressive syndrome preceding the evolution of immobility and mutism, with such symptoms as depressed mood, anergia, anhedonia, and changes in sleep and appetite.

The persistent vegetative state may also appear similar to akinetic mutism; however, in this condition the eye movements – although at times seeming purposeful – are less consistently 'lively'; furthermore, in patients with the persistent vegetative state one always finds a history of coma secondary to severe traumatic brain injury, global hypoxia, etc.

The locked-in syndrome, occurring secondary to high brainstem infarction or other lesions, such as central pontine myelinolysis, is characterized by tetraparesis, bilateral facial paresis, and mutism, and thus may appear similar to akinetic mutism. Examination of eye movements, however, will enable the correct diagnosis. In contrast with akinetic mutism, wherein extraocular movements are full, in the locked-in syndrome there is a paralysis of lateral gaze, with only vertical gaze being left intact. Furthermore, and again in contrast with akinetic mutism, in the locked-in syndrome the patient is often desperate for communication and will attempt to do so by utilizing the remaining vertical eye movements in a sort of 'Morse code'.

Stupor of various causes may leave patients immobile and mute; however, in stupor patients are not alert and eye movements, rather than being 'lively', are generally roving or dysconjugate.

Abulia may also be considered on the differential; however, the distinction is readily apparent upon merely instructing the patient to do something. When left undisturbed, the abulic patient is mute and immobile like the akinetic mute; however, when the abulic patient is given directions he or she follows them, in contrast with the akinetic mute, who remains immobile.

Treatment

Anecdotally, bromocriptine is effective (Psarros *et al.* 2003; Ross and Stewart 1981); treatment may be initiated at 2.5 mg/day (given in two divided doses: once in the early morning and once in the early afternoon), and increased in similar increments every few days until significant improvement or limiting side-effects occur or a maximum dose of 40 mg is reached.

4.3 STUTTERING

Stuttering, a speech dysfluency familiar to most ears, although most commonly seen on a developmental basis, may also, as noted below, occur on an acquired basis.

Clinical features

The phenomenology of stuttering differs according to whether it occurs on a developmental or an acquired basis (Helm *et al.* 1978).

In developmental stuttering, patients find themselves 'blocked' as they attempt to speak the first letter or syllable of a word and have particular difficulty getting past the letters

B, D, K, P, and T. Unable to surmount the sound, patients repeat it again and again, often with progressively increasing force and volume; with these ever-more vigorous attempts, there may be associated features, such as facial grimacing, blinking, hissing, and fist-clenching. The block is eventually overcome and there is often a cascade of words, all clearly and unhesitatingly pronounced, as if the dam had broken. Interestingly, patients with developmental stuttering may find themselves unblocked if they sing, read aloud, or are quite angry.

Although acquired stuttering may be clinically similar to developmental stuttering, it tends to differ in several ways. First, the block may be as likely to occur on the second or subsequent letter as on the first. Second, although patients may be annoyed at being blocked, and do engage in repeated attempts to make the sound, the effort to do so is rarely as vigorous or as forceful as in developmental stuttering. Finally, when a patient with acquired stuttering does get beyond the block, it is unusual to see a subsequent 'cascade' of words.

Etiology

The various causes of stuttering are listed in Table 4.2, where they arc divided into developmental and acquired types.

Developmental stuttering, as noted earlier, is the most common cause of stuttering. Here, as discussed in more detail in Section 9.20, stuttering usually appears between the ages of 2 and 10 years; although such developmental stuttering may persist into adulthood, most cases undergo a spontaneous remission by early teenage years.

Table 4.2   Causes of stuttering

Developmental stuttering

Acquired stuttering
 Medications (Bar *et al.* 2004; Brady 1998; Christensen *et al.* 1996; Lee *et al.* 2001; Nurnberg and Greenwald 1981)
  Tricyclic antidepressants
  Selective serotonin reuptake inhibitors (SSRIs)
  Antipsychotics
  Alprazolam
  Theophylline
 Stroke
  Frontal cortex (Freedman *et al.* 1984) or subcortical white matter (Ludlow *et al.* 1987)
  Parietal cortex (Turgut *et al.* 2002)
  Putamen (Ciabarra *et al.* 2000)
  Caudate nucleus (Caplan *et al.* 1990)
  Corpus callosum (Hamano *et al.* 2005)
 Parkinsonian conditions
  Parkinson's disease (Koller 1983)
  Progressive supranuclear palsy (Kluin *et al.* 1993; Koller 1983)
 Dialysis dementia (O'Hare *et al.* 1983)

Of the various causes of acquired stuttering, medications are the most common: among these, the tricyclic antidepressants and selective serotonin reuptake inhibitors (SSRIs) are the most frequent offenders, followed by the antipsychotics – including both first- and second-generation agents. Alprazolam and theophylline only rarely have been reported to cause stuttering.

Stroke may be accompanied by stuttering and this has been noted with infarction of the frontal cortex, the subcortical white matter of the frontal lobe, the parietal cortex, the putamen, and the caudate nucleus; there is also a case report of stuttering with infarction of the body of the corpus callosum. Although most cases of stuttering due to cerebral infarction occur with left-sided infarcts, there are rare cases of 'crossed' stuttering wherein stuttering occurred with a right-sided infarction in a right-handed patient (Fleet and Heilman 1985).

Parkinsonian conditions, such as Parkinson's disease and progressive supranuclear palsy may cause *de novo* stuttering, and in the case of Parkinson's disease, the onset of parkinsonism may be associated with a relapse of childhood stuttering (Shahed *et al.* 2001). Stuttering also constitutes the classic presentation of the now vanishingly rare dialysis dementia.

Differential diagnosis

Palilalia is distinguished by the fact that the last word (or phrase) of a statement is repeated, in contrast with stuttering wherein typically it is the first letter or syllable which is repeated. The effortful speech of patients with motor aphasia may suggest stuttering; however, in aphasia one also finds 'telegraphic' speech, with an absence of conjugations, which stands in contrast with stuttering wherein grammar is preserved.

Treatment

Treatment of developmental stuttering is discussed in Section 9.20; there are few data regarding treatment of stuttering as seen in stroke or parkinsonian conditions.

4.4 PALILALIA

Palilalia, first described by Souques in 1908, is characterized, according to Kinnier Wilson, by 'the repetition of words or short phrases perhaps at increasing speed with decreasing audibility' (Wilson 1954, p. 138).

Clinical features

Palilalic patients involuntarily repeat the last phrase or word, and do so with increasing rapidity, but with diminishing distinctness: 'One patient (Serra-Mestres *et al.* 1996), when asked "How are you today?" replied "I am very well, thank you, thank you, thank you, thank you . . ." up to six times with increasing speed and decreasing volume.'

Etiology

Palilalia occurs in Parkinson's disease (Benke *et al.* 2000), progressive supranuclear palsy (Kluin *et al.* 1993), Tourette's syndrome (Cardoso *et al.*), and in advanced Alzheimer's disease (Cummings *et al.* 1985). There are also rare case reports of palilalia in multi-infarct dementia (Serra-Mestres *et al.* 1996), thalamic infarction (Yasuda *et al.* 1990), and as one manifestation of complex partial status epilepticus (Linetsky *et al.* 2000).

Differential diagnosis

Verbal perseveration is distinguished by the fact that the repeated word or phrase is spoken without the distinctive increasing rapidity and decreasing distinctness.

Stuttering is distinguished by the fact that it is the first letter of a word that is repeated, and echolalia by the fact that in echolalia what is repeated is not something the patient spoke but rather what the examiner or another person said.

Treatment

Treatment is directed at the underlying condition. In a case of palilalia occurring as part of a multi-infarct dementia, trazodone was effective (Serra-Mestres *et al.* 1996); whether this would carry over into other conditions is not known.

4.5 PERSEVERATION

Perseverative speech or behavior (Sandson and Albert 1987) is commonly seen in a variety of conditions, most notably dementia.

Clinical features

Perseverative speech generally occurs in one of two forms. In one, termed *recurrent*, patients supply the same response to repeated, but different, questions. For example, one patient, when asked where she was, replied 'Louisville;' when asked next what year it was, she perseverated in her response, and again said 'Louisville.' The other form is termed *continuous* and here, without being prompted, patients repeat the same word or phrase again and again. One of Kinnier Wilson's (Wilson 1954) patients with Pick's disease 'repeated endlessly, "I want my husband and my children and I don't know where they are." '

Perseverative behavior may involve drawing, writing, or other motor activity. After being asked to draw a stick figure one patient did so and then drew multiple others until the page was filled. Another patient who was asked to write his name wrote out 'Paul' and then perseverated with the letter 'l', until he reached the edge of the page. In another case, a patient, after being asked to get dressed, went to the closet, took out a pair of pants, then paused and hung them back up, then took them out again, and repeated the sequence until being asked to stop.

Etiology

Perseveration is common in dementia (Bayles *et al.* 1985), especially frontotemporal dementia (Thompson *et al.* 2005), Alzheimer's disease (Bayles *et al.* 2004), and diffuse Lewy body disease (Doubleday *et al.* 2002). It is commonly seen in delirium, and is also an integral part of the frontal lobe syndrome. Other conditions characterized by perseveration include aphasia (Albert and Sandson 1986), autism (Rumsey *et al.* 1986), schizophrenia (Siegel *et al.* 1976), and traumatic brain injury (Hotz and Helm-Estabrooks 1995).

Differential diagnosis

Palilalia is distinguished by the fact that the verbal repetition has a distinctive character to it, in that the repeated word or phrase is said with increasing speed and decreasing distinctness.

Stereotypies represent a subset of perseverative motor behavior wherein the repeated behaviors are distinctly purposeless and monotonous. In many patients with dementia, schizophrenia or autism, both purposeful and stereotypical perseveration may appear.

Treatment

Perseverative behavior may lessen or remit with treatment of the underlying condition. In one unblinded study, bromocriptine reduced perseverative behavior in dementia (Imamura *et al.* 1998).

4.6 PRIMITIVE REFLEXES

Normal infancy is characterized by numerous reflexes that, in the usual course of events, tend to fade or disappear with development; these may, however, be found in adults, and in such cases they are known as 'primitive' reflexes. Although these reflexes are found in certain pathologic conditions, such as dementia, they may also, as noted below, be found in normal individuals, and hence care must be taken in their interpretation.

Primitive reflexes are also known as developmental reflexes; 'frontal release signs' constitutes another synonym.

Clinical features

Four primitive reflexes are considered here, namely the palmomental reflex, the snout reflex, the grasp reflex, and the grope reflex.

The palmomental reflex (Blake and Kunkle 1951; Jacobs and Gossman 1980) is elicited by repeatedly and rapidly dragging an object, such as the tip of the reflex hammer, across the thenar eminence from the lateral aspect medially toward the center of the palm: the contact should be definite, and slightly disagreeable, but not painful. When the reflex is present, one sees a wrinkling of the ipsilateral *mentum*, or chin.

The snout reflex (Jacobs and Gossman 1980) is elicited by placing one's index finger just above the patient's upper lip, in the midline, centered upon the philtrum, and then either gently pressing the finger in or gently tapping it with the reflex hammer: a positive reflex is indicated by a puckering or protruding of the lips.

The grasp reflex is tested for by laying one's index finger flat across the palm of the patient's hand (with the tip of the finger pointing toward the hypothenar eminence and the base of the finger resting between the patient's thumb and index finger) and then slowly withdrawing one's finger between the patient's thumb and index finger (Adie and Critchley 1927; Seyffarth and Denny-Brown 1948). When present, the reflex consists of the patient's fingers involuntarily closing upon the examiner's finger, as if grasping it. Once the finger has been grasped, attempts by the examiner to pull it free often result in a stronger grasp, but if the examiner ceases all effort to remove the finger the patient's hand typically relaxes (Walshe and Robertson 1933). If there is any doubt as to the involuntary nature of the grasp the test may be repeated, but only after first instructing the patient to not grab the examiner's finger. Interestingly, such a grasping reflex may be present in a hemiplegic limb, such that although the patient is unable to flex the fingers voluntarily, grasping occurs with the appropriate stimulation (Stewart-Wallace 1939).

The grope reflex (also known as 'instinctive grasping') is a truly remarkable clinical phenomenon. Testing is accomplished by simply touching the patient's hand: when the reflex is present, the patient's hand will involuntarily reach out in a groping fashion to grasp the examiner's finger (Mori and Yamadori 1985). In some cases, one may also demonstrate the 'magnet' reaction, wherein by successive touches of the patient's hand from successively different positions one may lead the patient's hand through space, much as if it were being attracted by a magnet (Seyffarth and Denny-Brown 1948). When fully developed, actual touch may not be required to elicit the reflex, and the patient's hand may automatically begin groping at the mere sight of another object (Mori and Yamadori 1985).

The presence of a grope reflex may significantly interfere with the patient's day-to-day life. One patient, whenever passing through a doorway, found that his 'left hand clung to [the] door handle . . . with such tenacity that he had to use his right hand to free himself' (Seyffarth and Denny-Brown 1948). In another case (Stewart-Wallace 1939), the patient's right hand 'developed a habit of clutching hold of objects of its own accord, such as the lapel of his coat, the edge of his trouser pocket, or the bed-clothes. This distressed him so much that in order to prevent it, he used to wear a glove most of the time. At other times he would keep his hand in his pocket, holding a coin or a key'. Another patient (Walshe and Hunt 1936), questioned about the experience, noted that 'I can't leave things alone. If I see anything lying near me, my hand seems to want it.'

Etiology

Primitive reflexes, as noted earlier, may be found in normal individuals, especially the elderly (Jacobs and Gossman 1980; Koller *et al.* 1982); indeed the palmomental reflex has been noted in anywhere from 11 (Jensen *et al.* 1983) to 37 percent (Jacobs and Gossman 1980) of normal people; consequently finding one primitive reflex is of uncertain clinical significance. Finding more than one primitive reflex, however, is uncommon and finding three in one patient should raise strong suspicions regarding disease of the frontal lobe (Brown *et al.* 1998; Di Legge *et al.* 2001).

As a group, primitive reflexes are commonly found in parkinsonian conditions, such as Parkinson's disease (Maartens de Noordhout and Delwaide 1988; Vreeling *et al.* 1993), diffuse Lewy body disease (Boroni *et al.* 2006), and progressive supranuclear palsy (Brodsky *et al.* 2004), and in various dementias (Tweedy *et al.* 1981; Waite *et al.* 1996), such as frontotemporal dementia (Sjogren *et al.* 1997), Alzheimer's disease (Vreeling *et al.* 1995), multi-infarct dementia (Vreeling *et al.* 1995), and AIDS dementia (Marder *et al.* 1995); they have also been noted in patients with schizophrenia (Barnes *et al.* 1995; Hyde *et al.* 2007; Lohr 1985).

Primitive reflexes are associated with frontal lobe pathology, and this is especially the case with the grasp and grope reflexes: although they have been noted with infarction of the motor and premotor cortex, they appear to be more common with infarction of the medial aspect of the frontal lobe, particularly the cingulate gyrus in its anterior portion, and the supplemental motor area (De Renzi and Barbieri 1992; Hashimoto and Tanaka 1998; Mori and Yamadori 1985; Stewart-Wallace 1939; Walshe and Robertson 1933; Walshe and Hunt 1936).

Differential diagnosis

The grope reflex must be distinguished from the alien hand sign, a distinction made possible by attending to the seeming 'intent' of the moving hand. In groping, the hand reaches for whatever may be nearby, whether a doorknob or the examiner's hand, and simply grabs hold. In the alien hand sign, however, the left hand does something with the object, something, which, importantly, is at cross-purposes with what the patient is intentionally doing with the right hand.

Treatment

Except for the grope reflex, treatment is not required; in cases when the grope reflex interferes with activities of daily living, occupational therapy may assist in developing strategies to prevent the reflex from happening.

4.7 PSEUDOBULBAR PALSY

Pseudobulbar palsy is a syndrome that occurs secondary to interruption of the corticobulbar tracts.

Clinical features

When fully developed (Langworthy and Hesser 1940; Tilney 1912), the syndrome of pseudobulbar palsy consists of 'emotional incontinence', dysarthria, dysphagia, a stiff and shuffling gait, an exaggerated jaw jerk and gag reflex, and a variable degree of paresis of the tongue; the corticospinal tracts are often also involved, as evidenced by exaggerated deep tendon reflexes and bilateral Babinski signs.

Emotional incontinence (also known as 'pathologic laughing and crying' or 'pseudobulbar affect') is the most striking aspect of the syndrome, and is characterized by either laughter or crying, occurring either spontaneously or in response to some otherwise trivial stimulus, such as someone approaching the bed (Lieberman and Benson 1977). After suffering bilateral strokes, one of Kinnier Wilson's patients:

> was seen to have a distinctly vacant, apathetic facial expression at rest. She was able to move facial muscles voluntarily on both sides, although there was the slightest weakness of the left corner of the mouth. On the slightest stimulus, even when the observer simply came to her bedside, she at once assumed a most lugubrious expression, her mouth opened widely, and a long, almost noiseless bout of weeping ensued, lasting for many seconds, even minutes, at a time.
>
> (Wilson 1924)

Another of Wilson's patients, again after bilateral strokes:

> exhibited characteristic involuntary laughing. Whatever the emotional stimulus, and however slight, he at once began to laugh and laugh loudly. Thus, on reading the war news he at once began to smile, and the more serious and anxious the news, the more he laughed. On examination, there was some voluntary facial paresis on both sides, especially the left, some dysarthria, and some dysphagia, but during the laughing the facial movements were in no way restricted. A double extensor response was present.
>
> (Wilson 1924)

Importantly, these emotional displays are not accompanied by any corresponding feeling of sadness or mirth. In one case (Davison and Kelman 1939), a patient, although feeling no mirth, experienced such 'gales of laughter' that he 'felt foolish and ashamed, and had tears in his eyes, because he could not 'control the laughter'. The paroxysms of laughter or crying tend to last on the order of minutes and then resolve spontaneously; in some cases there may be only laughter, or only crying; however, in others one may see laughter succeeded by crying, or vice versa, in the same episode.

Etiology

As noted earlier, pseudobulbar palsy occurs secondary to interruption of the corticobulbar tract. This tract originates in the cortex and descends, in concert with corticospinal fibers, inferiorly, through the internal capsule, the crus cerebri, the basis pontis, and, finally, the medullary pyramids (Besson et al. 1991). Throughout its course in the brainstem, fibers leave the tract to head toward various brainstem nuclei. Most brainstem nuclei are innervated bilaterally and in most cases bilateral interruption of the corticobulbar tracts is required before significant symptomatology occurs. Of the many disorders capable of causing emotional incontinence, vascular disease is the most common.

Emotional incontinence has been noted after bilateral infarction of the posterior frontal cortex (Colman 1894; Davison and Kelman 1939; Wilson 1924), bilateral lacunar infarctions affecting the posterior limbs of the internal capsule (Helgason et al. 1988), and bilateral lacunar infarctions of the basis pontis (Asfora et al. 1989; Bassetti et al. 1996). In many cases of stroke-related emotional incontinence, one finds a history of a stroke wherein there was damage to the corticobulbar fibers on one side, with the current stroke completing the picture by damaging fibers on the other side (Wilson 1924). There are, however, rare cases of emotional incontinence occurring after isolated unilateral infarction of the internal capsule (Ceccaldi et al. 1994; Derex et al. 1997): the mechanism by which emotional incontinence occurs in such cases is not clear and may involve congenital abnormalities.

Other disorders capable of causing bilateral interruption of the corticobulbar tracts and emotional incontinence include amyotrophic lateral sclerosis (ALS) (Gallagher 1989; Ironside 1956; Ziegler 1930), multiple sclerosis (Feinstein et al. 1997), central pontine myelinolysis (van Hilten et al. 1988), progressive supranuclear palsy (Behrman et al. 1969; Menza et al. 1995), and multiple system atrophy (Parvizi et al. 2007). Emotional incontinence may also be seen in disorders characterized by widespread damage to the cortex or subcortical areas, including traumatic brain injury (Tateno et al. 2004; Zelig et al. 1996), Binswanger's disease (Caplan and Schoene 1978), and, in advanced stages, Alzheimer's disease (Starkstein et al. 1995).

Finally, emotional incontinence has been noted with intrinsic brainstem tumors (Achari and Colover 1976;

Cantu and Drew 1966) and also with compression of the brainstem, as for example by a meningioma (Motomura *et al.* 1980).

Differential diagnosis

'Emotionalism' is not at all uncommon after strokes but it is readily distinguished from the emotional incontinence of pseudobulbar palsy by the fact that 'emotional' patients experience an affect congruent with their facial expression, whereas the emotionally incontinent patient feels neither sadness nor mirth and is often as surprised at the emotional display as is the observer.

Lability of affect, as may be seen in mania, is, like emotionalism, distinguished from emotional incontinence by the presence of an affect congruent with the facial expression.

Episodes of mirthless laughter may also occur in an isolated fashion as *le fou rire prodromique* and as a simple partial seizure in gelastic epilepsy. *Le fou rire prodromique*, as discussed in Section 4.9, represents a prodrome to stroke and is distinguished from the emotional incontinence of pseudobulbar palsy in that the mirthless laughter of emotional incontinence occurs after stroke. Gelastic seizures are suggested by a history of other seizure types, such as grand mal or complex partial seizures.

Treatment

In placebo-controlled, double-blind studies, several medications have been shown to be effective for emotional incontinence. For cases occurring secondary to infarction nortriptyline (in doses of from 50 to 100 mg) (Robinson *et al.* 1993), imipramine (in doses of 10–20 mg) (Lawson and McLeod 1969), and citalopram (in doses of 10–20 mg) (Andersen *et al.* 1993) are each effective. For emotional incontinence in ALS (Brooks *et al.* 2004) a combination of dextromethorphan (30 mg) and quinidine (30 mg), given twice daily, is also effective: in this preparation, quinidine is used merely in order to inhibit the metabolism of dextromethorphan, which is the active agent. In cases of MS, both amitriptyline (Schiffer *et al.* 1985) and the combination of dextromethorphan and quinidine are effective (Panitch *et al.* 2006).

It must be stressed that although amitriptyline, nortriptyline, imipramine, and citalpram are all antidepressants, they are effective regardless of whether patients are depressed or not; furthermore, although the response to both amitriptyline and nortriptyline may take weeks, the response to citalopram may be very rapid, with some patients getting relief within a day or two.

It is not clear whether the agents that are found to be effective in stroke cases would be effective in amyotrophic lateral sclerosis or multiple sclerosis, and vice versa, and it is not clear whether any of these agents would be effective in emotional incontinence of other causes. In choosing among these agents, amitriptyline, nortriptyline and imipramine

are probably second choices, given their side-effect burdens; citalopram, in contrast, is extraordinarily easy to use. In cases when citalopram is ineffective, one might consider dextromethorphan or one of the other antidepressants; nortriptyline would probably be the best of these, given its lower side-effect burden.

4.8 EMOTIONAL FACIAL PALSY

Most central facial palsies are of the 'voluntary' sort, in that when patients are asked to voluntarily perform a facial maneuver, such as showing their teeth, there is a droop evident on one side; less commonly one finds an 'emotional' facial paresis wherein, although voluntary movements are intact, a 'droop' becomes evident when the patient smiles in response, say, to a joke. This emotional facial paresis has also been termed 'mimetic' or 'involuntary' facial paresis.

Clinical features

Facial palsies may be either peripheral or central. In a peripheral facial palsy, there is no movement in either the forehead or the lower face, whether on voluntary command or in response to a joke. Central facial palsies are immediately distinguished from peripheral palsies in that this palsy affects only the lower half of the face, with forehead movements being spared.

The two forms of central facial palsy, namely voluntary and emotional, may be distinguished by first noting facial movements when patients are instructed to voluntarily show their teeth and then, at some point in the examination, by closely observing facial movements when the patient spontaneously smiles, for example in response to a joke or recollection of some happy memory (Monrad-Krohn 1924).

In voluntary central facial paresis there is a droop of one side of face when patients are asked to show their teeth; however, when these patients are observed smiling at a joke, one sees full facial movements on both sides.

In emotional facial paresis there is full movement bilaterally when patients are asked to show their teeth; however, when one observes these patients smiling at a joke, there is drooping of one side of the face; this produces what might be called a 'hemismile'.

Etiology

Voluntary and emotional facial paresis are dissociated because the corticobulbar fibers subserving these two functions are separate.

Corticobulbar fibers for voluntary facial movement arise in the posterior portion of the frontal cortex, descend through the corona radiata to the posterior limb of the internal capsule and then travel through the ventral mesencephalon in the crus cerebri to the basis pontis. At this point most of these fibers then cross to travel directly to the contralateral facial nucleus, whereas a minority of them descend further into the medulla, cross and 'loop' back up into the pons, and continue to the facial nucleus.

Corticobulbar fibers for emotional facial movements have widespread origins in the cerebrum, including the supplemental motor area on the medial aspect of the frontal lobe and temporal lobe structures (e.g., the amygdala); the thalamus also plays a role. Fibers descend in the anterior limb of the internal capsule, pass through the tegmentum of the mesencephalon and into the dorsal pons. At this point, most fibers then cross to end in the contralateral facial nerve; however, a minority of fibers proceed down into the medulla, crossing in this structure and then looping back up into the pons to contact the facial nucleus.

Emotional facial paresis has been reported with contralateral lesions, generally infarctions, of a large number of structures (Hopf et al. 1992), including the supplemental motor area (Gelmers 1983), temporal lobe (Remillard et al. 1977), thalamus (Bogousslavsky et al. 1988; Graff-Radford et al. 1984; Ross and Mathiesen 1998), anterior limb of the internal capsule (Trosch et al. 1990), mesencephalic tegmentum (Wilson 1924), and the dorsal pons (Hopf et al. 2000); a case has also been reported of emotional facial paresis with an ipsilateral medullary lesion (Cerrato et al. 2003).

Emotional facial paresis has also been noted in patients with chronic complex partial seizures of temporal lobe origin, and in these cases the emotional facial paresis is generally contralateral to the side with the seizure focus (Jacob et al. 2003). The theory here is that repetitive ictal activity leads to damage of the amygdala.

Differential diagnosis

Some individuals have a congenital 'lopsided' grin; the differential rests here on determining that the 'lopsidedness' has been present since earliest childhood.

Treatment

Specific treatment is not required.

4.9 LE FOU RIRE PRODROMIQUE

Very rarely, uncontrollable, mirthless laughter may occur as the prodrome to an ischemic infarction; this phenomenon was first described by Fere in 1903, who named it le fou rire prodromique.

Clinical features

Le fou rire prodromique manifests as a paroxysmal, uncontrollable fit of laughter, lasting for minutes to a half hour, during which there is full preservation of consciousness and, critically, no corresponding sense of mirth.

In one case (Wali 1993), a 35-year-old woman, 'after a warm shower suddenly began to laugh. The laughter was inappropriate to the situation and continued for nearly 15 minutes at the end of which it became a low grade giggle. This lasted for another 15 minutes and ended abruptly when she collapsed'. On admission she was found to have suffered a bilateral pontine infarction, and was left in a 'locked-in' state. In another case (Martin 1950), the patient's first attack occurred at his mother's funeral, and, much to his distress, recurred and recurred, without any apparent cause, until he collapsed and died several days later; autopsy revealed an interpeduncular aneurysm that had ruptured.

Etiology

Such prodromal laughter has been noted with infarction of the following structures: parietotemporal cortex (Lago 1998), external and extreme capsules (Kumral and Calli 2006); striatum (Carel et al. 1997), genu (Uzunca et al. 2005) or posterior limb (Ceccaldi and Milandre 1994) of the internal capsule, and the basis pontis (Assal et al. 2000; de AA Gondin et al. 2001; Wali 1993).

Differential diagnosis

Mirthless laughter may be seen in the 'emotional incontinence' of pseudobulbar palsy and during gelastic seizures. Pseudobulbar palsy is distinguished by the clinical course, in that in pseudobulbar palsy the episodes of mirthless laughter occur after the stroke, whereas in le fou rire prodromique the episodes occur beforehand. Gelastic seizures are suggested by the occurrence, at other times, of other seizure types, for example grand mal or complex partial.

Treatment

Treatment for the laughter per se is not required as it eventually remits spontaneously; of obviously greater importance is recognizing mirthless laughter as a possible stroke prodrome and proceeding accordingly.

4.10 ABULIA

The term abulia is derived from the Greek, and means 'a lack of will or drive'; synonyms include pure psychic akinesia and athymormia.

Clinical features

Abulic patients, to a greater or lesser degree, lack 'will' in that they fail to experience any initiative or sense of drive: there are no impulses of action, no desires, angers, or longings; one patient commented that there was 'a blank in my mind' (Laplane *et al.* 1984). Importantly, these patients are not depressed or bored; rather they experience a benign sort of emptiness.

Abulic patients, thus volitionally impoverished, may be content to sit or lie quietly, doing nothing and saying nothing, and thus present a picture of immobility and mutism. Importantly, however, if they are asked to do something or to speak, one finds that they are able to perform and complete tasks in a timely and successful fashion: once left to themselves, however, they rapidly lapse back into a placid quietude.

Etiology

Pure abulia may be seen with bilateral or unilateral infarction or hemorrhage of various subcortical structures including the caudate nucleus (Bhatia and Marsden 1994; Caplan *et al.* 1990; Kumral *et al.* 1999; Mendez *et al.* 1989), globus pallidus (Bhatia and Marsden 1994; Giroud *et al.* 1997; Laplane *et al.* 1984), thalamus (Bogousslavsky *et al.* 1991; Van Der Werf *et al.* 1999), or genu of the internal capsule (Yamanaka *et al.* 1996).

Abulia has also been noted as a sequela to carbon monoxide intoxication with bilateral necrosis of the globus pallidus (Laplane *et al.* 1984; Lugaresi *et al.* 1990).

Finally, abulia occurs commonly in schizophrenia, especially simple schizophrenia. Kraepelin (1921) noted that such patients 'experience no tediousness, have no need to pass the time . . . but can lie in bed unoccupied for days and weeks, stand about in corners, "stare into a hole", (or) watch the toes of their boots'.

Differential diagnosis

Akinetic mutism and catatonia enter the differential as in each of these syndromes the patients, like those with abulia, are immobile and mute. Differentiating them from abulia is quite readily done, however, by simply urging the patient to do something, and providing some ongoing supervision: akinetic mutes and catatonics will not respond, whereas the abulic patient does, and will continue to do so until supervision stops.

Apathy and depression are both distinguished by the presence of dysphoria. Abulic patients experience nothing except an untroubled sense of emptiness; depressed or apathetic patients, by contrast, experience a more or less oppressive mood.

Abulia may be seen as part of the frontal lobe syndrome, wherein it may be accompanied by perseveration.

Treatment

Bromocriptine, anecdotally, has been effective (Barrett 1991); treatment may be commenced at a low dose of 2.5 mg in total per day, and increased in similar increments every few days until satisfactory improvement or unacceptable side-effects occur, or a maximum dose of perhaps 40 mg is reached; in all cases, dosage is generally divided into two doses: one in the morning and the next in the early afternoon.

4.11 ENVIRONMENTAL DEPENDENCY SYNDROME

This rare syndrome was initially described in 1983 by Lhermitte, who named it 'utilization behavior'; in a subsequent paper, he changed the name to the 'environmental dependency syndrome' (Lhermitte 1986).

Clinical features

In this syndrome, patients appear to lose their autonomy, becoming 'dependent' on their environment such that they feel compelled to pick up and 'utilize' whatever may come to their attention. For example, one patient upon seeing a pair of glasses put them on, even though they were not his; another patient, upon seeing a toothbrush, picked it up and began brushing, even though there was no need to do so. At times, the utilization behavior can be more complex. For example, in describing one of his patients Lhermitte noted that both he and the patient:

> sat down in my office. I put some medical instruments on my desk. She immediately picked up the blood pressure gauge and very meticulously took my blood pressure . . . After this she took the tongue depressor and placed it in front of my mouth, which I opened, and she examined my throat . . . Last, she picked up the reflex tester and, to make sure she tested the ankle jerks, I knelt down on the chair. When I asked her what she thought, she said she was satisfied with my state of health.
>
> Lhermitte (1983)

Importantly, patients engage in this behavior without being invited, asked or told to, and some may even persist in the behavior despite being asked to stop.

Etiology

The syndrome has been noted most commonly with bilateral or unilateral lesions of the inferior frontal lobe (De Renzi *et al.* 1996; Lhermitte 1983, 1986; Lhermitte *et al.* 1986; Shallice *et al.* 1989); cases have also been reported with infarction of the white matter subjacent to the superior frontal gyrus (Ishihara *et al.* 2002) and with infarction of the thalamus (Eslinger *et al.* 1991; Hashimoto *et al.* 1995). Frontotemporal dementia may also exhibit this syndrome.

Differential diagnosis

One of the primitive reflexes, namely the grasp reflex, appears similar to the environmental dependency syndrome in that in both cases patients will involuntarily reach and grasp objects. The difference lies in what the patient does with the grasped object: the patient with forced grasping simply holds on, whereas the patient with the environmental dependency syndrome will utilize the object and do something with it.

The alien hand sign also appears similar to utilization behavior in that the alien hand involuntarily reaches out and does things with objects: the difference here is that what the alien hand does is at cross-purposes with what the patient is attempting to do with the 'good' hand, whereas in utilization behavior, the two hands act in concert, without any conflict.

Echopraxia or 'imitation behavior' is said to be present when patients involuntarily and automatically imitate what the examiner is doing. This is fundamentally different from environmental dependency, for in the environmental dependency syndrome the examiner does nothing except perhaps place objects in the patient's view.

Delirious patients may take hold of and use nearby objects but here one also finds confusion, a sign that is absent in the environmental dependency syndrome.

Treatment

Depending on the dangerousness of objects in the patient's environment, supervision may or may not be required.

4.12 KLUVER–BUCY SYNDROME

In 1939, Kluver and Bucy reported striking behavioral changes in monkeys subjected to bilateral temporal lobectomy. This Kluver–Bucy syndrome has subsequently been noted in humans, wherein its most prominent clinical manifestations are hyperorality and hypersexuality.

Clinical features

In the full form of the human Kluver–Bucy syndrome, one finds a heightened, but indiscriminate, interest in nearby objects coupled with hyperorality, hypersexuality, and a certain placidity marked by an absence of fear. Patients appear to take an almost equal interest in all nearby objects and may appear restless as they reach out for one object on the bedside table after another, or pace about the room, again, from one thing to another. Hyperorality comes to light in that there is a strong tendency on the patients' part to put anything into their mouths, whether it is edible or not: patients may eat Styrofoam cups, drink urine out of urinals, or stuff their mouths full of tissue papers. Hypersexuality may be very problematic: patients may display no gender preference and may proposition males and females alike; there may be excessive masturbation, sometimes done publicly. The placidity of these patients is at times remarkable: they seem to have no fear, and pointing out the consequences of their behavior to them typically does nothing to disturb them.

Some examples from the literature may help to fix this clinical picture in the reader's mind. In one case, a 57-year-old professor suffered head trauma that led to a maceration of the inferior surface of both temporal lobes. After recovering from the trauma, the patient:

> failed to recognize objects placed in front of him or into his hand. He ate voraciously and, in fact, had a tendency to place almost everything that came into view in his mouth. For instance, after one meal he drank a cup of tea and then ate the teabag. He wandered aimlessly and did not know the location of his room. He made inappropriate sexual advances, rather indiscriminately; both male and female attendants were cautious in his presence. In general, however, his affect was flat and unconcerned. He was readily distracted and there was a constant shifting of his attention. If restrained, he became agitated, but when his attention was diverted, he immediately calmed down.
>
> (Lilly et al. 1983)

In another case, a 46-year-old man had a complex partial seizure wherein:

> he was awake and alert, but almost mute and lacking facial expression. He was observed grabbing for objects on his bedside table, and he masturbated in front of the nursing staff. He also placed objects in his mouth, chewed on tissue paper, and attempted to drink from his own urine container.
>
> (Nakada et al. 1984)

Finally, another patient, after recovering from an episode of complex partial status epilepticus, displayed:

> a voracious appetite and indiscriminate eating habits which included paper towels, plants, styrofoam cups, and even faeces. At one point he drank urine from a catheter bag. The patient was no longer his assertive self and had become quite docile. He tended to wander about the ward touching objects or people and made inappropriate comments of a sexual nature ... On the day of his death, the patient had a respiratory arrest after stuffing his mouth with surgical gauze. He had wandered about the ward picking up whatever he could find and putting it into his mouth.
>
> (Mendez and Foti 1997)

Kluver and Bucy (1939), as noted above, first described this syndrome in monkeys and their descriptions are of interest. The terminology they utilized is somewhat cumbersome but is still at times seen in the literature.

The heightened interest of the monkeys (which they termed 'hypermetamorphosis') was manifest by 'an excessive tendency to take notice of and to attend and react to every visual stimulus . . . the monkey seems to be dominated by only one tendency, namely the tendency to contact every object as soon as possible [and] . . . when turned loose in a room, the monkey often behaves as if it were ceaselessly "pulled" from one object to another'.

According to Kluver and Bucy's terminology, the indiscriminate nature of this heightened interest represented a kind of 'psychic blindness' in that the monkey would approach and examine objects 'no matter whether they are very large or very small, dead or alive, edible or inedible, moving or stationary . . . The monkey seems to be just as eager to examine the tongue of a hissing snake, the mouth of a cat, feces, a wire cage or a wagon as a piece of bread'.

Hyperorality (or, as Kluver and Bucy termed it, 'oral tendencies') was manifest by a 'strong tendency to examine all objects by mouth', for example 'putting the object into the mouth, biting gently, chewing, licking, touching with the lips and smelling . . . the object'.

Hypersexuality was referred to as 'changes in sexual behavior' and was manifest by a general 'increase in sexual behavior' that could involve other monkeys, regardless of their gender, or masturbation.

Placidity was termed 'emotional changes' by Kluver and Bucy and was marked by 'absence of all emotional reactions . . . generally associated with anger and fear'. For example, 'after being attacked and bitten by another animal, (the monkey) may approach this animal again and again in an attempt to examine it'.

Etiology

As with monkeys, it appears that in humans the Kluver–Bucy syndrome generally appears only with bilateral damage or dysfunction of the temporal lobes – I could find only one case report of the syndrome occurring with unilateral involvement, namely in a case of unilateral temporal lobectomy (Ghika-Schmid et al. 1995). Table 4.3 lists the various causes reported in the literature.

Bilateral ablation or injury to the temporal lobes is most obvious after bilateral temporal lobectomy. Traumatic brain injury, with contusions of the inferior surfaces of both temporal lobes, may also cause the syndrome, as may a late-delayed radiation encephalopathy after irradiation, say, for a pituitary tumor or nasopharyngeal carcinoma. Herpes simplex viral encephalitis classically involves both temporal lobes, and the syndrome may appear as a sequela in those who survive. Finally, there are rare cases of infarction of both temporal lobes (as for example secondary to a vasculopathy of systemic lupus erythematosus) with a resulting Kluver–Bucy syndrome.

Table 4.3   Causes of the Kluver-Bucy syndrome

Bilateral ablation or injury to the temporal lobes
Temporal lobectomy (Terzian and Dalle Ore 1955)
Traumatic brain injury (Formisano et al. 1995; Lilly et al. 1983)
Late-delayed radiation encephalopathy (Lam and Chiu 1997; Thajeb 1995)
Post-herpes simplex viral encephalitis (Greenwood et al. 1983; Marlowe et al. 1975; Shoji et al. 1979)
Infarction (Oliveira et al. 1989)

Epileptic conditions
Complex partial seizure (Nakada et al. 1984)
Post-ictal, after either a grand mal seizure (Anson and Kuhlman 1993) or complex partial status epilepticus (Mendez and Foti 1997; Varon et al. 2003)

Neurodegenerative disorders
Pick's disease (Cummings and Duchen 1981; Mendez et al. 1993)
Frontotemporal dementia (Gydesen et al. 2002; Heutink et al. 1997; Mendez and Perryman 2002)
Alzheimer's disease (Mendez et al. 1993; Teri et al. 1988)

Miscellaneous causes
Adrenoleukodystrophy (Powers et al. 1980)
Heatstroke (Pitt et al. 1995)

Epileptic conditions may be characterized by the Kluver–Bucy syndrome, either ictally during a complex partial seizure or post-ictally after either a grand mal seizure or an episode of complex partial status epilepticus.

Neurodegenerative disorders may cause a Kluver–Bucy syndrome of gradual onset and progression, and this is most characteristic of those disorders such as Pick's disease and frontotemporal dementia, which preferentially involve the temporal lobes early on. Other neurodegenerative disorders, such as Alzheimer's disease, may, late in their course, also cause the syndrome.

Miscellaneous, and very rare, causes of the syndrome include adrenoleukodystrophy and heat stroke.

Differential diagnosis

When a patient presents with disinhibition, the frontal lobe syndrome may come to mind; in this syndrome, as in the Kluver–Bucy syndrome, one may see inappropriate sexual advances. The differential lies in finding features such as hyperorality and a heightened and indiscriminate interest in nearby objects, features which are not found in the frontal lobe syndrome.

Treatment

There are no controlled studies of the treatment of the Kluver–Bucy syndrome. Anecdotally, overall improvement has been noted with carbamazepine (Stewart 1985), sertraline (Mendhekar and Duggal 2005), or antipsychotics (Carrol *et al.* 2001); should an antipsychotic be chosen, a second-generation agent, such as risperidone or quetiapine, may be considered. Hypersexuality has also been reduced by treatment with leuprolide (Ott 1995). As noted in one of the examples above, hyperorality may be lethal and appropriate precautions must be taken.

4.13 ALIEN HAND SIGN

The alien hand sign represents one of the most remarkable phenomena seen in neuropsychiatric practice, or for that matter, in the practice of medicine at large. Here, one of the patient's hands, almost always the left one, begins to act as if it had an independent will of its own, often engaging in complex activity that thwarts what the patient is attempting to do with the right hand.

This sign was first described by the German physician Kurt Goldstein in 1908; Akelaitis, in 1941, described it in patients who had been subjected to corpus callosotomy for epilepsy, and named it 'diagonistic dyspraxia'. The current name, 'alien hand sign', is derived from a French paper by Brion and Jedynak (1972), who termed it '*le signe de la main étrangère*': although the authors translated this as the 'strange hand' sign (which is indeed a more faithful translation from the French), English-speaking authors have universally favored translating it as 'alien hand sign'. Another synonym, seen infrequently, is 'anarchic hand' (Della Sala 1994).

Clinical features

The alien hand sign is said to be present when one of the patient's hands (almost, as noted above, always the left one) spontaneously and autonomously acts in a way that is at definite cross-purposes to what the patient is intending to do with the right hand (Bogen 1985a). This 'intermanual conflict', as it has been termed, is not merely a matter of a clumsy or apraxic left hand 'getting in the way', or of reflexive groping or grasping by the left hand, but rather of the appearance of complex and seemingly purposeful activity of the left hand, activity that is at definite cross-purposes with the patient's consciously experienced will and intent. Patients may be astonished to see the left hand acting independently and outside their control, and may comment that it is as if the left hand had 'a mind of its own'.

Some examples of the alien hand sign will serve to flesh out this definition. The complexity of the behavior engaged in by the alien hand ranges from relatively simple activities, such as buttoning or unbuttoning, to very complex behaviors, even to the point of 'murderous' behavior. Examples of relatively simple alien hand behavior include the case of a patient, who, after an infarction of the corpus callosum, found that after he buttoned 'a shirt with the right hand the left hand would proceed to unbutton it and if pulling a cup

of coffee toward him with the right hand the left hand would push it away' (Gottlieb *et al.* 1992). Similarly, subsequent to a corpus callosotomy, 'one patient was seen buttoning up his shirt with one hand while the other hand was following along behind it undoing the buttons' (Bogen 1985b). Akelaitis (1945) noted that one of his patients, also after a corpus callosotomy, 'would be putting on her clothes with her right hand and pulling them off with her left hand, opening a door or drawer with the right hand and simultaneously pushing it shut with the left hand'.

More complex behavior is illustrated in the case of a patient who, after suffering an infarction of the corpus callosum, 'told the story of herself frying a steak, turning it over in the frying pan with her right hand and, immediately after, finding herself turning it over once again with her left hand' (Barbizet *et al.* 1974; Degos *et al.* 1987). Another patient, after suffering an infarction of the anterior portion of the corpus callosum and adjacent medial aspects of both frontal lobes, found, 'while playing checkers on one occasion, [that] the left hand made a move that he did not wish to make, and he corrected the move with the right hand; however, the left hand, to the patient's frustration, repeated the false move' (Banks *et al.* 1989).

Finally, there are examples of a 'murderous' alien hand. The first reported case of the alien hand sign, described by Kurt Goldstein (1908), was just such an example: the patient was a 57-year-old female with a callosal infarction whose 'left hand attempted to choke [her] ... and this hand had to be pulled away. Furthermore the left hand did other unpleasant acts, such as tearing the bedclothes off the bed' (Geschwind 1981). The patient herself 'complained, "Es muss wohl ein boser Geist in der Hand sein" [There must be a devil in my hand]' (Hanakita and Nishi 1991). In another case, a patient who had suffered a callosal infarction treated her left arm 'as an alien presence with hostile motivations . . . she complained that the arm moved on its own and that it struck her and tried to choke her . . . often the hand reached for the neckline of her gown, pinched her right arm or leg, or knocked her glasses off' (Levine and Rinn 1986). Finally, there is the case of a patient who had suffered a callosal infarction (Geschwind *et al.* 1995) who 'awoke several times with her left hand choking her, and while she was awake her left hand would unbutton her gown, crush cups on her tray, and fight with the right hand while she was using the phone'.

Patients' reactions to the presence of the alien hand vary. One patient commented that 'my hands don't agree with each other' (Degos *et al.* 1987), and another, that her hand 'disobeyed her' (Goldenberg *et al.* 1985), whereas a third felt 'as if someone "from the moon" were controlling her hand' (Geschwind *et al.* 1995). Patients also adopt different strategies to control the alien hand: one, 'to keep her left hand from doing mischief, . . . would subdue it with her right hand' (Geschwind *et al.* 1995); another found the behavior 'so astonishing and uncontrollable that he occasionally hit his left [hand] ... with the right one' (Leiguarda *et al.* 1989). Another patient, 'encouraged to "make friends" with the arm by talking to it, . . . soon came to treat it as a misbehaving child, fondling and talking to it: 'There, there, behave yourself now . . . Don't be naughty"' (Levine and Rinn 1986).

As noted earlier, the alien hand sign is almost always found on the left: indeed, of all the cases of strictly defined alien hand sign that I could find, in only one was the sign found on the right in a right-handed patient (Della Sala et al. 1994).

Etiology

Once one is certain that the clinical phenomenon in question is in fact the alien hand sign, one can be reasonably assured that in all likelihood the patient has a lesion in the corpus callosum. In addition to occurring after section of the corpus callosum (Akelaitis 1941, 1945; Akelaitis et al. 1942; Ay et al. 1998; Bogen 1985a,b; Ferguson et al. 1985; Gazzaniga et al. 1962; Nishikawa et al. 2001, Rayport et al 1983; Smith and Akelaitis 1942; Sperry 1966; Van Waggenen and Herrin 1940; Wilson et al. 1977), the alien hand sign has also been noted in various pathologic lesions of the corpus callosum, including infarction (Banks et al. 1989; Barbizet et al. 1974; Beukelman et al. 1980; Chan and Ross 1988, 1997; Chan et al. 1996; Degos et al. 1987; Geschwind et al. 1995; Goldberg and Bloom 1990; Goldenberg et al. 1985; Goldstein 1908, 1909; Hanakita and Nishi 1991; Jason and Pajurkova 1992; Nishikawa et al. 2001, Suwanwela and Leelacheavasit 2002; Tanaka et al. 1990, 1996; Watson and Heilman 1983; Watson et al. 1985), hemorrhage (Leiguarda et al. 1989; Starkstein et al. 1988), and tumor or angioma (Brion and Jedynak 1972).

I could find only three cases of strictly defined alien hand sign that appeared to occur secondary to focal lesions that spared the corpus callosum. Levine and Rinn (1986) described a case secondary to infarction of the basal aspect of the temporo-occipital area, but the only imaging performed was with computed tomography (CT) scanning and the authors admitted that they could not exclude damage to either the splenium or the adjacent white matter. Gottlieb et al. (1992) described a case occurring with infarction of the medial aspect of the frontoparietal area. Again, only CT scanning was performed, but it appeared that the infarction was in the watershed area between the distributions of the anterior and middle cerebral arteries, and thus may truly have spared the corpus callosum. Perhaps the most convincing case comes from Dolado et al. (1995), who described a patient with an old infarction in the left parietal lobe who went on to develop the alien hand sign after a fresh infarction in the right parietal lobe.

It is commonly said that the alien hand sign may also be found in corticobasal ganglionic degeneration, but a close reading of detailed reports reveals, rather than the alien hand sign, a variety of other signs, such as 'wandering' and grasping (Rinne et al. 1994), and levitation (Gibb et al. 1989; Riley et al. 1990).

Creutzfeldt–Jakob disease may, very rarely, present with a combination of myoclonus and the alien hand sign (MacGowan et al. 1997). In one case, the alien left hand 'would grab [the patient's] throat or hit her in the face and she usually limited its activity by holding it in her right hand's grasp'. In another case presented by the same authors, the alien hand, again on the left, unbuttoned the patient's blouse and removed a hair pin. In both cases, the eventual appearance of periodic complexes on the EEG and dementia suggested the correct diagnosis. There is also one case report of an alien hand sign occurring due to Alzheimer's disease (Green et al. 1995).

Differential diagnosis

The alien hand sign must be differentiated from the grasp and grope reflexes, asomatagnosia, the 'levitation' phenomenon, 'mirror' movements and utilization behavior (as seen in the environmental dependency syndrome).

The grasp reflex is easily distinguished from the alien hand sign if one attends to what the hand does when it comes into contact with an object: the grasping hand merely holds tight and goes no further, whereas the alien hand takes hold and does something with the object. The grope reflex may be a little harder to distinguish, as here the hand appears to be purposefully 'groping' for something. The distinction is again made possible by attending to what the groping hand does once it reaches the object: the groping hand, like the grasping hand, merely holds tight, again in contrast with the alien hand, which does something complex with the object. The failure to distinguish these primitive reflexes from the 'intermanual conflict' seen in the alien hand sign has led to some unfortunate confusion in terminology, namely a proposal, made by Feinberg et al. (1992) (and further elaborated by Chan et al. [1997]) that, rather than only one alien hand syndrome, there are in fact two: namely a 'frontal' alien hand sign and a 'callosal' alien hand sign. Close reading of these papers, however, reveals that the 'frontal' alien hand was merely grasping and groping; the 'callosal' type, however, corresponded to the clinical features noted above. Given this terminological controversy, it is incumbent on the reader to examine closely any literature on the subject to see whether the patients described had mere grasping or groping or a true alien hand sign.

Asomatagnosia is said to be present when patients deny that a limb belongs to them. Although patients with asomatagnosia and the alien hand sign both experience the limb as foreign, the phenomena are easily distinguished in that whereas the 'foreign' limb of the patient with asomatagnosia does nothing independently, and generally nothing purposeful, the alien hand acts 'on its own'.

The levitation phenomenon, seen in patients with parietal lesions (Denny-Brown et al. 1952), as well as in a small minority of patients with progressive supranuclear palsy (Barclay et al. 1999), consists of the upper extremity spontaneously rising up, or 'levitating'. This differs from the alien hand sign in that the levitated arm or hand does not do anything further, engaging in no complex behavior but simply staying 'levitated'.

Mirror movements are said to be present when patients who are doing something with one limb then find the contralateral limb involuntarily engaging in a more or less faithful imitation. Such mirror movements are more likely when the intended movement is very forceful or sudden; a common example is when one very tightly clenches one fist and finds that the fingers on the other hand are involuntarily flexing. Mirror movements are normal in early childhood and, in a minority of individuals, may persist into adult life (Haerer and Currier 1966; Regli *et al.* 1967). They may be associated with agenesis of the corpus callosum (Schott and Wyke 1981) and may also occur in patients with hemiplegia, wherein they are generally found in the paretic limb (Berlin 1951; Walshe 1923). Mirror movements may 'get in the way' and thus seem to be at cross-purposes; a closer inspection, however, will reveal that the abnormal movement does in fact 'mirror' the intended movement in the other limb and that its 'interference' is merely accidental.

Utilization behavior appears similar to the alien hand sign, given that patients with utilization behavior involuntarily utilize objects. The difference between utilization behavior and the alien hand sign lies in the fact that in utilization behavior there is no intermanual conflict between the hands, which act in concert and with cooperation, whereas in the alien hand sign the left hand acts at definite cross-purposes with the right.

Treatment

A mitt placed on the alien hand may mitigate its effects; in some cases, the entire extremity must be restrained.

4.14 BALINT'S SYNDROME

This syndrome, first described in 1907 by a Hungarian neurologist, Rezso Balint (Husain and Stein 1988), is characterized by the triad of simultanagnosia, optic ataxia, and optic apraxia.

Clinical features

Simultanagnosia, discussed further in Section 2.9, may be tested for by asking the patient to look at a drawing of a complex scene, and asking for a description of each of the objects in the drawing: typically, patients will fail to mention one or more of the objects.

Optic ataxia is characterized by an inability to voluntarily reach and touch an object with the hand. Testing may be accomplished by holding up your index finger and asking the patient to touch it. When optic ataxia is present, the patient behaves almost as if he were blind, missing the examiner's finger by a wide margin. Interestingly, despite this inability, patients are still able to accurately touch parts of their own body.

Optic apraxia, also known as 'sticky fixation' or 'psychic paralysis of visual fixation', represents a peculiar difficulty in eye movement wherein patients are unable to voluntarily look from one fixation point to another. Testing for this may be performed by first having the patient fix his gaze on an object and then commanding him to look at another one. When optic apraxia is present there is a peculiar 'stickiness', as if the patient is unable to withdraw his gaze from the initial object to fix it on the next one. Interestingly, this 'stickiness' is present only with voluntary eye movements: should someone walk unexpectedly into the room, the patient may spontaneously shift his gaze without difficulty to fix it on this new object of interest.

Etiology

Most cases of Balint's syndrome occur secondary to bilateral infarctions in the parieto-occipital areas (Montero *et al.* 1982; Perez *et al.* 1996), commonly watershed infarctions seen after cardiac arrest. Balint's syndrome may also constitute part of a syndrome known as posterior cortical atrophy. In this syndrome, one may see a gradually progressive, more or less isolated, Balint's syndrome; the underlying neuropathology may include corticobasal ganglionic degeneration or Alzheimer's disease (Hof *et al.* 1993; McMonagle *et al.* 2006; Mendez 2000; Renner *et al.* 2004; Tang-Wai *et al.* 2004). Balint's syndrome has also been noted in Creutzfeldt–Jakob disease (Victoroff *et al.* 1994) and progressive multifocal leukoencephalopathy (Ayuso-Peralta *et al.* 1994).

Differential diagnosis

Before deciding that Balint's syndrome is present, one must determine that the visual difficulties are not due to hemineglect, hemianopia, visual agnosia or, with regard to optic ataxia, cerebellar dysmetria.

Treatment

Various rehabilitation techniques, anecdotally, have been helpful (Perez *et al.* 1996; Roselli *et al.* 2001).

4.15 PHANTOM AND SUPERNUMERARY LIMBS

The phantom limb phenomenon and the supernumerary limb phenomenon are similar in that, in both cases, patients experience the presence of limbs which, in fact, are not present. These two phenomena differ, however, in that whereas phantom limb follows amputation and is characterized by a re-experiencing of the limb that has been lost, supernumerary limb occurs with cerebral lesions, such as infarctions, and is characterized by the experience of an extra limb, over and above the normal complement already present.

Phantom limb occurs in the vast majority of patients after amputation, and typically appears within the first few days post-operatively; in about three-quarters of cases, it is also accompanied by phantom limb pain. The supernumerary limb phenomenon, in contrast, is quite rare and is not painful.

Clinical features

Phantom limb (Carlen *et al.* 1978; Ephraim *et al.* 2005; Haber 1956; Henderson and Smythe 1948; Jensen *et al.* 1984; Shukla *et al.* 1982) is a tactile experience, rather than a visual one: although patients do not see the limb, they 'feel' it and have a sense of its presence, and in some cases report being able to move it. Importantly, patients retain insight here and do not, in fact, believe that a limb is actually present. Phantom limb pain is variously described as burning, electric, throbbing, cramping, tearing or crushing, and can be quite severe. Over time, most patients experience what is known as 'telescoping': here, it is as if the phantom were being gradually absorbed back into the remaining limb, the most proximal part of the phantom disappearing first and the remaining portions telescoping after it, with the most distal portion, usually the fingers or toes, disappearing last. In some cases, the phantom may disappear entirely after months or longer, whereas in others it may be permanent.

Childhood amputations, before the age of 4 years, are only rarely followed by phantoms (Simmel 1962). The congenital absence of a limb may, interestingly, be followed in a small minority by the development of a phantom 'replacement' (Weinstein and Sersen 1961), generally around the age of 9 years (Melzak *et al.* 1997).

The phantom phenomenon, although most common after amputation of a limb, also occurs after mastectomy in one-fifth (Ackerly *et al.* 1955; Jarvis 1967) to two-thirds of women (Bressler *et al.* 1956) and may, in a small minority, be accompanied by pain. Phantom eye has also been reported after enucleation (Soros *et al.* 2003).

Supernumerary limb is characterized by the experience of having an extra arm or leg. One patient felt the extra arm lying across his abdomen (Mayeux and Benson 1979), another experienced it growing out of his forearm (Brock and Merworth 1957), and one patient, after suffering bilateral parietal lobe infarctions, experienced four legs, two on each side (Vuilleumier *et al.* 1997). Although in some cases patients may retain insight, at times this may be lost and patients may insist that, in fact, an extra limb is present (Halligan *et al.* 1993; Weinstein *et al.* 1954).

Etiology

The phantom limb phenomenon probably represents persistent activity of those structures, such as the parietal cortex, which maintain the body schema.

Supernumerary limbs have been noted with lesions of the parietal lobe (Vuilleumier *et al.* 1997; Weinstein *et al.* 1954), the medial aspect of the frontal cortex (McGonigle *et al.* 2002), the basal ganglia (Halligan *et al.* 1993), thalamus (Miyazawa *et al.* 2004), and pons (Brock and Merwarth 1957). Although most supernumerary limbs appear on the left side, right-sided occurrence has also been noted (Mayeux and Benson 1979). Supernumerary limbs may also occur as a manifestation of a sensory simple partial seizure, a diagnosis immediately suggested by the paroxysmal onset and relatively brief duration of the experience. One patient, for a few seconds, would experience a supernumerary arm next to his actual left arm (Riddoch 1941); another had such a strong sense that an extra right arm was over his head that he asked his wife to help him pull it down (Russell and Whitty 1953).

Differential diagnosis

The phantom limb appearing after amputation is not mimicked by other conditions. It must be kept in mind, however, that, albeit rarely, not all pain experienced in the phantom limb is 'phantom limb pain' resulting from cortical or subcortical reorganization. For example, one patient, who experienced a non-painful phantom after amputation of a lower extremity, subsequently developed disk disease with typical sciatic pain radiating down into the phantom (King 1956).

Treatment

The optimum treatment of phantom limb pain is not clear. Opioids are used, and provide some relief (Huse *et al.* 2001) but are certainly not universally effective. Gabapentin in high dosage was effective in one double-blind study (Bone *et al.* 2002) but not in another (Smith *et al.* 2005). Similarly, memantine, in a dose of 30 mg/day, was effective in one double-blind study (Schley *et al.* 2006) but ineffective in two others (Maier *et al.* 2003; Wiech *et al.* 2004). Infusions of salmon calcitonin were effective in one double-blinded study (Jaeger and Maier 1992). Anecdotally, patients have responded to treatment with a TENS unit (on the contralateral extremity) (Carabelli and Kellerman 1985), deep brain stimulation (Bittar *et al.* 2005), clonazepam (Bartusch *et al.* 1996), carbamazepine (Patterson 1988), chlorpromazine (Logan 1983), and, despite an absence of depression, to fluoxetine (Power-Smith and Turkington 1993), and to ECT (Rasmussen and Rummans 2000).

4.16 DEPERSONALIZATION

Depersonalization is a common experience that is found not only in normal individuals, but also in patients with epilepsy and various other disorders.

Clinical features

In depersonalization, patients feel uncannily detached from themselves. Although they may continue to engage in some activity, whether it be talking, walking, or driving a car, it seems to them as if they are not really doing it but observing it being done, as if it were being carried out by a robot or an automaton. In some cases, visual distortions may occur: arms or legs may appear misshapen or shrunken. Patients may occasionally have the experience of 'floating' above the scene, watching themselves do things from a distance.

Etiology

The various causes of depersonalization are listed in Table 4.4.

Depersonalization is most commonly seen as a normal, transient reaction to extreme danger, as may occur in combat, assaults, traumatic accidents, etc.

Intoxication with marijuana or MDMA (3,4 methylene-dioxymethamphetamine, 'Ecstasy') is very commonly associated with depersonalization, and in some cases patients may subsequently re-experience depersonalization as a 'flashback' when not intoxicated. Certain medications may also, albeit very rarely, cause depersonalization, including quetiapine, fluoxetine, minocycline, and indomethacin.

Table 4.4 Causes of depersonalization

Normal response to danger (Morgan *et al.* 2001; Noyes and Kletti 1977; Noyes *et al.* 1977; Sedman 1966)

Intoxicants or medications
 Marijuana (Mathew *et al.* 1993, Melges *et al.* 1970)
 MDMA (Ecstasy) (Vollenweider *et al.* 1998)
 Quetiapine (Sarkar *et al.* 2001)
 Fluoxetine (Black and Wojcieszek 1991)
 Minocycline (Cohen 2004)
 Indomethacin (Schwartz and Moura 1983)

In association with migraine or seizures
 Migraine aura (Lippman 1953)
 Aura to complex partial or grand mal seizure (Devinsky *et al.* 1989; Ionasescu 1960)
 Simple partial seizure (Williams 1956)

Traumatic brain injury (Grigsby and Kaye 1993; Hillbom 1960)

Panic attack (Cassano *et al.* 1989)

Depression (Noyes *et al.* 1977)

Depersonalization disorder (Baker *et al.* 2003; Davison 1964; Shorvon 1946; Simeon *et al.* 1997, 2003)

Migraine headaches may be preceded by an aura of depersonalization, and the diagnosis is immediately suggested by the succeeding headache. Depersonalization may also occur as an aura to either a complex partial or grand mal seizure, and here again the diagnosis is immediately indicated by the subsequent seizure. Depersonalization may also constitute the sole symptomatology of a simple partial seizure, and here a high index of suspicion may be required to make the diagnosis. One important clue, of course, would be a history of other seizure types; however, this may not be universally present as in some cases epilepsy may be characterized only by simple partial seizures, without other seizure types: in such cases, an exquisitely paroxysmal onset of the depersonalization may be the only clue.

Traumatic brain injury is very commonly accompanied by depersonalization, especially in those who have suffered relatively mild trauma.

Panic attacks may have depersonalization as part of their symptomatology, and here the diagnosis is suggested by the associated anxiety and other autonomic symptoms such as tremor, tachycardia and diaphoresis.

Depression may be complicated by depersonalization; here the occurrence of depersonalization within the setting of chronic depressive symptoms indicates the correct diagnosis.

Finally, when all other causes have been ruled out, one is left with a diagnosis, by exclusion, of depersonalization disorder. This is an idiopathic disorder, with an onset in late adolescence or early adult years, characterized by depersonalization that may either persist in a chronic, waxing and waning fashion, or be episodic, with the duration of the episodes exhibiting an enormous variation that may last from seconds to days.

Differential diagnosis

Autoscopy is a kind of visual hallucination wherein patients hallucinate a 'double' and see themselves as vividly as if looking in a mirror. Depersonalization differs from this in that there is always an 'as if' quality to the experience of depersonalization, accompanied by the sense of 'floating' over the scene that one is actually in.

Treatment

Treatment is directed toward the underlying cause; in the case of depersonalization occurring in traumatic brain injury or depersonalization disorder, however, there are no established treatments.

4.17 OBSESSIONS AND COMPULSIONS

True obsessions and compulsions, once considered rare oddities, are now known to be quite common, occurring not only in idiopathic obsessive–compulsive disorder, but in a large number of other conditions.

Clinical features

Obsessions are involuntary, unwanted, and often distressing thoughts that persistently recur despite attempts on the part of patients to stop them. Although the subject matter may at times be neutral, it more often than not concerns sexual or violent acts, acts in which the patient would never voluntarily engage. Compulsions represent an overwhelming and anxious need to do something, something that patients realize is more or less nonsensical. The compulsion is typically intimately connected with an apprehension on the part of patients that they have done something that they ought not to have done, or that they have left undone something that they ought to have done, and the compulsive act serves in some fashion either to undo what was done or to make good something that ought to have been done.

An example of an obsession is found in the case of the mother of a newborn infant, who was horrified to find herself recurrently having thoughts of 'stabbing the child, putting the infant in the microwave, or sexually abusing the newborn' (Sichel et al. 1993). In another case, the obsession was, per se, of a neutral character, consisting of 'silly poems that kept running through his consciousness': what 'appalled' the patient was the fact that he could not stop them (Mulder et al. 1951).

Common compulsions include compulsions to wash, to pray, or to check. Tuke (1894) described a 'young lady', who feared 'infecting herself' if she touched anything that might have germs on it, with the result that 'the act of washing her hands in the morning is repeated, immediately, again and again' such that the hands 'are quite rough and discoloured afterward', and Gordon (1950) described a patient who felt compelled to repeat his prayers again and again for fear each time that he had left a word out. Finally, Bleuler (1924), in commenting on a patient with a checking compulsion, noted that the anxious apprehension that the door had been left unlocked 'compels the patient to try it over and over again'.

Etiology

Table 4.5 lists the various causes of obsessions and compulsions.

By far the most common cause is the idiopathic disorder known as obsessive-compulsive disorder. This disorder, characterized primarily by obsessions and compulsions, has an onset in adolescence or early adult years, and generally pursues a chronic course. A depressive episode of a major depressive disorder may also cause obsessions and compulsions; however, here the occurrence of these symptoms in the setting of a typical depressive episode suggests the correct diagnosis. Schizophrenia, likewise, may be accompanied by obsessions and compulsions; however, here also it is the setting, in this case a chronic psychosis, which allows the correct diagnosis. Importantly,

Table 4.5 Causes of obsessions and compulsions

Idiopathic disorders and medication side-effects
Obsessive–compulsive disorder (Rasmussen and Tsuang 1986)
Major depressive disorder (Kraepelin 1921)
Schizophrenia (Byerly et al. 2005)
Second-generation antipsychotic medications (clozapine [Baker et al. 1992], olanzapine [Mottard and de la Sablonniere 1999], risperidone [Alevizos et al. 2002], quetapine [Stamouli and Lykouras 2006])

Movement disorders
Tourette's syndrome (Frankel et al. 1986, Miguel et al. 1995, Robertson et al. 1988)
Sydenham's chorea (Maia et al. 2005, Swedo et al. 1989, 1993)
Huntington's disease (Cummings and Cunningham 1992)
Parkinson's disease (Alegret et al. 2001)

With precipitating events
Post-encephalitic (encephalitis lethargica [Jelliffe 1929] and western equine encephalitis [Mulder et al. 1951])
Post-anoxic (Escalona et al. 1997; Laplane et al. 1984, 1989)
Traumatic brain injury (Hillbom 1960; McKeon et al. 1984)

Miscellaneous causes
Fahr's syndrome (Lopez-Villegas et al. 1996)
Infarction of the globus pallidus (Giroud et al. 1997)
Infarction of the parietal cortex (Simpson and Baldwin 1995)
Complex partial (Mendez et al. 1996) or simple partial (Kroll and Drummond 1993) seizures
Systemic lupus erythematosus (Slatterly et al. 2004)
Velocardiofacial syndrome (Gothelf et al. 2004)
Normal pressure hydrocephalus (Mendhekar et al. 2007)

second-generation antipsychotic medications, as used in the treatment of schizophrenia, may also cause obsessions and compulsions as a side-effect: clozapine is most likely to do this; however, cases have also been reported secondary to olanzapine, risperidone, and quetiapine.

Obsessions and compulsions may also occur secondary to disorders characterized by abnormal movements, such as the tics of Tourette's syndrome, the chorea of Sydenham's chorea or Huntington's disease, and the parkinsonism of Parkinson's disease. Sydenham's chorea is of special interest here in that obsessions or compulsions are seen in the majority of patients and, interestingly, tend to appear prior to the onset of the chorea.

Of the precipitating events capable of causing obsessions and compulsions, the classic one is encephalitis lethargica, wherein these symptoms occurred as chronic sequelae, often in association with oculogyric crises. Other encephalitides, such as western equine encephalitis, have also been implicated. Both anoxic encephalopathy and traumatic brain injury may also leave obsessions and compulsions in their wake.

Of the miscellaneous causes, Fahr's syndrome, with calcification of the basal ganglia, stands out; infarction of the globus pallidus or the right parietal cortex has also rarely been at fault. Obsessions and compulsions may also constitute part of the symptomatology of a complex partial seizure or a simple partial seizure. In the case of a complex partial seizure the associated defect of consciousness suggests the correct diagnosis; however, with simple partial seizures there may not be any other symptomatology besides the obsession or compulsion, and in this case the diagnosis may rest on a history of other seizure types. Finally, there is also an association of obsessions and compulsions with systemic lupus erythematosus, the velocardiofacial syndrome, and normal pressure hydrocephalus.

In reviewing these various causes of obsessions and compulsions, it is interesting to note the involvement of the basal ganglia, especially the globus pallidus. Thus, in Fahr's syndrome, one sees calcification of the basal ganglia bilaterally (Lopez-Villegas *et al.* 1996), and in Sydenham's chorea the caudate is heavily involved (Husby *et al.* 1976). Post-anoxic lesions preferentially involve the globus pallidus bilaterally (Escalona *et al.* 1997; Laplane *et al.* 1989), and unilateral infarction of the globus pallidus has also been implicated (Giroud *et al.* 1997). Given these findings, it may be appropriate to consider obsessions and compulsions as having some localizing value to the basal ganglia.

Differential diagnosis

The adjectives 'obsessive' and 'compulsive' have been used not only to refer to true obsessions and compulsions, as described above, but also to other symptoms, and it is important to clearly distinguish 'true' obsessions and compulsions from these other symptoms. Thus, one hears of 'compulsive' spending, shopping, eating, or sex; however, one clinical feature clearly distinguishes all these from 'true' compulsions, namely the fact that patients with compulsive spending, shopping, eating, or sex enjoy the behavior they feel 'compelled' to partake in, in clear contrast with patients with 'true' compulsions who take no pleasure in their compulsive behavior, whether it be washing, praying, checking, or whatever.

Obsessive–compulsive personality traits must also be distinguished from obsessions and compulsions. Individuals with these personality traits are 'obsessed' with detail and feel 'compelled' to do things perfectly. These traits, however, are quite different from 'true' obsessions and compulsions in that individuals with these traits typically see nothing wrong with them (and in fact may even value them), in contrast with patients with 'true' obsessions and compulsions who see these experiences as more or less senseless and wish to be rid of them.

Perseverations, as may be seen in some patients with frontal lesions, are distinguished from compulsive behaviors by the patients' attitude toward the behavior in question. Perseverative patients can often offer no reason for their repetitive behavior and do not resist engaging in it: by contrast, patients with compulsions engage in their compulsive behavior for a definite purpose and often attempt to resist the urge. An allied symptom is 'compulsive' hoarding or collecting, as may be seen in various dementias (Hwang *et al.* 1998) and, rarely, with focal lesions of the frontal lobe (Anderson *et al.* 2005).

Treatment

Treatment is directed, if possible, at the underlying cause; if this is ineffective, consideration may be given to an empirical trial of one of the medications useful in obsessive–compulsive disorder, such as an SSRI.

4.18 REDUPLICATIVE PARAMNESIA

Reduplicative paramnesia, described in 1903 by Pick (Pick 1903) is a syndrome in which patients believe that their location has somehow been duplicated, such that, for example, the house they are in is not actually theirs or, conversely, that their house has been relocated at some distance, perhaps to another city. This syndrome has also been referred to as 'double orientation' or 'delusional disorientation'.

Clinical features

In some cases, patients may correctly identify the city they are in, but may maintain that the building they are in is not, in fact, what it appears to be. Some may admit that it perhaps looks like their home, but maintain that, in fact, it is not and, in fact, is rather a replica or duplicate of their actual home (Hudson and Grace 2000).

In other cases, patients may accurately identify the building they are in, for example University Hospital, but may maintain that the building, in fact, is not in the city, but has been transported or duplicated in another locale (Benson *et al.* 1976), perhaps their home town.

Etiology

Reduplicative paramnesia may occur in the setting of a dementia, for example Alzheimer's disease (von Gunten *et al.* 2005), in the setting of a delirium as after a closed head injury (Benson *et al.* 1976), or in a psychosis, for example delusional disorder or schizophrenia. Occasionally, the syndrome may occur in a more or less isolated fashion, and in such cases lesions, such as infarctions, have been noted in the right frontal lobe (Kapur *et al.* 1988) and in the right fusiform gyrus (Hudson *et al.* 2000).

Differential diagnosis

Reduplicative paramnesia must be distinguished from disorientation to place. The differential here rests on the patient's reaction when corrected: the disoriented patient may either accept the correction or simply make no comment; the patient with 'delusional disorientation', however, will stoutly maintain his or her belief, and may even argue with the physician about it.

Treatment

Apart from treatment of the underlying cause, no confident recommendations can be made. Should the syndrome persist and be troubling, a case could be made for treatment with an antipsychotic.

4.19 CONFABULATION

At times, patients with amnesia will report experiences, which, though plausible-sounding, in fact did not occur. These confabulations seem, as it were, to 'fill in the blanks' of those portions of the patient's past that cannot be recalled because of the amnesia.

Clinical features

Confabulations generally appear in response to questions about the recent past. Patients, although not confused, relate experiences which, upon examination, clearly did not occur. For example, one patient, hospitalized for 3 days, when asked what he had done the evening before, replied that he'd been out with friends at a restaurant, where everyone had enjoyed a fine meal, etc. Most patients, when pressed about their confabulated responses, do not persist in them, but may offer other confabulated responses. For example, the patient in question, when told that, according to the nurse, he had been in the hospital on the evening in question, hesitated a moment, then responded that, yes, that was the case, and that he must have been mistaken. Asked then what he had, in fact, done the night before, he went on to relate how family members had come to visit and had spent the night with him, an event that did not, according to the nurse, in fact happen.

Further examination reveals that although patients are neither confused nor incoherent, they do, however, have short-term memory loss, as manifested by an inability to recall all out of three test words after 5 minutes and by some disorientation to date or place.

Etiology

Confabulations are most commonly seen in patients with Korsakoff's syndrome (Benson *et al.* 1996) and are discussed further in Section 13.5. They may also occur in the amnestic states following rupture of aneurysms of the anterior communicating artery (DeLuca and Cicernone 1991; Schnider *et al.* 2005), and may also be seen in patients with dementia, for example frontotemporal dementia (Nedjam *et al.* 2004).

Differential diagnosis

Simple lying is distinguished by the presence of a motivation for the false statement and by the fact that liars tend to persist in their lies, in contrast with confabulators who, generally, when challenged, renounce their statements without much ado.

Delusions about the past, as may be seen in psychosis (e.g., schizophrenia), delirium or advanced dementia, are generally implausible on their face. For example, a report by a patient that the night before he had been tortured and that the nurses had ripped his skin off should be considered a delusion and not a confabulation. In these cases, the patient's speech is often rambling and more or less incoherent, being composed of disconnected statements.

Treatment

Treatment is directed at the underlying condition.

4.20 AMUSIA

Amusia, also known as amelodia, is characterized by an inability to either recognize or produce a melody, and may occur on either an acquired or a developmental basis.

Clinical features

Amusia occurs in both receptive and expressive forms.

In receptive amusia, patients are, to a greater or lesser degree, 'tone deaf'. In such a case, if the patient were to listen to a singer simply humming the tune to a song he might be unable to recognize it, whereas if the singer actually sang the song, the lyrics would immediately allow the patient to recognize the song. As might be expected, if patients with receptive amusia listen to instrumental music they would have difficulty 'naming the tune' and might complain that the music sounded flat.

Patients with expressive amusia have great difficulty in 'carrying a tune', and if such patients hum a tune, listeners have great difficulty recognizing it; should these patients sing the lyrics, however, listeners are able to recognize the song but may comment that the singing is quite poor. Patients with expressive amusia also have great difficulty playing instruments.

In some cases, both receptive and expressive components are present, producing a global amusia.

Etiology

Most cases of acquired amusia occur secondary to infarction or hemorrhage. Receptive amusia has been noted with lesions of the temporal lobe (Mazzucchi *et al.* 1982; Sparr 2002). Expressive amusia has been noted with lesions of the superior temporal cortex (McFarland and Fortin 1982) and of the frontal cortex (Botez and Werheim 1959). Global amusia has been seen with lesions of the superior temporal cortex (Piccirilli *et al.* 2000) and also of Heschl's gyrus (Russell and Golfinos 2003). Typically, lesions are found in the non-dominant hemisphere.

Expressive amusia has also been reported as a manifestation of a simple partial seizure, with the seizure focus being found in the right temporo-occipital region (Bautista and Ciampetti 2003).

Global acquired amusia of gradual onset and slow progression has also been reported secondary to a neurodegenerative disorder characterized by bilateral atrophy of the frontotemporal cortices (Confavreux *et al.* 1992).

Developmental, or 'congenital' amusia, is not uncommon and such 'tone deaf' individuals have a variable degree of difficulty in recognizing tunes and singing/playing instruments (Ayotte *et al.* 2001).

Differential diagnosis

Aprosodia is distinguished from amusia by the fact that aprosodia is related to the emotional tone with which one speaks, whether happy, angry or sad, whereas amusia is related to the tune with which one sings.

Treatment

There are no established treatments.

4.21 FOREIGN ACCENT SYNDROME

The foreign accent syndrome, wherein patients speak with an accent foreign to their native tongue, is a rare syndrome that typically evolves out of either a motor aphasia, or an aphemia, in stroke patients.

Clinical features

As noted, patients present initially with either a motor aphasia (Christoph *et al.* 2004) (or its transcortical variant [Graff-Radford *et al.* 1986]) or an aphemic mutism (Schiff *et al.* 1983; Takayama *et al.* 1993): as the motor aphasia or the mutism resolve, patients begin to speak intelligibly but with a foreign accent. One native English speaker spoke with an Irish brogue (Seliger *et al.* 1992), another with a French accent (Hall *et al.* 2003), and another with a Chinese accent (Schiff *et al.* 1983). In one most unfortunate case, a Norwegian, who developed the syndrome during World War II, spoke in such a convincing German accent that she was suspected of being a traitor (Monrad-Krohn 1947).

Etiology

Lesions are found in the left hemisphere, typically in the posterior–inferior portion of the frontal cortex (Schiff *et al.* 1983; Takayama *et al.* 1993) or subjacent white matter (Blumstein *et al.* 1987); cases have also been reported secondary to infarction of the left basal ganglia (Fridriksson *et al.* 2005), and there is one report of the syndrome occurring with infarction of the mid-portion of the body of the corpus callosum (Hall *et al.* 2003).

There are also report of the syndrome occurring in the course of schizophrenia (Reeves and Norton 2001): in one such case the patient, who had the delusion that he was connected with British royalty, spoke with a British accent (Reeves *et al.* 2007).

Differential diagnosis

Motor aphasia is distinguished by the characteristic effortful speech that stands in contrast with the fluent and effortless speech of patients with the foreign accent syndrome; it is distinguished from dysarthria by the fact that in the foreign accent syndrome there is simply no slurring of speech.

Treatment

There is no known treatment.

4.22 CATAPLEXY

Cataplexy is a condition characterized by the occurrence of cataplectic attacks, that is to say episodes of a greater or lesser degree of muscle atonia.

Clinical features

Cataplectic attacks (Adie 1926; Dyken *et al.* 1996; Guilleminault *et al.* 1974; Kales *et al.* 1982; Parkes *et al.* 1975; Wilson 1928) are generally precipitated by some strong emotion, such as laughter or anger, and are characterized by the paroxysmal onset of more or less generalized weakness lasting on the order of seconds to a minute or so: subsequent recovery is rapid and complete. During the attack, all voluntary muscle power, with the exception of the diaphragm and, at times, the extraocular muscles, is lost, and patients may fall to the ground or slump in a chair. In some cases, the muscle weakness, although generalized, may be of minor degree, and such patients may merely experience their heads lolling forward, their jaws slackening, and their knees beginning to buckle. Limited attacks, confined perhaps to an arm or leg, have also been reported. Attacks that last much longer than a minute may be joined by visual or auditory hallucinations

(Van Den Hoed *et al.* 1979). Importantly, during the attack, patients remain completely alert and conscious.

Etiology

The overwhelming majority of cases of cataplexy occur secondary to narcolepsy. As discussed in Section 18.7, this disorder generally presents in late teenage or early adult years with narcoleptic sleep attacks; cataplectic attacks are seen in about three-quarters of patients, and although they typically occur within the first few years after the appearance of sleep attacks, in rare instances they may precede them (Parkes *et al.* 1975).

Isolated cataplectic attacks have also, very rarely, been reported to occur on an autosomal dominant (Gelardi and Brown 1967) or idiopathic basis (Van Dijk *et al.* 1991).

Cataplectic attacks, again very rarely, have also been noted with lesions, generally gliomas, of the hypothalamus (Anderson and Salmon 1977; Schwartz *et al.* 1984; Stahl *et al.* 1980), midbrain tegmentum (Fernandez *et al.* 1995) or dorsal pontomedullary junction (D'Cruz *et al.* 1994). There are also case reports of cataplexy occurring as sequelae to encephalitis lethargica (Adie 1926; Fournier and Helguera 1934), in association with paraneoplastic limbic encephalitis (Rosenfeld *et al.* 2001) in Niemann–Pick disease (Smit *et al.* 2006), and as a side-effect of clozapine (Desarkar *et al.* 2007).

Differential diagnosis

Cataplectic attacks must be distinguished from vertebrobasilar transient ischemic attacks, syncope, and atonic seizures, and one feature helps in distinguishing all of these from cataplexy, namely, (in contrast with cataplectic attacks) that none of these is typically provoked by strong emotion.

Attacks of vertebrobasilar insufficiency may be characterized by 'drop attacks' with preservation of consciousness. These are usually seen in elderly individuals, and may be accompanied by other evidence of brainstem ischemia, such as transient diplopia, dysarthria, or vertigo.

Syncopal attacks are immediately distinguished from cataplexy by loss of consciousness.

Atonic seizures may or may not be accompanied by loss of consciousness or by post-ictal confusion. In cases of atonic seizures with preserved consciousness and no post-ictal confusion, a history of other seizure types will suggest the correct diagnosis (Lipinski 1977; Pazzaglia *et al.* 1985).

Treatment

Treatment of cataplexy occurring in association with narcolepsy is discussed in Section 18.7; when symptomatic treatment is required for cataplexy occurring secondary to other causes, an empirical trial of these same treatments would be reasonable.

4.23 SYMPATHETIC STORM

Sympathetic storms, also known as acute autonomic crises, constitute episodes of severe sympathetic hyperactivity, and are usually seen after traumatic brain injury.

Clinical features

The episodes may occur either spontaneously or after some trivial precipitant, such as a change in position. During the episode one sees the acute onset of profuse diaphoresis, tachycardia, tachypnea, pupillary dilation, and, in some, rigid extensor posturing. The diaphoresis is indeed impressive, with beads of sweat dripping from the head. During the episode, patients may grimace as if in pain, and family members and other observers may become quite alarmed. The episodes themselves last from minutes to hours, and terminate slowly.

Etiology

These episodes probably represent disinhibition of the hypothalamus and related structures. Although most commonly seen after severe traumatic brain injury with prominent diffuse axonal injury (Baguley *et al.* 1999), they may also occur in the setting of acute hydrocephalus (Rossitch and Bullard 1988) and after cardiac arrest (Diamond *et al.* 2005).

Although these episodes were once considered to represent diencephalic seizures (Penfield and Jasper 1954), there is no evidence for epileptic activity during them, and antiepileptic drugs are not effective (Boeve *et al.* 1998).

Differential diagnosis

Complex partial seizures are distinguished by their exquisitely paroxysmal onset, over seconds. Furthermore, one rarely sees such sympathetic hyperactivity in a complex partial seizure: at most, there may be some modest tachycardia and modestly elevated blood pressure.

Malignant hyperthermia, the neuroleptic malignant syndrome and Stauder's lethal catatonia may all be considered (Thorley *et al.* 2001), however in each of these conditions, symptoms, rather than being episodic, are persistent. The setting, of course, also aids in differentiation, and one should look, respectively, for administration of an anesthetic or an antipsychotic, or pre-existing catatonia.

Treatment

The goal of treatment is prevention of future episodes, and in this regard chronic treatment with a beta-blocker, such as propranolol or labetalol (Do *et al.* 2000), constitutes a reasonable first approach. Both morphine sulfate and bromocriptine have also been used with success (Bullard

1987), as has gabapentin, in doses of 600–1800 mg/day (Baguley *et al.* 2007). Doses should be titrated to clinical effect or tolerance; in some cases a combination of agents, such as a beta-blocker plus bromocriptine, may be required. Should pharmacologic treatment fail, consideration may be given to intrathecal baclofen (Becker *et al.* 2000).

4.24 CATASTROPHIC REACTION

The catastrophic reaction, originally described by Kurt Goldstein (1939, 1942), is characterized by an extreme emotional reaction when patients are confronted with tasks that, since falling ill, they are no longer able to accomplish. This may not be an uncommon phenomenon, being described in 19 percent of patients with stroke (Starkstein *et al.* 1993) and 16 percent of those with Alzheimer's disease (Tilberti *et al.* 1998).

Clinical features

The reaction occurs when patients find themselves unable to accomplish a task which, prior to falling ill, would have occasioned them little or no difficulty. The task itself might be something as simple as making change, or something more formal, as for example answering questions regarding memory or calculations during a mental status examination. Finding themselves hopelessly unable to proceed, patients become frustrated, tearful, or angry; some may begin shouting or swearing, and aggressive behavior may occur. Carota *et al.* (2001) noted that when patients with expressive aphasia were given paper and pencil and asked to write they would 'start crying, showing unwillingness, tearing the paper or even throwing the pencil and other objects toward the examiner'. Typically, this catastrophic display of emotion passes soon after patients are relieved of the burdensome task.

Etiology

There has been debate as to whether the catastrophic reaction is merely an expected emotional reaction when patients find themselves failing at tasks that would have caused no difficulty in the past or whether it is perhaps related to specific brain pathologies. Although Goldstein held to the former theory, there is some evidence that catastrophic reactions, at least in patients with stroke, are related to the presence of a post-stroke depression and to infarctions in the anterior left hemisphere or the left basal ganglia (Starkstein *et al.* 1993). There is also some evidence of an association with expressive aphasia (Carota *et al.* 2001; Gainotti 1972) but not all studies support this (Starkstein *et al.* 1993).

Differential diagnosis

Catastrophic reactions, as defined here, are clinical events that occur in reaction to stressful demands, and thus are differentiated from more 'free-floating' agitation, as may be seen in various deliria or dementias.

Treatment

Apart from treatment, if possible, of the associated disease, such as stroke, and a modulation of environmental demands, there is no known treatment.

4.25 FLATTENED AFFECT

Clinical features

Flattened, or blunted, affect is characterized by a lifeless and wooden facial expression accompanied by an absence or diminution of feeling.

Etiology

Flattened affect is found very commonly in schizophrenia (Andreasen *et al.* 1979); it may also occur in other psychoses (Cornelius *et al.* 1991) and, rarely, in dementia secondary to infarction of the mesencephalon or thalamus (Katz *et al.* 1987).

Differential diagnosis

Motor aprosodia is characterized by a monotone voice but, in contrast with patients with flattened affect, who feel little, if anything, patients with aprosodia retain lively emotional feelings. The 'hypomimia' seen in parkinsonism is distinguished in the same way: although these patients' facial movements are more or less frozen and devoid of expression, they still may have strong feelings.

In depression, the play of emotions on the face is slowed and thus depressed affect may appear similar to flattened affect; however, these patients do experience a sense of sadness in contrast with patients with flattened affect, who, again, simply feel nothing.

Treatment

Treatment is directed at the underlying cause.

4.26 INAPPROPRIATE AFFECT

The term 'affect' refers both to what is felt and to what shows in facial expression. Normally, there is a congruence between these two, as, for example, when sad feelings are accompanied by a sad facial expression. In cases when there is an involuntary incongruence between these two components of affect – a mismatch as it were between what is felt and what shows – one speaks of inappropriate affect.

Clinical features

Examples may help fix this sign in the reader's mind. When attending his brother's funeral, one patient, while feeling nothing but grief and sadness, was noted to have a strange grin on his face; another, although reporting pleasure at receiving a gift, was noted to grimace as if in pain.

Etiology

By far the most common condition in which inappropriate affect is seen is schizophrenia (John *et al.* 2003) and the closely allied schizotypal personality disorder (Fossati *et al.* 2001). Such affect has also been noted during intoxication with hallucinogens, such as ketamine and dimethyltryptamine (Gouzoulis-Mayfrank *et al.* 2005), and in the very rare velocardiofacial syndrome (Sachdev 2002).

Differential diagnosis

Inappropriate affect, as defined here, must be distinguished from the far more common 'socially' inappropriate affect. For example, smiling at a funeral, although certainly socially inappropriate would not be considered pathologic if the person smiling felt a sense of triumph at the death of a hated rival, for here there is no mismatch between what is felt and what is displayed.

'Nervous laughter', for example when someone laughs to cover up a feeling of sadness, although indeed representing a mismatch is distinguished by the fact that the covering laughter can be easily dispelled with a few sympathetic questions, after which the laughter is replaced by an appropriate look of sadness.

Aprosodia of the sensory type, as discussed in Section 2.7, is quite similar to inappropriate affect in that in both these signs there is an incongruence, or mismatch, between what the patient feels and the tone of voice with which that feeling is expressed. The difference is that in sensory aprosodia, patients also have difficulty in comprehending what others feel by listening to the tone of voice with which others speak, whereas in inappropriate affect patients retain this ability.

Treatment

Treatment is directed at the underlying condition.

4.27 MANNERISMS

Manneristic transformation of gestures or speech, or of activities such as walking or eating, although most common in schizophrenia, may occur in other disorders. The resulting mannerisms often strike others as peculiar or bizarre.

Description

Kraepelin (1907) noted that patients with mannerisms may '... walk with a peculiar gait, drag one foot, go in straight lines or in circles, hold their spoons at the very end, eat in a definite rhythm, and shake hands with extended fingers'. He felt that mannerisms were '... especially common in speech (with) ... grunts, lisping, peculiar words, phrases and inflection'.

Bleuler (1924) commented further regarding the manneristic transformation that gestures may undergo, noting that '... every conceivable stilted gesture occurs. Shaking hands is done very stiffly with the hand turned or only the little finger is presented; the hand may be shot forward quickly and withdrawn just as rapidly'.

Etiology

Although mannerisms are most commonly seen in schizophrenia they may also occur in mental retardation (Leudar *et al.* 1984), autism (Sears *et al.* 1999), ketamine intoxication (Krystal *et al* 2005), and in cases of dementia occurring in the elderly (Rabinowitz *et al.* 2004).

Differential diagnosis

Stereotypies are distinguished by their monotonous repetitiveness.

In patients treated chronically with antipsychotics, mannerisms must be distinguished from tardive dyskinesia (Granacher 1981). One clue to the differential lies in the presence or absence of a motivation for the behavior in question: mannerisms represent intentional behaviors that have undergone a bizarre transformation; the abnormal movements of tardive dyskinesias, in contrast, are involuntary and occur in the absence of any motivation.

Treatment

Treatment is directed at the underlying etiology.

4.28 STEREOTYPIES

Stereotypies represent a kind of perseverative motor activity in which behaviors are repeated again and again in a purposeless, monotonous, and thoroughly stereotyped fashion: they may range from such simple behaviors as hand flapping to complex activities such as repeatedly taking apart and then putting back together a small machine. Importantly, although some of these stereotypies appear, on the surface, to be purposeful, patients are unable to adequately explain why they repeatedly engage in the behavior.

Clinical features

As noted, stereotypical behaviors can range from simple to complex. Simple stereotypies might consist of hand-flapping, shoulder-shrugging or hand-wringing. More complex stereotypies include folding and unfolding a towel, repeatedly putting on, then taking off, an article of clothing, or repeatedly sitting down and standing up.

Stereotypies may persist for anywhere from minutes to hours, days, or even longer. Importantly, patients, provided they are not severely or profoundly retarded, are generally able to voluntarily stop the behavior.

Etiology

Among adults, stereotypies are seen in schizophrenia and in dementia, most particularly front-temporal dementia and Alzheimer's disease (Nyatsanza et al. 2003). Both mental retardation and autism (with or without mental retardation) are characterized by frequent stereotypies (Bodfish et al. 2000), and stereotypies may also occur in a small percentage of children with attention-deficit disorder or learning disabilities (Mahone et al. 2004).

Stereotypies may be seen during intoxication with amphetamines (where they are classically referred to as 'punding') or with cocaine (Brady et al. 1991) and, interestingly, may also occur with treatment with levodopa (Evans et al. 2000); they may also constitute part of tardive dyskinesia (Stacy et al. 1993). Finally, lesions of the lenticular nuclei may also cause stereotypies (Laplane et al. 1989).

Differential diagnosis

As noted above, stereotypies represent a kind of perseveration, and, as noted in Section 4.5, are distinguished from other perseverations by their purposelessness and monotonous character.

Tics are generally not repetitious and although they can be suppressed this is done only with great effort, and eventual failure. Compulsions are distinguished by the fact that there is a motivation for the behavior: if you ask a patient who repeatedly goes to and from the stove, each time touching the gas knob, why he or she is acting so, the patient with a compulsion might explain that it is because of an overwhelming anxiety that the stove might not have been turned off, whereas the patient with a stereotypy will not be able to offer a reason.

Treatment

In patients with schizophrenia, antipsychotics are effective; the optimal treatment for stereotypies in dementia is not clear.

In patients with mental retardation, low-dose antipsychotics, such as risperidone, are useful and clomipramine is also effective (Lewis et al. 1996). Risperidone (McDougle et al. 2005) and haloperidol are effective in autism, as is clomipramine but this is not as well tolerated as haloperidol (Remington et al. 2001); a recent study also suggested effectiveness for divalproex (Hollander et al. 2006). Various behavioral therapies may also be effective.

4.29 ECHOLALIA AND ECHOPRAXIA

Echolalia and echopraxia represent, respectively, the repetition or mirroring of what others say or do (Ford 1989). Importantly, these echophenomena are not under voluntary control and occur regardless of whether patients wish them or not.

Clinical features

In echolalia, patients automatically repeat, parrot-like, what others have said: in some cases only single words are repeated, whereas in other whole phrases or sentences may be echoed. In echopraxia, patients, again automatically and without being instructed to do so, will mirror what others do. For example, if the physician crosses his or her arms, the echopractic patient will do the same thing; likewise, if the physician stands, the patient will also stand.

Etiology

Echophenomena apparently do not occur in isolation but are seen as part of a larger syndrome, as for example catatonia (e.g., catatonic schizophrenia [Kraepelin 1971, p. 142]), autism (Roberts 1989), and Tourette's syndrome (Comings and Comings 1987). Echophenomena have also been noted in post-encephalitic parkinsonism (Wilson 1954), frontotemporal dementia (e.g., Pick's disease [Wilson 1954]), and in the later stages of Alzheimer's disease (Cummings et al. 1985). Transcortical aphasia, including transcortical motor aphasia (Hadano et al. 1998) and transcortical mixed aphasia (Mendez 2002), may also be characterized by echolalia.

Differential diagnosis

Palilalia is distinguished from echolalia by the fact that the repetition in palilalia involves not words spoken by others but words spoken by the patient. The environmental dependency syndrome is distinguished from echopraxia by the fact that the patient's automatic behavior represents not a mirroring of what others do but rather an involuntary utilization of objects at hand.

Treatment

Treatment is directed at the syndrome of which the echophenomenon is a part.

4.30 HALLUCINATIONS AND DELUSIONS

Hallucinations are said to be present when patients have the experience of something that is in fact not actually present. Thus, a patient who hallucinates a dog in the hospital room might report seeing a dog, and even reach down to pat it, whereas others in the room see nothing.

Delusions are false beliefs that cannot be explained on the basis of either the patients' culture or religion and that persist despite evidence and reasonable argument to the contrary. Thus, in evaluating patients with false beliefs it is critical to take into account their culture and religion. Although a belief in zombies would not generally be considered to be a delusion in poor and uneducated Haitians, for example, any well-acculturated American who maintained such a belief would generally be considered delusional. Although some physicians make much of the 'contextual' nature of beliefs, most delusions are in practice so bizarre and unbelievable that there is no question of their status. Thus, there is but little debate about the status of such beliefs that bodies of family members are inhabited by malevolent aliens or that telepathic listening devices have been implanted inside the spleen.

A group of specific hallucinations and delusions, known as Schneiderian first rank symptoms, is discussed separately in Section 4.31. As pointed out there, these Schneiderian first rank symptoms, although found in diverse disorders, are highly suggestive of schizophrenia.

Clinical features

The various types of hallucinations and delusions are noted in Table 4.6. As noted there, hallucinations are categorized according to the sensory modality affected, and delusions according to their content. Specific descriptions of hallucinations and delusions follow.

HALLUCINATIONS

Visual hallucinations range from simple to complex in form. Simple hallucinations include such phenomena as 'zigzag linear patterns' (Panayiotopoulos 1994) and 'dancing lights, rings and circles' (Parkinson *et al.* 1952). Complex phenomena may be quite detailed: one patient, a war veteran, saw 'stretcher bearers walking past him and then the figures of nurses whom he would recognize' (Russell and Whitty 1955); another saw 'the Queen, with a bag over her arm [who] walked from the left to the centre of the ward, then vanished' (Lance 1976).

In some cases, autoscopy may occur, wherein patients hallucinate an image of themselves (Lukianowicz 1958): one 74-year-old woman 'suddenly noticed a figure seated on [her] left. "It wasn't hard to realize that it was I myself who was sitting there. I looked younger and fresher than I do now. My double smiled at me in a friendly way, as though she wanted to tell me something"' (Kolmel 1985).

Table 4.6 Types of hallucinations and delusions

Hallucinations
Visual
Autoscopy
Lilliputian
Palinopsia
Polyopia
Auditory
Tactile
Olfactory
Gustatory
Delusions
Delusions of persecution
Capgras syndrome
Fregoli syndrome
Delusions of grandeur
Delusions of jealousy
Erotomanic delusions (De Clerambault syndrome)
Nihilistic delusions
Cotard's syndrome
Delusions of sin
Delusions of reference

'Lilliputian' hallucinations are said to be present when the hallucinated figures are quite small, much as in the novel *Gulliver's Travels* (Alexander 1926; Goldin 1955; Leroy 1922).

Palinopsia represents a peculiar kind of visual hallucination that Critchley (1951) considered to be a type of 'visual perseveration'. Here, objects originally actually seen by the patient are subsequently recurrently hallucinated out of place. For example (Michel and Troost 1980), one patient reported that 'each person she saw had the face of someone she had just seen on television. She later peeled a banana and in a few minutes saw multiple vivid images of bananas projected over the wall. She realized they were only images, and not real. Next, after putting a 20-dollar bill in her purse, she saw heaps of 20-dollar bills everywhere'.

Another patient (Meadows and Munro 1977), after seeing someone costumed as Santa Claus at a Christmas party, 'noticed that a replica of the white beard of . . . Santa Claus was superimposed upon the face of everyone she spoke to'.

Polyopsia refers to a condition in which patients, rather than simply seeing 'double', see multiple reduplications of the same image (Lopez *et al.* 1993). Whether or not this should be considered to be a variant of palinopsia is unclear.

Hallucinations that occur upon falling asleep or upon awakening are known, respectively, as hypnagogic and hypnopompic (Zarcone 1973).

Auditory hallucinations may range from such simple phenomena as 'grinding noises' or a noise 'like a freight train' (Cascino and Adams 1986) to complex experiences such as hearing music (Hammeke *et al.* 1983) or voices. Voices, the most compelling type of auditory hallucination, may be soft, mere whisperings, or quite clear and distinct. They may come from an internal organ or have their source outside the patient, in 'the air', or perhaps electronic devices or simply the walls. Some patients seem able to ignore them, whereas others will talk back to them. There may occasionally be 'command' hallucinations, which, as noted by Kraepelin (1921), 'in certain circumstances are very precisely obeyed. They forbid the patient to eat and to speak, to work, to go to church . . . "Go on, strike him, beat him".'

Tactile hallucinations (Berrios 1982) are extraordinarily varied. Kraepelin (1921), in describing a tactually hallucinated patient, noted that he 'feels himself laid hold of, touched over his whole body, he feels tickling in his thigh and right up to his neck, pricking in his back and in his calves, a curious feeling in his neck, heat in his face'. When patients hallucinate the feeling of ants or insects crawling on the skin, one speaks of 'formication'.

Olfactory hallucinations, although at times consisting of such pleasant aromas as perfume, are generally unpleasant, even repulsive: Kraepelin (1921) noted 'a smell of sulphur; of corpses and chloride of lime, of blood, of fire, of the fumes of hell'.

Gustatory hallucinations are perhaps the least common of all types: Kraepelin (1921) reported patients who tasted 'petroleum or arsenic' in the food.

DELUSIONS

Delusions of persecution take the most varied of forms: patients are spied on and followed; a conspiracy has been set up, and the police, FBI, or even the mafia are involved. Neighbors and co-workers, even family members, have turned on them: poison gas surrounds them, and their food, indeed even their medicine, has been adulterated.

The Capgras syndrome (Alexander *et al.* 1979; Christodoulou 1977; Enoch 1963) represents a particular kind of delusion of persecution wherein patients believe that malevolent 'imposters' have somehow entered and taken over the bodies of familiar persons, such as family members or neighbors. In one case (Merrin and Silberfarb 1976), the patient believed that 'the "substitution" first occurred on [her] wedding day, when her husband went to the men's room and an imposter took his place'. Although others could not see anything amiss with her husband, the patient felt able to differentiate the husband from the imposter given that the imposter 'had a rotten green toenail. Once she even went so far as calling the police and demanding that her husband remove his shoe to expose the green toenail to the police'. In some cases of the Capgras syndrome, patients may turn on the 'imposter', in the process assaulting innocent parties (Thompson and Swan 1993).

In a related kind of delusion of persecution, known as the Fregoli syndrome, patients believe that the body of a stranger has somehow been invaded and taken over by a familiar person (O'Sullivan and Dean 1991).

Delusions of grandeur may involve various themes: the patient 'is "something better", born to a higher place, the

"Glory of Israel", an inventor, a great singer, can do what he will' (Kraepelin 1921).

Delusions of jealousy (Soyka *et al.* 1991) fuel patients' jealousies: the infidelities of spouses or lovers are revealed and their 'playing around' is no longer hidden. Protestations of faithfulness have no effect as patients find evidence for their suspicions: the spouse is late coming home; the phone rings at odd times; the sheets are rumpled in a suggestive way.

Erotomanic delusions are characterized by a belief in an 'amorous communication with a person of much higher rank who has been the first to fall in love and the first to make advances' (Gillett *et al.* 1990). Also known as De Clerambault's syndrome (Ellis and Mellsop 1985), these delusions often impel patients to attempt contact with these supposed lovers, even to the point of stalking and kidnapping them.

Nihilistic delusions entail the belief that animate objects, such as other people, animals or such living things as trees, are in fact dead. In a variant of this, known as Cotard's syndrome (Joseph and O'Leary 1986), patients come to believe that they themselves are in fact dead: in one case (Cohen *et al.* 1997), a 13-year-old girl had the 'absolute conviction that she was already dead, waiting to be buried, and that she had no teeth and no hair and that her uterus was malformed'.

Delusions of sin give form to the patients' sense that they have committed unpardonable acts: they have cursed God, engaged in unspeakable practices, betrayed those close to them and violated all their sacred principles. Such a patient 'is a damned soul, the refuse of humanity' (Kraepelin 1921).

Delusions of reference embody a sense that seemingly unrelated and chance events in some fashion pertain to or refer to the patient. 'Indifferent remarks and chance looks, the whispering of other people, appear suspicious to the patient' (Kraepelin 1921). In many cases, such delusions of reference serve, as it were, to bolster or reinforce other delusions. Thus, patients with delusions of persecution, on seeing police officers talking, might immediately believe that the conversation was about them and that it was evidence that the conspiracy had begun in earnest. To take another example, patients with delusions of grandeur might, upon seeing the sun break radiantly through the storm clouds, assume that it was a sign of God's special grace for them.

Etiology

The causes of delusions or hallucinations are listed in Table 4.7. In the vast majority of cases, the delusions or hallucinations occur in the context of a major syndrome, and the first task is to determine whether one of those syndromes is present. Dementia (Section 5.1) is suggested by co-existent cognitive deficits, such as disorientation or short-term memory loss, and delirium (Section 5.3) by similar cognitive deficits with the all-important addition of confusion.

Table 4.7   Causes of delusions or hallucinations

Delusions or hallucinations occurring in the context of a major syndrome	Blindness (Charles Bonnet Syndrome) (Schultz and Melzack 1993; Teunisse *et al.* 1995, 1996)

Delusions or hallucinations occurring in the context of a major syndrome
Dementia
Delirium
Depression
Mania
Psychosis

Isolated hallucinations occurring with preserved insight
Visual hallucinations
    Medications
        Dopaminergics (Banerjee *et al.* 1989; Barnes *et al.* 2001, Fenelon *et al.* 2000; Goetz *et al.* 2005, Shaw *et al.* 1980)
        Digoxin (Closson 1983)
        Quinidine (Fisher 1981)
        Propranolol (Shopsin *et al.* 1975)
        Acyclovir (Rashiq *et al.* 1993)
        Imipramine (Kane and Keeler 1964; Klein 1964)
        Amitriptyline (Hemmingsen and Rafaelsen 1980)
        Maprotiline (Albala *et al.* 1983)
        Bupropion (Golden *et al.* 1985)
        Trazodone (Hughes and Lessell 1990)
        Selective serotonin reuptake inhibitors (SSRIs) (Marcon *et al.* 2004)
        Mirtazapine (Ihde-Scholl and Jefferson 2001)
        Risperidone (Lauterbach *et al.* 2000)
        Methylphenidate (Gross-Tsur *et al.* 2004)
    Intoxicants
        Hallucinogens
            Mescaline (Mitchell 1896)
            LSD (Bercel *et al.* 1956; Isbell *et al.* 1956)
            Psilocybin (Hollister *et al.* 1960)
            Phencyclidine (Meyer *et al.* 1959)
        Cocaine (Siegel 1978)
        Solvents (Channer and Stanley 1983; Evans and Raistrick 1987)
    Partial seizures
        Simple partial seizures (Penfield and Perot 1963; Russell and Whitty 1955; Sowa and Pituck 1989; Williams 1956)
        Complex partial seizures (Mulder and Daly 1952)
        Aura to complex partial or grand mal seizures (Lee *et al.* 2005)
    Migraine (Hachinski *et al.* 1973; Selby and Lance 1960)

Blindness (Charles Bonnet Syndrome) (Schultz and Melzack 1993; Teunisse *et al.* 1995, 1996)
Focal intracerebral lesions
    Occipital lobe or occipitotemporal and occipitoparietal areas (Kolmel 1985; Parkinson *et al.* 1952)
    Thalamus (Noda *et al.* 1993; Serra Catafau *et al.* 1992)
    Mesencephalon ('peduncular hallucinations') (Lhermitte 1922, 1932; McKee *et al.* 1990)
    Pontine tegmentum ('Pick's visions') (Bing 1940)
Miscellaneous causes
    Narcolepsy (Zarcone 1973)
    Guillain–Barré syndrome (Cochen *et al.* 2005)
    Bereavement (Grimby 1993)
    Sleep deprivation (Kollar *et al.* 1968)
    Normal (McDonald 1971)

Auditory hallucinations
    Medications
        Dopaminergics (Goetz *et al.* 2005)
        Pentoxyfylline (Gilbert 1993)
    Partial seizures
        Simple partial seizures (Williams 1956)
        Complex partial seizures (Currie *et al.* 1971)
    Deafness (Griffiths 2000; Hammeke *et al.* 1983; Miller and Crosby 1979; Ross *et al.* 1975)
    Focal intracerebral lesions
        Temporal lobe (Keschner *et al.* 1936)
        Putamen (Cerrato *et al.* 2001)
        Mesencephalon (Cascino and Adams 1986)
        Pontine tegmentum (Cascino and Adams 1986; Murata *et al.* 1994; Schielke *et al.* 2000)
Tactile hallucinations
    Cocaine (Siegel 1978)
    Amphetamines (Bell 1973)
Olfactory hallucinations
    Simple partial seizures (Mauguire and Courjon 1978)
    Complex partial seizures ('uncinate fits') (Jackson and Stewart 1899)
    Migraine (Fuller and Guiloff 1987; Wolberg and Ziegler 1982)
    Olfactory bulb or tract (Kaufman *et al.* 1988; Paskind 1935)
Gustatory hallucinations
    Simple partial seizures (Mulder and Daly 1952)
    Complex partial seizures (Daly 1958; Hausser-Hauw and Bancaud 1987)

Depression (Section 6.1) is indicated by depressed mood, anergia, anhedonia, and changes in appetite and sleep, and mania (Section 6.3) by heightened mood, hyperactivity, pressured speech, increased energy, and a decreased need for sleep. Should the delusions or hallucinations be occurring in the context of any one of these, the differential for that syndrome should be pursued, as described in the respective chapter.

In cases where the foregoing syndromes are absent, one other syndrome must be considered, namely psychosis.

In this syndrome, despite generally intact orientation and memory, and in the absence of significant depression or mania, patients exhibit a 'loss of reality testing' as evidenced by the presence of delusions or the presence of hallucinations without insight. Thus, all patients with isolated delusions are considered to have a psychosis, and in such cases the differential for that syndrome, as described in Section 7.1, should be pursued. Isolated hallucinations may occur either with or without insight, and it is critical to determine which is the case. Happily, this is not terribly difficult. 'Insight', a much belabored term, refers here not to some sophisticated level of psychological understanding, but rather simply to whether or not the patient recognizes that the hallucination is 'not real'. Sometimes simple observation will enable one to determine whether the patient experiences the hallucination as 'real': for example, should a patient report seeing a dog in the room and then reach down to pat it, one may reasonably assume that the patient has no insight into the hallucinatory nature of the experience. In doubtful cases, further inquiry may be required. Although one might simply ask whether or not the patient thinks the 'dog' is 'really' there in the room, such questions may offend some patients, and a more diplomatic approach is often better accepted. Thus, one might say, in an off-handed way, 'I don't see it. Could you tell me where it is?' In cases where insight has been preserved, the patient might respond, 'Oh, there's not a dog here. I must be seeing things.' Conversely, in cases where insight has been lost the patient might point emphatically to a corner of the room and say 'It's right over there. Can't you see it?' In cases of hallucinations where insight has been lost, the syndromal diagnosis of psychosis is reasonable, and should be pursued as in Section 7.1. In cases of isolated hallucinations occurring with preserved insight, however, the diagnosis should proceed as described below.

In determining the cause of isolated hallucinations occurring with preserved insight, the differential is different for each of the different kinds of hallucinations, and thus each type is discussed in turn, beginning with visual hallucinations, and proceeding to auditory, tactile, olfactory, and, finally, gustatory hallucinations.

Visual hallucinations are by far the most common type, and of the various causes of these, medications and intoxicants stand out. Of the medications capable of causing hallucinations, by far the most common are dopaminergic agents when used in the treatment of Parkinson's disease. After five or more years of treatment with levodopa, for example, visual hallucinations occur in a little over one-fifth of all patients (Friedman and Sienkiewicz 1991; Graham *et al.* 1997). The hallucinations themselves may, at times, be quite elaborate: in one case (Graham *et al.* 1997) a patient had 'hallucinations of miniature people and domestic animals ... the figures were non-threatening, laughed and talked among themselves, and had a male leader who organized them into purposeful activities'. It is important to note that although parkinsonian patients with levodopa-induced visual hallucinations retain insight initially, over many years insight tends to be lost and the syndrome of psychosis emerges (Goetz *et al.* 2006). The other medications listed in Table 4.7 are far less likely to be at fault.

Of the intoxicants capable of causing hallucinations, the aptly named hallucinogens immediately stand out. Of note, in this group, one of the earliest descriptions was provided by the eminent neurologist S. Weir Mitchell, who, in 1896, reported his own experiences with mescaline. Although the hallucinogen-induced hallucinations are, in most cases, fairly simple, for example geometric forms, they may sometimes be complex (e.g. with lysergic diethylamide [LSD] [Bercel *et al.* 1956]). Hallucinogen-induced visual hallucinations may also occur as 'flashbacks', wherein long after hallucinogen intoxication the patient spontaneously re-experiences some of the visual phenomena that occurred during the intoxication (Abraham 1983; Horowitz 1969).

Partial seizures may present with visual hallucinations: in simple partial seizure the visual hallucination may constitute the entire symptomatology of the seizure, whereas in complex partial seizures, it will be accompanied by some defect of consciousness.

Migraine headaches are typically preceded by an aura consisting of a visual hallucination; these tend to be simple, consisting of flashing lights or zigzagging lines (Panayiotopoulos 1994; Russell and Olesen 1996). An aura may, very rarely, persist long after the headache has cleared, sometimes for years (Liu *et al.* 1995).

Blindness, whether partial or complete, may be associated with either simple or complex visual hallucinations in what is known as the Charles Bonnet syndrome (Santhouse *et al.* 2000; White 1980). This syndrome has been noted with visual loss caused by cataracts (Bartlett 1951), macular degeneration (Holroyd *et al.* 1992), and lesions of the optic nerve, chiasm, tract and optic radiations (Lepore 1990). Although classically the hallucinations of the Charles Bonnet syndrome are said to be 'Lilliputian' in character, it in fact appears that such miniaturization occurs in only a minority of patients with this syndrome (Teunisse *et al.* 1994). The onset of the Charles Bonnet syndrome can at times be quite dramatic: in one case (White 1980), a 69-year-old man, while listening to music, 'suddenly saw a brightly coloured circus troupe burst through the window'.

Focal intracerebral lesions, usually infarctions, may cause hallucinations, and this has been noted with lesions of the occipital lobe and adjacent temporal and parietal lobes, and with lesions of the thalamus, mesencephalon or pons.

Lesions of the occipital cortex may, of course, also cause a hemianopia, and in such cases the hallucinations tend to occur in the hemianopic field (Kolmel 1985; Vaphiades *et al.* 1996). The clinical presentation in such cases may be quite remarkable: one patient (Lance 1976) with a left hemianopia saw animals appearing: 'from the left one at a time. At various times he saw dogs, goats, a lion and a horse as well as birds and butterflies. The animals would emerge from a door on the left side of the room and walk to the mid-line. If he looked to the left the animals retreated towards the door but would advance again as he looked to the front'.

Another patient, a neurologist, after suffering an infarction of the medial left occipital lobe, developed a right hemianopia in which he experienced vivid visual hallucinations: he noted that 'often there was a pony with his head cradled in my right arm' (Cole 1999).

Hallucinations occurring secondary to mesencephalic lesions are often referred to as 'peduncular' hallucinations, given that the lesion typically involves one of the cerebral peduncles. These peduncular hallucinations are typically complex and vivid: one patient (Geller and Bellor 1987) saw 'cats running about the floor, flowery outdoor scenes in bright purple colors, and the faces of neighbors and friends', whereas another (De La Fuente Fernandez *et al.* 1994) saw 'motorbikes . . . dogs, horses . . . and people . . . entering and driving silently around the room'. Although insight is preserved, and patients recognize the unreality of these peduncular hallucinations, their vivid character can nonetheless have a profound effect: in one case (Dunn *et al.* 1983), a patient saw 'snakes . . . that appeared from any direction' and although 'he knew the snakes were not real (nevertheless) during the examination he frequently jumped because he was pulling away from the perceived snakes'. The mesencephalic location of the responsible lesions usually entails 'neighborhood' symptoms of localizing value: thus, a right mesencephalic infarction affecting both the right cerebral peduncle and the midbrain tegmentum also caused left hemiplegia and bilateral ptosis (Geller and Bellor 1987); a left mesencephalic infarction that primarily involved the substantia nigra also caused a parkinsonian syndrome with prominent tremor on the right (De La Fuente Fernandez *et al.* 1994).

Hallucinations occurring secondary to pontine infarction have been referred to as 'Pick's visions', and have a distinctive character in that they often consist of hallucinating people walking through walls (Bing 1940).

Of the miscellaneous causes of visual hallucinations, narcolepsy is the most common and in this disorder they occur on either a hypnogogic or hypnopompic basis. Guillain–Barré syndrome, at its height, may cause visual hallucinations, possibly due to direct central nervous system involvement. Normal individuals may experience hallucinations during bereavement, with sleep deprivation, or, occasionally, on a hypnogogic basis. Hallucinations seen in bereavement are often of the deceased and the grieving person often finds them comforting; they tend to clear spontaneously within a few months.

Before leaving this section on visual hallucinations, a few extra words are in order regarding palinopsia as its differential is quite limited. Palinopsia has been noted with treatment with trazodone (Hughes and Lessell 1990), mirtazapine (Ihde-Scholl and Jefferson 2001) and risperidone (Lauterbach *et al.* 2000), as a manifestation of a simple partial seizure (Muller *et al.* 1995), and with lesions of the occipital lobe (Michel and Troost 1980), occipitotemporal region (Meadows and Munro 1977), occipitoparietal region (Bender *et al.* 1968), and the parietal lobe (Critchley 1951).

Auditory hallucinations occurring with preserved insight are relatively uncommon, and may be seen as side-effects to medications, manifestations of partial seizures, with deafness, or with focal intracerebral lesions.

Levodopa, used in the treatment of parkinsonism, may cause auditory hallucinations, but these are less common than the visual hallucinations discussed earlier. There is also a case report of hallucination secondary to pentoxyfylline.

Partial seizures may manifest with auditory hallucinations. In one case of a simple partial seizure (Williams 1956) the patient heard 'a buzz' that was quickly followed by 'music like a loudspeaker in which he heard clearly a recognized section of Veni Creator'. One of Penfield and Perot's (1963) patients, during a complex partial seizure, 'heard voices which seemed to come from her right side' as if she were in the middle of a 'crowd of people'.

Deafness may be followed by auditory hallucinations, thus constituting, as it were, the 'auditory' equivalent of the Charles Bonnet syndrome. Interestingly, the hallucinations seen here tend to be musical.

Focal intracerebral lesions, very rarely, may cause isolated auditory hallucinations, and these have been noted with lesions of the temporal cortex, putamen, mesencephalon, and pontine tegmentum.

Tactile hallucinations may be seen with intoxication with either cocaine or amphetamines, and typically consist of formication.

Olfactory hallucinations may represent either the sole symptomatology of a simple partial seizure or be part of the symptomatology of a complex partial seizure. Classically, they indicate a focus in the temporal lobe, particularly the uncus, and the resulting seizures are sometime referred to as 'uncinate fits'. They may also appear as a migraine aura or, very rarely, secondary to lesions of the olfactory bulb or tract.

Gustatory hallucinations with preserved insight have been reported during simple or complex partial seizures.

Differential diagnosis

As noted earlier, delusions must be distinguished from culturally or religiously sanctioned beliefs. Hallucinations, in turn, must be distinguished from illusions. Illusions are distorted experiences of actual objects, as for example the experience of a shimmering pool of water floating above a distant hot pavement, a pool that 'disappears' as one approaches closer.

Treatment

Treatment is directed, wherever possible, at the underlying cause. In the case of the Charles Bonnet syndrome, although there are no controlled studies, anecdotal reports attest to the efficacy of generally low-dose treatment with various medications including valproate (Hori *et al.* 2000), gabapentin (Paulig *et al.* 2001), carbamazepine (Batra *et al.* 1997), donepezil (Ukai *et al.* 2004), venlafaxine (Lang *et al.* 2007), risperidone (Maeda *et al.* 2003), and olanzapine (Coletti Moja *et al.* 2005). In the case of hallucinations occurring with focal intracerebral lesions, an empirical trial of a low-dose antipsychotic may be justified.

4.31 SCHNEIDERIAN FIRST RANK SYMPTOMS

Kurt Schneider (1887–1967) was a very influential German psychiatrist whose classic text *Clinical Psychopathology* went through multiple revisions from its first edition in 1939 up to the fifth, and last, edition, published in 1959. In this text, Schneider described a number of hallucinations and delusions that he believed were of 'first rank' importance in the diagnosis of schizophrenia. Although these Schneiderian first rank symptoms are, indeed, most commonly seen in schizophrenia, they may also, as pointed out by Schneider himself, occur in 'diverse' other conditions, as described below.

Clinical features

The various Schneiderian first rank symptoms, as noted in Table 4.8, may be divided into those which are auditory hallucinations and those which represent delusions.

Audible thoughts are said to occur when patients hear their own thoughts as if they were spoken out loud and indeed as if others might be able to hear them also. One of Schneider's (1959) patients said, 'I hear my own thoughts. I can hear them when everything is quiet.'

Voices commenting on what the patient does, keep up, as it were, a running commentary on the patient's behavior. One of Schneider's (1959) patients 'heard a voice say, whenever she wanted to eat, "Now she is eating, here she is munching again,"' and one of Kraepelin's (1921) patients heard a voice telling her, 'Mary, you're talking nonsense, the policeman has seen you already.'

Voices arguing with each other, or, as Schneider (1959) elaborated, merely 'conversing with one another', may engage patients' attention, as if the voices were carrying on a debate about them.

Delusions of passivity or influence are said to be present when 'feelings, impulses (drives) and volitional acts . . . are experienced by the patient as the work or influence of others' (Schneider 1959). Such patients believe that their thoughts, feelings or behavior are under the direct and unmediated control of some outside force or agency. Thus passively played upon by these forces, patients feel as if they were robots or automatons. Patients will typically elaborate on this delusion of influence and express a belief as to the source of the influence, for example an 'electrical device', 'distant computers', or 'powerful magnets'.

Table 4.8   Schneiderian first rank symptoms

Auditory hallucinations
Audible thoughts
Voices commenting on what the patient does
Voices arguing with each other

Delusions
Delusions of passivity or influence
Thought withdrawal
Thought insertion
Thought broadcasting

Thought withdrawal represents a delusion wherein patients experience their thoughts being directly removed and withdrawn from their minds. One of Kraepelin's (1921) patients spoke of his thoughts being 'drawn off'. This is quite different from simply losing track of what one was thinking: those who lose track have a sense of having forgotten or lost something, whereas those with thought withdrawal have, as emphasized by Schneider (1959), a definite sense that some other agency or person has directly removed the thought.

Thought insertion represents the delusional belief of patients that the thoughts occurring in their minds are not their own but rather originate from, as Schneider (1959) put it, 'other people, who intrude their thoughts upon the patient'. Such inserted thoughts are quite different from obsessions: obsessions are recognized by patients as their own thoughts and as originating within them, whereas inserted thoughts are experienced as a kind of cognitive 'foreign body'.

Thought broadcasting represents the delusion that others can know what a patient is thinking without the patient in any way relating those thoughts. This 'thought diffusion' led one of Schneider's (1959) patients to complain that, 'if I think of anything, at once those opposite me know it and it is embarrassing.' As she believed that 'the doctor too knew exactly what she was thinking, . . . she suggested that she would stop talking and (the physician) could just listen'. In some cases, patients will elaborate on this delusion, developing further beliefs about how such thought transfer is possible: Kraepelin (1921) noted that some patients believe that 'their thoughts are conveyed by a machine, there is a "mechanical arrangement", "a sort of little conveyance", telepathy'.

Etiology

It has, at times, been felt that Schneiderian first rank symptoms were virtually pathognomonic of schizophrenia, occurring in virtually no other condition. The source of this belief is not clear: it certainly does not come from Schneider, who clearly stated that these first rank symptoms could occur secondary to a 'number of diverse morbid cerebral processes' (Schneider 1959).

The various causes of the first rank symptoms are listed in Table 4.9. Of all of these, schizophrenia is, by far, the most common cause, with first rank symptoms being found in anywhere from one-third (Radhakrishnan et al. 1983) to over one-half (Tandon and Greden 1987) of such patients. Among patients with schizophrenia, it appears that thought broadcasting and thought insertion are probably most common out of all the first rank symptoms (Mellor 1970). Schizoaffective disorder is probably the next most common cause, with symptoms noted in about one-quarter of these patients (Tandon and Greden 1987). Mania, as seen in bipolar disorder, during stage II or III, may also cause first rank symptoms, and the diagnosis here

Table 4.9   Causes of Schneiderian first rank symptoms

Schizophrenia (Tandon and Greden 1987)
Schizoaffective disorder (Koehler and Seminario 1979)
Mania (Gonzales-Pinto *et al.* 2003; Jampala *et al.* 1989)
Depression (Tandon and Greden 1987)
Substance or medication-related
    Intoxications
        Amphetamines (Angrist and Gershon 1970; Bell 1973;
         Janowsky and Risch 197)
        Cocaine (Harris and Batki 2000; Rosse *et al.* 1994)
        Phencyclidine (Rosse *et al.* 1994)
        Alcohol hallucinosis (Marneros 1988)
        Benzodiazepine withdrawal (Roberts and Vass 1986)
        Fluvoxamine (Ueda *et al.* 2003)
Epileptic conditions
    Simple partial seizures (Mesulam 1981)
    Chronic interictal psychosis (Kido and Yamaguchi 1989;
     Slater and Beard 1963)
Miscellaneous causes
    Cushing's syndrome (Trethowan and Cobb 1952)
    New-variant Creutzfeldt–Jakob disease (Zeidler *et al.* 1997)
    Subacute sclerosing panencephalitis (Duncalf *et al.* 1989)
    Fahr's syndrome (Cummings *et al.* 1983)
    Metrizamide myelography (Davis *et al.* 1986)

is suggested by typical manic symptoms seen in stage I, such as pressured speech, hyperactivity, increased energy, decreased need for sleep, etc. Depression, as seen in major depressive disorder, is only rarely associated with first rank symptoms, and hence the appearance of such a symptom in a depressed patient should make one pause before giving a diagnosis of major depression; in such cases a diagnosis of schizoaffective disorder may be more likely.

The other causes noted in Table 4.9, although rare, must be kept in mind. Of these, intoxications with amphetamines, cocaine, or phencyclidine are perhaps most common. Chronic, severe, alcoholism may be associated with alcohol hallucinosis, which may be characterized by first rank symptoms, and there are case reports of these symptoms occurring during benzodiazepine withdrawal and as a side-effect to fluvoxamine.

Epileptic conditions associated with first-rank symptoms include simple partial seizures and the chronic interictal psychosis. In one case of a simple partial seizure, the patient, during the ictus, had 'blurry vision, abdominal discomfort, sensation of imminent death, intense fear, and the conviction that his body (was) controlled by external forces' (Mesulam 1981). The chronic interictal psychosis, discussed further in Section 7.1, is seen only in patients with chronic, severe, uncontrolled epilepsy: one of Slater and Beard's (1963) patients believed that there was a 'pick-up' device in his body 'which transmitted thoughts from the brain, and also made the brain receive'.

The remaining miscellaneous causes listed in Table 4.9 only very rarely cause first rank symptoms.

Treatment

Treatment is directed at the underlying condition.

REFERENCES

Abraham HD. Visual phenomenology of the LSD flashback. *Arch Gen Psychiatry* 1983; **40**:884–9.

Achari AN, Colover J. Posterior fossa tumors with pathological laughter. *JAMA* 1976; **235**:1469–71.

Ackerly W, Lhamom W, Fitts WT. Phantom breast. *J Nerv Ment Dis* 1955; **121**:177–8.

Adie WJ. Idiopathic narcolepsy: a disease *sui generis*, with remarks on the mechanism of sleep. *Brain* 1926; **49**:257–306.

Adie WJ, Critchley M. Forced grasping and groping. *Brain* 1927; **50**:142–70.

Akelaitis AJ. Psychobiological studies following section of the corpus callosum. *Am J Psychiatry* 1941; **97**:1147–57.

Akelaitis AJ. Studies on the corpus callosum. IV. Diagionistic dyspraxia in epileptics following partial and complete section of the corpus callosum. *Am J Psychiatry* 1945; **101**:594–9.

Akelaitis AJ, Risteen WA, Herren RY *et al.* Studies on the corpus callosum. III. A contribution to the study of dyspraxia and apraxia following partial and complete section of the corpus callosum. *Arch Neurol Psychiatry* 1942; **47**:971–1008.

Albala AA, Weinberg N, Allen SM. Maprotilene induced hyonopompic hallucinations. *J Clin Psychiatry* 1983; **44**:149–50.

Albert ML, Sandson J. Perseveration in aphasia. *Cortex* 1986; **22**:103–15.

Alevizos B, Lykouras L, Zervas IM *et al.* Risperidone-induced obsessive-compulsive symptoms. A review of six cases. *J Clin Psychopharmacol* 2002; **22**:461–7.

Alexander MC. Lilliputian hallucinations. *J Ment Sci* 1926; **72**:187–91.

Alexander MP, Schmitt MA. The aphasia syndrome of stroke in the left anterior cerebral artery territory. *Arch Neurol* 1980; **37**:97–100.

Alexander MP, Stuss DT, Benson DF. Capgras syndrome: a reduplicative phenomenon. *Neurology* 1979; **29**:334–9.

Andersen G, Vestergaard K, Riis JO. Citalopram for post-stroke pathological crying. *Lancet* 1993; **342**:837–9.

Anderson M, Salmon MV. Symptomatic cataplexy. *J Neurol Neurosurg Psychiatry* 1977; **40**:186–91.

Anderson SW, Damasio H, Damasio AR. A neural basis for collecting behavior in humans. *Brain* 2005; **128**:201–18.

Andreasen NC. Affective flattening and criteria for schizophrenia. *Am J Psychiatry* 1979; 136: 944–7.

Angrist B, Gershon S. The phenomenology of experimentally induced amphetamine psychosis. *Biol Psychiatry* 1970; **2**:95–107.

Anson JA, Kuhlman DT. Post-ictal Kluver–Bucy syndrome after temporal lobectomy. *J Neurol Neurosurg Psychiatry* 1993; **56**:311–13.

Asfora WT, DeSalles AAF, Masamitsu ABE *et al.* Is the syndrome of pathological laughing and crying a manifestation of pseudobulbar palsy? *J Neurol Neurosurg Psychiatry* 1989; **52**:523–5.

Assal F, Valenza N, Landis T. Clinicoanatomic correlates of a Fou rire prodromique in a pontine infarction. *J Neurol Neurosurg Psychiatry* 2000; **69**:697–8.

Ay H, Buoanno S, Price BH *et al.* Sensory alien hand syndrome: case report and review of the literature. *J Neurol Neurosurg Psychiatry* 1998; **65**:366–9.

Ayotte J, Peretz I, Hyde K. Congenital amusia. A group study of adults afflicted with a music-specific disorder. *Brain* 2001; **125**:238–51.

Ayuso-Peralta L, Jimenez-Jimenez FJ, Tejeiro J *et al.* Progressive multifocal leukoencephalopathy in HIV infection presenting as Balint's syndrome. *Neurology* 1994; **44**:1339–40.

Baguley IJ, Nicholls JL, Felmingham KL *et al.* Dysautonomia after traumatic brain injury: a forgotten syndrome? *J Neurol Neurosurg Psychiatry* 1999; **67**:39–43.

Baguley IJ, Heriseanu RE, Gurka JA *et al.* Gabapentin in the management of dysautonomia following severe traumatic brain injury: a case series. *J Neurol Neurosurg Psychiatry* 2007; **78**:539–41.

Baker D, Hunter E, Lawrence E *et al.* Depersonalization disorder: clinical features of 204 cases. *Br J Psychiatry* 2003; **182**:428–33.

Baker RW, Chengappa R, Baird JW *et al.* Emergence of obsessive compulsive symptoms during treatment with clozapine. *J Clin Psychiatry* 1992; **53**:439–42.

Banerjee AJ, Falkai PG, Savidge M. Visual hallucinations in the elderly associated with the use of levodopa. *Postgrad Med J* 1989; **65**:358–61.

Banks G, Short P, Martinez AJ *et al.* The alien hand syndrome: clinical and postmortem findings. *Arch Neurol* 1989; **46**:456–9.

Bar KJ, Hager F, Sauer H. Olanzapine- and clozapine-induced stuttering. A case series. *Pharmacopsychiatry* 2004; **37**:131–4.

Barbizet J, Degos JD, Duizabo Ph *et al.* Syndrome de deconnexion interhemispherique d'origine ischemique. *Rev Neurol* 1974; **130**:127–42.

Barclay CL, Bergeron C, Lang AE. Arm levitation in progressive supranuclear palsy. *Neurology* 1999; **52**:879–82.

Barnes J, David AS. Visual hallucinations in Parkinson's disease: a review and phenomenological survey. *J Neurol Neurosurg Psychiatry* 2001; **70**:72–3.

Barnes TR, Crichton P, Nelson HE *et al.* Primitive (developmental) reflexes, tardive dyskinesia and intellectual impairment in schizophrenia. *Schizophr Res* 1995; **16**:47–52.

Barrett K. Treating organic abulia with bromocriptine and lisuride: four case studies. *J Neurol Neurosurg Psychiatry* 1991; **54**:718–21.

Barris RW, Schuman HR. Bilateral anterior cingulate gyrus lesions: syndrome of the anterior cingulate gyri. *Neurology* 1953; **3**:44–52.

Bartlett JEA. A case of organized visual hallucinations in an old man with cataract, and their relationship to the phenomenology of the phantom limb. *Brain* 1951; **79**:363–73.

Bartusch SL, Sander BJ, D'Alessio JG *et al.* Clonazepam for the treatment of lancinating phantom limb pain. *Clin J Pain* 1996; **12**:59–62.

Bassetti C, Bogousslavsky J, Barth A *et al.* Isolated infarcts of the pons. *Neurology* 1996; **46**:165–75.

Batra A, Bartels M, Wormstall H. Therapeutic options in Charles Bonnet Syndrome. *Acta Psychiatr Scand* 1997; **96**:129–33.

Bautista RE, Ciampetti MZ. Expressive aprosody and amusia as a manifestation of right hemisphere seizures. *Epilepsia* 2003; **44**:466–7.

Bayles KA, Tomoeda CK, Kaszniak AW *et al.* Verbal perseveration of dementia patients. *Brain Lang* 1985; **25**:102–16.

Bayles KA, Tomoeda CK, McKnight PE *et al.* Verbal perseveration in individuals with Alzheimer's disease. *Semin Speech Lang* 2004; **25**:335–47.

Becker R, Benes L, Sure U *et al.* Intrathecal baclofen alleviates autonomic dysfunction in severe brain injury. *J Clin Neurosci* 2000; **7**:316–19.

Behrman S, Carroll JD, Janota I *et al.* Progressive supranuclear palsy. *Brain* 1969; **92**:663–78.

Bell DS. The experimental reproduction of amphetamine psychosis. *Arch Gen Psychiatry* 1973; **29**:35–40.

Benke T, Hohenstein C, Poewe W *et al.* Repetitive speech phenomena in Parkinson's disease. *J Neurol Neurosurg Psychiatry* 2000; **69**:319–24.

Bender MB, Feldman M, Sobin AJ. Palinopsia. *Brain* 1968; **91**:321–38.

Benegal V, Hingorani S, Khanna S *et al.* Is stupor by itself a catatonic symptom? *Psychopathology* 1992; **25**:229–31.

Benson DF, Gardner H, Meadows JC. Reduplicative paramnesia. *Neurology* 1976; **26**:147–51.

Benson DF, Djenderedjian A, Miller A *et al.* Neural basis of confabulation. *Neurology* 1996; **46**:1239–43.

Bercell NA, Travis LE, Olinger LB *et al.* Model psychoses induced by LSD-25 in normals. I. Psychophysiological investigations, with special reference to the mechanism of the paranoid reaction. *Arch Neurol Psychiatry* 1956; **75**:588–611.

Berlin I. Mirror movements. Report of two cases. *Arch Neurol Psychiatry* 1951; **66**:394.

Berrios GE. Tactile hallucinations: conceptual and historical aspects. *J Neurol Neurosurg Psychiatry* 1982; **45**:285–93.

Besson G, Bogousslavsky J, Regli F *et al.* Acute pseudobulbar or suprabulbar palsy. *Arch Neurol* 1991; **48**:501–7.

Beukelman DR, Flowers CR, Swanson PD. Cerebral disconnection associated with anterior communicating aneurysm: implications for evaluation of symptoms. *Arch Phys Med Rehabil* 1980; **61**:18–23.

Bhatia K, Marsden CD. The behavioral and motor consequences of focal lesions of the basal ganglia in man. *Brain* 1994; **117**:859–76.

Bing R. *Compendium of regional diagnosis in lesions of the brain and spinal cord*, 11th edn, translated by Haymaker W. St Louis: CV Mosby, 1940.

Bird GLA, Meadows J, Goka J *et al.* Cyclosporin-associated akinetic mutism and extrapyramidal syndrome after liver transplantation. *J Neurol Neurosurg Psychiatry* 1990; **53**:1068–71.

Bittar RG, Otero S, Carter H *et al.* Deep brain stimulation for phantom limb pain. *J Clin Neurosci* 2005; **12**:399–404.

Black DW, Wojcieszek J. Depersonalizaton syndrome induced by fluoxetine. *Psychosomatics* 1991; **32**:468–9.

Blake JR, Kunkle EC. The palmomental reflex. A physiological and clinical analysis. *Arch Neurol Psychiatry* 1951; **65**:337–45.

Bleuler E. *Textbook of psychiatry*, 1924, translated by Brill AA. New York: Arno Press, 1976.

Blumstein SE, Alexander MP, Ryalls JH *et al.* On the nature of the foreign accent syndrome; a case study. *Brain Lang* 1987; **31**:215–44.

Bodfish JW, Symons FJ, Parker DE *et al.* Varieties of repetitive behavior in autism: comparisons to mental retardation. *J Autism Dev Disorder* 2000; **30**:237–43.

Boeve BF, Wijdicks EF, Benarroch EE *et al.* Paroxysmal sympathetic storms ('diencephalic seizures') after severe diffuse axonal head injury. *Mayo Clin Proc* 1998; **73**:148–52.

Bogen JE. The callosal syndrome. In: Heilmann KM, Valenstein E eds. *Clinical neuropsychology*, 2nd edn. New York: Oxford University Press, 1985a.

Bogen JE. Split-brain syndromes. In: Vinken PJ, Bruyn GW, Klawans HL eds. *Handbook of clinical neurology*, 2nd edn. Amsterdam: Elsevier, 1985b.

Bogousslavsky J, Regli F. Anterior cerebral artery territory infarction in the Lausanne stroke registry: clinical and etiologic patterns. *Arch Neurol* 1990; **47**:144–50.

Bogousslavsky J, Regli F, Uske A. Thalamic infarcts: clinical syndromes, etiology, and prognosis. *Neurology* 1988; **38**:837–48.

Bogousslavsky J, Delayoe-Bischof A, Assal G. Loss of psychic self-activation with bithalamic infarction: neurobehavioral, CT, MRI and SPECT correlates. *Acta Neurol Scand* 1991; **83**:309–26.

Bone M, Critchley P, Buggy DJ. Gabapentin in postamputation phantom limb pain: a randomized, double-blind, placebo-controlled, cross-over study. *Reg Anesth Pain Med* 2002; **27**:481–6.

Borroni B, Broli M, Costanzi C *et al.* Primitive reflex evaluation in the clinical assessment of extrapyramidal syndromes. *Eur J Neurol* 2006; **13**:1026–8.

Botez MI, Werheim N. Expressive aphasia and amusia following right frontal lesion in a right-handed man. *Brain* 1959; **82**:187–202.

Brady JP. Drug-induced stuttering: a review of the literature. *J Clin Psychopharmacol* 1998; **18**:50–4.

Brady TK, Lydiard RB, Malcom R *et al.* Cocaine-induced psychosis. *J Clin Psychiatry* 1991; **52**:509–12.

Bressler B, Cohen SI, Magnussen F. The problem of phantom breast and phantom pain. *J Nerv Ment Dis* 1956; **123**:181–7.

Brion S, Jedynak CP. Troubles de transport interhemispherique: a propos de trois observations de tumeurs du corps calleux. *Rev Neurol* 1972; **126**:257–66.

Brock S, Merwarth HR. The illusory awareness of body parts in cerebral disease. *Arch Neurol Psychiatry* 1957; **77**:366–75.

Brodsky H, Vuong KD, Thomas M *et al.* Glabellar and palmomental reflexes in parkinsonian disorders. *Neurology* 2004; **63**:1096–8.

Brooks BR, Thisted RA, Appel SH *et al.* Treatment of pseudobulbar affect in ALS with destromethorphan/quidine. A randomized trial. *Neurology* 2004; **63**:1364–70.

Brown DL, Smith TL, Knepper LE. Evaluation of five primitive reflexes in 240 young patients. *Neurology* 1998; **51**:322.

Bullard DE. Diencephalic seizures: responsiveness to bromocriptine and morphine. *Ann Neurol* 1987; **21**:609–11.

Byerly M, Goodman W, Acholonu W *et al.* Obsessive compulsive symptoms in schizophrenia: frequency and clinical features. *Schizophr Res* 2005; **76**:309–16.

Cairns H, Oldfield RC, Pennybacker JB *et al.* Akinetic mutism with an epidermoid cyst of the 3rd ventricle. *Brain* 1941; **64**:273–90.

Cantu RC, Drew JH. Pathological laughing and crying associated with a tumor ventral to the pons. *J Neurosurg* 1966; **24**:1024–6.

Caplan LR, Schoene WC. Clinical features of subcortical arteriosclerotic encephalopathy (Binswanger's disease). *Neurology* 1978; **28**:1206–15.

Caplan LR, Schmahmann JD, Kase CS *et al.* Caudate infarcts. *Arch Neurol* 1990; **47**:133–43.

Carabelli RA, Kellerman WC. Phantom limb pain: relief by application of TENS to contralateral extremity. *Arch Phys Med Rehabil* 1985; **66**:466–7.

Cardoso F, Veado CC, de Oliveira JT. A Brazilian cohort of patients with Tourette's syndrome. *J Neurol Neurosurg Psychiatry* 1996; **60**:209–12.

Carel C, Albucher JF, Manelfe C *et al.* Fou rire prodromique heralding a left internal carotid artery occlusion. *Stroke* 1997; **28**:2081–3.

Carlen PL, Wall PD, Nadvorna H *et al.* Phantom limbs and related phenomena in recent traumatic amputations. *Neurology* 1978; **28**:211–17.

Carota A, Rossetti AO, Karapanayiotides T *et al.* Catastrophic reaction in acute stroke: a reflex behavior in aphasic patients. *Neurology* 2001; **57**:1902–5.

Carroll BT, Goforth HW, Raimonde LA. Partial Kluver-Bucy syndrome: two cases. *CNS Spectr* 2001; **6**:329–32.

Cascino GD, Adams RD. Brainstem auditory hallucinosis. *Neurology* 1986; **36**:1042–7.

Cassano GB, Petracca A, Perugi G *et al.* Derealization and panic attacks: a clinical evaluation on 150 patients with panic disorder/agoraphobia. *Compr Psychiatry* 1989; **30**:5–12.

Catsman-Berrevoets CE, Van Dongen HR, Mulder PG *et al.* Tumor type and size are high risk factors for the syndrome of 'cerebellar' mutism and subsequent dysarthria. *J Neurol Neurosurg Psychiatry* 1999; **67**:755–7.

Ceccaldi M, Milandre L. A transient fit of laughter as the inaugural symptom of capsular-thalamic infarction. *Neurology* 1994; **44**:1762.

Ceccaldi M, Poncet M, Milandre L *et al.* Temporary forced laughter after unilateral strokes. *Eur Neurol* 1994; **34**:36–9.

Cerrato P, Imperiale D, Giraudo M *et al.* Complex musical hallucinosis in a professional musician with a left subcortical hemorrhage. *J Neurol Neurosurg Psychiatry* 2001; **71**:280–1.

Cerrato P, Imperilae D, Bergoni M *et al.* Emotional facial paresis in a patient with a lateral medullary infarction. *Neurology* 2003; **60**:723–4.

Chan JL, Ross ED. Left-handed mirror writing following right anterior cerebral artery infarction: evidence for non-mirror transformations of motor programs by right supplementary motor area. *Neurology* 1988; **38**:59–63.

Chan J-L, Ross ED. Alien hand syndrome: influence of neglect on the clinical presentation of frontal and callosal variants. *Cortex* 1997; **33**:287–99.

Chan JL, Chen RS, Ng KK. Leg manifestations in alien hand syndrome. *J Formosan Med Assoc* 1996; **45**:342–6.

Channer KS, Stanley S. Persistent visual hallucinations secondary to chronic solvent encephalopathy: case report and review of the literature. *J Nerv Ment Dis* 1983; **46**:83–6.

Christensen RC, Byerly MJ, McElroy RA. A case of sertraline-induced stuttering. *J Clin Psychopharmacol* 1996; **16**:92–3.

Christodoulou GN. The syndrome of Capgras. *Br J Psychiatry* 1977; **130**:556–64.

Christoph DH, de la Freias GR, Dos Santos DP *et al*. Different perceived foreign accents in one patient after prerolandic hematoma. *Eur Neurol* 2004; **52**:198–201.

Ciabarra A, Elkino MS, Roberts JK *et al*. Subcortical infarction resulting in acquired stuttering. *J Neurol Neurosurg Psychiatry* 2000; **69**:546–9.

Closson RG. Visual hallucinations as the earliest symptom of digoxin intoxication. *Arch Neurol* 1983; **40**:386.

Cochen V, Arnulf I, Demeret S *et al*. Vivid dreams, hallucinations, psychosis and REM sleep in Guillian-Barre syndrome. *Brain* 2005; **128**:2535–45.

Cohen D, Cottias C, Basquin M. Cotard's syndrome in a 15-year-old girl. *Acta Psychiatr Scand* 1997; **95**:164–5.

Cohen PR. Medication-associated depersonalization symptoms: report of transient depersonalization symptoms induced by monocycline. *South Med J* 2004; **97**:70–3.

Cole M. When the left brain is not right the right brain may be left: report of personal experience of occipital hemianopia. *J Neurol Neurosurg Psychiatry* 1999; **67**:169–73.

Coletti Moja M, Milano E, Gasverde S *et al*. Olanzapine therapy in hallucinatory visions related to Bonnet syndrome. *Neurol Sci* 2005; **26**:168–70.

Colman WS. A case of pseudo-bulbar paralysis, due to lesions in each internal capsule; degeneration of direct and crossed pyramidal tracts. *Brain* 1894; **17**:88–9.

Comings DE, Comings BG. A controlled study of Tourette syndrome, IV: obsession, compulsion, and schizoid behavior. *Am J Med Genet* 1987; **41**:782–803.

Confavreux C, Croisile B, Garassus P *et al*. Progressive amusia and aprosody. *Arch Neurol* 1992; **49**:971–6.

Cornelius JR, Day NL, Fabrega H *et al*. Characterizing organic delusional syndrome. *Arch Gen Psychiatry* 1991; **48**:997–9.

Critchley M. Types of visual perseveration: 'palinopsia' and 'illusory visual spread'. *Brain* 1951; **74**:267–99.

Cummings JL, Cuningham K. Obsessive-compulsive disorder in Huntington's disease. *Biol Psychiatry* 1992; **31**:263–70.

Cummings JL, Duchen LW. Kluver–Bucy syndrome in Pick disease: clinical and pathologic correlations. *Neurology* 1981; **31**:1415–22.

Cummings JL, Gosenfeld LF, Houlihan JP *et al*. Neuropsychiatric disturbnces associated with idiopathic calcification of the basal ganglia. *Biol Psychiatry* 1983; **18**:591–601.

Cummings JL, Benson F, Hill MA *et al*. Aphasia in dementia of Alzheimer's type. *Neurology* 1985; **35**:394–7.

Currie S, Heathfield KW, Henson RA *et al*. Cinical course and prognosis of temporal lobe epilepsy. A survey of 666 patients. *Brain* 1971; **94**:173–90.

Daly D. Ictal affect. *Am J Psychiatry* 1958; **115**:97–108.

David AS, Bone I. Mutism following left hemisphere infarction. *J Neurol Neurosurg Psychiatry* 1984; **47**:1342–4.

Davis RE, Cummings JL, Malin BD *et al*. Prolonged psychosis with first-rank symptoms following metrizamide myelography. *Psychosomatics* 1986; **27**:373–5.

Davison C, Kelman H. Pathologic laughing and crying. *Arch Neurol Psychiatry* 1939; **42**:595–643.

Davison K. Episodic depersonalization: observations on 7 patients. *Br J Psychiatry* 1964; **110**:505–13.

D'Cruz OF, Vaughn BV, Gold SH *et al*. Symptomatic cataplexy in ponto-medullary lesions. *Neurology* 1994; **44**:2189–91.

Degos JD, Gray F, Louarn F *et al*. Posterior callosal infarction: clinicopathological correlations. *Brain* 1987; **110**:1155–71.

De La Fuente Fernandez R, Lopez JM, Del Corral PR *et al*. Peduncular hallucinosis and right hemiparkinsonism caused by left mesencephalic parkinsonism. *J Neurol Neurosurg Psychiatry* 1994; **57**:870.

Della Sala S, Mrachetti C, Spinnler H. The anarchic hand: a fronto-mesial sign. In: Boller F, Grafman J eds. *Handbook of neuropsychology*, vol. 9. Amsterdam: Elsevier Science, 1994.

DeLuca J, Cicerone KD. Confabulation following aneurysm of the anterior communicating artery. *Cortex* 1991; **27**:417–23.

Denny-Brown D, Meyer JS, Horenstein S. The significance of perceptual rivalry resulting from parietal lesions. *Brain* 1952; **75**:433–71.

De Renzi E, Barbieri C. The incidence of the grasp reflex following hemispheric lesion, and its relation to frontal damage. *Brain* 1992; **115**:293–313.

De Renzi E, Cavalleri F, Facchini S. Imitation and utilization behavior. *J Neurol Neurosurg Psychiatry* 1996; **61**:396–400.

Derex L, Ostrowsky K, Nighoghossian N *et al*. Severe pathological crying after left anterior choroidal artery infarct. Reversibility with paroxetine treatment. *Stroke* 1997; **28**:1464–6.

Desarkar P, Goyan N, Khess CRJ. Clozapine-induced cataplexy. *J Neuropsychiatry Clin Neurosci* 2007; **19**:87–8.

Devinsky O, Lemann W, Evans AC *et al*. Akinetic mutism in a bone marrow transplant recipient following total-body irradiation and amphotericin-B chemoprophylaxis. *Arch Neurol* 1987; **44**:414–17.

Devinsky O, Felmann E, Burrowes K *et al*. Autoscopic phenomenon with siezures. *Arch Neurol* 1989; **46**:1080–8.

Diamond AL, Callison RC, Shokri J *et al*. Paroxysmal sympathetic storm. *Neurocrit Care* 2005; **2**:288–91.

DiLegge S, Di Piero V, Altieri M *et al*. Usefulness of primitive reflexes in demented and non-demented cerebrovascular patients in daily clinical practice. *Eur Neurol* 2005; **41**;104–10.

Do D, Sheen VL, Bromfield E. Treatment of paroxysmal sympathetic storm with labetalol. *J Neurol Neurosurg Psychiatry* 2000; **69**:832–3.

Dolado AM, Castrillo C, Urra DG *et al*. Alien hand sign or alien hand syndrome? *J Neurol Neurosurg Psychiatry* 1995; **59**:100–1.

Doubleday EK, Snowden JS, Varma AR *et al*. Qualitative performance characteristics differentiate dementia with Lewy bodies and Alzheimer's disease. *J Neurol Neurosurg Psychiatry* 2002; **72**:602–7.

Dummit ES, Klein RG, Tancer NK *et al*. Systematic assessment of 50 children with selective mutism. *J Am Acad Child Adolesc Psychiatry* 1997; **36**:653–60.

Duncalf CM, Kent JNG, Harbord M *et al.* Subacute sclerosing panencephalitis presenting as schizophreniform psychosis. *Br J Psychiatry* 1989; **155**:557–9.

Dunn DW, Weisberg LA, Nadell J. Peduncular hallucinations caused by brainstem compression. *Neurology* 1983; **33**:1360–1.

Dyken ME, Yamada T, Lin-Dyken DC *et al.* Diagnosing narcolepsy through the simultaneous clinical and electrophysiologic analysis of cataplexy. *Arch Neurol* 1996; **53**:456–60.

Ellis P, Mellsop G. De Clerambault's syndrome – a nosological entity? *Br J Psychiatry* 1985; **146**:90–5.

Elson A, Pearson C, Jones CD *et al.* Follow-up study of childhood elective mutism. *Arch Gen Psychiatry* 1965; **13**:182–7.

Enoch MD. The Capgras syndrome. *Acta Psychiatr Scand* 1963; **39**:437–62.

Ephraim PL, Wegener ST, MacKenzie EJ *et al.* Phantom pain, residual limb pain, and back pain in amputees: results of a national survey. *Arch Phys Med Rehabil* 2005; **86**:1910–19.

Escalona PR, Adair JC, Roberts BB *et al.* Obsessive-compulsive disorder following bilateral globus pallidus infarction. *Biol Psychiatry* 1997; **42**:410–12.

Eslinger PJ, Warner GC, Grattan LM *et al.* 'Frontal lobe' utilization behavior associated with paramedian thalamic infarction. *Neurology* 1991; **41**:450–2.

Evans AC, Raistrick D. Phenomenology of intoxication with toluene-based adhesives and butane gas. *Br J Psychiatry* 1987; **150**:769–73.

Faris AA. Limbic system infarction: a report of two cases. *Neurology* 1969; **19**:91–6.

Feinberg TE, Schindler RJ, Flanagan NG *et al.* Two alien hand syndromes. *Neurology* 1992; **42**:19–24.

Feinstein A, Feinstein K, Gray T *et al.* Prevalence and neurobehavioral correlates of pathological laughing and crying in multiple sclerosis. *Arch Neurol* 1997; **54**:1116–21.

Fenelon G, Mahieux F, Huon R *et al.* Hallucinations in Parkinson's disease: prevalence, phenomenonology and risk factors. *Brain* 2000; **123**:733–45.

Fere C. Le fou rire prodromique. *Rev Neurol* 1903; **11**:353–8.

Ferguson SM, Rayport M, Corrie WS. Neuropsychiatric observations of corpus callosum section for seizure control. In: Reeves AJ ed. *Epilepsy and the corpus callosum.* New York: Plenum Press, 1985.

Fernandez JM, Sadaba F, Villaverde FJ *et al.* Cataplexy associated with midbrain lesion. *Neurology* 1995; **45**:393–4.

Fisher CM. Visual disturbances associated with quinidine and quinine. *Neurology* 1981; **31**:1569–71.

Fleet WS, Heilman KM. Acquired stuttering from a right hemisphere lesion in a right-hander. *Neurology* 1985; **35**:1343–6.

Ford RA. The psychopathology of echophenomena. *Psychol Med* 1989; **19**:627–35.

Formisano R, Saltuari L, Gerstendbrand F. Prevalence of Kluver-Bucy syndrome as a positive prognostic feature for the remission of traumatic prolonged disturbances of consciousness. *Acta Neurol Scand* 1995; **91**:54–7.

Fossati A, Maffei C, Battaglia M *et al.* Latent class analysis of DSM-IV schizotypal personality disorder criteria in psychiatric patients. *Schizophr Bull* 2001; **27**:59–71.

Fournier JCM, Helguera RAL. Postencephalitic narcolepsy and cataplexy: muscle and motor nerves electrical inexcitability during the attack of cataplexy. *J Nerv Ment Dis* 1934; **80**:159–62.

Frankel M, Cummings JL, Robertson MM *et al.* Obsessions and compulsions in Gilles de la Tourette's syndrome. *Neurology* 1986; **36**:378–82.

Freedman M, Alexander MP, Naeser MA. Anatomic basis of transcortical motor aphasia. *Neurology* 1984; **34**:409–17.

Freemon FR. Akinetic mutism and bilateral anterior cerebral artery occlusion. *J Neurol Neurosurg Psychiatry* 1971; **34**:693–8.

Fridriksson J, Ryalls J, Rorden C *et al.* Brain damage and cortical compensation in foreign accent syndrome. *Neurocase* 2005; **11**:319–24.

Friedman A, Sienkiewicz J. Psychotic complications of long-term levodopa treatment of Parkinson's disease. *Acta Neurol Scand* 1991; **84**:111–13.

Fuller GN, Guiloff RJ. Migrainous olfactory hallucinations. *J Neurol Neurosurg Psychiatry* 1987; **50**:1688–90.

Gainotti G. Emotional behavior and hemispheric side of lesion. *Cortex* 1972; **8**:41–55.

Gallagher JP. Pathologic laughter and crying in ALS: a search for their origin. *Acta Neurol Scand* 1989; **80**:114–17.

Gazzaniga MS, Bogen JE, Sperry RW. Some functional effects of sectioning the cerebral commissures in man. *Proc Nat Acad Sci* 1962; **48**:1765–9.

Gelardi J-A M, Brown JW. Hereditary cataplexy. *J Neurol Neurosurg Psychiatry* 1967; **30**:455–7.

Geller TJ, Bellor SN. Peduncular hallucinosis: magnetic resonance imaging confirmation of mesencephalic infarction during life. *Ann Neurol* 1987; **21**:602–4.

Gelmers HJ. Non-paralytic motor disturbance and speech disorders: the role of the supplementary motor area. *J Neurol Neurosurg Psychiatry* 1983; **46**:1052.

Geschwind DH, Iacoboni M, Mega MS *et al.* Alien hand syndrome: interhemispheric motor disconnection due to a lesion in the midbody of the corpus callosum. *Neurology* 1995; **45**:802–8.

Geschwind N. The perverseness of the right hemisphere. *Behav Brain Sci* 1981; **4**:106–7.

Ghika-Schmid F, Assal G, De Tribolet N *et al.* Kluver-Bucy syndrome after left anterior temporal resection. *Neuropsychologia* 1995; **33**:101–13.

Gibb WRC, Luthert PJ, Marsden CD. Corticobasal degneration. *Brain* 1989; **112**:1171–92.

Gilbert GJ. Pentoxifylline-induced musical hallucinations. *Neurology* 1993; **43**:1621–2.

Gillett T, Eminson SR, Hassanyeh F. Primary and secondary erotomania. Clinical characteristics and follow-up. *Acta Psychiatr Scand* 1990; **82**:65–9.

Giroud M, Lemesle M, Madinier G *et al.* Unilateral lenticular infarcts: radiological and clinical syndromes, etiology, and prognosis. *J Neurol Neurosurg Psychiatry* 1997; **63**:611–15.

Goetz CG, Wuu J, Curgian LM *et al.* Hallucinations and sleep disorders in PD. Six-year prospective longitudinal study. *Neurology* 2005; **64**:81–6.

Goetz CG, Fan W, Leurgans S et al. The malignant course of 'benign hallucinations' in Parkinson disease. Arch Neurol 2006; 63:713–16.

Goldberg G, Bloom KK. The alien hand syndrome: localization, lateralization, and recovery. J Phys Med Rehab 1990; 69:228–38.

Golden RN, James SP, Sherer MA et al. Psychoses associated with bupropion treatment. Am J Psychiatry 1985; 42:1459–62.

Goldenberg G, Wimmer A, Holzner F et al. Apraxia of the left limb in a case of callosal disconnection: the contribution of medial frontal lobe damage. Cortex 1985; 21:135–48.

Goldin S. Lilliputian hallucinations. J Ment Sci 1955; 101:569–76.

Goldstein K. Sur Lehre der motorischen Apraxia. J fur Psychologie und Neurologie 1908; 11:169–87.

Goldstein K. Der makroskopische Hirnbefund in meinem Falle von linksseitiger motorischer Apraxie. Neurol Centralbl 1909; 28:898–906.

Goldstein K. The organism: a holistic approach to biology derived from pathological data in man. New York: American Books, 1939.

Goldstein K. After effects of brain injuries in war. New York: Grune and Stratton, 1942.

de AA Gondin F, Parks BJ, Cruz-Flores S. 'Fou rire prodromique' as the presentation of pontine ischemia secondary to vertebrobasilar stenosis. J Neurol Neurosurg Psychiatry 2001; 71:802–4.

Gonzales-Pinto A, van Os J, Perez de Heredia JL et al. Age-dependence of Schneiderian psychotic symptoms in bipolar patients. Schizophren Res 2003; 61:157–62.

Gordon A. Transition of obsessions into delusions. Am J Psychiatry 1950; 107:455–8.

Gorno-Tempini ML, Ogar JM, Brambati SM et al. Anatomical correlates of early mutism in progressive nonfluent speech. Neurology 2006; 67:1849–51.

Granacher RP. Differential diagnosis of tardive dyskinesias: an overview. Am J Psychiatry 1981; 38:1288–97.

Gothelf D, Presburger G, Zohar AH et al. Obsessive-compulsive disorder in patients with velocardiofacial (22q11 deletion) syndrome. Am J Med Genet Neuropsychiatr Genet 2004;126:99–105.

Gottlieb D, Robb K, Day B. Mirror movements in the alien hand syndrome. Am J Phys Med Rehabil 1992; 71:297–300.

Gouzoulis-Mayfrank E, Heekeren K, Neukirch A et al. Psychological effects of (S)-ketamine and N,N-dimethyltryptamine (DMT): a double-blind, cross-over study in healthy volunteers. Pharmacopsychiatry 2005; 38:301–11.

Graff-Radford NR, Eslinger PJ, Damasio AR et al. Nonhemorrhagic infarction of the thalamus: behavioral, anatomic, and physiologic correlates. Neurology 1984; 34:14–23.

Graff-Radford NR, Cooper WE, Colsher PL et al. An unlearned foreign 'accent' in a patient with aphasia. Brain Lang 1986; 28:86–94.

Graham JM, Gruenwald RA, Sagar HJ. Hallucinosis in idiopathic Parkinson's disease. J Neurol Neurosurg Psychiatry 1997; 63:434–40.

Green RC, Goldstein FC, Mirra SS et al. Slowly progressive apraxia in Alzheimer's disease. J Neurol Neurosurg Psychiatry 1995; 59:312–15.

Greenwood R, Bhalla A, Gordon A et al. Behavior disturbances during recovery from herpes simplex encephalitis. J Neurol Neurosurg Psychiatry 1983; 46:809–17.

Griffiths TD. Musical hallucinosis in acquired deafness. Phenomenology and brain substrate. Brain 2000; 123:2065–76.

Grigsby J, Kaye K. Incidence and correlates of depersonalization following head trauma. Brain Inj 1993; 7:507–13.

Grimby A. Bereavement among elderly people: grief reactions, post-bereavement hallucinations and quality of life. Acta Psychiatr Scand 1993; 87:72–80.

Gross-Tsu V, Joseph A, Shlev RS. Hallucinations during methylphenidate therapy. Neurology 2004; 63:753–4.

Guilleminault C, Wilson RA, Dement WC. A study on cataplexy. Arch Neurol 1974; 31:255–61.

von Gunten A, Miklossy J, Suva ML et al. Environmental reduplicative paramnesia in a case of atypical Alzheimer's disease. Neurocase 2005; 11:216–26.

Gydesen S, Brown JN, Brun A et al. Chromosome 3 linked frontotemporal dementia (FTD-3). Neurology 2002; 59:1585–94.

Haber WB. Observations on phantom-limb phenomena. Arch Neurol Psychiatry 1956; 75:624–36.

Hachinski VC, Porchawka J, Steele JC. Visual symptoms in the migraine syndrome. Neurology 1973; 23:570–9.

Hadano K, Nakamura H, Hamanaka T. Effortful echolalia. Cortex 1998; 34:67–82.

Haerer AE, Currier RD. Mirror movements. Neurology 1966; 16:757–60.

Hall DA, Anderson CA, Filley CM et al. A French accent after corpus callosum infarct. Neurology 2003; 60:1551–2.

Halligan PW, Marshall JC, Wade DT. Three-arms: a case study of supernumerary phantom limbs after right hemisphere stroke. J Neurol Neurosurg Psychiatry 1993; 56:159–66.

Hamano T, Hiraki S, Kawamur Y et al. Acquired stuttering secondary to callosal infarction. Neurology 2005; 64:1092–3.

Hammeke TA, McQuillen MP, Cohen BA. Musical hallucinations associated with acquired deafness. J Neurol Neurosurg Psychiatry 1983; 46:570–2.

Hanakita J, Nishi S. Left alien hand sign and mirror writing after left anterior cerebral artery infarction. Surg Neurol 1991; 35:290–3.

Harris DL, Batki SL. Stimulant psychosis: symptom profile and acute clinical course. Am J Addict 2000; 9:28–37.

Hashimoto R, Tanaka Y. Contribution of the supplmentary motor area and anterior cingulate gyrus to pathological grasping phenomena. Eur Neurol 1998; 40:151–8.

Hashimoto R, Yoshida M, Tanaka Y. Utilization behavior after right thalamic infarction. Eur Neurol 1995; 35:58–62.

Hause-Hauw C, Bancaud J. Gustatory hallucinations in epileptic seizures. Electrophysiological, clinical and anatomical correlates. Brain 1987; 110:39–59.

Helgason C, Wilbur A, Weiss A et al. Acute pseudobulbar mutism due to discrete bilateral capsular infarction in the territory of the anterior choroidal artery. Brain 1988; 111:507–24.

Helm NA, Butler RB, Benson DF. Acquired stuttering. Neurology 1978; 28:1159–65.

Hemmingsen R, Rafaelsen OJ. Hypnagogic and hypnopompic hallucinations during amitriptyline treatment. *Acta Neurol Scand* 1980; **62**:364–8.

Henderson WR, Smythe GE. Phantom limbs. *J Neurol Neurosurg Psychiatry* 1948; **11**:89–112.

Heutink P, Stevens M, Rizzu P *et al*. Hereditary frontotemporal dementia is linked to chromosome 17q21–q22: a genetic and clinicopathological study of three Dutch families. *Ann Neurol* 1997; **41**:150–9.

Hillbom E. After-effects of brain-injuries. *Acta Psychiatr Neurol Scand* 1960; **142**(suppl.):1–195.

Hof PR, Archin N, Osmand AP *et al*. Posterior cortical atrophy in Alzheimer's disease: analysis of a new case and re-evaluation of a historical report. *Acta Neuropathol* 1993; **86**:215–23.

Hollander E, Soorya L, Wasserman S *et al*. Divalproex sodium vs. placebo in the treatment of repetitive behaviors in autism spectrum disorder. *Int J Neuropsychopharmacol* 2006; **9**:209–13.

Hollister LE, Prusmack JJ, Paulsen JA *et al*. Comparison of three psychotropic drugs (psilocybin, JB-329, IT-290) in volunteer subjects. *J Nerv Ment Dis* 1960; **131**:428–34.

Holroyd S, Rabins PV, Finkelstein D *et al*. Visual hallucinations in patients with macular degeneration. *Am J Psychiatry* 1992; **149**:1701–6.

Hopf HC, Muller-Forell W, Hopf NJ. Localization of emotional and volitional facial paresis. *Neurology* 1992; **42**:1918–23.

Hopf HC, Fitzek C, Mark J *et al*. Emotional facial paresis of pontine origin. *Neurology* 2000; **54**:1217.

Hori H, Terao T, Shiraishi Y *et al*. Treatment of Charles Bonnet syndrome with valproate. *Int Clin Psychopharmacol* 2000; **15**:117–19.

Horowitz MJ. Flashbacks: recurrent intrusive images after the use of LSD. *Am J Psychiatry* 1969; **126**:565–9.

Hotz G, Helm-Estabrooks N. Perseveration. Part II: A study of perseveration in closed-head injury. *Brain Inj* 1995; **9**:161–72.

Hudson AJ, Grace GM. Misidentification syndromes related to face specific area in the fusiform gyrus. *J Neurol Neurosurg Psychiatry* 2000; **69**:645–8.

Hughes MS, Lessell S. Trazodone-induced palinopsia. *Arch Ophthalmol* 1990; **108**:359.

Husain M, Stein J. Rezso Balint and his most celebrated case. *Arch Neurol* 1988; **45**:89–93.

Huse E, Larbig W, Flor H *et al*. The effect of opioids on phantom limb pain and cortical reorganization. *Pain* 2001; **90**:47–55.

Husby G, van de Rijn I, Zabriskie JB *et al*. Antibodies reacting with cytoplasm of subthalamic and caudate neurons in chorea and acute rheumatic fever. *J Exp Med* 1976; **144**:1094–110.

Hwang JP, Tsai SJ, Yang CH *et al*. Hoarding behavior in dementia. A preliminary report. *Am J Geriatr Psychiatry* 1998; **6**:285–9.

Hyde TM, Goldberg TE, Egan MF *et al*. Frontal release signs and cognition in people with schizophrenia, their siblings and healthy controls. *Br J Psychiatry* 2007; **191**:120–5.

Ihde-Scholl T, Jefferson JW. Mirtazapine-associated palinopsia. *J Clin Psychiatry* 2001; **62**:373.

Imamura T, Takanashi M, Hattori N *et al*. Bromocriptine treatment for perseveration in demented patients. *Alzheimer Dis Assoc Disord* 1998; **12**:109–13.

Ionasescu V. Paroxysmal disorders of the body image in temporal lobe epilepsy. *Acta Psychiatr Neurol Scand* 1960; **35**:171.

Ironside R. Disorders of laughter due to brain lesions. *Brain* 1956; **79**:589–609.

Isbell H, Belleville RE, Fraser HF *et al*. Studies on lysergic acid diethylamide (LSD-25). *Arch Neurol Psychiatry* 1956; **76**:468–78.

Ishihara K, Nishino H, Maki T *et al*. Utilization behavior as a white matter disconnection syndrome. *Cortex* 2002; **38**:379–87.

Jackson JH, Stewart P. Epileptic attacks with a warning of a crude sensation of smell and with the intellectual aura (dreamy state) in a patient who had symptoms pointing to gross organic disease of the right temporo-sphenoidal lobe. *Brain* 1899; **32**:209.

Jacobs L, Gossman MD. Three primitive reflexes in normal adults. *Neurology* 1980; **30**:184–8.

Jaeger H, Maier C. Calcitonin in phantom limb pain: a double-blind study. *Pain* 1992; **48**:21–7.

Jampala VC, Taylor MA, Abrams R. The diagnostic implication of formal thought disorder in mania and schizophrenia: a reassessment. *Am J Psychiatry* 1989; **146**:459–63.

Janowsky DS, Risch C. Amphetamine psychosis and psychotic symptoms. *Psychopharmacology* 1979; **65**:73–7.

Jaob A, Cherian PJ, Radhakrishnan K *et al*. Emotional facial paresis in temporal lobe epilepsy: its prevalence and lateralizing value. *Seizure* 2003; **12**:60–4.

Jarvis JH. Post-mastectomy breast phantoms. *J Nerv Ment Dis* 1967; **144**:266–72.

Jason GW, Pajurkova EM. Failure of metacontrol: breakdown of behavioral unity after lesions of the corpus callosum and inferomedial frontal lobes. *Cortex* 1992; **28**:241–60.

Jelliffe SE. Oculogyric crises as compulsion phenomena in postencephalitis: their occurrence, phenomenology and meaning. *J Nerv Ment Dis* 1929; **69**:59–68, 165–84, 278–97, 415–26, 531–51, 666–79.

Jensen JPA, Gron U, Pakkenberg H. Comparison of three primitive reflexes in neurological patients and in normal volunteers. *J Neurol Neurosurg Psychiatry* 1983; **46**:162–7.

Jensen TS, Krebs B, Nielsen J *et al*. Non-painful phantom limb phenomena in amputees: incidence, clinical characteristics and temporal course. *Acta Neurol Scand* 1984; **70**:407–14.

John JP, Khanna S, Thennarasau K *et al*. Exploration of dimensions of psychopathology in neuroleptic-naive patients with recent-onset schizophrenia/schizophreniform disorder. *Psychiatry Res* 2003; **121**:11–20.

Joseph AB, O'Leary DH. Brain atrophy and interhemispheric fissure enlargement in Cotard's syndrome. *J Clin Psychiatry* 1986; **47**:518–20.

Kales A, Cadieux RJ, Soldatos CR *et al*. Narcolepsy–cataplexy. I. Clinical and electrophysiologic characteristics. *Arch Neurol* 1982; **39**:164–8.

Kane FT, Keeler MH. Visual hallucinations while receiving imipramine. *Am J Psychiatry* 1964; **121**:611–12.

Kapur N, Turner A, King C. Reduplicative paramnesia: possible anatomical and neuropsychological mechanisms. *J Neurol Neurosurg Psychiatry* 1988; **51**:579–81.

Katz DI, Alexander MP, Mandell AM. Dementia following strokes in the mesencephalon and diencephalons. *Arch Neurol* 1987; **44**:1127–33.

Kaufman MD, Lassiter KR, Shenoy BV. Paroxysmal unilateral dysosmia: a cured patient. *Ann Neurol* 1988; **24**:450–1.

Keschner M, Bender MB, Strauss I. Mental symptoms in cases of tumor of the temporal lobe. *Arch Neurol Psychiatry* 1936; **35**:572–96.

Kido H, Yamaguchi N. Clinical studies of schizophrenia-like state in epileptic patients. *Jpn J Psychiatry Neurol* 1989; **43**:433–8.

King AB. 'Phantom' sciatica. *Arch Neurol Psychiatry* 1956; **76**:72–4.

Klein DF. Visual hallucinations with imipramine. *Am J Psychiatry* 1964; **121**:911–14.

Kluin KJ, Norman LF, Berent S *et al.* Perceptual analysis of speech disorders in progressive supranuclear palsy. *Neurology* 1993; **43**:563–6.

Kluver H, Bucy PC. Preliminary analysis of functions of the temporal lobes in monkeys. *Arch Neurol Psychiatry* 1939; **42**:979–1000.

Koehler K, Seminario I. Research diagnosable 'schizo-affective' disorder in Schneiderian 'first rank' schizophrenia. *Acta Psychiatr Scand* 179; **60**:347–54.

Kollar EJ, Namerow N, Pasnau RO *et al.* Neurological findings during prolonged sleep deprivation. *Neurology* 1968; **18**:836–40.

Koller WC. Dysfluency (stuttering) in extrapyramidal disease. *Arch Neurol* 1983; **40**:175–7.

Koller WC, Glatt S, Wilson RS *et al.* Primitive reflexes and cognitive function in the elderly. *Ann Neurol* 1982; **12**:302–4.

Kolmel HW. Complex visual hallucinations in the hemianopic field. *J Neurol Neurosurg Psychiatry* 1985; **48**:29–38.

Kraepelin E. *Clinical psychiatry.* Translated by Diefendorff, R. New York: MacMillan Company, 1907, p. 86.

Kraepelin E. *Dementia praecox and paraphrenia.* Translated by Barclay RM, Robert E. Huntington, NY: Krieger Publishing, 1971.

Kraepelin E. *Manic-depressive insanity and paranoia*, 1921. New York: Arno Press, 1976.

Kraepelin E. *Psychiatry. A textbook for students and physicians*, 6th edn, 1899. Translated by Metoui H, Ayed S. Canton, MA: Science History Publications, 1990.

Kroll L, Drummond LM. Temporal lobe epilepsy and obsessive-compulsive symptoms. *J Nerv Ment Dis* 1993; **181**:457–8.

Krystal JH, Perry EB, Gueorguieva R *et al.* Comparative and interactive human psychopharmacologic effects of ketamine and amphetamine: implications for gluatamatergic and dopaminergic model psychoses and cognitive function. *Arch Gen Psychiatry* 2005; **62**:985–94.

Kumral E, Calli C. External and extreme capsular stroke: clinical, topographical and etiologic patterns. *Cerebrovasc Dis* 2006; **21**:217–22.

Kumral E, Evyapan D, Balkir K. Acute caudate vascular lesions. *Stroke* 1999; **30**:100–8.

Lago A. *Fou Rire Prodromique* and ischemic stroke. *Stroke* 1998; **29**:1067–8.

Lam LC, Chiu HF. Kluver-Bucy syndrome in a patient with nasopharyngeal carcinoma: a late complication of radiation brain injury. *J Geriatr Psychiatry Neurol* 1997; **10**:111–13.

Lance JW. Simple formed hallucinations confined to the area of a specific visual field defect. *Brain* 1976; **99**:719–34.

Lang UE, Stogowski D, Schulze D *et al.* Charles Bonnet syndrome: successful treatment of visual hallucinations due to vision loss with selective serotonin reuptake inhibitors. *J Psychopharmacol* 2007; **21**:553–5.

Langsworthy OR, Hesser FH. Syndrome of pseudobulbar palsy. *Arch Int Med* 1940; **65**:106–21.

Laplane D, Baulac M, Widocher D *et al.* Pure psychic akinesia with bilateral lesion of basal ganglia. *J Neurol Neurosurg Psychiatry* 1984; **47**:377–85.

Laplane D, Levasseur M, Pillon B *et al.* Obsessive-compulsive and other behavioral changes with bilateral basal ganglia lesions. A neuropsychological, magnetic resonance imaging and positron tomography study. *Brain* 1989; **112**:699–725.

Lauterbach EC, Abdlhamid A, Annandale JB. Posthallucinogen-like visual illusions (palinopsia) with risperidone in a patient without previous hallucinogen exposure: possible relation to serotonin 5-HT2A blockade. *Pharmacopsychiatry* 2000; **33**:38–41.

Lawson IR, McLeod RD. The use of imipramine ('Tofranil') and other psychotropic drugs in organic emotionalism. *Br J Psychiatry* 1969; **115**:281–5.

Lee HJ, Lee HS, Kim L *et al.* A case of risperidone-induced stuttering. *J Clin Psychopharmacol* 2001; **21**:115–16.

Lee SK, Lee SL, Kim D-W *et al.* Occipital lobe epilepsy: clinical characteristics, surgical outcome, and role of diagnostic modalities. *Epilepsia* 2005; **46**:688–95.

Leiguarda R, Starkstein S, Berthier M. Anterior callosal hemorrhage. A partial interhemispheric disconnection syndrome. *Brain* 1989; **112**:1019–37.

Lepore FE. Spontaneous visual phenomena with visual loss: 104 patients with lesions of retinal and visual afferent pathways. *Neurology* 1990; **40**:444–7.

Leroy R. The syndrome of Lilliputian hallucinations. *J Nerv Ment Dis* 1922; **56**:325–33.

Leudar I, Fraser WI, Jeeves MA. Behavior disturbances and mental handicap: typology and longitudinal trends. *Psychol Med* 1984; **14**:923–35.

Levine DN, Rinn WE. Opticosensory ataxia and alien hand syndrome after posterior cerebral artery territory infarction. *Neurology* 1986; **36**:1094–7.

Lewis MH, Bodfish JW, Powell SB *et al.* Clomipramine treatment for self-injurious behavior of individuals with mental retardation: a double-blind comparison with placebo. *Am J Ment Retard* 1996; **100**:654–65.

Lhermitte F. 'Utilization behavior' and its relation to lesions of the frontal lobes. *Brain* 1983; **106**:237–55.

Lhermitte F. Human anatomy and the frontal lobes. II. Patient behavior in complex and social situations: the 'environmental dependency syndrome'. *Ann Neurol* 1986; **19**:335–43.

Lhermitte F, Pillon B, Serdaru M. Human anatomy and the frontal lobes. I. Imitation and utilization behavior: a neuropsychological study of 75 patients. *Ann Neurol* 1986; **19**:326–44.

Lhermitte J. Syndrome de la calotte du pedoncule cerebral. Les troubles psycho-sensoriels dans les lesions du mesocephale. *Rev Neurol* 1922; **38**:1359–65.

Lhermitte J. L'hallucinose pedonculaire. *Encephale* 1932; **27**:422–35.

Lieberman A, Benson DF. Control of emotional expression in pseudobulbar palsy. *Arch Neurol* 1977; **34**:717–19.

Lilly R, Cummings JL, Benson DF *et al*. The human Kluver-Bucy syndrome. *Neurology* 1983; **33**:1141-5.

Linetsky E, Planer D, Ben-Hur T. Echolalia-palilalia as the sole manifestation of nonconvulsive status epilepticus. *Neurology* 2000; **55**:733-4.

Lipinski CG. Epilepsies with astatic seizures of late onset. *Epilepsia* 1977; **18**:13-20.

Lippman CO. Hallucinations of physical disability in migraine. *J Nerv Ment Dis* 1953; **117**:345-50.

Liu GT, Scatz NJ, Galetta SL *et al*. Persistent positive visual phenomena in migraine. *Neurology* 1995; **45**:664-8.

Logan TP. Persistent phantom limb pain: dramatic response to chlorpromazine. *South Med J* 1983;**76**:1585.

Lohr JB. Transient grasp reflexes in schizophrenia. *Biol Psychiatry* 1985; **20**:172-5.

Lopez JR, Adornato BT, Hoyt WF. 'Entomopia': a remarkable case of cerebral polyopia. *Neurology* 1993; **43**:2145-6.

Lopez-Villegas D, Kulisevsky J, Deus J *et al*. Neuropsychological alterations in patients with computed tomography-detected basal ganglia calcification. *Arch Neurol* 1996; **53**:251-6.

Ludlow CL, Rosenberg J, Salazar A *et al*. Site of penetrating brain lesion causing chronic acquired stuttering. *Ann Neurol* 1987; **22**:60-6.

Lugaresi A, Montagna P, Morreale A *et al*. 'Psychic akinesia' following carbon monoxide poisoning. *Eur Neurol* 1990; **30**:167-9.

Lukianowicz N. Autoscopic phenomena. *Arch Neurol Psychiatry* 1958; **80**:199-220.

MacGowan DJL, Delanty N, Petito F *et al*. Isolated myoclonic alien hand as the sole presentation of pathologically established Creutzfeldt-Jakob disease: a report of two patients. *J Neurol Neurosurg Psychiatry* 1997; **63**:404-7.

Maeda K, Shirayama Y, Nukima S *et al*. Charles Bonnet syndrome with visual hallucinations of childhood experience: successful treatment of 1 patient with risperidone. *J Clin Psychiatry* 2003; **64**:1131-2.

Maertens de Noordhout AM, Delwaide PJ. The palmomental reflex in Parkinson's disease: comparisons with normal subjects and clinical relevance. *Arch Neurol* 1988; **45**:425-7.

Mahone EM, Bridges D, Prahme C *et al*. Repetitive arm and hand movements (complex motor stereotypies) in children. *J Pediatr* 2004; **145**:391-5.

Maia DP, Teixeira AL, Cunningham MCQ *et al*. Obsessive-compulsive behavior, hyperactivity, and attention deficit disorder in Sydnham chorea. *Neurology* 2005; **64**:1799-801.

Maier C, Derwinkel R, Mansourian N *et al*. Efficacy of NMDA-receptor antagonist memantine in patients with chronic phantom limb pain: results of a randomized double-blinded, placebo-controlled trial. *Pain* 2003; **103**:277-83.

Marcon G, Cancelli I, Zamarian L *et al*. Visual hallucinations with sertraline. *J Clin Psychiatry* 2004; **65**:446-7.

Marder K, Liu X, Stern Y *et al*. Neurologic signs and symptoms in a cohort of homosexual men followed for 4.5 years. *Neurology* 1995; **45**:261-7.

Marlowe WB, Mancall EL, Thomas TJ. Complete Kluver-Bucy syndrome in man. *Cortex* 1975; **11**:53-9.

Marneros A. Schizophrenia first-rank symptoms in organic mental disorders. *Br J Psychiatry* 1988; **152**:625-8.

Martin JP. Fits of laughter (sham-mirth) in organic cerebral disease. *Brain* 1950; **73**:453-64.

Masdeu JC, O'Hara RJ. Motor aphasia unaccompanied by faciobrachial weakness. *Neurology* 1983; **33**:519-21.

Mathew RJ. Wilson WH, Humphreys D *et al*. Depersonalization after marijuana smoking. *Biol Psychiatry* 1993; **33**:431-41.

Mauguire F, Courjon J. Somatosensory epilepsy: a review of 127 cases. *Brain* 1978; **101**:307-32.

Mayeux R, Benson DF. Phantom limb and multiple sclerosis. *Neurology* 1979; **29**:724-6.

Mayeux R, Stern Y, Spanton S. Heterogeneity in dementia of the Alzheimer type: evidence of subgroups. *Neurology* 1985; **35**:453-61.

Mazzucchi A, Marchini C, Budai R *et al*. A case of receptive amusia with prominent timbre perception defect. *J Neurol Neurosurg Psychiatry* 1982; **45**:644-7.

McDonald C. A clinical study of hypnagogic hallucinations. *Br J Psychiatry* 1971; **118**:543-7.

McDougle CJ, Scahill L, Aman MG *et al*. Risperidone for the core symptom domains of autism: results from the study by the autism network of the research units on pediatric psychopharmacology. *Am J Psychiatry* 2005; **162**:1142-8.

McFarland HR, Fortin D. Amusia due to right temporoparietal infarct. *Arch Neurol* 1982; **39**:725-7.

McGonigle DJ, Hanninen R, Salenius S *et al*. Whose arm is it anyway? An fMRI study of supernumerary phantom limb. *Brain* 2002; **125**:1265-74.

McKee AC, Levine DN, Kowall NW *et al*. Peduncular hallucinosis associated with isolated infarction of the substantia nigra pars reticulata. *Ann Neurol* 1990; **27**:500-4.

McKeon J, McGuffin P, Robinson P. Obsessive-compulsive neurosis following head injury. A report of four cases. *Br J Psychiatry* 1984; **144**:190-2.

McMonagle P, Deering F, Berliner Y *et al*. The cognitive profile of posterior cortical atrophy. *Neurology* 2005; **66**:331-8.

Meadows JL, Munro SSF. Palinopsia. *J Neurol Neurosurg Psychiatry* 1977; **40**:5-8.

Melges FT, Tinklenberg JR, Hollister LE *et al*. Temporal disintegration and depersonalization during marijuana intoxication. *Arch Gen Psychiatry* 1970; **23**:204-10.

Mellor CS. First rank symptoms of schizophrenia. I. The frequency in schizophrenics on admission to hospital. II. Differences between individual first rank symptoms. *Br J Psychiatry* 1970; **117**:15-23.

Melzak R, Israel R, Lacroix R *et al*. Phantom limbs in people with congenital limb deficiency or amputation in early childhood. *Brain* 1997; **120**:1603-20.

Mendez MF. Corticobasal ganglionic degeneration with Balint's syndrome. *J Neuropsychiatry Clin Neurosci* 2000; **12**:273-5.

Mendez MF. Prominent echolalia from isolation of the speech area. *J Neuropsychiatry Clin Neurosci* 2002; **14**:56-7.

Mendez MF, Foti DJ. Lethal hyperoral behavior from the Kluver-Bucy syndrome. *J Neurol Neurosurg Psychiatry* 1997; **62**:293-4.

Mendez MF, Perryman KM. Neuropsychiatric features of frontotemporal dementia: evaluation of consensus criteria and review. *J Neuropsychiatry Clin Neurosci* 2002; **14**:424-9.

Mendez MF, Adams NL, Lewandowski KS. Neurobehavioral changes associated with caudate lesions. *Neurology* 1989; **39**:349–54.

Mendez MF, Selwood A, Mastri AR *et al.* Pick's disease versus Alzheimer's disease: a comparison of clinical characteristics. *Neurology* 1993; **43**:289–92.

Mendez MF, Cherrier MM, Perryman KM. Epileptic forced thinking from left frontal lesions. *Neurology* 1996; **47**:79–83.

Mendhekar DN, Duggal HS. Sertraline for Kluver-Bucy syndrome in an adolescent. *Eur Psychiatry* 2005; **20**:355–6.

Mendhekar DN, Sharma A, Inamdar A. Obsessive-compulsive disorder with hydrocephalus: effect of ventricular shunting. *J Neuropsychiatry Clin Neurosci* 2007; **19**:84.

Menza MA, Cocchiola J, Golbe LI. Psychiatric symptoms in progressive supranuclear palsy. *Psychosomatics* 1995; **36**:550–4.

Merrin EL, Silberfarb PM. The Capgras phenomenon. *Arch Gen Psychiatry* 1976; **33**:965–8.

Messert B, Henke TK, Langheim W. Syndrome of akinetic mutism associated with obstructive hydrocephalus. *Neurology* 1966; **16**:635–49.

Mesulam M-M. Dissociative states with abnormal temporal lobe EEG. *Arch Neurol* 1981; **38**:176–81.

Meyer JS, Greifenstein F, Devault M. A new drug causing symptoms of sensory deprivation. *J Nerv Ment Dis* 1959; **129**:54–61.

Michel EM, Troost BT. Palinopsia: cerebral localization with computed tomography. *Neurology* 1980; **30**:887–9.

Miguel EC, Coffey BJ, Baer L *et al.* Phenomenology of intentional repetitive behavior in obsessive-compulsive disorder and Tourette's disorder. *J Clin Psychiatry* 1995; **56**:246–55.

Miller TC, Crosby TW. Musical hallucinations in a deaf elderly patient. *Ann Neurol* 1979; **5**:301.

Mitchell SW. The effects of *Anhelonium lewinii* (the mescal button). *BMJ* 1896; **2**:1625–9.

Miyazawa N, Hayashi M, Komiya K *et al.* Supernumerary phantom limbs associated with left hemispheric stroke: case report and review of the literature. *Neurosurgery* 2004; **54**:228–31.

Monrad-Krohn GH. On the dissociation of voluntary and emotional innervation in facial paresis of central origin. *Brain* 1924; **47**:22–35.

Monrad-Krohn GH. Dysprosody or altered 'melody of language'. *Brain* 1947; **70**:405–15.

Montero J, Pena J, Genis D *et al.* Balint's syndrome. Report of four cases with watershed parieto-occipital lesions from vertebrobasilar ischemia or systemic hypotension. *Acta Neurol Belg* 1982; **82**:270–80.

Morgan CA, Hazlett G, Wang S *et al.* Symptoms of dissociation in humans experiencing acute uncontrollable stress: a prospective investigation. *Am J Psychiatry* 2001;**158**: 1239–47.

Mori E, Yamadori A. Unilateral hemispheric injury and ipsilateral instinctive grasp reaction. *Arch Neurol* 1985; **42**:485–8.

Motomura S, Tabira T, Kuroiwa Y. A clinical comparative study of multiple sclerosis and neuro-Behçet's syndrome. *J Neurol Neurosurg Psychiatry* 1980; **43**:210–13.

Mottard J-P, de la Sablonniere J-F. Olanzapine-induced obsessive-compulsive disorder. *Am J Psychiatry* 1999; **156**:799–800.

Mulder DW, Daly D. Psychiatric symptoms associated with lesions of temporal lobe. *J Am Med Assoc* 1952; **150**:173–6.

Mulder DW, Parrott M, Thaler M. Sequelae of western equine encephalitis. *Neurology* 1951; **1**:318–27.

Muller T, Buttner TH, Kuhn W *et al.* Palinopsia as sensory epileptic phenomenon. *Acta Neurol Scand* 1995; **91**:433–6.

Murata S, Naritomi H, Sawada T. Musical auditory hallucinations caused by a brainstem lesion. *Neurology* 1994; **44**:156–8.

Nakada T, Lee H, Kwee IL *et al.* Epileptic Kluver–Bucy syndrome: case report. *J Clin Psychiatry* 1984; **45**:87–8.

Neary D, Snowden JS, Mann DMA. Familial progressive atrophy: its relationship to other forms of lobar atrophy. *J Neurol Neurosurg Psychiatry* 1993; **56**:1122–5.

Nedjam Z, Devouche E, Della Barabara G. Confabulation, but not executive dysfunction discriminate AD from frontotemporal dementia. *Eur J Neurol* 2004; **11**:728–33.

Nielsen JM. The cortical components of akinetic mutism. *J Nerv Ment Dis* 1951; **114**:459–61.

Nishkawa T, Okuda J, Mizuta I *et al.* Conflict of intentions due to callosal disconnection. *J Neurol Neurosurg Psychiatry* 2001; **63**:462–71.

Noda S, Mizoguchi M, Yamamoto A. Thalamic experiential hallucinosis. *J Neurol Neurosurg Psychiatry* 1993; **56**:1224–6.

Nordgren RE, Markesbery WR, Fukada K *et al.* Seven cases of cerebromedullospinal disconnection: the 'locked-in' syndrome. *Neurology* 1971; **21**:1140–8.

Noyes R, Kletti R. Depersonalization in accident victims and psychiatric patients. *Compr Psychiatry* 1977; **18**:375–84.

Noyes R, Hoenk P, Kuperman S *et al.* Depersonalization in accident victims and psychiatric patients. *J Nerv Ment Dis* 1977; **164**:401–7.

Nurnberg HG, Greenwald B. Stuttering: an unusual side-effect of phenothiazines. *Am J Psychiatry* 1981; **138**:386–7.

Nyatsanza S, Shetty T, Gregory C *et al.* A study of stereotypic behaviors in Alzheimer's disease and frontal and temporal variant frontotemporal dementia. *J Neurol Neurosurg Psychiatry* 2003; **74**:1398–402.

O'Hare JA, Callaghan NM, Murnaghan DJ. Dialysis encephalopathy. Clinical, electroencephalographic, and interventional aspects. *Medicine* 1983; **62**:129–41.

Oliveira V, Ferro JM, Foreid JP *et al.* Kluver-Bucy syndrome in systemic lupus erythematosus. *J Neurol* 1989; **236**:55–6.

O'Sullivan D, Dean C. The Fregoli syndrome and puerperal psychosis. *Br J Psychiatry* 1991; **159**:274–7.

Ott BR. Leuprolide treatment of sexual aggression in a patient with dementia and the Kluver-Bucy syndrome. *Clin Neuropharmacol* 1995; **18**:443–7.

Panayiotopoulos CP. Elementary visual hallucinations in migraine and epilepsy. *J Neurol Neurosurg Psychiatry* 1994; **57**:1371–4.

Panitch HS, Thisted RA, Smith RA *et al.* Randomized controlled trial of dextromethorphan/quinidine for pseudobulbar affect in multiple sclerosis. *Ann Neurol* 2006; **59**:780–7.

Parkes JD, Baraitser M, Marsden CD *et al.* Natural history, symptoms and treatment of the narcoleptic syndrome. *Acta Neurol Scand* 1975; **52**:337–53.

Parkinson D, Rucker CW, McK Craig W. Visual hallucinations associated with tumors of the occipital lobe. *Arch Neurol Psychiatry* 1952; **68**:60–8.

Parvizi J, Joseph J, Press DZ *et al.* Pathological laughter and crying in patients with multiple system atrophy-cerebellar type. *Mov Disord* 2007; **22**:798–803.

Paskind HA. Parosmia in tumorous involvement of olfactory bulbs and nerves. *Arch Neurol Psychiatry* 1935; **33**:835–8.

Patterson JF. Carbamazepine in the treatment of phantom limb pain. *South Med J* 1988;**81**:1100–2.

Paulig M, Mentrup H. Charles Bonnet's syndrome: complete remission of complex visual hallucinations treated by gabapentin. *J Neurol Neurosurg Psychiatry* 2001; **70**:813–14.

Pazzaglia P, D'Alessandro R, Ambrosetto G *et al.* Drop attacks: an ominous change in the evolution of partial epilepsy. *Neurology* 1985; **35**:1725–30.

Penfield W, Jasper H. *Epilepsy and the functional anatomy of the human brain.* Boston: Little, Brown and Company, 1954, pp. 383–4.

Penfield W, Perot P. The brain's record of auditory and visual experience. *Brain* 1963; **86**:595.

Perez FM, Tunkel RS, Lachmann EA *et al.* Balint's syndrome arising from bilateral posterior cortical atrophy or infarction: rehabilitation strategies and their limitation. *Disabil Rehabil* 1996; **18**:300–4.

Piccirilli M, Sciarma T, Luzzi S. Modularity of music: evidence from a case of pure amusia. *J Neurol Neurosurg Psychiatry* 2000; **69**:541–5.

Pick A. On reduplicative paramnesia. *Brain* 1903; **26**:260–7.

Pitt DC, Kriel RL, Wagner NC *et al.* Kluver–Bucy syndrome following heat stroke in a 12-year-old girl. *Pediatr Neurology* 1995; **13**:73–6.

Powers JM, Schaumburg HH, Gaffney CL. Kluver–Bucy syndrome caused by adrenoleukodystrophy. *Neurology* 1980; **30**:1131–2.

Power-Smith P, Turkington D. Fluoxetine in phantom limb pain. *Br J Psychiatry* 1993; **163**:105–6.

Psarros T, Zours A, Coimbra C. Bromocriptine-responsive akinetic mutism following endoscopy for ventricular neurocysticercosis. Case report and review of the literature. *J Neurosurg* 2003; **99**:397–401.

Rabinowitz J, Katz JR, De Deyn PP *et al.* Behavioral and psychological symptoms in patients with dementia as a target for pharmacotherapy with risperidone. *J Clin Psychiatry* 2004; **65**:1329–34.

Radhakrishnan J, Mathew K, Richard J *et al.* Schneider's first rank symptoms – prevalence, diagnostic use and prognostic implications. *Br J Psychiatry* 1983; **142**:557–9.

Rashiq S, Briewa L, Moooney M *et al.* Distinguishing aclovir neurotoxicity from encephalomyelitis. *J Int Med* 1993; **234**:507–11.

Rasmussen KG, Rummans TA. Electroconvulsive therapy for phantom limb pain. *Pain* 2000; **85**:297–9.

Rasmussen SA, Tsuang MT. Clinical characteristics and family history in DSM-III obsessive-compulsive disorder. *Am J Psychiatry* 1986; **143**:317–22.

Rayport M, Ferguson SM, Corrie WS. Outcomes and indications of corpus callosum section for intractable seizure control. *Appl Neurophysiol* 1983; **46**:47–51.

Reeves RR, Norton JW. Foreign accent-like syndrome during psychotic exacerbations. *Neurpsychiatry Neuropsychol Behav Neurol* 2001; **14**:135–8.

Reeves RR, Burke RS, Parker JD. Characterization of psychotic patients with foreign accent syndrome. *J Neuropsychiatry Clin Neurosci* 2007; **19**:70–6.

Regli F, Filippa G, Wiesendanger M. Hereditary mirror movements. *Arch Neurol* 1967; **16**:620.

Remillard GM, Andermann F, Rhi-Sausa A *et al.* Facial asymmetry in patients with temporal lobe epilepsy. *Neurology* 1977; **27**:109–14.

Remington G, Sloman L, Konstantareas M *et al.* Clomipramine versus haloperidol in the treatment of autistic disorder: a double-blind, placebo-controlled, crossover study. *J Clin Psychopharmacol* 2001; **21**:440–4.

Renner JA, Burns JM, Hou CE *et al.* Progressive posterior cortical dysfunction. A clinicopathologic series. *Neurology* 2004; **63**:1175–80.

Riddoch G. Phantom limbs and body shape. *Brain* 1941; **64**:197–222.

Riley DE, Lang AE, Resch L *et al.* Cortico-basal ganglionic degeneration. *Neurology* 1990; **40**:1203–12.

Rinne JO, Lee MS, Thompson PD *et al.* Cortico-basal degeneration. *Brain* 1994; **117**:1183–96.

Roberts JM. Echolalia and comprehension in autistic children. *J Autism Dev Disord* 1989; **19**:271–81.

Roberts K, Vass N. Schneiderian first-rank symtoms caused by benzodiazepine withdrawal. *Br J Psychiatry* 1986; **148**:593–4.

Robertson MM, Trimble MR, Lees AJ. The psychopathology of Gilles de la Tourette's syndrome: a phenomenological analysis. *Br J Psychiatry* 1988; **182**:388–90.

Robinson RG, Parikh RM, Lipsey JR *et al.* Pathological laughing and crying following stroke; validation of a measurement scale and a double-blind treatment study. *Am J Psychiatry* 1993; **150**:286–93.

Rosenfeld MR, Eichen JG, Wade DF *et al.* Molecular and clinical diversity in paraneoplastic immunity to Ma proteins. *Ann Neurol* 2001; **50**:339–48.

Ross ED, Stewart RM. Akinetic mutism from hypothalamic damage: successful treatment with dopamine agonists. *Neurology* 1981; **31**:1435–9.

Ross ED, Jossman PB, Bell B *et al.* Musical hallucinations in deafness. *JAMA* 1975; **231**:620–1.

Ross RT, Mathiesen R. Images in clinical medicine: volitional and emotional supranuclear facial weakness. *N Engl J Med* 1998; **338**:1515.

Rosse RB, Collins JP, Fay-McCarthy M *et al.* Phenomenologic comparison of the idiopathic psychosis of schizophrenia and drug-induced cocaine and phencyclidine psychoses: a retrospective study. *Clin Neuropharmacol* 1994; **17**:359–69.

Rosselli M, Ardila A, Beltran C. Rehabilitation of Balint's syndrome: a single case report. *Appl Neuropsychol* 2001; **8**:242–7.

Rossitch E, Bullard DE. The autonomic dysfunction syndrome: aetiology and treatment. *Br J Neurosurg* 1988; **2**:471–8.

Rumsey JM, Andreasen NC, Rapoport JL. Thought, language, communication and affective flattening in autistic adults. *Arch Gen Psychiatry* 1986; **43**:771–7.

Russell MB, Olesen J. A nosographic analysis of the migraine aura in a general population. *Brain* 1996; **119**:355–61.

Russell SM, Golfinos JG. Amusia following resection of Heschl gyrus glioma. Case report. *J Neurosurg* 2003; **98**:1109–12.

Russell WR, Whitty CWM. Studies in traumatic epilepsy. 2. Focal motor and somatic sensory fits: a study of 85 cases. *J Neurol Neurosurg Psychiatry* 1953; **16**:73–97.

Russell WR, Whitty CWM. Studies in traumatic epilepsy. 3. Visual fits. *J Neurol Neurosurg Psychiatry* 1955; **18**:79–96.

Sachdev P. Schizophrenia-like illness in velo-cardio-facial syndrome: a genetic subsyndrome of schizophrenia? *J Psychosom Res* 2002; **53**:721–7.

Sandson J, Albert ML. Perseveration in behavioral neurology. *Neurology* 1987; **37**: 1736–41.

Santhouse AM, Howard RJ, ffytche DH. Visual hallucinatory syndrome and the anatomy of the visual brain. *Brain* 2000;**123**:2055–64.

Sarkar J, Jones N, Sulivan G. A case of depersonalization-derealization syndrome during treatment with quetiapine. *J Psychopharmacol* 2001; **15**:209–11.

Schielke E, Reuter U, Hoffmnn O et al. Musical hallucinations with dorsal pontine lesions. *Neurology* 2000; **55**:454–5.

Schiff HB, Alexander MP, Naeser MA et al. Aphemia: clinical-anatomic correlations. *Arch Neurol* 1983; **40**:720–7.

Schiffer RB, Herndon RM, Rudick RA. Treatment of pathologic laughing and weeping with amitriptyline. *N Engl J Med* 1985; **312**:1480–2.

Schley M, Topfner S, Wiech K et al. Continuous brachial plexus blockade in combination with the NMDA receptor antagonist memantine prevents phantom limb pain in acute traumatic upper limb amputees. *Eur J Pain* 2007; **11**:299–308.

Schneider K. *Clinical psychopathology.* London: Grune & Stratton, 1959.

Schnider A, Bonvallat J, Emond H et al. Reality confusion in spontaneous confabulation. *Neurology* 2005; **65**:1117–19.

Schott GD, Wyke MA. Congenital mirror movements. *J Neurol Neurosurg Psychiatry* 1981; **44**:586–99.

Schultz G, Melzack R. Visual hallucinations and mental state: a study of 14 Charles Bonnet syndrome hallucinations. *J Nerv Ment Dis* 1993; **181**:639–43.

Schwartz JI, Moura RJ. Severe depersonalization and anxiety associated with indomethacin. *South Med J* 1983; **76**:679–80.

Schwartz W, Stakes JW, Jobson JA. Transient cataplexy after removal of a craniopharyngioma. *Neurology* 1984; **34**:1372–5.

Sears LL, Vest C, Mohamed S et al. An MRI study of the basal ganglia in autism. *Prog Neuropsychopharmacol Biol Psychiatry* 1999; **23**:613–24.

Sedman G. Depersonalization in a group of normal subjects. *Br J Psychiatry* 1966; **112**:907–12.

Selby G, Lance JW. Observations on 500 cases of migraine and allied vascular headache. *J Neurol Neurosurg Psychiatry* 1960; **23**:23–32.

Seliger GM, Abrams GM, Horton A. Irish brogue after stroke. *Stroke* 1992; **23**:1655–6.

Serra Catafau J, Rubio R, Peres Serra J. Peduncular halucinosis associated with posterior thalamic infarction. *J Neurol* 1992; **239**:89–90.

Serra-Mestres J, Shapleske J, Tym E. Treatment of palilalia with trazodone. *Am J Psychiatry* 1996; **153**:580–1.

Seyffarth H, Denny-Brown D. The grasp reflex and the instinctive grasp reflex. *Brain* 1948; **71**:109–83.

Shahed J, Jankovic J. Re-emergence of childhood stuttering in Parkinson's disease: an hypothesis. *Mov Disord* 2001; **16**:114–18.

Shallice T, Burgess PW, Schon F et al. The origins of utilization behavior. *Brain* 1989; **112**:1587–98.

Shaw KM, Lees AJ, Stern GM. The impact of treatment with levodopa on Parkinson's disease. *Q J Med* 1980; **49**:283–93.

Shoji H, Teramoto H, Satowa S et al. Partial Kluver–Bucy syndrome following probable herpes simplex encephalitis. *J Neurol* 1979; **221**:163–7.

Shopsin B, Hirsch J, Gershon S. Visual hallucinations and propranolol. *Biol Psychiatry* 1975; **10**:105–7.

Shorvon H. The depersonalization syndrome. *Proc R Soc Med* 1946; **39**:779–92.

Shukla GD, Sahu SC, Tripathi RP et al. Phantom limb: a phenomenological study. *Br J Psychiatry* 1982; **141**:54–8.

Sichel DA, Cohen LS, Dimmock JA et al. Postpartum obsessive compulsive disorder: a case series. *J Clin Psychiatry* 1993; **54**:156–9.

Siegel A, Harrow M, Reilly FE et al. Loose associations and disordered speech patterns in chronic schizophrenia. *J Nerv Ment Dis* 1976; **162**:105–12.

Siegel RK. Cocaine hallucinations. *Am J Psychiatry* 1978; **135**:309–14.

Simeon D, Gross C, Guralnik O et al. Feeling unreal: 30 cases of DSM-III-R depersonalization disorder. *Am J Psychiatry* 1997; **154**:1107–13.

Simeon D, Knutelska M, Nelson O et al. Feeling unreal: a depersonalization disorder update of 117 cases. *J Clin Psychiatry* 2003; **64**:990–7.

Simmel ML. Phantom experiences following amputation in childhood. *J Neurol Neurosurg Psychiatry* 1962; **25**:69–78.

Simpson S, Baldwin B. Neuropsychiatry and SPECT of an acute obsessive-compulsive syndrome patient. *Br J Psychiatry* 1995; **166**:390–7.

Sjogren M, Wallin A, Edman A. Symptomatological differences distinguish between frontotemporal dementia and vascular dementia with a dominant frontal lobe syndrome. *Int J Geriatr Psychiatry* 1997; **12**:656–61.

Slater E, Beard AW. The schizophrenia-like psychoses of epilepsy. i. Psychiatric aspects. *Br J Psychiatry* 1963; **109**:95–112.

Slatterly MJ, Dubbert BK, Allen AJ et al. Prevalence of obsessive-compulsive disorder in patients with systemic lupus erythematosus. *J Clin Psychiatry* 2004; **65**:301–6.

Smit LS, Lammers GJ, Catsman-Berrevoets CE. Cataplexy leading to the diagnosis of Niemann-Pick disease type C. *Pediatr Neurol* 2006; **35**:82–4.

Smith DG, Ehds DM, Hanley MA et al. Efficacy of gabapentin in treating chronic phantom limb and residual limb pain. *J Rehabil Res Dev* 2005; **42**:645–54.

Smith KU, Akelaitis AJ. Studies on the corpus callosum. I. Laterality in behavior and bilateral motor organization in man before and after section of the corpus callosum. *Arch Neurol Psychiatry* 1942; **47**:519–43.

Snowden JS, Neary D, Mann DMA *et al.* Progressive language disorder due to lobar atrophy. *Ann Neurol* 1992; **31**:174–83.

Soros P, Vo G, Husstedt I-W *et al.* Phantom eye syndrome. Its prevalence, phenomenology and putative mechanisms. *Neurology* 2003; **60**:1542–3.

Souques A. Palilalia. *Rev Neurol* 1908; **16**:340–3.

Sowa MV, Pituck S. Prolonged spontaneous complex visual hallucinations and illusions as ictal phenomena. *Epilepsia* 1989; **30**:524–6.

Soyka M, Naber G, Volcker A. Prevalence of delusional jealousy in different psychiatrc disorders. *Br J Psychiatry* 1991; **158**:549–53.

Sparr SA. Receptive amelodia in a trained musician. *Neurology* 2002; **59**:1659–60.

Sperry RW. Brain bisection and mechanisms of consciousness. In: Eccles JC ed. *Brain and conscious experience.* New York: Springer-Verlag, 1966.

Stacy M, Cardoso F, Jankovic J. Tardive stereotypy and other movement disorders in tardive dyskinesias. *Neurology* 1993; **43**:937–41.

Stahl SM, Layzer RB, Aminoff MJ *et al.* Continuous cataplexy in a patient with a midbrain tumor: the limp man syndrome. *Neurology* 1980; **30**:1115–18.

Stamouli S, Lykouras L. Quetiapine-induced obsessive-compulsive symptoms: a series of five cases. *J Clin Psychopharmacol* 2006; **26**:396–400.

Starkstein SE, Berthier M, Leiguarda R. Disconnection syndrome in a right-handed patient with right hemispheric speech dominance. *Eur Neurol* 1988; **28**:187–90.

Starkstein SE, Federoff JP, Price TR *et al.* Catastrophic reaction after cerebrovascular lesions: frequency, correlates, and validation of a scale. *J Neuropsychiatry Clin Neurosci* 1993; **5**:189–94.

Starkstein SE, Migliorelli R, Teson A *et al.* Prevalence and clinical correlates of pathological affective display in Alzheimer's disease. *J Neurol Neurosurg Psychiatry* 1995; **59**:55–60.

Steinhausen H-C, Juzi C. Elective mutism: an analysis of 100 cases. *J Am Acad Child Adolesc Psychiatry* 1996; **35**:606–14.

Stewart JT. Carbamazepine treatment of a patient with Kluver-Bucy syndrome. *J Clin Psychiatry* 1985; **46**:496–7.

Stewart-Wallace AM. An unusual case of the grasp reflex, with some observations on the volitional and reflex components. *J Neurol Neurosurg Psychiatry* 1939; **2**:149–53.

Suwanwela NC, Leelacheavasit N. Isolated corpus callosal infarction secondary to pericallosal artery disease presenting as alien hand syndrome. *J Neurol Neurosurg Psychiatry* 2002; **72**:533–6.

Swedo SE, Rapoport JL, Cheslow DL *et al.* High prevalence of obsessive-compulsive symptoms in patients with Sydenham's chorea. *Am J Psychiatry* 1989; **146**:246–9.

Swedo SE, Leonard HL, Schapiro MB *et al.* Sydenham's chorea: physical and psychological symptoms of St. Vitus dance. *Pediatrics* 1993; **91**:706–13.

Takayama Y, Sugishita M, Kido T *et al.* A case of foreign accent syndrome without aphasia caused by a lesion of the left precentral gyrus. *Neurology* 1993; **43**:1361–3.

Tanaka Y, Iwasa H, Yoshuida M. Diagonistic dyspraxia: case report and movement-related potentials. *Neurology* 1990; **40**:657–61.

Tanaka Y, Yoshida A, Kawahata N *et al.* Diagnostic dyspraxia: clinical characteristics, responsible lesions and possible underlying mechanism. *Brain* 1996; **119**:859–74.

Tandon R, Greden JF. Schneiderian first rank symptoms: reconfirmation of high specificity for schizophrenia. *Acta Psychiatr Scand* 1987; **75**:392–6.

Tang-Wai DF, Graff-Radford NR, Boeve BF *et al.* Clinical, genetic, and neuropathologic characteristics of posterior cortical atrophy. *Neurology* 2004; **63**:1168–74.

Tateno A, Jorge RE, Robinson RG. Pathological laughing and crying following traumatic brain injury. *J Neuropsychiatry Clin Neurosci* 2004; **16**:426–34.

Teri L, Larson EB, Reifler BV. Behavioral disturbance in dementia of the Alzheimer's type. *J Am Ger Soc* 1988; **36**:1–6.

Terzian H, Dalle Ore G. Syndrome of Kluver and Bucy: reproduced in man by bilateral removal of the temporal lobes. *Neurology* 1955; **5**:373–80.

Teunisse RJ, Zitman FG, Raes DCM. Clinical evaluation of 14 patients with the Charles Bonnet syndrome (isolated visual hallucinations). *Compr Psychiatry* 1994; **35**:70–5.

Teunisse RJ, Cruysberg JRM, Verbeek A *et al.* The Charles Bonnet syndrome: a large prospective study in the Netherlands. *Br J Psychiatry* 1995; **166**:234–57.

Teunisse RJ, Cruysberg JR, Hoefnagels WH *et al.* Visual hallucinations in psychologically normal people: Charles Bonnet's syndrome. *Lancet* 1996; **347**:794–7.

Thajeb P. Progressive late delayed postirradiation encephalopathy with Kluver-Bucy syndrome. Serial MRI and clinico-pathological studies. *Clin Neurol Neurosurg* 1995; **97**:264–8.

Thompson AE, Swan M. Capgras syndrome presenting with violence following heavy drinking. *Br J Psychiatry* 1993; **162**:692–4.

Thompson JC, Stopford CL, Snowden JS *et al.* Qualitative neuropsychological performance characteristics in frontotemporal dementia and Alzheimer's disease. *J Neurol Neurosurg Psychiatry* 2005; **76**:920–7.

Thorley RR, Wertsch JJ, Kingbell GE. Acute hypothalamic instability in traumatic brain injury: a case report. *Arch Phys Med Rehabil* 2001; **82**:246–9.

Tilberti C, Sabe L, Kuzis G *et al.* Prevalence and correlates of the catastrophic reaction in Alzheimer's disease. *Neurology* 1998; **50**:546–8.

Tilney F. Pseudobulbar palsy clinically and pathologically considered with the clinical report of five cases. *J Nerv Ment Dis* 1912; **39**:505–35.

Trethowan WH, Cobb S. Neuropsychiatric aspects of Cushing's syndrome. *Arch Neurol Psychiatry* 1952; **67**:283–309.

Trosch RM, Sze G, Brass LM *et al.* Emotional facial paresis with striatocapsular infarction. *J Neurol Sci* 1990; **98**:195–201.

Tuke DH. Imperative ideas. *Brain* 1894; **17**:179–97.

Turgut N, Utku U, Balci K. A case of acquired stuttering resulting from left parietal infarction. *Acta Neurol Scand* 2002; **105**:408–10.

Tweedy J, Reding M, Garcia C *et al.* Significance of cortical disinhibition signs. *Neurology* 1981; **31**:169–73.

Ueda N, Tarao T, Ohmori O *et al.* Schneiderian first-rank symptoms associated with fluvoxamine treatment: a case report. *Hum Psychopharmacol* 2003; **18**:477–8.

Ukai S, Yamamoto M, Tanaka M *et al*. Treatment of typical Charles Bonnet syndrome with donepezil. *Int Clin Psychopharmacol* 2004; **19**:355–7.

Uzunca I, Utku U, Asil T *et al*. 'Fou rire prodromique' associated with simultaneous bilateral capsular genu infarction. *J Clin Neurosci* 2005; **12**:174–5.

Valldeoriola F, Graus F, Rimola A *et al*. Cyclosporine-induced mutism in liver transplant patients. *Neurology* 1996; **46**:252–4.

Van den Hoed J, Lucas EA, Dement WC. Hallucinatory experiences during cataplexy in patients with narcolepsy. *Am J Psychiatry* 1979; **136**:1210–11.

Van Der Werf YD, Weerts JGE, Jolles J *et al*. Neuropsychological correlates of a right unilateral lacunar thalamic infarction. *J Neurol Neurosurg Psychiatry* 1999; **66**:36–42.

Van Dijk JG, Lammers GJ, Blansjaar BA. Isolated cataplexy of more than 40 years duration. *Br J Psychiatry* 1991; **154**:719–21.

Van Dongen HR, Catsman-Berrevoets CE, van Mourik M. The syndrome of 'cerebellar' mutism and subsequent dysarthria. *Neurology* 1994; **44**:2040–6.

Van Hilten JJ, Buruma OJ, Kessing P *et al*. Pathologic crying as a prominent behavioral manifestation of central pontine myelinolysis. *Arch Neurol* 1988; **45**:936.

Van Waggenen WP, Herren RY. Surgical division of commisural pathways in the corpus callosum: relation to spread of an epileptic attack. *Arch Neurol Psychiatry* 1940; **44**:740–57.

Vaphiades MS, Celesia GG, Brigell MG. Positive spontaneous visual phenomena limited to the hemianopic field in lesions of central visual pathways. *Neurology* 1996; **47**:408–17.

Varon D, Pritchard PB, Wagner MT *et al*. Transient Kluver-Bucy syndrome following complex partial status epilepticus. *Epilepsy Behav* 2003; **4**:348–51.

Victoroff J, Ross GW, Benson DF *et al*. Posterior cortical atrophy. Neuropathologic correlations. *Arch Neurol* 1994; **51**:269–74.

Vollenweider FX, Gamma A, Liechti M *et al*. Psychological and cardiovascular effects and short-term sequelae of MDMA ('ecstasy') in MDMA-naive healthy volunteers. *Neuropsychopharmacology* 1998; **19**:241–51.

Vreeling FW, Verhey FR, Houx PJ *et al*. Primitive reflexes in Parkinson's disease. *J Neurol Neurosurg Psychiatry* 1993; **56**:1323–6.

Vreeling FW, Houx PJ, Jolles J *et al*. Primitive reflexes in Alzheimer's disease and vascular dementia. *J Geriatr Psychiatr Neurol* 1995; **8**:111–17.

Vuilleumier P, Reverdin A, Landis T. Four legs: illusory reduplication of the lower limbs after bilateral parietal lobe damage. *Arch Neurol* 1997; **54**:1543–7.

Waite LM, Broe GA, Creasey H *et al*. Neurological signs, aging, and the neurodegenerative syndromes. *Arch Neurol* 1996; **53**:498–502.

Wali GM. 'Fou rire prodromique' heralding a brainstem stroke. *J Neurol Neurosurg Psychiatry* 1993; **56**:209–10.

Walshe FMR. On certain tonic or postural reflexes in hemiplegia with special reference to the so-called 'associated movements'. *Brain* 1923; **46**:1–37.

Walshe FMR, Hunt JH. Further observations upon grasping movements and reflex tonic grasping. *Brain* 1936; **59**:315–23.

Walshe FMR, Robertson EG. Observations upon the form and nature of the 'grasping' movements and 'tonic innervation' seen in certain cases of lesions of the frontal lobe. *Brain* 1933; **56**:40–70.

Watson RT, Heilman KM. Callosal apraxia. *Brain* 1983; **106**:391–403.

Watson RT, Heilman KM, Bowers D. Magnetic resonance imaging (MRI, NMR) scan in a case of callosal apraxia and pseudoneglect. *Brain* 1985; **108**:535–6.

Weinstein EA, Kahn RL, Malitz S *et al*. Delusional reduplication of parts of the body. *Brain* 1954; **77**:45–60.

Weinstein S, Sersen EA. Phantoms in cases of congenital absence of limbs. *Neurology* 1961; **11**:905–11.

Wergeland H. Elective mutism. *Acta Psychiatr Scand* 1979; **59**:218–28.

White NJ. Complex visual hallucinations in partial blindness due to eye disease. *Br J Psychiatry* 1980; **136**:284–6.

Wiech K, Kiefer RT, Topfner S *et al*. A placebo-controlled randomized crossover trial of the N-methyl-D-aspartate acid receptor antagonist, memantine, in patients with chronic phantom limb pain. *Anesth Analg* 2004; **98**:408–13.

Wijdicks EF, Wiesner RH, Dahlke LJ *et al*. FK506-induced neurotoxicity in liver transplantation. *Ann Neurol* 1994; **35**:498–501.

Williams D. The structure of emotions reflected in epileptic experiences. *Brain* 1956; **79**:29–67.

Wilson DH, Reeves A, Gazzaniga M. Cerebral commisurotomy for control of intractable seizures. *Neurology* 1977; **27**:708–15.

Wilson SAK. Some problems in neurology. II. Pathological laughing and crying. *J Neurol Psychopathology* 1924; **4**:299–333.

Wilson SAK. The narcolepsies. *Brain* 1928; **51**:63–109.

Wilson SAK. *Neurology*, 2nd edn. London: Butterworth & Co, 1954.

Wolberg FL, Ziegler DK. Olfactory hallucinations in migraine. *Arch Neurol* 1982; **39**:382.

Yamamaka K, Fukuyama H, Kimura J. Abulia from unilateral capsular genu infarction: report of two cases. *J Neurol Sci* 1996; **143**:181–4.

Yasuda Y, Akiguchi I, Ino M *et al*. Paramedian thalamic and midbrain infarcts associated with palilalia. *J Neurol Neurosurg Psychiatry* 1990; **53**:797–9.

Zarcone V. Narcolepsy. *N Engl J Med* 1973; **288**:1154–66.

Zeidler M, Johnstone EC, Bamber RWK *et al*. New variant Creutzfeldt–Jakob disease: psychiatric features. *Lancet* 1997; **350**:908–10.

Zelig G, Drubach DA, Katz-Zelig M *et al*. Pathological laughter and crying in patients with closed traumatic brain injury. *Brain Inj* 1996; **10**:591–7.

Ziegler LH. Psychotic and emotional phenomena associated with amyotrophic lateral sclerosis. *Arch Neurol Psychiatry* 1930; **24**:930–6.

5

Syndromes of cognitive impairment

5.1 DEMENTIA

The dementias constitute one of the most common syndromes seen in neuropsychiatric practice. Accurate diagnosis is critical not only for prognostic purposes, but also because a not insignificant number of the diseases capable of causing dementia are treatable.

Clinical features

Dementia is a syndrome of multiple different etiologies characterized by a global decrement in cognitive functioning occurring in a clear sensorium, without significant confusion (Cummings 1987). When the condition is fully developed, patients display deficits in memory, abstracting abilities, calculations, and judgment.

Memory impairment is manifest most prominently with short-term memory loss, as manifest during examination by an inability to recall all out of three words after 5 minutes; this memory loss may be apparent as one obtains a history and finds that patients have forgotten where they put their keys or wallets, or tend to forget what family members have told them earlier. Long-term memory also suffers, although not as severely as does the short-term type: patients may be unable to recall public facts, such as the names of the last four presidents, or biographical facts, such as where they last worked, or where they went to school. Whenever memory impairment is present, one also typically finds partial or complete disorientation to time and, albeit less commonly, to place.

Abstracting ability is tested formally by asking patients to interpret familiar proverbs, such as 'don't count your chickens before they hatch' and watching for a 'concrete' response, such as 'well, they might not all hatch', rather than an 'abstract' one, such as 'don't count on things'. Difficulty with abstract thinking may also be evident in the patient's daily life, depending on the cognitive demands

occasioned by the patient's day-to-day life. For example, an accountant may find it no longer possible to understand complex accounting formulae or a chess player may find it impossible to think out moves.

Calculating ability is tested for by asking patients to do simple arithmetic, such as subtracting 8 from 12, and, if they perform well at this task, asking them to perform 'serial 7's' by first subtracting 7 from 100, then 7 from that answer, etc. Any deficits here must be judged in light of the patients' educational experience and their premorbid abilities. Difficulties with calculations may be evident in day-to-day life as patients have trouble making change or balancing a checkbook.

A loss of good judgment is often what first calls patients to medical attention. Patients may make ruinous financial agreements or allow themselves to be misled in a variety of ways.

Some patients, impaired by these cognitive deficits, may experience a 'catastrophic reaction'. As discussed in more detail in Section 4.24, these patients become acutely agitated when they find themselves unable to accomplish a cognitive task that, premorbidly, would have caused no difficulty.

In addition to these symptoms one often sees a personality change. This may be of a specific type, such as the frontal lobe syndrome, but is more often non-specific. In some cases, previously maladaptive traits may become accentuated, as when an overly thrifty person becomes miserly. In other cases, new traits may appear: a previously shy person may become overly familiar or a well-mannered person may become sloppy and crude.

Other deficits, such as aphasia, apraxia, or agnosia, may or may not be present, depending on the underlying cause of the dementia.

Dementia may also be accompanied by agitation and delusions or hallucinations. The delusions tend to be persecutory and patients may accuse others of stealing from them. Delusions of infidelity may also occur and patients may accuse spouses of having affairs. One may also encounter the 'phantom boarder' delusion wherein patients believe that someone is hiding in the house, perhaps in the basement or attic. Hallucinations tend to be visual and may be quite complex: patients may see animals or people. Auditory hallucinations, although less common, may also occur, and patients may hear music, voices, or bells.

Depression is common, and insomnia, with or without depression, may also occur.

Etiology

The causes of dementia are numerous, as indicated by the lengthy list provided in Table 5.1. In an attempt to bring some order to the differential task, the various causes are divided into several groups. The first group to consider contains those disorders which may cause a dementia *of gradual or subacute onset, often lacking in distinctive features*, such as Alzheimer's disease. Next is a group of vascular disorders, all of which may cause a dementia *in the setting of a history of strokes*, for example multi-infarct dementia. Following this is a group of disorders that tend to present with a dementia *characterized by a frontal lobe syndrome*, as may be seen in frontotemporal dementia. The next group contains those disorders that may present *with a progressive aphasia*, which, subsequently, and gradually, evolves into a dementia, as may be seen in a variety of neurodegenerative disorders.

The next groups are each marked by dementia occurring in concert with a movement disorder. Such abnormal movements must be carefully sought for in the examination as they provide very valuable diagnostic clues: these groups include dementia occurring *with parkinsonism* (e.g., Parkinson's disease), *chorea* (e.g., Huntington's disease), *dystonia* (e.g., corticobasal ganglionic degeneration), *myoclonus* (e.g., Creutzfeldt–Jakob disease), and *ataxia* (e.g., multiple system atrophy).

The next group in the list is a heterogeneous one, containing a number of disorders, each *with distinctive features*, for example the tendon enlargement seen in cerebrotendinous xanthomatosis. Following this is a group characterized by dementias occurring *with obvious precipitating events*, such as traumatic brain injury with subdural hematoma or diffuse axonal injury.

Next is a group of disorders, each causing dementia *in the setting of mental retardation*, as may be seen in Down's syndrome. Finally, there is a group of *miscellaneous causes*, for example systemic lupus erythematosus.

In working up a patient with dementia, it is reasonable to keep in mind the most common causes: Alzheimer's disease, diffuse Lewy body disease, multi-infarct dementia, Parkinson's disease and traumatic brain injury. Furthermore, given the frequency with which these occur, it is not at all uncommon to find patients with a 'mixed' dementia, for example a combination of Alzheimer's disease and multi-infarct dementia (Molsa *et al.* 1985).

If, after a thorough history and examination, the cause of the dementia is still not clear, one may consider choosing from among the following 'screening' tests: complete blood count (CBC) chemistry survey, magnetic resonance (MR) scanning, thyroid profile, vitamin B12 and folate levels, fluorescent treponemal antibody (FTA), anti-nuclear antibody (ANA), and erythrocyte sedimentation rate (ESR).

OF GRADUAL OR SUBACUTE ONSET, OFTEN LACKING IN DISTINCTIVE FEATURES

Of all the disorders capable of causing a dementia of more or less gradual onset without distinctive features, Alzheimer's disease is the most common, followed by diffuse Lewy body disease and two vascular disorders, namely Binswanger's disease and lacunar dementia. Other disorders to keep in mind, in large part because they are eminently treatable, include hypothyroidism, hyperthyroidism, vitamin B12 deficiency, folate deficiency, depression, and, in some cases, tumors and hydrocephalus. Infectious disorders that may or may not yield to treatment include AIDS dementia, Lyme disease and neurosyphilis. The other disorders listed in this section are all relatively rare causes of dementia presenting in this fashion.

Alzheimer's disease is typically of gradual or insidious onset, often presenting with a gradually worsening amnesia (Goodman 1953; Linn *et al.* 1995), which is eventually joined by various 'cortical' signs such as aphasia, apraxia, and primitive reflexes (Huff *et al.* 1987; Price *et al.* 1993).

Diffuse Lewy body disease may present with a gradually progressive dementia that, early on, may be difficult to distinguish from that seen in Alzheimer's disease. Helpful differential clues include visual hallucinations, spontaneously appearing episodes of confusion, and the eventual appearance of parkinsonism. Visual hallucinations are prominent early on, and may be quite vivid (Byrne *et al.* 1989; McKeith *et al.* 1994a; Tiraboschi *et al.* 2006). Episodes of confusion last on the order of hours and, in contrast with the confusional episodes that may occur in patients with other dementias when patients are confronted with cognitively demanding tasks, the episodes seen in diffuse Lewy body disease appear spontaneously, without any obvious precipitating factors (Ballard *et al.* 2001; Bradshaw *et al.* 2004). Parkinsonism eventually appears in almost all patients, and generally within a year of the onset of the dementia. Even before the onset of parkinsonism, patients may display a pronounced 'neuroleptic sensitivity', when treated with an antipsychotic, developing severe antipsychotic-induced parkinsonism (McKeith *et al.* 1992).

Binswanger's disease, occurring on the basis of a vascular microangiopathy with diffuse white matter disease, as noted by Binswanger (Blass *et al.* 1991) himself, may present with a slowly progressive dementia, which, although often accompanied by strokes (Caplan and Schoene 1978), may lack them entirely (Kinkel *et al.* 1985; Yoshitake *et al.* 1995).

Lacunar dementia, like Binswanger's disease, may also present with a gradually progressive dementia and although this is more likely to be accompanied by stroke (of the

Table 5.1   The causes of dementia

Of gradual or subacute onset, often lacking in distinctive features
Alzheimer's disease
Diffuse Lewy body disease
Binswanger's disease
Lacunar dementia
Hypothyroidism
Hyperthyroidism
Vitamin B12 deficiency
Folate deficiency
Depression
Tumors
Hydrocephalus
Acquired autoimmune deficiency syndrome (AIDS)
Lyme disease
Neurosyphilis
Pick's disease
Cerebral amyloid angiopathy
Creutzfeldt–Jakob disease
Multiple sclerosis
Huntington's disease
Amyotrophic lateral sclerosis
Systemic lupus erythematosus
Granulomatous angiitis

In the setting of a history of strokes
Multi-infarct dementia
Lacunar dementia
Binswanger's disease
Cranial arteritis
Cerebral amyloid angiopathy
Cerebral autosomal dominant arteriopathy with subcortical infarcts and leukoencephalopathy (CADASIL)
Mitochondrial myopathy, encephalopathy, lactic acidosis, and stroke (MELAS)

Characterized by a frontal lobe syndrome
Frontotemporal dementia
Pick's disease
Amyotrophic lateral sclerosis
Tumors

With a progressive aphasia
Alzheimer's disease
Pick's disease
Frontotemporal dementia
Corticobasal ganglionic degeneration
Progressive supranuclear palsy
Tumors

With parkinsonism
Parkinson's disease
Diffuse Lewy body disease
Multiple system atrophy
Progressive supranuclear palsy
Corticobasal ganglionic degeneration
Frontotemporal dementia with parkinsonism
Vascular parkinsonism

Dementia pugilistica
Fahr's syndrome
Carbon monoxide intoxication
Manganese intoxication
Methanol intoxication
Valproic acid
Hypoparathyroidism
Pantothenate kinase-associated neurodegeneration
Huntington's disease of juvenile onset
Systemic lupus erythematosus

With chorea
Huntington's disease
Choreoacanthocytosis
Dentatorubropallidoluysian atrophy
Acquired hepatocerebral degeneration

With dystonia
Corticobasal ganglionic degeneration
Wilson's disease
Pantothenate kinase-associated neurodegeneration

With myoclonus
Creutzfeldt–Jakob disease
Post-anoxic dementia
Dialysis dementia
AIDS dementia
Diffuse Lewy body disease
Multiple system atrophy
Corticobasal ganglionic degeneration
Dentatorubropallidoluysian atrophy
Alzheimer's disease
Subacute sclerosing panencephalitis
Juvenile-onset Huntington's disease
Whipple's disease
Idiopathic hemochromatosis
Thalamic degeneration

With ataxia
Multiple system atrophy
Spinocerebellar ataxia
Fragile X-associated tremor/ataxia syndrome (FXTAS)
Dentatorubropallidoluysian atrophy
Creutzfeldt–Jakob disease
Gerstmann–Sträussler–Scheinker disease
Lithium intoxication
Mercury intoxication
Tin intoxication
Inhalant abuse
Dementia pugilistica
Acquired hepatocerebral degeneration
Metachromatic leukodystrophy
Progressive rubella panencephalitis

With distinctive features
Cerebrotendinous xanthomatosis (tendon enlargement)
Myotonic dystrophy (myotonia)
Thallium intoxication (painful polyneuropathy and alopecia)

(continued)

Table 5.1 *(Continued)*

Arsenic intoxication (painful polyneuropathy and alopecia)	**In the setting of mental retardation**
Pellagra (diarrhea and dermatitis)	Down's syndrome
Behçet's syndrome (aphthous oral and genital ulcers)	Sturge–Weber syndrome
Sjögren's syndrome (dry eyes and mouth)	Congenital rubella syndrome
Polymyalgia rheumatica (polymyalgia)	
Sneddon's syndrome (livedo reticularis)	**Miscellaneous causes**
	Systemic lupus erythematosus
With obvious precipitating events	Polyarteritis nodosa
Subdural hematoma	Anti-phospholipid syndrome
Diffuse axonal injury	Sarcoidosis
Dementia pugilistica	Progressive multifocal
Post-anoxic encephalopathy	leukoencephalopathy
Delayed post-anoxic encephalopathy	Kufs' disease
Radiation encephalopathy	Metachromatic leukodystrophy
Post-encephalitic	Adrenoleukodystrophy
Status epilepticus	Pantothenate kinase-associated
Dialysis dementia	neurodegeneration
Hypoglycemia	Hypoparathyroidism
Prednisone	Whipple's disease
Valproic acid	Lead intoxication
Disulfiram	Thalamic degeneration
Lithium	Sleep apnea
Methanol	Bilateral carotid occlusion
Heroin vapor	Hyperviscosity syndrome
Alcoholic dementia	Hypereosinophilia
Inhalant dementia	Hypertriglyceridemia

'lacunar' variety), its presentation may be confined to a dementia (Ishii *et al.* 1986; Yoshitake *et al.* 1995).

Hypothyroidism may cause a dementia (Asher 1949) marked by sluggishness (de Fine Olivarious and Roder 1970). In most cases, one will also see other, typical symptoms of hypothyroidism, such as myxedema, cold sensitivity, constipation, and hair loss.

Hyperthyroidism may cause dementia: although this is only rarely reported in typical cases, wherein it is accompanied by autonomic signs such as tremor and tachycardia (Bulens 1981), it is not uncommon in elderly patients with the 'apathetic' variant, wherein the only clue may be atrial fibrillation (Martin and Deam 1996).

Vitamin B12 deficiency may cause dementia (Lurie 1919) and although this is usually accompanied by a macrocytic anemia, cases have occurred that lacked both anemia and macrocytosis (Chatterjee *et al.* 1996; Lindenbaum *et al.* 1988).

Folate deficiency can clearly cause dementia. Cases have been reported of folate deficiency dementia occurring with subacute combined degeneration (Pincus *et al.* 1972) or spasticity (Reynolds *et al.* 1973), or in the absence of any other symptoms (Strachan and Henderson 1967).

Depression, as may be seen in major depression, is a not uncommon cause of dementia (Reding *et al.* 1985). The dementia of depression used to be called a 'pseudo-dementia' (Caine 1981; Wells 1979), but this is inappropriate as the dementia of depression is no more 'pseudo' than any

other dementia and may indeed be very severe. Clues to the correct diagnosis include the presence of significant depressive symptoms, such as disturbances in sleep and appetite, and, above all, a history of past depressive episodes (Rabins *et al.* 1984). Furthermore, the appearance of depression in a patient with a pre-existing dementia may worsen the patient's cognitive deficits (Greenwald *et al.* 1989). It must be borne in mind that these elderly patients are still liable to other dementing disorders and may indeed develop a dementia of another cause in the future (Alexopoulus *et al.* 1993).

Tumors of the frontal lobe (Sachs 1950), corpus callosum (Alpers and Grant 1931; Ironside and Guttmacher 1929), thalamus (Smyth and Stern 1938), and hypothalamus (Alpers 1937; Liss 1958; Lobosky *et al.* 1984; Strauss and Globus 1931) may all cause a gradually progressive dementia without striking distinctive features: tumors in other locations may of course cause dementia, but these are often accompanied by focal deficits, such as hemiplegia, which are also gradually progressive and strongly suggest a space-occupying lesion. Some hypothalamic tumors capable of causing dementia may also be accompanied by other symptoms (Lobosky *et al.* 1984) such as hypersomnolence (Strauss and Globus 1931), massive weight gain (Liss 1958), or diabetes insipidus (Alpers 1937).

Chronic hydrocephalus (Gustafson and Hagberg 1978; Harrison *et al.* 1974; McHugh 1964; Messert and Baker 1966), including normal pressure hydrocephalus (Adams *et al.* 1965; Hill *et al.* 1967), may present primarily with a dementia, but this may be accompanied by other symptoms and signs, such as urinary incontinence, and a broad-based shuffling gait often marked by a 'magnetic' aspect wherein the feet seem to be magnetically 'stuck' to the floor.

AIDS dementia, although generally occurring with other symptoms suggestive of AIDS (e.g. *Pneumocystis* pneumonia, Kaposi's sarcoma, and thrush) may, in a small minority, be the presenting symptom of AIDS (Navia and Price 1987; Navia *et al.* 1986a,b).

Lyme disease, during its third stage, may cause a mild dementia (Halperin *et al.* 1989; Logigian *et al.* 1990). The history may or may not reveal the original tick bite and erythema chronica migrans of stage I or the polyarthralgia of stage II, and patients may or may not have the oligoarthritis that typifies stage III.

Neurosyphilis, presenting as general paresis of the insane, although much less common than early in the twentieth century, when it filled hospital wards, is still with us and making something of a comeback, especially in connection with AIDS. The dementia may be non-specific or may be accompanied by dysarthria and pupillary changes, including the classic Argyll Robertson pupil (Gomez and Aviles 1984; Storm-Mathisen 1969).

Pick's disease, although typically presenting with a personality change, often of the frontal lobe type (Munoz *et al.* 1993), may occasionally present in a fashion quite similar to that of Alzheimer's disease (Wisniewski *et al.* 1972).

Cerebral amyloid angiopathy, although classically marked by a gradually progressive dementia punctuated by lobar intracerebral hemorrhages, may cause a progressive dementia alone without any strokes (Bornebroek *et al.* 1996; Cosgrove *et al.* 1985; Haan *et al.* 1990; Nobuyoshi *et al.* 1984). In some cases, however, there may be transient events similar to transient ischemic attacks (Greenberg *et al.* 1993).

Creutzfeldt–Jakob disease may present with a dementia with few distinguishing features (Brown *et al.* 1984; Will and Mathews 1984), although in approximately 80 percent of cases, myoclonus eventually appears (Brown *et al.* 1986; Roos *et al.* 1973), thus suggesting the correct diagnosis. It must be borne in mind, however, that not all cases will develop myoclonus (Zochodne *et al.* 1988); the relative rapidity of the progression, measured in months, may suggest the diagnosis.

Multiple sclerosis may cause dementia, which is in most cases seen to occur in the context of a history of signs and symptoms indicating white matter lesions 'disseminated in time and space'. In a minority the dementia may be the primary expression of multiple sclerosis, being accompanied by few other symptoms (Jennekens-Schinkel and Sanders 1986; Mendez and Frey 1992) and, very rarely, it may constitute the presentation of the disease without any other symptoms or signs (Fontaine *et al.* 1994; Hotopf *et al.* 1994).

Huntington's disease, although typically presenting with either a personality change or chorea, may rarely present with a dementia, as has been noted in juvenile Huntington's

disease (Hansotia *et al.* 1968) and in a 60-year-old patient (Case records 1992): in both cases, chorea eventually appeared after a number of years.

Amyotrophic lateral sclerosis may present with a combination of dementia and typical upper and lower motor neuron signs (i.e., fasciculations, hyper-reflexia, and pseudobulbar palsy) (Horoupian *et al.* 1984; Robertson 1953; Wechsler and Davison 1932) or may rarely present with dementia alone (Ferrer *et al.* 1991).

Systemic lupus erythematosus may, very rarely, present with a gradually progressive dementia: in one patient, who recovered with steroid treatment, the diagnosis was delayed until the development of a fever and pleural effusion suggested the correct diagnosis (MacNeill *et al.* 1976).

Granulomatous angiitis may present with a dementia (Case records 1989) and, although headache is often prominent, it is not invariable.

IN THE SETTING OF A HISTORY OF STROKES

In the evaluation of a patient with dementia, a history of repeated stroke is of great diagnostic import. Large 'territorial' infarctions may be associated with multi-infarct dementia, and small subcortical lacunar infarctions with lacunar dementia. Binswanger's disease, as noted earlier, is characterized by a vascular microangiopathy and hence generally does not cause clinically discernible stroke; Binswanger's disease, however, is often associated with other vascular pathology, such as small vessel disease that can cause stroke (of the lacunar variety) and hence is also considered in this section. Cranial arteritis should be considered in any patient with stroke, especially when there is a history of temporal headache or visual loss. Cerebral amyloid angiopathy is suggested by a history of lobar intracerebral hemorrhages. Finally, consideration may be given to two rare disorders, CADASIL (*c*erebral *a*utosomal *d*ominant *a*rteriopathy with subcortical *i*nfarcts and *l*eukoencephalopathy) and MELAS (*m*itochondrial *e*ncephalopathy with *l*actic *a*cidosis and stroke-like episodes), both of which are associated with migrainous headaches.

Multi-infarct dementia is typically characterized by a dementia that progresses in a 'stepwise' fashion, each step corresponding to a fresh, large, cortical, or subcortical infarction. Critically, in between the 'steps', the patient experiences a clinical plateau without any between-step deterioration (Erkinjunti *et al.* 1988; Tomlinson *et al.* 1970; Yoshitake *et al.* 1995). An examination of such patients typically reveals various focal findings, such as hemiplegia, aphasia, and apraxia, corresponding to the location of the prior infarctions. Rarely, a dementia will result from one large or strategically placed infarction: clearly, subsuming these cases under the rubric of 'multi-infarct' constitutes something of a semantic trespass but a term equivalent to 'single-infarct dementia' has simply not found its way into current usage. Examples of such 'single' infarctions include large cortical infarctions or strategically placed subcortical infarctions (Yoshitake *et al.* 1995).

Lacunar dementia may also pursue a classic 'stepwise' course; however, several features serve to distinguish it from multi-infarct dementia. First, one typically finds a history of 'lacunar syndromes', such as pure motor stroke, pure sensory stroke, etc. Second, as noted earlier, in lacunar dementia, one may also find a progressive downhill course in between the obvious strokes (Ishii *et al.* 1986; Yoshitake *et al.* 1995). Third, and finally, lacunar dementia is often marked clinically by a frontal lobe syndrome (Ishii *et al.* 1986; Wolfe *et al.* 1990). Eventually, however, the diagnosis is often made on MR scanning, which reveals multiple subcortical lacunes.

Binswanger's disease classically presents with a dementia that pursues a gradual downhill course; this disease, however, often is accompanied by small vessel disease and lacunar strokes (Caplan and Schoene 1978; Kinkel *et al.* 1985; Revesz *et al.* 1989) and is difficult to distinguish from lacunar dementia on a clinical basis. MR scanning will reveal, however, the leukoencephalopathy typical of Binswanger's disease, thus making the diagnosis.

Cranial arteritis may rarely cause a dementia, of either the multi-infarct or lacunar type (Caselli 1990, Nightingale *et al.* 1982). Diagnostic clues include unilateral headache (generally temporal in location), amaurosis fugax, and polymyalgia rheumatica.

Cerebral amyloid angiopathy classically presents with a gradually progressive dementia punctuated by lobar intracerebral hemorrhages (Cosgrove *et al.* 1985; Gilles *et al.* 1984), demonstrable on computed tomography (CT) or magnetic resonance imaging (MRI) and suggested clinically by the prominent headache associated with the lobar hemorrhage.

CADASIL presents in a fashion similar to that of Binswanger's disease. Distinguishing features include migrainous headaches and a family history consistent with an autosomal dominant inheritance (Dichgans *et al.* 1998; Jung *et al.* 1995; Malandrini *et al.* 1996).

MELAS syndrome is a rare maternally inherited disorder that, although generally presenting in the childhood years, may present in adulthood with stroke-like episodes, progressive dementia, migraine-like headaches, and hearing loss (Clark *et al.* 1996).

CHARACTERIZED BY A FRONTAL LOBE SYNDROME

The frontal lobe syndrome, as discussed further in Section 7.2, is marked by varying degrees of affective changes (euphoria or irritability), disinhibition and perseveration, and its appearance early on in a dementing disorder is strongly suggestive of frontal pathology, as may be seen with various tumors and in certain neurodegenerative disorders, such as Pick's disease, frontotemporal dementia, and amyotrophic lateral sclerosis.

Frontotemporal dementia, like Pick's disease, typically presents with a frontal lobe syndrome. A distinguishing feature in some cases is the early appearance of an aphasic disturbance of the motor or anomic type (Heutink *et al.* 1997; Mann *et al.* 1993; Neary *et al.* 1993).

Pick's disease classically presents with the frontal lobe syndrome (Bouton 1940; Ferraro and Jervis 1936), and it is indeed this presentation that most strongly distinguishes it from Alzheimer's disease (Litvan *et al.* 1997a; Mendez *et al.* 1993).

Amyotrophic lateral sclerosis, once thought to spare the cortex outside the precentral gyrus, is now known to involve the frontal lobes. In a minority, the disease may present with a frontal lobe syndrome followed by a dementia and typical upper and lower motor neuron signs (Cavalleri and De Renzi 1994; Neary *et al.* 1990; Peavy *et al.* 1992).

Tumors of the frontal lobe may present with a dementia marked by a frontal lobe syndrome (Avery 1971; Frazier 1936; Williamson 1896), which is true not only of tumors confined to the frontal lobe, but also of those tumors of the corpus callosum that extend laterally into the adjacent frontal lobes (Moersch 1925).

WITH A PROGRESSIVE APHASIA

A number of different neurodegenerative diseases may present with an isolated aphasia in a syndrome known as 'primary progressive aphasia'. In such cases, the aphasia progressively worsens and is eventually joined by a dementia. Such a scenario has been noted in Alzheimer's disease (Green *et al.* 1990, 1996; Karbe *et al.* 1993), Pick's disease (Kertesz *et al.* 1994), and frontotemporal dementia (Neary *et al.* 1993; Snowden *et al.* 1992; Turner *et al.* 1996); other, much less common, causes include corticobasal ganglionic degeneration (Ikeda *et al.* 1996), progressive supranuclear palsy (Knibb *et al.* 2000), and Creutzfeldt–Jakob disease (Mandell *et al.* 1989). It must be borne in mind that a similar picture may occur with slowly growing appropriately situated tumors.

WITH PARKINSONISM

The combination of dementia and parkinsonism may occur secondary to a large number of disorders, of which certain neurodegenerative disorders are the most common. Of these neurodegenerative disorders, the most frequent causes are Parkinson's disease, diffuse Lewy body disease, and multiple system atrophy, each one of which, in addition to dementia, may cause a fairly 'classic' parkinsonism; other neurodegenerative disorders to consider include progressive supranuclear palsy, corticobasal ganglionic degeneration, and frontotemporal dementia; however, as detailed below, the parkinsonism seen in these disorders tends to have some distinctive atypical features. Some other disorders that present in a fashion similar to these neurodegenerative ones include vascular parkinsonism, dementia pugilistica, and Fahr's syndrome.

Less common disorders to consider include those with more or less obvious precipitating factors, such as intoxications (carbon monoxide, manganese, methanol) and treatment with valproic acid. Miscellaneous, and rare, causes include hypoparathyroidism, pantothenate kinase-associated neurodegeneration, juvenile-onset Huntington's disease, and systemic lupus erythematosus.

Parkinson's disease may cause dementia but this is a late development, generally not appearing until five or more years after the parkinsonism has been well established. The prevalence of dementia in patients with Parkinson's disease increases with age (Biggins et al. 1992; Marder et al. 1995) and overall, in population-based studies, the prevalence of dementia ranges from 18 percent (Tison et al. 1995) to 41 percent (Mayeux et al. 1992).

Diffuse Lewy body disease may present with parkinsonism; however, within a year of the onset of the parkinsonism, patients develop a dementia, and it is this 'one year rule' that most reliably distinguishes diffuse Lewy body disease from Parkinson's disease. Other, helpful differential features include the presence of hallucinations and spontaneous episodes of confusion in the dementia of diffuse Lewy body disease, features that are generally not as prominent in Parkinson's disease (Burkhardt et al. 1988; Klatka et al. 1996; McKeith et al. 1994).

Multiple system atrophy of the striatonigral degeneration type presents with a typical parkinsonism but it is generally accompanied by evidence of either autonomic failure or cerebellar involvement (Colosimo et al. 1995; Litvan et al. 1997b; Wenning et al. 1994, 1995). The autonomic failure may include postural hypotension and dizziness, urinary incontinence or retention, fecal incontinence, and erectile dysfunction; cerebellar signs include ataxia and intention tremor. A minority of these patient will eventually develop a dementia (Robbins et al. 1992).

Progressive supranuclear palsy typically presents with postural instability and frequent unexplained falls; over time, parkinsonism develops, marked by rigidity, bradykinesia, and, notably, a dystonic axial extension, which may also be evident in the neck (Collins et al. 1995; Daniel et al. 1995; Litvan et al. 1996a,b,c, 1997c). Most, but not all, patients eventually demonstrate the hallmark of this disease, namely supranuclear ophthalmoplegia for vertical gaze. Most patients also eventually become demented and many will also develop a pseudobulbar palsy with emotional incontinence (Menza et al. 1995).

Corticobasal ganglionic degeneration typically presents with a strikingly asymmetric rigid–akinetic parkinsonism, generally in an arm, which may be accompanied by a dystonic rigidity. Apraxia is a common accompaniment, and some patients may also develop myoclonus (Litvan et al. 1997d; Riley et al. 1990; Rinne et al. 1994). A minority may eventually become demented. Uncommonly, the disease may present with dementia (Grimes et al. 1999), and in such cases, parkinsonism may appear later (Schneider et al. 1997).

Frontotemporal dementia, specifically frontotemporal dementia with parkinsonism linked to chromosome 17 (FTDP-17) (Pickering-Brown et al. 2002) typically presents with a dementia marked by a personality change with frontal lobe features that may, over years, be joined by parkinsonism in a minority of cases.

Vascular parkinsonism is characterized by a gradually progressive rigidity, bradykinesia, and gait abnormality, all notably in the absence of tremor. This parkinsonism is typically accompanied by signs of damage to the corticospinal and corticobulbar tracts, such as spasticity, hyper-reflexia, and pseudobulbar palsy. In some cases, a dementia may appear (Bruetsch and Williams 1954; Keschner and Sloane 1931).

Dementia pugilistica has a gradual onset anywhere from 5 to 40 years after repeated head trauma (e.g., as in boxing), with a combination of parkinsonism, dysarthria, ataxia, and dementia (Harvey and Davis 1974; Martland 1928).

Fahr's syndrome (Margolin et al 1980; Mathews 1957; Nyland and Skre 1977) may present with parkinsonism and dementia. Cerebellar signs such as dysarthria, intention tremor, and ataxia may also be present, but the distinctive finding is calcification of the basal ganglia, which is best demonstrated on CT scanning.

Carbon monoxide intoxication may, after a lucid interval of from days to weeks, be followed in a minority of cases by the subacute onset of dementia and parkinsonism (Choi 1983; Min 1986).

Manganese intoxication, as may occur in those working in manganese mines, steel mills, or battery factories, may cause a gradually progressive parkinsonism that may be joined by a dementia (Cook et al. 1974). The parkinsonism in these cases is often marked by dystonic rigidity of the neck and face and by ankle dystonia, which results in the classic 'cock-walk' gait.

Methanol intoxication, as may occur in desperate alcoholics, may, as a sequela, leave patients with dementia, parkinsonism, and blindness (McLean et al. 1980).

Valproic acid, with chronic use, as for epilepsy or bipolar disorder, may cause a combination of dementia and parkinsonism, which is potentially reversible on discontinuation of the drug (Armon et al. 1996; Shill and Fife 2000); importantly, this side-effect of valproic acid may take from 6 months to 4 years to appear (Ristic et al. 2006).

Hypoparathyroidism may cause parkinsonism and dementia but this is usually in the context of Fahr's syndrome, which, as noted above, includes calcification of the basal ganglia. In one rare case, however, dementia and parkinsonism occurred with hypoparathyroidism in the absence of calcification and with a normal serum calcium level. The only clue to the diagnosis was cataracts; the parathyroid hormone level was low and the patient recovered with dihydroxycholecalciferol (Stuerenburg et al. 1996).

Pantothenate kinase-associated neurodegeneration of the late-onset type may present with a slowly progressive parkinsonism that is eventually joined by dementia and dystonia (Jankovic et al. 1985, Murphy et al. 1989).

Huntington's disease of juvenile onset, seen in late childhood or adolescence, may present with parkinsonism and dementia (Bird and Paulson 1971; Campbell et al. 1961; Siesling et al. 1997).

Systemic lupus erythematosus very rarely presents with a combination of dementia and parkinsonism (Dennis et al. 1992).

WITH CHOREA

The prototypical cause of dementia occurring in the setting of chorea is Huntington's disease; two other neurodegenerative conditions that present in a somewhat similar fashion are choreoacanthocytosis and dentatorubropallidoluysian atrophy. Other disorders to consider are acquired hepatocerebral degeneration and Wilson's disease.

Huntington's disease, as noted by George Huntington himself (Brody and Wilkins 1967), typically presents with chorea which, over years, is joined by a dementia (Pflanz et al. 1991).

Choreoacanthocytosis may also present with chorea and dementia. A diagnostic clue is involuntary lip biting or other self-injurious behavior (Critchley et al. 1968; Hardie et al. 1991), although this is not seen in all patients.

Dentatorubropallidoluysian atrophy may likewise present with chorea and dementia; diagnostic clues include elements of ataxia and dystonia (Becher et al. 1997; Warner et al. 1994, 1995).

Acquired hepatocerebral degeneration, occurring after repeated bouts of hepatic encephalopathy, is seen most often in chronic alcoholics and may present with a dementia accompanied by a complex movement disorder, with chorea and tremor (Finlayson and Superville 1981; Victor et al. 1965).

WITH DYSTONIA

Corticobasal ganglionic degeneration, as noted earlier, typically presents with parkinsonism and dementia; however, in some cases the dominant movement disorder may be a unilateral dystonia.

Wilson's disease may present with dystonia, later to be joined by a dementia (Walshe and Yealland 1992). The fact that this disease is treatable mandates testing in any young person who presents with a compatible clinical picture.

Pantothenate kinase-associated neurodegeneration typically presents in childhood or adolescence with a progressive dystonia and dementia (Dooling et al. 1974, 1980; Hayflick et al. 2003).

WITH MYOCLONUS

Myoclonus, when prominent in the overall clinical picture, is a very important diagnostic sign and, although more commonly associated with delirium (as described in Section 6.3), it may also be a significant clue in the diagnosis of dementia in adults. Of the dementing disorders associated with myoclonus, the most important is Creutzfeldt–Jakob disease (including the 'new-variant' type) and two other disorders: post-anoxic dementia and dialysis dementia. Myoclonus may also appear in AIDS dementia and in various neurodegenerative disorders; however, here it plays only a minor role and is overshadowed by other clinical features.

Among children or adolescents, myoclonus is an important sign in subacute sclerosing panencephalitis and may also be seen in the juvenile form of Huntington's disease.

Finally, myoclonus may also be seen in certain rare disorders such as Whipple's disease, idiopathic hemochromatosis, and thalamic degeneration.

Creutzfeldt–Jakob disease is the classic example of a disease causing dementia with myoclonus: approximately 80 percent of patients eventually display this sign (Brown et al. 1986, 1994; Roos et al. 1973). New-variant Creutzfeldt–Jakob disease, contracted by eating beef from cows with 'mad cow' disease (bovine spongiform encephalopathy), like Creutzfeldt–Jakob disease also eventually causes myoclonus in most patients (Zeidler et al. 1997).

Post-anoxic dementia, appearing after an anoxic coma, may be accompanied by myoclonus, which is often of the intention type (Werheran et al. 1997).

Dialysis dementia is immediately suggested by the appearance of dementia after several years of hemodialysis. Myoclonus is common and helps to confirm the diagnosis (Burks et al. 1976; Lederman and Henry 1978).

AIDS dementia, once well established, may, in a minority, be accompanied by myoclonus (Navia et al. 1986b), and myoclonus may also play a minor role in the dementia seen in diffuse Lewy body disease (Louis et al. 1997), multiple system atrophy (Rodriguez et al. 1994), corticobasal ganglionic degeneration (Litvan et al. 1997d), dentatorubropallidoluysian atrophy (of childhood onset) (Becher et al. 1997), and in end-stage Alzheimer's disease (Benesch et al. 1993; Chen et al. 1991).

Subacute sclerosing panencephalitis, typically with an onset in childhood or adolescence, presents with dementia that is eventually joined by myoclonus (Dawson 1934).

Juvenile-onset Huntington's disease is distinguished by parkinsonism and dementia, as noted above. In a minority of cases myoclonus may also appear (Siesling et al. 1997).

Whipple's disease may cause a dementia and, although a history of abdominal complaints (especially diarrhea) and arthopathy is generally most helpful diagnostically, about one-quarter of these patients will also have myoclonus (Louis et al. 1996).

Idiopathic hemochromatosis may present, very rarely, with dementia and myoclonus (Jones and Hedley-Whyte 1983). Other, suggestive clinical features include hepatic failure, diabetes mellitus, and cardiomyopathy.

Thalamic degeneration is a very rare syndrome that may present with dementia and myoclonus (Little et al. 1986).

WITH ATAXIA

Dementia occurring in the setting of ataxia may be seen in neurodegenerative disorders such as multiple system atrophy, spinocerebellar atrophy, fragile X-associated tremor/ataxia syndrome (FXTAS) and dentatorubropallidoluysian atrophy, and in prion diseases such as Creutzfeldt–Jakob disease and Gerstmann–Sträussler–Scheinker disease. A similar constellation may occur with more or less obvious precipitating factors such as intoxications with lithium, mercury, or tin, long-term inhalant use, repeated head trauma, and cirrhosis. Finally, when this clinical picture occurs in childhood or adolescence, one must consider metachromatic leukodystrophy and the very rare progressive rubella panencephalitis.

Multiple system atrophy of the olivopontocerebellar type may present with ataxia (Wenning *et al.* 1994) and may also cause dementia (Robbins *et al.* 1992). The presence of evidence of autonomic failure (e.g., postural hypotension and dizziness, urinary incontinence or retention, fecal incontinence, or erectile dysfunction) or mild parkinsonism is an important diagnostic clue.

Spinocerebellar ataxia presents with a progressive ataxia, which, in a minority, is eventually joined by dementia (Carter and Sukavajuna 1956; Chandler and Bebin 1956; Goldfarb *et al.* 1989; Lasek *et al.* 2006; Modi *et al.* 2000; Sasaki *et al.* 1996; Zhou *et al.* 1998).

FXTAS is characterized by the gradual onset of a progressive ataxia and tremor in middle or later years, with, in a minority, the eventual development of a dementia (Hagerman *et al.* 2001).

Dentatorubropallidoluysian atrophy may rarely present with a combination of ataxia and dementia (Potter *et al.* 1995).

Creutzfeldt–Jakob disease may present with ataxia, followed within weeks or months by a dementia (Brown *et al.* 1986, 1994; de Villemeur *et al.* 1996).

Gerstmann–Sträussler–Scheinker disease, an inherited prion disease, typically presents with ataxia and dementia (Barbanti *et al.* 1996; Brown *et al.* 1991).

Lithium intoxication, if severe, may leave patients permanently ataxic and demented (Schou 1984).

Mercury, in large amounts, may cause dementia and ataxia: this has been noted with mercury salts (as found in a laxative [Davis *et al.* 1974]), methyl mercury (as used in a fungicide for wheat [Rustam and Hamri 1974]), and ethyl mercury (as occurred with industrial exposure [Hay *et al.* 1963]).

Tin intoxication, in one case, caused a coma from which the patient emerged with dementia and ataxia (Wu *et al.* 1990).

Inhalant abuse may, if chronic, cause a dementia accompanied by ataxia and other cerebellar signs such as intention tremor, nystagmus, and titubation (Escobar and Aruffo 1980; Fornazzari *et al.* 1983; Holmes *et al.* 1986; Lazar *et al.* 1983; Rosenberg *et al.* 1988).

Dementia pugilistica, occurring 5–40 years after repeated head trauma, as, for example, in boxers, may present with dementia and prominent ataxia, a sign that accounts for the colloquial name for this disorder: 'punch-drunk' (Harvey and Davis 1974; Martland 1928).

Acquired hepatocerebral degeneration, generally occurring in the setting of alcoholic cirrhosis after repeated bouts of hepatic encephalopathy, may present with a dementia and a complex movement disorder: although chorea and tremor are most common, in some cases ataxia may dominate the clinical picture (Raskin *et al.* 1984; Victor *et al.* 1965).

Metachromatic leukodystrophy typically causes a dementia that may be accompanied by ataxia in both juvenile- (Haltia *et al.* 1980) and adult-onset cases (Hirose and Bass 1972; Rauschka *et al.* 2006; Reider-Grosswasser and Bornstein 1987).

Progressive rubella panencephalitis, although usually occurring in the setting of the congenital rubella syndrome with mental retardation, may occasionally present in the late teenage years in patients of normal premorbid intelligence. One patient had cataracts and microphthalmos due to congenital rubella (Townsend *et al.* 1976), whereas another had contracted rubella in childhood but had no sequelae at the time (Wolinsky *et al.* 1976); in both cases, the dementia was accompanied by ataxia.

WITH DISTINCTIVE FEATURES

The following disorders are all relatively rare causes of dementia which, in each case, have certain distinctive features, as described below.

Cerebrotendinous xanthomatosis, when fully developed, manifests with dementia, tendon enlargement, cataracts, and ataxia. Tendon enlargement is the most distinctive feature, and although it may appear in a variety of areas, it is most commonly, and classically, found in the Achilles tendon. The disease evolves very slowly and may present with any one of these features anywhere from childhood or adolescence to the adult years (Berginer *et al.* 1988; Farpour and Mahloudji 1975; Watts *et al.* 1996).

Myotonic dystrophy typically presents with myotonia in late adolescence or early adult years. Over time, a 'myopathic facies', with frontal baldness, ptosis, and temporal wasting appears, as does weakness and atrophy, most prominent distally. In a small minority, a dementia may also occur (Huber *et al.* 1989; Perini *et al.* 1989).

Thallium intoxication may be followed by dementia with a painful polyneuropathy and prominent alopecia (Thompson *et al.* 1988; Reed *et al.* 1963).

Arsenic intoxication with organic arsenicals may cause a picture similar to that of thallium intoxication but with less prominent hair loss.

Pellagra of the chronic, gradual onset type classically presents with the 'three Ds': diarrhea, dermatitis, and dementia (Langworthy 1931; Pierce 1924).

Behçet's syndrome causes dementia in only a small minority of patients, virtually all of whom have both oral and genital aphthous ulcers (Serdaroglu *et al.* 1989). The dementia may follow upon numerous prior attacks (Rubinstein and Urich 1963) or may be slowly progressive (Borson 1982).

Sjörgen's syndrome is an autoimmune disorder that typically involves the exocrine glands, producing the 'sicca syndrome' with dry eyes and a dry mouth. Rarely, a dementia (Kawashima *et al.* 1993) may occur, probably secondary to a cerebral vasculitis (Caselli *et al.* 1991).

Polymyalgia rheumatica, distinguished by severe pain and stiffness of the proximal muscle groups, is rarely associated with a dementia, both the dementia and the polymyalgia responding to treatment with steroids (Nightingale *et al.* 1982).

Sneddon's syndrome is a rare disorder characterized in adults by livedo reticularis, strokes, transient ischemic attacks, and, in some, dementia (Adair *et al.* 2001; Tourbah *et al.* 1997).

WITH OBVIOUS PRECIPITATING EVENTS

Dementia may appear as a sequela to obvious precipitating events such as traumatic brain injury, anoxia, radiation, encephalitis, status epilepticus, chronic dialysis, and hypoglycemia. Various medications, even when taken at normal doses, may also cause dementia, and these include prednisone, valproic acid, and disulfiram. Intoxications with lithium, methanol, or heroin vapor may have dementia as a sequela, and chronic alcoholics or chronic inhalant abusers may also eventually become demented.

Subdural hematoma of the chronic type may cause a dementia (Arieff and Wetzel 1964; Black 1984), but there may be an interval lasting anywhere from months to years between the initial trauma and the onset of the dementia. In some cases, the trauma itself may have been forgotten.

Diffuse axonal injury, occurring secondary to violent acceleration–deceleration during a 'closed head' injury may, depending on its severity, leave patients in a coma, a persistent vegetative state, or a dementia of varying severity (Strich 1956).

Dementia pugilistica (Harvey and Davis 1974; Martland 1928) is one of the sequelae of repeated head trauma, as may occur in boxers, and appears after a latent interval of anywhere from 5 to 40 years. As noted above, it is often accompanied by a combination of parkinsonism and ataxia.

Post-anoxic encephalopathy (Richardson *et al.* 1959) occurs after global hypoxic–ischemic injury. Those who survive and emerge from coma are initially delirious; as the delirium gradually resolves, a dementia is left in its wake.

Delayed post-anoxic leukoencephalopathy presents with a delirium generally within weeks of recovery from an anoxic insult. Although most patients eventually recover, some, after the confusion clears, are left with a dementia (Plum *et al.* 1962).

Radiation encephalopathy of the late-delayed type may present with a gradually progressive dementia anytime from months to decades after brain irradiation. Interestingly, this sequela may occur after either whole-brain (Correa *et al.* 2004; DeAngelis *et al.* 1989; Duffy *et al.* 1996) or focal irradiation; note that in the case of focal irradiation it is essential that critical structures such as the temporal lobes have been exposed (Crompton and Layton 1961; Shewmon and Masdeu 1980).

Post-encephalitic dementia has been noted after both herpes simplex encephalitis and arbovirus encephalitis (Przelomski *et al.* 1988; Richter and Shimojyo 1961).

Status epilepticus, whether grand mal or complex partial, has been reported to leave patients demented (Krumholz *et al.* 1995); however, this is not at all inevitable with most patients surviving without cognitive sequelae.

Dialysis dementia may appear gradually after approximately 3 years of hemodialysis, often presenting with a stuttering type of aphasia (Garrett *et al.* 1988; O'Hare *et al.* 1983).

Hypoglycemia, if severe (e.g., a glucose level of less than 1.11–1.37 mmol/L [20–25 mg/dL]) and prolonged, may cause neuronal death, leaving the patient demented (Kalimo and Olsson 1980).

Prednisone, in doses of 60 mg or more, has been reported to cause a dementia that cleared on discontinuation of the drug (Varney *et al.* 1984).

Valproic acid may, with chronic use, cause a dementia, which, as noted earlier, may be accompanied by parkinsonism (Armon *et al.* 1996) or may occur without any distinguishing features (Guerrini *et al.* 1998; Papazian *et al.* 1995).

Disulfiram, taken over decades at a therapeutic dosage, in one case caused a dementia and polyneuropathy (Borrett *et al.* 1985).

Lithium intoxication, if severe, may leave patients with a dementia, which, as noted above, may be accompanied by ataxia (Schou 1984).

Methanol intoxication, when severe, may leave patients demented with, as previously noted, parkinsonism (McLean *et al.* 1980).

Heroin vapor, produced by heating heroin on aluminum foil, may cause dementia accompanied by a varying degree of bradykinesia and ataxia (Kriegstein *et al.* 1999)

Alcoholic dementia appears in the setting of chronic, severe and ongoing alcoholism, and is distinguished by apathy and an overall coarsening of the personality (Lee *et al.* 1979; Lishman 1981).

Inhalant-induced dementia makes a gradual appearance in the setting of chronic, ongoing inhalant use and, as noted earlier, is often accompanied by ataxia and other cerebellar signs (Escobar and Aruffo 1980; Fornazzari *et al.* 1983; Holmes *et al.* 1986; Lazar *et al.* 1983; Rosenberg *et al.* 1988).

IN THE SETTING OF MENTAL RETARDATION

Certain forms of mental retardation may, in the natural course of events, be complicated years or decades later by dementia, including Down's syndrome, Sturge–Weber syndrome, and the congenital rubella syndrome.

Down's syndrome, in those who survive past the age of 40, is eventually complicated by the development of Alzheimer's disease in over one-half of all patients (Lai and Williams 1989). In those with pre-existing mild mental retardation, the dementia presents with a typical loss of cognitive function; in those with a moderate or more severe degree of retardation, a loss of cognitive ability may be difficult to appreciate, and the dementia may instead come to attention because of apathy and decreased social interaction.

Sturge–Weber syndrome is characterized by a unilateral facial port-wine stain, seizures, hemiplegia, and mental retardation. In those with frequent seizures, a dementia may supervene with a drop in cognitive ability below the baseline that characterized the pre-existing mental retardation (Lichtenstein 1954; Petermann *et al.* 1958; Sujanksy and Conradi 1995).

Congenital rubella syndrome is characterized by cataracts, deafness, and mental retardation; in a minority, a dementia may appear in childhood or adolescence secondary to progressive rubella panencephalitis (Townsend *et al.* 1975; Weil *et al.* 1975).

MISCELLANEOUS CAUSES

Systemic lupus erythematosus may cause a dementia (Brey *et al.* 2002; Johnson and Richardson 1968; Kirk *et al.* 1991) via a number of different mechanisms (Devinsky *et al.* 1988a), including infarctions and an autoimmune cerebritis. In most cases, the dementia is accompanied by such systemic symptoms as arthralgia, rash, pleural effusion, and constitutional symptoms such as fever, fatigue, and weight loss.

Polyarteritis nodosa may cause a dementia (MacKay *et al.* 1950), but, as with lupus, this is usually in the setting of systemic symptoms such as renal or gastrointestinal disease or constitutional symptoms.

Anti-phospholipid antibody syndrome is characterized by recurrent arterial and venous thrombosis and, in women, by a history of recurrent miscarriage. Strokes may occur, producing a multi-infarct dementia (Coull *et al.* 1987). In some cases, however, the dementia may occur without specific MRI findings, suggesting a direct antineuronal effect (Van Horn *et al.* 1996).

Sarcoidosis may cause dementia (Camp and Frierson 1962; Sanson *et al.* 1996) but only in a very small minority (fewer than 1 percent) of patients (Oksanen 1986); in such cases, granulomata have been found in the cerebrum (Cordingly *et al.* 1981; Miller *et al.* 1988). A clue to the diagnosis is a chest radiograph finding of either bilateral hilar lymphadenopathy or bilateral reticulonodular infiltrates.

Progressive multifocal leukoencephalopathy, as may be seen in AIDS or other immunocompromised states, typically presents with a focal sign such as hemiplegia or aphasia, which is eventually joined by a gradually progressive dementia (Krupp *et al.* 1985; Richardson 1961); rarely, the presentation may be with dementia alone (Sellal *et al.* 1996; Zunt *et al.* 1997).

Kufs' disease, or the adult form of neuronal ceroid lipofuscinosis may present with a dementia which may or may not be accompanied by myoclonus and ataxia (Burneo *et al.* 2003)

Metachromatic leukodystrophy may, in addition to ataxia (as noted above), also cause dementia associated with seizures, spasticity, or chorea (Alves *et al.* 1986; Haltia *et al.* 1980; Wulff and Trojaborg 1985); polyneuropathy may also be obvious (Bosch and Hart 1978). Personality change is also prominent, especially in adults, with aggressiveness and irritability (Hageman *et al.* 1995) and 'frontal lobe' symptoms such as disinhibition, poor judgment, and socially inappropriate behavior (Shapiro *et al.* 1994).

Adrenoleukodystrophy may present in childhood, adolescence, or adulthood. Childhood- or adolescent-onset often occurs with a personality change and dementia accompanied by hemianopia or cortical blindness and spasticity of the lower extremities (Moser *et al.* 1984; Schaumberg *et al.* 1975). Adult-onset adrenoleukodystrophy may likewise be accompanied by visual symptoms such as blindness (Powers *et al.* 1980) or Balint's syndrome (Uyama *et al.* 1993) but, in some cases, visual symptoms are lacking: in one patient, the clue to the correct diagnosis was generalized hyper-reflexia (Coria *et al.* 1993), whereas in another it was bronzing of the skin (Weller *et al.* 1992).

Pantothenate kinase-associated neurodegeneration, as noted above, typically presents with dementia in the setting of dystonia or, less commonly, parkinsonism. There are, however, adult-onset cases that are marked by other signs, such as a fine tremor (Dooling *et al.* 1974) or dysarthria and clumsiness (Rozdilsky *et al.* 1968).

Hypoparathyroidism, without basal ganglia calcification, may present with a dementia accompanied by seizures and cataracts (Mateo and Gimenez-Roldan 1982).

Whipple's disease, although typically presenting with diarrhea and arthropathy, very rarely may affect the central nervous system in isolation, and in such cases these typical symptoms may be absent. One case was marked by hypothalamic involvement with hypersomnia (Adams *et al.* 1987) and another by seizures (Romanul *et al.* 1977).

Lead intoxication may initially cause a delirium and upon recovery patients may be left demented (Jenkins and Mellins 1957).

Thalamic degeneration, a rare syndrome, may present with dementia alone (Moosy *et al.* 1987) or dementia accompanied by somnolence (Stern 1939).

Sleep apnea, in one extraordinary case, presented with a dementia: the only clue to the diagnosis was the presence of daytime sleepiness and a history of prominent snoring (Scheltens *et al.* 1991).

Bilateral carotid occlusion, the brain being perfused primarily by only one vertebral artery, has been shown to cause a dementia that was reversed by intracranial–extracranial bypass surgery (Tatemichi *et al.* 1995).

Very rare causes include the hyperviscosity syndrome (as occurred in one case secondary to multiple myeloma [Mueller *et al.* 1983]), hypereosinophilia (92 percent eosinophils) (Kaplan *et al.* 1990), and extreme hypertriglyceridemia (with values of at least 10 times the normal value) (Heilman and Fisher 1974; Mas *et al.* 1985).

Differential diagnosis

Dementia must be distinguished from mild cognitive impairment, delirium, mental retardation, and amnesia.

Mild cognitive impairment is a syndrome characterized, as the name clearly suggests, by cognitive impairments that, although similar to those seen in dementia, are so mild that they cause little in the way of impairment. As noted in

Section 5.2, this may or may not be a syndrome *sui genereis* – it might just as well be thought of as a prodrome to a dementia.

Delirium is distinguished from dementia by the presence of prominent confusion; here, however, one must keep in mind that some diseases may be characterized by both dementia and intermittent delirium. In multi infarct dementia, for example, each fresh stroke may be heralded by an episode of delirium that, once having cleared spontaneously, leaves the patient not confused but more demented. Furthermore, some diseases, albeit characterized primarily by dementia, may also cause intermittent, brief, episodes of confusion, as may occur in diffuse Lewy body disease.

Mental retardation is distinguished primarily by its course: in mental retardation, the intellectual development of patients proceeds only to a certain point, at which it 'stalls', leaving patients on an intellectual 'plateau' beyond which they do not progress. Importantly, there is no decrement in intellectual ability but merely a plateauing. In contrast, there is in dementia a definite decrement from a previously acquired level of intellectual ability. Importantly, as noted above, some disorders may cause both mental retardation and a dementia: for example, in the setting of mental retardation secondary to Down's syndrome, a dementia eventually develops in most patients who survive past the age of 40.

Amnesia is distinguished from dementia by the restricted nature of the cognitive deficit: in amnestic disorders, one finds only a deficit in memory, whereas in dementia, in addition to a defective memory, one also finds other cognitive deficits, for example in abstracting or calculating abilities. It must be borne in mind, however, that some dementing conditions, such as Alzheimer's disorder, may present with a pure amnesia that persists for a prolonged period before being joined by other cognitive deficits.

Treatment

Treatment, if possible, is directed at the underlying condition, as discussed in the respective chapters. What follows here are general measures, applicable in most cases.

Patients' liberty should be circumscribed proportionate to their reduced abilities; thus, financial affairs should usually be managed by others and guardianship may be required. Driving privileges are often retained by patients with great tenacity, but these too must eventually be withdrawn. Visiting nurses, 'meals on wheels' and adult daycare centers should each be considered, as they help patients maintain functional abilities and enable them to stay at home longer. Cognitively stimulating activities should also be encouraged (Olazaran *et al.* 2004) and patients should be encouraged to do crossword puzzles, play card games, etc., as these all help to preserve cognitive abilities.

If patients have to move, for example to a retirement/nursing home, efforts should be made to make the patient feel 'at home', for example by bringing in familiar photographs and, where possible, furniture, and by subscribing to the patient's home-town paper. If patients are admitted to hospital, the same measures should be undertaken; furthermore, the room should have a large calendar and clock and, whenever possible, a window with a view.

The need for prosthetic devices (e.g., glasses, hearing aids, dentures, and 'quad canes') should be assessed, and medical regimens should be kept as simple as possible. Although many patients eventually require a wheelchair, ambulation should be encouraged and maintained for as long as possible.

Rigorous internal medical follow-up is essential, and it must be kept in mind that, in patients with dementia, even trivial intercurrent illnesses, such as an uncomplicated urinary tract infection, may cause dramatic cognitive decrements.

In addition to implementing treatment, where possible, of the underlying cause of the dementia, consideration may also be given to symptomatic treatment of various clinical features such as agitation, delusions or hallucinations, depression, and insomnia.

Agitation in dementia, as discussed in detail in Section 6.4, may respond to either risperidone or olanzapine, in low doses, for example 0.25–1 mg of risperidone or 2.5–7.5 mg of olanzapine; the same medications may also be effective in the treatment of delusions or hallucinations. It must be borne in mind, however, that, although safer than the first-generation antipsychotics (e.g., haloperidol) (Wang *et al.* 2005), these second-generation agents still carry with them an increased risk of death or stroke, especially in those patients who are 80 years or older, or those treated concurrently with benzodiazepines (Kryzhanovskaya *et al.* 2006), and, consequently, they must be used cautiously and continued only if the benefits are substantial.

Depression may be treated with an antidepressant, and consideration may be given to either citalopram or escitalopram, as these tend to be the best tolerated of the available agents.

Insomnia may be treated with melatonin or ramelteon; if these are ineffective, consideration may be given to agents such as zolpidem, with careful monitoring for any daytime sedation.

5.2 MILD COGNITIVE IMPAIRMENT

Mild cognitive impairment (MCI) (Gautier *et al.* 2006; Portet *et al.* 2006; Winblad *et al.* 2004) is a recently described syndrome seen in elderly patients, characterized, as the name suggests, by an impairment in cognitive ability that, although clearly representing a departure from the patient's premorbid baseline, is not severe enough to cause significant impairment in day-to-day activities; among those patients of 65 years or older, the prevalence of such impairment ranges anywhere from 3 to 19 percent.

As noted below, neuropathologic studies indicate that most of these patients suffer from an early stage of one or more of the common causes of dementia, most notably Alzheimer's disease. Given this, it may be just as accurate to refer to these patients as being in the prodromal stage of a dementia.

Clinical features

Cognitive impairments seen in MCI include deficits in short-term memory, calculating ability, abstracting ability, visuospatial ability, etc. Of all these deficits, short-term memory loss is the most common and, when this is seen in isolation, one speaks of the 'amnestic' type of MCI. When two or more deficits are present (which may or may not include difficulty with short-term memory), the term 'mixed domain' MCI is used; when memory is intact but some other deficit is present, one speaks of 'single-domain non-memory' MCI.

Cognitive impairment typically occurs gradually, and should be present for roughly a year before the diagnosis is made. In all three types, although patients or others report the cognitive impairment, which in turn is demonstrable on clinical evaluation, there is nevertheless no significant disruption to the patients' routine daily functioning.

Although most cases of MCI demonstrate a gradual progression over the years, in a minority the impairment remains stable or undergoes improvement.

Etiology

In autopsy studies (Bennett et al. 2005; Guillozet et al. 2003; Jicha et al. 2006; Petersen et al. 2006; Storandt et al. 2006), the most common findings are changes typical of Alzheimer's disease in medial temporal structures; other pathologies found include infarcts and diffuse Lewy body disease.

There is also an association with pre-existing depression (Barnes et al. 2006; Geda et al. 2006) and with chronic use of medications with anticholinergic properties (Ancelin et al. 2006).

Differential diagnosis

MCI must be distinguished from dementia and amnesia. One differential feature that distinguishes MCI from both of these is the severity of the cognitive deficits and their effect on activities of daily living. As noted earlier, in MCI the deficits are mild and tend to have little or no effect on day to day functioning; in contrast, in dementia and amnesia the deficits are of sufficient severity to cause obvious difficulties in patients' abilities to function. Importantly, in many, if not most, cases, long-term follow-up reveals a progression of both the severity and number of cognitive deficits to the point when a diagnosis of dementia is justified (Tschanz et al. 2006).

Delirium is immediately distinguished from MCI by the presence of confusion, which, by definition, is absent in MCI.

Treatment

The overall treatment of patients with MCI should begin with a thorough diagnostic evaluation, as discussed in the chapters on dementia and amnesia, with every attempt being made to determine the underlying cause; treatment should then proceed as for that cause. In cases of amnestic MCI, most of which represent 'incipient' Alzheimer's disease, donepezil may be given (Petersen et al. 2005); in cases preceded by depression wherein depressive symptoms persist, a case may be made for treatment with an antidepressant; and when toxic factors are present, for example anticholinergic medications, these, obviously, should be discontinued.

5.3 DELIRIUM

Delirium is one of the most common neuropsychiatric disorders seen in general hospital practice and is especially common among the hospitalized elderly (Francis 1992). Prompt diagnosis is critical as, in many cases, the underlying cause of the syndrome, untreated, carries a grave prognosis (Cameron et al. 1987; Pompeii et al. 1994; Rabins and Folstein 1982).

Clinical features

Delirium, as reviewed by Lipowski (1983, 1987, 1989), is characterized by confusion, disorientation, memory loss, and often other symptoms such as hallucinations and delusions. The syndrome is typically of acute or subacute onset, and most patients develop the full syndrome within a day or two (Levkoff et al. 1992).

Confusion, or, as it is also known, 'clouding of the sensorium', is the cardinal symptom of delirium and is present in all cases. Patients may appear dazed, their attention wanders, and they often seem to drift off. In most cases, a varying degree of incoherence will also be seen (Johnson et al. 1992; Sirois 1988). Disorientation, found in almost all cases (Morse and Litin 1971) may be for both place and time together, or merely in one of these spheres. Memory loss is typically of the short-term or anterograde type: patients are unable to remember all of three words after 5 minutes and consequently have grave difficulty in keeping track of what happens around them. Retrograde amnesia may also be present but is generally less prominent: patients may have trouble recalling clearly what happened in the days or weeks prior to the onset of the delirium.

Hallucinations are seen in about one-half of all cases (Morse and Litin 1971) and may be either visual or, less commonly, auditory (Cutting 1987; Sirois 1988). Patients may see family members in the hospital room, and bugs or small animals may hide in the sheets. Auditory hallucinations range from such simple phenomena as bells or sirens to hearing voices.

Delusions are generally fragmentary and unsystematized. One typically finds evidence of delusions of persecution (Morse and Litin 1971; Sirois 1988), and patients may report that family members are trying to get rid of them or that the medicine given by the nurse is actually poison.

The overall behavior of patients with delirium may be characterized by either agitation or quietude. Although, in a minority of cases, patients are either consistently hyperactive or consistently hypoactive, one sees in most a mix – patients now agitated, now quiet (Johnson et al. 1992; Liptzin and Levkoff 1992). In some cases, one may see an 'occupational delirium' wherein patients act as if they were at work (Wolff and Curran 1935): one patient, a former truck driver, was found with his hands held out in front of him as if gripping a steering wheel, busily 'driving' his bed around the ward. Sleep reversal is common (Johnson et al. 1992), and many patients display the phenomenon of 'sundowning', wherein their confusion markedly worsens with the coming of darkness. In some mild cases of delirium, patients may be relatively lucid in the morning, with obvious symptoms only appearing later in the day and as night falls: this is an important fact to keep in mind, for such 'lucid intervals' may deceive the physician making morning rounds into thinking that the patient is cognitively intact.

Etiology

For practical diagnostic purposes, it is useful, as laid out in Table 5.2, to subdivide delirium into various types. First, there is *toxic* delirium, occurring secondary to *medications* (e.g., opioids) or actual *intoxicants* (e.g., cocaine). After this, there is *metabolic* delirium, due to *specific metabolic derangements* (e.g., uremia), *systemic effects of infections* (e.g., pneumonia), or *vitamin deficiencies* (e.g., Wernicke's encephalopathy). Following this is *substance withdrawal delirium* (e.g., delirium tremens during alcohol withdrawal). Next one considers delirium secondary to *intracranial disorders* (e.g., *stroke*). At this point attention is shifted to a syndrome known as *post-operative delirium*: this is a very common disorder, and, in most cases, represents, etiologically, a combination of toxic, metabolic, or intracranial pathologies. Finally, there is a group of *other causes*, each of them relatively uncommon, including, for example, *autoimmune disorders*, *endocrinologic disorders*, and *epileptic disorders*.

In general hospital practice, the vast majority of deliria are toxic or metabolic in character; withdrawal delirium and delirium due to intracranial disorders are somewhat less common. In working up a case, it must be kept in mind, however, that very often the etiology is multifactorial, and that the various factors involved may be simultaneous or sequential.

In the physical examination it is very important to take note of the presence of certain abnormal movements, namely, postural tremor (Section 3.1), myoclonus (Section 3.2), and asterixis (Section 3.12), as they are very suggestive of certain etiologies. Postural tremor may be seen in toxic deliria (e.g., the serotonin and neuroleptic malignant syndromes), metabolic deliria (e.g., uremic and hepatic encephalopathy, hypoglycemia), and all of the substance withdrawal deliria. Myoclonus, likewise, may be seen in toxic deliria (e.g., the serotonin syndrome), metabolic deliria (e.g., uremic encephalopathy, hyperglycemia), and certain others (e.g., Hashimoto's encephalopathy). Asterixis is highly suggestive of one of three metabolic deliria, namely uremic encephalopathy, hepatic encephalopathy, and respiratory failure.

When, after a through history and examination, the cause of the delirium is not clear, one may consider a laboratory 'screen'. To begin with, this should include a complete blood count, a urinalysis, a chemistry survey (including sodium, blood urea nitrogen (BUN), creatinine, glucose, calcium, magnesium, liver enzymes, and bilirubin) and an ammonia level; an ANA and ESR may be ordered if an autoimmune disorder is suspected, and a drug screen may be considered if intoxication seems likely. If there is any suspicion of pneumonia a chest radiograph is ordered and, if respiratory failure is suspected, oximetry or arterial blood gases should be considered. Neuroimaging, preferably with MR scanning, is in order if an intracranial disorder is suspected. An electroencephalogram (EEG) is often ordered but, with the exception of delirium secondary to status epilepticus, often does not add much; as discussed in Section 1.5, generalized slowing or FIRDA (frontal intermittent delta activity) is common in toxic and metabolic deliria and in various of the intracranial disorders; periodic complexes are somewhat more specific, indicating such disorders as hepatic encephalopathy, uremic encephalopathy, or herpes simplex viral encephalitis. Lumbar puncture is reserved for suspected encephalitis.

These various etiologic types of delirium are now considered in turn, beginning with toxic delirium.

TOXIC DELIRIUM

Toxic delirium, as noted above, may occur due to the toxicity of certain medications, most notably opioids, or to the effects of intoxicants *per se*, such as cocaine. Medications are considered first.

Medications

In evaluating the role medications may play in a delirium it is essential to have an accurate listing of all of the patient's medications, including both those taken on a regular basis and those administered as needed; furthermore, one must note when each medication was started, and, importantly, whether there have been any recent changes in dosage. In this regard, when evaluating hospitalized patients, it is also essential to obtain a list of home medications from a reliable historian, such as a close family member. Although, as noted further on, certain medications are more likely to cause delirium than others, virtually any medicine can be at fault: this is particularly the case in elderly patients or those with pre-existing brain disease, who may be exquisitely sensitive to medications which, when taken by a younger person with an intact brain, are generally innocuous. Confirmation of a medicine's etiologic role rests on demonstrating a temporal relationship between the onset of the delirium and the initiation (or substantial dosage increase) of a medicine, and the resolution of the delirium subsequent to a discontinuation (or substantial dose decrease) of the selfsame medicine. In assessing this temporal relationship one must keep in mind that although the delirium may appear fairly promptly, often within a day or so, the resolution of the delirium may be gradual, corresponding not only to the gradual 'washout' of the offending medication, but also to the diminution of the medication's pharmacodynamic effects, which may persist for some time longer.

Of the medications listed in Table 5.2, by far the most common offenders are the opioid analgesics (Lawlor et al. 2000; Tuma and DeAngelis 2000); although both propoxyphene and tramadol can also cause delirium they are very much less likely to do so. Medications with anticholinergic effects, most notably diphenhydramine and scopolamine, run a close second to the opioid analgesics: although in some cases, they may produce a full anticholinergic syndrome, with, as described in Section 22.6, mydriasis and dry skin, these additional features may not be present. Following this is a group of medicines, such as baclofen, which, although not carrying a high risk are so commonly prescribed in some settings that they must be kept clearly in mind. With regard to baclofen it must be remembered that delirium may occur not only during treatment with baclofen, but also after long-term use, with its discontinuation.

Next are two specific syndromes, namely the serotonin syndrome and the neuroleptic malignant syndrome, which, although not common, must, given their lethality, be considered. The serotonin syndrome occurs secondary to pharmacologically enhanced serotoninergic tone, which, in turn, generally requires the administration of a combination of serotoninergic agents. Of the various combinations of medications reported to cause this syndrome (discussed in detail in Section 22.5), the most toxic is the combination of a selective serotonin reuptake inhibitor (SSRI) and a monoamine oxidase inhibitor. Clinically, the serotonin syndrome presents with a combination of delirium, myoclonus, dysarthria or ataxia, and hyper-reflexia (Feighner et al. 1990; Sternbach 1991). The neuroleptic malignant syndrome occurs secondary to any pharmacologic manipulation that leads to an abrupt diminution in dopaminergic tone. Most commonly, such a diminution occurs secondary to the use of a dopamine blocker, such as one of the first-generation antipsychotics. Second-generation antipsychotics, such as risperidone and clozapine, may also be at fault. The neuroleptic malignant syndrome will occasionally be seen secondary not to dopamine blockade but to an abrupt discontinuation of a dopaminergic agent. Thus, the neuroleptic malignant syndrome has been seen after an abrupt discontinuation of long-term treatment with levodopa or with amantadine. Clinically, within a day or two of the abrupt diminution of dopaminergic tone, patients develop varying combinations of delirium, fever, rigidity, and autonomic instability (Pope et al. 1986; Rosebush and Stewart 1989; Velamoor et al. 1994).

The remaining medications in the list are grouped under customary headings (dopaminergic medications, cardiac medications, antimetabolites, antimicrobials, anti-epileptics, antidepressants and mood stabilizers, and a miscellaneous group); for the most part these medications have only rarely been implicated in delirium and hence a fairly strong case would have to be made before ascribing a delirium to any one of them, not only by demonstrating a clear temporal relationship, but also by ruling out other, more likely causes. With regard to delirium secondary to valproate, it must be kept in mind that in some cases this is associated with elevated ammonia levels (Eyer et al. 2005), and that in these cases carnitine may be an effective treatment.

It must be kept in mind that this list is not presented as being comprehensive; new case reports continue to appear and both new and old medicines (even those long considered to be innocuous) continue to be implicated.

Intoxicants

Delirium secondary to intoxication with illicit substances is not uncommonly seen in the emergency room. Delirium secondary to cocaine or amphetamine is suggested by agitation, hypertension, and mydriasis. Delirium secondary to phencyclidine, cannabis, inhalants, and methanol is typically accompanied by cerebellar signs, such as dysarthria and ataxia.

METABOLIC DELIRIUM

Metabolic deliria, as indicated earlier, may be due not only to specific metabolic derangements, such as uremia, but also to the systemic effects of infection and to vitamin deficiencies. Each of these types is considered in turn.

Specific metabolic derangements

The specific metabolic deliria are so common that in the evaluation of delirious patients it is almost customary to order a screening chemistry survey. In general, acute derangements are more likely to cause symptoms; gradual changes are much better tolerated.

Uremic encephalopathy, as discussed in Section 13.18, is generally accompanied by both asterixis and myoclonus. In renal failure of acute onset, a BUN of over 100 is generally sufficient to cause delirium; however, in those cases where the renal failure is gradually progressive, much higher levels may be tolerated before a delirium supervenes.

Hepatic encephalopathy, discussed further in Section 13.19, may likewise be accompanied by asterixis and myoclonus, and one may, clinically, appreciate a characteristic bad breath or fetor hepaticus. Importantly, although the ammonia level is generally elevated, cases have been reported with normal levels.

Table 5.2 Causes of delirium

Toxic delirium
Medications
  Analgesics
    Opioids (Crawford and Baskoff 1980; Eisendrath *et al.* 1987;
      Morisy and Platt 1986; Steinberg *et al.* 1992)
    Propoxyphene (Nomdedeu *et al.* 2001)
    Tramadol (Kunig *et al.* 2006)
  Anticholinergics
    Diphenhydramine (Agostini *et al.* 2001)
    Scopolamine (Minagar *et al.* 1999; Ziskind 1988)
    Benztropine (De Smet *et al.* 1982)
  Commonly prescribed
    Baclofen (Lee *et al.* 1992)
    Baclofen withdrawal (Leo and Bar 2005)
    Metoclopramide (Fishbain and Rogers 1987)
    Cyclobenzaprine (Engel and Chapron 1993)
    Amantadine (Postma and Van Tilburg 1975)
    Benzodiazepines (Marcantano *et al.* 1994)
    Dextromethorphan (Lotrich *et al.* 2005)
  Specific syndromes
    Serotonin syndrome
      Combination of serotoninergic medications (Bodner
        et al. 1995)
    Neuroleptic malignant syndrome
      First-generation (Keck *et al.* 1987; Pope *et al.* 1986;
        Rosebush and Stewart 1989) and second-generation
        (Meterissian 1996, Miller *et al.* 1991; Sachdev *et al.* 1995)
        antipsychotics
    Discontinuation of dopaminergic agents (e.g., levodopa
      [Sechi *et al.* 1984; Toru *et al.* 1981], amantadine
      [Cunningham *et al.* 1991; Harsch 1987])
  Dopaminergic medications
    Levodopa (Friedman and Sienkiewicz 1991)
    Bromocriptine (Serby *et al.* 1978)
    Lergotrile (Serby *et al.* 1978)
  Cardiac medications
    Amiodarone (Anastasiou-Nana *et al.* 1986; Athwal
      et al. 2003; Barry and Franklin 1999)
    Digoxin (Eisendrath and Sweeney 1987; Shear and
      Sacks 1978)
    Quinidine (Qunitanilla 1957)
  Antimetabolites
    Tacrolimus (Buis *et al.* 2002)
    Cyclosporine (Buis *et al.* 2002)
  Antimicrobials
    Acyclovir (Rashiq *et al.* 1993; Tomson *et al.* 1985)
    Gancyclovir (Davis *et al.* 1990)
    Vidarabine (Cullis and Cushing 1984)
    Trimethoprim (Antonen *et al.* 1999)
    Cefipime (Capparelli *et al.* 2005)
    Ciprofloxacin (Altes *et al.* 1989)
    Oflaxacin (Fennig and Mauas 1992)
    Clarithromycin (Mermelstein 1997)
    Metronidazole (Kusumi *et al.* 1980)
    Ketoconazole (Fisch and Lahad 1989)

  Anti-epileptics
    Valproic acid (Beversdorf *et al.* 1996)
    Carbamazepine (Horvath *et al.* 2005)
    Gabapentin (Zhang *et al.* 2005)
  Antidepressants and mood stabilizers
    Amitriptyline (Preskorn and Simpson 1982)
    Imipramine (Goodwin 1983)
    Bupropion (Ames *et al.* 1992)
    Lithium (DePaulo *et al.* 1982; Kaplan *et al.* 2006; Simard
      et al. 1989)
    Valproic acid (Beversdorf *et al.* 1996)
  Miscellaneous
    Propranolol (Topliss and Bond 1977)
    Verapamil (Jacobsen *et al.* 1987)
    Interleukin 2 (Illowsky *et al.* 1996)
    Disulfiram (Hotson and Langston 1976; Kirubakaran *et al.*
      1983; Knee and Razani 1974; Laplane *et al.* 1992)
    Gold (McCauley *et al.* 1977)
    Aspirin (in overdose [Steele and Morton 1986])
    Bismuth (Gordon *et al.* 1995; Jungreis and Shaumberg
      1993; Molina *et al.* 1989; Supino-Viterbo *et al.* 1977)
    Bromide (Curran 1938; Palatucci 1978)
    Metrizamide (Elliot *et al.* 1984)
Intoxicants
  Cocaine (Fischman *et al.* 1976)
  Amphetamine (Hollister and Gillespie 1970)
  Phencyclidine (Allen and Young 1978; Pearlson 1981)
  Cannabis (Chopra and Smith 1974; Palsson *et al.* 1982)
  Inhalants (Evans and Raistrick 1987)
  Methanol (Bennett *et al.* 1953; Erlanson *et al.* 1965;
    Wood and Buller 1904)

Metabolic delirium
Specific metabolic derangements
  Uremic encephalopathy (Raskin and Fishman 1976;
    Stenback and Haapanen 1967; Tyler 1968)
  Hepatic encephalopathy (Fraser and Arieff 1985; Read
    et al. 1961; Summerskill *ct al.* 1956)
  Respiratory failure (Austen *et al.* 1957; Bacchus 1958; Dulfano
    and Ishikawa 1965; Westlake *et al.* 1955)
  Obstructive sleep apnea (Lee 1998; Munoz *et al.* 1998; Whitney
    and Gannon 1996)
  Hyponatremia (Karp and Laureno 1993; Swanson and Iseri
    1958; Welti 1956)
  Hypernatremia (Jana and Romano-Jana 1973)
  Hypoglycemia (Case records 1988a; Hart and Frier 1998;
    Malouf and Brust 1985; Moersch and Kernohan 1938)
  Hyperglycemia (Gomez Diaz *et al.* 1996; Khardori and
    Soler 1984)
  Hypocalcemia (Denko and Kaelbling 1962, Hossain 1970)
  Hypercalcemia (Karpati and Frame 1964; Weizman *et al.*
    1979)
  Hypomagnesemia (Fishman 1965; Hall and Joffe 1973)
  Hypermagnesemia (Clark and Bowen 1992)
Systemic effects of infection
  Sepsis (Eidelman *et al.* 1996)

(continued)

Table 5.2   *(Continued)*

Pneumonia (Johnson *et al.* 2000)
Urinary tract infection (Manepalli *et al.* 1990)
Vitamin deficiencies
Wernicke's encephalopathy (Harper 1983)
Encephalopathic pellagra (Ishii and Nishihara 1981;
Serdaru *et al.* 1988)

Substance withdrawal delirium

Delirium tremens (Isbell *et al.* 1955; Lundquist 1961;
Nielsen 1965; Rosenbaum *et al.* 1941)
Benzodiazepine withdrawal (Heritch *et al.* 1987. Levy 1984,
Zipursky *et al.* 1985)
Barbiturate withdrawal (Fraser *et al.* 1958; Isbell *et al.* 1950)
Gamma-hydroxybutyric acid (Snead *et al.* 2005)
1-4 butanediol and gamma butyrolactone withdrawal
(Catalano *et al.* 2001)
Gabapentin withdrawal (Pittenger and Desan 2007)

Intracranial disorders

Stroke (see text for references)
Microembolism syndromes
Cardiac catheterization (Karalis *et al.* 1996) or coronary
artery bypass grafting (McKhann *et al.* 2002; Wityk
et al. 2001)
Multiple cholesterol emboli syndrome (Ezzeddine
et al. 2000)
Fat embolism syndrome (Jacobson *et al.* 1986)
Infectious and related disorders
Acute encephalitis (Chaudhuri and Kennedy 2002)
Abscess (e.g., bacterial [Jefferson and Keogh 1977])
Acute disseminated encephalomyelitis (Dolgopol *et al.*
1955; Giffin *et al.* 1948; Miller *et al.* 1956; Tenenbaum
et al. 2002)
Progressive multifocal leukoencephalopathy (Astrom *et al.* 1958;
Davies *et al.* 1973; Richardson 1961; Sponzilli *et al.* 1975)
Global hypoxic-ischemic disorders
Cardiac arrest, severe hypotension (Barcroft 1920)
Carbon monoxide intoxication (Finck 1966)
Delayed post-anoxic encephalopathy (Choi 1983;
Gottfried *et al.* 1997; Norris *et al.* 1982; Plum *et al.* 1962)
Traumatic brain injury (Rao and Lyketsos 2000)
Miscellaneous disorders
Tumors
Temporal lobe (Keschner *et al.* 1936)
Hypothalamus (Alpers 1940)
Brainstem (Wallack *et al.* 1977)
Hypertensive encephalopathy (Chester *et al.* 1978; Healton
et al. 1982; Oppenheimer and Fishberg 1928)
Reversible posterior leukoencephalopathy (Hinchey *et al.* 1996)
Thrombotic thrombocytopenic purpura (Bakshi *et al.* 1999;
Druscky *et al.* 1998; Silverstein 1968)
Central pontine myelinolysis (Adams *et al.* 1959;
Brunner *et al.* 1990; Karp and Laureno 1993)

Post-operative delirium (see text for references)

Other causes

Autoimmune disorders
Systemic lupus erythematosus (Ainiala *et al.* 2001; Johnson and
Richardson 1968; O'Connor and Musher 1966)
Polyarteritis nodosa (Ford and Siekert 1965)
Hashimoto's encephalopathy (Bohnen *et al.* 1997;
Ghika-Schmid *et al.* 1996; Henchey *et al.* 1995; Shaw
et al. 1991; Thrush and Boddie 1974)
Limbic encephalitis (Alamowitch *et al.* 1997; Antoine *et al.*
1995; Brennan and Craddock 1983; Case records 1988b;
Glaser and Pincus 1969)
Endocrinologic disorders
Adrenocortical insufficiency (Engel and Margolin 1941;
Fang and Jaspan 1989)
Cushing's syndrome (Kelly 1996; Kawashima *et al.* 2004)
Thyroid storm (Friedman and Kanzer 1937)
Epileptic disorders
Complex partial status epilepticus (Mayeux and Lueders
1978; Narayanan *et al.* 2007; Rennick *et al.* 1969; Sheth
et al. 2006; Tomson *et al.* 1992)
Petit mal status epilepticus (Narayanan *et al.* 2007; Tucker
and Forster 1958, Zappoli 1955)
Post-ictal state (after grand mal or complex partial
seizure)
Miscellaneous causes
Migraine (Gardner *et al.* 1997)
Heat stroke (Yaqub and Al Deeb 1998)
Malaria (Blocker *et al.* 1968)
Hepatic porphyria (Cross 1956; Goldberg 1959; Hierons
1957; Maramattom *et al.* 2005)
Pancreatitis (Estrada *et al.* 1979; Menza and Murray 1989)
Heavy metal intoxication
Lead (Akelaitis 1941; Morris *et al.* 1964; Whitfield *et al.*
1972)
Thallium (Bank *et al.* 1972; Reed *et al.* 1963)
Arsenic (Freeman and Couch 1978; Jenkins 1966)
Tin (Feldman *et al.* 1993; Wu *et al.* 1990)
Inherited disorders of urea cycle metabolism with
hyperammonemia (ornithine transcarbamylase deficiency
[Hu *et al.* 2007] and citrullinemia [Wong *et al.* 2007])
Celiac disease (Hadjivassiliou *et al.* 2001; Hu *et al.*
2006)
Marchiafava–Bignami disease (Bohrod 1942; Ironside
et al. 1961; Kamaki *et al.* 1993; Koeppen and Barron 1978;
Rosa *et al.* 1991)
Behçet's syndrome (Akman-Demir *et al.* 1993; Serdaroglu
et al. 1989)
Wegener's granulomatosus (Nishino *et al.* 1993; Weinberger
et al. 1993)
Granulomatous angiitis (Hughes and Brownell 1966; Koo
and Massey 1988; Vollmer *et al.* 1993)
Sarcoidosis (Douglas and Maloney 1973; Silverstein and
Siltzbach 1965; Wiederholdt and Siekert 1965)
Rheumatoid arthritis with pachymeningitis (Starosta and
Brandwein 2007)

Respiratory failure, as may be seen in pneumonia or decompensated chronic obstructive pulmonary disease (COPD), generally produces a delirium when the P_aO_2 falls below 50 mmHg; CO_2 levels are not as reliable a guide in this regard: although acute rises to 70 mmHg may be associated with delirium, levels of 90 mmHg or more may be tolerated if reached gradually. In cases where the delirium is secondary to elevated CO_2 levels, patients may appear intoxicated, a phenomenon that accounts for the old term for this condition, namely 'CO_2 narcosis'.

Obstructive sleep apnea may be accompanied by delirium, not only during nocturnal awakenings, but also while the patient is awake during the day, and this appears to be particularly common in stroke patients early in their recovery (Sandberg *et al.* 2001). Although the mechanism underlying the daytime delirium is not clear, it is probably related to nocturnal hypoxemia and hypercarbia.

Hyponatremia, most commonly seen, in hospital settings at least, as part of the syndrome of inappropriate antidiuretic hormone (ADH) secretion, generally is not associated with delirium until the sodium level falls to 120 mEq/L; although gradually developing falls to this level may be tolerated, falls below 110 mEq/L are generally symptomatic.

Hypernatremia, typically seen in the setting of dehydration, may, if of acute onset, cause a delirium when the sodium level reaches 160 mEq/L; gradual rises are better tolerated, and some patients may not experience delirium even with levels of 170 mEq/L.

Hypoglycemia may cause autonomic symptoms, such as anxiety, tremor, and diaphoresis, but these may or may not be present in cases of hypoglycemia-associated delirium; in any case, cognitive dysfunction generally does not appear until the blood glucose level falls below 50 mg/dL, or lower, if the fall is gradual.

Hyperglycemia of sufficient degree to cause delirium is generally only found in either diabetic ketoacidosis or the hyperglycemic, hyperosmolar, non-ketotic syndrome. In diabetic ketoacidosis delirium may appear with blood glucose levels in the range of 300 to 700 mg/dL, whereas in the hyperglycemic, hyperosmolar, non-ketotic syndrome the range associated with cognitive dysfunction is higher, from 600 mg/dL up to an astounding 2000 mg/dL.

Hypocalcemia of sufficient degree to cause delirium is generally associated with muscle cramping and tetany. Acute falls to 8 mg/dL may cause symptoms, whereas gradual falls to 6 mg/dL may be well tolerated.

Hypercalcemia is typically associated with nausea, vomiting, constipation, and abdominal pain; delirium may supervene when the level rises above 16 mg/dL.

Hypomagnesemia typically does not cause symptoms until the level falls below 1.2 mg/dL; given that magnesium is required for the release of parathyroid hormone, there is often an associated hypocalcemia.

Hypermagnesemia, generally occurring only with increased magnesium intake in the presence of renal failure, may cause delirium at a level of 6 mg/dL if reached acutely, whereas levels as high as 18 mg/dL may be tolerated if reached very gradually.

Systemic effects of infection

Although an association between sepsis and delirium is well known, it is perhaps not as well appreciated that less severe infections can also cause delirium. This is especially the case in the elderly, as for example in the case of pneumonia or even uncomplicated urinary tract infections. Indeed, in the author's experience, several cases of urinary tract infection have presented with delirium. In all likelihood, the delirium is mediated by cytokines (Reichenberg *et al.* 2001).

Vitamin deficiencies

Of the vitamin deficiencies seen in malnourished patients, two are typified by delirium: namely Wernicke's encephalopathy and encephalopathic pellagra.

Wernicke's encephalopathy, occurring secondary to thiamine deficiency, although most commonly seen in alcoholics, may occur secondary to thiamine deficiency of any cause, including fasting (Frantzen 1966), prolonged vomiting (as in post-gastric restriction surgery [Abarbanel *et al.* 1987; Paulson *et al.* 1985]), or prolonged intravenous feeding without adequate thiamine supplementation (Vortmeyer *et al.* 1992). Although most of us were taught to look for the classic 'triad' of delirium, ataxia, and nystagmus, this combination is, in fact, the exception (Cravioto *et al.* 1961), and most patients with Wernicke's encephalopathy present with delirium alone (Harper *et al.* 1986). The recognition of this syndrome is critical: treated promptly, patients may survive without sequelae; untreated, or with delayed treatment, patients may recover but be left with a permanent Korsakoff's syndrome (Malamud and Skillicorn 1956).

Pellagra, due to niacin deficiency, occurs in two forms. The chronic form is characterized by the classic 'three Ds' of dementia, dermatitis, and diarrhea. By contrast, the acute, 'encephalopathic' form is marked by delirium, mild parkinsonism, and dysarthria.

SUBSTANCE WITHDRAWAL DELIRIUM

Withdrawal from alcohol, benzodiazepines, or barbiturates may produce a syndrome of delirium accompanied by autonomic signs such as postural tremor, diaphoresis, and tachycardia. This diagnosis, sadly, is often missed. Alcoholics in delirium tremens may deny using alcohol to excess, and their relatives are often complicit in this denial, and the same holds true for those abusing benzodiazepines or barbiturates. Both benzodiazepines and barbiturates may also be taken in high doses for therapeutic reasons, and when writing admission orders it is not uncommon for physicians not to order these home medications, even although aware of them, on the belief that they are 'not needed'.

Gamma hydroxybutyrate is now available on prescription for treatment of cataplexy, but it is not appreciated by many physicians that a withdrawal delirium, similar to delirium tremens, may occur upon its abrupt discontinuation. Two related compounds, namely 1-4 butanediol and gamma butyrolactone, taken illicitly, carry the same liability.

Gabapentin, used chronically and in high dosage, may also, if abruptly discontinued, cause delirium.

INTRACRANIAL DISORDERS

Various intracranial disorders may present with delirium, including *stroke*, various *microembolic syndromes* (e.g., after coronary artery bypass grafting), *infectious and related disorders*, *global hypoxic-ischemic disorders*, *traumatic brain injury*, and a group of *miscellaneous disorders*, such as tumors. Stroke will be considered first.

Stroke

In cases of delirium of acute onset wherein there is no obvious cause, consideration should be given to stroke. Delirium has been noted with territorial infarction in the area of distribution of the following arteries: right middle cerebral artery (primarily the inferior division with infarction of the temporal cortex [Caplan *et al.* 1986], but also the superior division with infarction of the frontal cortex [Mori and Yamdori 1987]), the left posterior cerebral artery (with infarction of the inferomedial aspect of the left temporal lobe [Medina *et al.* 1974]), and the right posterior cerebral artery (with infarction of the inferomedial aspect of the right temporal lobe) (Devinsky *et al.* 1988b; Medina *et al.* 1974). Delirium has also been noted with lacunar infarction of the thalamus (Fromm *et al.* 1985; Kumral *et al.* 2001; Perren *et al.* 2005), either unilaterally (on the left [Graff-Radford *et al.* 1984] or the right [Friedman 1985]) or bilaterally (Bogousslavsky *et al.* 1988; Giannopoulos *et al.* 2006).

The diagnosis of delirium due to infarction is typically suspected when there are associated deficits, such as hemiplegia. Unfortunately for the diagnostician, in many cases, especially when it is the temporal lobe that is infarcted, there may be no obvious signs, such as hemiplegia, and, although patients may indeed have other signs (such as hemianopia or various agnosias) their confusion may be so great as to preclude examination. It cannot be stressed enough that delirium, in itself, may at times be a 'focal' sign, indicating acute damage to the temporal lobe.

Microembolism syndromes

A 'shower' of microemboli to the cerebrum may cause multiple microinfarcts and present as a delirium, with or without obvious focal signs, such as hemiplegia. The emboli themselves may be composed of various materials: atherosclerotic debris may be released from plaques of the ascending aorta during cardiac catheterization or coronary bypass graft surgery; cholesterol emboli may be released during coronary or carotid catheterization to produce the multiple cholesterol emboli syndrome; and fat emboli may be released into the venous circulation with fractures of the long bones to produce the fat embolism syndrome.

Cardiac catheterization or coronary artery bypass graft surgery may be followed by an encephalopathy. In these cases, the ascending aorta is generally severely arteriosclerotic, and multiple minute emboli are released either as a catheter scrapes by or during cross-clamping of the aorta. Typically, patients are found to be delirious upon recovery from anesthesia, and diffusion-weighted MRI will reveal multiple small infarcts.

The multiple cholesterol emboli syndrome may occur after cardiac catheterization, coronary artery bypass grafting, or carotid catheterization. In this syndrome, multiple cholesterol crystals embolize from atherosclerotic plaques and eventually lodge in the brain. This syndrome, clinically, differs from that seen with embolization of atherosclerotic debris in that the onset of the encephalopathy is typically delayed for a day or so, corresponding to the time required for the development of an inflammatory response to these crystals; furthermore, one typically also finds evidence of embolization to the kidneys, with renal failure, and to the lower extremities, with livedo reticularis.

The fat embolism syndrome represents an uncommon complication of fractures of the long bones or trauma to fatty tissues; in both instances, globules of fat pass via the venous circulation first to the lungs, causing dyspnea, and thence to the brain, causing multiple microinfarcts and an encenphalopathy.

Infectious and related disorders

The acute appearance of a delirium in the context of headache and fever, especially if accompanied by seizures or focal signs, should immediately suggest the diagnosis of acute encephalitis, cerebral abscess, or post-infectious encephalomyelitis.

Acute encephalitis, as discussed further in Section 7.6., is generally due a viral infection, such as herpes simplex or one of the arboviruses; rarely one may see a bacterial encephalitis, as for example with Rocky Mountain spotted fever.

Abscesses, whether bacterial or mycotic, may also cause delirium, and this is more likely in cases of multiple abscesses.

Acute disseminated encephalomyelitis is probably an autoimmune disorder, triggered by a preceding, usually viral, infection. Within days to weeks after the infection, patients develop an illness very similar to that seen with acute encephalitis.

Another disorder to consider here is progressive multifocal leukoencephalopathy. This is an uncommon disorder, generally seen only in immunosuppressed patients, occurring secondary to infection by the JC virus; the onset, in contrast with the disorders just discussed, is generally subacute or gradual, and is characterized, initially, by progressively worsening focal signs; delirium supervenes only in a small minority of cases.

Global hypoxic–ischemic disorders

Global hypoxia or ischemia, if sustained for more than a few minutes, will cause a variable degree of cortical necrosis. In those who survive and emerge from coma, a delirium is seen; over time the confusion gradually resolves either leaving patients completely recovered or with a dementia known as post-anoxic encephalopathy. In general hospital practice the most common causes of such global hypoxia or ischemia are cardiac arrest or severe and sustained hypotension, as may be seen intraoperatively or during sepsis.

Carbon monoxide, by binding with hemoglobin and displacing oxygen, also leads to tissue hypoxia, causing delirium and headache.

Those who recover from a global hypoxic insult are at risk for the development of a delayed post-anoxic leuko-encephalopathy. This is an autoimmune disorder, triggered by cellular damage during the preceding hypoxic insult; clinically, within days to months after the initial hypoxic delirium, patients redevelop a delirium, often accompanied by incontinence, extensor plantar responses, and a movement disorder – either parkinsonism or, less commonly, chorea or dystonia.

Traumatic brain injury

Traumatic brain injury, as discussed in Section 7.5, is characterized pathologically by various intracranial injuries, including diffuse axonal injury, cerebral contusions, subdural hematomas, etc. Clinically, patients who do recover consciousness will be delirious for a variable period of time and may, eventually, be left with a dementia.

Miscellaneous disorders

Tumors, if appropriately situated, for example in the temporal lobe, hypothalamus or brainstem, may cause a delirium, which, in contrast with most other deliria, will be of subacute or gradual onset, in keeping with the relatively slow growth of the responsible tumor. Focal signs may or may not be present.

Hypertensive encephalopathy may occur in the setting of an acute elevation of diastolic pressure, generally to 130 mmHg or more; patients present over a day or so with headache, nausea and vomiting, delirium, blindness (or mere visual blurring) and, in many cases, seizures.

The reversible posterior leukoencephalopathy syndrome presents in a fashion similar to hypertensive encephalopathy, and is strongly associated with use of various antimetabolites, such as tacrolimus, cyclosporine, vincristine, and others.

Thrombotic thrombocytopenic purpura (TTP), generally seen in young or middle-aged adults, is characterized by delirium, transient focal signs and thrombocytopenia, with a platelet count below 30 000; other features include fever, renal failure, and purpura. The delirium itself typically shows a marked fluctuation in severity throughout the day.

Central pontine myelinolyis, occurring days after the overly rapid correction of chronic hyponatremia, typically presents with delirium and a flaccid quadriparesis; uncommonly, the presentation may be with delirium alone.

Post-operative delirium

Delirium is seen in a significant minority of patients after major operations. The term 'post-operative delirium', although in common usage, may be a little misleading as it appears to designate a specific entity, whereas in fact delirium seen post-operatively, rather than being an entity *sui generis*, merely results, as noted earlier, from one or more toxic, metabolic, or intracranial disorders occurring intra- or post-operatively.

Although post-operative delirium can occur in any patient, regardless of age or premorbid status, it is most commonly seen in the elderly and in those with pre-existing cognitive impairment (Litaker et al. 2001).

It is imperative to determine the etiology of the delirium, and in this regard it must be kept in mind that most cases are multifactorial. Toxicity secondary to medications is very common, being seen especially with opioids and benzodiazepines (Marcantoni et al. 1994) and with any medications with anticholinergic properties (Mach et al. 1995; Tune et al. 1981). Metabolic factors (Yildizeli et al. 2005) commonly seen include uremia, hepatic failure, respiratory failure, and significant elevations or depressions of sodium or glucose. Pneumonia, line infections, or urinary tract infections may contribute to the delirium via their systemic effects. Unrecognized alcoholism or benzodiazepine dependence is not uncommon, and patients may develop withdrawal delirium; furthermore, malnourished alcoholics are at risk for Wernicke's encephalopathy.

Intracranial disorders, seen particularly after cardiac surgery, such as valve replacement or coronary artery bypass grafting, include stroke and microembolism of atherosclerotic debris or cholesterol crystals. Hypoxic–ischemic injury is not uncommon and the operative report should be inspected for any episodes of significant hypotension or blood loss.

Other causes

The other causes of delirium may be heuristically grouped into autoimmune disorders, endocrinologic disorders, epileptic disorders, and, finally, a large, heterogeneous group of miscellaneous causes.

Of the *autoimmune disorders*, the most important to keep in mind is systemic lupus erythematosus. In this disease, delirium may occur secondary to infarction or to a lupus cerebritis, and this diagnosis should be considered whenever a delirium occurs in the setting of constitutional symptoms, arthralgia, rashes, pleurisy, pericarditis, and various cytopenias. Polyarteritis nodosa may cause delirium secondary to multiple cerebral infarctions and, as in lupus, the delirium generally occurs in the context of constitutional symptoms. Hashimoto's encephalopathy is a very important cause of delirium, given its treatability, and should be suspected when delirium occurs concurrent with myoclonus, ataxia, or stroke-like episodes. Limbic encephalitis, a paraneoplastic syndrome, may present with delirium alone, and, importantly, may constitute the presentation of the underlying malignancy; the diagnosis is often entertained in cases of delirium of unknown cause in middle-aged or elderly patients, especially those at risk for cancer.

Endocrinologic disorders only rarely directly cause delirium. Adrenocortical insufficiency is suggested by postural dizziness and nausea and vomiting, Cushing's syndrome by moon facies, truncal obesity, and violaceous abdominal striae, and thyroid storm by proptosis, postural tremor, tachycardia, and restlessness.

Epileptic disorders characterized by delirium include status epilepticus of the complex partial or petit mal types, and the post-ictal state. Status epilepticus is suggested by the exquisitely paroxysmal onset of the delirium, over seconds, and a history of epilepsy, and is confirmed by an ictal EEG. It is important to keep in mind that these episodes of status can last for hours, days, or even longer. The post-ictal state, after either a grand mal or a complex partial seizure, is immediately suggested by the preceding seizure.

The *miscellaneous causes* listed in Table 5.2 constitute rare causes of delirium but should be considered when the diagnostic work-up has been unrevealing.

DIFFERENTIAL DIAGNOSIS

Delirium must be distinguished from dementia, sensory aphasia, amnesia, and psychosis.

Dementia is distinguished by an absence of significant confusion. As noted earlier, confusion is the cardinal symptom of delirium: both delirium and dementia are characterized by memory deficits, disorientation, etc., but only in delirium does one find prominent and persistent confusion. At times, however, one may find dementia and delirium in the same patient. Pre-existing brain damage of any sort makes patients more sensitive to various toxic and metabolic insults (Koponen and Riekkinen 1993; Koponen *et al.* 1989; Layne and Yudofsky 1971; O'Keefe and Lavan 1997), and it is not uncommon to find a patient with dementia, for example due to Alzheimer's disease or multi-infarct dementia, promptly becoming delirious upon coming being given an opioid analgesic or coming down with pneumonia. Furthermore, some disorders capable of causing dementia may also, at times, of themselves, cause confusion. This is perhaps most problematic, from a diagnostic point of view, in cases of diffuse Lewy body disease, wherein patients, once demented, are prone to develop transient episodes of confusion, lasting perhaps hours, which then resolve spontaneously. Another common example is multi-infarct dementia, wherein the dementia is, as it were, punctuated by an episode of confusion occurring with each fresh infarction: as the peri-infarct edema resolves, the delirium clears, leaving the patient one cognitive 'step' further down. Finally, in the end-stage of most neurodegenerative disorders, most patients gradually develop a persistent confusion: whether, nosologically, this should be considered merely an extension of the dementing process or the transition of a dementia into a delirium, may be a moot point.

Sensory aphasia is characterized by incoherence and hence these patients with this condition appear similar to those delirious patients who also demonstrate incoherence.

A differential point is confusion: aphasic patients, despite their incoherence, are generally focused and appear attuned to events in their environment; in contrast, delirious patients, with their confusion, appear dazed and have great difficulty attending to events around them.

Amnesia, like dementia and sensory aphasia, is distinguished by an absence of confusion. In some cases, however, a single underlying pathology may initially present with a delirium, which, upon resolution, leaves the patient with an amnesia. A familiar example is thiamine deficiency, which, acutely, causes the delirium of Wernicke's encephalopathy, and which, upon resolution, leaves the patient with the amnestic Korsakoff's syndrome.

Psychosis, although primarily characterized by delusions and hallucinations, may, when severe, also be characterized by confusion. A common example is the psychosis of schizophrenia: here, during periods of exacerbation, confusion may be quite severe. It is not clear whether or not one should consider this development of confusion, nosologically, as merely part of the psychosis, or whether one should make a diagnosis of psychosis with superimposed delirium. Certainly, if the confusion persists after treatment of the psychosis when the delusions and hallucinations have cleared then it would be appropriate to consider a 'dual' diagnosis and proceed with a work-up as described above.

Treatment

Concurrent with symptomatic treatment, as described below, it is imperative to pursue a vigorous diagnostic investigation and, if possible, treat the underlying cause.

Symptomatic treatment, in all cases, involves environmental measures; symptomatic pharmacologic treatment may also be required in 'noisy' deliria when agitation is prominent, and in cases where delusions or hallucinations impel patients to dangerous behaviors.

Environmental measures are aimed at enabling patients, as much as possible, to stay 'in touch' with the environment and the current situation. Large calendars and digital clocks should be kept in full view, and the importance of having a window in the room cannot be overstated (Wilson 1972). At night, the room should be as quiet as possible, and nursing procedures that can be delayed to the daylight hours should be. A night-light should be left on, and a nurse's call button should be within easy reach. In some cases, for example when confused patients are apt to get out of bed and either wander off, or perhaps slip and fall, sitters may be required.

Pharmacologic treatment, as discussed further in Section 6.4, may involve use of either risperidone or haloperidol. In emergent situation, one may begin with either risperidone (as the concentrate) in a dose of from 0.25 to 1 mg, or haloperidol, 1–5 mg (either as the concentrate or parenterally, using roughly half the oral dose), with repeat doses every 1–2 hours until the patient is out of danger, limiting side-effects occur, or one reaches a maximum dose (approximately 5 mg of risperidone or 20 mg or haloperidol). The patient should then be started on a regular daily dose, roughly equivalent to the total amount required in p.r.n. doses, with an order for repeat doses on as needed basis; on subsequent days, the total daily dose should be adjusted based on the clinical situation and on the amount required in p.r.n. doses over the preceding 24 hours. In non-emergent situations, one may begin with risperidone in a dose of 0.5–1 mg or haloperidol in doses of from 2 to 5 mg, with subsequent dosage adjustments made on a daily basis. Other antipsychotics, for example, quetiapine, although not as yet proven effective in blinded studies, are, in fact, used with success, and may be considered. Quetiapine may be given in emergent situations in doses of 25 mg orally every 2–3 hours until one of the end-points just described, with the maximum total dose being roughly 200 mg; in non-emergent situations one may begin with quetiapine in a dose of from 25 to 75 mg, with subsequent daily adjustments. Lorazepam is often used in general hospital practice; however, as pointed out in Section 6.4, blinded work suggests that the side-effects of lorazepam may outweigh any benefits.

In some cases, restraints may be required: one should not be shy about ordering these, as they may be life-saving.

5.4 AMNESIA

Memory is technically divided into two broad types: memory for how things are done (known as procedural memory) and memory for things that have happened in the past (known as declarative memory). An example of procedural memory would be one's ability to remember how to ride a bicycle or play a piano, and examples of declarative memory include one's ability to remember what happened 5 minutes earlier, a day earlier, or years ago. These two types of memory are quite distinct, and procedural memory may remain intact in cases of profound deficits in declarative memory (Cavaco et al. 2004). From a clinical point of view, disorders of declarative memory are most important, and this section focuses on these.

Defective memory may or may not be accompanied by other cognitive deficits, such as confusion or deficits in abstracting or calculating abilities; when other deficits are present, consideration, as discussed below under 'Differential diagnosis', should be given to a diagnosis of syndromes such as delirium or dementia. This section focuses on amnesia as a specific syndrome, characterized by a more or less isolated and 'pure' memory deficit.

Clinical features

New memories are formed on an ongoing basis and this process may occur either automatically or as a matter of effort, for example when one 'pays attention' to something in an attempt to 'commit' it to memory. Once memories are formed, and, as it were 'stored', they may, with a greater or lesser degree of difficulty, be recalled. Amnesia may affect either one of these aspects of memory: when there is difficulty in forming new memories, one speaks of 'anterograde' amnesia, and when there is difficulty in summoning up memories one speaks of 'retrograde' amnesia.

Anterograde amnesia is often also referred to as 'short-term' memory loss, and is tested for, formally, by giving patients three words to remember, having them repeat them once, and then, after 5 minutes spent on other items, coming back and asking patients to recall the three words, noting how many are accurately recalled: normally, all three are remembered. Informally, one may find during the interview that patients with short-term memory loss repeat the same question they asked minutes earlier, as they have no recall of the answer that had been provided.

Retrograde amnesia is also referred to as 'long-term' memory loss, and is tested for during the interview by a series of questions, focusing on memories of autobiographic events successively more distant in the past. Thus, one may ask patients what they had for breakfast, what brought them to the hospital, how they had spent the past few weeks, where they lived, went to school, etc.; long-term memory for public events may similarly be tested by asking about current newsworthy events or by asking patients to name the last four presidents.

There are three different types of amnestic syndromes. The first is constituted by transient episodes characterized by anterograde amnesia with a variable retrograde component. The second type is chronic and characterized not only by an anterograde component but also by a prominent retrograde one. The third is quite rare, and is characterized primarily by a deficit in retrograde memory. Each of these is now considered in turn.

EPISODIC ANTEROGRADE AMNESIA

Episodes of anterograde amnesia typically begin abruptly and generally resolve in less than a day. During the episode, patients are unable to keep track of what is happening, and are unable to recall three out of three words after 5 minutes. There may also be a retrograde component, in that patients may have difficulty recalling what happened in the minutes or hours (and sometimes months or years) just prior to the onset of the episode. Once the episode terminates, patients are once again able to keep track of ongoing events, and are able to recall three out of three words after 5 minutes; furthermore, they are able to recall events that happened up until, or just before, the episode began. Notably, however, they are unable to recall what happened while they were in the episode: looking back, it is as if there is an 'island' of amnesia, a period of time for which they have no recall.

CHRONIC ANTEROGRADE AMNESIA WITH A RETROGRADE COMPONENT

Depending on the underlying cause, as discussed further on, this type of amnesia may have either a relatively acute onset (e.g., after infarction of the temporal lobes) or a gradual one (e.g., when due to a neurodegenerative disorder such as Alzheimer's disease). Upon examination one finds that patients are unable to keep track of ongoing events and unable to recall three out of three words after 5 minutes. Furthermore, they will have difficulty recalling events of the more distant past, events which, before falling ill, they were able to recall without difficulty. This retrograde component often exhibits a 'temporal gradient' in that the patients' recall, although perhaps quite poor for relatively recent events, becomes progressively better for events progressively more distant in the past (Albert *et al.* 1979; Seltzer and Benson 1974).

RETROGRADE AMNESIA

This is a very rare, and quite unusual, type of amnesia. Premorbidly, patients have no difficulty in remembering events of their past; once having fallen ill, however, they are unable to summon up memories of past events: one patient commented that it was as if his memories had been 'destroyed'. Remarkably, in the face of this severe retrograde memory deficit, patients retain anterograde capabilities, and are able to keep track of ongoing events and to recall all three out of three words after 5 minutes.

Etiology

The various causes of amnesia are listed in Table 5.3, and discussed in detail below, beginning with the episodic anterograde amnesias.

EPISODIC ANTEROGRADE AMNESIA

Transient global amnesia (discussed further in Section 10.18) is the prototype of episodic anterograde amnesia. This condition usually has an onset in the seventh decade of life and is characterized by the appearance of one or more episodes, lasting anywhere from 4 to 18 hours, and sometimes longer, during which there is a dense anterograde amnesia coupled with a retrograde amnesia of variable duration, from hours to decades (Hodges and Ward 1989; Kritchevsky and Squire 1989; Kushner and Hauser 1985; Miller *et al.* 1987; Quinette *et al.* 2006; Shuttleworth and Morris 1966). Characteristically during the episode, patients, although not confused, may repeatedly ask what is happening. Recovery is typically complete except for an 'island' of amnesia extending backwards in time from when the episode resolved to perhaps an hour or two before the episode began. In some cases, it appears that the episode is precipitated by some emotionally laden event, such as sexual intercourse or an argument (Fisher 1982; Kushner and Hauser 1985).

Pure epileptic amnesia (discussed further in Section 7.3) represents a partial seizure characterized solely by a combination of anterograde and variable retrograde amnesia

Table 5.3   Causes of amnesia

Episodic anterograde amnesia
Transient global amnesia
Pure epileptic amnesia
Blackouts
Concussion
Transient ischemic attacks
'Transient tumor attacks'

Chronic anterograde amnesia with a retrograde component
Korsakoff's syndrome
Stroke
  Temporal lobe
  Thalamus
Tumors
Limbic encephalitis
Neurodegenerative disorders
  Alzheimer's disease
  Pick's disease
  Frontotemporal dementia
Traumatic brain injury
Global hypoxic injury
Encephalitis
Status epilepticus
Certain neurosurgical procedures

Retrograde amnesia
Epileptic
Traumatic brain injury
Herpes simplex encephalitis

(Butler *et al.* 2007; Lee *et al.* 1992; Palmini *et al.* 1992; Stracciari *et al.* 1990). These amnestic episodes differ from those of transient global amnesia in that they are of hyperacute, or paroxysmal, onset, relatively brief, and may not be accompanied by anxious questioning on the patient's part. Furthermore one typically finds evidence of either complex partial or grand mal seizures in the history.

Blackouts (Goodwin 1971; Goodwin *et al.* 1969a,b) may complicate moderate or severe alcohol intoxication, and although characteristic of chronic alcoholism, they may at times be seen in normal subjects. The patients themselves are generally not aware anything is amiss, and apart from other evidence of intoxication (e.g., dysarthria), others may not be able to discern any problem either. The next day, however, patients may find that they have no memory of the night before, and may anxiously (and often circumspectly) ask others what happened. Importantly, although alcohol is the usual culprit, blackouts may also occur with benzodiazepines, especially those of high potency, such as triazolam (Greenblatt *et al.* 1991).

Concussion, as may occur after minor head injury (Fisher 1966) or whiplash (Miller 1982), may be accompanied by a dense anterograde and variable retrograde amnesia, and upon recovery, the patient is left with the typical 'island' of amnesia, extending back from the time of recovery to, generally, either the injury itself or a short time before that. In one famous example (as reported in the New York *Daily News* of 3 August 1928), Gene Tunney, a heavyweight contender, recalled nothing of a boxing match even though he won the fight. He later decided to quit boxing before a blow would, as he put it, 'permanently hurt my brain'.

Transient ischemic attacks may be characterized in whole or in part by an episode of amnesia. This has been noted with ischemia of the left thalamus (Gorelick et al. 1988) and in the area of distribution of the posterior cerebral arteries; in the latter case, the presence of visual problems, such as hemianopia or cortical blindness, served to indicate the cortical areas involved (Benson et al. 1974). In another case, an episode occurred during cardiac angiography, presumably on an embolic basis (Shuttleworth and Wise 1973). Distinguishing between amnesia resulting from a transient ischemic attack and that caused by transient global amnesia may be difficult unless there are associated symptoms such as hemianopia.

'Transient tumor attacks' occur in association with cerebral tumors and may happen either because of transient compression of a nearby artery or because of a tumor-related seizure. In one case of a left-sided temporoparietal mass, the attack was characterized by an episode of amnesia (Lisak and Zimmerman 1977).

CHRONIC ANTEROGRADE AMNESIA WITH A RETROGRADE COMPONENT

As this type of amnesia localizes reasonably well to the circuit of Papez, a review of the relevant neuroanatomy may be helpful. The circuit of Papez involves the mamillary body, thalamus, hippocampus, and fornix. Fibers from the mamillary body project to the anterior thalamic nuclei via the mamillothalamic tract. The anterior thalamic nuclei, in turn, project to the cingulate cortex and its cingulum, which in turn projects to the entorhinal and subicular cortices on the medial aspect of the temporal lobe. Fibers from the entorhinal cortex extend, via the perforant pathway, to terminate in the dentate gyrus, from where fibers arise that project to the pyramidal cells of the hippocampus proper. In turn, hippocampal fibers become incorporated into the fornix, which also receives fibers directly from the subicular cortex. The fornix then proceeds posteriorly and superiorly, arching up under the splenium to course anteriorly under the corpus callosum, eventually turning inferiorly, as the columns of the fornix, to dive down into and through the hypothalamus, finally coming to rest in the mamillary body and thus completing the circuit.

This type of amnesia has been noted with lesions in most portions of the circuit of Papez, beginning with the mamillary bodies (Kahn and Crosby 1971; Tanaka et al. 1997). Amnesia has also occurred with thalamic lesions but it has been difficult to pinpoint exactly which tracts or nuclei in the thalamus are involved. Lesion studies strongly implicate the mamillothalamic tract (Graff-Radford et al.

1990; Malamut et al. 1992; von Cramon et al. 1985), the anterior thalamic nuclei (Pepin and Auray-Pepin 1993), and perhaps the mediodorsal nucleus (Clarke et al. 1994; Gorelick et al. 1988). Turning next to the temporal lobes, temporal lobectomy may cause amnesia (Penfield and Mathieson 1974), and lesions confined to the hippocampus (Duyckaerts et al. 1985), specifically fields CA1 and CA2 of the hippocampus (Kartsounis et al. 1995) or CA1 alone (Zola-Morgan et al. 1986), have also been responsible. Lesions of the fornix have been implicated (D'Esposito et al. 1995; Gaffan et al. 1991; Sweet et al. 1958), including those located beneath the splenium (Heilman and Sypert 1977) and those involving the columns (Calabrese et al. 1995; Hodges and Carpenter 1991).

Although these lesions have in most cases been bilateral, it appears that a properly situated unilateral lesion may also be to blame. Thus, amnesia has occurred with unilateral lesions of the thalamus, either on the left (Choi et al. 1983; Clarke et al. 1994; Gorelick et al. 1988; Landi et al. 1982) or on the right (Pepin and Auray-Pepin 1993), and with unilateral lesions of the temporal lobes, with either temporal lobectomy (Scoville and Milner 1957; Walker 1957) or infarction (Gaffan et al. 1991).

Specific disorders capable of producing such lesions of the circuit of Papez are now discussed, beginning with the prototype, namely, Korsakoff's syndrome.

Korsakoff's syndrome occurs as a sequela to Wernicke's encephalopathy (Malamud and Skillicorn 1956; Victor and Yakovlev 1955). Wernicke's encephalopathy occurs secondary to thiamine deficiency and is characterized, pathologically, by hemorrhage in the mammillary bodies and dorsomedial nuclei of the thalamus. Clinically, patients with Wernicke's encephalopathy present with delirium (with or without nystagmus and ataxia); as the delirium clears, patients are left with an amnesia. Of note, from a nosologic point of view, the term 'Korsakoff's syndrome' is often used to refer to all cases of chronic anterograde amnesia with a retrograde component; in this text, however, it refers only to the form occurring secondary to thiamine deficiency.

Stroke may be characterized by amnesia, this having been noted with infarction of the medial aspect of the temporal lobe or the medial portion of the thalamus. Infarction of the medial aspect of the temporal lobe, in the area of distribution of the posterior cerebral artery, involves, among other structures, the hippocampus, and it is from this lesion that the amnesia arises (DeJong et al. 1969; Victor et al. 1961). The involvement of other 'downstream' structures may lead to symptoms that suggest the correct diagnosis, including hemianopia, cortical blindness, or alexia without agraphia (Benson et al. 1974). In the case of thalamic infarction, the stroke may be initially characterized by coma (Hodges and McCarthy 1993; Malamut et al. 1992) or delirium (Clarke et al. 1994); as alertness returns and confusion clears, the patient is left with an amnesia. In two remarkable cases, however, amnesia was the dominant and initial manifestation of the infarction (Pepin and Auray-Pepin 1993; Warren et al. 2000).

Thalamic hemorrhage may also be at fault with, in one such case, an amnesia emerging after the clearing of a delirium (Choi *et al.* 1983). Amnesia has also been noted as a sequela of infarction of the fornices (Fukatsu *et al.* 1998; Park *et al.* 2000).

Tumors, if properly situated, may cause a progressive amnesia, which has been noted with the following: craniopharyngiomas (which compress the overlying mamillary bodies) (Kahn and Crosby 1971; Palmai *et al.* 1967; Tanaka *et al.* 1997; Williams and Pennybacker 1954), thalamic tumors (Ziegler *et al.* 1977), large tumors affecting structures such as the corpus callosum, fornices, and thalami (Sprofkin and Sciarra 1952), and a subsplenial tumor, which damaged both fornices (Heilman and Sypert 1977).

Limbic encephalitis results from an autoimmune assault on the limbic system, including the hippocampus. Although most patients present with delirium, the delirium will, in a small minority, be preceded by an amnestic syndrome (Alamowitch *et al.* 1997; Bak *et al.* 2001; Nokura *et al.* 1997, Scheid *et al.* 2004).

Neurodegenerative disorders may present with an amnesia that evolves very slowly into a dementia; in a sense, the amnesia represents a 'prodrome' to the dementia. This is most commonly seen with Alzheimer's disease (Crystal *et al.* 1989; Didic *et al.* 1998; Linn *et al.* 1995; Sim *et al.* 1966), but has also been noted with Pick's disease (Wisniewski *et al.* 1972) or frontotemporal dementia (Graham *et al.* 2005).

Traumatic brain injury characteristically causes coma, and upon recovery from the coma, the patient may be left with various cognitive deficits, prominent among which may be an amnesia. The amnesia has both anterograde and retrograde components, and the duration of the anterograde amnesia generally (but not always) correlates well with the severity of the injury itself (Russell and Smith 1961; Wilson *et al.* 1994). The retrograde amnesia exhibits a temporal gradient (Levin *et al.* 1988), and as the patient experiences some recovery, the period of time covered by the retrograde amnesia gradually shrinks (Russell and Nathan 1946). Importantly, neither missile nor crush injuries are associated with much in the way of amnesia, and indeed, in some cases, there may be none at all (Russell 1951; Russell and Schiller 1949).

Global hypoxic injury, as may occur with attempted hanging (Berlyne and Strachan 1968; Medalia *et al.* 1991), carbon monoxide intoxication (Alison 1961), cardiorespiratory arrest (Broman *et al.* 1997; Cummings *et al.* 1984), or after inhalation anesthesia (Muramoto *et al.* 1979), may, upon the recovery of consciousness, be followed by an amnesia.

Encephalitis may have an amnesia as one of its sequelae (Rose and Symonds 1960); this is particularly true of herpes simplex encephalitis, which often affects medial temporal structures (Hokkanen *et al.* 1996; Kapur *et al.* 1994; McGrath *et al.* 1997; Young *et al.* 1992).

Status epilepticus may leave an amnesia in its wake, as occurred in one case after grand mal status (Meierkord *et al.* 1997).

Certain neurosurgical procedures may have amnesia as a complication. Unilateral temporal lobectomy may be at fault (Walker 1957), but in some cases at least, this appears to be because the remaining temporal lobe had already been damaged in some fashion (Penfield and Mathieson 1974). Surgery for an anterior communicating artery aneurysm may be followed by an amnesia (Abe *et al.* 1998; Phillips *et al.* 1987; Talland *et al.* 1967), and this appears to be not uncommon when preceded by actual rupture of the aneurysm (Lindquist and Norlen 1966). Neurosurgical intervention directed toward the third ventricle, as in an attempt to remove a colloid cyst, may cause injury to the fornices, with a resulting amnesia (Hodges and Carpenter 1991).

RETROGRADE AMNESIA

Pure retrograde amnesia, without any anterograde component, may occur on either an episodic or a chronic basis.

Episodic retrograde amnesia occurred, in one case, as a manifestation of a seizure: the patient experienced the sudden onset of an inability to recall any events of his life, but was able, even during the seizure, to keep track of ongoing events; once the seizure terminated, he was again able to recall his past (Venneri and Caffarra 1998).

Chronic retrograde amnesia appears to localize to the anterior portions of the temporal lobes, as may be seen in traumatic brain injury (Kroll *et al.* 1997; Markowitsch *et al.* 1993) or after herpes simplex encephalitis (Calabrese *et al.* 1996). In one traumatic brain injury case, a young woman, despite being eventually able to recall most of the events that had occurred after the head trauma, was unable to remember anything that happened before the trauma, all the way back to early childhood (Kapur *et al.* 1992). Further, after resolution of a herpes simplex encephalitis, a patient, although able to recall events that occurred subsequent to her recovery from the encephalitis, could not recall autobiographical events that occurred before the encephalitis, such as her own wedding (Tanaka *et al.* 1999).

Before leaving this discussion of retrograde amnesia, note must be made of a condition known as dissociative amnesia. Here, patients report a chronic inability to recall some, or all, of their past. However, in this condition, in contrast with cases of chronic retrograde amnesia occurring with, for example, traumatic brain injury, patients with psychotherapy are generally able to recover these memories (Abeles and Schilder 1935; Kanzer 1939). This is a controversial condition and there is some doubt regarding whether it actually exists.

Differential diagnosis

Amnesia must be distinguished from delirium and dementia. Although both of these syndromes include difficulty with memory, they are distinguished by the presence of additional features, not seen in amnesia, such as confusion in delirium, and in dementia deficits in abstracting and calculating ability.

MCI may manifest with a chronic deficit in anterograde memory and the differential here is based on severity: in MCI, the memory deficit is not severe enough to interfere with activities of daily living, whereas in amnesia it is. It must be kept in mind, as discussed earlier in Section 5.2, that in most instances MCI constitutes merely a prodrome to a full syndrome of either amnesia or dementia.

Depression may mimic an amnestic condition, especially when the task of recall is effortful (Cohen *et al.* 1982; Roy-Byrne *et al.* 1986): such depressed patients essentially 'give up' on the task. The presence of other depressive symptoms, such as depressed mood, fatigue, and insomnia, suggests the correct diagnosis.

Treatment

Where available, treatment is directed at the underlying condition. Supervision of a variable degree is often required during the amnesia, and this may suffice for the transient forms. In the case of persistent amnesias, various techniques, such as the use of mnemonics and lists, may enable the patient to better navigate the temporal landscape.

5.5 MENTAL RETARDATION

Mental retardation is characterized by a failure to progress, despite adequate educational opportunity, beyond a certain developmental point, in both an intellectual and a social sense. This is a very common disorder, seen in about 1 percent of the general population.

Clinical features

Mental retardation is divided, according to its severity, into four grades, namely mild, moderate, severe, and profound. Thus, those with mild mental retardation generally progress no further than an elementary school level, those with moderate mental retardation a second-grade level, those with severe mental retardation a pre-school level, and those with profound mental retardation the level seen in infants or very small children. By convention, these various grades of mental retardation are also demarcated by IQ level and these are presented in Table 5.4, along with the

Table 5.4 Grades of mental retardation

Grade	Developmental age (years)	IQ
Mild	7–11	50–55 to 65–75
Moderate	3–7	35–40 to 50–55
Severe	1–3	20–25 to 35–40
Profound	<1	<20–25

'developmental' age at which the patient's intellectual and social progress generally stalls. Mild mental retardation is most common, seen in about 80–85 percent of cases; 10–12 percent are moderate, 3–7 percent are severe, and roughly 1 percent are profoundly retarded. Among the mildly retarded, males outnumber females; however, as the grade of retardation increases, the sex ratio approaches unity. Each of these grades is described below in more detail.

Mild mental retardation may not become apparent until the child is in elementary school. These children have difficulty in learning to read, write, and do arithmetic, and at best they may progress academically to a fourth-, fifth-, or perhaps sixth-grade level. Thinking is more or less concrete, and seeing things from another's point of view or appreciating the importance of anything that lies outside of their immediate concerns is difficult. These patients fail to grasp social nuances and may appear 'immature'. Affects tend to be exaggerated, with little or no shading: a patient may slip from joyful exuberance to profound, seemingly inconsolable, despair within moments. Judgment tends to be poor and a certain degree of gullibility is often displayed. Sudden changes or new situations often catch these patients helpless and render them in need of direct, one-on-one supervision if they are to make it successfully through the transition. In tranquil circumstances, however, many of these patients are able to work at simple jobs and to live independently or with only minimal supervision.

Moderate mental retardation is generally apparent during pre-school years. These children are often able to talk but have great difficulty in learning to read, write, or do arithmetic and at best may progress academically to a second-grade level. Thinking is sparse, very concrete, and limited to immediate needs. These patients fail to understand ordinary social conventions and have great difficulty in getting along with others. With close supervision they may be able to perform simple work and live outside of an institution, perhaps in a group home.

Severe mental retardation is generally apparent during the first several years of life. Malformations may be apparent at birth and seizures are not uncommon. These infants are slow to laugh, have difficulty in imitating others, and at best acquire only limited speech. They do not learn to read or write, and at best may be able to count on their fingers. Some may be able to live with family or in closely supervised group homes; however, many are unable to survive outside of an institution.

Profound mental retardation is usually apparent during the first year of life. Malformations are common, as are seizures. These infants are generally unable to walk, and some may be unable to stand or even sit. Speech is generally not acquired, and vocalizations are generally limited to grunts, cries, or some expression of pleasure. Constant close supervision is required to maintain adequate nutrition and hygiene, and institutional care is generally required.

In addition to these specific aspects, patients with mental retardation often display a number of associated features.

Aggression, impulsivity, a low frustration tolerance, and an insistence on routine may be seen in all grades. Among those with moderate and higher grades, feeding difficulties, stereotypies and self-injurious behaviors may be seen, and among the severely and profoundly retarded, rectal digging and coprophagia may occur.

Feeding difficulties include pica, rumination, and food refusal. Food refusal at times may be related to conditions such as pharyngeal or esophageal dysmotility, or to reflux, but at times appears to have no other cause than the mental retardation.

Common stereotypies include rocking, head-rolling, waving or hand-flapping, finger-sucking, or repeated, meaningless utterances.

Self-injurious behaviors may include slapping, scratching, head-banging, hair-pulling, biting, and eye-gouging.

Rectal digging, as noted, is generally seen only in the severely and profoundly retarded, and generally only in those who are institutionalized. Although it may be related to conditions such as hemorrhoids or pinworms, at times it seems simply to stem from the mental retardation. In addition to coprophagia, fecal smearing may also occur.

Other neuropsychiatric disorders are seen in one-half or more of patients with mental retardation (Gillberg et al. 1986; Gostason 1985) and may include attention-deficit/hyperactivity, major depressive disorder, bipolar disorder, or schizophrenia. In instances where another disorder does occur the mental retardation itself modifies the presentation of the new disorder, occasionally making it almost unrecognizable. Thus, depression may present merely with insomnia, weight loss, and psychomotor change, and mania may present as irritability, agitation, and sleeplessness. Schizophrenia may manifest only with bizarre behavior.

Etiology

Although there are over a thousand different causes of mental retardation, only several dozen account for the vast majority of cases. Common causes are noted in Table 5.5, where they are divided into three groups: genetic and chromosomal abnormalities, intrauterine insults, and peri-natal or post-natal factors. In the United States, by far the most common causes of mental retardation are Down's syndrome, fragile X syndrome, and fetal alcohol syndrome.

These common causes are discussed below; in working up a case, if the clinical and laboratory results fail to support one of these then referral to a specialist is in order.

GENETIC AND CHROMOSOMAL ABNORMALITIES

Polygenic inheritance is of particular importance, especially in cases of mild mental retardation (Thapar et al. 1994).

Down's syndrome is suggested by a characteristic appearance with narrowed palpebral fissures, epicanthal folds, a broad nasal root, and an often-protruding tongue. Importantly, as noted in the Section 5.1, a dementia may supervene in adults with Down's syndrome. Although typically in such cases autopsy reveals pathology characteristic of Alzheimer's disease (Evenhuius 1990), these patients are also prone to hypothyroidism, which, of itself, may also cause dementia (Lai and Williams 1989).

Fragile X syndrome may cause mental retardation in affected males, and is suggested by facial dysmorphism with a long, narrow face, prognathism, and, in those who have passed puberty, macro-orchidism (Finelli et al. 1985; Wisniewski et al. 1985).

Klinefelter's syndrome may also cause mental retardation and is suggested by a tall stature, small testicular size, and, in some, gynecomastia (Ratcliffe et al. 1982).

Tuberous sclerosis commonly causes mental retardation and is suggested by the presence of adenoma sebaceum and seizures (Lagos and Gomez 1967; Pampiglione and Moynahan 1976; Ross and Dickerson 1943).

Sturge–Weber syndrome is suggested by a facial port-wine stain, a contralateral hemiplegia, and in some, mental retardation; in those with seizures, a dementia, as noted in Section 5.1, may supervene (Lichtenstein 1954; Pascual-Castroviejo et al. 1993; Petermann et al. 1958).

Von Recklinghausen's disease, suggested by café au lait spots and neurofibromas (Huson et al. 1988) may, in a minority, also cause mental retardation (Rosman and Pearce 1967).

Both the Prader–Willi syndrome and the Bardet–Biedl syndrome may cause mental retardation, both being characterized by massive obesity and hypogonadism. Distinguishing characteristics for the Prader–Willi syndrome

Table 5.5   Common causes of mental retardation

Genetic and chromosomal abnormalities
Polygenic inheritance
Down's syndrome
Fragile X syndrome
Klinefelter's syndrome
Tuberous sclerosis
Sturge–Weber syndrome
Von Recklinghausen's syndrome
Prader–Willi syndrome
Bardet–Biedl syndrome
Lesch–Nyhan syndrome
Rett's syndrome
Phenylketonuria

Intrauterine insults
Fetal alcohol syndrome
Anti-epileptic drugs
Rubella
Toxoplasmosis

Peri-natal or post-natal factors
Cerebral palsy
Prematurity
Malnutrition

(Bray *et al.* 1983; Hall and Smith 1972; Robinson *et al.* 1992) include a characteristic dysmorphism, with almond-shaped eyes, and for the Bardet–Biedl syndrome (Rathmell and Burns 1938; Roth 1947), retinitis pigmentosa and either polydactyly or syndactyly.

The Lesch–Nyhan syndrome often causes mental retardation and is suggested by choreoathetosis and self-mutilating lip- or finger-biting (Jankovic *et al.* 1988; Lesch and Nyhan 1964; Nyhan 1972).

Rett's syndrome is seen virtually only in females and is suggested by a characteristic history (Hagberg 1993; Hagberg *et al.* 1983): at around the age of 1.5 years, mental retardation becomes apparent, along with a characteristic stereotyped hand movement, much like hand-washing. Microcephaly also gradually becomes apparent. At around the age of 3 years, there may be some partial recovery of communicative ability, and seizures often appear. Patients may then remain stable until the adult years, when scoliosis and dystonia gradually ensue.

Phenylketonuria as a cause of mental retardation is uncommon today, thanks to newborn screening. Importantly, however, adherence to the low-phenylalanine diet should be lifelong in order to prevent deterioration. It is especially critical that mothers with phenylketonuria adhere strictly to the diet during pregnancy in order to prevent neurologic damage to the fetus. Mothers who are heterozygous for the gene should also adopt the diet during pregnancy in order to prevent fetal damage (Lenke and Levy 1980).

INTRAUTERINE INSULTS

The fetal alcohol syndrome, a very common cause of mental retardation (Abel and Sokol 1986; Spohr *et al.* 1993), is characterized by short stature, microcephaly, and a characteristic facies, with shortened palpebral fissures, epicanthal folds, a thin upper lip with a smooth philtrum, maxillary hypoplasia, and a degree of micrognathia.

Anti-epileptic drugs, notably phenytoin (Hanson and Smith 1975) and valproate, taken during pregnancy may cause retardation.

Maternal infection with either rubella (Miller *et al.* 1982) or toxoplasmosis (Desmonts and Couvrer 1974) may cause severe mental retardation.

PERI-NATAL OR POST-NATAL FACTORS

Of all the disorders of peri-natal origin that may cause mental retardation, cerebral palsy (Nicholson and Alberman 1992) is the most important. Both prematurity (Collin *et al.* 1991; Volpe 1991) and malnutrition (Chase and Martin 1970) may also cause the syndrome.

Differential diagnosis

In evaluating an individual who never progressed, in an academic sense, beyond levels expected in elementary school years, consideration must first be given to whether the environment was such that, given normal intelligence, these skills could be acquired. Thus, in cases of severe deprivation or inadequate educational opportunity, the failure to acquire these skills may not reflect mental retardation at all. Observing an individual's social behavior may offer a clue here: those of normal intelligence who failed to progress academically due to a lack of educational opportunity may yet display a keen and subtle grasp of social nuances: here, this demonstration of 'native' intelligence is a more accurate reflection of intellectual capacity than is performance on tests of academic ability.

Various other conditions may, even in the presence of adequate educational resources, prevent the acquisition of academic skills, including significant deafness or reduced visual acuity, developmental disabilities (such as developmental dyslexia or developmental dysphasia), attention-deficit/hyperactivity, schizophrenia, and significant depression.

Dementia is clearly distinguished from mental retardation by its course. In mental retardation, there is no falling off or decrement in intellectual ability from a previously acquired level: rather, there is, as noted above, a 'stalling' of development wherein patients reach a plateau, significantly below that expected for their age, beyond which there is no further progress. By contrast, there is in dementia a definite falling off from a previously acquired level, this decrement being more or less profound.

Treatment

In addition to any treatment specific for the condition responsible, several measures are generally applicable for mental retardation, regardless of the cause.

Educational and training measures are especially important for those with mild and moderate mental retardation, and family members generally will benefit from counseling; in genetic or chromosomal cases, genetic counseling should be offered.

Aggressiveness and impulsivity may respond to low-dose risperidone (Aman *et al.* 2002, Vanden Borre *et al.* 1993); lithium may also be effective (Craft *et al.* 1987; Spreat *et al.* 1989); troublesome stereotypies may respond to behavioral programs and in some cases risperidone may also be effective. Self-injurious behaviors may also respond to behavioral programs; antipsychotics appear less responsive here, but clomipramine may be effective (Lewis *et al.* 1996).

Attention-deficit/hyperactivity may be treated with stimulants in the usual fashion (Gadow 1985; Handen *et al.* 1990; Payton *et al.* 1989); however, careful attention must be paid to any worsening of stereotypies with stimulant treatment; should this occur, alternatives, as discussed in Section 9.15, should be considered.

Mood disorders and schizophrenia may also be treated in the usual way.

REFERENCES

Abarbanel JM, Berginer VM, Osimani A *et al.* Neurologic complications after gastric restriction surgery for morbid obesity. *Neurology* 1987; **37**:196–200.

Abe K Inokawa A, Yanagihara T. Amnesia after a discrete basal forebrain lesion. *J Neurol Neurosurg Psychiatry* 1998; **65**:126–30.

Abel EL, Sokol RJ. Fetal alcohol syndrome is now leading cause of mental retardation. *Lancet* 1986; **2**:1222.

Abeles M, Schilder P. Psychogenic loss of personal identity. *Arch Neurol Psychiatry* 1935; **34**:587–604.

Adair JC, Digre KB, Swanda RM *et al.* Sneddon's syndrome: a cause of cognitive decline in young adults. *Neuropsychiatry Neuropsychol Behav Neurol* 2001; **14**:197–204.

Adams M, Rhyner PA, Day J *et al.* Whipple's disease confined to the central nervous system. *Ann Neurol* 1987; **21**:104–8.

Adams RD, Victor M, Mancall EL. Central pontine myelinolysis: a hitherto undescribed disease occurring in the alcoholic and malnourished patient. *Arch Neurol Psychiatry* 1959; **81**:154–72.

Adams RD, Fisher CM, Hakim S *et al.* Symptomatic occult hydrocephalus with 'normal' cerebrospinal fluid pressure. *N Engl J Med* 1965; **273**:117–26.

Agostini JV, Leo-Summers LS, Inouye SK. Cognitive and other adverse effects of diphenhydramine in hospitalized older adults. *Arch Int Med* 2001; **161**:2091–7.

Ainiala H, Loukkola J, Peltola J *et al.* The prevalence of neuropsychiatric syndromes in systemic lupus erythematosus. *Neurology* 2001; **57**:496–500.

Akelaitis AJ. Lead encephalopathy in children and adults. *J Nerv Ment Dis* 1941; **93**:313–32.

Akman-Demir G, Baykan-Kurt B, Serdaroglu P *et al.* Seven-year follow-up of neurologic involvement in Behçet's syndrome. *Arch Neurol* 1993; **53**:691–4.

Alamowitch S, Graus F, Uchuya M *et al.* Limbic encephalitis and small cell lung cancer: clinical and immunological features. *Brain* 1997; **120**:923–8.

Albert MS, Butters N, Levin J. Temporal gradients in the retrograde amnesia of patients with alcoholic Korsakoff's disease. *Arch Neurol* 1979; **36**:211–16.

Alexopoulus GS, Meyers BS, Young RC *et al.* The course of geriatric depression with 'reversible dementia': a controlled study. *Am J Psychiatry* 1993; **150**:1693–9.

Allen RM, Young SJ. Phencyclidine induced psychosis. *Am J Psychiatry* 1978; **135**:1081–4.

Alison RS, Chronic amnesic syndromes in the elderly, *Proc R Soc Med* 1961; **54**:961–5.

Alpers BJ. Relation of the hypothalamus to disorders of personality: report of a case. *Arch Neurol Psychiatry* 1937; **38**:291–303.

Alpers BJ. Personality and emotional disorders associated with hypothalamic lesions. In: Fulton JF, Ranson SW, Frantz AM eds. *Research publications. Association for Research in Nervous and Mental Disease.* Volume XX. *The hypothalmus and central levels of autonomic function.* Baltimore, MD: Williams & Wilkins, 1940.

Alpers BJ, Grant FC. The clinical syndrome of the corpus calosum. *Arch Neurol Psychiatry* 1931; **25**:67–86.

Altes J, Gasco J, de Antonio J *et al.* Ciprofloxacin and delirium. *Ann Int Med* 1989; **110**:170–1.

Alves D, Pires MM, Guimaraes A *et al.* Four cases of late onset metachromatic leukodystrophy in a family: clinical, biochemical and neuropathological studies. *J Neurol Neurosurg Psychiatry* 1986; **49**:1417–22.

Aman MG, De Smedt G, Derivan A *et al.* Double-blind, placebo-controlled study of risperidone for the treatment of disruptive behaviors in children with subaverage intelligence. *Am J Psychiatry* 2002; **159**:1337–46.

Ames D, Wirshing WC, Szuba MP. Organic mental disorders associated with bupropion in three patients. *J Clin Psychiatry* 1992; **53**:53–5.

Anastasiou-Nana MI, Anderson JL, Nanas JS *et al.* High incidence of clinical and subclinical toxicity associated with amiodarone treatment of refractory tachyarrhythmias. *Can J Cardiol* 1986; **2**:138–45.

Ancelin ML, Artero S, Portet F *et al.* Non-degenerative mild cognitive impairment in elderly people and use of anticholinergic drugs: longitudinal cohort study. *BMJ* 2006; **332**:455–9.

Antoine JC, Honnorat J, Anterion CT *et al.* Limbic encephalitis and immunological perturbations in two patients with thymoma. *J Neurol Neurosurg Psychiatry* 1995; **58**:706–10.

Antonen JA, Markula KP, Pertovaara MI *et al.* Adverse drug reactions in Sjogren's syndrome. Frequent allergic drug reactions and a specific trimethoprim-associated systemic reaction. *Scand J Rheumatol* 1999; **38**:157–9.

Arieff AJ, Wetzel N. Subdural hematoma following epileptic convulsion. *Neurology* 1964; **14**:731–2.

Armon C, Shin C, Miller P *et al.* Reversible parkinsonism and cognitive impairment with chronic valproate use. *Neurology* 1996; **47**:626–35.

Asher R. Myxoedematous madness. *BMJ* 1949; **2**:555–62.

Astrom K-E, Mancall EL, Richardson EP. Progressive multi-focal leuko-encephalopathy: a hitherto unrecognized complication of chronic lymphocytic leukaemia and Hodgkin's disease. *Brain* 1958; **81**:93–111.

Athwal H, Murphy G, Chun S. Amiodarone-induced delirium. *Am J Geriatr Psychiatry* 2003; **11**:696–7.

Austen FK, Carmichael MW, Adams RD. Neurologic manifestations of chronic pulmonary insufficiency. *N Engl J Med* 1957; **257**:579–90.

Avery TL. Seven cases of frontal tumor with psychiatric presentation. *Br J Psychiatry* 1971; **111**:19–23.

Bacchus M. Encephalopathy and pulmonary disease. *Arch Int Med* 1958; **102**:194–8.

Bak TH, Antoun N, Balan KK *et al.* Memory lost, memory regained: neuropsychological findings and neuroimaging in two cases of paraneoplastic limbic encephalitis with radically different outcomes. *J Neurol Neurosurg Psychiatry* 2001; **71**:40–7.

Bakshi R, Shaikh ZA, Bates VE *et al.* Thrombotic thrombocytopenic purpura: brain CT and MRI findings in 12 patients. *Neurology* 1999; **52**:1285–8.

Ballard C, O'Brien J, Gray A *et al.* Attention and fluctuating attention in patients with dementia wih Lewy bodies and Alzheimer's disease. *Arch Neurol* 2001; **58**:977–82.

Bank WJ, Pleasure DE, Suzuki K *et al.* Thallium poisoning. *Arch Neurol* 1972; **26**:456–64.

Barbanti P, Fabrini G, Salvatore M *et al.* Polymorphism at codon 129 or codon 219 of PRNP and clinical heterogeneity in a previously unreported family with Gerstmann–Sträussler–Scheinker disease (PrP-P102L mutation). *Neurology* 1996; **47**:734–41.

Barcroft J. Anoxemia. *Lancet* 1920; **2**:485–9.

Barnes DE, Alexopoulos GS, Lopez EL *et al.* Depressive symptoms, vascular disease, and mild cognitive impairment: findings from the Cardiovascular Health Study. *Arch Gen Psychiatry* 2006; **63**: 273–9.

Barry JJ, Franklin K. Amiodarone-induced delirium. *Am J Psychiatry* 1999; **156**:1119.

Becher MW, Rubinsztein DC, Leggo J *et al.* Dentatorubral and pallidoluysian atrophy (DRPLA): clinical and neuropathological findings in genetically confirmed North American and European pedigrees. *Mov Disord* 1997; **12**:519–30.

Benesch CG, McDaniel KD, Cox C *et al.* End-stage Alzheimer's disease: Glasgow coma scale and neurologic examination. *Arch Neurol* 1993; **50**:1309–15.

Bennett DA, Schneider JA, Bienias JL *et al.* Mild cognitive impairment is related to Alzheimer disease pathology and cerebral infarctions. *Neurology* 2005; **64**: 834–41.

Bennett IL, Cary FM, Mitchell GL *et al.* Acute methyl alcohol poisoning: a review based on experience in an outbreak of 323 cases. *Medicine* 1953; **32**:431–63.

Benson DF, Marsden CD, Meadows JC. The amnesia syndrome of posterior cerebral artery occlusion. *Acta Neurol Scand* 1974; **50**:133–45.

Berginer VM, Foster NL, Sadowsky M *et al.* Psychiatric disorders in patients with cerebrotendinous xanthomatosis. *Am J Psychiatry* 1988; **145**:354–7.

Berlyne N, Strachan M. Neuropsychiatric sequelae of attempted hanging. *Br J Psychiatry* 1968; **114**:411–22.

Beversdorf D, Allen C, Nordgren R. Valproate induced encephalopathy treated with carnitine in an adult. *J Neurol Neurosurg Psychiatry* 1996; **61**:211.

Biggins CA, Boyd JL, Harrop FM *et al.* A controlled, longitudinal study of dementia in Parkinson's disease. *J Neurol Neurosurg Psychiatry* 1992; **55**:566–71.

Bird MT, Paulson GW. The rigid form of Huntington's chorea. *Neurology* 1971; **21**:271–6.

Black DW. Mental changes resulting from subdural hematoma. *Br J Psychiatry* 1984; **145**:200–3.

Blass JP, Hoyer S, Nitsch R. A translation of Otto Binswanger's article ' The deliniation of the generalized progressive paralyses'. *Arch Neurol* 1991; **48**:961–72.

Blocker WW, Kastl AJ, Daroff RB. The psychiatric manifestations of cerebral malaria. *Am J Psychiatry* 1968; **125**:192–6.

Bodner RA, Lynch T, Lewis L *et al.* Serotonin syndrome. *Neurology* 1995; **45**:219–23.

Bogousslavsky J, Ferrazzini M, Regli F *et al.* Manic delirium and frontal-like syndrome with paramedian infarction of the right thalamus. *J Neurol Neurosurg Psychiatry* 1988; **51**:116–19.

Bohnen NILJ, Parnell KJ, Harper CM. Reversible MRI findings in a patient with Hashimoto's encephalopathy. *Neurology* 1997; **49**:246–7.

Bohrod MG. Primary degeneration of the corpus callosum (Marchiafava's disease): report of the second American case. *Arch Neurol Psychiatry* 1942; **47**:465–73.

Bornebroek M, Haan J, van Buchem MA *et al.* White matter lesions and cognitive deterioration in presymptomatic carriers of the amyloid precursor protein gene codon 693 mutation. *Arch Neurol* 1996; **53**:43–8.

Borrett D, Ashby P, Bilbao J *et al.* Reversible, late-onset disulfiram-induced neuropathy and encephalopathy. *Ann Neurol* 1985; **17**:396–9.

Borson S. Behçet's disease as a psychiatric disorder: a case report. *Am J Psychiatry* 1982; **139**:1348–9.

Bosch EP, Hart MN. Late adult-onset metachromatic leukodystrophy: dementia and polyneuropathy in a 63-year-old man. *Arch Neurol* 1978; **35**:475–7.

Bouton SM. Pick's disease. *J Nerv Ment Dis* 1940; **91**:9–30.

Bradshaw J, Saling M, Hopwood M *et al.* Fluctuating cognition in dementia with Lewy bodies and Alzheimer's disease is qualitatively distinct. *J Neurol Neurosurg Psychiatry* 2004; **75**:382–7.

Bray GA, Dahms WT, Swerdloff RS *et al.* The Prader–Willi syndrome: a study of 40 patients and a review of the literature. *Medicine* 1983; **62**:59–88.

Brennan LV, Craddock PR. Limbic encephalopathy as a non-metastatic complication of oat cell cancer: its reversal after treatment of the primary lung lesion. *Am J Med* 1983, **75**:518–20.

Brey RL, Holliday SL, Saklad AR *et al.* Neuropsychiatric syndromes in lupus. Prevalence using standardized definitions. *Neurology* 2002; **58**:1214–20.

Brody IA, Wilkins RH. Huntington's chorea. *Arch Neurol* 1967; **17**:331–3.

Broman M, Rose AL, Hotson G *et al.* Severe anterograde amnesia with onset in childhood as a result of anoxic encephalopathy. *Brain* 1997; **120**:417–33.

Brown P, Rodgers-Johnson P, Cathala F *et al.* Creutzfeldt–Jacob disease of long duration: clinicopathological characteristics, biotransmissibility, and differential diagnosis. *Arch Neurol* 1984; **16**:295–304.

Brown P, Cathala F, Castaigne P *et al.* Creutzfeldt–Jakob disease: clinical analysis of a consecutive series of 230 neuropathologically verified cases. *Ann Neurol* 1986; **20**:597–602.

Brown P, Goldfarb LG, Brown WT *et al.* Clinical and molecular genetic study of a large German kindred with Gerstmann–Sträussler–Scheinker syndrome. *Neurology* 1991; **41**:375–9.

Brown P, Gibbs CJ, Rodgers-Johnson P *et al.* Human spongiform encephalopathy: the National Institutes of Health series of 300 cases of experimentally transmitted disease. *Ann Neurol* 1994; **35**:513–29.

Bruetsch WL, Williams CL. Arteriosclerotic rigidity with special reference to gait disturbances. *Am J Psychiatry* 1954; **111**:332–6.

Brunner JE, Redmond JM, Haggar AM *et al*. Central pontine myelinolysis and pontine lesion after rapid correction of hyponatremia: a prospective magnetic resonance imaging study. *Ann Neurol* 1990; **27**:61–6.

Buis CI, Wiesner RH, Ruud AF *et al*. Acute confusional state following liver transplantation for alcoholic liver disease. *Neurology* 2002; **59**:601–5.

Bulens C. Neurologic complications of hyperthyroidism: remission of spastic paraplegia, dementia and optic neuropathy. *Arch Neurol* 1981; **38**:669–70.

Burkhardt CR, Filley CM, Kleineschmidt-DeMasters BK *et al*. Diffuse Lewy body disease and progressive dementia. *Neurology* 1988; **38**:1520–8.

Burks JS, Alfrey AC, Huddlestone J *et al*. A fatal encephalopathy in chronic hemodialysis patients. *Lancet* 1976; **1**:764–8.

Burneo JG, Arnold T, Palemr CA *et al*. Adult-onset neuronal ceroid lipofuscinosis (Kufs' disease) with autosomal dominant inheritance in Alabama. *Epilepsia* 2003; **44**:841–6.

Butler CR, Graham KS, Hodges JR *et al*. The syndrome of transient epileptic amnesia. *Ann Neurol* 2007; **61**:587–98.

Byrne EJ, Lennox G, Lowe J *et al*. Diffuse Lewy body disease: clinical features in 15 cases. *J Neurol Neurosurg Psychiatry* 1989; **52**:709–17.

Caine ED. Pseudodementia: current concepts and future directions. *Arch Gen Psychiatry* 1981; **38**:1359–64.

Calabrese P, Markowitsch HJ, Harders AG *et al*. Fornix damage and memory: a case report. *Cortex* 1995; **31**:555–64.

Calabrese P, Markowitsch HJ, Widlitzek H *et al*. Right temporofrontal cortex as a critical locus for the ecphory of old episodeic memories. *J Neurol Neurosurg Psychiatry* 1996; **61**:304–12.

Cameron DJ, Thomas RI, Mulvihill M *et al*. Delirium: a test of DSM-III criteria on medical inpatients. *J Am Geriatr Soc* 1987; **35**:1007–10.

Camp WA, Frierson JG. Sarcoidosis of the central nervous system. *Arch Neurol* 1962; **7**:432–41.

Campbell AMG, Corner B, Norman RM *et al*. The rigid form of Huntington's disease. *J Neurol Neurosurg Psychiatry* 1961; **24**:71–7.

Caplan LR, Schoene WC. Clinical features of subcortical arteriosclerotic encephalopathy (Binswanger disease). *Neurology* 1978; **28**:11206–15.

Caplan LR, Kelly M, Kase CS *et al*. Infarcts of the inferior division of the right middle cerebral artery: mirror image of Wernicke's aphasia. *Neurology* 1986; **36**:1015–20.

Capparelli FJ, Diaz MF, Hlavnika A *et al*. Cefipine- and cefixime-induced encephalopathy in a patient with normal renal function. *Neurology* 2005; **65**:1840.

Carter HR, Sukavajuna C. Familial cerebello-olivary degeneration with the late development of rigidity and dementia. *Neurology* 1956; **6**:876–84.

Caselli RJ. Giant cell (temporal) arteritis: a treatable cause of multi-infarct dementia. *Neurology* 1990; **40**:753–5.

Caselli RJ, Scheithauer BW, Bowles CA *et al*. The treatable dementia of Sjorgen's syndrome. *Ann Neurol* 1991; **30**:98–101.

Case records of the Massachusetts General Hospital. Case 23–1988. *N Engl J Med* 1988; **318**:1523–7.

Case records of the Massachusetts General Hospital. Case 39–1988. *N Engl J Med* 1988; **319**:849–60.

Case records of the Massachusetts General Hospital. Case 8–1989. *N Engl J Med* 1989; **320**:514–24.

Case records of the Massachusetts General Hospital. Case 2–1992. *N Engl J Med* 1992; **326**:117–25.

Catalano MC, Glass JM, Catalano G *et al*. Gamma butyrolactone withdrawal syndromes. *Psychosomatics* 2001; **42**:83–8.

Cavaco S, Anderson SW, Allen JS *et al*. The scope of preserved procedural memory in amnesia. *Brain* 2004; **127**:1853–67.

Cavalleri F, De Renzi E. Amyotrophic lateral sclerosis with dementia. *Acta Neurol Scand* 1994; **89**:391–4.

Chandler JH, Bebin J. Hereditary cerebellar ataxia: olivopontocerebellar type. *Neurology* 1956; **6**:187–95.

Chase HP, Martin HP. Undernutrition and child development. *N Engl J Med* 1970; **282**:933–9.

Chatterjee A, Yapundich R, Palmer CA *et al*. Leukoencephalopathy associated with cobalmin deficiency. *Neurology* 1996; **46**:832–4.

Chaudhuri A, Kennedy PG. Diagnosis and treatment of viral encephalitis. *Postgrad Med J* 2002; **78**:575–83.

Chen J-Y, Stern Y, Sano M *et al*. Cumulative risks of developing extrapyramidal signs, psychosis, or myoclonus in the course of Alzheimer's disease. *Arch Neurol* 1991; **48**:1141–3.

Chester EM, Agamanolis DP, Banker BP *et al*. Hypertensive encephalopathy: a clinicopathologic study of 20 cases. *Neurology* 1978; **28**:928–39.

Choi D, Sudarsky L, Schacter S *et al*. Medial thalamic hemorrhage with amnesia. *Arch Neurol* 1983; **40**:611–13.

Choi IS. Delayed neurologic sequelae in carbon monoxide intoxication. *Arch Neurol* 1983; **40**:433–5.

Chopra GS, Smith JW. Psychotic reactions following cannabis use in East Indians. *Arch Gen Psychiatry* 1974; **30**:24–7.

Clark BA, Bowen RS. Unsuspected morbid hypermagnesemia in elderly patients. *Am J Nephrol* 1992; **12**:336–43.

Clark JM, Marks MP, Adalsteinsson E *et al*. MELAS: clinical and pathologic correlation with MRI, xenon/CT, and MR spectroscopy. *Neurology* 1996; **46**:223–7.

Clarke S, Assal G, Bogousslavsky J *et al*. Pure amnesia after unilateral left polar thalmic infarct: topographic and sequential neurophysiological and metabolic (PET) correlations. *J Neurol Neurosurg Psychiatry* 1994; **57**:27–34.

Cohen RM, Weingartner H, Smallberg SA *et al*. Effort and cognition in depression. *Arch Gen Psychiatry* 1982; **39**:593–7.

Collin MF, Halsey CL, Anderson CL. Emerging developmental sequelae in the 'normal' extremely low birthweight infant. *Pediatrics* 1991; **88**:115–20.

Collins SJ, Ahlskog JE, Parisi JE *et al*. Progressive supranuclear palsy: neuropathologically based diagnostic clinical criteria. *J Neurol Neurosurg Psychiatry* 1995; **58**:167–73.

Colosimo C, Albanese A, Hughes AJ *et al*. Some specific clinical features differentiate multiple system atrophy (striatonigral variety) from Parkinson's disease. *Arch Neurol* 1995; **52**:294–8.

Cook DG, Fahn S, Brait KA. Chronic manganese intoxication. *Arch Neurol* 1974; **30**:59–64.

Cordingly G, Navarro C, Brust JCM *et al*. Sarcoidosis presenting as senile dementia. *Neurology* 1981; **31**:1148–51.

Coria F, Garcia-Viejo MA, Delgado JA *et al*. Diagnosis of X-adrenoleukodystrophy phenotypic variants. *Acta Neurol Scand* 1993; **87**:499–502.

Correa DD, DeAngelis LM, Shi W *et al*. Cognitive functions in survivors of primary central nervous system lymphoma. *Neurology* 2004; **62**:548–55.

Cosgrove CR, Leblanc R, Meagher-Villemure K *et al*. Cerebral amyloid angiopathy. *Neurology* 1985; **35**:625–31.

Coull BM, Bourdette DN, Goodnight SH *et al*. Multiple cerebral infarctions and dementia associated with anticardiolipin antibodies. *Stroke* 1987; **18**:1107–12.

Craft M, Ismail IA, Krishnamurti D *et al*. Lithium in the treatment of aggression in mentally handicapped patients: a double-blind trial. *Br J Psychiatry* 1987; **150**:685–9.

von Cramon DY, Hebel N, Schuri U. A contribution to the anatomical basis of thalamic amnesia. *Brain* 1985; **108**:993–1008.

Cravioto H, Korein J, Silberman J. Wernicke's encephalopathy: a clinical and pathological study of 28 autopsied cases. *Arch Neurol* 1961; **4**:510–19.

Crawford RD, Baskoff JD. Fentanyl-associated delirium in man. *Anesthesiology* 1980; **53**:168–9.

Critchley EMR, Clark DB, Wikler A. Acanthocytosis and neurological disorder without abetalipoproteinemia. *Arch Neurol* 1968; **18**:134–40.

Crompton MR, Layton DD. Delayed radionecrosis of the brain following therapeutic X-irradiation of the pituitary. *Brain* 1961; **84**:85–101.

Cross TN. Porphyria – a deceptive syndrome. *Am J Psychiatry* 1956; **112**:1010–14.

Crystal HA, Grober E, Masur D. Preservation of visual memory in Alzheimer's disease. *J Neurol Neurosurg Psychiatry* 1989; **52**:1415–16.

Cullis PA, Cushing R. Vidarabine encephalopathy. *J Neurol Neurosurg Psychiatry* 1984; **47**:1351–4.

Cummings JL. Dementia syndrome: neurobehavioral and neuropsychiatric features. *J Clin Psychiatry* 1987; **48**(suppl. 5):3–8.

Cummings JL, Tomiyasu U, Read S *et al*. Amnesia with hippocampal lesions after cardiopulmonary arrest. *Neurology* 1984; **34**:679–81.

Cunningham MA, Darby DG, Donnan GA. Controlled-release delivery of L-dopa associated with nonfatal hyperthermia, rigidity and autonomic dysfunction. *Neurology* 1991; **41**:942–3.

Curran FJ. A study of fifty cases of bromide psychosis. *J Nerv Ment Dis* 1938; **88**:163–92.

Cutting J. The phenomenology of acute organic psychosis: comparison with acute schizophrenia. *Br J Psychiatry* 1987; **151**:324–32.

Daniel SE, de Bruin VMS, Lees AJ. The clinical and pathological spectrum of Steele–Richardson–Olszewski syndrome (progressive supranuclear palsy): a reappraisal. *Brain* 1995; **118**:759–70.

Davies JA, Hughes JT, Oppenheimer DR. Richardson's disease (progressive multifocal leukoencephalopathy). *Q J Med* 1973; **42**:481–93.

Davis CL, Springmeyer S, Gmerek BJ. Central nervous system side-effects of ganciclovir. *N Engl J Med* 1990; **322**:933–4.

Davis LE, Wands JR, Weiss SA *et al*. Central nervous system intoxication from mercurous chloride laxatives. *Arch Neurol* 1974; **30**:428–31.

Dawson JR. Cellular inclusions in cerebral lesions of epidemic encephalitis. *Arch Neurol Psychiatry* 1934; **31**:685–700.

DeAngelis LM, Delattre J-Y, Posner JB. Radiation-induced dementia in patients cured of brain metastases. *Neurology* 1989; **39**:172–7.

DeJong RN, Itabashi HH, Olson JR. Memory loss due to hippocampal lesions. *Arch Neurol* 1969; **20**:339–48.

Denko J, Kaelbling R. The psychiatric aspects of hypoparathyroidism. *Acta Psychiatr Scand* 1962; (suppl. 164):1–70.

Dennis MS, Byrne EJ, Hopkinson N *et al*. Neuropsychiatric systemic lupus erythematosus in elderly people. *J Neurol Neurosurg Psychiatry* 1992; **55**:1157–61.

DePaulo JR, Folstein MF, Correa EI. The course of delirium due to lithium intoxication. *J Clin Psychiatry* 1982; **43**:447–9.

De Smet Y, Ruberg M, Serdaru M *et al*. Confusion, dementia and anticholinergics in Parkinson's disease. *J Neurol Neurosurg Psychiatry* 1982; **45**:1161–4.

Desmonts G, Couvrer J. Congenital toxoplasmosis. *N Engl J Med* 1974; **290**:1110–16.

D'Esposito M, Verfaellie M, Alexander MP *et al*. Amnesia following traumatic bilateral fornix transection. *Neurology* 1995; **45**:1546–50.

Devinsky O, Petito CK, Alonso DR. Clinical and neuropathological findings in systemic lupus erythematosus: the role of vasculitis, heart emboli and thrombotic thrombocytopenic purpura. *Ann Neurol* 1988a; **23**:380–4.

Devinsky O, Bear D, Volpe BT. Confusional states following posterior cerebral artery infarction. *Arch Neurol* 1988b; **45**:160–3.

Dichgans M, Mayer M, Uttner I *et al*. The phenotypic spectrum of CADASIL: clinical findings in 102 cases. *Ann Neurol* 1998; **44**:731–9.

Didic M, Cherif AA, Gambarelli D *et al*. A permanent pure amnestic syndrome of insidious onset related to Alzheimer's disease. *Ann Neurol* 1998; **43**:526–30.

Dolgopol VB, Greenberg M, Aronoff R. Encephalitis following smallpox vaccination. *Arch Neurol Psychiatry* 1955; **73**:216–23.

Dooling EC, Schoene WC, Richardson EP. Hallervorden–Spatz syndrome. *Arch Neurol* 1974; **30**:70–83.

Dooling EC, Richardson EP, Davis KR. Computed tomography in Hallervorden–Spatz disease. *Neurology* 1980; **30**:1128–30.

Douglas AC, Maloney AFJ. Sarcoidosis of the central nervous system. *J Neurol Neurosurg Psychiatry* 1973; **36**:1024–33.

Druscky A, Erbguth F, Strauss R et al. Central nervous system involvement in thrombotic thrombocytopenic purpura. Eur Neurol 1998; 40:220–4.

Duffy P, Chari G, Cartlidge NEF et al. Progressive deterioration of intellect and motor function occurring several decades after cranial irradiation. Arch Neurol 1996; 53:814–18.

Dulfano MJ, Ishikawa S. Hypercapnia: mental changes and extrapulmonary complications. Ann Int Med 1965; 63:829–41.

Duyckaerts C, Derouesne C, Signoret JL et al. Bilateral and limited amygdalohippocampal lesions causing a pure amnestic syndrome. Ann Neurol 1985; 18:314–19.

Eidelman LA, Putterman D, Putterman C et al. The spectrum of septic encephalopathy: definitions, etiologies and mortalities. JAMA 1996; 275:470–3.

Eisendrath SJ, Sweeney MA. Toxic neuropsychiatric effects of digoxin at therapeutic serum concentrations. Am J Psychiatry 1987; 144:506–7.

Eisendrath SJ, Goldman B, Douglas J et al. Meperidine-induced delirium. Am J Psychiatry 1987; 144:1062–5.

Elliott RL, Wild JH, Snow WT. Prolonged delirium after metrizamide myelography. JAMA 1984; 252:2057–8.

Engel GL, Margolin SG. Neuropsychiatric disturbances in Addison's disease and the role of impaired carbohydrate metabolism in production of abnormal cerebral function. Arch Neurol Psychiatry 1941; 45:881–4.

Engel PA, Chapron D. Cyclobenzaprine-induced delirium in two octogenarians. J Clin Psychiatry 1993; 54:39.

Erkinjunti T, Haltia M, Palo J et al. Accuracy of the clinical diagnosis of vascular dementia: a prospective clinical and post-mortem study. J Neurol Neurosurg Psychiatry 1988; 51:1037–44.

Erlanson P, Fritz H, Hagstam KE et al. Severe methanol intoxication. Acta Med Scand 1965; 177:393–408.

Escobar A, Aruffo C. Chronic thinner intoxicaton: clinico-pathologic report of a human case. J Neurol Neurosurg Psychiatry 1980; 43:986–94.

Estrada RV, Moreno J, Martinez E et al. Pancreatic encephalopathy. Acta Neurol Scand 1979; 59:135–9.

Evans AC, Raistrick D. Phenomenology of intoxication with toluene-based adhesives and butane gas. Br J Psychiatry 1987; 150:769–73.

Evenhuius HM. The natural history of dementia in Down's syndrome. Arch Neurol 1990; 47:263–7.

Eyer F, Felgenhauer N, Gempel K et al. Acute valproate poisoning. J Clin Psychopharmacol 2005; 25:376–80.

Ezzeddine MA, Primavera JM, Rosand J et al. Clinical characteristics of pathologically proved cholesterol emboli to the brain. Neurology 2000; 54:1681–3.

Fang VBS, Jaspan JB. Delirium and neuromuscular symptoms in an elderly man with isolated corticotroph deficiency syndrome completely reversed with glucocorticoid replacement. J Clin Endocrinol Metab 1989; 69:1073–7.

Farpour H, Mahloudji M. Familial cerebrotendinous xanthomatosis: report of a new family and review of the literature. Arch Neurol 1975; 32:223–5.

Feighner JP, Boyer WF, Tyler DL et al. Adverse consequences of fluoxetine–MAOI combination therapy. J Clin Psychiatry 1990; 51:222–5.

Feldman RG, White RF, Eriator II. Trimethyltin encephalopathy. Arch Neurol 1993; 50:132–4.

Fennig S, Mauas L. Oflaxacin-induced delirium. J Clin Psychiatry 1992; 53:137–8.

Ferraro A, Jervis GA. Pick's disease: clinicopathologic study with report of two cases. Arch Neurol Psychiatry 1936; 36:738–67.

Ferrer I, Roig C, Espino A et al. Dementia of the frontal lobe type and motor neuron disease: a Golgi study of the frontal cortex. J Neurol Neurosurg Psychiatry 1991; 54:932–4.

Finck MA. Exposure to carbon monoxide: review of the literature and 567 autopsies. Mil Med 1966; 131:1513–19.

de Fine Olivarius B, Roder E. Reversible psychosis and dementia in myxedema. Acta Psychiatr Scand 1970; 46:1–13.

Finelli PF, Pueschel SM, Padre-Mendoza T et al. Neurological findings in patients with the fragile-X syndrome. J Neurol Neurosurg Psychiatry 1985; 48:150–3.

Finlayson MH, Superville B. Distribution of cerebral lesions in acquired hepatocerebral degeneration. Brain 1981; 104:79–95.

Fisch RZ, Lahad A. Adverse psychiatric reaction to ketoconazole. Am J Psychiatry 1989; 146:939–40.

Fischman MW, Schuster CR, Resnekov L et al. Cardiovascular and subjective effects of intravenous cocaine administration in humans. Arch Gen Psychiatry 1976; 33:983–9.

Fishbain DA, Rogers A. Delirium secondary to metoclopramide hydrochloride. J Clin Psychopharmacol 1987; 7:281–2.

Fisher CM. Concussion amnesia. Neurology 1966; 16:826–30.

Fisher CM. Transient global amnesia: precipitating activities and other observations. Arch Neurol 1982; 39:605–8.

Fishman RA. Neurological aspects of magnesium metabolism. Arch Neurol 1965; 12:562–9.

Fontaine B, Seilhean D, Tourbah A et al. Dementia in two histologically confirmed cases of multiple sclerosis: one case with isolated dementia and one case associated with psychiatric symptoms. J Neurol Neurosurg Psychiatry 1994; 57:353–9.

Ford RG, Siekert RG. Central nervous system manifestations of periarteritis nodosa. Neurology 1965; 15:114–22.

Fornazzari L, Wilkinson DA, Kapur BM et al. Cerebellar, cortical and functional impairment in toluene abusers. Acta Neurol Scand 1983; 67:319–29.

Francis J. Delirium in older patients. J Am Geriatr Soc 1992; 40:829–38.

Francis J, Martin D, Kapoor W. A prospective study of delirium in hospitalized elderly. JAMA 1990; 263:1097–101.

Frantzen E. Wernicke's encephalopathy: 3 cases occurring in connection with severe malnutrition. Acta Neurol Scand 1966; 42:426–41.

Fraser CL, Arieff AI. Hepatic encephalopathy. N Engl J Med 1985; 313:865–73.

Fraser HF, Wiler A, Essig CF et al. Degree of physical dependence induced by secobarbital or pentobarbital. J Am Med Assoc 1958; 166:126–9.

Frazier CH. Tumor involving the frontal lobe alone: a symptomatic survey of one hundred and five verified cases. Arch Neurol Psychiatry 1936; 35:525–71.

Freeman JW, Couch JR. Prolonged encephalopathy with arsenic poisoning. Neurology 1978; 28:853–5.

Friedman A, Sienkiewicz J. Psychotic complications of long-term levodopa treatment of Parkinson's disease. *Acta Neurol Scand* 1991; **84**:111–13.

Friedman JH. Syndrome of diffuse encephalopathy due to non-dominant thalamic infarction. *Neurology* 1985; **35**:1524–6.

Friedman JH, Kanzer M. Thyrotoxicosis with psychosis: clinico-neuropathologic observations in a case. *J Nerv Ment Dis* 1937; **85**:30–5.

Fromm D, Holland AL, Swindell CS *et al.* Various complications of subcortical stroke: prospective study of 16 consecutive cases. *Arch Neurol* 1985; **42**:943–50.

Fukatsu R, Yamadori A, Fujii T. Impaired recall and preserved encoding in prominent amnesic syndrome: a case of basal forebrain amnesia. *Neurology* 1998; **50**:539–41.

Gadow KD. Prevalence and efficacy of stimulant drug use with mentally retarded children and youth. *Psychopharmacol Bull* 1985; **21**:291–303.

Gaffan EA, Gaffan D, Hodges JR. Amnesia following damage to the left fornix and to other sites. *Brain* 1991; **114**:1297–13.

Gardner K, Barmada M, Ptacek LJ *et al.* A new locus for hemiplegic migraine maps to chromsome /q3/. *Neurology* 1997; **49**:1231–8.

Garrett PJ, Mulcahy D, Carmody M *et al.* Aluminium encephalopathy: clinical and immunologic features. *Q J Med* 1988; **69**:775–83.

Gautier S, Reisberg B, Zaudig M *et al.* Mild cognitive impairment. *Lancet* 2006; **367**: 1262–70.

Geda YA, Knopman DS, Mrazek DA *et al.* Depression, apolipoprotein E genotype, and the incidence of mild cognitive impairment: a prospective cohort study. *Arch Neurol* 2006; **63**:435–40.

Ghika-Schmid F, Ghika J, Regli F. Hashimoto's myoclonic encephalopathy: an underdiagnosed treatable condition? *Mov Disord* 1996; **11**:555–62.

Giannopoulos S, Kostadima V, Selvi A *et al.* Bilateral paramedian thalamic infarcts. *Arch Neurol* 2006; **63**:1625.

Giffin ME, Rogers HM, Kernohan JW. Postvaccinial (typhoid) encephalitis. *Arch Neurol Psychiatry* 1948; **59**:233–40.

Gillberg C, Persson E, Grufman M *et al.* Psychiatric disorders in mildly and severely mentally retarded urban children and adolescents. Epidemiological aspects. *Br J Psychiatry* 1986; **149**:68–74.

Gilles C, Brucher JM, Khoubesserian P *et al.* Cerebral amyloid angiopathy as a cause of multiple intracerebral hemorrhages. *Neurology* 1984; **34**:730–5.

Glaser G, Pincus JH. Limbic encephalitis. *J Nerv Ment Dis* 1969; **149**:59–67.

Goldberg A. Acute intermittent porphyria. *Q J Med* 1959; **28**:183–209.

Goldfarb LG, Chumakov MP, Petrov PA *et al.* Olivopontocerebellar atrophy in a large Iakut kinship in eastern Siberia. *Neurology* 1989; **39**:1527–30.

Gomez EA, Avilens M. Neurosyphilis in community mental health clinics: a case series. *J Clin Psychiatry* 1984; **45**:127–9.

Gomez Diaz RA, Rivera Moscosco R, Ramos Rodriguez R *et al.* Diabetic ketoacidosis in adults: clinical and laboratory features. *Arch Med Res* 1996; **27**:177–81.

Goodman L. Alzheimer's disease: a clinico-pathologic analysis of twenty-three cases with a theory on pathogenesis. *J Nerv Ment Dis* 1953; **118**:97–130.

Goodwin CD. Case report of tricyclic-induced delirium at a therapeutic drug concentration. *Am J Psychiatry* 1983; **140**:1517–18.

Goodwin DW. True species of alcoholic 'blackout'. *Am J Psychiatry* 1971; **127**:1665–70.

Goodwin DW, Crane JB, Guze SB. Alcoholic 'blackout': a review and clinical study of 100 alcoholics. *Am J Psychiatry* 1969a; **126**:191–8.

Goodwin DW, Crane JB, Guze SB. Phenomenological aspects of the alcoholic 'blackout'. *Br J Psychiatry* 1969b; **115**:1033–8.

Gordon MF, Abrams RI, Rubin DB *et al.* Bismuth subsalicylate toxicity as a cause of prolonged encephalopathy with myoclonus. *Mov Disord* 1995; **10**:220–2.

Gorelick PB, Amico LL, Ganellen R *et al.* Transient global amnesia and thalamic infarction. *Neurology* 1988; **38**:496–9.

Gostason R. Psychiatric illness among mentally retarded: a Swedish population study. *Acta Psychiatr Scand* 1985; (suppl. 318):1–117.

Gottfried JA, Mayer SA, Shungu DC *et al.* Delayed posthypoxic demyelination: association with arylsulfatase A deficiency and lactic acidosis and proton MR spectroscopy. *Neurology* 1997; **49**:140–4.

Graff-Radford NR, Eslinger PJ, Damasio AR *et al.* Nonhemorrhagic infarction of the thalamus: behavioral, anatomic, and physiologic correlates. *Neurology* 1984; **34**:14–23.

Graff-Radford NR, Tranel D, Van GW *et al.* Diencephalic amnesia. *Brain* 1990; **113**:1–25.

Graham A, Davies R, Xuereb J *et al.* Pathologically proven frontotemporal dementia presenting with severe amnesia. *Brain* 2005; **128**:597–605.

Green J, Morris JC, Sandson J *et al.* Progressive aphasia: a precursor of global dementia? *Neurology* 1990; **40**:423–9.

Greenberg SM, Vonsattel JPG, Stakes JW *et al.* The clinical spectrum of cerebral amyloid angiopathy: presentations without lobar hemorrhage. *Neurology* 1993; **43**:2073–9.

Greenblatt DJ, Harmatz JS, Shapiro L *et al.* Sensitivity to triazolam in the elderly. *N Engl J Med* 1991; **324**:1691–8.

Greene JBW, Patterson K, Xuereb J *et al.* Alzheimer disease and nonfluent progressive aphasia. *Arch Neurol* 1996; **53**:1072–8.

Greenwald BS, Kramer-Ginsberg E, Marin DB *et al.* Dementia with coexistent major depression. *Am J Psychiatry* 1989; **146**:1472–8.

Grimes DA, Lang AE, Bergeron CB. Dementia as the most common presentation of cortical-basal ganglionic degeneration. *Neurology* 1999; **53**:1969–74.

Guerrini R, Belmonte A, Canapicchi R *et al.* Reversible pseudoatrophy of the brain and mental deterioration associated with valproate treatment. *Epilepsia* 1998; **39**:27–32.

Guillozet AL, Weintraub S, Mash DC *et al.* Neurofibrillary tangles, amyloid, and memory in aging and mild cognitive impairment. *Arch Neurol* 2003; **60**:729–36.

Gustafson L, Hagberg B. Recovery in hydrocephalic dementia after shunt operation. *J Neurol Neurosurg Psychiatry* 1978; **41**:940–7.

Haan J, Lanser JBK, Zijderveld I *et al.* Dementia in hereditary cerebral hemorrhage with amyloidosis – Dutch type. *Arch Neurol* 1990; **47**:965–7.

Hadjivassiliou M, Grunewald RA, Lawden M *et al.* Headache and CNS white matter abnormalities associated with luten sensitivity. *Neurology* 2001; **56**:385–8.

Hagberg B (ed.). *Rett syndrome: clinical and biological aspects.* London: MacKeith Press, 1993.

Hagberg B, Aicardi J, Dias K *et al.* A progressive syndrome of autism, dementia, ataxia, and loss of purposeful hand movements: Rett's syndrome: report of 35 cases. *Ann Neurol* 1983; **14**:471–9.

Hageman ATM, Gabreels FJM, de Jong JGN *et al.* Clinical symptoms of adult metachromatic leukodystrophy and arylsulfatase A pseudodeficiency. *Arch Neurol* 1995; **52**:408–13.

Hagerman RJ, Leehey M, Heinrichs W *et al.* Intention tremor, parkinsonism, and generalized brain atrophy in male carriers of fragile X. *Neurology* 2001; **57**:127–30.

Hall BD, Smith DW. Prader–Willi syndrome. A resume of 32 cases including an instance of affected first cousins, one of whom is of normal stature and intelligence. *J Pediatrics* 1972; **81**:286–93.

Hall RCW, Joffe JR. Hypomagnesemia: physical and psychiatric symptoms. *J Am Med Assoc* 1973; **224**:1749–51.

Halperin JJ, Luft BJ, Anand AK *et al.* Lyme neuroborreliosis: central nervous system manifestations. *Neurology* 1989; **39**:753–9.

Haltia T, Palo J, Haltia M *et al.* Juvenile metachromatic leukodystrophy: clinical, biochemical, and neuropathologic studies in nine new cases. *Arch Neurol* 1980; **37**:42–6.

Handen BL, Beaux AM, Gosling A *et al.* Efficacy of methylphenidate among mentally retarded children with attention deficit hyperactivity disorder. *Pediatrics* 1990; **86**:922–30.

Hanson JW, Smith DW. The fetal hydantoin syndrome. *J Pediatrics* 1975; **87**:285–90.

Hansotia P, Cleeland CS, Chun RWM. Juvenile Huntington's chorea. *Neurology* 1968; **18**:217–24.

Hardie RJ, Pullon HWH, Harding AE *et al.* Neuroacanthocytosis: a clinical, haemotological and pathological study of 19 cases. *Brain* 1991; **114**:13–49.

Harper C. The incidence of Wernicke's encephalopathy in Australia – a neuropathologial study of 131 cases. *J Neurol Neurosurg Psychiatry* 1983; **46**:593–8.

Harper CG, Giles M, Finlay-Jones R. Clinical signs in the Wernicke–Korsakoff complex: a retrospective analysis of 131 cases diagnosed at necropsy. *J Neurol Neurosrug Psychiatry* 1986; **49**:341–5.

Harrison MJG, Robert CM, Uttley D. Benign aqueductal stenosis in adults. *J Neurol Neurosurg Psychiatry* 1974; **37**:1322–8.

Harsch HH. Neuroleptic malignant syndrome: physiological and laboratory findings in a series of nine cases. *J Clin Psychiatry* 1987; **48**:328–33.

Hart SP, Frier BM. Causes, management and morbidity of acute hypoglycemia in adults requiring hospital admission. *Q J Med* 1998; **91**:505–10.

Harvey PKP, Davis JN. Traumatic encephalopathy in a young boxer. *Lancet* 1974; **2**:928–9.

Hay WJ, Rickards AG, McMenemy WH *et al.* Organic mercurial encephalopathy. *J Neurol Neurosurg Psychiatry* 1963; **26**:199–202.

Hayflick SJ, Westaway SK, Levinson B *et al.* Genetic, clinical, and radiographic delineation of Hallervorden–Sptaz syndrome. *N Engl J Med* 2003; **348**:33–40.

Healton EB, Brust JC, Feinfeld DA *et al.* Hypertensive encephalopathy and the neurologic manifestations of malignant hypertension. *Neurology* 1982; **32**:127–30.

Heilman KM, Fisher WR. Hyperlipidemic dementia. *Arch Neurol* 1974; **31**:67–8.

Heilman KM, Sypert GW. Korakoff's syndrome resulting from bilateral fornix lesion. *Neurology* 1977; **27**:490–3.

Henchey R, Cibula J, Helveston W *et al.* Electroencephalographic findings in Hashimoto's encephalopathy. *Neurology* 1995; **45**:977–81.

Heritch AJ, Capwell R, Roy-Byrne PR. A case of psychosis and delirium following withdrawal from triazolam. *J Clin Psychiatry* 1987; **48**:168–9.

Heutink P, Stevens M, Rizzu P *et al.* Hereditary frontotemporal dementia is linked to chromosome 17q21–q22: a genetic and clinicopathological study of three Dutch families. *Ann Neurol* 1997; **41**:150–9.

Hierons R. Changes in the nervous system in acute porphyria. *Brain* 1957; **80**:176–92.

Hill ME, Lougheed WM, Barnett HJM. A treatable form of dementia due to normal pressure, communicating hydrocephalus. *Can Med Assoc J* 1967; **97**:1309.

Hinchey J, Chaves C, Appignani B *et al.* A reversible posterior leukoencephalopathy syndrome. *N Engl J Med* 1996; **334**:494–500.

Hirose G, Bass NH. Metachromatic leukodystrophy in the adult: a biochemical study. *Neurology* 1972; **22**:312–20.

Hodges JR, Carpenter K. Anterograde amnesia with fornix damage following removal of IIIrd ventricle colloid cyst. *J Neurol Neurosurg Psychiatry* 1991; **54**:633–8.

Hodges JR, McCarthy RA. Autobiographical amnesia resulting from bilateral paramedian thalamic infarction: A case study in cognitive neurobiology. *Brain* 1993; **116**:921–40.

Hodges JR, Ward CD. Observations during transient global amnesia: a behavioral and neuropsychological study of five cases. *Brain* 1989; **112**:595–620.

Hokkanen L, Salonen O, Launes J. Amnesia in acute herpetic and nonherpetic encephalitis. *Arch Neurol* 1996; **53**:972–8.

Hollister LE, Gillespie HK. Marijuana, ethanol, and dextroamphetamine: mood and mental function alterations. *Arch Gen Psychiatry* 1970; **23**:199–203.

Holmes JT, Filley CM, Rosenberg NL. Neurologic sequelae of chronic solvent vapor abuse. *Neurology* 1986; **36**:698–702.

Horoupian DS, Thal L, Katzman R *et al.* Dementia and motor neuron disease: morphometric, biochemical, and golgi studies. *Ann Neurol* 1984; **16**:305–13.

Horvath J, Coeytax A, Jallow P *et al.* Carbamazepine encephalopathy masquerading as Creutzfeldt–Jakob disease. *Neurology* 2005; **65**:650–1.

Hossain M. Neurological and psychiatric manifestations in idiopathic hypoparathyroidism: response to treatment. *J Neurol Neurosurg Psychiatry* 1970; **33**:153–6.

Hotopf MH, Pollock S, Lishman WA. An unusual presentation of multiple sclerosis. *Psychol Med* 1994; **24**:525–8.

Hotson JR, Langston JW. Disulfiram-induced encephalopathy. *Arch Neurol* 1976; **33**:141–2.

Hu WT, Murray JA, Greenaway MC *et al.* Cognitive impairment and celiac disease. *Arch Neurol* 2006; **63**:1440–6.

Hu WT, Kantarc OH, Meritt JL *et al.* Ornithine transcarbamylase deficiency presenting as encephalopathy during adulthood following bariatric surgery. *Arch Neurol* 2007; **64**:126–8.

Huber SJ, Kissel JT, Shuttleworth EC *et al.* Magnetic resonance imaging and clinical correlates of intellectual impairment in myotonic dystrophy. *Arch Neurol* 1989; **46**:536–40.

Huff FJ, Boller F, Lucchelli F *et al.* The neurologic examination in patients with probable Alzheimer's disease. *Arch Neurol* 1987; **44**:929–32.

Hughes JT, Brownell B. Granulomatous giant-celled angiitis of the central nervous system. *Neurology* 1966; **16**:293–8.

Huson SM, Harper PS, Compston DAS *et al.* Von Recklinghausen neurofibromatosis: A clinical and population study in south-east Wales. *Brain* 1988; **111**:1355–81.

Ikeda K, Akiyama H, Iritani S *et al.* Corticobasal degeneration with primary progressive aphasia and accentuated cortical lesion in superior temporal gyrus: case report and review. *Acta Neuropathol* 1996; **92**:534–9.

Illowsky B, Yang JC, Khorsand M *et al.* Multiple cerebral lesions complicating therapy with interleukin-2. *Neurology* 196; **47**:417–24.

Ironside R, Guttmacher M. The corpus callosum and its tumors. *Brain* 1929; **52**:442–83.

Ironside R, Bosanquet FD, McMenemy WH. Central demyelination of the corpus callosum (Marchaifava-Bignami disease): with report of a second case in Great Britian. *Brain* 1961; **84**:212–30.

Isbell H, Alstschul S, Kornetsky CH *et al.* Chronic barbiturate intoxication. *Arch Neurol Psychiatry* 1950; **64**:1–28.

Isbell H, Fraser HF, Wickler A *et al.* An experimental study of etiology of 'rum fits' and delirium tremens. *Q J Stud Alcohol* 1955; **16**:1–33.

Ishii N, Nishihara Y. Pellagra among chronic alcoholics: clinical and pathological study of 20 necropsy cases. *J Neurol Neurosurg Psychiatry* 1981; **44**:209–15.

Ishii N, Nishihara Y, Imamura T. Why do frontal lobe symptoms predominate in vascular dementia with lacunes? *Neurology* 1986; **36**:340–5.

Jacobsen FM, Sack DA, James SP. Delirium induced by verapamil. *Am J Psychiatry* 1987; **144**:248.

Jacobson DM, Terrance CF, Reinmuth OM. The neurologic manifestations of fat embolism. *Neurology* 1986; **36**:847–51.

Jana DK, Romano-Jana L. Hypernatremic psychosis in the elderly: case reports. *J Am Ger Soc* 1973; **21**:473–7.

Jankovic J, Kirkpatrick JB, Blomquist KA *et al.* Late-onset Hallervorden–Spatz disease presenting as familial parkinsonism. *Neurology* 1985; **35**:227–34.

Jankovic J, Caskey TC, Stout T *et al.* Lesch–Nyhan syndrome: a study of motor behavior and cerebrospinal fluid neurotransmitters. *Ann Neurol* 1988; **23**:466–9.

Jefferson AA, Keogh AJ. Intracranial abscesses: a review of treated patients over 20 years. *Q J Med* 1977; **46**:389–400.

Jenkins CD, Mellins RB. Lead poisoning in children: a study of forty-six cases. *Arch Neurol Psychiatry* 1957; **77**:70–8.

Jenkins RB. Inorganic arsenic and the nervous system. *Brain* 1966; **89**:479–98.

Jennekens-Schinkel A, Sanders EACM. Decline of cognition in multiple sclerosis: dissociable deficits. *J Neurol Neurosurg Psychiatry* 1986; **49**:1354–60.

Jicha GA, Parisi JE, Dickson DW *et al.* Neuropathologic outcome of mild cognitive impairment following progression to clinical dementia. *Arch Neurol* 2006; **63**:674–81.

Johnson JC, Kerse NM, Gottleib G *et al.* Prospective versus retrospective methods of identifying patients with delirium. *J Am Geriatr Soc* 1992; **40**:316–19.

Johnson JC, Jayadevappa R, Baccash PD *et al.* Nonspecific presentation of pneumonia in hospitalized people: age effect or dementia? *J Am Geriatr Soc* 2000; **48**:1316–20.

Johnson RI, Richardson EP. The neurological manifestations of systemic lupus erythematosus. *Medicine* 1968; **47**:337–69.

Jones HR, Hedley-Whyte T. Idiopathic hemochromatosis (IHC): dementia and ataxia as presenting signs. *Neurology* 1983; **33**:1479–83.

Jung HH, Bassetti C, Tournier-Lasserve E *et al.* Cerebral autosomal dominant arteriopathy with subcortical infarcts and leukoencephalopathy: a clinicopathological and genetic study of a Swiss family. *J Neurol Neurosurg Psychiatry* 1995; **59**:138–43.

Jungreis AC, Shaumberg HH. Encephalopathy from abuse of bismuth subsalicylate (Pepto-Bismol). *Neurology* 1993; **43**:1265.

Kahn EA, Crosby EC. Korsakoff's syndrome associated with surgical lesions involving the mammillary bodies. *Neurology* 1971; **21**:117–25.

Kalimo H, Olsson Y. Effect of severe hypoglycemia on the human brain. *Acta Neurol Scand* 1980; **62**:345–56.

Kamaki M, Kawamura M, Moriya H *et al.* 'Crossed homonymous hemianopia' and 'crossed left hemispatial neglect' in a case of Marchiafava-Bignami disease. *J Neurol Neurosurg Psychiatry* 1993; **56**:1027–32.

Kanzer M. Amnesia: a statistical study. *Am J Psychiatry* 1939; **96**:711–16.

Kaplan PW, Birbeck G. Lithium-induced confusional states: nonconvulsive status epilepticus or triphasic encephalopathy? *Epilepsia* 2006; **47**:2071–7.

Kaplan PW, Waterbury L, Kawas C *et al.* Reversible dementia with idiopathic hypereosinophilia. *Neurology* 1990; **40**:1388–91.

Kapur N, Ellison D, Smith MP *et al.* Focal retrograde amnesia following isolated bilateral temporal lobe pathology. *Brain* 1992; **115**:73–85.

Kapur N, Barker S, Burrows EH *et al.* Herpes simplex encephalitis: long-term magnetic resonance imaging and neuropsychological profile. *J Neurol Neurosurg Psychiatry* 1994; **57**:1334–42.

Karalis DG, Quinn V, Victor MF et al. Risk of catheter-related emboli in patients wth atherosclerotic debris in the thoracic aorta. Am Heart J 1996; 131:1149-55.

Karbe H, Kertesz A, Polk M. Profiles of language impairment in primary progressive aphasia. Arch Neurol 1993; 50:192-201.

Karp BI, Laureno R. Pontine and extrapontine myelinolysis: a neurologic disorder following rapid correction of hyponatremia. Medicine 1993; 72:359-73.

Karpati G, Frame B. Neuropsychiatric disorders in primary hyperparathyroidism: clinical analysis with review of the literature. Arch Neurol 1964; 10:387-97.

Kartsounis LD, Rudge P, Stevens JM. Bilateral lesions of CA1 and CA2 fields of the hippocampus are sufficient to cause a severe amnesia syndrome in humans. J Neurol Neurosurg Psychiatry 1995; 59:95-8.

Kawashima N, Shindo R, Kohno M. Primary Sjorgen's syndrome with subcortical dementia. Intern Med 1993; 32:561-4.

Kawashima T, Oda M, Kund T et al. Metyrapone for delirium due to Cushing's syndrome induced by occult ectopic adrenocorticotrophic hormone secretion. J Clin Psychiatry 2004; 65:1019-20.

Keck PE, Pope HG, McElroy SL. Frequency and presentation of neuroleptic malignant syndrome: a prospective study. Am J Psychiatry 1987; 144:1344-6.

Kelly WF, Psychiatric aspects of Cushing's syndrome. Q J Med 1996; 89:543-51.

Kertesz A, Hudson L, MacKenzie IRA et al. The pathology and nosology of primary progressive aphasia. Neurology 1994; 44:2065-72.

Keschner M, Sloane P. Encephalitis, idiopathic and arteriosclerotic parkinsonism: a clinicopathologic study. Arch Neurol Psychiatry 1931; 25:1011-45.

Keschner M, Bender MB, Strauss I. Mental symptoms in cases of tumor of the temporal lobe. Arch Neurol Psychiatry 1936; 35:572-96.

Khardori R, Soler NG. Hyperosmolar hyperglycemic nonketotic syndrome. Report of 22 cases and brief review. Am J Med 1984; 77:899-904.

Kinkel WR, Jacobs L, Polachino I et al. Subcortical arteriosclerotic encephalopathy (Binswanger's disease): computed tomographic, nuclear magnetic resonance, and clinical correlations. Arch Neurol 1985; 42:951-9.

Kirk A, Kertesz A, Polk MJ. Dementia with leukoencephalopathy in systemic lupus erythematosus. Can J Neurol Sci 1991; 18:344-8.

Kirubakaran V, Liskow B, Mayfield D et al. Case report of acute disulfiram overdose. Am J Psychiatry 1983; 140:1513-14.

Klatka LA, Louis ED, Schiffer RB. Psychiatric features in diffuse Lewy body disease: a clinicopathologic study using Alzheimer's disease and Parkinson's disease comparison groups. Neurology 1996; 47:1148-52.

Knee ST, Razani J. Acute organic brain syndrome: a complication of disulfiram therapy. Am J Psychiatry 1974; 131:1281-2.

Knibb J, Xuereb JH, Patterson K et al. Clinical and pathological characterization of progressive aphasia. Ann Neurol 2006; 59:156-65.

Koeppen AH, Barron KD. Marchaifava-Bignami disease. Neurology 1978; 28:290-4.

Koo EH, Massey EW. Granulomatous angiitis of the central nervous system: protean manifestations and response to treatment. J Neurol Neurosurg Psychiatry 1988; 51:1126-33.

Koponen HJ, Riekkinen PJ. A prospective study of delirium in elderly patients admitted to a psychiatric hospital. Psychol Med 1993; 23:103-9.

Koponen H, Stenback U, Mattila E et al. Delirium among elderly persons admitted to a psychiatric hospital: clinical course during the acute stage and one-year follow-up. Acta Psychiatr Scand 1989; 79:579-85.

Kriegstein AR, Shungu DC, Millar WS et al. Leukoencephalopathy and raised brain lactate from heroin vapor inhalation ('chasing the dragon'). Neurology 1999; 53:1765-73.

Kritchevsky M, Squire LR. Transient global amnesia: evidence for extensive, temporally graded retrograde amnesia. Neurology 1989; 39:213-18.

Kroll NEA, Markowitsch HJ, Knight RT et al. Retrieval of old memories: the temporofrontal hypothesis. Brain 1997; 120:1377-99.

Krupp LB, Lipton RB, Swerdlow ML et al. Progressive multifocal leukoencephalopathy: clinical and radiographic features. Ann Neurol 1985; 17:344-9.

Kryzhanovskaya LA, Jeste PV, Young CA et al. A review of treatment-emergent adverse events during olanzapine clinical trials in elderly patients with dementia. J Clin Psychiatry 2006; 67:933-45.

Kumral E, Evyapan D, Balkir K et al. Bilateral thalamic infarction: clinical, etiological and MRI correlates. Acta Neurol Scand 2001; 103:35-42.

Kunig G, Datwyler S, Eschen A et al. Unrecognized long-lasting tramadol-induced delirium in two elderly patients. A case report. Pharmacopsychiatry 2006; 39:194-9.

Kushner MJ, Hauser WA. Transient global amnesia: a case-control study. Ann Neurol 1985; 18:684-91.

Kusumi RK, Plouffe JF, Wyatt RH et al. Central nervous system toxicity associated with metronidazole therapy. Ann Int Med 1980; 93:59-60.

Lagos JC, Gomez MR. Tuberose sclerosis: reappraisal of a clinical entity. Mayo Clin Proc 1967; 42:26-49.

Lai F, Williams RS. A prospective study of Alzheimer's disease in Down syndrome. Arch Neurol 1989; 46:849-53.

Landi G, Giusti MC, Guidotti M. Transient global amnesia due to left temporal hemorrhage. J Neurol Neurosurg Psychiatry 1982; 45:1062-3.

Langworthy OR. Lesions of the central nervous system characteristic of pellagra. Brain 1931; 54:291-302.

Laplane D, Attal N, Sauron B et al. Lesions of basal ganglia due to disulfiram. J Neurol Neurosurg Psychiatry 1992; 55:925-9.

Lasek K, Lencer R, Gaser C et al. Morphological basis for the spectrum of clinical deficits in spinocerebellar ataxia 17 (SCA 17). Brain 2006; 129:2341-52.

Lawlor PG, Gagnon B, Mancini IL et al. Occurrence, causes, and outcome of delirium in patients with advanced cancer: a prospective study. Arch Int Med 2000; 160:786-94.

Layne OL, Yudofsky SC. Postoperative psychosis in cardiotomy patients: the role of organic and psychiatric features. *N Engl J Med* 1971; **284**:518–20.

Lazar RB, Ho SU, Melen O *et al.* Multifocal central nervous system damage caused by toluene abuse. *Neurology* 1983; **33**:1337–40.

Lederman RJ, Henry CE. Progressive dialysis encephalopathy. *Ann Neurol* 1978; **4**:199–204.

Lee BI, Lee BC, Hwang YM *et al.* Prolonged ictal amnesia with transient focal abnormalities on magnetic resonance imaging. *Epilepsia* 1992; **33**:1042–6.

Lee JW. Recurrent delirium associated with obstructive sleep apnea. *Gen Hosp Psychiatry* 1998; **30**:120–2.

Lee K, Moller L, Hardt F *et al.* Alcohol induced brain damage and liver damage in young males. *Lancet* 1979; **2**:759–61.

Lee TH, Chen SS, Su SL *et al.* Baclofen intoxication: report of four cases and review of the literature. *Clin Neuropharmacol* 1992;**15**:56–62.

Lenke RR, Levy HL. Maternal phenylketonuria and hyperphenylalanemia: an international survey of the outcome of treated and untreated pregnancies. *N Engl J Med* 1980; **303**:1202–8.

Leo RJ, Baer D. Delirium associated with baclofen withdrawal: a review of common presentations and management strategies. *Psychosomatics* 2005; **46**:503–7.

Lesch M, Nyhan WL. A familial disorder of uric acid metabolism and central nervous system dysfunction. *Am J Med* 1964; **36**:561–70.

Levkoff SE, Evans DA, Liptzin B *et al.* Delirium: the occurrence and persistence of symptoms among elderly hospitalized patients. *Arch Intern Med* 1992; **152**:334–40.

Levin HS, High WM, Eisenberg HM. Learning and forgetting during post-traumatic amnesia in head injured patients. *J Neurol Neurosurg Psychiatry* 1988; **51**:14–20.

Levy AB. Delirium and seizures due to abrupt alprazolam withdrawal: case report. *J Clin Psychiatry* 1984; **45**:38–9.

Lewis MH, Bodfish JW, Powell SB *et al.* Clomipramine treatment for self-injurious behavior of individuals with mental retardation: a double-blind comparison with placebo. *Am J Ment Retard* 1996; **100**:654–65.

Lichtenstein BW. Sturge–Weber–Dimitri syndrome: cephalic form of neurocutaneous hemangiomatosus. *Arch Neurol Psychiatry* 1954; **71**:291–301.

Lindenbaum J, Healton EB, Savage DG *et al.* Neuropsychiatric disorders caused by cobalamin deficiency in the absence of anemia or macrocytosis. *N Engl J Med* 1988; **318**:1720–8.

Lindquist G, Norlen G. Korsakoff's syndrome after operation on ruptured aneurysm of the anterior communicating artery. *Acta Psychiatr Scand* 1966; **42**:24–34.

Linn RT, Wolf PA, Bachman DL *et al.* The 'preclinical phase' of probable Alzheimer's disease. *Arch Neurol* 1995; **52**:485–90.

Lipowski ZJ. Transient cognitive disorders (delirium, acute confusional states) in the elderly. *Am J Psychiatry* 1983; **140**:1426–36.

Lipowski ZJ. Delirium (acute confusional state). *JAMA* 1987; **258**:1789–92.

Lipowski ZJ. Delirium in the elderly patient. *N Engl J Med* 1989; **320**:578–82.

Liptzin B, Levkoff SE. An empirical study of delirium subtypes. *Br J Psychiatry* 1992; **161**:843–5.

Lisak RP, Zimmerman RA. Transient global amnesia due to a dominant hemisphere tumor. *Arch Neurol* 1977; **34**:317–18.

Lishman WA. Cerebral disorder in alcoholism: syndromes of impairment. *Brain* 1981; **104**:373–410.

Liss L. Pituicytoma, a tumor of the hypothalamus. *Arch Neurol Psychiatry* 1958; **80**:567–76.

Litaker D, Locala J, Franco K *et al.* Preoperative risk factors for postoperative delirium. *Gen Hosp Psychiatry* 2001; **23**:84–9.

Little BW, Brown PW, Rodgers-Johnson P *et al.* Familial myoclonic dementia masquerading as Creutzfeldt–Jakob disease. *Ann Neurol* 1986; **20**:231.

Litvan I, Mangone CA, McKee A *et al.* Natural history of progressive supranuclear palsy (Steele–Richardson–Olszewski syndrome) and clinical predictors of survival: a clinicopathologic study. *J Neurol Neurosurg Psychiatry* 1996a; **61**:615–20.

Litvan I, Agid Y, Jankovic J *et al.* Accuracy of clinical criteria for the diagnosis of progressive supranuclear palsy (Steele–Richardson–Olszewski syndrome). *Neurology* 1996b; **46**:922–30.

Litvan I, Mega MS, Cumings JL *et al.* Neuropsychiatric aspects of progressive supranuclear palsy. *Neurology* 1996c; **47**:1184–9.

Litvan I, Agid Y, Sastrj N *et al.* What are the obstacles for an accurate clinical diagnosis of Pick's disease? *Neurology* 1997a; **49**:62–9.

Litvan I, Goetz G, Jankovic J *et al.* What is the accuracy of the clinical diagnosis of multiple system atrophy? A clinicopathologic study. *Arch Neurol* 1997b; **54**:937–44.

Litvan I, Campbell G, Mangone CA *et al.* Which clinical features differentiate progressive supranuclear palsy (Steele–Richardson–Olszewski syndrome) from related disorders? A clinicopathologic study. *Brain* 1997c; **120**:65–74.

Litvan I, Agid Y, Goetz C *et al.* Accuracy of the clinical diagnosis of corticobasal degeneration: a clinicopathologic study. *Neurology* 1997d; **48**:119–25.

Lobosky JM, Vangilder JC, Damasio AR. Behavioral manifestations of third ventricular colloid cysts. *J Neurol Neurosurg Psychiatry* 1984; **47**:1075–80.

Logigian EL, Kaplan RF, Steere AC. Chronic neurologic manifestations of Lyme disease. *N Engl J Med* 1990; **323**:1438–44.

Lotrich FE, Rosen J, Pollock BG. Dextromethorphan-induced delirium and possible methadone interaction. *Am J Geriatr Pharmacother* 2005; **3**:17–20.

Louis ED, Lynch T, Kaufmann P *et al.* Diagnostic guidelines in central nervous system Whipple's disease. *Ann Neurol* 1996; **40**:561–8.

Louis ED, Klatka LA, Liu Y *et al.* Comparison of extrapyramidal features in 31 pathologically confirmed cases of diffuse Lewy body disease and 34 pathologically confirmed cases of Parkinson's disease. *Neurology* 1997; **48**:376–80.

Lundquist G. Delirium tremens: a comparative study of pathogenesis, course and prognosis with delirium tremens. *Acta Psychiatr Neurol Scand* 1961; **36**:443–66.

Lurie LA. Pernicious anemia with mental symptoms: observations on the variable extent and probable duration of central nervous system lesions in four necropsied cases. *Arch Neurol Psychiatry* 1919; **2**:67–109.

Mach J, Dysken M, Richards H *et al*. Serum anticholinergic activity in hospitalized older persons with delirium: a preliminary study. *J Am Geriatr Soc* 1995; **43**:491–5.

MacKay ME, McLardy T, Harris C. A case of periarteritis nodosa of the central nervous system. *J Ment Sci* 1950; **96**:470–5.

MacNeill A, Grennan DM, Ward D *et al*. Psychiatric problems in systemic lupus erythematosus. *Br J Psychiatry* 1976; **128**:442–5.

McCauley DLF, Lecky BRF, Earl CJ. Gold encephalopathy. *J Neurol Neurosurg Psychiatry* 1977; **40**:1021–2.

McHugh PR. Occult hydrocephalus. *Q J Med* 1964; **33**:297–308.

McKeith IG, Fairbairn A, Perry RH. Neuroleptic sensitivity with senile dementia of the Lewy body type. *BMJ* 1992; **305**:673–8.

McKeith IG, Fairbairn AF, Bothwell RA *et al*. An evaluation of the predictive ability and inter-rater reliability of clinical diagnostic criteria for senile dementia of the Lewy body type. *Neurology* 1994a; **44**:872–7.

McKeith IG, Fairbairn AF, Perry RH *et al*. The clinical diagnosis and misdiagnosis of senile dementia of Lewy body type (SDLT). *Br J Psychiatry* 1994b; **165**:324–32.

McKhann GM, Grega MA, Borowicz LM *et al*. Encephalopathy and stroke after coronary artery bypass grafting: incidence, consequences, and prediction. *Arch Neurol* 2002; **59**:1422–8.

McLean DR, Jacobs H, Mielke BW. Methanol poisoning: a clinical and pathological study. *Ann Neurol* 1980; **8**:161–7.

Malamud N, Skillicorn SA. Relationship between the Wernicke and the Korsakoff syndrome. *Arch Neurol Psychiatry* 1956; **76**:585–91.

Malamut BL, Graff-Radford N, Chawluk J *et al*. Memory in a case of bilateral thalamic infarction. *Neurology* 1992; **42**:163–9.

Malandrini A, Carrera P, Palmeri ST *et al*. Clinicopathological and genetic studies of two further Italian families with cerebral autosomal dominant arteriopathy. *Acta Neuropathol* 1996; **92**:115–22.

Malouf R, Brust JCM. Hypoglycemia: causes, neurological manifestations, and outcome. *Ann Neurol* 1985; **17**:421–30.

Mandell AM, Alexander MP, Carpenter S. Creutzfeldt–Jakob disease presenting as isolated aphasia. *Neurology* 1989; **39**:55–8.

Manepalli J, Grossberg GT, Mueller C. Prevalence of delirium and urinary tract infection in a psychogeriatric unit. *J Geriatr Psychiatry Neurol* 1990; **3**:198–202.

Mann DMA, South PW, Snowden JS *et al*. Dementia of the frontal lobe type: neuropathology and immunohistochemistry. *J Neurol Neurosurg Psychiatry* 1993; **56**:605–14.

Maramattom BV, Zaldivar RA, Glynn SM *et al*. Acute intermittent porphyria presenting as a diffuse encephalopathy. *Ann Neurol* 2005; **57**:51–4.

Marcantino ER, Juarez G, Goldman L *et al*. The relationship of postoperative delirium with psychoactive medications. *JAMA* 1994; **272**:1518–22.

Marder K, Ming-Xin T, Cote L *et al*. The frequency and associated risk factors for dementia in patients with Parkinson's disease. *Arch Neurol* 1995; **52**:695–701.

Margolin D, Hammerstad J, Orwoll E *et al*. Intracranial calcification in hyperparathyroidism associated with gait apraxia and parkinsonism. *Neurology* 1980; **30**:1005–7.

Markowitsch HJ, Calabrese P, Liess J *et al*. Retrograde amnesia after traumatic injury of the fronto-temporal cortex. *J Neurol Neurosurg Psychiatry* 1993; **56**:988–92.

Martin FI, Deam DR. Hyperthyroidism in elderly hospitalized patients. Clinical features and treatment outcomes. *Med J Aust* 1996; **164**:200–3.

Martland HS. Punch drunk. *J Am Med Assoc* 1928; **91**:1103–7.

Mas J-L, Bousser M-G, Lacombe C *et al*. Hyperlipidemic dementia. *Neurology* 1985; **35**:1385–7.

Mateo D, Gimenez-Roldan S. Dementia in idiopathic hypoparathyroidism: rapid efficacy of alfacalcidol. *Arch Neurol* 1982; **39**:424–5.

Mathews WB. Familial calcification of the basal ganglia with response to parathormone. *J Neurol Neurosurg Psychiatry* 1957; **20**:172–7.

Mayeux R, Lueders H. Complex partial status epilepticus: case report and proposal for diagnostic criteria. *Neurology* 1978; **28**:957–61.

Mayeux R, Denaro J, Hemenegildo N *et al*. A population-based investigation of Parkinson's disease with and without dementia: relationship to age and gender. *Arch Neurol* 1992; **49**:492–7.

Medalia AA, Merriam AE, Ehrenreich JH. The neuropsychological sequelae of attempted hanging. *J Neurol Neurosurg Psychiatry* 1991; **54**:546–8.

Medina, JL, Rubino FA, Ross E. Agitated delirium caused by infarctions of the hippocampal formation and fusiform and lingual gyri. *Neurology* 1974; **24**:1181–4.

Medina JL, Sudhansu C, Rubino FA. Syndrome of agitated delirium and visual impairment: a manifestation of medial temporo-occipital infarction. *J Neurol Neurosurg Psychiatry* 1977; **40**:861–4.

Meierkord H, Wieshman U, Niehaus L *et al*. Structural consequences of status epilepticus with serial magnetic resonance imaging. *Acta Neurol Scand* 1997; **96**:127–32.

Mendez MF, Frey WH. Multiple sclerosis dementia. *Neurology* 1992; **42**:696.

Mendez MF, Selwood A, Mastri AR *et al*. Pick's disease versus Alzheimer's disease: a comparison of clinical characteristics. *Neurology* 1993; **43**:289–92.

Menza M, Murray GB. Pancreatic encephalopathy. *Biol Psychiatry* 1989; **25**:781–4.

Menza MA, Cocchiola J, Golbe LI. Psychiatric symptoms in progressive supranuclear palsy. *Psychosomatics* 1995; **36**:550–4.

Mermelstein HT. Clarithromycin-induced delirium in a general hospital. *Psychosomatics* 1997; **39**:540–2.

Messert B, Baker NH. Syndrome of progressive spastic ataxia and apraxia associated with occult hydrocephalus. *Neurology* 1966; **16**:440–52.

Meterissian GB. Risperidone-induced neuroleptic malignant syndrome: a case report and review. *Can J Psychiatry* 1996; **41**:52–4.

Miller CM. Whiplash amnesia. *Neurology* 1982; **32**:667–8.

Miller DD, Sharafuddin MJA, Kathol RG. A case of clozapine-induced neuroleptic malignant syndrome. *J Clin Psychiatry* 1991; **52**:99–101.

Miller DH, Kendall BE, Barter S *et al*. Magnetic resonance imaging in central nervous system sarcoidosis. *Neurology* 1988; **38**:378–83.

Miller E, Craddock-Watson JE, Pollock TM. Consequences of confirmed maternal rubella at successive stages of pregnancy. *Lancet* 1982; **2**:781–4.

Miller HG, Stanton JB, Gibbons JL. Para-infectious encephalomyelitis and related syndromes. *Q J Med* 1956; **25**:427–505.

Miller JW, Petersen RC, Metter EJ. Transient global amnesia: clinical characteristics and prognosis. *Neurology* 1987; **37**:733–7.

Min SK. A brain syndrome associated with delayed neuropsychiatric sequelae following acute carbon monoxide intoxication. *Acta Psychiatr Scand* 1986; **73**:80–6.

Minagar A, Shulman LM, Weiner WJ. Transderm-induced psychosis in Parkinson's disease. *Neurology* 1999; **53**:433–4.

Modi G, Modi M, Martinus R *et al*. The clinical and genetic characteristics of spinocerebellar ataxia type 7 (SCA7) in three black South African families. *Acta Neurol Scand* 2000; **101**:177–82.

Moersch FP. Psychic manifestations in cases of brain tumors. *Am J Psychiatry* 1925; **81**:707–24.

Moersch FP, Kernohan JW. Hypoglycemia: neurologic and neuropathologic studies. *Arch Neurol Psychiatry* 1938; **39**:242–57.

Molina JA, Calandre L, Bermejo F. Myoclonic encephalopathy due to bismuth salts: treatment with dimercaprol and analysis of CSF transmitters. *Acta Neurol Scand* 1989; **79**:200–3.

Molsa PK, Paljarvi L, Rinne JO *et al*. Validity of clinical diagnosis in dementia: a prospective clinico-pathological study. *J Neurol Neurosurg Psychiatry* 1985; **48**:1085–90.

Moosy J, Martinez AJ, Hanin I *et al*. Thalamic and subcortical gliosis with dementia. *Arch Neurol* 1987; **44**:510–13.

Mori E, Yamadori A. Acute confusional state and acute agitated delirium: occurrence after infarction in the right middle cerebral artery territory. *Arch Neurol* 1987; **44**:1139–43.

Morisy L, Platt D. Hazards of high-dose meperidine. *JAMA* 1986; **255**:467–8.

Morris LE, Heyman A, Pozersky T. Lead encephalopathy caused by ingestion of illicitly distilled whiskey. *Neurology* 1964; **14**:493–9.

Morse RM, Litin EM. The anatomy of delirium. *Am J Psychiatry* 1971; **128**:111–16.

Moser HU, Moser AE, Singh I *et al*. Adrenoleukodystrophy: survey of 303 cases: biochemistry, diagnosis and therapy. *Ann Neurol* 1984; **16**:628–41.

Mueller J, Hotson JR, Langston JW. Hyperviscosity-induced dementia. *Neurology* 1983; **33**:101–3.

Munoz MF, Selwood A, Mastri AR *et al*. Pick's disease versus Alzheimer's disease: a comparison of clinical abnormalities. *Neurology* 1993; **43**:289–92.

Munoz X, Marti S, Sumalla J *et al*. Acute delirium as a manifestation of obstructive sleep apnea syndrome. *Am J Respir Crit Care Med* 1998; **158**:1306–7.

Muramoto O, Kuru Y, Sugishita M *et al*. Pure memory loss with hippocampal lesions: a pneumoencephalographic study. *Arch Neurol* 1979; **36**:54–6.

Murphy MA, Feldman JA, Kilburn G. Hallervorden–Spatz disease in a psychiatric setting. *J Clin Psychiatry* 1989; **50**:66–8.

Narayanan ST, Murthy JMK. Nonconvulsive status epilepticus in a neurological intensive care unit: profile in a developing country. *Epilepsia* 2007; **48**:900–6.

Navia BA, Price RW. The acquired immunodeficiency syndrome dementia complex as the presenting or sole manifestation of human immunodeficiency infection. *Arch Neurol* 1987; **44**:65–9.

Navia BA, Petito CK, Gold JWM *et al*. Cerebral toxoplasmosis complicating the acquired immune deficiency syndrome: clinical and neuropathological findings in 27 patients. *Ann Neurol* 1986a; **19**:224–38.

Navia BA, Jordan BD, Price RW. The AIDS–dementia complex: I. Clinical features. *Ann Neurol* 1986b; **19**:517–24.

Neary D, Snowden JS, Mann DMA *et al*. Frontal lobe dementia and motor neuron disease. *J Neurol Neurosurg Psychiatry* 1990; **53**:23–32.

Neary D, Snowden JS, Mann DMA. Familial progressive atrophy: its relationship to other forms of lobar atrophy. *J Neurol Neurosurg Psychiatry* 1993; **56**:1122–5.

Nichelli P, Bahmanian-Behbahani G, Gentilini M *et al*. Preserved memory abilities in thalamic amnesia. *Brain* 1988; **111**:1337–53.

Nicholson A, Alberman E. Cerebral palsy – an increasing contributor to severe mental retardation. *Arch Dis Child* 1992; **67**:1050–5.

Nielsen J. Delirium tremens in Copenhagen. *Acta Psychiatr Scand* 1965; **41**(suppl. 187):1–92.

Nightingale S, Venables GS, Bates D. Polymyalgia rheumatica with diffuse cerebral disease responding rapidly to steroid therapy. *J Neurol Neurosurg Psychiatry* 1982; **45**:841–3.

Nishino H, Rubino FA, Parisi JE. The spectrum of neurologic involvement in Wegener's granulomatosis. *Neurology* 1993; **43**:1334–7.

Nobuyoshi I, Nishihara Y, Horie A. Amyloid angiopathy and lobar cerebral hemorrhage. *J Neurol Neurosurg Psychiatry* 1984; **47**:1203–10.

Nokura K, Yamamoto H, Okawara Y *et al*. Reversible limbic encephalitis caused by ovarian teratoma. *Acta Neurol Scand* 1997; **95**:367–73.

Nomdedeu M, Miro O, Nogue S *et al*. Hallucinatory delirium and psychomotor agitation as a paradoxical manifestation of acute propoxyphene poisoning. *Med Clin* 2001; **116**:318.

Norris CR, Trench JM, Hook R. Delayed carbon monoxide encephalopathy: clinical and research implications. *J Clin Psychiatry* 1982; **43**:294–5.

Nyhan WL. Clinical features of the Lesch–Nyhan syndrome. *Arch Int Med* 1972; **130**:186–92.

Nyland H, Skre H. Cerebral calcinosis with late onset encephalopathy – unusual type of pseudo-pseudohypoparathyroidism. *Acta Neurol Scand* 1977; **56**:309–25.

O'Connor JF, Musher DM. Central nervous system involvement in systemic lupus erythematosus. *Arch Neurol* 1966; **14**:157–64.

O'Hare JA, Callaghan NM, Murnaghan DJ. Dialysis encephalopathy. Clinical, electroencephalographic, and interventional aspects. *Medicine* 1983; **62**:129–41.

O'Keefe S, Lavan J. The prognostic significance of delirium in older hospital patients. *J Am Geriatr Soc* 1997; **45**:174–8.

Oksanen V. Neurosarcoidosis: clinical presentations and course in 50 patients. *Acta Neurol Scand* 1986; **73**:283–90.

Olazaran J, Muniz R, Reisberg B *et al.* Benefits of cognitive-motor intervention in mild to moderate Alzheimer's disease. *Neurology* 2004; **63**:2348–53.

Oppenheimer BS, Fishberg AM. Hypertensive encephalopathy. *Arch Int Med* 1928; **41**:264–78.

Palatucci DM. Paradoxical halide levels in bromide intoxication. *Neurology* 1978; **28**:1189–92.

Palmai G, Taylor DC, Falconer MA. A case of craniopharyngioma presenting as Korsakoff's psychosis. *Br J Psychiatry* 1967; **113**:619–23.

Palmini AL, Gloor P, Jones-Gotman M. Pure amnestic seizures in temporal lobe epilepsy. *Brain* 1992; **115**:749–69.

Palsson A, Thulin SO, Tunving K. Cannabis psychosis in south Sweden. *Acta Psychiatr Scand* 1982; **66**:311–21.

Pampiglione G, Moynahan EJ. The tuberous sclerosis syndrome: clinical and EEG studies in 100 children. *J Neurol Neurosurg Psychiatry* 1976; **39**:666–73.

Papazian O, Canizales E, Alfonso I *et al.* Reversible dementia and apparent brain atrophy during valproate therapy. *Ann Neurol* 1995; **38**:687–91.

Park SA, Hahn JH, Kim JI *et al.* Memory deficits after bilateral anterior fornix infarction. *Neurology* 2000; **54**:1379–82.

Pascual-Castroviejo I, Diaz-Gonzalez C, Garcia-Melian RM *et al.* Sturge–Weber syndrome: study of 40 patients. *Pediatr Neurol* 1993; **9**:283–8.

Paulson GW, Martin EW, Mojzisik C *et al.* Neurologic complications of gastric partitioning. *Arch Neurol* 1985; **42**:675–7.

Payton JB, Burkhart JE, Hersen M *et al.* Treatment of ADDH in mentally retarded children: a preliminary study. *J Am Acad Child Adolesc Psychiatry* 1989; **28**:761–7.

Pearlson GD. Psychiatric and medical symptoms associated with phencyclidine (PCP) abuse. *Johns Hopkins Med J* 1981; **148**:25–33.

Peavy GM, Herzog AG, Rubin NP *et al.* Neuropsychological aspects of motor neuron disease: a report of two cases. *Neurology* 1992; **42**:1004–8.

Penfield W, Mathieson G. Memory: autopsy findings and comments on the role of hippocampus in experiential recall. *Arch Neurol* 1974; **31**:145–54.

Penfield W, Milner B. Memory deficit produced by bilateral lesions in the hippocampal zone. *Arch Neurol Psychiatry* 1958; **79**:475–97.

Pepin EP, Auray-Pepin L. Selective dorsolateral frontal lobe dysfunction associated with diencephalic amnesia. *Neurology* 1993; **43**:733–41.

Perini GI, Colombi G, Armani M *et al.* Intellectual impairment and cognitive evoked potentials in myotonic dystrophy. *J Nerv Ment Dis* 1989; **177**:750–4.

Perren F, Clarke S, Bogousslavsky J. The syndrome of combined polar and paramedian thalamic infarction. *Arch Neurol* 2005; **62**:1212–16.

Perry JR, Warner E. Transient encephalopathy after paclitaxel (Taxol) infusion. *Neurology* 1996; **46**:1596–9.

Petermann AF, Hayles AB, Dockerty MB *et al.* Encephalotrigeminal angiomatosis (Sturge–Weber disease). Clinical study of thirty-five cases. *J Am Med Assoc* 1958; **167**:2169–76.

Petersen RC, Thomas RG, Grundman M *et al.* Vitamin E and donepezil for the treatment of mild cognitive impairment. *N Engl J Med* 2005; **352**:2379–88.

Petersen RC, Parisi JE, Dickson DW *et al.* Neuropathologic features of amnestic mild cognitive impairment. *Arch Neurol* 2006; **63**:665–72.

Pflanz S, Besson JAO, Ebmeier KP *et al.* The clinical manifestations of mental disorders in Huntington's disease: a retrospective case record study of disease progression. *Acta Psychiatr Scand* 1991; **83**:53–60.

Phillips S, Sangalang V, Sterns G. Basal forebrain infarction: a clinicopathologic corelation. *Arch Neurol* 1987; **44**:1134–8.

Pickering-Brown SM, Richardson AMT, Snowden JS *et al.* Inherited frontotemporal dementia in nine British families associated with intronic mutations in the tau gene. *Brain* 2002; **125**:732–51.

Pierce LB. Pellagra: report of a case. *Am J Psychiatry* 1924; **81**:237–43.

Pincus JH, Reynolds EH, Glaser GH. Subacute combined system degeneration with folate deficiency. *J Am Med Assoc* 1972; **221**:496–7.

Pittinger C, Desan PH. Gabapentin abuse, and delirium tremens upon gabapentin withdrawal. *J Clin Psychiatry* 2007; **68**:483–4.

Plum F, Posner JB, Hain RF. Delayed neurological deterioration after anoxia. *Arch Int Med* 1962; **110**:56–63.

Pompeii P, Foreman M, Rudberg MA *et al.* Delirium in hospitalized older persons: outcomes and predictors. *J Am Geriatr Soc* 1994; **42**:809–15.

Pope HG, Keck PE, McElroy SL. Frequency and presentation of neuroleptic malignant syndrome in a large psychiatric hospital. *Am J Psychiatry* 1986; **143**:1227–33.

Portet F, Ousset PJ, Visser PJ *et al.* Mild cognitive impairment in medical practice: critical review of the concept and new diagnostic procedure. Report of the MCI working group of the European Consortium on Alzheimer's disease (EADC). *J Neurol Neurosurg Psychiatry* 2006; **77**:714–18.

Postma JU, Van Tilburg W. Visual hallucinations and delirium during treatment with amantadine (Symmetrel). *J Am Geriatr Soc* 1975; **23**:212–15.

Potter NT, Meyer MA, Zimmerman AW *et al.* Molecular and clinical findings in a family with dentatorubral-pallidoluysian atrophy. *Ann Neurol* 1995; **37**:273–7.

Powers JM, Schaumburg HH, Gafney CL. Kluver–Bucy syndrome caused by adrenoleukodystrophy. *Neurology* 1980; **30**:1131–2.

Preskorn SH, Simpson S. Tricyclic-antidepressant-induced delirium and plasma drug concentration. *Am J Psychiatry* 1982; **139**:822–3.

Price BH, Gurvit H, Weintraud S *et al.* Neuropsychological patterns and language deficits in 20 consecutive cases of autopsy-confirmed Alzheimer's disease. *Arch Neurol* 1993; **50**:931–7.

Przelomski MM, O'Rourke E, Grady GF *et al.* Eastern equine encephalitis in Massachusetts. *Neurology* 1988; **38**:736–9.

Quinette P, Guillery-Giraud B, Dayan J *et al.* What does transient global amnesia really mean? Review of the literature and thorough study of 142 cases. *Brain* 2006; **129**:1640–58.

Qunitanilla J. Psychosis due to quinidine intoxication. *Am J Psychiatry* 1957; **113**:1031–2.

Rabins PV, Folstein MF. Delirium and dementia: diagnostic criteria and fatality rates. *Br J Psychiatry* 1982; **140**:149–53.

Rabins PV, Merchant A, Nestadt G. Criteria for diagnosing reversible dementia caused by depression: validation by 2-year follow-up. *Br J Psychiatry* 1984; **144**:488–92.

Rao V, Lyketsos C. Neuropsychiatric sequelae of traumatic brain injury. *Psychosomatics* 2000; **41**:95–103.

Rashiq S, Briewa L, Mooney M *et al.* Distinguishing acyclovir neurotoxicity from encephalomyelitis. *J Intern Med* 1993; **234**:507–11.

Raskin NH, Fishman RA. Neurologic disorders in renal failure. *N Engl J Med* 1976; **294**:143–8.

Raskin NH, Bredesen D, Ehrenfeld WK *et al.* Periodic confusion caused by congenital extrahepatic portocaval shunt. *Neurology* 1984; **34**:666–9.

Ratcliffe SG, Bancroft J, Axworthy D *et al.* Klinefelter's syndrome in adolescents. *Arch Dis Child* 1982; **57**:6–12.

Rathmell TK, Burns MA. The Laurence–Moon–Biedl syndrome occurring in a brother and a sister. *Arch Neurol Psychiatry* 1938; **39**:1033–42.

Rauschka H, Colsch B, Baumann N *et al.* Late-onset metachromatic leukodystrophy. Genotype strongly influences phenotype. *Neurology* 2006; **67**:859–63.

Read AE, Laidlaw J, Sherlock S. Neuropsychiatric complications of portocaval anastamosis. *Lancet* 1961; **1**:961–4.

Reding M, Haycox J, Blass J. Depression in patients referred to a dementia clinic: a three-year prospective study. *Arch Neurol* 1985; **42**:894–6.

Reed D, Crawley J, Faro SN *et al.* Thallotoxicosis. *J Am Med Assoc* 1963; **183**:516–22.

Reichenberg A, Yirmiya R, Schuld A *et al.* Cytokine-associated emotional and cognitive disturbances in humans. *Arch Gen Psychiatry* 2001; **58**:445–52.

Reider-Grosswasser I, Bornstein N. CT and MRI in late-onset metachromatic leukodystrophy. *Acta Neurol Scand* 1987; **75**:64–9.

Rennick PM, Perez-Borja C, Rodin EA. Transient mental deficits associated with recurrent prolonged epileptic clouded state. *Epilepsia* 1969; **10**:397–405.

Revesz T, Hawkins CP, du Boulay EPGH *et al.* Pathological findings correlated with magnetic resonance imaging in subcortical arteriosclerotic encephalopathy (Binswanger's disease). *J Neurol Neurosurg Psychiatry* 1989; **52**:1337–44.

Reynolds EH, Rothfeld P, Pincus JH. Neurological disease associated with folate deficiency. *BMJ* 1973; **2**:398–400.

Richardson EP. Progressive multifocal leukencephalopathy. *N Engl J Med* 1961; **265**:815–23.

Richardson JC, Chambers RA, Heywood PM. Encephalopathies of anoxia and hypoxemia. *Arch Neurol* 1959; **1**:178–90.

Richter RW, Shimojyo S. Neurologic sequelae of Japanese B encephalitis. *Neurology* 1961; **1**:553–9.

Riley DE, Lang AE, Lewis A *et al.* Cortical-basal ganglionic degeneration. *Neurology* 1990; **40**:1203–12.

Rinne JO, Lee MS, Thompson PD *et al.* Corticobasal degeneration: a clinical study of 36 cases. *Brain* 1994; **117**:1183–96.

Ristic AJ, Vojvodic N, Jankovic S *et al.* The frequency of reversible parkinsonism and cognitive decline associated with valproate treatment: a study of 364 patients with different types of epilepsy. *Epilepsia* 2006; **47**:2183–5.

Robbins TW, James M, Lance TW *et al.* Cognitive performance in multiple system atrophy. *Brain* 1992; **115**:271–91.

Robertson EE. Progressive bulbar paralysis showing heredofamilial incidence and intellectual impairment. *Arch Neurol Psychiatry* 1953; **69**:197–207.

Robinson WP, Bottani A, Yagang X. Molecular, cytogenetic, and clinical investigations of Prader–Willi syndrome patients. *Am J Hum Genet* 1992; **49**:1219–34.

Rodriguez ME, Artieda J, Zubieta JL *et al.* Reflex myoclonus in olivopontocerebellar atrophy. *J Neurol Neurosurg Psychiatry* 1994; **57**:316–19.

Romanul FCA, Radvany J, Rosales RK. Whipple's disease confined to the brain: a case confirmed clinically and pathologically. *J Neurol Neurosurg Psychiatry* 1977; **40**:901–9.

Roos R, Cajdusek DC, Gibbs CJ. The clinical characteristics of transmissible Creutzfeldt–Jakob disease. *Brain* 1973; **96**:1–20.

Rosa A, Demiati M, Cartz L *et al.* Marchiafava–Bignami disease, syndrome of interhemispheric disconnection, and right handed agraphia in a left-hander. *Arch Neurol* 1991; **48**:986–8.

Rose FC, Symonds CP. Persistent memory defect following encephalitis. *Brain* 1960; **83**:195–212.

Rosebush P, Stewart T. A prognostic analysis of 24 episodes of neuroleptic malignant syndrome. *Am J Psychiatry* 1989; **146**:717–25.

Rosenbaum M, Lewis M, Piker P *et al.* Convulsive seizures in delirium tremens. *Arch Neurol Psychiatry* 1941; **45**:486–93.

Rosenberg NL, Kleineschmidt-DeMasters BK, Davis KA *et al.* Toluene abuse causes diffuse central nervous system white matter changes. *Ann Neurol* 1988; **23**:611–14.

Rosman NP, Pearce J. The brain in multiple neurofibromatosis (Von Recklinghausen's disease): a suggested neuropathological basis for the associated mental defect. *Brain* 1967; **90**:829–37.

Ross AT, Dickerson WW. Tuberous sclerosis. *Arch Neurol Psychiatry* 1943; **50**:233–57.

Roth A. Familial eunuchoidism: the Laurence-Moon–Biedl syndrome. *J Urol* 1947; **57**:427–42.

Roy-Byrne PR, Weingartner H, Bierer LM *et al.* Effortful and automatic cognitive processes in depression. *Arch Gen Psychiatry* 1986; **43**:265–7.

Rozdilsky B, Cummings JN, Huston AF. Hallervorden–Spatz disease: late infantile and adult types, report of two cases. *Acta Neuropathol* 1968; **10**:1–16.

Rubinstein LJ, Urich H. Meningo-encephalitis of Behçet's disease: case report with pathological findings. *Brain* 1963; **86**:151–60.

Russell WR. Disability caused by brain wounds. *J Neurol Neurosurg Psychiatry* 1951; **14**:35–9.

Russell WR, Nathan PW. Traumatic amnesia. *Brain* 1946; **68**:280–300.

Russell WR, Schiller F. Crushing injuries to the skull. *J Neurol Neurosurg Psychiatry* 1949; **12**:52–60.

Russell WR, Smith A. Post-traumatic amnesia in closed head injury. *Arch Neurol* 1961; **5**:4–17.

Rustam H, Hamri T. Methyl mercury poisoning in Iraq. *Brain* 1974; **97**:499–510.

Sachdev P, Kruk J, Kneebone M *et al.* Clozapine-induced neuroleptic malignant syndrome: review and report of new cases. *J Clin Psychopharmacol* 1995; **15**:365–71.

Sachs E. Meningiomas with dementia as the first and presenting feature. *J Ment Sci* 1950; **96**:998–1007.

Sandberg O, Franklin KA, Bucht G *et al.* Sleep apnea, delirium, depressed mood, cognition and ADL ability after stroke. *J Am Geriatr Soc* 2001; **49**:391–7.

Sanson M, Duyckaerts C, Thibault J-L *et al.* Sarcoidosis presenting as late-onset dementia. *J Neurol* 1996; **243**:484–7.

Sasaki H, Fukazawa T, Yanagihara T *et al.* Clinical features and natural history of spinocerebellar ataxia type 1. *Acta Neurol Scand* 1996; **93**:64–71.

Schaumberg HH, Powers JM, Raine CS *et al.* Adrenoleukodystrophy: a clinical and pathological study of 17 cases. *Arch Neurol* 1975; **32**:577–91.

Scheid R, Honnarat J, Delmont E *et al.* A new anti-neuronal antibody in a case of paraneoplastic limbic encephalitis associated with breast cancer. *J Neurol Neurosurg Psychiatry* 2004; **75**:338–40.

Scheltens P, Visscher F, Van Keimpema ARJ *et al.* Sleep apnea syndrome presenting with cognitive impairment. *Neurology* 1991; **41**:155.

Schneider JA, Watts RL, Gearing M *et al.* Corticobasal degeneration neuropathologic and clinical heterogenity. *Neurology* 1997; **48**:959–69.

Schou M. Long-lasting neurological sequelae after lithium intoxication. *Acta Neurol Scand* 1984; **70**:594–602.

Scoville WB, Milner B. Loss of recent memory after bilateral hippocampal lesion. *J Neurol Neurosurg Psychiatry* 1957; **20**:11–21.

Sechi GP, Tanda F, Mutani R. Fatal hyperpyrexia after withdrawal of levodopa. *Neurology* 1984; **34**:249–51.

Sellal F, Mohr M, Collard M. Dementia in a 58-year-old woman. *Lancet* 1996; **347**:236.

Seltzer B, Benson DF. The temporal pattern of retrograde amnesia in Korsakoff's disease. *Neurology* 1974; **24**:527–30.

Serby M, Angrist B, Lieberman A. Mental disturbance during bromocriptine and lergotrile treatment of Parkinson's disease. *Am J Psychiatry* 1978; **135**:1227–9.

Serdaroglu P, Yazici H, Ozdemir C *et al.* Neurologic involvement in Behçet's syndrome: a prospective study. *Arch Neurol* 1989; **46**:265–9.

Serdaru M, Hausser-Hauw C, Laplane D *et al.* The clinical spectrum of alcoholic pellagra encephalopathy. *Brain* 1988; **111**:829–42.

Shapiro EG, Lockman LA, Knopman D *et al.* Characteristics of the dementia in late-onset metachromatic leukodystrophy. *Neurology* 1994; **44**:662–5.

Shaw PJ, Walls TJ, Newman PK *et al.* Hashimoto's encephalopathy: a steroid-responsive disorder associated with high anti-thyroid antibody titers: report of 5 cases. *Neurology* 1991; **41**:228–33.

Shear MK, Sacks MH. Digitalis delirium: report of two cases. *Am J Psychiatry* 1978; **135**:109–10.

Sheth RD, Drazkowski JF, Sirven JI. Protracted ectal confusion in elderly patients. *Arch Neurol* 2006; **63**:529–32.

Shewmon DA, Masdeu JC. Delayed radiation necrosis of the brain contralateral to original tumor. *Arch Neurol* 1980; **37**:592–4.

Shill HA, Fife TD. Valproic acid toxicity mimicking multiple system atrophy. *Neurology* 2000; **55**:1936–7.

Shuttleworth EC, Morris CE. The transient global amnesia syndrome. *Arch Neurol* 1966; **15**:515–20.

Shuttleworth EC, Wise GR. Transient global amnesia due to arterial embolism. *Arch Neurol* 1973; **29**:340–2.

Siesling S, Vester-van der Vlis M, Roos RAC. Juvenile Huntington's disease in the Netherlands. *Pediatr Neurology* 1997; **17**:34–43.

Silverstein A. Thrombotic thrombocytopenic purpura: the initial neurologic manifestations. *Arch Neurol* 1968; **18**:358–62.

Silverstein A, Siltzbach LE. Neurologic sarcoidosis: study of 18 cases. *Arch Neurol* 1965; **12**:1–11.

Sim M, Turner E, Smith WR. Cerebral biopsy in the investigation of presenile dementia. I. Clinical aspects. *Br J Psychiatry* 1966; **112**:119–25.

Simard M, Gumbiner B, Lee A *et al.* Lithium carbonate intoxication: a case report and review of the literature. *Arch Int Med* 1989; **149**:36–46.

Sirois F. Delirium: 100 cases. *Can J Psychiatry* 1988; **33**:375–8.

Smyth GE, Stern K. Tumours of the thalamus – a clinicopathological study. *Brain* 1938; **61**:339–74.

Snead OC, Gibson KM. Gamma-hydroxybutyric acid. *N Engl J Med* 2005; **352**:2721–32.

Snowden JS, Neary D, Mann DMA *et al.* Progressive language disorder due to lobar atrophy. *Ann Neurol* 1992; **31**:174–83.

Spohr HL, Willms J, Steinhausen HC. Prenatal alcohol exposure and long-term developmental consequences. *Lancet* 1993; **341**:907–10.

Sponzilli EE, Smith JK, Malamud N *et al.* Progressive multifocal leukoencephalopathy: a complication of immunosuppressive treatment. *Neurology* 1975; **25**:664–8.

Spreat S, Behar D, Reneski B *et al.* Lithium carbonate for aggression in mentally retarded persons. *Compr Psychiatry* 1989; **30**:505–11.

Sprofkin BE, Sciarra D. Korsakoff's psychosis associated with cerebral tumor. *Neurology* 1952; **2**:427–34.

Starosta MA, Brandwein SR. Clinical manifestation and treatment of rheumatoid pachymeningitis. *Neurology* 2007; **68**:1079–80.

Steele TE, Morton WA. Salicyclate-induced delirium. *Psychosomatics* 1986; **27**:455–6.

Steinberg RB, Gilman DE, Johnson F. Acute toxic delirium in a patient using transdermal fentanyl. *Anesth Analg* 1992; **75**:1014–16.

Stenback A, Haapanen E. Azotemia and psychosis. *Acta Psychiatr Scand* 1967; (suppl. 197):1–65.

Stern K. Severe dementia associated with bilateral symmetric degeneration of the thalamus. *Brain* 1939; **62**:157–71.

Sternbach H. The serotonin syndrome. *Am J Psychiatry* 1991; **148**:705 13.

Storandt M, Grant EA, Miller P *et al.* Longitudinal course and neuropathologic outcome in original versus revised MCI and in pre-MCI. *Neurology* 2006; **67**:467–73.

Storm-Mathisen A. General paresis: a follow-up study of 203 patients. *Acta Psychiatr Scand* 1969; **45**:118–32.

Stracciari A, Ciucci G, Bianchedi G *et al.* Epileptic transient amnesia. *Eur Neurol* 1990; **30**:176–90.

Strachan RW, Henderson JG. Dementia and folate deficiency. *Q J Med* 1967; **36**:189–204.

Strauss I, Globus JH. Tumor of the brain with disturbance in temperature regulation. *Arch Neurol Psychiatry* 1931; **25**:506–22.

Strich SJ. Diffuse degeneration of the cerebral white matter in severe dementia following head injury. *J Neurol Neurosurg Psychiatry* 1956; **19**:163–85.

Stuerenburg HJ, Hansen HC, Thie A *et al.* Reversible dementia in idiopathic hypoparathyroidism associated with normocalcemia. *Neurology* 1996; **47**:474–6.

Sujanski E, Conradi S. Sturge-Weber syndrome: age of onset of seizures and glaucoma and the prognosis for affected children. *J Child Neurol* 1995; **10**:49–58.

Summerskill WHJ, Davidson EA, Sherlock S *et al.* The neuropsychiatric syndrome associated with hepatic cirrhosis and extensive portal collateral circulation. *Q J Med* 1956; **25**:245–52.

Supino-Viterbo V, Sicard C, Risvegliato M *et al.* Toxic encephalopathy due to ingestion of bismuth salts: clinical and EEG studies of 45 patients. *J Neurol Neurosurg Psychiatry* 1977; **40**:748–52.

Swanson AG, Iseri OA. Acute encephalopathy due to water intoxication. *N Engl J Med* 1958; **258**:831–4.

Sweet WH, Talland GA, Erwin FR. Loss of recent memory following section of the fornix. *Trans Am Neurol Assn* 1958; **84**:76–82.

Talland GH, Sweet WH, Ballantine HT. Amnesic syndrome with anterior communicating artery aneurysm. *J Nerv Ment Dis* 1967; **145**:179–92.

Tanaka Y, Miyazawa Y, Akaoka F *et al.* Amnesia following damage to the mammillary bodies. *Neurology* 1977; **48**:160–5.

Tanaka Y, Miyazawa Y, Hashimoto R *et al.* Postencephalitic focal retrograde amnesia after bilateral anterior temporal lobe damage. *Neurology* 1999; **53**:344–50.

Tatemichi TK, Desmond DW, Prohovnik I *et al.* Dementia associated with bilateral carotid occlusions: neuropsychological and haemodynamic course after extracranial to intracranial bypass surgery. *J Neurol Neurosurg Psychiatry* 1995; **38**:633–6.

Tenenbaum S, Chamoles N, Fejerman N. Acute disseminated encephalomyelitis. A long-term follow-up of 84 pediatric patients. *Neurology* 2002; **59**:1224–31.

Thapar A, Gottesman II, Owen MJ *et al.* The genetic mental retardations. *Br J Psychiatry* 1994; **164**:747–58.

Thompson C, Dent J, Saxby P. Effects of thallium poisoning on intellectual function. *Br J Psychiatry* 1988; **153**:396–9.

Thrush DC, Boddie HG. Episodic encephalopathy associated with thyroid disorders. *J Neurol Neurosurg Psychiatry* 1974; **37**:696–700.

Tiraboschi P, Salmon DP, Hansen LA *et al.* What best differentiates Lewy body from Alzheimer's disease in early-stage dementia? *Brain* 2006; **129**:729–35.

Tison F, Dartigues JF, Auriacombe S *et al.* Dementia in Parkinson's disease: a population-based study in ambulatory and institutionalized individuals. *Neurology* 1995; **45**:705–8.

Tomlinson BE, Blessed GE, Roth M. Observations on the brains of demented old people. *J Neurol Sci* 1970; **11**:205–42.

Tomson CR, Goodship TH, Rodger RS. Psychiatric side-effects of acyclovir in patients with chronic renal failure. *Lancet* 1985; **2**:385–6.

Tomson T, Lindbom U, Nilsson BY. Nonconvulsive status epilepticus in adults: thirty-two consecutive patients from a general hospital population. *Epilepsia* 1992; **33**:829–35.

Topliss D, Bond R. Acute brain syndrome after propranolol treatment. *Lancet* 1977; **2**:1133–4.

Toru M, Matsuda O, Makiguchi K *et al.* Single case study: neuroleptic malignant-like state following a withdrawal of antiparkinsonian drugs. *J Nerv Ment Dis* 1981; **169**:324–7.

Tourbah A, Piette JC, Iba-Zizen MT *et al.* The natural course of cerebral lesions in Sneddon's syndrome. *Arch Neurol* 1997; **54**:53–60.

Townsend JJ, Baringer JR, Wolinsky JS *et al.* Progressive rubella panencephalitis: late onset after congenital rubella. *N Engl J Med* 1975; **292**:990–3.

Townsend JJ, Wolinsky JS, Baringer JR. The neuropathology of progressive rubella panencephalitis of late onset. *Brain* 1976; **99**:81–90.

Trzepacz PT, Teague GB, Lipowski ZJ. Delirium and other organic mental disorders in a general hospital. *Gen Hosp Psychiatry* 1985; **7**:101–6.

Tschanz JT, Welsh-Bohmer KA, Lyketsos CG *et al.* Conversion to dementia from mild cognitive disorder. The Cache County study. *Neurology* 2006; **67**:229–34.

Tucker WM, Forster FM. Petit mal epilepsy occurring in status. *Arch Neurol Psychiatry* 1958; **64**:823–7.

Tuma R, DeAngelis LM. Altered mental status in patients with cancer. *Arch Neurol* 2000; **57**:1727–31.

Tune L, Damlouji NF, Holland A *et al.* Association of postoperative delirium with raised serum levels of anticholinergic drugs. *Lancet* 1981; **2**:651–3.

Tune L, Carr S, Cooper T *et al.* Association of anticholinergic activity of prescribed medications with postoperative delirium. *J Neuropsychiatry Clin Neurosci* 1993; **5**:208–10.

Turner RS, Kenyon LC, Trojanowski JQ *et al.* Clinical, neuroimaging, and pathologic features of progressive nonfluent aphasia. *Ann Neurol* 1996; **39**:166–73.

Tyler RH. Neurologic disorders in renal failure. *Am J Med* 1968; **44**:734–8.

Uyama E, Iwagoe H, Maeda J *et al.* Presenile-onset cerebral adrenoleukodystrophy presenting as Balint's syndrome and dementia. *Neurology* 1993; **43**:1249–51.

Vandenn Borre R, Vermote R, Buttiens M et al. Risperidone as add-on therapy in behavioral disturbances in mental retardation: a double-blind placebo-controlled cross-over study. Acta Psychiatr Scand 1993; 87:167–71.

Van Horn G, Arnett FC, Dimachkie MM. Reversible dementia and chorea in a young woman with the lupus anticoagulant. Neurology 1996; 46:1599–603.

Varney NR, Alexander B, MacIndoe JH. Reversible steroid dementia in patients without steroid psychosis. Am J Psychiatry 1984; 141:369–73.

Velamoor VR, Norman RMG, Caroff SN et al. Progression of symptoms in neuroleptic malignant syndrome. J Nerv Ment Dis 1994; 182:168–73.

Venneri A, Caffarra P. Transient autobiographic amnesia: EEG and single-photon emission CT evidence of an organic etiology. Neurology 1998; 50:186–91.

Victor M, Yakovlev PI. S.S. Korsakoff's psychic disorder in conjunction with peripheral neuritis: a translation of Korsakoff's original article with brief comments on the author and his contribution to clinical medicine. Neurology 1955; 5:394–406.

Victor M, Angevine JB, Mancall EL et al. Memory loss with lesions of the hippocampal formation. Arch Neurol 1961; 5:244–63.

Victor M, Adams RD, Cole M. The acquired 'non-Wilsonian' type of chronic hepatocerebral degeneration. Medicine 1965; 44:345–96.

de Villemeur TB, Deslys J-P, Pradel A et al. Creutzfeldt–Jacob disease from contaminated growth hormone extracts in France. Neurology 1996; 47:690–5.

Vollmer TL, Guarnaccia J, Harrington W et al. Idiopathic granulomatous angiitis of the central nervous system: diagnostic challenges. Arch Neurol 1993; 50:925–30.

Volpe JJ. Cognitive deficits in premature infants. N Engl J Med 1991; 325:276–8.

Vortmeyer AO, Hagel C, Laas R. Haemorrhagic thiamine deficient encephalopathy following prolonged parenteral nutrition. J Neurol Neurosurg Psychiatry 1992; 55:826–9.

Walker AE. Recent memory impairment in unilateral temporal lesions. Arch Neurol Psychiatry 1957; 78:543–57.

Wallack EM, Reavis WM, Hall CD. Primary brain stem reticulum sarcoma causing dementia. Dis Nerv Syst 1977; 38:744–7.

Walshe JM, Yealland M. Wilson's disease: the problem of delayed diagnosis. J Neurol Neurosurg Psychiatry 1992; 55:692–6.

Wamboldt FS, Jefferson JW, Wamboldt MZ. Digitalis intoxication misdiagnosed as depression by primary care physician. Am J Psychiatry 1986; 143:219–21.

Wang PS, Schneeweiss S, Avorn J et al. Risk of death in elderly users of conventional vs. atypical antipsychotic medications. N Engl J Med 2005; 353:2335–41.

Warner TT, Lennox GG, Janota I et al. Autosomal-dominant dentatorubropallidoluysian atrophy. Mov Disord 1994; 9:289–96.

Warner TT, Williams LD, Walker RWH et al. A clinical and molecular genetic study of dentatorubropallidoluysian atrophy in four European families. Ann Neurol 1995; 37:452–9.

Warren JD, Thompson PD, Thompson PD. Diencephalic amnesia and apraxia after left thalamic infarction. J Neurol Neurosurg Psychiatry 2000; 68:248.

Watts GF, Mitchell WD, Bending JJ et al. Cerebrotendinous xanthomatosis: a family study of sterol 27–hydroxylase mutations and pharmacotherapy. Q J Med 1996; 89:55–63.

Wechsler IS, Davison C. Amyotrophic lateral sclerosis with mental symptoms: a clinicopathologic study. Arch Neurol Psychiatry 1932; 327:859–80.

Weil ML, Itabashi H, Cramer NE et al. Chronic progressive panencephalitis due to rubella virus simulating subacute sclerosing panencephalitis. N Engl J Med 1975; 292:994–8.

Weinberger LM, Cohen ML, Remler BF et al. Intracranial Wegener's granulomatosis. Neurology 1993; 43:1831–4.

Weizman A, Eldar M, Shoenfeld Y et al. Hypercalcemia-induced psychopathology in malignant diseases. Br J Psychiatry 1979; 135:363–6.

Weller M, Liedtke W, Petersen D et al. Very-late-onset adrenoleukodystrophy: possible precipitation of demyelination by cerebral contusion. Neurology 1992; 42:367–70.

Wells CE. Pseudodementia. Am J Psychiatry 1979; 136:895–900.

Welti W. Delirium with low serum sodium. Arch Neurol Psychiatry 1956; 76:559–64.

Wenning GK, Shlomo YB, Magalhaes M et al. Clinical features and natural history of multiple system atrophy: an analysis of 100 cases. Brain 1994; 117:835–45.

Wenning GK, Ben-Shlomo Y, Magalhaes M et al. Clinicopathological study of 35 cases of multiple system atrophy. J Neurol Neurosurg Psychiatry 1995; 58:160–6.

Werheran KJ, Brown P, Thompson PD et al. The clinical features and prognosis of chronic posthypoxic myoclonus. Mov Disord 1997; 12:216–20.

Westlake EK, Simpson T, Kaye M. Carbon dioxide narcosis in emphysema. Q J Med 1955; 24:155–73.

Whitfield CL, Ch'ien LT, Whitehead LD. Lead encephalopathy in adults. Am J Med 1972; 52:289–98.

Whitney JF, Gannon DE. Obstructive sleep apnea presenting as acute delirum. Am J Emerg Med 1996; 14:370–1.

Wiederholdt WL, Siekert RG. Neurological manifestations of sarcoidosis. Neurology 1965; 15:1147–54.

Wilkins RH, Brody IA. Encephalitis lethargica. Arch Neurol 1968; 18:324–8.

Will RG, Mathews WB. A retrospective study of Creutzfeldt–Jakob disease in England and Wales 1970–1979. I. Clinical features. J Neurol Neurosurg Psychiatry 1984; 47:134–40.

Williams M, Pennybacker J. Memory disturbances in third ventricle tumours. J Neurol Neurosurg Psychiatry 1954; 17:115–23.

Williamson RT. On the symptomatology of gross lesions (tumours and abscesses) involving the pre-frontal regions of the brain. Brain 1896; 19:346–65.

Wilson JTL, Teasdale GM, Hadley DM et al. Post-traumatic amnesia: still a valuable yardstick. J Neurol Neurosurg Psychiatry 1994; 57:198–201.

Wilson LM. Intensive care delirium: the effect of outside deprivation in a windowless unit. Arch Intern Med 1972; 130:225–6.

Winblad B, Palmer K, Kivipelto M et al. Mild cognitive impairment: beyond controversies, towards a consensus: report of the International Working Group on Mild Cognitive Impairment. J Intern Med 2004; 256: 240–6.

Wisniewski HM, Coblentz JM, Terry RD. Pick's disease: a clinical and ultrastructural study. *Arch Neurol* 1972; **26**:97–108.

Wisniewski KE, Frency JH, Fernando S *et al.* Fragile X syndrome: associated neurological abnormalities and developmental disabilities. *Ann Neurol* 1985; **18**:665–9.

Wityk RJ, Goldsborough MA, Hillis A *et al.* Diffusion- and perfusion-weighted brain magnetic resonance imaging in patients with neurologic complications after cardiac surgery. *Arch Neurol* 2001; **58**:571–6.

Wolfe HG, Curran D. Nature of delirium and allied states. *Arch Neurol Psychiatry* 1935; **33**:1175–215.

Wolfe N, Linn R, Babikian VL *et al.* Frontal system impairment following multiple lacunar infarcts. *Arch Neurol* 1990; **47**:129–32.

Wolinsky JS, Berg BO, Maitland CJ. Progressive rubella panencephalitis. *Arch Neurol* 1976; **33**:722–3.

Wong Y-C, Au WL, Xu M *et al.* Magnetic resonance spectroscopy in adult-onset citrullinemia. Elevated glutaime levels in comatose patients. *Arch Neurol* 2007; **64**:1034–7.

Wood CA, Buller F. Poisoning by wood alcohol. Cases of death and blindness from Columbian spirits and other methylated preparations. *J Am Med Assoc* 1904; **43**:972–7, 1058–62, 1117–23, 1213–21.

Wu R-M, Chang Y-L, Chiu H-C. Acute triphenyltin intoxication: a case report. *J Neurol Neurosurg Psychiatry* 1990; **53**:356–7.

Wulff CH, Trojaborg W. Adult metachromatic leukodystrophy: neuropsychologic findings. *Neurology* 1985; **35**:1776–8.

Yaqub B, Al Deeb S. Heat stroke; aetiopathogenesis, neurological characteristics, treatment and outcome. *J Neurol Sci* 1998; **156**:144–51.

Yildizeli B, Ozyurtkan MO, Batirel HF *et al.* Factors associated with postoperative delirium after thoracic surgery. *Ann Thorac Surg* 2005; **79**: 1004–9.

Yoshitake T, Kiyohara Y, Kato I *et al.* Incidence and risk factors of vascular dementia and Alzheimer's disease in a defined elderly Japanese population: the Hisayama study. *Neurology* 1995; **45**:1161–8.

Young CA, Humphrey DM, Ghadiali EJ *et al.* Short-term memory impairment in an alert patient as a presentation of herpes simplex encephalitis. *Neurology* 1992; **42**:260–1.

Zappoli R. Two cases of prolonged twilight state with almost continuous 'wave-spikes'. *Electroencephalogr Clin Neurophysiol* 1955; **7**:421–3.

Zeidler M, Stewart GE, Barraclough CR *et al.* New variant Creutzfeldt–Jakob disease: neurological features and diagnostic tests. *Lancet* 1997; **350**:903–7.

Ziegler DK, Kaufman A, Marshall HE. Abrupt memory loss associated with thalamic tumor. *Arch Neurol* 1977; **34**:545–8.

Zhang C, Glenn DG, Bell WL *et al.* Gabapentin-induced myoclonus in end stage renal disease. *Epilepsia* 2005; **46**:156–8.

Zhou Y-X, Wang G-X, Tang B-S *et al.* Spinocerebellar ataxia type 2 in China: molecular analysis and genotype–phenotype correlation in nine families. *Neurology* 1998; **51**:595–8.

Zipursky RB, Baker RW, Zimmer B. Alprazolam withdrawal delirium unresponsive to diazepam: case report. *J Clin Psychiatry* 1985; **46**:344–5.

Ziskind AA. Transdermal scopolamine-induced psychosis. *Postgrad Med* 1988; **84**:73–6.

Zochodne DW, Young GB, McLachlan RS *et al.* Creutzfeldt–Jakob disease without periodic sharp wave complexes: a clinical, electroencephalographic, and pathologic study. *Neurology* 1988; **38**:1056–60.

Zola-Morgan S, Squire LR, Amaral DG. Human amnesia and the medial temporal region: enduring memory impairment following a bilateral lesion limited to field CA1 of the hippocampus. *J Neurosci* 1986; **6**:2950–67.

Zunt JR, Tu RK, Anderson DM *et al.* Progressive multifocal leukoencephalopathy presenting as human immunodeficiency virus type 1 (HIV)-associated dementia. *Neurology* 1997; **49**:263–5.

Syndromes of disturbances of mood and affect

6

6.1 DEPRESSION

Depression, as conceived of here, is a syndrome that may result from any one of a large number of underlying causes. Although the most common cause of depression is major depressive disorder, it is critical to subject each depressed patient to a thorough diagnostic evaluation before concluding that major depressive disorder, or perhaps one of the other idiopathic disorders discussed below, is the cause.

Clinical features

The syndrome of depression, in its fully developed form, includes not only a depressed or irritable mood, but also other symptoms, as listed in Table 6.1; each one of these is considered in turn.

Mood is depressed or sometimes irritable; some, in addition to these symptoms, may also complain of anxiety. At times patients may deny a depressed mood, but rather complain of a sense of discouragement, or perhaps lassitude and a sense of being weighted down. The patient's affect generally mirrors the mood, and there may be copious tears. At times, and especially in those with anxiety, there may be a 'pained' facial expression. Occasionally, patients may attempt to hide their depressed mood by feigning a 'happy' affect, thus creating a 'smiling depression'.

Self-esteem typically sinks during depression, and the workings of conscience may become so prominent as to create an almost insupportable burden of guilt: patients may see their sins multiply in front of them, and in reviewing their past may be blind to their accomplishments and see only their misdeeds. Pessimism settles in and patients see no hope for themselves, either now or in the future.

Suicidal ideation is typically present, and may be either passive or active. Patients may say that they would not mind if they were in a fatal accident or died of some disease.

Others may actively seek death, perhaps by hanging, shooting, jumping from bridges, or taking overdoses.

Difficulty with concentration may be profound. Patients may complain that it is as if a 'fog' had settled in, and that they feel dull and heavy headed. Memory seems to fail, and patients may be unable to recall where they put things or what was said. Attempts at cognitive activities often end in failure: patients, in trying to read a book, may read the same paragraph again and again, and find themselves unable to absorb or understand what they have read. Things seem too complex and making decisions may be impossible.

The remaining symptoms, namely anhedonia, anergia, sleep disturbance, appetite change, and psychomotor change, are often referred to, collectively, as the 'vegetative' symptoms of depression, in that they represent disturbances in the basic vegetative functions critical for survival.

Anhedonia represents an inability to take pleasure in things, and patients may complain that nothing arouses or attracts them. Thus unable to experience pleasure, patients lose interest in formerly pleasurable activities and must force themselves to get through their days, which, to them, seem desolate and lifeless. Libido is especially lost, and patients may withdraw entirely from any sexual activities.

Anergia, or a dearth of energy, may leave patients complaining of fatigue, tiredness, and exhaustion, or of being 'drained'. The anergia may be so extreme that patients are unable to complete routine tasks; some may even be unable to find the energy to get dressed.

Sleep disturbance may manifest with either insomnia or hypersomnia. Insomnia is more common, and may be a particular torment to the patient. Although some complain of what is technically known as 'initial' insomnia, that is to say trouble initiating or falling asleep, a more characteristic complaint is 'middle' insomnia, wherein patients awaken in the middle of the night, and have great difficulty in falling back asleep; some complain that their 'mind' simply won't 'shut off'. Some may also experience 'terminal' insomnia, or, as it is also known, 'early morning awakening', wherein they

Table 6.1   Symptoms of depression

Depressed or irritable mood
Low self-esteem, guilt, pessimism
Suicidal ideation
Difficulty with concentration or forgetfulness
Anhedonia (lack of interest in formerly pleasurable activities)
Anergia (lack of energy)
Sleep disturbance (insomnia or hypersomnia)
Appetite disturbance (anorexia or increased appetite)
Psychomotor change (agitation or retardation)

awaken well before the desired time of arousal and then are unable to fall back asleep. When morning finally does come, patients arise unrefreshed and exhausted, sometimes feeling as if they had not slept at all. Hypersomnia is relatively uncommon: here, patients may sleep 12, 16, or even 18 hours a day. Remarkably, despite such extremes of sleep, patients do not feel refreshed during their waking hours.

Appetite is typically lost and this anorexia may be accompanied by an altered taste. Patients may complain that their food has no taste or has perhaps become unpalatable; some may say their food tastes like cardboard. Although some patients may force themselves to eat, most cannot and weight loss is typical, possibly extreme. Increased appetite is relatively uncommon but when it does occur the accompanying weight gain may be impressive.

Psychomotor change tends more to agitation than to retardation. Agitation, when slight, may be confined to a certain sense of inner restlessness. When more severe, there may be hand-wringing and restless pacing: patients may complain of being unable to keep still; they may loudly lament their fate, and some may give way to wailing and miserable pleas for help. The tension experienced by these patients may be almost palpable to the observer and yet, despite their pleas, these patients cannot be comforted no matter what is done for them. Psychomotor retardation is less common. Patients may speak slowly and haltingly, and some may become mute, as if the effort to speak were simply too great; if asked, they may report that their thoughts are sluggish and come very slowly. These patients may move very little, and some may become almost completely immobile: efforts to get them up may be met with reluctance, even irritation, and some patients, if left to themselves, may neither bathe nor change their clothes.

There is debate as to how many of these symptoms must be present before a syndromal diagnosis of depression is warranted. Some authorities insist on a large number and although such an approach yields a relatively 'pure' group it runs the risk of ignoring patients whose symptoms, although few in number, are severe, even disabling. I recommend, as a preliminary approach, reserving the diagnosis for those who, in addition to a depressed mood, also have at least three of the remaining symptoms noted in Table 6.1.

There is also debate as to the duration of symptoms before the diagnosis is given. Although it is customary to withhold the diagnosis until symptoms have persisted for about 2 weeks, some judgment is required here as there are clearly cases wherein patients have severe and numerous depressive symptoms, which, however, are relatively brief in duration. Examples include the premenstrual dysphoric disorder, some medication-induced depressions, and ictal depressions. In practice, most clinicians will relax the time duration in proportion to the increasing severity and number of symptoms.

Etiology

The various causes of depression are listed in Table 6.2, in which they are divided into several groups. The first group includes the *primary or idiopathic disorders*, such as major depressive disorder: the disorders in this group account, by far, for the most cases of depression. The next group includes *toxic depressions*, which may be either *medication induced*, for example the depression seen with high-dose prednisone, or due to *substances of abuse or toxins*, as may be seen in chronic alcoholism. *Metabolic depressions* are considered next, including such disorders as obstructive sleep apnea. *Medication or substance withdrawal depressions* follow, and include depressions occurring upon discontinuation of long-term treatment with anticholinergic medications or as may be seen during withdrawal from stimulants. *Endocrinologic disorders* constitute a very important cause of depression, and include such familiar conditions as hypothyroidism and Cushing's syndrome. Various *neurodegenerative and dementing disorders* may cause depression, and indeed approximately one-third of patients with Parkinson's disease will be so affected. Depression may also be seen in a large number of *other intracranial disorders*, for example in the syndrome of post-stroke depression. Each of these groups is considered in more detail below, beginning with the primary or idiopathic disorders.

PRIMARY OR IDIOPATHIC DISORDERS

As noted earlier, the disorders in this group constitute, by far, the most common causes of depression. As a group, however, they constitute 'rule-out' diagnoses, and a diagnosis of one of these disorders should generally not be made until one is reasonably certain that the depressive syndrome in question is not caused by one of the other disorders in Table 6.2. It must also be kept in mind that it is not at all uncommon that in any given patient more than one disorder may be present. For example, a patient with well-established major depressive disorder, with a long history of recurrent depressions, may come down with a depression during a course of prednisone treatment, which remits shortly after treatment is discontinued. Furthermore, some depressions may be multifactorial: consider a patient, again with well-established major depressive disorder, who, shortly after treatment with metoclopramide, develops a depression that persists for weeks, or longer, rather than remitting after

Table 6.2 Causes of depression

Primary or idiopathic disorders	Pellagra
Major depressive disorder	Pancreatic cancer
Bipolar disorder	
Dysthymia	**Medication or substance withdrawal**
Premenstrual dysphoric disorder	Cholinergic rebound
Post-partum blues	Stimulants
Post-partum depression	Anabolic steroids
Schizoaffective disorder	
Post-psychotic depression in schizophrenia	**Endocrinologic disorders**
	Hypothyroidism
Toxic depressions	Hyperthyroidism
Medication-induced	Cushing's syndrome
Prednisone (Wolkowitz *et al.* 1990)	Adrenocortical insufficiency
Alpha-interferon (Fried *et al.* 2002; Krauss *et al.* 2003;	Hyperaldosteronism
Raison *et al.* 2005; Torriani *et al.* 2004)	Hyperprolactinemia
Beta 1b-interferon (Neilley *et al.* 1996)	
Metoclopramide (Friend and Young 1997)	**Neurodegenerative and dementing disorders**
Pimozide (Bloch *et al.* 1997b)	Parkinson's disease
Propranolol (Petrie *et al.* 1982; Pollack *et al.* 1985)	Diffuse Lewy body disease
Nifedipine (Hullett *et al.* 1988)	Hereditary mental depression with parkinsonism
Cimetidine (Billings *et al.* 1981)	Huntington's disease
Ranitidine (Billings and Stein 1986)	Alzheimer's disease
Subdermal estrogen–progestin (Wagner 1996; Wagner and	Multi-infarct dementia
Berenson 1994)	
Alpha-methyl dopa (DeMuth and Ackerman 1983)	**Other intracranial disorders**
Reserpine (Jensen 1959; Quetsch *et al.* 1959)	Stroke
Levetiracetam (Mula *et al.* 2003; Wier *et al.* 2006)	Traumatic brain injury
Isotretinoin (Wysowski *et al.* 2001)	Multiple sclerosis
Bismuth (Supino-Viterbo *et al.* 1977)	Epilepsy-associated depression
Substances of abuse or toxins	Ictal depression
Chronic alcoholism	Interictal depression
Lead intoxication	Tumors
	Hydrocephalus
Metabolic depressions	Fahr's syndrome
Obstructive sleep apnea	Systemic lupus erythematosus
Chronic hypercalcemia	Limbic encephalitis
Vitamin deficiencies	Tertiary neurosyphilis
Vitamin B12 deficiency	New-variant Creutzfeldt–Jakob disease
	Down's syndrome

the metoclopramide is discontinued. In this instance, it is reasonable to assume that the medication triggered a new depressive episode of the major depressive disorder, which then persisted.

Major depressive disorder and bipolar disorder are both characterized by recurrent episodes of depression, the two disorders being distinguished by the fact that in bipolar disorder one also sees, at some point in the patient's history, a manic episode, whereas in major depressive disorder, manic episodes never occur. Given that bipolar disorder may commence with one, or several, episodes of depression before the first episode of mania occurs, one must, in evaluating a patient who has had only depressive episodes, allow a lengthy period of observation to pass before making a firm diagnosis of major depression. Statistically speaking, in patients with bipolar disorder, the first episode of mania

will, in over 90 percent of cases, occur within 10 years of the first depressive episode or by the time five or more episodes of depression have occurred, whichever comes first (Dunner *et al.* 1976).

Although not as reliable, certain clinical characteristics of the depressive episode may also suggest whether that depressive episode is occurring on a basis of bipolar disorder or major depression. Specifically, depressive episodes of bipolar disorder are, in contrast with those of major depression, more likely to have an acute onset (over weeks rather than months) (Winokur *et al.* 1993) and are also more likely to be accompanied by delusions or hallucinations (Guze *et al.* 1975).

Dysthymia is characterized by chronic, low-level, and generally fluctuating depressive symptoms. This condition is of uncertain nosologic status. In many cases, there will be an exacerbation of symptoms to the degree found in a depressive episode (Devanand *et al.* 1994), and, from my point of view, it may be appropriate to think of dysthymia simply as a chronic, low-level depressive episode that could be part of either major depression or bipolar disorder.

Premenstrual dysphoric disorder is characterized by relatively brief depressions that occur with each menstrual cycle, beginning anywhere from hours to one and a half weeks before the onset of menses and remitting spontaneously 2–3 days after menstrual flow begins. The depression is typically characterized by prominent lability of mood (Bloch *et al.* 1997a).

Post-partum blues is immediately suggested by its onset within the first few days post-partum and by its characteristic lability of affect (Pitt 1973; Rohde *et al.* 1997; Yalom *et al.* 1968).

Post-partum depression is distinguished from the post-partum blues by its later onset, with a latency of at least several weeks between delivery and the onset of the depression.

Schizoaffective disorder is characterized by chronic, persistent psychotic symptoms with the 'superimposition' of episodes of either depression or of mania, during either of which the pre-existing psychotic symptoms undergo a significant exacerbation. Differentiating schizoaffective disorder from bipolar disorder may be difficult (Pope *et al.* 1980), and the reader is directed to Section 20.2 for a discussion of this.

Post-psychotic depression in schizophrenia is seen in about one-third of patients with schizophrenia. In these patients, after a more or less complete remission of psychotic symptoms (whether occurring spontaneously or by virtue of antipsychotic treatment), a depressive episode occurs, typically within a matter of months (Mandel *et al.* 1982). In contrast with schizoaffective disorder, however, there is during this post-psychotic depression *no* exacerbation of psychotic symptoms.

TOXIC DEPRESSIONS

Toxic depressions may be either medication induced or secondary to substances of abuse or actual toxins. Medications are considered first.

Of the various medications listed in Table 6.2, the most common offender is prednisone, given in relatively high doses of 40–60 mg/day or more; similar effects may be expected with other corticosteroids. Alpha-interferon, as used in the treatment of hepatitis C and melanoma, is another major offender, inducing depression within a few weeks in approximately one-third of all patients: the effect here is so profound that prophylactic treatment is recommended, with one study demonstrating effectiveness for paroxetine (Musselman *et al.* 2001). Depression has also been associated with beta-1b-interferon, but this is comparatively rare. Metoclopramide, although producing depression in only a very small percentage of patients who take it, is, however, so commonly prescribed that it too

emerges as a frequent cause. The other medications listed in Table 6.2 only rarely cause depression, and before one ascribes any given depression to them it is necessary to demonstrate a close temporal relationship between the initiation of treatment and the onset of the depression and, ideally, a similarly close relationship between discontinuation and remission of the depression. This list of medicines should not be considered comprehensive, and the clinician should maintain a high index of suspicion for a medication-induced depression whenever such temporal relationships can be established, and other, more common, causes of depression appear absent.

Chronic alcoholism is commonly associated with depression, indeed a majority of newly admitted alcoholics will be so affected (Davidson 1995). Importantly, the symptoms typically resolve spontaneously during the first 4 weeks of abstinence (Brown *et al.* 1995).

Lead intoxication may be characterized by depression (Schottenfeld and Cullen 1984), and the diagnosis should be considered in cases wherein the depression is accompanied by a motor peripheral neuropathy with wrist or, less commonly, foot drop.

METABOLIC DEPRESSIONS

Obstructive sleep apnea may cause a depression marked by tiredness, indecisiveness, irritability, and complaints of insomnia (Millman *et al.* 1989). The diagnosis is suggested by a history of prominent snoring, and by a relief of symptoms upon successful treatment of the sleep apnea, as for example with continuous positive airway pressure.

Chronic hypercalcemia, as seen in hyperparathyroidism, may be accompanied by depression (Linder *et al.* 1988; Petersen 1968; Reinfrank 1961) and may in some cases present with depression (Gatewood *et al.* 1975; Karpati and Frame 1964).

Both vitamin B12 deficiency and niacin deficiency may, rarely, cause depression. In one case of B12 deficiency-induced depression, the only clue was a concurrent macrocytic anemia (Fraser 1960). Chronic niacin deficiency causes pellagra, which, in one case, presented with a combination of depression and the familiar rash/diarrhea (Hardwick 1943).

Pancreatic cancer is associated with depression (Holland *et al.* 1986; McDaniel *et al.* 1995) and may indeed present with depression (Fras *et al.* 1967; Rickles 1945). The eventual appearance of abdominal pain suggests the correct diagnosis.

MEDICATION OR SUBSTANCE WITHDRAWAL

Cholinergic rebound may occur after abrupt discontinuation of long-term treatment with anticholinergic agents, such as tricyclic antidepressants: shortly thereafter, patients fairly abruptly develop a depression accompanied by nausea (Dilsaver *et al.* 1983).

Stimulant withdrawal, for example after extended use of either amphetamines (Watson *et al.* 1972) or cocaine (Weddington *et al.* 1990), is typically characterized by a depression that tends to resolve in a few weeks.

Anabolic steroids may be taken chronically by athletes; abrupt discontinuation may be followed by a depression (Pope and Katz 1988) that tends to remit spontaneously within weeks or months.

ENDOCRINOLOGIC DISORDERS

The endocrinologic disorders constitute a particularly important group not only because they are a relatively common cause of depression, but also because they are eminently treatable. Of them, hypothyroidism is perhaps the most important.

Hypothyroidism may cause severe depression (Tonks 1964; Whybrow *et al.* 1969). In addition to such features as weight gain, hair loss, dry skin, and voice change, the condition is also suggested by prominent fatigue, sluggishness, and drowsiness (Nickel and Frame 1958).

Hyperthyroidism, although generally associated with anxiety and agitation, appears just as likely to cause depression (Kathol and Delahunt 1986; Trzepacz *et al.* 1988) and the correct diagnosis may be suggested by the presence of weight loss in the face of increased appetite (Trzepacz *et al.* 1988) or autonomic signs such as tremor and tachycardia (Taylor 1975). Apathetic hyperthyroidism is a condition seen in elderly patients with hyperthyroidism, and is distinguished from the more common presentation of hyperthyroidism seen in younger patients by marked apathy and the relative absence of tremor (Lahey 1931; Thomas *et al.* 1970). In some cases, rather than apathy, however, one may see depression (Thomas *et al.* 1970). Important clues to the correct diagnosis include atrial fibrillation or congestive heart failure (Arnold *et al.* 1974; Thomas *et al.* 1970).

Cushing's syndrome, as seen with pituitary or adrenal tumors (Haskett 1985), may be characterized by depression, as noted by Cushing himself (Cushing 1932), and this has been noted in over one-half of all cases (Cohen 1980; Haskett 1985; Kelly 1996; Starkman 1981). Suggestive features include weight gain, moon facies, hirsutism, acne, a buffalo hump, violaceous abdominal striae, hypertension, and diabetes mellitus (Haskett 1985; Spillane 1951). Cushing's syndrome may also occur on a paraneoplastic basis, and, in one case secondary to Hodgkin's disease, the patient presented with depression and slight facial puffiness (Anderson and McHugh 1971).

Adrenocortical insufficiency, when chronic, may cause depression (Engel and Margolin 1941; Varadaraj and Cooper 1986) and is suggested by associated features such as nausea, vomiting, abdominal pain, and postural dizziness.

Hyperaldosteronism, as may occur with adrenal tumors, very rarely, may cause depression: in one case the diagnosis was suggested by hypokalemia and weakness and cramping of the legs (Malinow and Lion 1979).

Hyperprolactinemia, as may be seen with prolactinomas, may cause depression, which, in turn, remits with treatment with bromocriptine (Cohen 1995; Mattox *et al.* 1986). The diagnosis may be suggested by galactorrhea or erectile dysfunction.

NEURODEGENERATIVE AND DEMENTING DISORDERS

Depression may occur in the context of various neurodegenerative and dementing disorders.

Parkinsonian disorders capable of causing depression include Parkinson's disease, diffuse Lewy body disease, and a very rare disorder known as hereditary mental depression with parkinsonism. Parkinson's disease, in most (but not all [Hantz *et al.* 1994]) studies, is associated with depression of varying degrees of severity in up to 40 percent of cases (Mayeux *et al.* 1986; Starkstein *et al.* 1990a). Diffuse Lewy body disease (distinguished from Parkinson's disease by the occurrence, within a year of the onset of parkinsonism, of dementia) is characterized by depression in about one-half of patients (Klatka *et al.* 1996). Hereditary mental depression with parkinsonism is a very rare familial disorder that presents with depression, followed, years later, by parkinsonism (Perry *et al.* 1975).

Huntington's disease not uncommonly causes depression (Caine and Shoulson 1983) and the suicide rate in this disorder is particularly elevated.

Alzheimer's disease, suggested by the gradual onset of a dementia with prominent amnestic features, is accompanied by prominent depressive symptoms in about one-fifth of all cases (Burns *et al.* 1990a; Starkstein *et al.* 1997, 2005a).

Multi-infarct dementia, suggested by its stepwise course and prominent focal findings, produces depression in over one-half of all sufferers (Cummings *et al.* 1987).

OTHER INTRACRANIAL DISORDERS

Of the other intracranial disorders capable of causing depression, the most common are stroke and traumatic brain injury. Other somewhat less common causes are multiple sclerosis and epilepsy. Finally, there is a miscellaneous group, including tumors, hydrocephalus, etc.

Post-stroke depression, which can be quite severe (Lipsey *et al.* 1986), may develop in the weeks or months after stroke in up to one-half of all patients. Most (Hermann *et al.* 1993; Robinson *et al.* 1983, 1984, 1985), but not all (House *et al.* 1990; MacHale *et al.* 1998; Stern and Bachman 1991), studies note that such depression is more likely with infarctions in the left frontal lobe than elsewhere. Such patients typically recover within a year (Astrom *et al.* 1993; Robinson *et al.* 1987). Post-stroke depression has also been associated with infarction of the left basal ganglia (Morris *et al.* 1996; Starkstein *et al.* 1987a, 1988a).

Traumatic brain injury may be associated with depression in up to one-half of all patients (Federoff *et al.* 1992).

Multiple sclerosis is more likely to cause depression than are other comparably debilitating disorders such as amyotrophic lateral sclerosis (Schiffer and Babigian 1984;

Whitlock and Siskind 1980). Although this depression is correlated with overall disability early in the course of the disease (Millefiorini *et al.* 1992), this correlation vanishes as the disease progresses (Fassbender *et al.* 1998; Moller *et al.* 1994); in more chronic cases, by contrast, one finds that depression correlates with the extent of cerebral (rather than cord) involvement (Rabins *et al.* 1986; Schiffer *et al.* 1983), specifically with involvement of the left arcuate fasciculus (Pujol *et al.* 1997). As with other signs of multiple sclerosis, the depression may also have a relapsing and remitting course (Dalos *et al.* 1983).

Epilepsy may be associated with depression, not only in that certain partial seizures may manifest with depression, but also, and, from a numeric point of view, more importantly, in that patients with epilepsy may develop a chronic, interictal depression. Partial seizures (Weil 1956, 1959; Williams 1956) may manifest with the paroxysmal onset of depression, which may be severe, with psychomotor retardation or agitation, and which may last for from minutes to, in cases of complex partial status epilepticus, weeks. In addition to the paroxysmal onset, important clues to the diagnosis are the presence of olfactory hallucinations and a history of more typical seizures at other times. Interictal depression of epilepsy occurs in a large proportion of patients with recurrent seizures (Mendez *et al.* 1986), especially those with recurrent complex partial seizures (Indaco *et al.* 1992; Perini *et al.* 1996).

Intracerebral tumors may cause depression, as has been noted with tumors of the anterior portion of the corpus callosum (Ironside and Guttmacher 1929).

Hydrocephalus may present with depression (Jones 1993) and in a minority of cases of normal-pressure hydrocephalus, it may play a prominent part in the overall clinical picture (Pujol *et al.* 1989). The presence of an ataxic/apraxic or 'magnetic' gait may suggest the correct diagnosis.

Fahr's syndrome may, rarely, present with depression, which is eventually joined by more typical signs such as dementia (Slyter 1979) and parkinsonism (Trautner *et al.* 1988); calcification of the basal ganglia, apparent on computed tomography, strongly suggests this diagnosis.

Systemic lupus erythematosus can definitely cause depression (Dennis *et al.* 1992). What is disputed, however, is how frequently it does so: some have found depression to be common in lupus (Ainiala *et al.* 2001; Brey *et al.* 2002; Ganz *et al.* 1972; Lim *et al.* 1988; Miguel *et al.* 1994), whereas older studies have not (Guze 1967; Hugo *et al.* 1996). The diagnosis should be suspected in patients with arthralgia, rashes, and constitutional symptoms.

Limbic encephalitis may present with a depression, which is later joined by other, more typical evidence of the encephalitis, such as delirium (Glaser and Pincus 1969) or dementia (Corsellis *et al.* 1968).

Tertiary neurosyphilis may cause a dementia (general paresis of the insane, GPI) characterized not only by cognitive deficits, but also by depression (Dewhust 1969; Gomez and Aviles 1984) in almost one-fifth of all cases (Storm-Mathisen 1969).

New-variant Creutzfeldt–Jakob disease may present with depression (Zeidler *et al.* 1997a) but eventually, over weeks or months this will be joined by other symptoms, such as ataxia, delirium, or dementia (Zeidler 1997b).

Down's syndrome, immediately suggested by mental retardation and a characteristic facies, may, in adults, cause depression (Collacott *et al.* 1992), which may be very severe (Warren *et al.* 1989).

Differential diagnosis

Depression is a normal reaction to the adverse events of life, especially losses, and this normal depression must be distinguished from depression caused by one of the disorders described above. Several features of normal depression are helpful in this differential. First, the severity of normal depression is generally proportionate to the severity of the preceding adverse event, whether it be the loss of a loved one, serious illness, or financial reversals; thus, although severe symptoms are to be expected after the death of a child, they would not be normal after, say, getting a parking ticket. Second, normal depressions generally remit spontaneously and do so, in most cases, within 6 months or so, rarely, if ever, lasting more than a year (Harlow *et al.* 1991); thus, depression lasting longer, surely, than a year, should not be considered a 'normal' reaction, unless, of course, the adverse event were ongoing. Third, and finally, normal depressions generally lack severe vegetative symptoms and never are characterized by delusions; thus, the presence of severe middle or terminal insomnia, anorexia or psychomotor change, or any delusions, argues strongly against a normal depression. Clearly, the exercise of good clinical judgment is required in making this differential. Many patients (and their family members) seem offended at the suggestion that they might be depressed, and wounded pride may prompt such comments as 'well, wouldn't you be depressed if you'd gone through what I did?' Whether or not the physician would is immaterial; what is important is for the physician to determine whether the patient's depression is normal or not.

Akinesia must also be considered in the differential of depression. Akinesia is perhaps most commonly seen in patients treated with antipsychotics, especially first-generation agents, and is characterized by a sluggishness of thought and an overall dulling of emotion: some patients complain of feeling like a 'zombie' (Rifkin *et al.* 1975; Van Putten and May 1978). Two points serve to differentiate this from depression: first, there is little in the way of changes in sleep or appetite, and actually little depressed mood, either; second, akinesia responds promptly to treatment with anticholinergics, such as benztropine, which have no effect on depression.

Treatment

Treatment, wherever possible, is directed at the underlying cause. Where this is not possible, or is perhaps ineffective, consideration may be given to symptomatic treatment with an antidepressant. In general, given their overall effectiveness, and, most importantly, their safety, selective serotonin reuptake inhibitors (SSRIs) constitute a first choice. Some studies back this up. With regard to post-stroke depression, citalopram was found to be superior to placebo (Anderson *et al.* 1994), and depression occurring after traumatic brain injury may respond to sertaline (Fann *et al.* 2000). If an SSRI is used for depression in parkinsonian conditions, a careful watch should be kept for any aggravation of the parkinsonism as has been seen with both fluoxetine (Ernst and Steur 1993) and paroxetine (Jimenez-Jimenez *et al.* 1994); furthermore, if a monamine oxidase inhibitor (MAOI) is being used for the treatment of parkinsonism, SSRIs should not be prescribed, given the risk of a serotonin syndrome.

6.2 APATHY

Apathy, or indifference, is very common in geriatric patients, and, as noted below, may occur secondary to a variety of causes.

Clinical features

Normally, thoughts of doing something, whether thinking a problem through, getting dressed, going to a movie, or whatever, when they appear, are invested with a greater or lesser degree of motivation to carry out the plan. In apathetic patients, however, such thoughts come, as it were, stillborn, and without sufficient associated motivation to impel the thinker to carry them into action. In apathetic patients, there is such a pervasive sense of not 'caring' enough that many lapse into inactivity, and appear detached and indifferent.

Etiology

Apathy may appear in a more or less isolated fashion or may occur as part of another syndrome, such as dementia, the frontal lobe syndrome, or depression.

Apathy in a more or less isolated form may be seen in stroke, acquired autoimmune deficiency syndrome (AIDS) (Paul *et al.* 2005), myotonic muscular dystrophy (Rubinsztein *et al.* 1998), and hyperthyroidism in the elderly ('apathetic' hyperthyroidism [Brenner 1978]). In the case of stroke, apathy has been associated with ischemic infarction involving the posterior limb of the internal capsule (Starkstein *et al.* 1993), both thalami (Catsman-Berrevoets and von Harskamp 1988), and the right frontosubcortical circuitry (Brodaty *et al.* 2005). Apathy has also been noted as a side-effect of treatment with antipsychotics, and, with chronic use, SSRIs (Hoehn-Saric *et al.* 1990). Finally, isolated apathy may occur in geriatric nursing home patients in whom it appears to result from chronic understimulation.

Dementia may be accompanied by apathy and this has been noted in various neurodegenerative disorders (Levy *et al.* 1998), most notably Alzheimer's disease (Starkstein *et al.* 2001, 2005b, 2006), frontotemporal dementia (Levy *et al.* 1996), Parkinson's disease (Isella *et al.* 2002, Pluck and Brown 2002), progressive supranuclear palsy (Litvan *et al.* 1996), and Huntington's disease (Burns *et al.* 1990b). Although in many of these demented patients apathy appears in association with a depressive syndrome, there is a definite, although minority, group, wherein apathy appears without any associated depressed mood, lack of energy, or other symptoms typical of a depressive syndrome. Apathy is seen commonly after traumatic brain injury, and, in these cases, is more common when the right hemisphere is involved, especially its subcortical portions (Andersson *et al.* 1999).

The frontal lobe syndrome, as discussed in Section 7.2, may, along with disinhibition and perseveration, also include apathy.

Depressive syndromes often include apathy as a symptom along with depressed mood, fatigue, insomnia, etc. Such syndromes may, as noted above, be seen in various dementing disorders, or more commonly, may appear as a manifestation of major depressive disorder (Feil *et al.* 2003; Starkstein *et al.* 2001).

Psychosis, as for example schizophrenia (Roth *et al.* 2004), may also include apathy as a symptom, along with delusions, hallucinations, etc.

Differential diagnosis

Abulia, superficially, appears almost identical to apathy, in that in both cases, afflicted patients are inactive. There are, however, significant differences. In abulia, there simply are no thoughts, plans or inclinations: the 'mental horizon' is empty and undisturbed. By contrast, thoughts, etc., do occur with apathy but without sufficient associated motivation to carry the patient into action. Furthermore, when abulic patients are subject to supervision they do carry out tasks, and typically do so at a normal rate, provided that the supervision is ongoing; by contrast, apathetic patients may shirk or withdraw when told to do something, and comply only half-heartedly, if that, with ongoing supervision.

Bradyphrenia and bradykinesia, as seen in parkinsonian conditions, may also appear similar to apathy in that, to a brief inspection, there is little activity. The differential, however, is relatively easy if one only observes the patient for a while: given enough time, the bradykinetic patient will get the job done, as here it is not a lack of motivation but rather a slowing down of all activities, whereas, by contrast, the apathetic patient will remain inactive.

Depressed mood, when accompanied by anhedonia, may appear very similar to apathy. Depressed mood, however, is a definite mood: patients feel sad, 'blue', or internally oppressed. By contrast, apathetic patients typically experience an absence of any particular mood, except, of course, for a sense of indifference. Furthermore, depressed patients who have lost their hedonic capacity may nevertheless at times feel some motivation to act but then fail to carry through as they realize that there will be no pleasure in finishing the task. By contrast, apathetic patients, lacking any motivation to act at all, simple fail to get started.

Treatment

In cases where apathy appears as part of another syndrome, the first approach is to treat the larger syndrome, as successful treatment in this regard may, in some cases, be followed by substantial improvement of the apathy. Examples include: cholinesterase inhibitors for Alzheimer's disease and Parkinson's disease dementia; levodopa or direct-acting dopamine agonists for Parkinson's disease and progressive supranuclear palsy; antidepressants for depressive syndromes; and antipsychotics for psychoses. When SSRIs or antipsychotics (especially first-generation agents) are used, one must be alert to their potential, as noted earlier, to cause apathy.

In cases when treatment of a larger syndrome leaves associated apathy untouched, or in cases where apathy is occurring in an isolated fashion, consideration may be given to symptomatic treatment aimed at apathy itself. In this regard, the most commonly used medication is methylphenidate, which appears effective for apathy associated with dementia (e.g., due to Alzheimer's disease or multiple strokes [Galynker *et al.* 1997]), apathy occurring in an isolated fashion after subcortical infarction (Watanabe *et al.* 1995), and apathy occurring in institutionalized geriatric patients (Kaplitz 1975). Methylphenidate should be started at a low dose, for example 2.5 mg in the morning and 2.5 mg in the early afternoon, and increased gradually every 2 or 3 days, in similar increments until a response is seen, limiting side-effects occur, or a maximum dose of 60 mg/day is reached: in many elderly patients, a total daily dose of from 10 to 20 mg generally suffices.

Apathy occurring after traumatic brain injury may also respond to bromocriptine (Powell *et al.* 1996), amantadine (Van Reekum *et al.* 1995), or selegeline (Newburn and Newburn 2005).

When attempting pharmacologic treatment of apathy, it should be borne in mind that of the studies noted above all were open except that by Kaplitz *et al.* (for methylphenidate in institutionalized geriatric patients), which utilized a double-blind protocol with 44 patients, and that by Van Reekum *et al.* (for amantadine in traumatic brain injury patients), which was an 'N of 1' study that also utilized a double-blind protocol. Clearly, more work is needed.

6.3 MANIA

Mania is one of the most distinctive syndromes in neuropsychiatric practice: once seen, never forgotten. Although most commonly caused by bipolar disorder, mania may occur secondary to a host of other causes, as described below.

Clinical features

The syndrome of mania, following the elegant descriptive study of Carlson and Goodwin in 1973, may be divided into three stages. Stage I mania, also known as *hypomania*, is present in all cases, and, in its fully developed form includes all the symptoms listed in Table 6.3. Most patients, over time, will enter into stage II mania, known as *acute mania*, with this transition being marked by an exacerbation of the symptoms seen in hypomania and by the appearance of delusions. A minority of patients will progress further, into stage III mania, known also as *delirious mania*, and here one finds confusion, hallucinations, worsening delusions, and an overall disintegration of behavior. As the manic syndrome gradually resolves, patients tend, as it were, to retrace the symptomatic steps that marked the evolution of the syndrome: thus, a patient who reached stage III would gradually settle back into stage II, then stage I, only finally to experience a remission of symptoms. The onset of a manic syndrome tends to be fairly acute, over perhaps days to a week; the range here is wide, from gradual onsets spanning months to hyperacute ones lasting hours or less. The overall duration of a manic episode depends on the underlying cause: in bipolar disorder, the most common cause, episodes typically last from weeks to months.

Additional studies have largely backed up this division by Carlson and Goodwin into stage I (Abrams and Taylor 1976; Carlson and Strober 1978; Clayton *et al.* 1965; Taylor and Abrams 1973, 1977; Winokur and Tsuang 1975; Winokur *et al.* 1969), stage II (Loudon *et al.* 1977; Rosenthal *et al.* 1979, 1980; Taylor and Abrams 1973, 1977), and stage III (Black and Nasrallah 1989; Bowman and Raymond 1931; Brockington *et al.* 1980; Carlson and Strober 1978; Rosenthal *et al.* 1979, 1980; Taylor and Abrams 1973, 1977; Winokur 1984).

Each one of the three stages of mania is described further below; in several instances quotations are provided from Emil Kraepelin's (1921) masterful *Manic-Depressive Insanity and Paranoia*.

STAGE I MANIA: HYPOMANIA

Of the symptoms of hypomania listed in Table 6.3, a heightened mood is present in all cases and although most patients will have all of the others, some may play only a relatively minor part in the clinical picture.

Table 6.3 The symptoms of hypomania

Heightened mood (either euphoric or irritable)
Increased energy
Decreased need for sleep
Pressure of speech
Flight of ideas
Distractibility
Hyperactivity

Heightened mood

Heightened mood may be either predominantly euphoric or irritable.

Euphoric patients are full of jollity and cheerfulness. Although at times selfish and pompous, their mood is nevertheless quite 'infectious'. They joke, make wisecracks and delightful insinuations, and those around them often get quite caught up in the spirit, always laughing with these patients and not at them. Indeed, when physicians find themselves unable to suppress their laughter when interviewing a patient, the diagnosis of mania should be seriously considered. Self-esteem and self-confidence are greatly increased. Inflated with their own grandiosity, patients may boast of fabulous achievements and lay out plans for even grander accomplishments in the future. Such patients rarely recognize that anything is wrong with them, and although their judgment is obviously impaired they have little or no insight into their condition. Kraepelin noted that the manic patient:

> is in imperturbable good temper, sure of success, 'courageous', feels happy and merry, not rarely overflowingly so, wakes up every morning 'in excellent humor'. He sees himself surrounded by pleasant and aristocratic people, finds complete satisfaction in the enjoyment of friendship, of art, of humanity; he will make everyone happy, abolish social wretchedness, convert all in his surroundings. For the most part an exuberant unrestrained mood inclined to practical jokes of all kinds is developed. Occasionally there is developed a markedly humorous trait, the tendency to look at everything and every occurrence from the jocular side, to invent nicknames, to make fun of himself and others. A patient called himself a 'thoroughbred professional fool'; another declared that the hospital was a 'nerve-ruining institution'; a third stated that he was a 'poet, cattle-driver, author, tinker, teacher, popular reformer, chief anarchist and detective'.

> Kraepelin (1921)

Irritable patients are loud, insistent, demanding, and intolerant, and the threat of violence hangs about them as a malignant fog. Kraepelin noted that such a patient is:

> dissatisfied, intolerant, fault-finding, especially in intercourse with his immediate surroundings, where he lets himself go; he becomes pretentious, positive, regardless, impertinent and even rough, when he comes up against opposition to his wishes and inclinations; trifling external occasions may bring about extremely violent outbursts of rage. In his fury he thrashes his wife and children, threatens to smash everything to smithereens, to run amuck, to set the house on fire, abuses the 'tribe' of his relatives in the most violent language, especially when under the influence of alcohol.

> Kraepelin (1921)

Increased energy

Energy is greatly, even immensely increased: patients are on the go, busy, and involved throughout the day. They wish to be a part of life and to be more involved in the lives of those around them. They are strangers to fatigue and still quite active when their companions, exhausted, plead for sleep.

Decreased need for sleep

Decreased need for sleep typically accompanies this increased energy. The patient, as described by Kraepelin, 'cannot stay long in bed; early in the morning, even at four o'clock he gets up, he clears out lumber rooms, discharges business that was in arrears, undertakes morning walks, excursions'.

Pressure of speech

Patients with pressured speech, as noted by Kraepelin, 'talk a great deal, hastily, in loud tones, with great verbosity and prolixity'. Speech becomes imperious, incredibly rapid and almost unstoppable, and listeners may feel veritably deluged by the torrent of words. Occasionally, patients may succumb to others' protests to stop and may be able to keep silent and withhold their speech, but such respites typically do not hold long and soon the dam bursts once again.

Pressured speech is often accompanied by pressure of thought, and patients may complain of racing thoughts. Kraepelin noted that 'thoughts come of themselves, obtrude themselves, impose upon the patients. "I can't grasp all the thoughts which obtrude themselves," said a patient. "It is so stormy in my head," declared another, "everything goes pell-mell." "My thoughts are all tattered." "I am not master over my thoughts.".'

Flight of ideas

In flight of ideas the patients' train of thought is characterized by abrupt leaps from one topic to another. When mild, the connections between these various topics, although perhaps tenuous, may nevertheless by 'understandable' to the listener. In higher grades, however, the connections may seem to lack any logic, and may come to depend more and more on puns or word-plays.

Distractibility

For distractible patients, other conversations or events, are like glittering jewels that they must attend to, take as their own, or furiously admire, although peripheral to their present purposes. In listening to patients one may find that a fragment of another conversation has suddenly been interpolated into their flight of ideas or there may be an absolutely abrupt change of topic triggered by a seemingly irrelevant event: one patient, in the midst of an exultant tirade, suddenly stopped and declared his unbounded admiration for the physician's tie, paused for a matter of seconds in great satisfaction, then proceeded with his previous rush of speech.

Hyperactivity

Hyperactivity, which might just as well be termed pressure of activity, follows from the patients' grandiosity and increased energy. Patients may enter into business arrangements with unbounded and completely uncritical enthusiasm. Ventures are begun, stocks are bought on a hunch, money is loaned out without collateral, and when the family fortune is spent, manic patients, undaunted, may seek to borrow more money for yet another prospect. Spending sprees are also quite typical. Clothes, furniture, and cars may be bought; the credit card is pushed to the limit, and another one is obtained; checks, without any foundation in the bank account, are written with alacrity. Kraepelin noted that such a patient is swelled by a 'need to get out of himself, to be on more intimate terms with his surroundings, to play a part'. It causes him:

> to change about his furniture, to visit distant acquaintances, to take himself up with all possible things and circumstances, which formerly he never thought about. Politics, the universal language, aeronautics, the women's question, public affairs of all kinds and their need of improvement, give him employment. A physician advertised about 'original sin, Genesis, natural selection and breeding'. Another patient drove about in a cab and distributed pictures of the saints. The patient enters into numerous engagements, suddenly pays all his business debts without it being necessary, makes magnificent presents, builds all kinds of castles in the air, and with swift enthusiasm precipitates himself in daring undertakings much beyond his powers. He has 16,000 picture post-cards of his little village printed....
>
> Kraepelin (1921)

STAGE II MANIA: ACUTE MANIA

The transition from hypomania to acute mania is marked by a severe exacerbation of the symptoms seen in hypomania and by the appearance of delusions, typically delusions of grandeur. Kraepelin noted, 'The patient asserts that he is descended from a noble family, that he is a gentleman; he calls himself a genius, the Emperor William, the Emperor of Russia, Christ; he can drive out the devil. A patient suddenly cried out on the street that he was the Lord God ... '. Delusions of persecution may also occur, especially in patients with irritability. Patients may assert that their failures are not their own but the result of treacheries and betrayals by family members or business colleagues. They are persecuted by those jealous of their grandeur; they are pilloried and crucified by their enemies. Terrorists have set a watch on their houses and seek to destroy them before they can ascend their thrones. Occasionally, in addition to these delusions, there may be transitory hallucinations. Grandiose patients may hear a chorus of angels; persecuted patients may hear the resentful muttering of the envious crowd.

With the intensification of hypomanic symptoms and the appearance of delusions, the overall behavior of these patients may become quite extravagant. Kraepelin noted that patients may:

> run out of the house in a shirt, go to church in a petticoat, spend the night in a field of corn, give away their property, disturb the service in church by screaming and singing, kneel and pray on the street, fire a pistol in the waiting-room, put soap and soda in the food, try to force their way into the palace, throw objects out at the window. A female patient jumped into the carriage of a prince for a joke ... A male patient appropriated the property of others in taverns. Another appeared in the court of justice in order to catch a murderer.
>
> Kraepelin (1921)

STAGE III MANIA: DELIRIOUS MANIA

The transition to delirious mania is marked by the appearance of confusion, more hallucinations, and an intense exacerbation of all the symptoms seen in stage II. There may be a dream-like clouding of consciousness and patients may become unaware of where they are; incoherence may appear and, as described by Kraepelin, 'Their linguistic utterances alternate between inarticulate sounds, praying, abusing, entreating, stammering, disconnected talk, in which clang-associations, senseless rhyming, diversion by external impressions, persistence of individual phrases, are recognized'. Hallucinations become prominent, and as further described by Kraepelin, 'The patient sees heaven open, full of camels and elephants, the King, his guardian-angel, the Holy Ghost; the devil has assumed the form of the Virgin Mary. The ringing of bells is heard, shooting, the rushing of water, a confused noise; Lucifer is speaking; the voice of God announces to him the day of judgment, redemption from all sins'.

With this evolution into stage III, overall behavior becomes very fragmented, and patients may 'become stupefied, confused, bewildered', they may:

> dance about, perform peculiar movements, shake their head, throw the bedclothes pell-mell, are destructive, pass their movements under them, smear everything, make impulsive attempts at suicide, take off their clothes. A patient was found completely naked in a public park. Another ran half-clothed into the corridor and then into the street, in one hand a revolver in the other a crucifix.
>
> Kraepelin (1921)

Etiology

The various causes of mania are listed in Table 6.4, in which they are organized into several groups. The first group is

Table 6.4 Causes of mania

Primary, idiopathic disorders	**Endocrinologic**
Bipolar disorder	Cushing's syndrome
Cyclothymia	Hyperthyroidism
Schizoaffective disorder	
Post-partum psychosis	**Intracranial disorders**
	Infarctions
Toxic	Midbrain
Prednisone (Lyons *et al.* 1988, Minden *et al.* 1988, Wolkowitz *et al.* 1990)	Thalamus
Anabolic steroids (Pope and Katz 1988, 1994)	Caudate
Oral contraceptives (Sale and Kalucy 1981)	Frontal lobe
Levodopa (Ryback and Schwab 1971; Van Woert *et al.* 1971)	Temporal lobe
Pramipexole (Singh *et al.* 2005)	Tumors
Ropinirole (Singh *et al.* 2005)	Midbrain
Antidepressants (Shulman *et al.* 2001; Stoll *et al.* 1994)	Hypothalamus
Buspirone (Liegghid and Yeragani 1988; Price and Bielfeld 1989)	Thalamus
Alpha-interferon (Constant *et al.* 2005)	Frontal lobe
Zidovudine (Maxwell *et al.* 1988; O'Dowd and McKegney 1988; Wright *et al.* 1989)	Multiple sclerosis
Abacavir (Brouilette and Routy 2007)	
Clarithromycin (Abouesh and Hobbs 1998)	**As part of certain dementing disorders**
Ciprofloxacin (Bhalerao *et al.* 2006)	Alzheimer's disease
Isoniazid (Chaturvedi and Upadhyaya 1988; Jackson 1957)	Huntington's disease
Topiramate (Jochum *et al.* 2002)	Neurosyphilis
Phenytoin (Patten *et al.* 1989)	Creutzfeldt–Jakob disease
Zonisamide (Sullivan *et al.* 2006)	Metachromatic leukodystrophy
Procyclidine (in high dosage) (Coid and Strang 1982)	Adrenoleukodystrophy
Propafenone (Jack 1985)	
Procarbazine (Mann and Hutchinson 1967)	**Miscellaneous**
Disulfiram (Ceylan *et al.* 2007)	Traumatic brain injury
Aspartame (in high dosage) (Walton 1986)	Epileptic disorders
Bromide (Sayed 1976)	Ictal mania
Mannitol (Navarro *et al.* 2001)	Post-ictal mania
Metrizamide (Kwentus *et al.* 1984)	Systemic lupus erythematosus
Baclofen withdrawal (Kirubakaren *et al.* 1984)	Vitamin B12 deficiency
Tiagabine withdrawal (Pushpal and Shamshul 2006)	Sydenham's chorea
Reserpine withdrawal (Kent and Wilber 1982)	Chorea gravidarum
Alpha-methyldopa withdrawal (Labbatte and Holzgang 1989)	Encephalitis lethargica
	Acute disseminated encephalomyelitis
Metabolic	Fahr's syndrome
Hepatic encephalopathy	Dialysis dementia
Uremia	Tuberous sclerosis
	Velocardiofacial syndrome

composed of *primary, idiopathic disorders*, such as bipolar disorder, which by far constitute the most common causes of mania. The next group, the *toxic* causes, includes medications, for example prednisone, capable of inducing mania as a side-effect. *Metabolic* causes come next, and include both hepatic encephalopathy and uremia. *Endocrinologic* causes include Cushing's syndrome and hyperthyroidism. *Intracranial disorders* capable of causing mania are considered next, including infarctions and tumors. Mania may also occur *as part of certain dementing disorders*, for example Alzheimer's disease. Finally, there is a *miscellaneous* group of causes, including lupus and others.

PRIMARY, IDIOPATHIC DISORDERS

Bipolar disorder is by far the most common cause of mania and is characterized, in most cases, by recurrent episodes of mania and recurrent episodes of depression throughout the lifetime of the patient. Critically, in the intervals between these episodes, patients are either asymptomatic or experience only mild residual symptoms, tending toward either euphoria or depression. The first episode of illness may be either manic or depressive in character. In cases where the first episode is depressive, a manic episode generally occurs within either 10 years or, if there are recurrent depressive episodes, five depressive episodes, whichever comes first (Dunner *et al.* 1976). Importantly, however, although in the intervals *between* episodes, there may be mild disturbances of mood, as noted above, there are *never* any psychotic symptoms. Some variations on the typical course of bipolar disorder described earlier are worthy of note. First, it rarely appears that some patients (often referred to as 'unipolar manic') have only manic episodes during their lifetime (Pfohl *et al.* 1982; Shulman and Tohen 1994) and never experience a depressive one. Second, a minority of cases may also be characterized by 'rapid cycling', wherein four or more episodes of illness occur during a year (Dunner *et al.* 1977).

Cyclothymia is best thought of as a very mild form of bipolar disorder (Akiskal *et al.* 1977). Like bipolar disorder, it is characterized by episodes of mood disturbance but these are much milder in intensity and indeed may not bring the patient to clinical attention.

Schizoaffective disorder, bipolar type (Grossman *et al.* 1984; Pope *et al.* 1980; Rosenthal *et al.* 1980), possesses a distinctive overall course: patients with this illness are not only chronically psychotic, but also, in the context of this ongoing psychosis, experience episodes of mania and episodes of depression. The chronic psychosis, which leaves them with psychotic symptoms (such as delusions and hallucinations) in the intervals between mood disturbances, clearly distinguishes this illness from bipolar disorder, which is *free* of psychotic symptoms in the intervening periods.

Post-partum psychosis has an abrupt onset between 3 days and several weeks after delivery (Munoz 1985) and is, in many cases, characterized by manic symptoms (Brockington *et al.* 1981). Importantly, these patients are well at other times, and although they may have recurrent post-partum psychoses after subsequent deliveries (Hadley 1941; Kumar *et al.* 1983), they do not have manic symptoms *outside* the puerperium. This is the critical difference between post-partum psychosis and bipolar disorder, for although female patients with bipolar disorder may indeed have manic episodes in the puerperium, they *also* have them at other times in their lives (Bratfos and Haug 1966).

TOXIC

Of all the medications listed in Table 6.4, by far the most common causes are prednisone and levodopa. Prednisone, in doses of 80 mg or more per day, may produce mania in approximately three-quarters of patients. Levodopa, as used in Parkinson's disease, in turn may cause mania in about one-tenth of patients (Celesia and Barr 1970; O'Brien *et al.* 1971). Celesia and Barr (1970) noted that their patients became euphoric with 'excessive self-confidence, over optimism, buoyancy, lack of inhibition, exaggerated motor activity and drive. They made inappropriate jokes, were garrulous, and were often impudent'. In some cases, levodopa-induced mania may be accompanied by hallucinations (Lin and Ziegler 1976). In some cases, the mania is so appealing that patients may abuse levodopa in order to

remain manic (Giovannoni *et al.* 2000). Mania may also occur secondary to direct-acting dopaminergics, such as pramipxole and ropinirole but this is much less common. Antidepressants are notorious for inducing mania, but this generally only occurs in patients with pre-existing bipolar disorder, and in these cases it is appropriate to consider that the antidepressant 'triggered' a manic episode. Anabolic steroid abuse, as seen in athletes such as weight-lifters and American football players, may cause mania, which may be marked by extreme irritability and violence: manic symptoms occurring in a 'bulked-up' athlete should always suggest anabolic steroid use and prompt a search for corroborating clinical evidence, such as gynecomastia and testicular atrophy. The other medications listed in Table 6.4 only rarely cause mania, and before attributing any given case to one of them, one would want to be able to demonstrate not only a fairly close temporal relationship between starting the medication (or substantially increasing the dose) and the onset of the mania, but also an absence of other, more common causes.

Before ending consideration of these toxic causes of mania, further comments are in order regarding the last four entries, namely baclofen, tiagabine, reserpine, and alpha-methyldopa. For each of these medications, mania occurs, not during treatment, but rather within days to a week after discontinuation of long-term treatment; here the mania occurs as a withdrawal phenomenon.

METABOLIC

Hepatic encephalopathy is often characterized by manic symptomatology, with euphoria and gregariousness (Murphy *et al.* 1948). Uremia may rarely present with mania: in one case (El-Mallakh *et al.* 1987) the only sign of uremia, despite a blood urea nitrogen level of 100 mg/dL and a creatinine concentration of 5.0 mg/dL, was mania.

ENDOCRINOLOGIC

Cushing's syndrome may produce manic symptoms, which have been noted in from 11 percent (Starkman *et al.* 1981) to 30 percent (Haskett 1985) of cases. Other symptoms of Cushing's syndrome, such as weight gain, hypertension, diabetes mellitus, acne, hirsutism, and easy bruising, typically accompany these manic changes (Haskett 1985) and serve to suggest the correct diagnosis.

Thyrotoxicosis may be accompanied by mania (Lee *et al.* 1991; Trzepacz *et al.* 1988), and the correct diagnosis is usually suggested by such signs as proptosis, tremor, and tachycardia. In one case, however, the only clue as to the correct diagnosis was a tachycardia of 130 beats per minute (Ingham and Nielsen 1931).

INTRACRANIAL DISORDERS

Appropriately situated infarctions, tumors, or plaques of multiple sclerosis may all cause mania and, as noted below, it appears that mania, although not of much localizing value, may have some lateralizing value.

Infarctions of the midbrain, thalamus, anterior limb of the internal capsule and adjacent head of the caudate nucleus, or the frontal or temporal lobes may all cause mania. In the case of midbrain infarction not only has mania been seen, but also, remarkably, in these cases there were recurrent episodes of mania and of depression: this has been noted after an infarction secondary to a subarachnoid hemorrhage (Blackwell 1991) and after an ischemic lesion of the right mesencephalopontine area (Kulisevsky et al. 1995). In this latter case, the patient, a 59-year-old woman, suddenly lost consciousness and fell to the ground. After coming to, she experienced transient dizziness and right ptosis, and then did well for about 2 weeks. She subsequently developed a severe depression accompanied by left hemiparkinsonism, both of which persisted, only to spontaneously remit after 19 months. She progressed well for the next 5 months and then developed mania characterized by elation, heightened activity and sexual interest, logorrhea, intrusiveness, and decreased sleep. Eventually she was successfully treated with lithium. Thalamic infarctions capable of causing mania may be either unilateral – on the right side – or bilateral. Regarding unilateral lesions, Cummings and Mendez (1984) reported a case of mania accompanied by left-sided hemianesthesia and slight hemiparesis, and Bogousslavsky et al. (1988) described a sudden onset of delirium that cleared in a few days, leaving behind mania as the sole indication of a right paramedian thalamic infarction. Kulisevsky et al. (1993) reported a case of mania accompanied by chorea and ballismus occurring secondary to an infarction of the ventral tier nuclei on the right. Bilateral thalamic infarction caused mania in two cases. In the first case (McGilchrist et al. 1993), there was an acute onset of drowsiness, followed by a cycling of mania and depression. The depression lasted for weeks and was characterized by apathy and increased eating and sleeping. The manias were brief, lasting only 1–2 days and were characterized by elation, pressured speech, and flight of ideas. The second case (Gentilini et al. 1987) presented, like the first, with somnolence, which was accompanied by amnesia and a vertical gaze paresis. As the patient, a 66-year-old man, became more alert, he displayed hypersexuality and grandiosity, asserting that he had a Swiss bank account and was a General in the Air Force. After 7 months, the amnesia had cleared but not the mania: he was 'cheerful . . . garrulous . . . [and] looking for a young girl who, enticed by his wealth, would be willing to marry him'. Capsular infarction involving the anterior limb of the internal capsule and the adjacent head of the caudate nucleus has been noted to cause either depression followed within a month by mania, or mania alone (Starkstein et al. 1990b). Cortical or subcortical white matter infarction of the right frontoparietal region (Jampala and Abrams 1983; Starkstein et al. 1988), bilateral orbitofrontal areas, or the right basotemporal area (Starkstein et al. 1990b) has been associated with mania.

Tumors affecting the mesencephalon (Greenberg and Brown 1985), the hypothalamus (via compression from an underlying craniopharyngioma [Malamud 1967] or pituitary adenoma [Alpers 1940]), the right thalamus (Stern and Dancey 1942), the right cingulate gyrus (Angelini et al. 1980), the inferior right frontal lobe (Gross and Herridge 1988), or both frontal lobes (Starkstein et al. 1988b) have all been associated with mania. As an aside, it is worth noting the remarkable ability of hypothalamic disturbances to cause mania. In one case (Alpers 1940), the patient was undergoing surgery for the removal of a craniopharyngioma; when the surgeon produced traction on the hypothalamus, 'the patient burst forth in a push of speech, quoting passages in Latin, Greek and Hebrew . . . and with every word of the [surgeon] broke into a flight of ideas'.

Multiple sclerosis has long been associated with manic symptomatology; indeed, Cottrell and Wilson (1926), noted euphoria in 63 percent of their 100 patients. Subsequent case series have reported a lower rate, varying from 42 percent (Rabins et al. 1986) to 26 percent (Surridge 1969), and a nationwide survey in Israel found euphoria in only 5 percent of cases (Kahana et al. 1971). Of all reasons underlying the admission of patients with multiple sclerosis to a psychiatric hospital, mania is, however, one of the most common: in one study, of over 2000 psychiatric admissions, 10 had multiple sclerosis, and seven of these patients were admitted because of mania (Pine et al. 1995). Importantly, in patients with multiple sclerosis, the presence of mania correlates with brain, rather than spinal cord, involvement (Rabins et al. 1986).

A review of the cases of mania secondary to infarctions and tumors allows for some speculation regarding both the localizing and the lateralizing value of this syndrome. The localizing value of mania does not appear to be high, as it has been noted with lesions of the mesencephalon (Blackwell 1991; Greenberg and Brown 1985; Kulisevsky et al. 1995), thalamus (Bogousslavsky et al. 1988; Cummings and Mendez 1984; Gentilini et al. 1987; Kulisevsky et al. 1993; Liebson 2000; McGilchrist et al. 1993; Starkstein et al. 1988a; Stern and Dancey 1942), hypothalamus (Alpers 1940; Malamud 1967), anterior limb of the internal capsule and adjacent head of the caudate (Starkstein et al. 1990b), cingulate gyrus (Angelini et al. 1980), and frontal (Benjamin et al. 2000; Gross and Herridge 1988; Starkstein et al. 1988b, 1990b), and temporal lobes (Starkstein et al. 1990b). The lateralizing value of mania, however, may be higher. In all but one of the instances cited above, the lesion responsible for mania was either on the right side or bilateral: in only one case, namely after the excision of an arteriovenous malformation from the left frontal lobe (Benjamin et al. 2000), did mania occur secondary to a left-sided lesion. This impression is bolstered by some controlled studies: although not all agree (House et al. 1990), it appears that when the frontal, temporal, or limbic areas of the cerebrum are involved mania is more likely with right-sided lesions (Robinson et al. 1988; Starkstein et al. 1987b). This impression is further reinforced by a study of 19 patients who underwent hemispherectomy: of the 14 who had a right hemispherectomy, 12 became euphoric and none was depressed; of the five who had a left hemispherectomy, one was euphoric, one was depressed, and the other three showed no mood change (Sackeim *et al.* 1982).

AS PART OF DEMENTING DISORDERS

Alzheimer's disease may, in a small minority, be characterized by mild manic symptoms such as an elevated mood (Burns *et al.* 1990), but this is seen only long after the dementia has become well established.

Huntington's disease, in addition to chronic chorea and dementia, may also, in a small minority of patients, cause manic symptoms, which range from simple 'excitement' (Oliver 1970) or 'euphoria' (Tamir *et al.* 1969) to a fuller syndrome with delusions of grandeur (Bolt 1970; Heathfield 1967).

Neurosyphilis, when manifesting as parenchymatous general paresis of the insane, presents with a dementia that may be marked by mania (Merritt and Springlova 1932): indeed, in one large study of 203 patients, approximately one-half were euphoric and excited (Storm-Mathisen 1969). Rarely, neurosyphilis may present with mania (Binder and Dickman 1980). Whenever a diagnosis of neurosyphilis is entertained, it is critical to carry out a serum fluorescent treponemal antibody absorption test and, if that is positive, to proceed to lumbar puncture *regardless* of whether the serum Venereal Disease Research Laboratory (VDRL) test is positive or not.

Creutzfeldt–Jakob disease is rarely characterized by mania but in one very rare case the disease presented with mania (Lendvai *et al.* 1999).

Metachromatic leukodystrophy may, very rarely, present with mania. One patient, a 22-year-old woman (Besson 1980), was grandiose, 'spent money irresponsibly . . . and called out the fire brigade'; she eventually became demented after several years.

Adrenoleukodystrophy, when occurring in the adult years, often presents with a dementia, with the dementia in one case (Weller *et al.* 1992) being accompanied by mania.

MISCELLANEOUS

Of these miscellaneous disorders capable of causing mania, perhaps the most important is traumatic brain injury. Mania was found in 9 percent of 66 patients recovering from a traumatic injury over a 1-year follow-up, and there was a correlation between this sequela and damage to the inferior and polar regions of the temporal lobes, either on the left or on the right (Jorge *et al.* 1993a). In some cases, the mania may appear almost immediately after the patient recovers from the post-coma delirium (Bakchine *et al.* 1989; Bracken 1987), whereas in others there may be a latent interval, lasting up to several months, before the mania appears (Clark and Davison 1987; Nizamie *et al.* 1988). Although, in most cases the mania is either persistent or eventually remits without recurrence, there may rarely be an episodic course closely resembling that seen in bipolar disorder, with alternating episodes of mania and episodes of depression (Parker 1957). The manic syndrome following traumatic brain injury may be quite classic in character (Bakchine *et al.* 1989): one patient (Bracken 1987) with euphoria, pressured speech, and flight of ideas had the grandiose delusion that he was writing a 'best seller'.

Epileptic disorders characterized by mania include both ictal and post-ictal mania. Ictal mania may occur as an aura or as part of a complex partial seizure. Dostoyevsky described his ecstatic aura as follows: 'the air was filled with a big noise . . . I felt that Heaven was going down upon the Earth and that it had engulfed me. I have really touched God . . . healthy people . . . can't imagine the happiness which we epileptics feel during the second before our fit . . . for all the joys that life may bring, I would not exchange this one' (Alajouanine 1963). Complex partial seizures may themselves occasionally be characterized by manic symptoms: one patient (Mulder and Daly 1952), during her attack, 'was euphoric, talkative and pleasant. When asked how she felt, she replied "wonderful"'.

Post-ictal mania may be seen 1–2 days after a 'flurry' of complex partial seizures, and this may be characterized by either stage I or stage II mania (Barczak *et al.* 1988; Nishida *et al.* 2006).

Systemic lupus erythematosus may be marked by manic symptoms, and in such cases other typical symptoms, such as rash, arthralgia, pleurisy, pericarditis, nephritis, or cytopenia, suggest the diagnosis (Brey *et al.* 2002, Johnson and Richardson 1968).

Vitamin B12 deficiency may, very rarely, present with mania, as was reported in one 81-year-old man (Goggans 1984).

Sydenham's chorea may, in addition to the acute onset of chorea, be characterized by mania (often with prominent lability [Adams 1975; Gatti and Rosenheim 1969]), which may in turn be characterized by prominent hallucinations and delusions, typically of persecution (Powell 1889; Reaser 1940; Shaskan 1938; Van Der Horst 1947).

Chorea gravidarum, which essentially represents a recurrence of Sydenham's chorea during pregnancy, may also, in addition to chorea, be characterized by mania (Wilson and Preece 1932).

Velocardiofacial syndrome, a rare disorder suggested by a characteristic facial dysmorphism with hypertelorism, a large nose and micrognathia, may be characterized by mania in over one-half of all cases (Papalos *et al.* 1996).

Encephalitis lethargica, currently a very rare disorder, typically presents with headache, fever, sleep reversal, delirium, and oculomotor paralyses. In some cases, patients displayed euphoria, sometimes accompanied by lability and pressured speech (Hohman 1921).

Acute disseminated encephalomyelitis results from an autoimmune assault on the brain that is triggered by a preceding, usually viral, infection and generally has an acute onset within 2–21 days of the initial infection. Although the typical presentation is with delirium, a mania may occasionally appear. In one case (Moscovich *et al.* 1995), 2 weeks after an influenza infection, a 32-year-old woman developed mania, which remained the only indication of the underlying encephalitis for almost 2 weeks, after which she became delirious and incontinent. In another case (Paskavitz *et al.* 1995), a post-mononucleosis acute disseminated encephalitis presented with a combination of mania and a grand mal seizure.

Fahr's syndrome, suggested by calcification of the basal ganglia, may, very rarely present with mania (Trautner *et al.* 1988).

Dialysis dementia, also very rarely, may be characterized by mania (Jack *et al.* 1983).

Tuberous sclerosis, in a very rare case, presented with classic mania in a 5-year-old child (Khanna and Borde 1989).

Differential diagnosis

Hypomania is a distinctive syndrome, and very difficult to confuse with anything else; thus if the physician either sees the patient during stage I, or has a compatible history from a reliable historian, the diagnosis is generally straightforward. Difficulty can arise in cases where patients have progressed to stage II or stage III; but even here if one has a clear history of a preceding stage I, again the diagnosis remains relatively easy. However, if patients come to medical attention during stages II or III and there is no history available then one must consider other syndromes that may cause significant agitation, namely psychosis, catatonia, and delirium.

Psychosis, that is to say a syndrome marked by delusions and hallucinations, naturally enters into the differential for patients in stages II or III. Here, the differential rests on identifying the persisting hypomanic symptoms.

Catatonia of the excited subtype is characterized by bizarre and purposeless hyperactivity, and hence may, to a degree, resemble the behavior of patients in stage III mania. In stage III mania, however, one may still see distinctive stage I symptoms; moreover, although the behavior of patients in stage III is fragmented, individual fragments may still retain some purpose. Furthermore, whereas the hyperactive catatonic tends to remain withdrawn, the hyperactive stage III manic still retains an interest in others.

Delirium is marked by confusion and incoherence, symptoms also seen in stage III mania. Here again, one must rely on identifying fragments of stage I mania, symptoms typically not seen in delirium.

It cannot be stressed enough that the easiest way to make these differentials is to obtain a 'longitudinal' view of the patient's illness by repeatedly questioning family, acquaintances, nurses, and aides until one can reliably say that the typical symptoms of hypomania were, or were not, present.

Treatment

Treatment is directed at the underlying cause. In cases when this is not possible, or where the clinical situation requires urgent symptomatic treatment, one may consider use of one of the mood-stabilizing agents, with or without an antipsychotic (discussed further in Section 6.4).

Of the three mood-stabilizing agents (namely divalproex, carbamazepine, and lithium), divalproex is probably easiest to use and treatment may begin with a loading dose of from 20 to 25 mg/kg/day, with subsequent doses determined on the basis of clinical response, side-effects, and blood levels. Generally, at least a few days are required to see a salutary effect, and in the meantime one may use adjunctive haloperidol, risperidone, or olanzapine. Initially, haloperidol may be given in a dose of 5 mg (either as the concentrate or intramuscularly), risperidone in a dose of 2 mg (as the concentrate) or olanzapine 10 mg (as a tablet or intramuscularly), with repeat doses every 1–2 hours until the patient is calm, limiting side-effects occur or a maximum of approximately 20 mg of haloperidol, 6 mg of risperidone or 40 mg of olanzapine. In truly emergent cases, some authorities recommend combining lorazepam – 2 mg intramuscularly with either haloperidol or risperidone. If effective, the adjunctive regimen should be continued until the mood-stabilizer has controlled the situation, after which it may be tapered and discontinued, leaving the patient on a mood-stabilizer alone.

Mood-stabilizers have also been used prophylactically in situations wherein mania is expected: thus, both lithium (Falk *et al.* 1979; Siegal 1978) and valproic acid (Abbas and Styra 1994) have been used preventively in patients who have experienced mania during prior courses of steroid treatment.

6.4 AGITATION

Agitation is extraordinarily common in general hospital and nursing home work. It is, as noted below, a nonspecific symptom, being seen in a variety of conditions.

Clinical features

Agitated patients are tense and restless. If confined to bed, they may thrash about; intravenous lines and tubes may be pulled out. Ambulatory patients may pace their rooms or up and down the hall, perhaps shouting or cursing. Some may become violent, slamming doors or throwing furniture, and some, especially if attempts are made to restrain them, may become assaultive.

Etiology

Agitation, of sufficient degree to merit clinical attention, generally occurs as part of a large number of conditions, including dementia, delirium, psychosis, traumatic brain injury, alcohol withdrawal, mania, depression, and during various intoxications, for example with stimulants. Agitation may also occur as a side-effect to various medications, for example bupropion. Pain may also cause patients to become agitated and this is particularly the case in elderly patients with dementia.

Differential diagnosis

Anxious patients may appear quite tense but generally are not given to restless pacing, and certainly not to violent or destructive behavior.

Akathisia, seen primarily as a side-effect to antipsychotics, may appear very similar to agitation. Clues to the correct diagnosis include a worsening of symptoms when sitting or lying down and a tendency to 'march in place'.

Treatment

Environmental measures can sometimes be remarkably effective in calming an agitated patient (Alessi et al. 1999). Overall stimulation should be kept to a minimum, and patients should be provided with constructive and quietly engaging activities. Interactions with the patient should preferably be on a one-to-one basis and, if it is necessary to have two people with the patient, it is important to ensure that only one person does all the talking. When patients tend to roam, they should generally be allowed to do so, provided that their behavior endangers neither themselves nor others. A private room should be provided, and if that is not possible then a calm patient should be selected as a roommate; in all cases, the room should have a large clock and calendar, and a window. Visitors should be screened, as in some cases certain visitors will agitate patients further; in general, there should be only one visitor at a time. Sitters are often utilized, and may obviate the need for restraints but, like visitors, sitters should be carefully screened: although some have a good 'way' with agitated patients, others may simply worsen the situation. Seclusion or restraints may at times be required and one must not be shy about ordering them, as they may at times be life-saving.

In all instances of agitation, it is also necessary to dovetail the symptomatic treatment of agitation with other aspects of treatment of the parent syndrome, and the reader is directed to the appropriate chapter on dementia, delirium, etc.

Pharmacologic treatment is typically required: agents utilized include antipsychotics (e.g., risperidone, haloperidol, quetiapine, or olanzapine), anti-epileptic drugs (e.g., divalproex and carbamazepine), and benzodiazepines (e.g., lorazepam). As noted above, agitation usually occurs as part of a larger syndrome and the choice of pharmacologic agent is often dictated by the syndrome within which the agitation is occurring. In the following, each of the more common syndromes is considered in turn, with recommendations for both non-emergent and emergent treatment; all of the recommendations, except where otherwise

noted, are based on double-blind studies. Importantly, as noted under the concluding remarks, these recommendations are offered as guidelines only: clinical reality often dictates alternative approaches and good clinical judgment is absolutely required.

Dementia

For non-emergent care, effectiveness has been demonstrated for risperidone (Brodaty et al. 2003; De Deyn et al. 2005), quetiapine (Zhong et al. 2007), haloperidol (Allain et al. 2000), and olanzapine, with haloperidol being of equal effectiveness to olanzapine (Verhey et al. 2006) and risperidone of equal effectiveness to olanzapine (Fontaine et al. 2003). In a partially blinded study (Porsteinsson et al. 2001) divalproex was effective, but a double-blinded study found it to be no more effective than placebo (Sival et al. 2002). In addition, one study found trazodone to be of similar efficacy to haloperidol (Sultzer et al. 1997).

In looking at more specific kinds of dementia, the effectiveness of haloperidol in Alzheimer's disease is uncertain: one study (Devanand et al. 1998) supported its use, whereas another (Teri et al. 2001) did not. Olanzapine (Street et al. 2000) appeared effective in a comparison with placebo, and in a large study olanzapine and risperidone were more effective than either quetiapine or placebo (Schneider et al. 2006). Carbamazepine (Olin et al. 2001; Tariot et al. 1998) appears effective but valproic acid is not (Hermann et al. 2007; Tariot et al. 2005). Trazodone does not appear to be effective (Teri et al. 2001). There is an intriguing study suggesting that citalopram may be effective (Pollock et al. 2002). In Parkinson's disease and diffuse Lewy body disease, quetiapine was not effective (Kurlan et al. 2007).

Overall, for the non-emergent treatment of agitation in dementia, it may be best to begin with a low dose of risperidone, perhaps 0.25 or 0.5 mg/day, with a gradual titration up to a maximum of perhaps 2 mg. Should this be ineffective or not tolerated then consideration may be given to quetiapine, beginning at 25 mg and increasing the dose gradually, if necessary, to 200 mg, or to olanzapine, beginning with a low dose of perhaps 2.5 mg and titrating gradually, if necessary, to a maximum of 10 mg. Consideration may also be given to carbamazepine and, perhaps, divalproex: in either case, the initial dose should be low, with very gradual titration to effectiveness, limiting side-effects, or a blood level within the therapeutic range, whichever comes first.

In emergent cases, consideration may be given to intramuscular olanzapine in a dose of 5 mg (Meehan et al. 2002), with repeat doses if needed.

Before leaving this section, some words are in order regarding the risk of death or stroke in elderly demented patients treated with antipsychotics. Although these risks are indeed increased for second-generation agents (Kryzhanovskaya et al. 2006), and even more so for first-generation agents (Wang et al. 2005), this increased risk, as with any medical treatment, must be weighed against the benefits obtained with treatment.

Delirium

I could not find any double-blind studies regarding the non-emergent pharmacologic treatment of delirium. In practice, patients are treated with low doses of antipsychotics (e.g., risperidone, 0.5–1 mg or haloperidol, 2–5 mg), with dosage adjustments made every day or so as needed.

In emergent cases, risperidone and haloperidol (Breitbart et al. 1996) are both effective and probably equally so (Han and Kim 2004); chlorpromazine may also be considered (Breitbart et al. 1996); open studies also support use of olanzapine (Skrobik et al. 2004) and quetiapine (Sasaki et al. 2003). Valproic acid, in open studies, used as 'add-on' therapy with antipsychotics, reportedly decreased agitation (Bourgeois et al. 2005). Lorazepam, in one study (Breitbart et al. 1996), was ineffective and associated with severe side-effects (sedation, disinhibition, ataxia, and increased confusion).

In emergent situations, one may begin with either risperidone (as the concentrate) 0.25–1 mg, or haloperidol (either as the concentrate or intramuscularly or intravenously) 1–5 mg, with repeat doses every hour until the patient is calm, limiting side-effects occur, or a maximum dose is reached of either 5 mg of risperidone or 20 mg of haloperidol. Should the patient respond satisfactorily, a regular daily dose is started the next day, roughly equivalent to the total required for success on the first day, with provisions for repeat doses if required, and further adjustments being made to the regular daily dose until no further p.r.n. doses are required. This maintenance dose is then continued until the cause of the delirium has been effectively treated, at which point the dose may be tapered to discontinuation over a few days.

Psychosis

Studies regarding the treatment of agitated patients with psychosis for the most part involve patients with schizophrenia.

In non-emergent cases, one may simply begin with the antipsychotic judged most appropriate for the patient's case.

In emergent cases, rapid control of agitation has been achieved with a combination of haloperidol and lorazepam, with the combination being more effective than use of either agent alone (Bieniek et al. 1998); a combination of risperidone and lorazepam was also shown to be as effective as combined treatment with haloperidol and lorazepam (Currier et al. 2004). Aripiprazole is of similar effectiveness to haloperidol and better tolerated (Tran-Johnson et al. 2007). Olanzapine is also of similar effectiveness to haloperidol (Breier et al. 2002; Wright et al. 2001); a combination of olanzapine at a dose of 10 mg plus lorazepam as needed was less effective than simply using olanzapine alone at a higher dose of 25–30 mg (Baker et al. 2003). Blinded work comparing ziprasidone in doses of 20 mg (Daniel et al. 2001) or 10 mg (Lesem et al. 2001) with ziprasidone in a dose of 2 mg indicates effectiveness for the higher doses.

Overall, for emergent treatment, it seems reasonable to begin with either haloperidol (5 mg, as the concentrate or i.m.), risperidone (2 mg, as the concentrate), aripiprazole (9.75 mg, intramuscularly), or olanzapine (10 mg, i.m.), with repeat doses every 1–2 hours until the patient is calm, limiting side-effects occur, or maximum doses of approximately 20 mg haloperidol, 6 mg of risperidone, 39 mg of aripiprazole, or 40 mg of olanzapine are reached. Although monotherapy is generally preferred, in cases when very rapid control is essential, intramuscular lorazepam (2 mg), may be safely given along with doses of either haloperidol or risperidone; note that it is probably also safe to give lorazepam with olanzapine but this has not been demonstrated as yet.

Traumatic brain injury

In non-emergent situations, propranolol is effective (Brooke et al. 1992); open studies also suggest effectiveness for quetiapine (Kim and Bijlani 2006), valproic acid (Chatham-Showalter and Kimmel 2000; Wroblewski et al. 1997), carbamazepine (Azouvi et al. 1999) and lithium (Glenn et al. 1989), amantadine (Chandler et al. 1988), amitriptyline (Mysiw et al. 1988), and sertraline (Kant et al. 1998)

Given the dearth of studies in this area, it is difficult to make firm recommendations for non-emergent treatment; in my experience use of one of the antidepressants (especially mirtazapine) or carbamazepine has worked out well.

Regarding emergent treatment, there are no double-blind studies. In practice, patients are generally treated in a manner similar to that for the emergent treatment of delirium, as described above.

Alcohol withdrawal

In non-emergent cases, alcohol withdrawal may be treated with either divalproex (Reoux et al. 2001) or carbamazepine (Stuppacek et al. 1992). Loading doses may be utilized (20 mg/kg/day of divalproex, 600–800 mg/day of carbamazepine), with the total daily loading dose divided into two or three doses: subsequent adjustments are made based on effectiveness, side-effects, and blood levels.

In emergent cases, one may give lorazepam (Miller and McCurdy 1984): a typical protocol calls for lorazepam, 2 mg, orally or parenterally, every 2 hours until symptoms are controlled, limiting side-effects occur, or a maximum dose of approximately 20 mg is reached (it must be borne in mind, however, that some patients require much higher, even heroic, doses). The next day, the patient is treated with a regular daily dose of oral lorazepam in a total daily dose approximately equivalent to that required for control the first day, with the total daily dose divided into three or four doses. Provision is also made for p.r.n. doses of 1–2 mg lorazepam every 2 hours for breakthrough agitation, with the total daily dose being appropriately adjusted on a daily basis until no further p.r.n. doses are required. Early on in this process one should generally load the patient with either divalproex or carbamazepine. As soon thereafter as the agitation is controlled and the blood level is therapeutic, it is generally possible to rapidly taper the lorazepam without any loss of control. The anti-epileptic drug is then continued for a week or more until the withdrawal has run its course, at which time it may be tapered and discontinued over a few days.

Mania

In cases of mania wherein significant agitation has appeared, emergent care is almost always required, and treatment may be undertaken with either divalproex (McElroy *et al.* 1996) or an antipsychotic (e.g., haloperidol [McElroy *et al.* 1996], aripiprazole [Zimbroff *et al.* 2007], or olanzapine [Tohen *et al.* 2002]), or, often, with a combination of divalproex and an antipsychotic. Divalproex may be given in a loading dose of 20 mg/kg/day in two or three divided doses, with subsequent adjustments based on clinical response, side-effects, and blood levels. Haloperidol, aripiprazole, or olanzapine may be given as described above, under psychosis. Once the mania is controlled, it is often possible to taper and discontinue the antipsychotic.

Depression

In most cases of agitated depression, reassurance coupled with ongoing treatment with an antidepressant, will suffice.

Emergent treatment, occasionally, may be required when agitation is extreme. In such cases, case reports suggest an effectiveness for benzodiazepines such as alprazolam (Gilbert and Hendrie 1987), and case series, for low-dose divalproex (Debattista *et al.* 2005).

Concluding remarks

Good clinical judgment often dictates a course of treatment that differs from those recommended above. Doses must often be reduced in elderly or frail patients, and in those with significant hepatic dysfunction. Antipsychotics other than risperidone, haloperidol, and olanzapine are often used successfully, and haloperidol, given its tendency to cause extrapyramidal side-effects, is falling into disfavor. Lorazepam is used quite routinely, and its sedative effect is often quite welcome. In some cases, certain medications are relatively contraindicated: for example, in cases of dementia secondary to diffuse Lewy body disease haloperidol should probably not be used, given the risk of severe, even fatal, parkinsonism (McKeith *et al.* 1992).

6.5 ANXIETY

Pathologic anxiety occurs in two forms. In one, anxiety is more or less persistent, whereas in the other it occurs in discrete attacks.

Clinical features

Persistent anxiety tends to come on gradually, and waxes and wanes over time. The anxiety itself is typically accompanied by autonomic signs such as tremor, tachycardia, and diaphoresis. Patients complain of a sense of tremulousness, and the tremor itself is fine and postural. Tachycardic patients may complain that the heart is 'racing' and there may be palpitations. Diaphoresis may be evident when one shakes the patient's hand. The duration of this persistent form of anxiety depends on the underlying cause and may, for example, range from years or decades in the case of generalized anxiety disorder to weeks or less in alcohol withdrawal.

Anxiety attacks typically arise acutely, over minutes, and symptoms crescendo rapidly. In addition to the anxiety, which may be quite extreme, patients also typically experience a variety of other symptoms, including tremor, tachycardia, palpitations, diaphoresis, dyspnea, light-headedness, nausea, and parasthesiae. The duration of the attack, although determined by the underlying cause, is generally brief, lasting from minutes to an hour or more.

Etiology

The various causes of anxiety are listed in Table 6.5, where they are divided into those causing persistent anxiety and those causing anxiety attacks.

PERSISTENT ANXIETY

The most common cause of persistent anxiety is an idiopathic disorder, namely generalized anxiety disorder (Anderson *et al.* 1984; Nisita *et al.* 1990). This disorder generally has an onset in adolescence or early adult years, and the characteristic anxiety tends to persist, in a waxing and waning fashion, for from years to decades.

Toxic causes include caffeine (Greden 1974; Hughes *et al.* 1991a) and sympathomimetics such as ephedrine and phenylpropanolamine (Sawyer *et al.* 1982) and ephedra alkaloids, found in many 'herbal supplements' (Haller and Benowitz 2000). Others include theophylline (Trembath and Boobis 1979) and levodopa (Celesia and Barr 1970). Although, in general, anxiety only occurs with high doses, some patients may be quite sensitive to these medications and experience considerable anxiety at 'therapeutic' doses.

Metabolic causes include hypocalcemia, as may be seen in hypoparathyroidism (Carlson 1986; Denko and Kaelbling 1962; Lawlor 1988), and the hypoxia and hypercarbia associated with respiratory failure, as in advanced chronic obstructive pulmonary disease (Brenes 2003) and severe congestive heart failure.

Substance or medication withdrawals are considered next. Of the substance withdrawals, alcohol withdrawal (Isbell *et al.* 1955) probably constitutes one of the most common causes of persistent anxiety seen in general hospital practice, and the diagnosis is often missed, given that patients in withdrawal typically either minimize their alcohol use or deny it altogether. A similar scenario may occur in patients withdrawing from sedative/hypnotics, such as benzodiazepines (Rickels *et al.* 1990). Nicotine withdrawal is typified by anxiety, irritability, and a craving for a 'smoke' (Hughes and Hatsukami 1986; Hughes *et al.* 1991b), and

Table 6.5   Causes of anxiety

Persistent anxiety	Anxiety attacks
Primary, idiopathic anxiety	Idiopathic disorders
Generalized anxiety disorder	Panic disorder
Toxic	Phobias
Caffeine	Post-traumatic stress disorder
Sympathomimetics	Obsessive–compulsive disorder
Theophylline	Toxic
Levodopa	Cocaine
Metabolic	Cannabis
Hypocalcemia	Hallucinogens
Chronic obstructive pulmonary disease	Clozapine
Congestive heart failure	Metabolic
Substance or medication withdrawal	Hypoglycemia
Alcohol	Hyperventilation
Sedative/hypnotic	Endocrinologic
Nicotine	Pheochromocytoma
Anticholinergic	Miscellaneous
Endocrinologic	Simple partial seizures
Hyperthyroidism	Right temporal lobe tumor
Cushing's syndrome	Paroxysmal atrial tachycardia
Intracranial disorders	Angina or myocardial infarction
Post-stroke	Pulmonary embolus
Traumatic brain injury	Parkinson's disease

likewise may go undiagnosed, given the shame associated with smoking and patients' reluctance to admit it. Anticholinergic withdrawal, occurring after an abrupt discontinuation of drugs with strong anticholinergic properties such as benztropine or tricyclic antidepressants, may be followed by a cholinergic rebound, with anxiety, jitteriness, insomnia, and nausea (Dilsaver et al. 1983).

Endocrinologic causes include hyperthyroidism and Cushing's syndrome. Hyperthyroidism classically causes chronic anxiety and may be suggested by such signs and symptoms as heat intolerance, diaphoresis, and lid retraction (Dietch 1981; Greer et al. 1973; Kathol and Delahunt 1986; MacCrimmon et al. 1979; Trzepacz et al. 1988). Cushing's syndrome, although classically associated with depression, may at times be characterized by severe anxiety (Kelly 1996). The diagnosis is suggested by such features as a 'moon' facies, buffalo hump, acne, hirsutism, violaceous abdominal striae, hypertension, and diabetes mellitus.

Intracranial disorders associated with persistent anxiety include stroke and traumatic brain injury. Post-stroke anxiety occurs chronically in a minority of patients and appears to be more likely with a right hemisphere infarction (Castillo et al. 1993, 1995; Starkstein et al. 1990c). Traumatic brain injury may be associated with anxiety in a small minority of cases (Fann et al. 1995; Jorge et al. 1993b).

ANXIETY ATTACKS

By far the most common causes of anxiety attacks are certain idiopathic disorders, namely panic disorder, phobias,

post-traumatic stress disorder and obsessive–compulsive disorder. Panic disorder is the prototypical cause of anxiety attacks, which, when occurring in this disorder, are often referred to as 'panic attacks'. In this disorder, anxiety attacks typically occur first in adolescence or early adult years, and then recur, with variable frequency, over years or decades. Interestingly, the anxiety attacks seen in panic disorder may awaken patients from sleep (Mellman and Uhde 1989) and may, in a minority, be accompanied by such 'temporal lobe phenomena' as micropsia and macropsia (Coyle and Sterman 1986). Phobias, including specific phobia, social phobia, and agoraphobia, may all be characterized by anxiety attacks when patients are brought into close proximity to the phobic object, such as a snake for a specific phobic, speaking to an audience for the social phobic with a fear of public speaking, and venturing away from home for the agoraphobic. Post-traumatic stress disorder may also be characterized by anxiety attacks when patients are exposed to events or objects that remind them of the original trauma; thus, a combat veteran might be seized with anxiety if a combat scene appeared on a television program. Obsessive–compulsive disorder may likewise be characterized by anxiety attacks when patients attempt to resist their compulsions. Thus, patients with a hand-washing compulsion may experience unbearable anxiety if they attempt to resist the urge to wash.

Toxic causes of anxiety attacks are relatively rare, and include intoxication with cocaine (Louie et al. 1996), cannabis (Bromberg 1934), and hallucinogens, such as LSD (Isbell et al. 1956; Kuramochi and Takahashi 1964); anxiety attacks have also been reported secondary to treatment with clozapine (Bressan *et al.* 2000).

Metabolic causes include the classic examples of hypoglycemia and hyperventilation. Hypoglycemic-induced anxiety attacks are typically seen in diabetics on insulin who miss a meal, and are suggested by the associated hunger. The hyperventilation syndrome is suggested by prominent dyspnea and by a resolution of symptoms with rebreathing through a paper bag.

Endocrinologically caused anxiety attacks may occur in pheochromocytoma, and in such cases the anxiety attack is typically accompanied not only by an elevated blood pressure, but also by headache (Doust 1958; Modlin *et al.* 1979; Starkman *et al.* 1985; Thomas *et al.* 1966).

Of the miscellaneous causes of anxiety attacks, perhaps the most important are simple partial seizures, which, rarely, may manifest solely with anxiety attacks (Sazgar *et al.* 2003). Although such ictal anxiety often lasts only seconds or minutes (Williams 1956), the seizure may in rare cases be very prolonged: one patient for 12 hours endured ictal fear of such a degree that she 'continually looked back over her shoulder' (McLachlan and Blume 1980). There are two clues to the correct diagnosis of these simple partial seizures: first, the exquisitely paroxysmal nature of the onset, and second, the occurrence, at other times in the patient's life, of more obvious ictal phenomena such as complex partial or grand mal seizures.

Anxiety attacks have also, very rarely, been associated with mass lesions in the right temporal lobe (Ghadarian *et al.* 1986).

Cardiopulmonary conditions associated with anxiety attacks include paroxysmal atrial tachycardia, angina or myocardial infarction, and pulmonary embolus. Paroxysmal atrial tachycardia is suggested by the almost instantaneous onset of severe tachycardia, followed immediately by severe anxiety as the patient becomes aware of the fluttering in his or her chest. The onset with tachycardia is suggestive, and the ability of the patient to terminate the attack with a Valsalva maneuver is also suggestive of the diagnosis. Angina or myocardial infarction may, in a minority, present primarily with anxiety, with chest pain or dyspnea being relatively minor symptoms. A pulmonary embolus, at the moment of its lodging in a large artery, can produce severe anxiety and dyspnea. The diagnosis is suggested by the dyspnea and by such clinical settings as prolonged immobilization or deep venous thrombophlebitis.

Finally, Parkinson's disease will, in a significant minority of levodopa-treated patients, be characterized by anxiety attacks during the 'off' interval as the effectiveness of the previous dose of levodopa wanes (Vazquez *et al.* 1993).

Differential diagnosis

The first task in differential diagnosis is to decide whether or not the anxiety in question is normal or pathologic. Although the experience of anxiety is a normal reaction to threatening events, the clinician should suspect pathology in cases when either the severity of the anxiety, or its duration, seem out of proportion to the inciting event.

Consideration should also be given to the possibility that the anxiety in question is existing as part of a larger syndrome, such as depression or delirium. Depression is commonly accompanied by anxiety, and hence in evaluating any patient with anxiety one should enquire after depressive symptoms, such as insomnia (especially middle or terminal insomnia), anergia, anhedonia, anorexia, etc., and, if they are present then the differential for depression should be pursued, as discussed earlier under Depression. Delirious patients are often quite anxious, and hence the diagnostician should be alert to such symptoms as confusion, disorientation, short-term memory loss, etc., and if these are present the differential outlined in Section 5.3 should be pursued.

Treatment

Treatment is directed at the underlying cause; in cases of persistent anxiety when this is not possible or ineffective, consideration may be given to symptomatic treatment with a benzodiazepine, such as lorazepam or clonazepam, or, when these are relatively contraindicated, an antidepressant or an antipsychotic, such as quetiapine. With regard to anxiety attacks, symptomatic treatment is generally not indicated: most attacks are of such brevity that they resolve spontaneously before any pharmacologic effects could be obtained.

REFERENCES

Abbas A, Styra R. Valproate prophylaxis against steroid-induced psychosis. *Can J Psychiatry* 1994; **39**:188–9.

Abouesh A, Hobbs WR. Clarithromycin-induced mania. *Am J Psychiatry* 1998; **155**:1626.

Abrams R, Taylor MA. Mania and schizoaffective disorder, manic type: a comparison. *Am J Psychiatry* 1976; **133**:1445–7.

Adams J. Psychological correlates of the course of Sydenham's chorea. Repeat evaluation of a case. *J Abnormal Child Psychol* 1975; **3**:33–40.

Ainiala H, Loukkola J, Peltola J *et al.* The prevalence of neuropsychiatric syndromes in systemic lupus erythematosus. *Neurology* 2001; **57**:496–500.

Akiskal HS, Djenderedjian AH, Rosenthal RH *et al.* Cyclothymic disorder: validating criteria for inclusion in the bipolar affective group. *Am J Psychiatry* 1977; **134**:1227–33.

Alajouanine T. Dostoiewski's epilepsy. *Brain* 1963; **86**:209.

Alessi CA, Yoon EJ, Schnelle JF *et al.* A randomized trial of a combined physical activity and environmental intervention in nursing home residents: do sleep and agitation improve? *J Am Geriatr Soc* 1999; **37**:784–91.

Allain H, Dautzenberg PH, Maurere K *et al.* Double blind study of tiapride versus haloperidol and placebo in agitation and aggressiveness in elderly patients with cognitive impairment. *Psychopharmacology* 2000; **148**:361–6.

Alpers BJ. Personality and emotional disorders associated with hypothalamic lesions. In: Fulton JF, Ranson SW, Frantz AM eds. *Research publications. Association for Research in Nervous and Mental Disease.* Vol. XX. *The hypothalamus and central levels of autonomic function.* Baltimore, MD: Williams & Wilkins, 1940.

Anderson AE, McHugh PR. Oat cell carcinoma with hyper-cortisolemia presenting to a psychiatric hospital as a suicide attempt. *J Nerv Ment Dis* 1971; **152**:427–31.

Anderson G, Vestergaard K, Lauritzen L. Effective treatment of poststroke depression with the selective serotonin reuptake inhibitor citalopram. *Stroke* 1994; **25**:1099–104.

Anderson JD, Noyes R, Crowe RR. A comparison of panic disorder and generalized anxiety disorder. *Am J Psychiatry* 1984; **141**:572–5.

Andersson S, Krogstad JM, Finset A. Apathy and depressed mood in acquired brain damage: relationship to lesion localization and psychophysiological reactivity. *Psychol Med* 1999; **29**:447–56.

Angelini L, Mazzuchi A, Picciotto F *et al.* Focal lesion of the right cingulum: a case report in a child. *J Neurol Neurosurg Psychiatry* 1980; **43**:355–7.

Arnold BM, Casal G, Higgins HP. Apathetic thyrotoxicosis. *Can Med Assoc J* 1974; **111**:957–8.

Astrom M, Adolfsson R, Asplund K. Major depression in stroke patients: a 3-year longitudinal study. *Stroke* 1993; **24**:976–82.

Azouvi P, Jokic C, Attal N *et al.* Carbamazepine in agitation and aggressive behavior following severe closed-head injury: results of an open trial. *Brain Inj* 1999; **13**:797–804.

Baker RW, Kinon BJ, Maguire GA *et al.* Effectiveness of rapid initial dose escalation of up to 40 mg per day of oral olanzapine in acute agitation. *J Clin Psychopharmacol* 2003; **23**:342–8.

Bakchine S, Lacomblez L, Benoit N *et al.* Manic-like state after bilateral orbitofrontal and right temperoparietal injury: efficacy of clonidine. *Neurology* 1989; **39**:777–81.

Barczak P, Edmunds E, Betis T *et al.* Hypomania following complex partial seizures: a report of three cases. *Br J Psychiatry* 1988; **152**:137–9.

Benjamin S, Kirsch D, Visscher T *et al.* Hypomania from left frontal AVM resection. *Neurology* 2000; **54**:1389–90.

Besson JAO. A diagnostic pointer to adult metachromatic leukodystrophy. *Br J Psychiatry* 1980; **137**:186–7.

Bieniek SA, Ownby RL, Penalver A *et al.* A double-blind study of lorazepam versus the combination of haloperidol and lorazepam in managing agitation. *Pharmacotherapy* 1998; **18**:57–62.

Bhalerao S, Talsky A, Hansen K *et al.* Ciprofloxacin-induced manic episode. *Psychosomatics* 2006; **47**:539–40.

Billings RF, Stein MB. Depression associated with ranitidine. *Am J Psychiatry* 1986; **143**:915–16.

Billings RG, Tang SW, Rakoff VM. Depression associated with cimetidine. *Can J Psychiatry* 1981; **26**:260–1.

Binder RL, Dickman WA. Psychiatric manifestations of neurosyphilis in middle-aged patients. *Am J Psychiatry* 1980; **137**:741–2.

Black DW, Nasrallah H. Hallucinations and delusions in 1,715 patients with unipolar and bipolar affective disorders. *Psychopathology* 1989; **22**:28–34.

Blackwell MJ. Rapid-cycling manic-depressive illness following subarachnoid haemorrhage. *Br J Psychiatry* 1991; **159**:279–80.

Bloch M, Schmidt PJ, Rubinow DR. Premenstrual syndrome: evidence for symptom stability across cycles. *Am J Psychiatry* 1997a; **154**:1741–6.

Bloch M, Stager S, Braun A *et al.* Pimozide-induced depression in men who stutter. *J Clin Psychiatry* 1997b; **58**:433–6.

Bogousslavsky J, Ferrazzini M, Regli F *et al.* Manic delirium and frontal-like syndrome with paramedian infarction of the right thalamus. *J Neurol Neurosurg Psychiatry* 1988; **51**:116–19.

Bolt JMW. Huntington's chorea in the West of Scotland. *Br J Psychiatry* 1970; **116**:259–70.

Bourgeois JA, Koike AK, Simmons JE *et al.* Adjunctive valproic acid for delirium and/or agitation on a consultation-liaison service: a report of six cases. *J Neuropsychiatry Clin Neurosci* 2005; **17**:232–8.

Bowman KM, Raymond AF. A statistical study of hallucinations in the manic-depressive psychoses. *Am J Psychiatry* 1931; **88**:299–309.

Bracken P. Mania following head injury. *Br J Psychiatry* 1987; **150**:690–2.

Bratfos O, Haug JO. Puerperal mental disorders in manic-depressive females. *Acta Psychiatr Scand* 1966; **42**:285–94.

Breier A, Meehan K, Birkett M *et al.* A double-blind, placebo-controlled dose-response comparison of intramuscular olanzapine and haloperidol in the treatment of acute agitation in schizophrenia. *Arch Gen Psychiatry* 2002; **59**:441–8.

Breitbart W, Marotta R, Platt MM *et al.* A double-blind trial of haloperidol, chlorpromazine, and lorazepam in the treatment of delirium in hospitalized AIDS patients. *Am J Psychiatry* 1996; **153**:231–7.

Brenes GA. Anxiety and chronic obstructive pulmonary disease: prevalence, impact, and treatment. *Psychosom Med* 2003; **65**:963–70.

Brenner I. Apathetic hyperthyroidism. *J Clin Psychiatry* 1978; **39**:479–80.

Bressan RA, Monteiro VBM, Dias CC. Panic disorder associated with clozapine. *Am J Psychiatry* 2000; **157**:2056.

Brey RL, Holliday SL, Saklad AR *et al.* Neuropsychiatric syndromes in lupus. Prevalence using standardized definitions. *Neurology* 2002; **58**:1214–20.

Brockington IF, Wainwright S, Kendell RE. Manic patients with schizophrenic or paranoid symptoms. *Psychol Med* 1980; **10**:73–83.

Brockington IF, Cernik KF, Schofield EM *et al.* Puerperal psychosis: phenomenon and diagnosis. *Arch Gen Psychiatry* 1981; **38**:829–33.

Brodaty H, Ames D, Snowdon J *et al.* A randomized placebo-controlled trial of risperidone for the treatment of aggression, agitation, and psychosis of dementia. *J Clin Psychiatry* 2003; **64**:134–43.

Brodaty H, Sachdev PS, Withall A *et al.* Frequency and clinical, neuropsychological and neuroimaging correlates of apathy following stroke: the Sydney Stroke Study. *Psychol Med* 2005; **35**:1707–16.

Bromberg W. Marijuana intoxication. *Am J Psychiatry* 1934; **91**:303–30.

Brooke MM, Patterson DR, Questad KA *et al.* The treatment of agitation during initial hospitalization after traumatic brain injury. *Arch Phys Med Rehabil* 1992; **73**:917–21.

Brouilette M-J, Routy J-P. Abacavir sulfate and mania in HIV. *Am J Psychiatry* 2007; **164**:979–80.

Brown SA, Inaba RK, Gillin JC *et al.* Alcoholism and affective disorder: clinical course of depressive symptoms. *Am J Psychiatry* 1995; **152**:45–52.

Burns A, Jacoby R, Levy R. Psychiatric phenomena in Alzheimer's disease. III. Disorders of mood. *Br J Psychiatry* 1990a; **157**:81–6.

Burns A, Folstein S, Brandt J *et al.* Clinical assessment of irritability, aggression, and apathy in Huntington and Alzheimer disease. *J Nerv Ment Dis* 1990b; **178**:30–6.

Caine ED, Shoulson I. Psychiatric syndromes in Huntington's disease. *Am J Psychiatry* 1983; **140**:728–33.

Carlson GA, Goodwin FK. The stages of mania: a longitudinal analysis of the manic episode. *Arch Gen Psychiatry* 1973; **28**:221–8.

Carlson GA, Strober M. Affective disorders in adolescence: issues in misdiagnosis. *J Clin Psychiatry* 1978; **39**:59–66.

Carlson RJ. Longitudinal observations of two cases of organic anxiety syndrome. *Psychosomatics* 1986; **27**:529–31.

Castillo CS, Starkstein SE, Federoff JP *et al.* Generalized anxiety disorder following stroke. *J Nerv Ment Dis* 1993; **181**:100–6.

Castillo CS, Schultz SK, Robinson RG. Clinical correlates of early-onset and late-onset poststroke generalized anxiety. *Am J Psychiatry* 1995; **152**:1174–9.

Catsman-Berrevoets CE, von Harskamp F. Compulsive pre-sleep behavior and apathy due to bilateral thalamic stroke: response to bromocriptine. *Neurology* 1988; **38**:647–9.

Celesia GG, Barr AN. Psychosis and other psychiatric manifestations of levodopa therapy. *Arch Neurol* 1970; **23**:193–200.

Ceylan ME, Turkcan A, Mutlu E *et al.* Manic episode with psychotic symptoms associated with high dose disulfiram: a case report. *J Clin Psychopharmacol* 2007; **27**:224–5.

Chandler MC, Barnhill JL, Gualtieri CT. Amantadine for the agitated head-injury patient. *Brain Inj* 1988; **2**:309–11.

Chatham-Showalter PE, Kimmel DN. Agitated symptom response to divalproex following acute brain injury. *J Neuropsychiatry Clin Neurosci* 2000; **12**:395–7.

Chaturvedi SK, Upadhyaya M. Secondary mania in a patient receiving isonicotinic acid hydrazide and pyroxidine: case report. *Can J Psychiatry* 1988; **33**:675–6.

Clark AF, Davison K. Mania following head injury: a report of two cases and a review of the literature. *Br J Psychiatry* 1987; **150**:841–4.

Clayton P, Pitts FN, Winokur G. Affective disorder. IV. Mania. *Compr Psychiatry* 1965; **3**:313–22.

Cohen AJ. Bromocriptine for prolactinoma-related dissociative disorder and depression. *J Clin Psychopharmacol* 1995; **15**:144–5.

Cohen SI. Cushing's syndrome: a psychiatric study of 29 patients. *Br J Psychiatry* 1980; **136**:120–4.

Coid J, Strang J. Mania secondary to procyclidine ('Kemadrin') abuse. *Br J Psychiatry* 1982; **141**:81–4.

Collacott RA, Cooper S-A, McGrother C. Differential rates of psychiatric disorder in adults with Down's syndrome compared with other mentally handicapped adults. *Br J Psychiatry* 1992; **161**:671–4.

Constant A, Castera L, Dantzer R *et al.* Mood alterations during interferon-alfa therapy in patients with chronic hepatitis C: evidence for an overlap between manic/hypomanic and depressive symptoms. *J Clin Psychiatry* 2005; **66**:1050–7.

Corsellis JAN, Goldberg GJ, Norton AR. 'Limbic encephalitis' and its association with carcinoma. *Brain* 1968; **91**:481–96.

Cottrell SS, Wilson SAK. The affective symptomatology of disseminated sclerosis: a study of 100 cases. *J Neurol Psychopathology* 1926; **7**:1–30.

Coyle PK, Sterman AB. Focal neurologic symptoms in panic attacks. *Am J Psychiatry* 1986; **143**:648–9.

Cummings JL, Mendez MF. Secondary mania with focal cerebrovascular lesions. *Am J Psychiatry* 1984; **141**:1084–7.

Cummings JL, Miller B, Hill MA *et al.* Neuropsychiatric aspects of multi-infarct dementia and dementia of the Alzheimer type. *Arch Neurol* 1987; **44**:389–93.

Currier GW, Chou JC, Feifel D *et al.* Acute treatment of psychotic agitation: a randomized comparison of oral treatment with risperidone and lorazepam versus intramuscular treatment with haloperidol and lorazepam. *J Clin Psychiatry* 2004; **65**:386–94.

Cushing H. The basophil adenomas of the pituitary body and their clinical manifestations (pituitary basophilism). *Bull Johns Hopkins Hosp* 1932; **50**:137–95.

Dalos NP, Rabins PV, Brooks BR *et al.* Disease activity and emotional state in multiple sclerosis. *Ann Neurol* 1983; **13**:573–7.

Daniel DG, Potkin SG, Reeves KR *et al.* Intramuscular (IM) ziprasidone 20 mg is effective in reducing acute agitation associated with psychosis: a double-blind, randomized trial. *Psychopharmacology* 2001; **155**:128–34.

Davidson KM. Diagnosis of depression in alcohol dependence: changes in prevalence with drinking status. *Br J Psychiatry* 1995; **166**:199–204.

DeBattista C, Solomon A, Arnow B *et al.* The efficacy of divalproex sodium in the treatment of agitation associated with major depression. *J Clin Psychopharmacol* 2005; **25**:476–9.

De Deyn PP, Katz IR, Brodaty H *et al.* Management of agitation, aggression, and psychosis associated with dementia: a pooled analysis including three randomized, placebo-controlled double-blind trials in nursing home residents treated with risperidone. *Clin Neurol Neurosurg* 2005; **107**:497–508.

DeMuth GW, Ackerman SH. Alpha-methyldopa and depression: a clinical study and review of the literature. *Am J Psychiatry* 1983; **140**:534–8.

Denko J, Kaelbling R. The psychiatric aspects of hypoparathyroidism. *Acta Psychiatr Scand* 1962; (suppl. 164):1–70.

Dennis MS, Byrne EJ, Hopkinson N *et al.* Neuropsychiatric systemic lupus erythematosus in elderly people: a case series. *J Neurol Neurosurg Psychiatry* 1992; **55**:1157–61.

Devanand DP, Nobler MS, Singer T et al. Is dysthymia a different disorder in the elderly? Am J Psychiatry 1994; 151:1591–9.

Devanand DP, Marder K, Michaels KS et al. A randomized, placebo-controlled dose-comparison trial of haloperidol for psychosis and disruptive behaviors in Alzheimer's disease. Am J Psychiatry 1998; 155:1512–20.

Dewhurst K. The neurosyphilitic psychoses today: a survey of 91 cases. Br J Psychiatry 1969; 115:31–8.

Dietch JT. Diagnosis of organic anxiety disorders. Psychosomatics 1981; 22:661–9.

Dilsaver SC, Feinberg M, Greden JF. Antidepressant withdrawal symptoms treated with anticholinergic agents. Am J Psychiatry 1983; 140:249–51.

Doust BC. Anxiety as a manifestation of pheochromocytoma. Arch Int Med 1958; 102:811–55.

Dunner DL, Fleiss JL, Fieve R. The course of development of mania in patients with recurrent depression. Am J Psychiatry 1976; 133:905–8.

Dunner DL, Patrick V, Fieve RR. Rapid cycling manic depressive patients. Compr Psychiatry 1977; 18:561–6.

El-Mallakh RS, Shrader SA, Widger E. Single case study: mania as a manifestation of end-stage renal disease. J Nerv Ment Dis 1987; 175:243–5.

Engel GL, Margolin SG. Neuropsychiatric disturbances in Addison's disease and the role of impaired carbohydrate metabolism in the production of abnormal cerebral function. Arch Neurol Psychiatry 1941; 45:881–4.

Ernst NH, Steur J. Increase of parkinsonian disability after fluoxetine medication. Neurology 1993; 43:211–13.

Falk WE, Mahnke MD, Poskanzer MD. Lithium prophylaxis of corticotropin-induced psychosis. JAMA 1979; 241:1011–12.

Fann JR, Uomoto JM, Katon WJ. Sertaline in the treatment of major depression following mild traumatic brain injury. J Neuropsychiatry Clin Neurosci 2000; 12:226–32.

Fann KR, Katon WJ, Uomoto JM et al. Psychiatric disorders and functional disability in outpatients with traumatic brain injuries. Am J Psychiatry 1995; 152:1493–9.

Fassbender K, Schmidt R, Mofsner R et al. Mood disorders and dysfunction of the hypothalmic-pituitary-adrenal axis in multiple sclerosis. Arch Neurol 1998; 55:66–72.

Federoff PJ, Starkstein SE, Forrester AW et al. Depression in patients with acute traumatic brain injury. Am J Psychiatry 1992; 149:918–23.

Feil D, Razani J, Boone K et al. Apathy and cognitive performance in older adults with depression. Int J Geriatr Psychiatry 2003; 18:479–85.

Fontaine CS, Hynn LS, Koch K et al. A double-blind comparison of olanzapine versus risperidone in the acute treatment of dementia-related behavioral disturbances in extended care facilities. J Clin Psychiatry 2003; 64:726–30.

Fras I, Litin EM, Pearson JS. Comparison of psychiatric symptoms in carcinoma of the pancreas with those in some other intra-abdominal neoplasms. Am J Psychiatry 1967; 123:1553–62.

Fraser TN. Cerebral manifestations of addisonian pernicious anemia. Lancet 1960; 2:458–9.

Fried MW, Shiffman ML, Reddy KR et al. Peginterferon alfa-2a plus ribaverin for chronic hepatitis C infection. N Engl J Med 2002; 347:975–82.

Friend KD, Young RC. Late-onset major depression with delusions after metoclopramide treatment. Am J Geriatr Psychiatry 1997; 5:79–82.

Galynker I, Ieronimo C, Miner C et al. Methylphenidate treatment of negative symptoms in patients with dementia. J Neuropsychiatry Clin Neurosci 1997; 9:231–9.

Ganz VH, Gurland BJ, Deming WE et al. The study of psychiatric symptoms of systemic lupus erythematosus: a biometric study. Psychosom Med 1972; 34:207–20.

Gatewood JW, Organ CH, Mead BT. Mental changes associated with hyperparathyroidism. Am J Psychiatry 1975; 132:129–32.

Gatti FM, Rosenheim E. Sydenham's chorea associated with transient intellectual impairment. Am J Dis Child 1969; 118:915–18.

Gentilini M, De Renzi E, Crisi G. Bilateral paramedian thalamic artery infarcts: report of eight cases. J Neurol Neurosurg Psychiatry 1987; 50:900–9.

Ghadarian AM, Gauthier S, Bertrand S. Anxiety attacks in a patient with a right temporal lobe meningioma. J Clin Psychiatry 1986; 47:270–1.

Gilbert A, Hendrie HC. Treatment of agitated depression with alprazolam. Am J Psychiatry 1987; 144:688.

Giovannoni G, O'Sullivan JD, Turner K et al. Hedonistic homeostatic dysregulation in patients with Parkinson's disease on dopamine replacement therapies. J Neurol Neurosurg Psychiatry 2000; 68:423–8.

Glaser G, Pincus JH. Limbic encephalitis. J Nerv Ment Dis 1969; 149:59–67.

Glenn MB, Wroblewski B, Parziale J et al. Lithium carbonate for aggressive behavior of affective instability in ten brain-injured patients. Am J Phys Med Rehabil 1989; 68:221–6.

Goggans FC. A case of mania secondary to vitamin B12 deficiency. Am J Psychiatry 1984; 141:300–1.

Gomez EA, Aviles M. Neurosyphilis in community mental health clinics: a case series. J Clin Psychiatry 1984; 45:127–9.

Greden JF. Anxiety or caffeinism: a diagnostic dilemma. Am J Psychiatry 1974; 131:1089–92.

Greenberg DB, Brown GL. Single case study: mania resulting from brain stem tumor. J Nerv Ment Dis 1985; 173:434–6.

Greer S, Ramsey I, Bagley C. Neurotoxic and thyrotoxic anxiety: clinical, psychological and physiological measurements. Br J Psychiatry 1973; 122:549–54.

Gross RA, Herridge P. A maniclike illness associated with a right frontal arteriovenous malformation. J Clin Psychiatry 1988; 49:119–20.

Grossman LS, Harrow M, Fudala JL et al. The longitudinal course of schizoaffective disorders: a prospective follow-up study. J Nerv Ment Dis 1984; 172:140–9.

Guze SB. The occurrence of psychiatric illness in systemic lupus erythematosus. Am J Psychiatry 1967; 123:1562–70.

Guze SB, Woodrugg RA, Clayton PJ. The significance of psychotic affective disorders. Arch Gen Psychiatry 1975; 32:1147–50.

Hadley HG. A case of puerperal psychosis recovering from four attacks. J Nerv Ment Dis 1941; 94:540–1.

Haller CA, Benowitz NL. Adverse cardiovascular and central nervous system events associated with dietary supplements containing ephedra alakaloids. *N Engl J Med* 2000; **343**:1833–8.

Han CS, Kim YK. A double-blind trial of risperidone and haloperidol for the treatment of delirium. *Psychosomatics* 2004; **45**:297–301.

Hantz P, Caradoc-Davies G, Caradoc-Davies T *et al.* Depression in Parkinson's disease. *Am J Psychiatry* 1994; **151**:1010–14.

Hardwick SW. Pellagra in psychiatric patients: twelve recent cases. *Lancet* 1943; **2**:43–5.

Harlow SD, Goldberg EL, Constock GW. A longitudinal study of the prevalence of depressive symptomatology in elderly widowed and married women. *Arch Gen Psychiatry* 1991; **48**:1065–8.

Haskett RF. Diagnostic categorization of psychiatric disturbance in Cushing's syndrome. *Am J Psychiatry* 1985; **142**:911–16.

Heathfield KW. Huntington's chorea. Investigation into the prevalence of the disease in the area covered by the North East Metropolitan Regional Hospital Board. *Brain* 1967; **90**:203–32.

Hermann M, Bartels C, Wallesch C-W. Depression in acute and chronic aphasia: symptoms, pathoanatomical–clinical correlations and functional implications. *J Neurol Neurosurg Psychiatry* 1993; **56**:672–8.

Hoehn-Saric R, Lipsey JR, McLeod DR. Apathy and indifference in patients on fluvoxamine and fluoxetine. *J Clin Psychopharmacol* 1990; **10**:343–5.

Hohman LB. Epidemic encephalitis (lethargic encephalitis): its psychotic manifestations with a report of twenty-three cases. *Arch Gen Psychiatry* 1921; **6**:295–333.

Holland JC, Korzun AH, Tross S *et al.* Comparative psychological disturbance in patients with pancreatic and gastric cancer. *Am J Psychiatry* 1986; **143**:982–6.

House A, Dennis M, Warlow C *et al.* Mood disorders after stroke and their relation to lesion location. *Brain* 1990; 1113–29.

Hughes JR, Hatsukami D. Signs and symptoms of tobacco withdrawal. *Arch Gen Psychiatry* 1986; **43**:289–94.

Hughes JR, Higgins ST, Bickel WK *et al.* Caffeine self-administration, withdrawal, and adverse effects among coffee drinkers. *Arch Gen Psychiatry* 1991a; **48**:611–17.

Hughes JR, Gust SW, Skoog K *et al.* Symptoms of tobacco withdrawal: a replication and extension. *Arch Gen Psychiatry* 1991b; **48**:52–9.

Hugo FJ, Halland AM, Spangenberg JJ *et al.* DSM-III-R classification of psychiatric symptoms in systemic lupus erythematosus. *Psychosomatics* 1996; **37**:262–9.

Hullett FJ, Potkin SG, Levy AB *et al.* Depression associated with nifedipine-induced calcium channel blockade. *Am J Psychiatry* 1988; **145**:1277–9.

Indaco A, Carrieri PB, Nappi C *et al.* Interictal depression in epilepsy. *Epilepsy Res* 1992; **12**:45–50.

Ingham SD, Nielsen JM. Thyroid psychosis: difficulties in diagnosis. *J Nerv Ment Dis* 1931; **74**:271–7.

Ironside R, Guttmacher M. The corpus callosum and its tumors. *Brain* 1929; **52**:442–83.

Isbell H, Fraser HF, Wickler A *et al.* An experimental study of etiology of 'rum fits' and delirium tremens. *Q J Stud Alcohol* 1955, **16**:1–33.

Isbell H, Belleville RE, Fraser HF *et al.* Studies on lysergic acid diethylamide (LSD-25). *Arch Neurol Psychiatry* 1956; **76**:468–78.

Isella V, Melzi P, Grimaldi M *et al.* Clinical, neuropsychological, and morphometric correlates of apathy in Parkinson's disease. *Mov Disord* 2002; **17**:366–71.

Jack RA. A case of mania secondary to propafenone. *J Clin Psychiatry* 1985; **46**:104–5.

Jack RA, Rivers-Bulkeley NT, Rabin PL. Single case study: secondary mania as a presentation of progressive dialysis encephalopathy. *J Nerv Ment Dis* 1983; **171**:193–5.

Jackson SL. Psychosis due to isoniazid. *Br Med J* 1957; **2**:743–6.

Jampala VC, Taylor MA, Abrams R. The diagnostic implications of formal thought disorder in mania and schizophrenia: a reassessment. *Am J Psychiatry* 1989; **146**:459–63.

Jensen K. Depression in patients treated with reserpine for arterial hypertension. *Acta Psychiatr Neurol Scand* 1959; **34**:195–204.

Jimenez-Jimenez FJ, Tejeiro J, Martinez-Junquera G *et al.* Parkinsonism exacerbated by paroxetine. *Neurology* 1994; **44**:2406.

Jochum T, Bar KJ, Sauer H. Topiramate-induced manic episode. *J Neurol Neurosurg Psychiatry* 2002; **73**:208–10.

Johnson RJ, Richardson EP. The neurological manifestations of systemic lupus erythematosus. *Medicine* 1968; **47**:337–69.

Jones AM. Psychiatric presentation of a third ventricular colloid cyst in a mentally handicapped woman. *Br J Psychiatry* 1993; **163**:677–8.

Jorge RE, Robinson RG, Starkstein SE *et al.* Secondary mania following traumatic brain injury. *Am J Psychiatry* 1993a; **150**:916–21.

Jorge RE, Robinson RG, Starkstein SE *et al.* Depression and anxiety following traumatic brain injury. *J Neuropsychiatry Clin Neurosci* 1993b; **5**:369–74.

Kahana E, Liebowitz U, Alter M. Cerebral multiple sclerosis. *Neurology* 1971; 21:1179–85.

Kant R, Smith-Seemiller L, Zeiler D. Treatment of aggression and irritability after head injury. *Brain Inj* 1998; **12**:661–6.

Kaplitz SE. Withdrawn, apathetic geriatric patients responsive to methylphenidate. *J Am Geriatr Soc* 1975; **23**:271–6.

Karpati G, Frame B. Neuropsychiatric disorders in primary hyperparathyroidism. *Arch Neurol* 1964; **10**:387–97.

Kathol RG, Delahunt JW. The relationship of anxiety and depression to symptoms of hyperthyroidism using operational criteria. *Gen Hosp Psychiatry* 1986; **8**:23–8.

Kelly WF. Psychiatric aspects of Cushing's syndrome. *Q J Med* 1996; **89**:543–51.

Kent TA, Wilber RD. Single case study: reserpine withdrawal psychosis: the possible role of denervation supersensitivity of receptors. *J Nerv Ment Dis* 1982; **170**:502–4.

Khanna R, Borde M. Mania in a five-year-old child with tuberous sclerosis. *Br J Psychiatry* 1989; **155**:117–19.

Kim E, Bijlani M. A pilot study of quetiapine treatment of aggression due to traumatic brain injury. *J Neuropsychiatry Clin Neurosci* 2006; **18**:547–9.

Kirubakaren V, Mayfield D, Rengachary S. Dyskinesia and psychosis in a patient following baclofen withdrawal. *Am J Psychiatry* 1984; **141**:692–3.

Klatka LA, Louis ED, Schiffer RB. Psychiatric features in diffuse Lewy body disease: a clinicopathologic study using Alzheimer's disease and Parkinson's disease comparison groups. *Neurology* 1996; **47**:1148–52.

Krauss MR, Schafer A, Faller H *et al.* Psychiatric symptoms in patients with chronic hepatitis C receiving inteferon alfa–2b therapy. *J Clin Psychiatry* 2003; **64**:708–14.

Kraepelin E. *Manic depressive insanity and paranoia*, 1921, translated by Barclay RM. New York: Arno Press, 1976.

Kryzhanovskaya LA, Jeste DV, Young CA *et al.* A review of treatment emergent adverse events during olanzapine clinical trials in elderly patients with dementia. *J Clin Psychiatry* 2006; **67**:933–45.

Kulisevsky J, Berthier ML, Pujol J. Hemiballismus and secondary mania following right thalamic infarction. *Neurology* 1993; **43**:1422–4.

Kulisevsky J, Asuncion A, Berthier ML. Bipolar affective disorder and unilateral parkinsonism after a brainstem infarction. *Movement Disord* 1995; **10**:799–802.

Kumar R, Issacs S, Meltzer E. Recurrent post-partum psychosis: a model for prospective clinical investigation. *Br J Psychiatry* 1983; **142**:618–20.

Kuramochi H, Takahashi R. Psychopathology of LSD intoxication: study of experimental psychosis induced by LSD–25: description of LSD symptoms in normal oriental subjects. *Arch Gen Psychiatry* 1964; **11**:151–61.

Kurlan R, Cummings J, Raman R *et al.* Quetiapine for agitation or psychosis in patients with dementia and parkinsonism. *Neurology* 2007; **68**:1356–63.

Kwentus JA, Silverman JJ, Sprague M. Manic syndrome after metrizamide myelography. *Am J Psychiatry* 1984; **141**:700–2.

Labbatte LA, Holzgang AJ. Manic syndrome after discontinuation of methyldopa. *Am J Psychiatry* 1989; **146**:1075–6.

Lahey FH. Non-activated (apathetic) type of hyperthyroidism. *N Engl J Med* 1931; **204**:747–8.

Lawlor BA. Hypocalcemia, hypoparathyroidism, and organic anxiety syndrome. *J Clin Psychiatry* 1988; **49**:317–18.

Lee S, Chow CC, Wing Yk *et al.* Mania secondary to thyrotoxicosis. *Br J Psychiatry* 1991; **159**:712–13.

Lendvai I, Saravay SM, Steinberg MD. Creutzfeldt–Jakob disease presenting as secondary mania. *Psychosomatics* 1999; **40**:524–5.

Lesem MD, Zajecka JM, Swift RH *et al.* Intramuscular ziprasidone, 2 mg versus 10 mg, in the short-term management of agitated psychotic patients. *J Clin Psychiatry* 2001; **62**:12–18.

Levy ML, Miller BL, Cummings JL *et al.* Alzheimer disease and frontotemporal dementias. Behavioral distinctions. *Arch Neurol* 1996; **53**:687–90.

Levy ML, Cummings JL, Fairbanks LA *et al.* Apathy is not depression. *J Neuropsychiatry Clin Neurosci* 1998; **10**:314–19.

Liebson E. Anosognosia and mania associated with right thalamic hemorrhage. *J Neurol Neurosurg Psychiatry* 2000; **68**:107–8.

Liegghid NE, Yeragani VK. Buspirone-induced hypomania. *J Clin Psychopharmacol* 1988; **8**:226–7.

Lim L, Ron MA, Ormerod IEC *et al.* Psychiatric and neurological manifestations in systemic lupus erythematosus. *Q J Med* 1988; **66**:27–38.

Lin J T-Y, Ziegler DK. Psychiatric symptoms with initiation of carbidopa-levodopa treatment. *Neurology* 1976; **26**:699–700.

Linder J, Brismar K, Granberg P-O *et al.* Characteristic changes in psychiatric symptoms, cortisol and melatonin but not prolactin in primary hyperparathyroidism. *Acta Psychiatr Scand* 1988; **78**:32–40.

Lipsey JR, Spencer WC, Rabins PV *et al.* Phenomenological comparison of functional and post-stroke depression. *Am J Psychiatry* 1986; **143**:527–9.

Litvan I, Mega MS, Cummings JL *et al.* Neuropsychiatric aspects of progressive supranuclear palsy. *Neurology* 1996; **47**:1184–9.

Loudon JB, Blackburn IM, Ashworth CM. A study of the symptomatology and course of manic illness using a new scale. *Psychol Med* 1977; **7**:723–9.

Louie AK, Lannon RA, Rutzick EA *et al.* Clinical feaures of cocaine-induced panic. *Biol Psychiatry* 1996; **40**:938–40.

Lyons PR, Newman PK, Saunders M. Methylprednisolone therapy in multiple sclerosis: a profile of adverse effects. *J Neurol Neurosurg Psychiatry* 1988; **51**:285–7.

MacCrimmon DJ, Wallace JE, Goldberg WM *et al.* Emotional disturbances and cognitive deficits in hyperthyroidism. *Psychosom Med* 1979; **41**:331–40.

MacHale SM, O'Rourke SJ, Wardlaw JM *et al.* Depression and its relation to lesion location after stroke. *J Neurol Neurosurg Psychiatry* 1998; **64**:371–4.

McDaniel JS, Musselman DL, Proter MR. Depression in patients with cancer. *Arch Gen Psychiatry* 1995; **52**:89–99.

McElroy SL, Keck PE, Stanton SP *et al.* A randomized comparison of divalproex oral loading versus haloperidol in the initial treatment of acute psychotic mania. *J Clin Psychiatry* 1996; **57**:142–6.

McGilchrist I, Goldstein LH, Jadresic D *et al.* Thalamo-frontal psychosis: a case report. *Br J Psychiatry* 1993; **163**:113–15.

McKeith I, Fairbarin A, Perry R *et al.* Neuroleptic sensitivity in patients with senile dementia of Lewy body type. *BMJ* 1992; **305**:1158–9.

McLachlan RS, Blume WT. Isolated fear in complex partial status epilepticus. *Ann Neurol* 1980; **8**:639–41.

Malamud N. Psychiatric disorder with intracranial tumors of the limbic system. *Arch Neurol* 1967; **17**:113–23.

Malinow KC, Lion JR. Hyperaldosteronism (Conn's disease) presenting as depression. *J Clin Psychiatry* 1979; **40**:358–9.

Mandel MR, Severe JB, Schooler NR *et al.* Development and prediction of postpsychotic depression in neuroleptic-treated schizophrenia. *Arch Gen Psychiatry* 1982; **39**:197–203.

Mann AM, Hutchinson JL. Manic reaction associated with procarabazine hydrochloride therapy of Hodgkin's disease. *CM AJ* 1967; **97**:1350–3.

Mattox JH, Buckman MT, Bernstein J *et al.* Dopamine agonists for reducing depression associated with hyperprolactinemia. *J Reproduct Med* 1986; **31**:694–8.

Maxwell S, Scheftner WA, Kessler HA *et al.* Manic syndrome associated with zidovudine treatment. *JAMA* 1988; **259**:3406–7.

Mayeux R, Stern Y, Williams JBW *et al.* Clinical and biochemical features of depression in Parkinson's disease. *Am J Psychiatry* 1986; **143**:756–9.

Mehan KM, Wang H, David SR et al. Comparison of rapidly acting intramuscular olanzapine, lorazepam, and placebo: a double-blind, randomized study in acutely agitated patients with dementia. Neuropsychopharmacology 2002; 26:494–504.

Mellman TA, Uhde TW. Sleep panic attacks: new clinical findings and theoretical implications. Am J Psychiatry 1989; 146:1204–7.

Mendez MF, Cummings JL, Benson DF. Depression in epilepsy. Significance and phenomenology. Arch Neurol 1986; 43:766–70.

Merritt H, Springlova M. Lissauer's dementia paralytica: a clinical and pathologic study. Arch Neurol Psychiatry 1932; 27:987–1030.

Miguel EC, Rodriguez Pereira RM, de Braganca Pereira CA et al. Psychiatric manifestations of systemic lupus erythematosus: clinical features, symptoms, and signs of central nervous system activity in 43 patients. Medicine 1994; 73:224–32.

Millefiorini E, Padovani A, Pozzilli C et al. Depression in the early phase of MS: influence of functional disability, cognitive impairment and brain abnormalities. Acta Neurol Scand 1992; 86:354–8.

Miller WC, McCurdy L. A double-blind comparison of the efficacy and safety of lorazepam and diazepam in the treatment of the acute alcohol withdrawal syndrome. Clin Ther 1984; 6:364–71.

Millman RP, Fogel BS, McNamara ME et al. Depression as a manifestation of obstructive sleep apnea: reversal with nasal continuous positive airway pressure. J Clin Psychiatry 1989; 50:348–51.

Minden SL, Orav J, Schildkraut JJ. Hypomanic reactions to ACTH and prednisone treatment for multiple sclerosis. Neurology 1988; 38:1631–4.

Modlin IM, Farndon JR, Shepherd A et al. Pheochromocytomas in 72 patients: clinical and diagnostic features, treatment and long-term results. Br J Surg 1979; 66:456–65.

Moller A, Wiedemann G, Rohde U et al. Correlates of cognitive impairment and depressive mood disorder in multiple sclerosis. Acta Psychiatr Scand 1994; 89:117–21.

Morris RLP, Robinson RG, Raphael B et al. Lesion location and poststroke depression. J Neuropsychiatr Clin Neurosci 1996; 8:399–403.

Moscovich DG, Singh MB, Efa FJ et al. Acute disseminated encephalomyelitis presenting as an acute psychotic state. J Nerv Ment Dis 1995; 183:116–17.

Mula M, Trimble MR, Yuen A et al. Psychiatric adverse events during levetiracetam therapy. Neurology 2005; 61:704–6.

Mula PL, Robinson RG, Raphael B et al. Lesion location and poststroke depression. J Neuropsychiatry Clin Neurosci 1996; 8:399–403.

Mulder DW, Daly D. Psychiatric symptoms associated with lesions of temporal lobe. JAMA 1952; 150:173–6.

Munoz RA. Postpartum psychosis as a discrete entity. J Clin Psychiatry 1985; 46:182–4.

Murphy TL, Chalmers TC, Eckhardt RD et al. Hepatic coma: clinical and laboratory observations on 40 patients. N Engl J Med 1948; 239:605–12.

Musselman DL, Lawson DH, Gumnick JF et al. Paroxetine for the prevention of depression induced by high-dose interferon-alfa. N Engl J Med 2001; 344:961–6.

Mysiw WJ, Jackson RD, Corrigan JD. Amitryptiline for post-traumatic agitation. Am J Phys Med Rehabil 1988; 67:29–33.

Navarro V, Vieta E, Gasto C. Mannitol-induced acute manic state. J Clin Psychiatry 2001; 62:126.

Neilley LK, Goodin DS, Goodkin DE et al. Side effect profile of interferon beta-1b in MS: results of an open-label trial. Neurology 1996; 46:552–4.

Newburn G, Newburn D. Selegiline in the management of apathy following traumatic brain injury. Brain Inj 2005; 19:149–54.

Nickel SN, Frame B. Neurologic manifestations of myxedema. Neurology 1958; 8:511–17.

Nishida T, Kudo T, Inoue Y et al. Postictal mania versus postictal psychosis: differences in clinical features, epileptogenic zone, and brain functional changes during postictal period. Epilepsia 2006; 47:2104–14.

Nisita C, Petracca A, Akiskal HS et al. Delimitation of generalized anxiety disorder: clinical comparisons with panic and major depressive disorder. Compr Psychiatry 1990; 31:409–15.

Nizamie SH, Mizamie A, Borde M et al. Mania following head injury: case reports and neuropsychological findings. Acta Psychiatr Scand 1988; 77:637–9.

O'Brien CP, DiGiacomo JN, Fahn J et al. Mental effects of high-dose levodopa. Arch Gen Psychiatry 1971; 24:61–4.

O'Dowd MA, McKegney FP. Manic syndrome associated with zidovudine. JAMA 1988; 260:3587–8.

Oliver JE. Huntington's chorea in Northamptonshire. Br J Psychiatry 1970; 116:241–53.

Olin JT, Fox LS, Pawluczyk S et al. A pilot randomized trial of carbamazepine for behavioral symptoms in treatment-resistant outpatients with Alzheimer disease. Am J Geriatr Psychiatry 2001; 9:400–5.

Papolos DF, Faedda GL, Veit S et al. Bipolar spectrum disorders in patients diagnosed with velo-cardio-facial syndrome: does a hemizygous deletion of chromosome 22q11 result in bipolar affective disorder? Am J Psychiatry 1996; 153:1541–7.

Parker N. Manic-depressive psychosis following head injury. Med J Aust 1957; 2:20–2.

Paskavitz JF, Anderson CA, Filley CM et al. Acute arcuate fiber demyelinating encephalopathy following Epstein–Barr virus infection. Ann Neurol 1995; 38:127–31.

Patten SB, Klein GM, Lussier C et al. Organic mania induced by phenytoin: a case report. Can J Psychiatry 1989; 34:457.

Paul R, Flanigan TP, Tashima K et al. Apathy correlates with cognitive function but not CD4 status in patients with human immunodeficiency virus. J Neuropsychiatry Clin Neurosci 2005; 17:114–18.

Perini GI, Tosin C, Carraro C et al. Interictal mood and personality disorders in temporal lobe epilepsy and juvenile myoclonic epilepsy. J Neurol Neurosurg Psychiatry 1996; 61:601–5.

Perry TL, Bratty PJA, Hansen S et al. Hereditary mental depression and parkinsonism with taurine deficiency. Arch Neurol 1975; 32:108–13.

Petersen P. Psychiatric disorders in primary hyperparathyroidism. J Clin Endo Metab 1968; 28:1491–5.

Petrie WM, Maffucci RJ, Woosley RL. Propranolol and depression. Am J Psychiatry 1982; 139:93–4.

Pfohl B, Vasquez N, Nasrallah H. Unipolar vs. bipolar mania: a review of 247 patients. *Br J Psychiatry* 1982; **141**:453–8.

Pine DS, Douglas CJ, Charles E *et al.* Patients with multiple sclerosis presenting to psychiatric hospitals. *J Clin Psychiatry* 1995; **56**:297–306.

Pitt B. Maternity blues. *Br J Psychiatry* 1973; **122**:431–3.

Pluck GC, Brown RG. Apathy in Parkinson's disease. *J Neurol Neurosurg Psychiatry* 2002; **73**:636–42.

Pollack MH, Rosenbaum JF, Cassem NH. Brief communication: propranolol and depression revisited: three cases and a review. *J Nerv Ment Dis* 1985; **173**:118–19.

Pollock BG, Mulsant BH, Rosen J *et al.* Comparison of citalopram, perphenazine, and placebo for the acute treatment of psychosis and behavioral disturbances in hospitalized, demented patients. *Am J Psychiatry* 2002; **159**:460–5.

Pope HG, Katz DL. Affective and psychotic symptoms associated with anabolic steroid use. *Am J Psychiatry* 1988; **145**:487–90.

Pope HG, Katz DL. Homicide and near-homicide by anabolic steroid users. *J Clin Psychiatry* 1990; **51**:28–31.

Pope HG, Katz DL. Psychiatric and medical effects of anabolic-androgenic steroid use: a controlled study of 160 athletes. *Arch Gen Psychiatry* 1994; **51**:375–82.

Pope HG, Lipinski JF, Cohen BM *et al.* 'Schizoaffective disorder': an invalid diagnosis? A comparison of schizoaffective disorder, schizophrenia and affective disorder. *Am J Psychiatry* 1980; **137**:921–7.

Powell E. Two fatal cases of acute chorea with insanity. *Brain* 1889; **12**:157–60.

Powell JH, al-Adawi S, Morgan J *et al.* Motivational deficits after brain injury: effects of bromocriptine in 11 patients. *J Neurol Neurosurg Psychiatry* 1996; **60**:416–21.

Porsteinsson AP, Tariot PN, Erb R *et al.* Placebo-controlled study of divalproex for agitation in dementia. *Am J Geriatr Psychiatry* 2001; **9**:58–66.

Price WA, Bielfeld M. Buspirone-induced mania. *J Clin Psychopharmacol* 1989; **9**:150–1.

Pujol J, Leal S, Fluvia X *et al.* Psychiatric aspects of normal pressure hydrocephalus. *Br J Psychiatry* 1989; **154** (suppl. 4):77–80.

Pujol J, Bello J, Deus J *et al.* Lesions in the left arcuate fasciculus region and depressive symptoms in multiple sclerosis. *Neurology* 1997; **49**:1105–10.

Pushpal D, Shamhul HN. Tiagabine withdrawal-emergent mania. *Aust N Z J Psychiatry* 2006; **40**:719.

Quetsch RM, Achor RWP, Litin EM *et al.* Depressive reactions in hypertensive patients. *Circulation* 1959; **19**:366–75.

Rabins PV, Brooks BR, O'Donnell P *et al.* Structural brain correlates of emotional disorder in multiple sclerosis. *Brain* 1986; **109**:585–97.

Raison CL, Borisov AS, Broadwell SD *et al.* Depression during pegylated interferon-alpha plus ribaverin therapy: prevalence and presentation. *J Clin Psychiatry* 2005; **66**:41–8.

Reaser EF. Chorea of infectious origin. *South Med J* 1940; **33**:1324–8.

van Reekum R, Bayley M, Garner S *et al.* N of 1 study: amantadine for the amotivational syndrome in a patient with traumatic brain injury. *Brain Inj* 1995; **9**:49–53.

Reinfrank RF. Primary hyperparathyroidism with depression. *Arch Int Med* 1961; **108**:162–6.

Reoux JP, Saxon AJ, Malte CA *et al.* Divalproex sodium in alcohol withdrawal: a randomized double-blind placebo-controlled trial. *Alcohol Clin Exp Res* 2001; **25**:1324–9.

Rickels K, Schweizer E, Case W *et al.* Long-term therapeutic use of benzodiazepines. I: Effects of abrupt discontinuation. *Arch Gen Psychiatry* 1990; **47**:899–907.

Rickles NK. Functional symptoms as first evidence of pancreatic disease. *J Nerv Ment Dis* 1945; **101**:566–71.

Rifkin AR, Quitkin F, Klein DF. Akinesia: a poorly recognized drug-induced extrapyramidal behavioral disorder. *Arch Gen Psychiatry* 1975; **32**:672–4.

Robinson RG, Kubos KL, Starr LB *et al.* Mood changes in stroke patients: relationship to lesion location. *Compr Psychiatry* 1983; **24**:555–66.

Robinson RG, Kubos KL, Starr LB *et al.* Mood disorders in stroke patients. *Brain* 1984; **107**:81–93.

Robinson RG, Lipsey JR, Bolla-Wilson K *et al.* Mood disorders in left-handed stroke patients. *Am J Psychiatry* 1985; **142**:1424–9.

Robinson RG, Bolduc P, Price TR. A two year longitudinal study of post-stroke depression: diagnosis and outcome at one and two year follow-up. *Stroke* 1987; **18**:837–43.

Robinson RG, Boston JD, Starkstein SE *et al.* Comparison of mania and depression after brain injury: causal factors. *Am J Psychiatry* 1988; **145**:172–8.

Rohde LA, Busnello E, Wolf A *et al.* Maternity blues in Brazilian women. *Acta Psychiatr Scand* 1997; **95**:231–5.

Rosenthal NE, Rosenthal LN, Stallone F *et al.* Psychosis as a predictor of response to lithium maintenance treatment in bipolar affective disorder. *J Affect Disord* 1979; **1**:237–45.

Rosenthal NE, Rosenthal LN, Stallone F *et al.* Toward the validation of RDC schizoaffective disorder. *Arch Gen Psychiatry* 1980; **37**:804–10.

Roth RM, Flashman LA, Saykin AJ *et al.* Apathy in schizophrenia: reduced frontal lobe volume and neuropsychological deficits. *Am J Psychiatry* 2004; **161**:157–9.

Rubinsztein JS, Rubinsztein DC, Goodburn S *et al.* Apathy and hypersomnia are common features of myotonic dystrophy. *J Neurol Neurosurg Psychiatry* 1998; **64**:510–15.

Ryback RS, Schwab RS. Manic response to levodopa therapy: report of a case. *N Engl J Med* 1971; **285**:788–9.

Sackeim HA, Greenberg MS, Weman AI *et al.* Hemispheric asymmetry in the expression of positive and negative emotions: neurologic evidence. *Arch Neurol* 1982; **39**:210–18.

Sale I, Kalucy P. Psychosis associated with oral contraceptive-induced chorea. *Med J Aust* 1981; **1**:79–80.

Sasaki Y, Matsuyama T, Inoue S *et al.* A prospective, open-label, flexible-dose study of quetiapine in the treatment of delirium. *J Clin Psychiatry* 2003; **64**:1316–21.

Sawyer DR, Connor CS, Rumack BH. Managing acute toxicity from nonprescription stimulants. *Clin Pharm* 1982; **1**:529–33.

Sayed AJ. Mania and bromism: a case report and a look to the future. *Am J Psychiatry* 1976; **133**:228–9.

Sazgar M, Carlen PL, Wennberg R. Panic attack semiology in right temporal lobe epilepsy. *Epileptic Disord* 2003; **5**:93–100.

Schiffer RB, Babigian H. Behavioral disorders in multiple sclerosis, temporal lobe epilepsy, and amyotrophic lateral sclerosis: an epidemiologic study. *Arch Neurol* 1984; **41**:1067–9.

Schiffer RB, Caine ED, Bamford KA *et al*. Depressive episodes in patients with multiple sclerosis. *Am J Psychiatry* 1983; **140**:1498–500.

Schneider LS, Tariot PN, Dagerman KS *et al*. Effectiveness of atypical antipsychotic drugs in patients with Alzheimer's disease. *N Engl J Med* 2006; **355**:1525–38.

Schottenfeld RS, Cullen MR. Organic affective illness associated with lead intoxication. *Am J Psychiatry* 1984; **141**:1425–6.

Shaskan D. Mental changes in chorea minor. *Am J Psychiatry* 1938; **95**:193–202.

Shulman KI, Tohen M. Unipolar mania revisited: evidence from an elderly cohort. *Br J Psychiatry* 1994; **164**:547–9.

Shulman RB, Scheftner WA, Mayudu S. Velafaxine-induced mania. *J Clin Psychopharmacol* 2001; **21**:239–41.

Siegal FP. Lithium for steroid-induced psychosis. *N Engl J Med* 1978; **299**:155–6.

Singh A, Althoff R, Martineau RJ *et al*. Pramipexole, ropinirole, and mania in Parkinson's disease. *Am J Psychiatry* 2005; **162**:814–15.

Sival RC, Haffmans PM, Jansen PA *et al*. Sodium valproate in the treatment of aggressive behavior in patients with dementia: a randomized placebo controlled clinical trial. *Int J Geriar Psychiatry* 2002; **17**:579–85.

Skrobik YK, Bergeron N, Dumont M *et al*. Olanzapine vs halopcridol: treating delirium in a critical care setting. *Intensive Care Med* 2004; **30**:444–9.

Slyter H. Idiopathic hypoparathyroidism presenting as dementia. *Neurology* 1979; **29**:393–4.

Spillane JD. Nervous and mental disorders in Cushing's syndrome. *Brain* 1951; **74**:72–94.

Starkman MN, Schteingart DE, Schork MA. Depressed mood and other psychiatric manifestations of Cushing's syndrome: relationship to hormone levels. *Psychosom Med* 1981; **43**:3–18.

Starkman MN, Zelnick TC, Nesse RM *et al*. Anxiety in patients with pheochromocytomas. *Arch Int Med* 1985; **145**:248–52.

Starkstein SE, Robinson RG, Price TR. Comparison of cortical and subcortical lesions in the production of poststroke mood disorders. *Brain* 1987a; **110**:1045–59.

Starkstein SE, Pearlson GD, Boston J *et al*. Mania after brain injury: a controlled study of causative factors. *Arch Neurol* 1987b; **44**:1069–73.

Starkstein SE, Robinson RG, Berthier ML *et al*. Differential mood changes following basal ganglia versus thalamic lesions. *Arch Neurol* 1988a; **45**:725–30.

Starkstein SE, Boston JD, Robinson RG. Mechanism of mania after brain injury: 12 case reports and review of the literature. *J Nerv Ment Dis* 1988b; **176**:87–100.

Starkstein SE, Preziosis TJ, Bolduc PL *et al*. Depression in Parkinson's disease. *J Nerv Ment Dis* 1990a; **178**:27–31.

Starkstein SE, Mayberg HS, Berthier ML *et al*. Mania after brain injury: neuroradiological and metabolic findings. *Ann Neurol* 1990b; **27**:652–9.

Starkstein SE, Cohen BS, Federoff P *et al*. Relationship between anxiety disorders and depressive disorders in patients with cerebrovascular injury. *Arch Gen Psychiatry* 1990c; **47**:785–9.

Starkstein SE, Federoff JP, Price TR *et al*. Apathy following cerebrovascular lesions. *Stroke* 1993; **24**:1625–30.

Starkstein SE, Chemerinski E, Sabe L *et al*. Prognostic longitudinal study of depression and anosognosia in Alzheimer's disease. *Br J Psychiatry* 1997; **171**:47–52.

Starkstein SE, Petracca G, Chemerinski E *et al*. Syndromic validity of apathy in Alzheimer's disease. *Am J Psychiatry* 2001; **158**:872–7.

Starkstein SE, Jorge R, Mizrahi R *et al*. The construct of minor and major depression in Alzheimer's disease. *Am J Psychiatry* 2005a; **162**:2086–93.

Starkstein SE, Ingram L, Garau ML *et al*. On the overlap between apathy and depression in dementia. *J Neurol Neurosurg Psychiatry* 2005b; **76**:1070–4.

Starkstein WE, Jorge R, Mizrahi R *et al*. A propspective longitudinal study of apathy in Alzheimer's disease. *J Neurol Neurosurg Psychiatry* 2006; **77**:8–11.

Stern K, Dancey TE. Glioma of the diencephalon in a manic patient. *Am J Psychiatry* 1942; **98**:716–19.

Stern RA, Bachman DL. Depressive symptoms following stroke. *Am J Psychiatry* 1991; **148**:351–6.

Stoll Al, Mayer PV, Kolbrener M *et al*. Antidepressant-associated mania: a controlled comparison with spontaneous mania. *Am J Psychiatry* 1994; **151**:1642–5.

Storm-Mathisen A. General paresis: a follow-up study of 203 patients. *Acta Psychiatr Scand* 1969; **45**:118–32.

Street JS, Clark WS, Gannnon KS *et al*. Olanzapine treatment of psychotic and behavioral symptoms in patients with Alzheimer disease in nursing care facilities: a double-blind, randomized, placebo-controlled trial. The HGEU Study Group. *Arch Gen Psychiatry* 2000; **57**:968–76.

Stuppacek CH, Pycha R, Miller C *et al*. Carbamazepine versus oxazepam in the treatment of alcohol withdrawal: a double-blind study. *Alcohol Alcoholism* 1992; **27**:153–8.

Sullivan KL, Ward CL, Zesiewicz TA. Zonisamide-induced mania in essential tremor patient. *J Clin Psychopharmacol* 2006; **26**:439–40.

Sultzer DL, Gray KF, Gunay I *et al*. A double-blind comparison of trazodone and haloperidol for treatment of agitation in patients with dementia. *Am J Geriatr Psychiatry* 1997; **5**:60–9.

Supino-Viterbo V, Sicard C, Risvegliato M *et al*. Toxic encephalopathy due to ingestion of bismuth salts: clinical and EEG studies of 45 patients. *J Neurol Neurosurg Psychiatry* 1977; **40**:748–52.

Surridge D. An investigation into some psychiatric aspects of multiple sclerosis. *Br J Psychiatry* 1969; **115**:749–64.

Tamir A, Whittier J, Korenys C. Huntington's chorea: a sex difference in psychopathological symptoms. *Dis Nerv Syst* 1969; **30**:103.

Tariot PN, Erb R, Podgorski CA *et al*. Efficacy and tolerability of carbamazepine for agitation and aggression in dementia. *Am J Psychiatry* 1998; **155**:54–61.

Tariot PN, Raman R, Jakimovich L *et al*. Divalproex sodium in nursing home residents with possible or probably Alzheimer disease complicated by agitation: a randomized, controlled trial. *Am J Geriatr Psychiatry* 2005; **13**:942–9.

Taylor JW. Depression in thyrotoxicosis. *Am J Psychiatry* 1975; **132**:552–3.

Taylor MA, Abrams R. The phenomenology of mania: a new look at some old patients. *Arch Gen Psychiatry* 1973; **29**:520–2.

Taylor MA, Abrams R. Catatonia: prevalence and importance in the manic phase of manic-depressive illness. *Arch Gen Psychiatry* 1977; **34**:1223–5.

Teri L, Logsdon RG, Peskind E *et al.* Treatment of agitation in AD: a randomized, placebo-controlled trial. *Neurology* 2000; **55**:1271–8.

Thomas FB, Mazzaferri EL, Skillman TG. Apathetic thyrotoxicosis: a distinctive clinical and laboratory entity. *Ann Intern Med* 1970; **72**:679–85.

Thomas JE, Rooke ED, Kuale WF. The neurologist's experience with pheochromocytoma: a review of 100 cases. *J Am Med Assoc* 1966; **197**:754–8.

Tohen M, Ketter TA, Zarate CA *et al.* Olanzapine versus divalproex sodium in the treatment of acute mania. *Am J Psychiatry* 2002; **159**:1011–17.

Tonks CM. Mental illness in hypothyroid patients. *Br J Psychiatry* 1964; **110**:706–10.

Torriani FJ, Rodriguez-Turres M, Rockstroh JK *et al.* Peginterferon alfa-2a plus ribaverinfor chronic hepatitis C in HIV-infected patients. *N Engl J Med* 2004; **351**:438–50.

Tran-Johnson TK, Sack DA, Marcus RN *et al.* Efficacy and safety of intramuscular aripiprazole in patients with acute agitation: a randomized, double-blind, placebo-controlled trial. *J Clin Psychiatry* 2007; **68**:111–19.

Trautner RJ, Cummings JL, Read SL *et al.* Idiopathic basal ganglia calcification and organic mood disorder. *Am J Psychiatry* 1988; **145**:350–3.

Trembath PW, Boobis SW. Plasma theophylline levels after sustained-release aminophylline. *Clin Pharmacol Ther* 1979; **26**:654–9.

Trzepacz P, McCue M, Klein I *et al.* A psychiatric and neuropsychological study of patients with untreated Graves' disease. *Gen Hosp Psychiatry* 1988; **10**:49–55.

Van Der Hurst L. Rheumatism and psychosis. *Digest Neurol Psychiatry* 1947; **15**:399–416.

Van Putten T, May PRA. 'Akinetic depression' in schizophrenia. *Arch Gen Psychiatry* 1978; **35**:1101–7.

Van Woert MH, Ambani LM, Weintraub MI. Manic behavior and levodopa. *N Engl J Med* 1971; **285**:1326.

Varadaraj R, Cooper AJ. Addison's disease presenting with psychiatric features. *Am J Psychiatry* 1986; **143**:553–4.

Vazquez A, Jimenez-Jimenez FJ, Garcia-Ruiz P *et al.* 'Panic attacks' in Parkinson's disease. *Acta Neurol Scand* 1993; **87**:14–18.

Verhey FR, Verkaaik M, Lousberg R. Olanzapine versus haloperidol in the treatment of agitation in elderly patients with dementia: results of a randomized controlled double-blind trial. *Dement Geriatr Cogn Disord* 2006; **21**:1–8.

Wagner KD. Major depression and anxiety disorders associated with Norplant. *J Clin Psychiatry* 1996; **57**:152–7.

Wagner KD, Berenson AB. Norplant-associated major depression and panic disorder. *J Clin Psychiatry* 1994; **55**:478–80.

Walton RG. Seizure and mania after high intake of aspartame. *Psychosomatics* 1986; **27**:218–20.

Wang PS, Schneeweiss S, Avorn J *et al.* Risk of death in elderly users of conventional vs atypical antipsychotic medicines. *N Engl J Med* 2005; **353**:2335–41.

Warren AC, Holyroyd S, Folstein MF. Major depression in Down's syndrome. *Br J Psychiatry* 1989; **155**:202–5.

Watanabe MD, Martin EM, DeLeon OA *et al.* Successful methylphenidate treatment of apathy after subcortical infarcts. *J Neuropsychiatry Clin Neurosci* 1995; **7**:502–4.

Watson R, Hartmann E, Schildkraut JJ. Amphetamine withdrawal: affective state, sleep patterns, and MHPG excretion. *Am J Psychiatry* 1972; **129**:263–9.

Weddington WW, Brown BS, Haertzen CA *et al.* Changes in mood, craving, and sleep during short-term abstinence reported by male cocaine addicts. *Arch Gen Psychiatry* 1990; **47**:861–8.

Weil AA. Ictal depression and anxiety in temporal lobe disorders. *Am J Psychiatry* 1956; **113**:149–57.

Weller M, Liedtke W, Petersen D *et al.* Very-late-onset adrenoleukodystrophy: possible precipitation of demyelination by cerebral contusion. *Neurology* 1992; **42**:367–70.

Whitlock FA, Siskind MM. Depression as a major symptom of multiple sclerosis. *J Neurol Neurosurg Psychiatry* 1980; **43**:861–5.

Whybrow PC, Prange AJ, Treadway CR. Mental changes accompanying thyroid gland dysfunction. *Arch Gen Psychiatry* 1969; **20**:48–63.

Wier LM, Tavares SB, Tyrka AR *et al.* Levetiracetam-induced depression in a healthy adult. *J Clin Psychiatry* 2006; **67**:1159–60.

Williams D. The structure of emotions reflected in epileptic experiences. *Brain* 1956; **79**:29–67.

Wilson P, Preece AA. Chorea gravidarum. *Arch Int Med* 1932; **49**:671–97.

Winokur G. Psychosis in bipolar and unipolar affective illness with special reference to schizo-affective disorder. *Br J Psychiatry* 1984; **145**:236–42.

Winokur G, Tsuang MT. Elation versus irritability in mania. *Compr Psychiatry* 1975; **16**:435–6.

Winokur G, Clayton PJ, Reich T. *Manic-depressive illness*. St Louis, MA: CV Mosby, 1969.

Winokur G, Coryell W, Endicott J *et al.* Further distinctions between manic-depressive illness (bipolar disorder) and primary depressive disorder (unipolar depression). *Am J Psychiatry* 1993; **150**:1176–81.

Wolkowitz OM, Rubinow D, Doran AR *et al.* Prednisone effects on neurochemistry and behavior. *Arch Gen Psychiatry* 1990; **47**:963–8.

Wright JM, Sachdev PS, Perkins RJ *et al.* Zidovudine related mania. *Med J Aust* 1989; **150**:339–41.

Wright P, Birkett M, David SR *et al.* Double-blind, placebo-controlled comparison of intramuscular olanzapine and intramuscular haloperidol in the treatment of acute agitation in schizophrenia. *Am J Psychiatry* 2001; **158**:1149–51.

Wroblewski BA, Joseph AB, Kupfer J *et al.* Effectiveness of valproic acid on destructive and aggressive behaviors in patients with acquired brain injury. *Brain Inj* 1997; **11**:37–47.

Wysowski DK, Pitts M, Beiz J. Depression and suicide in patients treated with isotretinoin. *N Engl J Med* 2001; **344**:460.

Yalom ID, Lunde DT, Moos RH *et al.* 'Postpartum blues' syndrome: a description and related variables. *Arch Gen Psychiatry* 1968; **18**:16–27.

Zeidler M, Johnstone EC, Bamber RWK *et al.* New variant Creutzfeldt–Jakob disease: psychiatric features. *Lancet* 1997a; **350**:908–10.

Zeidler M, Stewart GE, Barraclough CR *et al.* New variant Creutzfeldt–Jakob disease: neurological features and diagnostic tests. *Lancet* 1997b; **350**:903–7.

Zhong KX, Tariot PN, Mintzer J *et al.* Quetiapine to treat agitation in dementia: a randomized, double-blind, placebo-controlled study. *Curr Alzheimer Res* 2007; **4**:81–93.

Zimbroff DL, Marcus RN, Manos G *et al.* Management of acute agitation in patients with bipolar disorder: efficacy and safety of intramuscular aripiprazole. *J Clin Psychopharmacol* 2007; **27**:171–6.

7

Other major syndromes

7.1 PSYCHOSIS

The term psychosis has been used differently by different authors, and this has led to some confusion in the literature. In this text, psychosis refers to a condition characterized by hallucinations (without insight) and/or delusions, in the absence of either significant cognitive deficits or pronounced disturbances of mood.

Clinical features

Delusions and hallucinations are discussed at length in Section 4.30, and readers unfamiliar with these are encouraged to consult that chapter. Although in most cases of psychosis both delusions and hallucinations are present, exceptions do occur; thus in some disorders, for example delusional disorder, one may find only delusions, whereas in the psychosis caused by levodopa in patients with parkinsonian conditions one may find only hallucinations. Critically, as discussed in Section 4.30, in cases characterized by only hallucinations the diagnosis of psychosis should be reserved for situations wherein insight is absent and patients react to their hallucinations as if they were real.

Depending on the cause of the psychosis, other symptoms may also be present; however, the part they play in the overall clinical picture is relatively minor compared with the delusions and hallucinations. Thus there may be some incoherence, minor mood changes, anxiety, or even agitation.

Etiology

The various causes of psychosis are listed in Table 7.1, in which they are divided into several groups. The first group, composed of *idiopathic disorders*, constitutes by far the most common causes of psychosis and of these schizophrenia is

the most frequent. Next are the *toxic psychoses*, for example those seen with stimulants such as amphetamine or cocaine. *Endocrinologic psychoses*, such as the 'myxedema madness' of hypothyroidism, are considered next, followed by various *intracranial disorders* capable of causing psychosis, such as stroke or tumors. Consideration is then given to the various *epileptic psychoses* and then to *encephalitic and post-encephalitic psychoses*. Finally, there is a *miscellaneous* group, including the 'megaloblastic madness' that may be seen with vitamin B12 deficiency.

IDIOPATHIC DISORDERS

Schizophrenia is by far the most common cause of chronic psychosis. The onset typically occurs in the late teens or early twenties with the subacute or gradual elaboration of a psychosis characterized by varying combinations of hallucinations, delusions, incoherence, and bizarre behavior. In many cases, the symptomatology will crystallize into an enduring and recognizable subtype: paranoid, hebephrenic, catatonic, or simple (Fenton and McGlashen 1991; Kendler *et al.* 1994). Although the symptoms gradually wax and wane over time, the illness is generally chronic and lifelong, probably never going into a spontaneous and full remission.

Schizoaffective disorder is, like schizophrenia, characterized by a chronic psychosis: the difference is that in schizoaffective disorder one also finds recurrent episodes of either depression or mania, during either of which the chronically present psychotic symptoms undergo a significant exacerbation.

Delusional disorder, also like schizophrenia, is characterized by a chronic psychosis: here, however, hallucinations, incoherence, and bizarre behavior are negligible or absent, with the primary or sole symptom of the illness being one or more delusions. Importantly, these delusions are not bizarre but indeed have a certain plausibility to

Table 7.1 Causes of psychosis

Idiopathic disorders	**Tumors**
Schizophrenia	Frontal lobe
Schizoaffective disorder	Corpus callosum
Delusional disorder	Temporal lobe
Post-partum psychosis	Multiple sclerosis
Obsessive–compulsive disorder	Traumatic brain injury
Body dysmorphic disorder	Heredodegenerative disorders:
Borderline personality disorder	Huntington's disease
	Dentatorubropallidoluysian atrophy
Toxic psychoses	Spinocerebellar ataxia
Amphetamine	Wilson's disease
Cocaine	Miscellaneous
Hallucinogens	Creutzfeldt–Jakob disease
Phencyclidine	Fatal familial insomnia
Cannabis	Fahr's syndrome
Anabolic steroids	Aqueductal stenosis
Chronic alcoholism (alcoholic paranoia, alcoholic hallucinosis)	
Neuroleptic-induced supersensitivity psychosis ('tardive psychosis')	**Epileptic psychoses**
	Ictal psychosis
Dopaminergics (levodopa, bromocriptine, lergotrile, pramipexole)	Post-ictal psychosis
	Chronic interictal psychosis
Levetiracetam	Psychosis of forced normalization
Topiramate	
Vigabatrin	**Encephalitic and post-encephalitic psychoses**
Phenylpropanolamine	Encephalitic
Phenylephrine	Herpes simplex encephalitis
Bupropion	Infectious mononucleosis
Fluoxetine	Encephalitis lethargica
Disulfiram	Post encephalitic
Methysergide	Herpes simplex encephalitis
Manganese intoxication	Encephalitis lethargica
Baclofen withdrawal	
	Miscellaneous
Endocrinologic psychoses	Vitamin B12 deficiency
Hypothyroidism	Neurosyphilis
Hyperthyroidism	AIDS
Cushing's syndrome	Systemic lupus erythematosus
Adrenocortical insufficiency	Sydenham's chorea
	Chorea gravidarum
Intracranial disorders	Hepatic porphyria
Stroke	Metachromatic leukodystrophy
Temporal lobe	Velocardiofacial syndrome
Frontal lobe	Vanishing white matter leukoencephalopathy
Thalamus	Subacute sclerosing panencephalitis
	Prader–Willi syndrome

them (Kendler 1980; Opjordsmoen and Rettersol 1991; Winokur 1977). Certain variants of this disorder deserve special mention: parasittosis is characterized by a persistent belief that one is infested by some parasitic bug or other (Andrews *et al.* 1986; Mitchell 1989) and the olfactory reference syndrome by a delusion that one is emitting a foul odor (e.g., as in halitosis or flatus) that others detect and comment on (Videbech 1966).

Post-partum psychosis may appear between several days and several months post-partum and is often characterized by prominent agitation (Bagedahl-Strindlund 1986). Importantly, it is not uncommon for certain disorders, such as schizophrenia, to undergo an exacerbation post-partum, and such patients should not receive an additional diagnosis of post-partum psychosis.

The following disorders, namely obsessive–compulsive disorder, body dysmorphic disorder, and borderline personality disorder, although generally not associated with delusions and hallucinations, may at times cause these symptoms and hence are included here.

Both obsessive–compulsive disorder (Eisen and Rasmussen 1993; Gordon 1950; Insel and Akiskal 1986) and body dysmorphic disorder (McElroy *et al.* 1993) may have psychotic subtypes wherein patients 'lose insight' and come to accept their troubling ideas as true. Thus, a patient with obsessive–compulsive disorder might come to believe that his troubling need to pray recurrently was, in fact, ordained by God (Gordon 1950) or a patient with body dysmorphic disorder may come to believe that his or her face was, in fact, deformed.

Patients with a borderline personality disorder may, when under great stress, develop transient auditory hallucinations or delusions of persecution (Chopra and Beatson 1986): such patients are distinguished by the chronic characteristic traits of intolerance of being alone, anger, impulsivity, and disturbed relationships (Gunderson and Kolb 1978).

TOXIC PSYCHOSES

Amphetamines, if taken in a sufficiently high dose, may cause a psychosis (Bell 1973; Griffith *et al.* 1972) that is typically characterized by delusions of persecution and often of reference. Hallucinations may also occur, being much more commonly auditory than visual. The psychosis typically clears within a week, but in some cases longer durations of up to 3 months have been reported (Iwanami *et al.* 1994).

Cocaine may cause a psychosis characterized by hallucinations, more often auditory than visual, and delusions of persecution and reference (Brady *et al.* 1991; Satel *et al.* 1991; Sherer *et al.* 1988). Although such a psychosis may occur in 'recreational' users (Siegel 1978), it is more characteristic of addicts, who often note that a progressively lower 'dose' becomes capable of inducing the psychosis (Brady *et al.* 1991). Although, in most cases, the psychosis clears either with the intoxication itself or shortly thereafter, it may persist in some until after the withdrawal 'crash' resolves (Satel *et al.* 1991).

Hallucinogens, such as LSD, typically cause visual hallucinations, but most patients remain aware of their unreality. In a minority, however, the intoxication will be complicated by delusions of persecution (Bercel *et al.* 1956; Kuramochi and Takahashi 1964).

Phencyclidine intoxication may render patients agitated and psychotic (Allen and Young 1978), with delusions of grandeur or persecution and auditory hallucinations. The finding of nystagmus is a very important diagnostic clue.

Cannabis intoxication, if a sufficiently high dose is taken, may be characterized by fearfulness and delusions of persecution and reference (Kroll 1975; Thacore and Shukla 1976) that may outlast the intoxication itself by a matter of days.

Anabolic steroids, as may be abused by athletes, may, in a small minority, cause a psychosis variously characterized by delusions of persecution or grandeur, delusions of reference, and auditory hallucinations (Pope and Katz 1988).

The appearance of a psychosis in a 'bulked-up' young person should suggest this diagnosis.

Chronic alcoholism may be complicated by two different psychoses: alcoholic paranoia and alcohol hallucinosis. Alcoholic paranoia (Albert *et al.* 1996; Soyka *et al.* 1991) is characterized by the gradual development of delusions, often of either jealousy or persecution. By contrast, alcohol hallucinosis typically appears as a sequela to an alcohol withdrawal delirium: whereas the other symptoms of the delirium tremens (DTs), such as tremor, clear, the auditory hallucinations, often accompanied by delusions of persecution, persist (Soyka 1990; Victor and Hope 1958).

Antipsychotic-induced supersensitivity psychosis appears in a very small minority of patients treated with antipsychotics for a year or more and is characterized by delusions and hallucinations, which may appear either while the patient is still taking the neuroleptic or shortly after discontinuation or a significant dose reduction (Chouinard and Jones 1980; Steiner *et al.* 1990). This psychosis probably has an etiology similar to that of tardive dyskinesia and hence is often referred to as 'tardive psychosis'; like tardive dyskinesia, it exists as a strong reminder not to use antipsychotics chronically unless they are absolutely necessary.

Dopaminergic drugs, such as levodopa or direct-acting agents, for example bromocriptine, ropinirole, or pramipexole, as used in the treatment of parkinsonism, may cause a psychosis. In the case of levodopa (Celesia and Barr 1970; Fenelon *et al.* 2000; Moskovitz *et al.* 1978), the psychosis may occur either upon the initiation of treatment (Lin and Ziegler 1976) or, much more commonly, after 3–4 years (Friedman and Sienkiewicz 1991). This levodopa-induced psychosis may be characterized by hallucinations, often visual but also auditory (Fenelon *et al.* 2000; Inzelberg *et al.* 1998), and, in a minority, delusions of persecution (Graham *et al.* 1997). In the overwhelming majority of cases, patients first experience hallucinations with preserved insight: however, over many months insight is gradually lost, thus producing the syndrome of psychosis (Barnes and David 2001; Goetz *et al.* 2006). Direct-acting dopaminergic drugs may also cause psychosis but this is much less common than with levodopa: bromocriptine, lergotrile (Serby *et al.* 1978), and pramipexole (Almeida and Ranjith 2006) have all been implicated.

The remaining drugs in the list only rarely cause psychosis. These include the anti-epileptic drugs levetiracetam (Mula *et al.* 2003), topiramate (Kober and Gabbard 2005), vigabatrin (Sander *et al.* 1991) (in the case of levetiracetam the onset may, as with the others, occur soon after starting the drug, or may be delayed for up to 3–9 months [Kossoff *et al.* 2001; Motamedi *et al.* 2003]), the sympathomimetics phenylpropanolamine and ephedrine (Lambert 1987), the antidepressants bupropion (Golden *et al.* 1985) and fluoxetine (Mandalos and Szarek 1990), and disulfiram (Bicknell and Moore 1960) and methysergide (Cittandi and Goadsby 2005).

A toxic psychosis may also occur with chronic manganese exposure. This 'manganese madness' may present with a combination of parkinsonism, excitation, delusions, and hallucinations (Abd El Naby and Hassanein 1965).

Finally, note should also be made of a psychosis associated with baclofen. Here, the psychosis occurs not during use of the drug but rather as a withdrawal phenomenon after chronic use. Here, about a week after discontinuation, one may see a psychosis with agitation, delusions of persecution, and hallucinations (Swigar and Bowers 1986), which, in one case, was accompanied by a complex movement disorder, with chorea, tremor, and dystonia being evident (Kirubakaren et al. 1984).

ENDOCRINOLOGIC PSYCHOSES

Hypothyroidism may present with psychosis in a condition known as 'myxedema madness', typically characterized by delusions of persecution and reference and by hallucinations, generally auditory (Asher 1949). The delusions of persecution may at times be so compelling that patients become assaultive (Reed and Bland 1977); in other cases, patients may be reduced to a seclusive 'mumbling' (Karnosh and Stout 1935). Pertinent clues to the correct diagnosis include slowness and a certain 'fogginess' of thought, cold intolerance, deepening of the voice, constipation, hair loss, and myxedema of the face, supraclavicular fossae, and dorsa of the hands and feet.

Hyperthyroidism may be accompanied by a psychosis, with prominent delusions of persecution: in one case, the hyperthyroid patient slashed his throat rather than let his 'persecutors' capture him (Ingham and Nielsen 1931). When the psychosis occurs in the setting of 'thyroid storm' (Bursten 1961; Greer and Parsons 1968), the prominent autonomic signs (increased temperature, tachycardia, and tremor) immediately suggest the diagnosis; however, when the responsible hyperthyroidism is milder, the diagnosis may be elusive (Hodgson et al. 1992).

Cushing's syndrome may be characterized by a psychosis, the diagnosis being suggested by the typical cushingoid habitus of moon facies, truncal obesity, buffalo hump, violaceous abdominal striae, and so on. One patient had classic Schneiderian first rank symptoms, including audible thoughts, thought broadcasting, and thought insertion (Trethowan and Cobb 1952), whereas another presented with auditory hallucinations and delusions of a grandiose and religious nature (Hertz et al. 1955).

Adrenocortical insufficiency is suggested by abdominal complaints (nausea, vomiting, diarrhea or constipation, and abdominal pain) and orthostatic hypotension with postural dizziness. A psychosis may rarely also be seen (Cleghorn 1951; McFarland 1963).

INTRACRANIAL DISORDERS

The various intracranial disorders capable of causing psychosis include stroke, tumors, multiple sclerosis, traumatic brain injury (TBI), various heredodegenerative disorders, such as Huntington's disease, and a miscellaneous group.

Stroke

Stroke may be characterized by the fairly sudden onset of psychosis: this has been noted with infarction of the temporal lobe (Peroutka et al. 1982); in one case (Thompson and Nielsen 1949), the patient, a 58-year-old man, suddenly began to hear 'unusual noises which he believed were caused by wires placed in his house', and soon after, 'while in a restaurant, he suddenly declared that someone had put ground glass into his food. He then ran out of the restaurant into the street, shouting that his son-in-law had been killed after having been held captive by a gang of criminals'. Frontal lobe involvement may also be found: in one case of a ruptured frontal lobe aneurysm, a 23-year-old woman presented acutely with auditory hallucinations, delusions of persecution, and loosening of associations (Hall and Young 1992). Finally, thalamic infarction involving the right dorsomedial area was, in one case (Feinberg and Rapcsak 1989), associated with vivid visual hallucinations; indeed, the patient 'reached down to pat the dog' that he had hallucinated at his side.

Tumors

Tumors may present with psychosis, as has been noted with tumors of the frontal lobe (Strauss and Keschner 1935), corpus callosum (Murthy et al. 1997), and especially the temporal lobe (Gal 1958; Keschner et al. 1936; Malamud 1967; Strobos 1953; Tucker et al. 1986). In contrast with stroke, the onset here is typically subacute or gradual.

Multiple sclerosis

Multiple sclerosis may cause psychosis (Geocaris 1957; Langworthy et al. 1941; Mathews 1979), generally in the company of signs suggestive of disseminated lesions (e.g., concurrent with nystagmus [Parker 1956]). Rarely, multiple sclerosis may present with a psychosis, as in one patient who developed 'mystic' hallucinations and religious delusions, who eventually was found to have compatible lesions on magnetic resonance (MR) scanning (Fontaine et al. 1994).

Traumatic brain injury

TBI may also be followed by psychosis (Buckley et al. 1993; Hillbom 1951; Nasrallah et al. 1981), and in some cases there may be a long delay, even up to years, between the injury and the onset of the psychosis (Fujii and Ahmed 2002; Sachdev et al. 2001).

Heredodegenerative disorders

Of the heredodegenerative disorders capable of causing psychosis, Huntington's disease is the classic example; others include dentatorubropallidoluysian atrophy, spinocerebellar ataxia, and Wilson's disease. Of note each of these is also characterized, at some point, by abnormal movements.

Huntington's disease is not uncommonly characterized by a combination of chorea and psychosis (Bolt 1970; Garron 1973; Heathfield 1967) and, albeit rarely, the disease may present with a psychosis (Caine and Shoulson 1983; Garron 1973; James *et al.* 1969): in such cases, the correct diagnosis may be suggested by a positive family history and confirmed by genetic testing.

Dentatorubropallidoluysian atrophy, another autosomal dominant disorder, may also present with psychosis, accompanied by ataxia and seizures (Adachi *et al.* 2001).

Spinocerebellar ataxia, also an autosomal dominant disorder characterized by ataxia, may also cause a psychosis with delusions of persecution (Chandler and Bebin 1956). In one family (Benton *et al.* 1998), the disorder presented with auditory hallucinations and delusions, eventually being joined by abnormal movements.

Finally, Wilson's disease must be considered in young adults with psychosis and a movement disorder (Beard 1959; Gysin and Cooke 1950; Jackson and Zimmerman 1919). It must also be kept in mind that, albeit rarely, the initial presentation of Wilson's disease may be with a psychosis, with a movement disorder appearing only much later, as indeed was the case with one of Wilson's first patients (Wilson 1912).

Miscellaneous

Of the miscellaneous disorders capable of causing psychosis, consideration may first be given to Creutzfeldt–Jakob disease (Brown *et al.* 1984; Dervaux *et al.* 2004; Zeng *et al.* 2001) (especially the new-variant type [Zeidler *et al.* 1997a]), which may present with psychosis, with the diagnosis finally being suggested by the appearance of myoclonus or a dementia. Fatal familial insomnia, a rare inherited prion disease, in one case also presented with a psychosis, accompanied, true to the name of the disease, by severe insomnia (Dimitri *et al.* 2006).

Fahr's syndrome, suggested by extensive calcification of the basal ganglia, may rarely present with psychosis, as in one familial case wherein the illness was manifest symptomatically with basal ganglia calcification on imaging and a chronic psychosis (Francis and Freeman 1984).

Aqueductal stenosis, one of the causes of noncommunicating hydrocephalus, has also been associated with a psychosis (Roberts *et al.* 1983).

EPILEPTIC PSYCHOSES

The various psychoses seen in epileptics may be distinguished by their relationship to the seizures experienced by the patient. Ictal psychoses are in fact seizures and are immediately suggested by their paroxysmal onset. Post-ictal psychoses, as the name suggests, follow seizures and, critically, are separated from the last seizure by a 'lucid' interval. The psychosis of forced normalization represents a paradoxical event in that it appears when the patient's seizures are finally brought under control with anti-epileptic treatment. Finally, chronic interictal psychosis occurs in the setting of a chronically uncontrolled seizure disorder.

Ictal psychosis consists of a complex partial seizure wherein, in addition to some defect of consciousness, there

are delusions and hallucinations (Ellis and Lee 1978; Wells 1975): the diagnosis is suggested by the paroxysmal onset of the psychosis and its relative brevity.

Post-ictal psychosis (Briellman *et al.* 2000; Kanner *et al.* 1996; Lancman *et al.* 1994; Leutmezer *et al.* 2003; Logsdail and Toone 1988; Nishida *et al.* 2006; Savard *et al.* 1991; Umbricht *et al.* 1995) may follow a bout of seizures and, critically, is separated from the last seizure by a 'lucid' interval, lasting from hours to days, during which the patient's mental status is 'clear'. The psychosis itself is characterized by delusions of persecution and hallucinations, most commonly auditory, and may last for hours or months, although most patients clear spontaneously within a matter of days. Most patients have a long history of recurrent complex partial seizures.

Chronic interictal psychosis may occur in the setting of chronic epilepsy, generally of over a decade in duration. Either insidiously or subacutely, patients develop a psychosis with delusions, often of persecution and reference, auditory hallucinations and various other symptoms, all of which occur in the setting of a clear sensorium (Fluger *et al.* 2006; Kristensen and Sindrup 1979; Perez and Trimble 1980; Slater and Beard 1963a,b).

Of note post-ictal psychosis and chronic interictal psychosis may exist in the same patient, and in such cases either the chronic interictal psychosis or post-ictal psychoses may appear first (Adachi *et al.* 2003).

Psychosis of forced normalization is a rare condition, first described by Landolt (1953, 1958) and characterized by the appearance of a psychosis *after* anti-epileptic drugs (Pakainis *et al.* 1987) or, in one case, vagus nerve stimulation (Gatzonis *et al.* 2000), have controlled the seizure disorder and 'normalized' the electroencephalogram (EEG).

ENCEPHALITIC AND POST–ENCEPHALITIC PSYCHOSES

Psychosis may either be directly caused by a viral encephalitis or occur as a sequela.

Viral encephalitis is suggested by fever, headache, and lethargy, and may in some cases present with psychosis, as has been noted with herpes simplex encephalitis (Drachman and Adams 1962; Johnson *et al.* 1972; Williams and Lerner 1978; Wilson 1976) and infectious mononucleosis (Raymond and Williams 1948). Encephalitis lethargica may present similarly (Kirby and Davis 1921; Meninger 1926; Sands 1928) and is suggested by sleep reversal and oculomotor pareses.

Viral encephalitis may also leave a psychosis in its wake, and such postencephalitic psychoses have been noted as sequelae to herpes simplex encephalitis (Rennick *et al.* 1973) and encephalitis lethargica (Fairweather 1947).

MISCELLANEOUS

A large number of miscellaneous causes of psychosis also exists, first among which is 'megaloblastic madness' due to vitamin B12 deficiency, with this colorful name being derived from the associated megaloblastic anemia. It must be borne in mind, however, that this anemia may not be present: in one case, the diagnosis became clear only when symptoms of subacute combined degeneration appeared (Smith 1929), and in another, the only evidence of vitamin B12 deficiency was the psychosis itself: there was no anemia and no evidence of spinal cord involvement (Evans et al. 1983).

Neurosyphilis rarely presents with a psychosis (Rothschild 1940; Schube 1934), and the diagnosis may remain elusive until other, more typical symptoms appear, such as a dementia, pupillary changes (e.g., Argyll Robertson pupil), tremor, or seizures.

Acquired immunodeficiency syndrome (AIDS) may cause a psychosis (Bulrich et al. 1988; Harris et al. 1991), and the presence of other AIDS-related illnesses, such as thrush or Pneumocystis pneumonia may serve to suggest the correct diagnosis. Rarely, AIDS may present with psychosis (Thomas and Szabadi 1987), and in such cases the diagnosis may prove elusive until other, more typical, features of AIDS make their appearance.

Systemic lupus erythematosus may also cause psychosis (Brey et al. 2002; Devinsky et al. 1988a; Johnson and Richardson 1968; Lim et al. 1988; Miguel et al. 1994) and although this usually occurs in the context of other symptoms, such as arthralgia, rash, pericarditis, or pleurisy, psychosis may rarely constitute the presenting feature of lupus (Agius et al. 1997).

Sydenham's chorea may rarely be complicated by a psychosis with hallucinations and delusions (Hammes 1922; Putzel 1879): the diagnosis is immediately suggested by the context of subacutely developing chorea in a child or adolescent.

Chorea gravidarum, Latin for 'chorea of pregnant women', may, rarely, be accompanied by psychosis (Beresford and Graham 1950; Wilson and Preece 1932). The diagnosis should be suspected in pregnant women with psychosis, chorea, and a history of Sydenham's chorea.

Hepatic porphyria typically presents in attacks accompanied by abdominal pain, often with vomiting and constipation or, less commonly, diarrhea. Rarely, such patients may also have a psychosis (Mandoki and Sumner 1994), which, in one case, was accompanied by bizarre behavior (Hirsch and Dunsworth 1955).

Metachromatic leukodystrophy, although rare, is of particular interest in that it can cause a psychosis that *very* closely resembles that caused by schizophrenia (Hyde et al. 1992; Muller et al. 1969). Indeed, in some cases, it was not initially possible to distinguish between the two disorders until other symptoms suggestive of metachromatic leukodystrophy, as for example a peripheral neuropathy (Manowitz et al. 1978) or a dementia (Betts et al. 1968a; Rauschka et al. 2006; Waltz et al. 1987) developed years later.

Velocardiofacial syndrome has also attracted great interest, as it too can cause a psychosis symptomatically quite similar to that caused by schizophrenia (Gothelf et al. 2007; Ivanov et al. 2003; Murphy et al. 1999). The diagnosis may be suggested by the characteristic dysmorphic facies with hypertelorism, a bulbous nose, and micrognathia.

Vanishing white matter leukoencephalopathy is an autosomal recessively inherited disorder, which, in adults, may present with a psychosis very similar to that seen in schizophrenia (Denier et al. 2007): the diagnosis may be suggested by evidence of bilateral corticospinal tract damage, and confirmed by finding extensive white matter disease in the cerebral hemispheres.

Subacute sclerosing panencephalitis, a vanishingly rare disease in developed countries thanks to measles vaccination, may cause psychosis and myoclonus (Cape et al. 1973; Salib 1988) or may present with a psychosis, the diagnosis only becoming clear with the later appearance of a delirium (Duncalf et al. 1989; Koehler and Jakumeit 1976).

Prader–Willi syndrome, a rare disorder characterized by massive obesity and dysmorphic facies, may rarely cause a psychosis with delusions and hallucinations (Clarke 1993).

Differential diagnosis

Delusions and hallucinations may be found in a number of other syndromes, namely dementia, delirium, depression, and mania, and thus the first task is to determine if one of these syndromes is present, and, if so, to then pursue the differential for that syndrome, as discussed in the respective chapters.

Dementia and delirium are both marked by significant cognitive deficits, such as decreased short-term memory and disorientation, and, in the case of delirium, confusion. Delusions and hallucinations are quite common in both syndromes, and in some instances, for example diffuse Lewy body disease, they may constitute a diagnostic hallmark.

Both depression and mania, when they are severe, may be characterized by delusions or hallucinations; however, in both these instances the delusions or hallucinations occur within the context of the mood syndrome, and, upon getting a reliable history, one always finds, prior to the onset of the delusions or hallucinations, a prominent and progressively worsening depressive or manic syndrome.

Finally, simulated psychoses, as seen in malingering, factitious illness, and *folie à deux* must be distinguished from 'true' psychoses. Malingerers may simulate a psychosis in order to avoid unpleasant consequences, as may occur in prisoners facing trial (Tsoi 1973). Factitious psychosis is said to occur when the simulation has the purpose of simply being a patient in the hospital (Pope et al. 1982). *Folie à deux* is said to occur when a person with a true psychosis, usually paranoid schizophrenia, exerts such a profound influence on close relatives or acquaintances that they come to adopt the patient's own delusional beliefs as true. Importantly, in such cases, if the 'truly' psychotic person is successfully treated or if a prolonged separation is enforced, the others gradually come to see the falseness of their beliefs (Dewhurst and Todd 1956; Kashiwase and Kato 1997; Partridge 1950; Waltzer 1963).

Treatment

Treatment is directed at the underlying cause; in cases when that is ineffective or where symptomatic treatment is required, an antipsychotic is indicated. In general, second-generation antipsychotics are more effective and better tolerated than first-generation agents and, of the second-generation agents, risperidone, olanzapine, or quetiapine are reasonable choices. In general, and especially in the elderly or medically frail, or patients with hepatic failure, it is appropriate to 'start low and go slow' with regard to initial dose and subsequent titrations. In the case of levodopa-induced psychosis wherein dose reduction is often not feasible, good success has been had with clozapine, in low doses of 6.25–25 mg/day. In cases where emergent treatment is required, one may proceed as described in Section 6.4.

7.2 PERSONALITY CHANGE

Every individual has a definite personality structure, which, once formed in childhood and adolescence, persists in a lifelong fashion, being very resistant to any modification. Thus, the appearance of a fundamental change in personality, that is to say a far-reaching transformation of the patient's characteristic personality traits, is an ominous clinical sign and demands prompt diagnostic evaluation.

Clinical features

The personality change may be non-specific and characterized either by a marked exaggeration of pre-existing personality traits or by the emergence of altogether new traits, previously foreign to the patient. For example, a characteristically financially prudent person may become stingy to the point of miserliness. In another example, a previously outgoing and generous person may gradually become withdrawn and miserly; or, conversely, a premorbidly shy and timid person may become freer in personal contacts and even outgoing. In addition to this non-specific personality change there are also two specific types of personality change, namely the frontal lobe syndrome and the inter-ictal personality syndrome, both discussed below. Regardless, however, of which kind of personality change occurs, those around the patient often make comments such as 'he's not himself anymore', and indeed it may be this realization that leads family members to bring the patient to medical attention.

FRONTAL LOBE SYNDROME

The frontal lobe syndrome is characterized by varying combinations of disinhibition, affective change (euphoria, irritability, or depressed mood), perseveration, and apathy.

Disinhibited patients seem to lose regard for customs or morals: they may eat with gluttony, curse with no regard for company, and tell coarse and crude jokes. Inappropriate sexual advances are not uncommon, and patients may, with no hint of shame, proposition much younger individuals, even at times children. Some may engage in reckless masturbation, at the dinner table or in the front yard.

Affective changes may have some lateralizing value: euphoria is seen more often with right-sided lesions and depressed mood with left-sided lesions. The euphoria may occasionally be accompanied by *witzelsucht*, or a tendency to make simple, silly puns.

Perseveration is characterized by a tendency to repeat the same behavior over and over: examples include repeatedly uttering the same phrase, opening and closing a book, or buttoning and unbuttoning a shirt.

Apathy is characterized by a lack of motivation. Although patients may experience some urges or consider some actions, their plans, if they occur at all, often come, as it were, stillborn, and, lacking in motivation, apathetic patients may either never come to the point of action or, if they do get started, soon find themselves indifferent, after which they give up.

These clinical features often, but not always, coalesce into one of two subtypes, namely the orbitofrontal and dorsolateral frontal lobe syndromes: the orbitofrontal subtype is characterized by disinhibition and affective changes (often either euphoria or irritability) and the dorsolateral type by perseveration and apathy.

The frontal lobe syndrome is also often accompanied by what is known as the 'dysexecutive syndrome', which represents, as one might expect from the name, a disturbance in 'executive' abilities. Thus, patients with these executive deficits have difficulty in the following areas: formulating and setting goals, developing plans to meet these goals, initiating planned behavior, and, lastly, monitoring and correcting activity when it gets 'off course'. Patients with these executive deficits may not come to attention until they are faced with new, and relatively complex, situations. Thus, patients whose lives are passed in fixed routines, where habit rules the day, may have little difficulty. However, if faced with an unaccustomed task, as for example planning a formal dinner or developing a financial plan, they may find themselves unable to successfully complete the work in front of them.

Some examples may help to fix the picture of the frontal lobe syndrome. The classic case is that of Phineas Gage (Neylan 1999), who manifested disinhibition and irritability. As reported by his physician (Harlow 1848), on 3 September 1848, while Gage was tamping down an explosive charge with a special 'tamping iron', the charge exploded, blowing the iron rod back up and through his skull, causing extensive frontal lobe damage. Prior to the injury, Gage had been a foreman, capable, well balanced, and an exemplary worker. Twenty years later, however, Harlow (1868) found him to be 'irreverent, indulging at times in the grossest profanity (which was not previously his custom), manifesting but little deference for his fellows, impatient of restraint or advice when it conflicts with his desires . . . In this regard his mind was so radically changed . . . that his friends and acquaintances said he was "no longer Gage." '

Mulder *et al.* (1951) reported another case marked by disinhibition and irritability. The patient's wife complained that the patient:

no longer cared about his appearance, that he drove through red lights, threw bills in the wastebasket remarking they were 'only bills', and frequently threatened to harm his family. He spilled his food on his clothing and on the floor, and to his family's dismay, he then picked it up and ate it. He did not wait for food to be served, but would snatch it off platters with his fingers as his wife neared the table. His sexual activity became uninhibited, and he sought intercourse with neighborhood children and prostitutes with no concern for possible consequences.

Another case (Moersch 1925) was marked by perseveration and apathy. The patient, a 54-year-old man was:

brought to the clinic . . . Because of loss of bladder and rectal control, and lack of interest. The patient himself made no complaint. About three months before, a gradually increasing mental change had been observed. The patient lost his ambition and interest in work, although he had continued at his trade of carpentry until two weeks before. He had become careless in his work, would forget what he was doing, and seemed little concerned about his short-comings. For two weeks before his examination he had been content to sit aimlessly at home, or to play with his children. He voided at any time and even defecated in his clothes . . . During general examination, the patient was indifferent and aimless, would sit and look at a newspaper, which might be upside down. He was oriented in all spheres, and his attention might be held for a few moments when aroused. He would follow his son about in a fairly good-natured manner, but always object to being examined, saying that he was not sick. He showed considerable perseveration, repeating movements at times for long periods. For example, one evening he sat before a wash bowl for over a half hour, turning the faucets on and off.

INTERICTAL PERSONALITY SYNDROME

The interictal personality syndrome, also known as the Geschwind syndrome, is said to appear insidiously in epileptics after years of uncontrolled complex partial seizures. It should be emphasized that this is a controversial entity and that it has not as yet been possible to prove conclusively that such a specific syndrome exists. Nevertheless, the clinical

impression of many is that it does occur and that it may have a profound effect on patients' lives.

The outstanding characteristic of this syndrome is a trait known variously as 'viscosity', 'adhesiveness' or 'stickiness' (Waxman and Geschwind 1975). In this, patients seem unable to break away from a train of thought or a certain emotion, thoughts and feelings plodding on and adhering to one another in a sort of viscous mass. Bleuler (1924), writing of epileptics in the early part of the twentieth century, asserted that:

the most conspicuous anomaly concerns the *affectivity*, which reacts to a morbid degree, and at the same time shows the peculiarity, that an existing affect lasts a long time and is difficult to divert by new impressions; *it is not merely irritability that shows itself in this manner but the other affects, as attachments, or joy, all take the same course* . . . In *speaking* and *writing* we have the same peculiarities: the patient does not get anywhere with his talking, not only because of its slowness, but especially because of its circumstantiality, which must depict all trivialities in repetition and in manifold expression of the same idea in different forms. Besides this the manner of speaking is verbose and clumsy, and always vague. (Italics in original.)

Bear *et al.* (1982), in addition to this viscosity of thought and emotion, also emphasized an 'interpersonal adhesiveness' manifest in 'interpersonal clinging' and a 'tendency to draw out interpersonal encounters'. In some cases, patients, on shaking hands while saying goodbye to the physician, will simply continue to 'hang on', requiring the physician to extricate him or herself.

The viscosity of thought may have a written expression in hypergraphia, wherein patients may write voluminous amounts, far and above what is required for any social or professional purposes (Hermann *et al.* 1988), often writing about philosophic or religious concerns (Waxman and Geschwind 1974).

In addition to viscosity, patients also tend to be preoccupied with religious, ethical, or philosophical concerns and to experience hyposexuality.

Religiosity is, according to Maudsley (1874) 'often very notable in epileptics' and Kraepelin (1902), writing in the early part of the twentieth century, noted that 'the religious content of [epileptic's] thought is another striking symptom, many patients spending a large part of their time in reading the Bible or praying aloud'. Bear *et al.* (1982) noted the 'nascent metaphysical or cosmological preoccupations' of patients.

Hyposexuality manifests primarily as a loss of libido (Blumer 1970; Blumer and Walker 1967).

As noted earlier, the interictal personality syndrome is a controversial entity. Early attempts to validate it (Bear 1979; Bear and Fedio 1977) made use of a complex rating instrument, and subsequent attempts to replicate these

Table 7.2 Criteria for the diagnosis of the interictal personality syndrome (all five elements, A–E, must be present)

A	The patient's behavior represents an enduring change in personality.
B	The disorder occurs after 3 or more years of repeated complex partial seizures.
C	The patient displays viscosity, as manifested by one or more of: deep and persistent affects; verbose, overly detailed, and circumstantial speech; or hypergraphia.
D	The patient displays either a preoccupation with religious, ethical ,or philosophical concerns, or hyposexuality.
E	There are no delusions or hallucinations.

earlier findings met with no success (Mungas 1982, 1983; Nielsen and Kristensen 1981; Rodin and Schmaltz 1984) or only partial success (Bear *et al.* 1982; Hermann and Reil 1981). Provisionally, as I have discussed elsewhere (Moore 1997), the diagnosis should probably be reserved for cases meeting the criteria listed in Table 7.2.

Etiology

The etiologies of the various types of personality change, namely the non-specific type, the frontal lobe syndrome and the interictal personality syndrome, differ, and hence each is discussed separately. As may be seen, however, in regard to the non-specific type and the frontal lobe syndrome, the most common causes are neurodegenerative disorders (e.g., frontotemporal dementia), tumors, and stroke.

NON-SPECIFIC PERSONALITY CHANGE

The various causes of non-specific personality change are listed in Table 7.3, which divides them into three groups. The first group contains those disorders capable of causing a personality change of *subacute or gradual onset*, such as neurodegenerative disorders, tumors, and others (e.g., normal pressure hydrocephalus). The next group recognizes personality change of *acute onset*, as may occur after stroke. Finally, there is a *miscellaneous* group of disorders, including, notably, TBI.

Subacute or gradual onset

Of the neurodegenerative disorders that may present with a personality change, perhaps the most important is frontotemporal dementia. Frontotemporal dementia occurs in two variants, namely the 'temporal variant' and the 'frontal variant'. The frontal variant is discussed below, under the frontal lobe syndrome. In the 'temporal variant', one may see either a Kluver–Bucy syndrome (as discussed in Section 4.12), or a personality change marked by hoarding or stereotyped, ritualistic behavior. Pick's disease may present

Table 7.3 Causes of non-specific personality change

Subacute or gradual onset
Neurodegenerative disorders
 Frontotemporal dementia (Seeley *et al.* 2005)
 Pick's disease (Mendez *et al.* 1993)
 Alzheimer's disease (Mendez *et al.* 1993)
 Huntington's disease (Pflanz *et al.* 1991)
 Wilson's disease (Bridgman and Smyth 1944; Dening and
  Berrios 1989; Starosta-Rubinstein *et al.* 1987; Walshe and
  Yealland 1992)
 Metachromatic leukodystrophy (Finelli 1985; Hageman
  et al. 1995)
 Adrenoleukodystrophy (Schaumburg *et al.* 1975)
Tumors
 Temporal lobe (Keschner *et al.* 1936; Strobos 1953)
 Thalamus (Partlow *et al.* 1992)
 Hypothalamus (Alpers 1937)
Other
 Normal pressure hydrocephalus (Rice and Gendelman 1973)
 Chronic subdural hematoma (Cameron 1978)
 Neurosyphilis (Storm-Mathisen 1969)
 Vitamin B12 deficiency (Lindenbaum *et al.* 1988)
 Limbic encephalitis (Alamowitch *et al.* 1997)
 Creutzfeldt–Jakob disease (Brown *et al.* 1994; Roos *et al.*
  1973; Zeidler *et al.* 1997a,b)
 Mercury intoxication (O'Carroll *et al.* 1995)
 Manganese intoxication (Abd El Naby and Hassanein 1965)

Acute onset
Stroke (Stone *et al.* 2004)

Miscellaneous
Traumatic brain injury (Brooks *et al.* 1986; Thomsen 1984)
Post-viral encephalitis (McGrath *et al.* 1997)

in a similar fashion. Alzheimer's disease may present with a very non-specific personality change. Huntington's disease, rarely, may present with personality change; however, the eventual appearance of chorea will indicate the correct diagnosis. Wilson's disease may also present with a personality change; however, in this case the development of various abnormal movements will also eventually suggest the diagnosis. It is of interest that Wilson's first case (Wilson 1912), a 25-year-old woman, presented with a personality change wherein she became 'restless, unable to settle to anything, easily provoked to laughter, constantly smiling and unnaturally cheerful'. Metachromatic leukodystrophy and adrenoleukodystrophy are two rare disorders that may present with a personality change in adolescence or early adult years.

Tumors productive of a non-specific personality change are most often found in the temporal lobe; rarely a similar presentation may occur with tumors of the thalamus or hypothalamus.

The other causes of non-specific personality change are relatively uncommon. Normal pressure hydrocephalus may be suggested by incontinence and a 'magnetic' gait. Patients with a chronic subdural hematoma may or may not recall any head trauma. Tertiary neurosyphilis may present solely with a personality change, and the diagnosis may only be suspected when the fluorescent treponemal antibody (FTA) test comes back positive. Vitamin B12 deficiency, likewise, may also present with a personality change, which may or may not be accompanied by a macrocytosis or a peripheral neuropathy. Both limbic encephalitis and Creutzfeldt–Jakob disease (especially the new-variant type) may present with a subacute personality change; however, in both cases cognitive changes, either delirium or dementia, supervene fairly quickly. Mercury intoxication with either elemental mercury (as may occur in factories making thermometers [Vroom and Greer 1972]) or organic mercury may cause a personality change known as erethism, with prominent timidity and irritability, often accompanied by tremulousness. Manganism, as may be seen in manganese miners, may present with a personality change marked by asthenia, fatigue, irritability, emotional lability, and a peculiar unmotivated laughter. One author (Charles 1927), in commenting on the laughter, noted that 'excessive smiling without any adequate cause is very common, and the patient, if asked any simple question, will not infrequently burst out into hilarious laughter'; parkinsonism, if not already present, generally supervenes.

Acute onset

Stroke may be followed by a non-specific personality change of relatively acute onset, and this may occur with both cortical and subcortical infarcts. By and large, patients become irritable, easily frustrated and overall less easy going.

Miscellaneous

Both TBI and viral encephalitis (e.g., herpes simplex viral encephalitis) may have personality change as a sequela, and in the case of TBI, this may be the most disabling sequela.

FRONTAL LOBE SYNDROME

As noted in Table 7.4, the various causes may be divided into those that produce a frontal lobe syndrome of *subacute or gradual onset*, as may be seen with various neurodegenerative disorders (e.g., frontotemporal dementia), tumors that produce a frontal lobe syndrome of *acute onset*, as may be seen in stroke, and a *miscellaneous* group, for example TBI.

Subacute or gradual onset

Of the neurodegenerative disorders capable of producing a frontal lobe syndrome, the two most important are frontotemporal dementia and Pick's disease, both of which may present with a frontal lobe syndrome, with the advent of significant cognitive deficits being delayed for months to

Table 7.4 Causes of the frontal lobe syndrome

Subacute or gradual onset
Neurodegenerative disorders
  Frontotemporal dementia (Brun *et al.* 1994; Heutink *et al.* 1997; Neary *et al.* 1993)
  Pick's disease (Boulon 1940; Litvan *et al.* 1997; Mendez *et al.* 1993)
  Alzheimer's disease (Mega *et al.* 1996; Petry *et al.* 1988)
  Amyotrophic lateral sclerosis (Massman *et al.* 1996)
  Corticobasal ganglionic degeneration (Bergeron *et al.* 1996)
  Progressive supranuclear palsy (Verny *et al.* 1996)
  Multiple system atrophy (olivopontocerebellar type) (Critchley and Greenfield 1948)
  Spinocerebellar ataxia (Zeman *et al.* 2004)
  Metachromatic leukodystrophy (Rauschka *et al.* 2006)
Tumors
  Frontal lobe (Avery 1971; Frazier 1936; Hunter *et al.* 1968; Strauss and Keschner 1935; Williamson 1896)
  Corpus callosum (Alpers and Grant 1931; Beling and Martland 1919; Moersch 1925)

Acute onset
Stroke
  Frontal lobe (Logue *et al.* 1968)
  Caudate nucleus (Mendez *et al.* 1989; Petty *et al.* 1996)
  Thalamus (Sandson *et al.* 1991)
  Mesencephalon (Adair *et al.* 1996)

Miscellaneous
Traumatic brain injury (Oder *et al.* 1992; Roberts 1976)
Gunshot wounds (Lishman 1973)
Multiple sclerosis (Blinkenberg *et al.* 1996)
Post-viral encephalitis (Friedman and Allen 1969; Mulder *et al.* 1951)

years. Alzheimer's disease may also present with a frontal lobe syndrome but this is often accompanied early on by the classic short-term memory loss. Amyotrophic lateral sclerosis (ALS) typically, of course, presents with upper and lower motor neuron signs, and in about one-tenth of such typical cases a frontal lobe syndrome will eventually follow; importantly, albeit rarely, ALS may also present with a frontal lobe syndrome (Cavalleri and De Renzi 1994; Neary *et al.* 1990; Peavy *et al.* 1992). The other neurodegenerative disorders in the list, relative to the foregoing, only rarely cause the syndrome. Corticobasal ganglionic degeneration and progressive supranuclear palsy both cause parkinsonism and dementia, and the dementia may be accompanied by a frontal lobe syndrome. Multiple system atrophy (of the olivopontocerebellar type) and spinocerebellar ataxia are both characterized by ataxia and both, rarely, may cause the frontal lobe syndrome. Finally, consideration may be given to the very rare late-onset form of metachromatic leukodystrophy that may present with a frontal lobe syndrome in early adult years and which is eventually superseded by a dementia.

As might be expected, tumors capable of causing the frontal lobe syndrome are found typically in the frontal lobes. Anteriorly placed tumors of the corpus callosum may also cause the syndrome; however, it is suspected that in these cases the syndrome does not occur as a result of damage to the corpus callosum but rather to lateral extension of the tumor into the adjacent medial aspects of the frontal lobes.

Acute onset

When the frontal lobe syndrome appears acutely, stroke should immediately be suspected. Thus, the syndrome may appear after infarction of the frontal lobe (as seen not uncommonly after subarachnoid hemorrhage [Alexander and Freedman 1984; Greene et al. 1995]). In addition, lacunar infarctions of the caudate nucleus, thalamus and, rarely, the mesencephalon, may also produce the syndrome.

Miscellaneous

TBI may leave a frontal lobe syndrome in its wake, often marked by disinhibition and irritability; indeed such a personality change may represent one of the most disabling sequelae of severe TBI (Thomsen 1984). Gunshot wounds to the frontal areas may also, as might be expected, create the syndrome. In one such case, the substitution of the euphoria of the frontal lobe syndrome for the depression that prompted the suicidal gunshot actually constituted an improvement (Lebensohn 1941).

Finally, the syndrome may occur secondary to appropriately situated plaques in multiple sclerosis and as a sequela to a viral encephalitis.

Comments on the localizing and lateralizing value of the frontal lobe syndrome

The frontal lobe exists in a 'circuit' involving the frontal cortex, the caudate nucleus, the lenticular nucleus, and the thalamus, which eventually sends fibers back to the frontal cortex. The frontal lobe syndrome, in general, localizes to this circuit, and may be seen with lesions of the frontal lobe (Frazier 1936; Williamson 1896), caudate nucleus (Mendez et al. 1989; Petty et al. 1996; Richfield et al. 1987), globus pallidus (Strub 1989), and thalamus (Sandson et al. 1991; Smyth and Stern 1938). The ventral tegmental area of the mesencephalon also projects to the frontal cortex and, as noted above, infarction of the mesencephalon may also cause the syndrome (Adair et al. 1996).

The syndrome may not have much lateralizing value: although in most cases, the lesions are bilateral, unilateral lesions may also cause the syndrome, this having been noted with lesions of either the right or left frontal lobe (Frazier 1936; Strauss and Keschner 1935; Williamson 1896), the

right caudate nucleus (Degos et al. 1993), and the left thalamus (Sandson et al. 1991; Smyth and Stern 1938).

INTERICTAL PERSONALITY SYNDROME

If indeed the interictal personality syndrome does exist as a discrete entity, it may then represent a 'functional hyperconnection' (Bear 1979; Bear and Fedio 1977) in the limbic system, which may in turn occur secondary to the 'kindling' effect of frequently repeated seizures (Adamec and Stark-Adamec 1983).

Differential diagnosis

Personality change must be distinguished from a personality *disorder*. Personality disorders, for example borderline personality disorder or antisocial personality disorder, do *not* represent a change in the patient's personality make-up, but rather have been present, at least in a nascent form, since childhood or adolescence. Rather than replacing a pre-existing personality structure, the personality disorder just does, in fact, constitute the patient's lifelong personality. Thus, in the history of an adult patient with a personality disorder, one finds that the various personality traits may be traced back into the patient's adolescence or childhood in a seamless and continuous fashion: by contrast, in a patient with a personality *change*, one finds a more or less distinct boundary in the history that separates the patient's original personality from that which currently exists. Relatives and friends may indicate such a change by saying that the patient is 'not himself' any more.

Dementia may be accompanied by an exaggeration of pre-existing personality traits, or by the emergence of new ones; however, the accompanying cognitive deficits indicate dementia as the primary syndrome, and the differential should then be pursued as discussed in Section 5.1. Importantly, certain dementing disorders, as noted above, may present not with cognitive deficits but with a personality change, and the diagnosis may be elusive until, with further progression, cognitive deficits make their appearance. This is particularly the case, as noted above, with some of the neurodegenerative disorders, most particularly frontotemporal dementia.

Many psychoses also are accompanied by an alteration in the sufferer's personality, this being particularly true of schizophrenia. The psychoses, however, are marked by delusions or hallucinations – symptoms that are not seen in personality change – and their presence should prompt the clinician to refer to the differential diagnosis for psychosis, as discussed in Section 7.1.

Mood syndromes, namely mania and depression, may suggest the frontal lobe syndrome. The euphoria seen in mania may, superficially, appear similar to the euphoria seen in some cases of the frontal lobe syndrome; however, there are some clear differences. The euphoria of mania is heightened, full, and quite infectious, and this is in marked contrast with the shallow, silly euphoria of the frontal lobe syndrome, which lacks any infectiousness. Furthermore, in mania one also sees pressured speech, increased energy, decreased need for sleep and hyperactivity – symptoms lacking in the frontal lobe syndrome. A depressed mood may suggest the syndrome of depression; however, in the frontal lobe syndrome one does not see the characteristic vegetative symptoms of the depressive syndrome, such as changes in sleep or appetite, anergia, or anhedonia.

With regard to the interictal personality syndrome, one must keep in mind that slowly growing tumors in the temporal lobe may present with epilepsy, followed, years later, by a personality change caused by the tumor itself. Thus, the appearance of a personality change in an epileptic should prompt consideration of an MR scan.

Finally, there are two syndromes, namely the environmental dependency syndrome (also known as 'utilization behavior') and the Kluver–Bucy syndrome, which are considered by some to be personality changes: to me, however, they are so dissimilar from any conceivable personality trait or type that they are discussed elsewhere, respectively in Sections 4.11 and 4.12. In the environmental dependency syndrome patients appear to lose their autonomy and become, as it were, 'dependent' on the environment such that they feel compelled to make use of whatever comes to their attention. Thus, if a pen and a piece of paper came to the patient's attention, he would feel compelled to pick them up and write, even although such activity was inappropriate to the ongoing situation. The Kluver–Bucy syndrome, in humans, typically manifests with the traits of hyperorality and hypersexuality. In hyperorality, patients put things into their mouths, whether edible or not, and thus may end up eating Styrofoam cups or drinking urine from urinals. Hypersexuality may manifest with public masturbation or sexual activity with others, regardless of their gender.

Treatment

If possible, treatment is directed at the underlying cause. Most patients require some form of supervision, and in some cases admission to a secure facility may be necessary. Regarding pharmacologic treatment, with the exception of utilizing carbamazepine for the disinhibition of the frontal lobe syndrome (Foster *et al.* 1989), little is known. In practice, antipsychotics (e.g., quetiapine) are also used for disinhibition, and antidepressants (e.g., a selective serotonin reuptake inhibitor, SSRI) or anxiolytics (e.g., lorazepam or clonazepam) are given when depressed mood or anxiety are prominent.

7.3 SEIZURES AND EPILEPSY

A seizure, or ictus, is paroxysmal in onset, generally brief in duration, and occurs secondary to an equally paroxysmal

Table 7.5 Types of seizures

Simple partial
Complex partial (also known as psychomotor)
Petit mal (also known as absence)
Grand mal (also known as generalized tonic–clonic)
Atonic (also known as astatic seizures or 'drop attacks')
Amnestic
Reflex
Status epilepticus

electrical discharge within the cerebral grey matter. Although, as detailed below, the actual symptomatology seen during a seizure and the cause of the responsible electrical discharge are both extraordinarily varied, the essential formal characteristic of the seizure, namely its 'paroxysmal-ness', remains. The term 'epilepsy' is generally reserved for cases in which there has been more than one seizure and the cause of the seizures is such that one may reasonably expect that the patient, in the absence of definitive treatment, will continue to have seizures. Thus, whereas it might not be proper to consider a patient who has only had but one seizure, and that during an episode of severe hypoglycemia, to have epilepsy, it would be appropriate in the case of a patient with recurrent seizures and mesial temporal sclerosis.

Clinical features

The classification of the various seizure types has changed over time, as evidenced by the evolution of criteria set forth by the International League Against Epilepsy (ILAE) in 1964 (Gastaut *et al.* 1964), 1970 (Gastaut 1970), 1981 (Commission of Classification and Terminology 1981), and 1989 (Commission of Classification and Terminology 1989). The 1981 ILAE criteria have proved the most enduring for clinical practice and, with some modification, are adhered to in this text.

The various seizure types are listed in Table 7.5. In differentiating among these types, the first step is to determine the patient's state of consciousness during the seizure. If consciousness remains clear, that is to say the patient remains alert, with intact memory, and without any clouding or confusion, a simple partial seizure is present. If, however, consciousness is in some fashion impaired, but not entirely lost, either a complex partial or a petit mal seizure is present. The distinction between complex partial and petit mal seizures, as elaborated further in the text, is based on the overall nature of the seizure: complex partial seizures are often preceded by an aura, last several minutes, and are typically followed by some post-ictal confusion; whereas petit mal seizures occur without an aura, are very brief – lasting only seconds – and terminate abruptly, without any post-ictal confusion. If consciousness is entirely lost, one is typically dealing with a grand mal seizure, with its accompanying tonic–clonic activity. Atonic seizures may or may not be accompanied by an impairment or loss of consciousness but they are always characterized by an abrupt loss of muscle tone with, in most cases, a resulting fall. Amnestic seizures are unusual in that they are characterized solely by a paroxysmal amnesia in a clear consciousness. Reflex seizures are said to be present when any of the foregoing types occurs on a 'reflexive' basis, being provoked by some specific stimulus, such as hearing music or reading. Finally, each of the foregoing seizure types may also occur over a prolonged time, in which case *status epilepticus* is said to be present.

Although any given patient with epilepsy may experience but one type of seizure during the entire course of the illness, the history more often than not reveals different seizure types at disparate times. Thus, the course of epilepsy may be marked by varying combinations of simple partial, complex partial, and grand mal seizures (Devinsky *et al.* 1988; Golub *et al.* 1951; Mauguire and Courjon 1978; Sperling *et al.* 1989); furthermore, patients with petit mal epilepsy often also experience grand mal seizures (Livingston *et al.* 1965; Sato *et al.* 1976). Of interest, among adults, partial seizures (either simple or complex) are more common than grand mal seizures (Gastaut *et al.* 1975; Kotsopoulos *et al.* 2002).

Importantly, in many cases, a given ictal event or seizure may in fact represent an amalgamation of two different seizure types, the first merging seamlessly into the following one. Thus, a simple partial seizure may immediately precede a complex partial seizure (Bare *et al.* 1994; Sperling *et al.* 1989) or, in other cases, a simple partial seizure may precede a grand mal seizure (Mauguire and Courjon 1978; Theodore *et al.* 1994). In such cases, it is customary no longer to refer to the ictal event that occurred in clear consciousness as a simple partial seizure but rather to speak of it as an 'aura' to the following seizure type. Furthermore, complex partial seizures may also transform without interruption into grand mal seizures (Theodore *et al.* 1994; Tinuper *et al.* 1996a), and in such cases one speaks of the complex partial seizure undergoing 'secondary generalization' into a grand mal seizure.

Each of the various seizure types noted in Table 7.5 is now considered in detail.

SIMPLE PARTIAL SEIZURES

Simple partial seizures usually last of the order of a minute or two, uncommonly extending for up to 5 minutes, and exceptionally persevering for as long as 15 minutes (Devinsky *et al.* 1988b; Mauguire and Courjon 1978). Following the 1981 ILAE criteria, they may be subdivided according to their predominant symptomatology into the following subtypes: simple partial seizures with motor signs, simple partial seizures with somatosensory or special sensory symptoms, simple partial seizures with autonomic symptoms or signs, and simple partial seizures with psychic symptoms. Furthermore, there is a group, not specified in the ILAE criteria, of miscellaneous simple partial seizures.

Simple partial seizures with motor signs

These seizures are most commonly characterized by unilateral clonic or tonic activity, or a combination of the two, such motor activity being seen most frequently in the hand, arm, or face and somewhat less so in the lower extremity (Russell and Whitty 1953). Jacksonian seizures represent a variety of simple partial seizure in which there is a 'march' of the ictal symptomatology from one part of the body to another. Such marches may begin variously in the hands or the fingers, proceed proximally to the face, and then march inferiorly; less commonly, they begin in the lower extremity. In most cases, the march is completed within a matter of minutes (Penfield and Jasper 1954; Russell and Whitty 1953). 'Versive' seizures represent a variety of motor simple partial seizure wherein there is a 'forced' tonic version of the head, and sometimes the trunk, to one side or the other (Mauguire and Courjon 1978; Russell and Whitty 1953). Motor aphasia may be seen in what the ILAE calls a 'phonatory' seizure. Such a motor aphasia may constitute the sole manifestation of the seizure (Labar *et al.* 1992) or may be accompanied by motor activity on the face. In one case (Williamson *et al.* 1985a), the seizure began with right-sided facial twitching followed by muteness: although the patient could follow commands and was still able to communicate by writing, she was unable, much to her distress, to speak. In another case (Walshe 1943), the seizure began with muteness and was 'followed by the advance of the tongue to the line of the teeth and the utterance of a rapid series of "D" sounds (D-D-D-D-D-D). The throat then "constricts", the mouth is drawn to the right and finally the head and eyes turn in a series of jerks to the right'.

Rarely, simple partial seizures with motor signs may be characterized by *bilateral* motor activity (Kanner *et al.* 1990; Tachibana *et al.* 1996). Such seizures often lead to diagnostic uncertainty as they 'break the rule' that bilateral epileptic motor activity is always accompanied by some impairment of consciousness (Morris *et al.* 1988). In one case (Tukel and Jasper 1952): 'seizures began with a stiffness in the right arm and leg. The patient then stared and the right arm raised to the level of the chest. This was followed by the extension of both arms. There was then adversive movement of the head and eyes to the right and vocalization. The patient remained conscious throughout … she heard herself vocalize but could not speak'.

Although the motor behavior in these seizures may be simple, as in the foregoing example, or perhaps involve non-directed thrashing (Salanova *et al.* 1995), it may at times be fairly complex (Chassagnon *et al.* 2003). In one case (Weinberger 1973), the patient's 'head and neck turned to the right. Both arms moved to the right and turned rhythmically on their axis at the wrist in a fashion best described as turning two door knobs, but in opposite directions': although the patient 'was aware of what was happening to her, and could understand what people were saying . . . she could only utter a phrase such as "uh-uh-uh"'. Although in almost all cases such simple partial seizures with bilateral motor signs arise from seizure foci in the supplemental motor area on the medial aspect of the frontal lobe, exceptions do occur, as in a case where the focus was in the parietal lobe (Bell *et al.* 1997).

Inhibitory motor simple partial seizures represent a kind of 'inverse' motor seizure, wherein, rather than seeing tonic or clonic muscle contraction, there is a paroxysmal paresis or paralysis. The hand, arm, or leg may be involved (Noachtar and Luders 1999; Russell and Whitty 1953; Villani *et al.* 2006), and in some cases hemiparesis may result (Globus *et al.* 1982; Hanson and Chodos 1978). The spread of epileptic electrical activity from the precentral gyrus to nearby areas may sometimes produce a more complex picture: in one case, a patient experienced not only ictal paresis of the right upper extremity, but also an associated motor aphasia (Lee and Lerner 1990).

Simple partial seizures with somatosensory or special sensory symptoms

Seizures with somatosensory symptoms are characterized by generally unilateral paresthesiae, numbness, pain, or a sensation of warmth or coldness. The hands and fingers are most frequently affected, followed by the face, foot, or entire upper or lower extremity (Mauguire and Courjon 1978). Ictal pain may be either diffuse (Wilkinson 1973) or localized (Young and Blume 1983, 1986) (as for example with muscle cramping in one extremity [Balkan 1995]) and may be quite severe (Russell and Whitty 1953). Although the vast majority of somatosensory seizures are unilateral, involving only one side of the body, there may rarely be bilateral involvement, for example simultaneous paresthesiae of both hands (Blume *et al.* 1992).

Somatosensory simple partial seizures may also undergo a Jacksonian 'march' (Lende and Popp 1976; Sittig 1925). These somatosensory Jacksonian marches tend to follow the same distribution as motor marches, most often beginning in the hand or fingers (Mauguire and Courjon 1978), but they are, unlike motor marches, generally quite rapid, completing their trek in a matter of seconds (Russell and Whitty 1953). One may at times encounter a kind of 'mixed' march with both somatosensory and motor components; interestingly, in such cases, one almost always finds the sensory component appearing first, followed by the motor one (Penfield and Jasper 1954; Russell and Whitty 1953, Villani *et al.* 2006).

Seizures with special sensory symptoms present with simple visual, auditory, olfactory, or gustatory hallucinations and, at times, with vertigo. Ictal visual hallucinations may consist of such crude phenomena as 'weaving patterns, zigzag lights, showers of sparks or coloured clouds' (Russell and Whitty 1955). One of William Gower's patients (Holmes 1927) had simple partial seizures that 'commenced with the appearance of several small spheres, white in the center with an intermediate zone of blue and outside this a ring of red . . . [which] moved either at a uniform rate or in jerks to the left and downwards'. Hemianopia or blindness may also occur on an ictal basis (Barry *et al.* 1985; Russell and Whitty 1955). Ictal auditory hallucinations may consist of such phenomena as buzzing or ringing noises (Mauguire and Courjon 1978). Ictal olfactory hallucinations (Mauguire and Courjon 1978) tend to be unpleasant, such as the smell of something rotten or burning: one of Jackson's patients (Jackson and Beevor 1890) had 'a very nasty smell – "burning dirty stuff"'. Ictal gustatory hallucinations tend likewise to be unpleasant, the taste being described as foul or metallic. Ictal vertigo may be characterized either by mere giddiness or by a classic sense of rotation (Kluge *et al.* 2000; Russell and Whitty 1953).

Simple partial seizures with autonomic symptoms or signs

Ictal autonomic phenomena include an ill-defined 'rising' epigastric sensation, vomiting (Mitchell *et al.* 1983; Shukla and Mishra 1985), or diarrhea with abdominal cramping (Zarling 1984).

Simple partial seizures with psychic symptoms

These seizures may consist of a variety of experiences: 'dysmnesic' phenomena (e.g., déjà vu); 'cognitive' disturbances such as depersonalization; affective experiences such as fear; illusions such as macropsia; and complex, 'structured' hallucinations in either the auditory or the visual realms.

Dysmnesic phenomena represent a disturbance in the sense of familiarity, and include déjà vu, jamais vu, déjà entendu and jamais entendu. In déjà vu, patients have the uncanny sense that they have already seen or experienced something that they are in fact encountering for the first time; in jamais vu, the opposite phenomenon occurs in that patients, although in the presence of something they 'intellectually' know they have experienced before, yet have the sense that it is entirely new. Déjà entendu and jamais entendu represent analagous experiences concerning not sight but hearing. A related phenomenon is the experience of prescience, wherein the seizure is characterize by a sense that the patient 'knew' beforehand what was going to happen (Sadler and Rahey 2004).

Cognitive disturbances most commonly involve depersonalization. One of Wilson's patients (Wilson 1930) noted that it was 'as if my mind were looking at myself from afar'. In another case (Daly 1958), the patient, while 'dissociated from his body' had the classic sense that he 'was looking down on the scene'. In other cases, the cognitive distortion may be difficult to categorize: one of Wilson's (1930) patients described her seizure as an experience wherein 'her "thoughts just stopped"'.

Affective experiences may include anxiety, depression or, rarely, euphoria. Anxiety and fear have been frequently noted (Kennedy 1911; Macrae 1954a,b; Weil 1959; Williams 1956) and may be quite severe, progressing to a full anxiety attack (Alemayehu *et al.* 1995). In one case, the seizures were characterized by anxiety, palpitations, dizziness, and pallor (Rush *et al.* 1977), and in another the patient was 'afraid, perspired and did not want to be left alone' (McLachlan and Blume 1980). As might be expected, some patients may become agoraphobic on the basis of such ictal anxiety attacks: one patient, whose ictal anxiety attacks lasted of the order of a minute, 'went to the emergency room', and, fearful 'she could have spells while driving, at work, or in social situations . . . confined herself to home' (Weilburg *et al.* 1987). Ictal depressions 'are characterized by rather sudden let-down of mood and psychomotor retardation . . . from simple listlessness and apathy to agitated depression with suicidal attempts' (Weil 1959). One patient's ictal depressions were ushered in by olfactory hallucinations, like 'stuffed cabbage in a dirty outhouse', and could last for hours, during which the patient 'felt paralyzed inside and couldn't follow through an act' (Weil 1955). Euphoria may occur (Williams 1956) but in one case was followed, after 10–20 seconds, by an intense depression (Mulder and Daly 1952). In another case (Dewhurst and Beard 1970) the patient had, rather than simple euphoria, a complex and ecstatic religious experience: 'he had a vision in which he was in the cockpit of an aeroplane . . . the aircraft gained altitude and brought him to a different land, a land of peace. He had no cares and no burdens. He felt that the power of God was upon him and changing him for the better'. The experience was so powerful that the patient later converted from Judaism to Pentecostalism.

Illusions may include macropsia, wherein objects appear larger than they are, micropsia, wherein they appear smaller, and various illusory movements of objects (Heilman and Howell 1980; Russell and Whitty 1955). Also possible are hyperacusis or hypoacusis, wherein sounds appear louder or fainter, respectively, than they in fact are. The supernumerary limb experience may also be included here: one patient had such a strong ictal sense that his arm was raised above his head that he asked his wife to pull it down even though he acknowledged that he could in fact see his actual arm at his side (Russell and Whitty 1953).

Structured hallucinations are characterized by complex visual or auditory experiences. One of Russell and Whitty's (1955) patients, wounded in the right occipital area, saw 'stretcher bearers walking past and then the figures of nurses whom he could recognize', all in the left hemifield; another, wounded in the right occipitoparietal area, 'felt that as if he was in a dream he was back in Khartoum during the war. He saw and recognized friends around him'. In another case (Sowa and Pituck 1989) the patient saw the 'right side of people's faces missing' and 'water coming out of a clock'. Of interest, such ictal visual hallucinations may

also reappear in the patient's dreams (Reami *et al.* 1991). Although, in most cases, these complex visual hallucinations occur in only one hemifield, they may at times spread to appear in the entire visual field (Russell and Whitty 1955). Palinopsia may also occur, and one patient's seizures were characterized by seeing 'non-existent pedestrians in an empty street, having seen these people minutes before in different surroundings' (Muller *et al.* 1995). Autoscopy may occur, in which patients hallucinate an image of themselves (Brugger *et al.* 1994; Devinsky *et al.* 1989a). Auditory structured hallucinations may consist of voices or music: one patient heard the same song, repeated over and over again (Wieser 1980).

Miscellaneous simple partial seizures

Various other signs and symptoms may occur on an ictal basis, including prosopagnosia (Agnetti *et al.* 1978), asomatognosia (Russell and Whitty 1955; So and Scauble 2004), and a combination of expressive aprosodia and amusia (Bautista and Ciampetti 2003).

Other miscellaneous types of simple partial seizures include unexplained urges, sexual experiences, involuntary laughing or crying, forced thoughts and, rarely, delusions.

Inexplicable urges have included impulses to laugh (Sturm *et al.* 2000) or to run (Strauss 1960).

Sexual experiences include strong sexual arousal (Erickson 1945) or orgasm (Reading and Will 1997; Ruff 1980).

Seizures characterized by involuntary laughing ('gelastic' seizures) or crying ('dacrystic' seizures) differ from those characterized by ictal emotion (e.g., anxiety or depression, as noted earlier) in that these patients, although laughing or crying, do not experience any associated mirth or sadness. One patient happened to see herself in the mirror in the midst of a gelastic seizure and 'was puzzled by the discrepancy between her facial expression and her feelings' (Arroyo *et al.* 1993); in another case, the smile accompanying the laughter reminded observers of a '"toothpaste advertisement" smile' (Lehtinen and Kivalo 1965). Dacrystic seizures manifest with a sad facial expression and tears (Luciano *et al.* 1993; Marchini *et al.* 1994), in one case capping off a sensory march that began in the left leg, ascended to the left shoulder and was then succeeded by weeping (Efron 1961).

Forced thoughts may occur and are quite similar to obsessions (Mendez *et al.* 1996).

Delusions noted during simple partial seizures include the Capgras phenomenon (delusion of doubles) (Kanemoto 1997) and a Schneiderian first rank symptom, namely a conviction on the patient's part 'that his body is being controlled by external forces' (Mesulam 1981).

COMPLEX PARTIAL SEIZURES

Complex partial seizures (Delgado-Escueta *et al.* 1982; Escueta *et al.* 1977; Golub *et al.* 1951; Holmes 1984; Theodore *et al.* 1983) generally last of the order of one to several minutes and may or may not be preceded by an aura. The seizure proper is characterized, in all cases, by some 'impairment' of consciousness, ranging in severity from the slightest degree of confusion to a more or less profound stupor.

Although, in some cases, the seizure manifests with this impairment of consciousness alone, one will in most cases also see a 'motionless stare' and/or automatisms. The 'motionless stare' is characterized by the abrupt appearance of a vacant stare and a complete arrest of all behavior, leaving the patient quite still and unmoving. This stare occupies only a portion of the seizure itself, and is typically either followed or, in some cases, preceded, by automatisms. Automatisms range in complexity from such simple, stereotyped behavior as lip-smacking or chewing to highly complex activity, which is, to a greater or lesser degree, 'reactive' to the environment. Such reactive automatisms may consist of a more or less faithful continuation of pre-ictal behavior or may represent behavior, which, although still reactive to the environment, represents a break with the patient's pre-ictal behavior.

After the seizure ends, most patients will display a degree of post-ictal confusion, lasting from one to several minutes, after which they gradually recover. Patients are subsequently totally, or sometimes only partially, amnestic for the events that occurred during the seizure.

Before discussing in detail the individual clinical aspects of complex partial seizures (i.e., aura, impairment of consciousness, motionless stare, and automatisms), some descriptions of more or less typical cases are provided to give an overall sense of what a complex partial seizure comprises. The first to be considered is Hughlings Jackson's famous patient, considered by many to be the 'paradigm of temporal lobe epilepsy' (Taylor and Marsh 1980), whom Jackson referred to as 'Dr Z' (Jackson 1889; Jackson and Colman 1898). Dr Z's first complex partial seizure was preceded by an aura of déjà vu, which was then followed by an impairment of consciousness. In Dr Z's own words:

> I was waiting at the foot of a college staircase, in the open air, for a friend who was coming down to join me. I was carelessly looking round me, watching people passing, etc., when my attention was suddenly absorbed in my own mental state, of which I know no more than that it seemed to me to be a vivid and unexpected 'recollection'; – of what, I do not know. My friend found me a minute or two later, leaning my back against the wall, looking rather pale, and feeling puzzled and stupid for the moment. In another minute or two I felt quite normal again, and was as much amused as my friend at finding that I could give no distinct account of what had happened …

In another case (Golub et al. 1951), the seizure was characterized by a motionless stare, followed by an impairment of consciousness and automatisms. The patient was in the physician's office when the seizure occurred. He:

> suddenly stopped talking, looked off into space, staring. He slumped down in his chair for a brief moment, then sat up and began to rub his abdomen with both hands. A flashlight was shined into his eyes and he turned away. He began to rummage about the desk as if looking for something. When questioned as to what he wanted, he said, 'I wanna, I wanna.' At this point he took a cigarette from his pocket, lit it and started to smoke. He then got up from his chair, walked out of the office, wandered down the hall opening all the doors saying 'I want a toilet.' Next he walked down the hall, but could not be distracted by any outside contact. He then lay down on the bed and appeared to regain contact gradually.

Aurae

As noted earlier, aurae are merely simple partial seizures that happen to evolve into complex partial seizures: they thus include all of the forms of simple partial seizure noted above. Several studies (Boon et al. 1991; Gupta et al. 1983; Kanemoto and Janz 1989; Sperling et al. 1989) provide a rough estimate of the frequency with which various aurae are found: the most common is a rising epigastric sensation; next come dysmnesic symptoms (déjà vu or jamais vu), affective symptoms (fear, anxiety, and depression), sensory symptoms (visual, tactile, gustatory, olfactory, or auditory hallucinations), vertigo, and nausea. Least common are illusions (macropsia, micropsia, hyperacusis, and hypoacusis) and various unclassified symptoms such as thirst or simply an 'indescribable' sensation. In some cases, the aura may be a combination of two or more symptoms: in an early report, Anderson (1886) noted an aura compounded of auditory and visual hallucinations and déjà vu, and Hughlings Jackson (Jackson and Stewart 1899) noted a combination of an olfactory hallucination with déjà vu. Although aurae are typically remembered, amnesia for the aura may be found in approximately one-fourth of all patients upon recovering from a complex partial seizure (Schulz et al. 1995).

Impairment of consciousness

An impairment of consciousness (or, as it is sometimes referred to, a defect of consciousness) of one sort or another, is present in all cases. As noted by Hughlings Jackson (Taylor 1931), this impairment may involve 'all degrees of obscuration of consciousness', from a profound clouding of the sensorium to the slightest trace of confusion or inattention. Indeed, determining the presence of an impairment of consciousness may in some cases be difficult: Murray Falconer (1954), in commenting on this, noted that a patient, during a seizure 'may carry on with what he is doing, such as playing the piano or driving a car.

His performance may seem without fault, or he may betray himself [only] by ignoring the traffic light.'

Motionless stare

Although appearing in most complex partial seizures, a motionless stare is certainly not seen in all (Delgado-Escueta *et al.* 1982; Holmes 1984). Some authors have categorized complex partial seizures into two types – 'type I' referring to those seizures that are characterized by the motionless stare, and 'type II' being those without one – and have gone on to assert that, in type I seizures, the stare always precedes automatisms (Delgado-Escueta *et al.* 1982; Escueta *et al.* 1977). It appears, however, that this sequencing may not be always present, as subsequent work (Theodore *et al.* 1983) has shown that, in type I seizures, the motionless stare may be preceded by automatisms.

Automatisms

Automatisms represent behavior that is performed in a more or less automatic way, such that the patient is, to a greater or lesser degree, left in a less adaptive 'fit' with the environment. Spratling (1902) felt that a patient in the midst of an automatism acted 'like a machine', and Kraepelin (1902) described patients as acting in 'a mechanical or automatic manner'. Penfield (Penfield and Jasper 1954) echoed these impressions, noting a range in the severity of the automatism such that 'when the condition is severe, the patient acts like an automaton or a robot', but when mild, the patient 'may be cooperative and only slightly confused, but still unable to deal with new problems normally'. Automatisms are currently roughly divided into those that are stereotyped and those that are still, to some or other degree, 'reactive' to the environment.

Stereotyped automatisms generally consist of simple, purposeless behavior. Table 7.6 lists various common stereotyped automatisms as noted in studies by Delgado-Escueta *et al.* (1982), Golub (1951), Holmes (1984), and Gibbs and Gibbs (1952), roughly arranged from most (top) to least (bottom) frequent. Chewing or lip-smacking, looking around and fumbling with sheets or clothing are fairly straightforward; the other stereotyped automatisms, however, deserve some comment.

Speaking or mumbling may consist of simple, but coherent, phrases, such as 'Oh my God', or may be characterized by varying degrees of incoherence (Bell *et al.* 1990; Serafetinides and Falconer 1963; van der Horst 1953), which may at times be extreme (Gillig *et al.* 1988; Knight and Cooper 1986). In one case, the patient simply repeated neologisms such as 'exeverdedeen' over and over again (Bell *et al.* 1990).

Laughing or crying may or may not be accompanied by a sense of mirth (Yamada and Yoshida 1977) and may or may not sound natural: in one case it was 'identical' to the patient's 'natural laughter', and in another, it was 'most contagious'. More commonly, however, the laughter is unnatural

Table 7.6 Common stereotyped automatisms

Chewing or lip-smacking
Looking around
Fumbling with sheets or clothing; groping, or searching
Speaking or mumbling
Laughing or crying
Sitting or standing up
Walking or running
Thrashing or kicking; 'bicycling' movements

(Ames and Enderstein 1975; Gascon and Lombroso 1971), not 'infectious' (Sethi and Surya 1976), and has been described as cackling (Gumpert *et al.* 1970; Lehtinen and Kivalo 1965). Also, dacrystic seizures may or may not be accompanied by a sense of sadness (Luciano *et al.* 1993).

Running, if prominent, may allow one to speak of 'cursive' epilepsy (Chen and Forster 1973; Sethi and Surya 1976; Sisler *et al.* 1953). The running is generally uncontrollable: one patient's seizure consisted of 'howling and running' (Marsh 1978).

Bicycling movements of the lower extremities exhibit varying degrees of coordination and may or may not be accompanied by rhythmic movements of the upper extremities (Sussman *et al.* 1989; Swartz 1994).

In addition to the foregoing stereotyped automatisms, one may, rarely, see other types. In some cases, automatisms may consist of sexual activity. There may be pelvic thrusting (Geyer *et al.* 2000), genital manipulation (Leutmezer *et al.* 1999), and sexual arousal and orgasm (Remillard *et al.* 1983): in one case (Spencer *et al.* 1983), the patient's seizure consisted of lip-smacking, snorting, grimacing, thrashing about, uttering obscenities, and masturbation. Coital movements have been noted (Freemon and Nevis 1969), and in one remarkable case (Currier *et al.* 1971), a 50-year-old woman:

> began having what her daughter and husband described as 'sexual' seizures. One was as follows. The patient was sitting at the kitchen table with her daughter making out a shopping list. She stopped making the list, appeared dazed, and gradually slumped to the floor helped by her daughter. She lay on the floor on her back, lifted up her skirt, spread her knees, and elevated her pelvis rhythmically. She made appropriate vocalizations for intercourse, such as 'it feels good' and 'further, further.' . . . Following these episodes the patient would appear confused and have no memory of them.

Other, rare, stereotyped automatisms include the Kluver–Bucy syndrome (Nakada *et al.* 1984) and stuporous catatonia with waxy flexibility (Shah and Kaplan 1980),

Reactive automatisms may, as noted earlier, consist either of behavior that represents a more or less faithful continuation of the patient's pre-ictal behavior or of behavior that, although still 'reactive' to the environment, represents a definite break with what the patient was doing before the seizure began.

Examples of 'continuation' reactive automatisms include delivering newspapers (Steegmann and Winer 1961) or continuing to drive a car (Falconer 1954). One of Hughlings Jackson's patients (Jackson 1889), if she suffered a seizure while serving tea, 'would go on pouring out but would pour out wrongly'. In another example, Forster and Liske (1963) described 'a patient, who worked in his father's shirt and pyjama factory as a sorter, [who] would, in the course of a seizure, continue to place the shirts, as they came off the line, into the same stack regardless of the size of the shirt. When the seizure ended, he would correctly place the shirts coming off the line'. In a similar example, Liddell (1953) described a 38-year-old clerk who was 'adding up a column of figures when the attack would occur. To other people he would appear to carry on as if nothing had happened. When he came to he would discover that he had written in something irrelevant or the wrong figures'.

Reactive automatisms that represent a break with pre-ictal behavior may be quite startling to observers. One patient, while walking down the street, began to 'throw away' his money (McCarthy 1900); another, a church organist, suddenly stopped playing the service music and broke out into 'hot jazz' (Forster and Liske 1963). One of Hughling Jackson's patients (Taylor 1931), in the middle of an interview, suddenly stopped responding. Jackson:

> waited a little time, and then, looking at him, I saw that he was grinning as if amused at something. Next, whilst sitting quietly in his chair, he tore a piece off a packet of prescriptions, and put it in his mouth. I took it away, but he picked up another piece from the floor and began to chew it. In about a minute more he came to himself, and then spat out into the fire a pellet of chewed paper.

In a further example, one of Penfield's patients (Penfield and Jasper 1954), a 16-year-old girl, had a complex partial seizure at a formal ball. During the seizure, she:

> proceeded to take her clothing down as though she were about to sit on the toilet. Her friends gathered round and tried to hide the performance but she seemed to come to herself and finding certain articles of apparel around her ankles, she said, 'well if they are off we had better take them off completely.' She did this and hid them in her handbag. Finally, as complete awareness returned, she was overwhelmed by shame and chagrin.

As a final example, consider a patient of Gloor's (1975), who, during a depth electrode-monitored seizure:

> got up from his chair and began to hum and sing . . . He suddenly looked very cheerful, which was in

marked contrast to the solemn expression which he had had prior to the attack. The radio in the room was on and some dance music was being broadcast. The patient now approached the female technician and started to dance with her to the tune coming over the radio. He continued to hum at the same time.

Before concluding this discussion of reactive automatisms, consideration must be given to the possibility of ictal violence. Violence during a complex partial seizure is a rare event, and usually only occurs with provocation, as when an attempt is made to restrain patients to protect them from harm (Delgado-Escueta et al. 1982). In one case (Rodin 1973), for example, a patient, during a seizure, 'suddenly lunged forward, having a bewildered and angry facial expression. An unsuccessful attempt to keep him in the chair by the attending physician resulted in making the patient angrier'; the patient then 'clenched [his] right fist . . . assumed a boxer-type stance, and violence [seemed] imminent. As soon as the patient was released, however, he merely got out of the chair, then sat down again and began typical fussing type behavior with the pillow'. In other cases, patients may engage in biting, but this is generally only when someone is injudicious enough to place his or her hand near the patient's face (Tassinari et al. 2005).

Spontaneous unprovoked violence is rare and in most of the reported cases the patient had been accused of a crime, thus raising the question of malingering. Nevertheless, there have been reports of violence occurring during monitored seizures (Delgado-Escueta et al. 1981): two patients 'shouted and spat at nurses' and another 'suddenly knelt on the bed and tried to scratch the psychologist's face'. Such violence may at times be extreme: in another report of monitored violence (Ashford et al. 1980), the patient:

> when unrestrained in his hospital room . . . would jump up and run around the room. On one occasion he grabbed the drapes next to his bed and kicked out from the wall on them. On another occasion he pulled the nurse's call button out of the wall, ran into the bathroom and swung it around his head so that it was crashing against the walls. In all observations, he was locked by himself in a closed room, having no opportunity to direct aggression against people.

Other clinical manifestations during complex partial seizures

Other manifestations that may occur during a complex partial seizure include abdominal pain (Peppercorn et al. 1978), vomiting (Kramer et al. 1988; Panayiotopoulus 1988), testicular pain (York et al. 1979), fever (Semel 1987), unilateral dystonia (Kotagal et al. 1989), and various arrhthymias, including bradycardia (Britton et al. 2006), complete A-V block (Wilder-Smith 1992) and asystole (Kiok et al. 1986; Roçamora et al. 2003; Rugg-Gunn et al. 2000), which may be followed by syncope (Schufle et al.

2007; Smaje *et al.* 1987): in such cases, if seizures cannot be controlled, placement of a pacemaker may be required.

PETIT MAL SEIZURES

Petit mal seizures (Delgado-Escueta 1979; Penry *et al.* 1975; Sadleir *et al.* 2006), also known as absence seizures, are abrupt in onset and occur without an aura; they are very brief, lasting of the order of 10 seconds, and generally consist of an arrest of all activity accompanied by a blank stare: the seizure ends as abruptly as it began, and there is no post-ictal confusion or drowsiness. To the observer, it may appear that the patient had a 'blank' spell or was merely momentarily 'out of it' then 'snapped to'. In some cases, there may be some myoclonic fluttering of the eyelids and occasionally some myoclonic jerks of the hands. Some patients will also experience a partial loss of muscle tone: the head may drop forwards, or the patient may slump somewhat, but falls are unusual. Many patients will also have some simple automatisms, such as lip-smacking, chewing or fumbling, during the absence (Fuster *et al.* 1954; Penry and Dreifuss 1969; So *et al.* 1984, Sadleir *et al.* 2006). There may very rarely be other features, such as auditory or visual hallucinations (Guinena and Taher 1955).

A variant of petit mal, known as 'atypical absence' may be seen, most commonly in patients with mental retardation. These atypical absences are of more gradual onset and offset, tend to last longer overall, and may be associated with prominent increased muscle tone (Holmes *et al.* 1987).

GRAND MAL SEIZURES

Grand mal seizures, often referred to as generalized tonic–clonic seizures, may be preceded by an aura composed of any of the symptoms or signs seen during simple partial seizures, or may evolve out of a complex partial partial seizure, a process known as secondary generalization. As discussed below, under Etiology, it is critical to determine whether or not grand mal seizures are preceded by an aura or a complex partial seizure: grand mal seizures preceded by such events may be assumed to have a 'focal' onset, that is to say to be due to a more or less localized lesion, whereas those that lack such preceding events are more likely to be occurring as part of one of the idiopathic generalized epilepsies. Caution must be exercised here, however, before deciding that no 'focal' features are present, given that many patients who did, under video–EEG monitoring, clearly have an aura, will be unable, after recovering from the grand mal seizure, to recall the aura (Schulz *et al.* 1995).

Typical grand mal seizures (Theodore *et al.* 1994) begin with an abrupt loss of consciousness, often accompanied by an inarticulate 'cry': immediately there is tonic activity in all four extremities. After perhaps 15–20 seconds, the tonic activity slowly fades to be gradually replaced by regular clonic activity, which, in turn, may last anywhere from 30 seconds to 1.5 minutes. In some cases, there may be variations, the tonic phase being preceded by a few clonic jerks, or the tonic phase constituting the majority of the seizure, with only a few clonic jerks trailing behind. During the tonic activity, respirations cease and cyanosis may appear. There is often incontinence of urine, and, during the clonic phase, the tongue may be bitten. Upon cessation of the seizure proper, most patients remain in a coma or stupor for a matter of minutes. A delirium then supervenes, with prominent confusion, lasting perhaps 15–30 minutes, after which most patients fall into a deep sleep.

ATONIC SEIZURES

Atonic seizures (Gambardella *et al.* 1994; Lipinski 1977; Pazzaglia *et al.* 1985), also known as astatic seizures or 'drop attacks', occur without prodrome or aura and are characterized by a sudden loss of motor tone. In most cases, this atonus is generalized, and patients fall or slump to the ground; occasionally, however, the lack of tone may be focal, with, for example, only an abrupt drooping of the head. The atonus itself generally lasts on the order of a few seconds and may or may not be associated with a loss of consciousness. After the restoration of normal tone, most patients arise immediately, without any post-ictal confusion; however, others may, for a minute or two, experience a more or less profound degree of post-ictal confusion.

Atonic seizures generally occur only in patients who have already suffered from complex partial or grand mal seizures for many years (Gambardella *et al.* 1994; Lipinski 1977; Tinuper *et al.* 1998).

AMNESTIC SEIZURES

Amnestic seizures, also known as 'pure epileptic amnesia', are characterized solely by the appearance of amnesia. As such, they differ from complex partial seizures in that there is no impairment of consciousness, no motionless stare, and no automatic behavior. Typically, the amnesia itself is primarily of the anterograde type but, in some cases, the amnesia represents a combination of anterograde and retrograde types. Rarely, the seizure will be characterized by retrograde amnesia alone. Examples of each type follow.

Amnestic seizures of the anterograde type

These seizures are characterized by the abrupt onset of a loss of short-term memory: patients are able to recall events that occurred up to the onset of the seizure, and behave normally during the seizure itself, but subsequent to the termination of the seizure, they have no or only spotty recall of the events that transpired concurrent with the seizure itself; they generally last from minutes up to an hour (Butler *et al.* 2007; Palmini *et al.* 1992). Palmini *et al.* (1992) provide some interesting examples. In one case, a waitress, during her seizure, 'was able to compute a customer's bill accurately and to bring him a correct amount of change'; later, upon recovery, 'she then realized she had a blank in her memory and could not recall her interaction with that customer'. In another case, the patient: 'was in the cafeteria at his work place, where he had to present a card and sign a register to pick up his meal. After having eaten he presented himself a second time and ate lunch twice. That same afternoon, the cook telephoned and upbraided him for having eaten two meals. He had no recollection of having done so'.

Finally, there is the case of a young woman, who, during a monitored seizure, answered a telephone, spoke with her cousin, and then went to sleep. 'The next morning she did not recall having received a phone call. When confronted with the video replay of her seizure, she was incredulous'. The investigators later contacted the cousin, who told them that 'their conversation had been entirely normal. He had not noticed anything amiss with the patient'.

Of some historical interest is the possibility that Hughlings Jackson's illustrious 'Dr Z' (Jackson 1889) may also have suffered from amnestic seizures of the anterograde type. In the midst of examining a patient, Dr Z remembered:

> taking out my stethoscope and turning away a little to avoid conversation. The next thing I recollect is that I was sitting at a writing-table in the same room, speaking to another person, and as my consciousness became more complete, recollected my patient, but saw that he was not in the room. I was interested to ascertain what had happened, and had an opportunity an hour later of seeing him in bed, with the note of a diagnosis I had made of 'pneumonia of the left base'. I gathered indirectly from conversation that I had made a physical examination, written these words, and advised him to take to bed at once. I re-examined him with some curiosity, and found that my conscious diagnosis was the same as my unconscious – or perhaps I should say, unremembered diagnosis had been. I was a good deal surprised, but not so unpleasantly as I should have thought probable.

Amnestic seizures of anterograde and retrograde types

In these seizures there is not only a defect of short-term memory, but also an inability, during the seizure itself, to recall events that occurred for a variable period of time before the onset of the seizure proper (Stracciari et al. 1990). Such patients may be quite alarmed at their retrograde amnesia and may ask others to fill them in (Zeman et al. 1998): one patient (Cole et al. 1987) suddenly became unable to recall whether he had gone to work that morning, long before the seizure began, and repeatedly asked others whether or not he had shown up for work. Upon termination of the seizure, the retrograde amnesia resolves, and patients are once again able to recall what events transpired up to the onset of the seizure and are also able to recall events that occurred after the termination of the seizure; those events, however, which transpired concurrent with

the seizure are in almost all cases lost to memory (Deisenhammer 1981).

Amnestic seizures characterized by retrograde amnesia alone

This type of pure epileptic amnesia is very rare. In these cases, although patients are able to keep track of events during the seizure itself, they are nevertheless unable to recall events that occurred before the seizure. In one case (Venneri and Caffarra 1998), the retrograde amnesia itself was limited to only autobiographical events. Thus, during the seizure, the patient, although able to recall public events, was unable to recall personal events from her own past. Once the seizure ended, her recall of personal events was restored, and she also was able to recall being in the seizure itself and having trouble recalling those personal events.

REFLEX SEIZURES

Reflex seizures, though uncommon, are of interest, from not only a therapeutic point of view, but also a general neuropsychiatric one. Therapeutically, they offer an obvious means of seizure reduction, namely avoiding the precipitating stimulus. In general, however, their interest lies in the fact that an experience, sometimes a very complex one (as in Penfield's example below), can 'spark' off an equally complex epileptic event. Various seizure types can be reflexively induced, including simple partial seizures, complex partial seizures, grand mal and petit mal, and atonic seizures.

Reflex simple partial seizures

Reflex simple partial seizures, albeit reported, appear to be uncommon. In one series, a startling stimulus, generally a loud noise, was noted to cause tonic activity (Manford et al. 1996), and in another, reading could induce motor phenomena such as myoclonic jerking of the jaw or, less frequently, alexia (Koutroumaniois et al. 1998). In one patient, voluntary movement was noted to induce ictal dystonia (Falconer and Driver 1963), and in another writing produced clonic activity in the involved upper extremity (Tanaka et al. 2006). In one patient, rubbing an arm produced a sensory Jacksonian march up the arm, immediately followed by a motor march up the same arm (Kanemoto et al. 2001), and in others toothbrushing produced numbness or tingling in the face or tongue followed by clonic movement of the face or upper extremity (D'Souza et al. 2007). In another case, listening to certain kinds of music-induced ictal structured visual hallucinations (Daly and Barry 1957), and ictal blindness has been induced by intermittent photic stimulation (Barry et al. 1985). Marchini et al. (1994) report the case of dacrystic seizures induced by speaking and, in a most unusual case (Falconer 1954; Mitchell et al. 1954), gazing at a safety pin was capable of precipitating a simple partial seizure characterized by a sense of profound, almost sexual, satisfaction.

Reflex complex partial seizures

Reflex complex partial seizures have, in some cases, earned specific names according to the provoking stimulus; thus one may speak of 'musicogenic', 'reading', and 'eating' epilepsy. Other stimuli, for example hearing certain people speak, may also be effective.

Musicogenic complex partial seizures, although extensively reported, are rare events (Critchley 1942; Forster 1977, Tayah et al. 2006). Critchley (1937) provided an illustrative case: the patient, after hearing 'a rather loud fox-trot with a well defined tempo ... suddenly became pale ... [and] leaned forward in her chair with a frightened look in her eyes ... and ... began smacking her lips'. In some cases, it appears that only specific kinds of music are capable of inducing seizures (Newman and Saunders 1980), for example the pealing of church bells (Poskanzer et al. 1962), organ music (Joynt et al. 1962), 'a large dance band playing "swing" music' (Daly and Barry 1957), emotionally laden music (Gastaut and Tassinari 1966), and 'Italian' songs (Wieser et al. 1997). This last case is of interest in that, upon hearing the Italian song, the patient's complex partial seizure was preceded by an aura composed of an auditory hallucination of 'pleasing female murmuring voices, which took increasing possession of her mind', following which she had a complex partial seizure with a motionless stare.

Reading-induced complex partial seizures may occur with 'silent' reading (Gastaut and Tassinari 1966) or only upon reading aloud (Forster et al. 1969a). In one case (Critchley et al. 1959), not just any reading material would do, but rather it was reading a newspaper, especially the patient's hometown newspaper, that constituted the effective stimulus.

Eating-induced complex partial seizures may occur regardless of what is eaten (Ahuja et al. 1980; Fiol et al. 1986; Forster 1971) or may occur only with eating certain foods, in one case, for example, apples (Abenson 1969).

Other stimuli capable of inducing complex partial seizures appear to be highly idiosyncratic: thus there are case reports of seizures induced by hearing the voices of certain specific radio announcers (Forster et al. 1969b), by answering the telephone (Michelucci et al. 2004), engaging in heartfelt prayer (Glass et al. 2007), hearing a vacuum cleaner (Carlson and St. Louis 2004), feeling sad (Fenwick and Brown 1989), arching the back (Jacome et al. 1980), exercising (Sturm et al. 2002), or experiencing orgasm (Ozkara et al. 2006). More remarkably, albeit very rarely, seizures may also be induced by thinking certain thoughts, as for example, in one case, thinking about home (Martinez et al. 2001). Finally, there is a fascinating case reported by Penfield (Penfield and Jasper 1954) wherein it appears that it was the evocation of a memory of a specific event that served as the trigger. The history is a bit lengthy and complex but worth retelling.

The patient, when 13 'was playing with a dog that belonged to a neighbor. He remembered grabbing a stick out of the mouth of the dog and throwing it to a distance.

The dog chased the stick and brought it back to him'. At the age of 17, the patient had his first seizure: 'he was in a crowd of people at the military school which he was attending [and] watched a demonstration of military tactics in which one of his classmates grabbed a rifle out of the hands of another man'. At that instant, 'there immediately came to the patient's mind' a memory of playing with the dog when he was 13, and 'in his mind he associated these two incidents and tried to put himself into the past memory. Following this, he became confused and was unable to speak for several seconds. Then he evidently lost consciousness and had a convulsive seizure'. The patient remained well until a half year later, when 'while in a night club, he heard a man saying, "Give me my hat." He saw him grab his hat from the hat-check girl. Immediately the memory of the dog chasing the stick, and the memory of grabbing the stick from the dog's mouth, came back to him. Following that he was confused and behaved in an automatic manner'.

Reflex grand mal and petit mal seizures

Both grand mal and petit mal seizures may be induced by such intermittent photic stimulation as with electronic video games (Quirk et al. 1995) or watching a flickering television set (Baykan et al. 2005).

Reflex atonic seizures

Atonic seizure were produced reflexively in the case of one girl, whose seizures could be 'triggered by laughing if she was told jokes or watched a comedy on television' (Jacome and Risko 1984).

STATUS EPILEPTICUS

Status epilepticus is said to be present when, for at least a half-hour, the patient is either undergoing a continuous seizure or has so many closely spaced seizures that there is no time for full recovery between them. Status epilepticus may be seen with simple partial, complex partial, petit mal, grand mal, and amnestic seizures, and, as the examples below demonstrate, may be very prolonged. Although most patients, upon recovery, are left without cognitive sequelae (Adachi et al. 2005), cognitive impairment, along with other sequelae, may, as noted below, be found after status, most especially after grand mal status.

Simple partial status epilepticus

Simple partial status epilepticus, although most commonly presenting with motor signs, has also been reported with psychic symptoms such as fear or structured hallucinations.

Motor simple partial status epilepticus is traditionally referred to as epilepsia partialis continua. These seizures typically consist of persistent clonic jerking involving the face, arm, or leg, and can last any time from hours to years (Cockerell et al. 1996; Scholtes et al. 1996a; Seshia et al. 2005); indeed in one series, the mean duration was 25 months, the longest seizure lasting 18 years (Thomas et al.

1977). Clonic activity may or may not persist into sleep (Cockerell *et al.* 1996; Thomas *et al.* 1977) and may be accompanied by other symptoms such as aphasia (Cockerell *et al.* 1996). Although the motor activity is, in the vast majority of cases, unilateral, there may in a small minority be bilateral involvement (Ashkenazi *et al.* 2000; Thomas *et al.* 1977). Rarely, inhibitory simple partial status epilepticus may occur, with prolonged ictal paresis (Smith *et al.* 1997).

Fear or anxiety may be the sole manifestation of simple partial status epilepticus and has been noted to last for between 10 days (Scott and Masland 1953) and 3 months (Henriksen 1973). Isolated ictal depression has also been noted; in one case (Weil 1956), the patient for 2 weeks 'felt "blue" and cried, and the smell of fat on a hot stove kept coming back'.

Structured hallucinations occurring in status have consisted of the auditory hallucination of a 'song' persisting for 3 hours (Wieser 1980) and a 5-day episode during which the patient experienced 'aphasia, acoustic hallucinations (strange sounds, music, voices), left sided headache, and visual hallucinations (red balls in the front of the right eye)'.

Complex partial status epilepticus

Complex partial status epilepticus is always characterized by a more or less profound impairment of consciousness, may or may not be accompanied by automatisms, and generally lasts from an hour or less up to days (Cockerell *et al.* 1994; Goldensohn and Gold 1960; Mayeux and Lueders 1978; Rennick *et al.* 1969; Sheth *et al.* 2006, Tomson *et al.* 1986, 1992; Van Rossum *et al.* 1985; Williamson *et al.* 1985b). Longer episodes, however, have been reported, up to 7.5 months in one case (Roberts and Humphrey 1988) and 18 months (Cockerell *et al.* 1994) in another.

Automatisms seen in complex partial status epilepticus may be either stereotyped or reactive. Reactive automatisms include such simple behavior as feeding oneself (Jaffe 1962) or wandering off. In one case (Coats 1876), immediately after the seizure began, the patient, a craftsman, 'laid aside his tools, took off and hung up his leather apron, and after muttering some unintelligible words to the foreman, left the shop. He himself remembers nothing of this, but woke to consciousness to find himself sitting on one of the benches in George Square'. When the wandering is quite prolonged, one speaks of 'poriomania': in one case the patient, after a seizure lasting 24 hours, came to find that he had travelled 'several hundred miles' (Mayeux *et al.* 1979).

In some cases of complex partial status epilepticus, hallucinations, delusions, and bizarre behavior may be prominent (Ballenger *et al.* 1983; Ellis and Lee 1978; Mikati *et al.* 1985). In one case (Drury *et al.* 1985), the patient, an elderly clergyman, 'became agitated and paranoid and had delusional thinking with religious overtones'; 2 days later he was still in status, and when seen 'was tremulous, had bizarre posturing and was masturbating'. In another case (Wells 1975): 'the patient became withdrawn . . . refused to eat . . . grew restless, fitful and irritable; episodes of violent anger requiring restraints followed. She appeared to be hallucinating, crying out on several occasions, "I am God." When placed on a stretcher for transfer . . . she became hostile and resistant, screaming "I'm dying" and "They're taking me to the morgue" '.

After 2 days, she was eventually treated with an antiepileptic drug, 'with prompt clearing. On recovery, she described her experience as though recovering from a bad dream'.

In other cases, stuporous catatonia has been reported (Engel *et al.* 1978): one patient (Lim *et al.* 1986) 'held his arms and legs rigidly in the air and would maintain his extremities in any bizarre posture indefinitely'.

Petit mal status epilepticus

Petit mal status epilepticus, which may occur in both childhood and the adult years (Belafsky *et al.* 1978; Michelucci *et al.* 1996; Nightingale and Welch 1982; Novak *et al.* 1971; Schwab 1953; Thompson and Greenhouse 1968; Tucker and Forster 1958; Zappoli 1955), is characterized by varying degrees of confusion, often accompanied by 'rhythmic blinking or small amplitude myoclonic jerking of the face and arms', and generally lasts anywhere from half an hour to 2 days (Andermann and Robb 1972). In some cases, the confusion may be very slight: in the case of one 30-year-old woman seen during petit mal status (Friedlander and Feinstein 1956), 'during the first minute or so of the examination nothing unusual in her manner was noted, but as she was questioned further it became apparent that there was slowness in comprehending certain questions', the presence of myoclonus of the eyelids and eyebrows suggested the correct diagnosis.

Rarely, there may be prominent automatisms. One patient went for a walk and took a bus while in petit mal status (Vizioli and Magliocco 1953), and in another case (Bornstein *et al.* 1956) a 16-year-old girl, while playing cards in her dormitory room, 'suddenly got up, walked out without a coat, went to the airport, and boarded a plane to New York without a ticket. Upon arrival in New York she was charged as a stowaway. She was found to be confused and incoherent'.

Grand mal status epilepticus

Grand mal status epilepticus (Aminoff and Simon 1980), the most dramatic and life-threatening of all forms of status, is characterized by closely spaced grand mal seizures. In some cases, the clinical presentation may evolve into an ictal coma, with no motor activity (Lowenstein and Aminoff 1992; Towne *et al.* 2000).

Amnestic status epilepticus

Amnestic status is rare, but has been noted, in some cases persisting for days (Zeman *et al.* 1998).

Sequelae of status

Enduring sequelae may be seen after simple partial, complex partial and, most especially, grand mal status epilepticus.

Simple partial status epilepticus may, albeit rarely, leave sequelae such as hemiparesis (Desbiens *et al.* 1993) (which may be permanent [Borchert and Labar 1995]) or a motor aphasia (Scholtes *et al.* 1996b).

Complex partial status epilepticus may also have permanent sequelae but this appears to be uncommon. Reported sequelae, after 1–3 days of status, include amnesia, with or without other cognitive deficits (Krumholz *et al.* 1995), and in one case hemianopia and receptive aphasia after an episode that lasted 8 days (Donaire *et al.* 2006); in this latter case, autopsy revealed laminar cortical necrosis in the left hemisphere involving the occipital, parietal, and temporal cortices.

Grand mal status may be followed by either a personality change or dementia of variable severity in approximately one-fourth of patients (Oxbury *et al.* 1971, Rowan and Scott 1970); these symptoms, may, in turn, be related to a loss of hippocampal pyramidal cells (DeGiorgio *et al.* 1992).

Etiology

The multiple causes of epilepsy and seizures are listed in Table 7.7, where they are divided into several groups. The first group, the *idiopathic generalized epilepsies* (e.g.,

Table 7.7   Causes of epilepsy and seizures

Idiopathic generalized epilepsies	Tin
Childhood absence epilepsy	Domoic acid
Juvenile absence epilepsy	Aspartame
Juvenile myoclonic epilepsy	
Idiopathic generalized epilepsy with tonic–clonic seizures only	**Alcohol or sedative/hypnotic withdrawal**
	Alcohol
Metabolic	Sedative/hypnotics
Hypoglycemia	
Hyperglycemia	**Common intracranial causes**
Hyponatremia	Mass lesions
Hypernatremia	Tumors
Hypocalcemia	Abscesses
Hypomagnesemia	Vascular malformations
Uremia	Cerebrovascular disorders
	Infarction
Toxic	Intracerebral hemorrhage
Medications	Subarachnoid hemorrhage
Clozapine	Neuronal migration disorders
Phenothiazines	Mesial temporal sclerosis
Bupropion	Traumatic brain injury
Tricyclic antidepressants	
Lithium	**Meningoencephalitis**
Tiagabine	Meningitis
Baclofen	Encephalitis
Penicillin	Acute disseminated encephalomyelitis
Cefipime	
Isoniazid	**In association with certain dementing and neurodegenerative disorders**
Busulfan	Multi-infarct dementia
Cyclosporine	Alzheimer's disease
Tacrolimus	Neurosyphilis
Theophylline	AIDS dementia
Meperidine	Progressive multifocal leukoencephalopathy
Bismuth	Toxoplasmosis
Intoxicants	Dentatorubropallidoluysian atrophy
Phencyclidine	Choreoacanthocytosis
Cocaine	McLeod syndrome
Miscellaneous toxins	Wilson's disease
Iodinated contrast dye	Spinocerebellar ataxia
Lead	Cerebrotendinous xanthomatosus

Table 7.7 (Continued)

Cerebral amyloid angiopathy
Creutzfeldt–Jakob disease
Granulomatous angiitis
Metachromatic leukodystrophy
Adrenoleukodystrophy
Pantothenate kinase-associated neurodegeneration
Juvenile Huntington's disease
Subacute sclerosing panencephalitis

Congenital disorders
Mental retardation
Autism
Down's syndrome
Fragile X syndrome
Klinefelter's syndrome
Sturge–Weber syndrome
Von Recklinghausen's disease
Rett's syndrome
Tuberous sclerosis
Prader–Willi syndrome

Miscellaneous causes
Systemic or autoimmune disorders
Hypertensive encephalopathy
Reversible posterior leukoencephalopathy syndrome
Hashimoto's encephalopathy
Limbic encephalitis

Systemic lupus erythematosus
Thrombotic thrombocytopenic purpura
Hyperthyroidism
Central pontine myelinolysis
Hepatic porphyria
Wernicke's encephalopathy
Sarcoidosis
Marchiafava–Bignami disease
Behçet's syndrome
Wegener's granulomatosus
Whipple's disease
Celiac disease
Autosomal dominant partial epilepsies
Multiple sclerosis
Disorders typically presenting in childhood or adolescence
Rasmussen's syndrome
Landau–Kleffner syndrome
Sydenham's chorea
Precipitating events
Post-anoxic encephalopathy
Radiation encephalopathy
Dialysis dysequilibrium syndrome
Dialysis dementia
Eclampsia
Post-electroconvulsive therapy

childhood absence epilepsy, with petit mal seizures), accounts for approximately one-third of all cases of epilepsy. The next three groups include seizures due to *metabolic* or *toxic* factors (such as hypoglycemia or treatment with a medication such as clozapine) or to *alcohol or sedative/hypnotic withdrawal*: in these cases, given that seizures generally do not recur if the underlying cause is treated, it is not appropriate to speak of epilepsy, a term generally reserved, as noted earlier, for cases in whom seizures, in the natural course of events, will, in all likelihood, continue to occur. The next group includes *common intracranial causes* of epilepsy, including mass lesions (e.g., tumors), cerebrovascular disorders (e.g., infarction), neuronal migration disorders (e.g., focal cortical dysplasia), mesial temporal sclerosis, and traumatic brain injury. Next are seizures occurring due to *meningoencephalitis*, which, although not a common cause, is a diagnosis that must not be missed. The next group includes epilepsy occurring *in association with certain dementing and neurodegenerative disorders*, such as multi-infarct dementia. Following this is a group of *congenital disorders*, such as mental retardation, also associated with epilepsy. Finally, there is a large *miscellaneous* group, including such disorders as hypertensive encephalopathy.

The diagnostic evaluation is simplified by attending to the kinds of seizures that the patient has. Petit mal seizures are seen only in the idiopathic generalized epilepsies. Grand mal seizures may occur either in idiopathic generalized epilepsies or secondary to some other cause: grand mal seizures of non-focal onset suggest one of the idiopathic generalized epilepsies or a toxic or metabolic factor, whereas focal-onset grand mal seizures indicate another cause. As noted earlier, the presence of an aura or a complex partial seizure immediately before the grand mal seizure indicates a focal onset. All the other seizure types, that is to say simple partial, complex partial, atonic and amnestic types, in almost all cases will be due to a focal lesion, and amongst adults by far the most frequent causes are found in the group of *common intracranial causes* (Currie *et al.* 1971; Dam *et al.* 1985; Jensen and Klinken 1976; King and Marsan 1977; Loiseau *et al.* 1990a; Mauguire and Courjon 1978; Rasmussen 1963, 1983; Sander *et al.* 1990; Zentner *et al.* 1995). Clearly, determining whether the seizures in question are 'focal' or 'non-focal' facilitates the diagnostic work-up.

In evaluating any given patient with seizures, the possibility must be kept in mind that multiple factors may be involved. Thus, patients with epilepsy, say, due to an intracranial cause such as an infarction, may also have seizures due to hypoglycemia occurring with over-vigorous treatment of diabetes mellitus. Or, to take another, not uncommon example, seizures in an alcoholic may be due not only to alcohol withdrawal but also to lesions sustained during the traumatic brain injuries that alcoholics are so prone to (Earnest *et al.* 1988).

After each of these groups is discussed, attention is then turned to a suggested *diagnostic work-up*.

IDIOPATHIC GENERALIZED EPILEPSIES

The idiopathic generalized epilepsies (IGEs) are genetically determined syndromes characterized by generalized seizures (petit mal, myoclonic, or grand mal) which usually first appear in childhood or adolescence, and which are usually, although not always, readily controlled by appropriate anti-epileptic drugs (AEDs), such as divalproex. Although there is some controversy as to how many, and what types, of IGE exist, most authorities describe the following: childhood absence epilepsy; juvenile absence epilepsy; juvenile myoclonic epilepsy; and, idiopathic generalized epilepsy with tonic–clonic seizures only. This is a very important group, accounting for approximately one-third of all epilepsies seen among adults.

Childhood absence epilepsy and juvenile absence epilepsy are similar in that in both disorders all patients have petit mal seizures, and most will also have grand mal seizures. These disorders differ in their age of onset, with childhood absence epilepsy appearing between the ages of 4 and 8 years, and juvenile absence epilepsy between the ages of 9 and 13 years. In all cases, the EEG shows typical interictal generalized spike and dome discharges, especially evident during hyperventilation.

Juvenile myoclonic epilepsy is characterized by generalized myoclonic seizures, and, in most, by either grand mal or petit mal seizures; onset is typically between the ages of 12 and 18 years. The EEG typically shows interictal generalized spike, polyspike, or polyspike and wave discharges.

Idiopathic generalized epilepsy with tonic–clonic seizures only is characterized, as the name suggests, by only grand mal seizures. Another name for this disorder is epilepsy with generalized tonic–clonic seizures on awakening, a synonym that calls attention to the fact that in this disorder the grand mal seizures, although able to occur at any time of the day, are most often seen early in the morning, soon after awakening. This disorder usually has an onset in adolescence or early adult years. As with juvenile myoclonic epilepsy, the EEG in this disorder typically shows interictal generalized spike, polyspike, or polyspike and wave discharges.

There is some evidence that all of these IGEs share a common genetic background, differing largely in their age of onset (Marini *et al.* 2004; Yenjun *et al.* 2003). From a general clinical point of view, the diagnosis should be suspected in all cases characterized by petit mal seizures or by non-focal grand mal seizures with onset between childhood and early adult years, and in any case when the EEG shows generalized interictal discharges of the spike and dome, spike, polyspike, or polyspike and wave types (Betting *et al.* 2006).

METABOLIC

Of the metabolic causes of seizures, hypoglycemia is perhaps most common, and although such seizures may be accompanied by autonomic signs (e.g., tremor) or delirium, it must be borne in mind that a seizure can be the presenting manifestation of hypoglycemia (Hoefer *et al.* 1946; Malouf and Brust 1985).

Hyperglycemia, occurring in the syndrome of non-ketotic hyperosmolar hyperglycemia, has been strongly associated with simple partial seizures with either sensory (Maccario *et al.* 1965) or, more commonly, motor symptoms (Grant and Warlow 1985; Hennis *et al.* 1992b): in some cases, these simple partial seizures with motor symptoms display a reflex character, being induced by motion (Brick *et al.* 1989). Occasionally, simple partial status epilepticus with motor symptoms (epilepsia partialis continua) may occur (Singh *et al.* 1973; Singh and Strobos 1980). Rarely, simple partial seizures may occur with hyperglycemia during diabetic ketoacidosis (Placidi *et al.* 2001).

Hyponatremia, with levels at 120 mEq/L or below may cause seizures, often in the context of a delirium (Swanson and Iseri 1958); seizures secondary to hypernatremia are very rare, and generally occur only with levels of 160 mEq/L or higher (Moder and Hurley 1990).

Hypocalcemia may provoke seizures that may or may not be accompanied by other signs, such as tetany (Glaser and Levy 1960). In cases of chronic hypocalcemia secondary to hypoparathyroidism, seizures may be the presenting sign (Berger and Ross 1981) or may be preceded by other signs, for example cataracts or parkinsonism (Eraut 1974).

Hypomagnesemia, in addition to causing delirium and myoclonus, may also lead to seizures (Hall and Joffe 1973).

Uremia may be accompanied by seizures (Tyler 1968), with one study finding this to be the case in approximately one-third of uremic patients (Locke *et al.* 1961). Rarely, seizures in uremia may be caused not so much by the uremia *per se*, but by aluminum intoxication, as occurred in some patients with renal failure who had chronically taken antacids (Russo *et al.* 1992).

TOXIC

Toxic seizures may occur secondary to *medications*, such as clozapine, *intoxicants*, such as cocaine, and *miscellaneous toxins*, such as iodinated contrast dye.

Medications

Of the medications capable of causing seizures perhaps the most notorious is clozapine. Clozapine, an atypical antipsychotic, causes seizures overall in 1.3 percent of patients (Pacia and Devinsky 1994), with a higher incidence found in patients with a history of seizures (Wilson and Claussen 1994): the risk increases with rapid dose titration (Baker and Conley 1991; Devinsky *et al.* 1991) and with high doses, rising to approximately 10 percent in those taking more than 600 mg daily (Haller and Binder 1990). Phenothiazine antipsychotics may also cause seizures (Olivier *et al.* 1982), especially with higher doses (Logothetis 1967). Of the antidepressants, bupropion is most likely to cause seizures: among patients treated with 600 mg or more daily, some

2 percent will have seizures; importantly, seizures are particularly common in patients with a history of bulimia nervosa (Davidson 1989; Johnston *et al.* 1991). Tricyclic antidepressants may cause seizures, as has been noted with amitriptyline (Betts *et al.* 1968b) and imipramine (Petti and Campbell 1975); maprotilene (Jabbari *et al.* 1985) and clomipramine (Clomipramine Collaborative Study Group 1991) are particularly likely to at therapeutic doses, and in the case of amoxapine, seizures are very common in overdose (Litovitz and Troutman 1983). Lithium may cause grand mal seizures (Wharton 1969) and may increase the frequency of seizures in those with petit mal epilepsy (Moore 1981). Interestingly, tiagabine, an AED, has been associated with complex partial status epilepticus (Koepp *et al.* 2005). Baclofen, in high dosage, caused complex partial status in one case (Zak *et al.* 1994). Antibiotics known to cause seizures include penicillin (Snavely and Hodges 1984), cefipine (Dixit *et al.* 2000, Fernandez-Torre *et al.* 2005), and isoniazid (Messing *et al.* 1984). Chemotherapeutic agents associated with seizures include busulfan (Murphy *et al.* 1992), cyclosporine (Appleton *et al.* 1989), and tacrolimus (Wijdicks *et al.* 1996). Other agents include theophylline (Messing *et al.* 1984), meperidine (Kaiko *et al.* 1983), and bismuth: bismuth, as may be used in the treatment of peptic ulcer, is known to cause delirium with myoclonus and either partial or grand mal seizures (Supino-Viterbo *et al.* 1977); uncommonly, bismuth intoxication may present with a seizure (Molina *et al.* 1989).

Intoxicants

Intoxicants noted to cause seizures include phencyclidine (Alldredge *et al.* 1989) and cocaine: in the case of cocaine, complex partial status epilepticus was noted (Merriam *et al.* 1988; Ogunyemi *et al.* 1989).

Miscellaneous toxins

Of the miscellaneous toxins, perhaps the most common offender is iodinated contrast dye, given intravenously (Aurahami *et al.* 1987), intra-arterially (Vickrey and Bahls 1989), or intrathecally (Greenberg and Vance 1980; Shiozawa *et al.* 1981). Lead intoxication in adults, when acute, often presents with delirium, abdominal pain, and seizures, as may be seen in adults who drink illicit 'moonshine' whiskey made in old radiators (Morris *et al.* 1964; Whitfield *et al.* 1972) or, in one case, where adults burned discarded lead storage battery boxes for fuel (Akelaitis 1941). Acute lead intoxication in children, as can be seen in those who ingest leaded paint chips, may, when severe, cause seizures and delirium or coma (Jenkins and Mellins 1957). Tin intoxication may cause a delirium with seizures, as has been noted with trimethyl (Fortemps *et al.* 1978) and triethyl tin (Alajouanine *et al.* 1958); in one case, upon recovery from trimethyl tin intoxication, a patient subsequently developed complex partial seizures (Feldman *et al.* 1993). Domoic acid intoxication, as may occur with the ingestion of mussels, is a very rare event but is noted here because the resulting neuropathology is similar to that of mesial temporal sclerosis. Domoic acid is an excitotoxin, similar to kainic acid, and in the reported case ingestion was followed by the development of hippocampal atrophy and complex partial seizures (Cendes *et al.* 1995). Finally, aspartame, taken in very high dose, has been noted, in a case report, to cause a seizure (Walton 1986).

ALCOHOL OR SEDATIVE/HYPNOTIC WITHDRAWAL

In general hospital practice, alcohol withdrawal seizures are quite common, especially among adults in their middle years (Sander *et al.* 1990); the diagnosis, however, often proves elusive as many patients (and their family members) may deny excessive alcohol use.

Alcohol withdrawal seizures are typically of the grand mal type, and are generally seen only in patients with a long history of heavy drinking (Lechtenberg and Worner 1992; Leone *et al.* 1997; Schuckitt *et al.* 1993). Seizures may occur either in an isolated fashion as 'rum fits' or in association with delirium tremens (Isbell *et al.* 1955). 'Rum fits' are generally restricted to the first 48 hours of abstinence, and although repeated seizures, even status, may occur, most patients have only one or two seizures (Earnest *et al.* 1988; Espir and Rose 1987; Victor and Brausch 1967). Delirium tremens, marked by delirium and prominent tremor, generally appears within the first few days of abstinence, and seizures, which may either 'usher in' the delirium or occur in the midst of it, are seen in between 10 percent (Rosenbaum *et al.* 1941) and 20 percent (Lundquist 1961) of patients. Importantly, although most seizures occurring in a newly abstinent alcoholic are related to the alcohol withdrawal *per se*, other epileptogenic factors, such as head trauma, hypoglycemia, hypomagnesemia, Wernicke's encephalopathy, or meningitis may also be present (Earnest *et al.* 1988; Lechtenberg and Worner 1992).

Withdrawal from other sedative/hypnotic agents such as benzodiazepines or barbiturates may also cause grand mal seizures (Kalinowsky 1942; Levy 1984), and in the case of barbiturates, status epilepticus is not uncommon.

COMMON INTRACRANIAL CAUSES

In cases when metabolic and toxic factors seem absent, withdrawal unlikely, and where the history is not compatible with idiopathic generalized epilepsy, consideration should be given to the presence of certain intracranial disorders, the most common of which are mass lesions (e.g., tumors), cerebrovascular disorders (e.g., infarction), mesial temporal sclerosis, neuronal migration disorders, and traumatic brain injury. Each of these is considered in turn.

Mass lesions

Tumors, abscesses, and vascular malformations may cause seizures, which may be simple or complex partial or grand mal.

Seizures occurring secondary to tumors are more likely to occur when the tumor involves the cerebral cortex, and less so when only the white matter or subcortical gray structures are involved (Hildebrand *et al.* 2005; Scott and Gibberb 1980). Given their frequency in adults (Dam *et al.* 1985), the clinical 'rule' that a new onset seizure disorder in an adult is, until proven otherwise, secondary to a tumor, is a sound clinical guide.

Cerebral abscesses, which may or may not be accompanied by fever and leukocytosis, are frequently associated with seizures, not only when acute, but also amongst those patients who survive (Legg *et al.* 1973); in this regard it may be noted that neurocysticercosis, a common cause of seizures in developing countries, may be emerging in developed countries, such as Portugal (Monteiro *et al.* 1995) and the United States (Wallin and Kurtzke 2004).

Vascular malformations, such as arteriovenous malformations and various angiomas, are a common cause of seizures, which may indeed constitute their sole clinical expression (Kramer and Awad 1994), even in the absence of any symptomatic hemorrhage.

Cerebrovascular disorders

Simple partial, complex partial, and grand mal seizures (Labovitz *et al.* 2001) may occur after infarction (Bogousslavsky *et al.* 1992; Daniele *et al.* 1989; Kilpatrick *et al.* 1990, 1992; Richardson and Dodge 1954; So *et al.* 1996), intracerebral hemorrhage (Passero *et al.* 2002), or subarachnoid hemorrhage and it is customary to divide these seizures into three types, depending on when they occur: (i) immediate seizures during the first day; (ii) early seizures during the following two weeks; and (iii) late seizures during the following months and years.

After cerebral infarction immediate and early seizures are seen in less than 3 percent of patients; late-appearing seizures are seen in a little more than 3 percent of cases, and generally appear within the first 2 years or so post stroke (Lamy *et al.* 2003): those with severe stroke seem at higher risk for late-appearing epilepsy (Lamy *et al.* 2003); the occurrence of an immediate or early seizure may (Lamy *et al.* 2003) or may not (Lossius *et al.* 2005) increase the likelihood of a late-appearing one.

Intracerebral hemorrhage is more likely to cause seizures when the hemorrhage is lobar, rather than subcortical (Passero *et al.* 2002), and immediate or early seizures are seen in up to 25 percent of cases.

Subarachnoid hemorrhage likewise may cause immediate or early seizures in some 25 percent of cases; late appearing seizures are seen in less than 10 percent, and appear more common in cases complicated by infarction (Claasen *et al.* 2003).

Neuronal migration disorders

Neuronal migration disorders comprise a large group of conditions, all of which result from defective neuronal migration during embryogenesis. In the normal course of embryogenesis, neurons migrate along radially oriented glial fibers from the periventricular area to the overlying cortical plate, where they come to rest in an orderly fashion, eventually resulting in a properly laminated and appropriately convoluted cortex.

Disordered migration, depending on its timing and degree, may result in a variety of morphologic changes (Raymond *et al.* 1995). In cases where migration stalls out, as it were, either at the periventricular area or in the white matter, one may find misplaced collections of neurons, known as heterotopias, in various locations (d'Orsi *et al.* 2004; Dubeau *et al.* 1995; Tassi *et al.* 2005): thus there may be periventricular nodular heterotopias (Battaglia *et al.* 2006; D'Agostino *et al.* 2002; Kothare *et al.* 1998) and what are known as 'band' or 'laminar' heteropias, wherein the heterotopia extends in a band through a greater or lesser portion of the white matter (Barkovich and Kjos 1992; Ono *et al.* 1997); in many cases one also finds an excessive number of isolated neurons scattered throughout the white matter. The overlying cortex may also be malformed, and this malformation may be either macroscopic or microscopic. Macroscopic malformations include pachygyria (a grossly thickened cortex), polymicrogyria (with multiple, small and highly convoluted gyri), or lissencephaly (a 'smooth' cortex, with little or no gyrification visible) (Brodtkorb *et al.* 1992). Microscopic abnormalities include microdysgenesis (with dyslamination) (Armstrong 1993; Meencke and Janz 1984) or focal cortical dysplasia (with dyslamination accompanied by dysmorphic neurons) (Fauser *et al.* 2006; Lawson *et al.* 2005; Palmini *et al.* 1991; Siegel *et al.* 2005; Sisodiya *et al.* 1995; Taylor *et al.* 1971).

Various seizure types may occur secondary to disordered neuronal migration, including complex partial, simple partial, and grand mal, and, with the advent of MRI, it has become apparent that disordered neuronal migration is one of the most common causes of focal epilepsy (Barkovich *et al.* 1995; Raymond *et al.* 1995; Sisodiya *et al.* 1996): in these cases the onset of seizures ranges from childhood to early adult years.

Before ending this discussion of disordered neuronal migration, mention should be made of a rare condition known as hypothalamic hamartoma. In this condition one finds one or more nodules, or hamartomas, composed of otherwise normal neurons, within the hypothalamus. Classically, these present in childhood with precocious puberty and simple partial seizures of the gelastic type (Ames and Enderstein 1980; Berkovic *et al.* 1988; Breningstall 1985; Cascino *et al.* 1993a; Kuzniecky *et al.* 1997). Further experience, however, has demonstrated that the onset may be delayed until adult years, that precocious puberty may not be present, and that various other seizure types, including complex partial and grand mal, may also be seen (Boudreau *et al.* 2005; Castro *et al.* 2007; Mullatti *et al.* 2003). The interictal EEG in hypothalamic hamartoma may show interictal epileptiform discharges in the temporal or frontal areas; importantly the ictal EEG during a gelastic seizure, as is the case in most simple partial seizures, is typically unremarkable (Leal *et al.* 2003). In reviewing the MRI in cases of gelastic seizures, although finding a nodular mass in the hypothalamus is highly suggestive of an hamartoma, one must keep in mind that other lesions, such as a ganglioglioma, may appear similar (List *et al.* 1958).

Mesial temporal sclerosis

Mesial temporal sclerosis is characterized by sclerosis of one or more of the structures on the medial aspect of the temporal lobe, including the hippocampus, amygdala, and parahippocampal gyrus (Cavenaugh *et al.* 1956; Cendes *et al.* 1993a; Falconer 1971; Hudson *et al.* 1993), as illustrated in Figure 7.1. Ammon's horn (cornu Ammonis) is an older term for the hippocampus, and some authors, rather than using the term 'hippocampal sclerosis', will speak of 'Ammon's horn sclerosis'.

Among patients with a seizure focus in the temporal lobe, mesial temporal sclerosis is the most common cause (Bruton 1988; Engel *et al.* 1975; Falconer 1971; Falconer *et al.* 1964; Margerison and Corsellis 1966; Sano and Malamud 1953). Given that most (but certainly not all) cases of complex partial seizures result from a focus in the temporal lobe, mesial temporal sclerosis turns out to be the most common cause of this type of seizure.

The etiology of mesial temporal sclerosis is not known with certainty. In some cases, albeit rare, it is familial (Kobayashi *et al.* 2002, 2003). With regard to the remaining large group of non-familial cases, a popular theory holds that seizures occurring secondary to other causes (e.g., childhood febrile seizures) may, via excitotoxic mechanisms, induce damage in the hippocampus, with the resulting sclerotic area then becoming epileptogenic in its own right. There is some evidence to support this. First, although certainly not all patients with mesial temporal sclerosis have a history of childhood febrile seizures, such events are more common in these patients than in the general population (Adam *et al.* 1994; Cendes *et al.* 1993b; French *et al.* 1993; Saygi *et al.* 1994). Second, among patients with focal cortical

dysplasia, a significant minority will also be found to have mesial temporal sclerosis (Fauser *et al.* 2006). Third, there are clearly documented cases wherein patients with normal hippocampi have developed mesial temporal sclerosis after experiencing seizures from other causes (Parmar *et al.* 2006; Worrell *et al.* 2002). Finally, although not all studies agree (Liu *et al.* 2002), there is evidence from prospective volumetric studies that progressive hippocampal atrophy occurs in patients who continue to experience complex partial or grand mal seizures (Briellmann *et al.* 2002; Fuerst *et al.* 2003; Salmenpara *et al.* 2005).

Traumatic brain injury

Seizures occurring after traumatic brain injury may appear early (within the first week) or late (at any time thereafter) (Jennett 1973; Jennett *et al.* 1973). Early seizures are seen in from 2 percent to 15 percent of cases, and late seizures, generally appearing within the first year post injury (Mazzini *et al.* 2003), in 5–10 percent of cases. Several factors increase the likelihood that patients will have late seizures, including the following: the occurrence of an early seizure; the presence of contusions or intracerebral hemorrhages; any intracranial operations; and dural penetration by metal fragments or by bone (Annegers *et al.* 1980; Annegers *et al.* 1998; Ashcroft 1941; Caveness 1976; Englander *et al.* 2003; Jennett 1975; Lishman 1968; McQueen *et al.* 1983; Mazzini *et al.* 2003; Russell and Whitty 1952; Salazar *et al.* 1985).

MENINGOENCEPHALITIS

The occurrence of a grand mal or, less commonly, simple partial or complex partial seizure in the context of an illness characterized by fever, headache and delirium should always raise the diagnostic possibility of meningitis or encephalitis (Annegers *et al.* 1988). Both arbovirus encephalitis, and

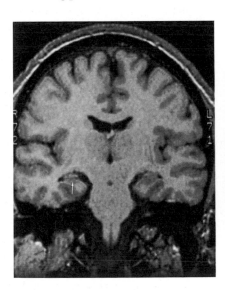
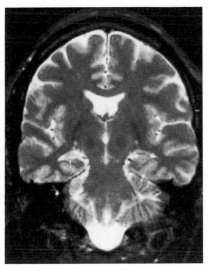

Figure 7.1 Coronal magnetic resonance imaging scan demonstrating mesial temporal sclerosis on the right. On the T1-weighted scan, atrophy of the hippocampus, indicated by the arrow, is fairly apparent, increased signal intensity being seen in the same area on the T2-weighted scan. (Reproduced from Hopkins *et al.* 1995.)

herpes simplex encephalitis may present in this fashion (Haymaker 1949; Kennedy 1988; Williams and Lerner 1978), and seizures have also been noted during infectious mononucleosis (Gautier-Smith 1965; Silverstein et al. 1972).

In those who survive, seizures may occur as sequelae (Marks et al. 1992), and this appears to be especially likely in cases in which the acute phase was characterized by seizures (Annegers et al. 1988) and when there are other sequelae indicative of cerebral damage (Pomeroy et al. 1990).

In this regard, it may also be noted that acute disseminated encephalomyelitis, occurring in the days or weeks following a viral illness, may also be characterized by seizures (Paskavitz et al. 1995; Tenenbaum et al. 2002).

IN ASSOCIATION WITH CERTAIN DEMENTING OR NEURODEGENERATIVE DISORDERS

Although partial and grand mal seizures may occur secondary to various dementing or neurodegenerative disorders, overall these disorders account for only a small minority of all seizure cases; furthermore, relative to other symptoms caused by these disorders, the seizures play but a minor role in the overall clinical picture.

Multi-infarct dementia may be associated with seizures at any point in its evolution (Rosenberg et al. 1979); in Alzheimer's disease, however, seizures typically occur only late in its course, and long after the dementia is well-established (Amatniek et al. 2006; Goodman 1953; Hauser et al. 1986; Romanelli et al. 1990).

Neurosyphilis, in particular general paresis of the insane (GPI), may cause either grand mal or partial seizures, most especially simple partial seizures with a Jacksonian march (Merritt et al. 1932; Storm-Mathisen 1969). Importantly, the Jarisch–Herxheimer reaction to penicillin treatment may also be characterized by seizures (Hahn et al. 1959; Zifko et al. 1994).

AIDS dementia may, late in its course, be accompanied by seizures (Navia et al. 1986a). Other disorders, often seen in association with AIDS, must also be considered, including progressive multifocal leukoencephalopathy and toxoplasmosis (Navia et al. 1986b; Porter and Sande 1992).

Various movement disorders, typically accompanied by dementia, may also cause partial or grand mal seizures, notably the choreiform disorders dentatorubropallidoluysian atrophy (Porter et al. 1995; Warner et al. 1995), choreoacanthocytosis (Feinberg et al. 1991; Hardie et al. 1991; Lossos et al. 2005) (which may present with complex partial seizures years before the onset of chorea [Al-Asmi et al. 2005]), and the McLeod syndrome (Danek et al. 2001). In the case of seizures occurring in a young person with a movement disorder (with chorea, parkinsonism, tremor), consideration must also always be given to Wilson's disease (Dening et al. 1988). Spinocerebellar ataxia, characterized by a slowly progressive ataxia, in certain of its types, may also cause seizures (Grewal et al. 2002; Rasmussen et al. 2001)

Cerebrotendinous xanthomatosis, typified by a combination of either mental retardation or dementia with Achilles tendon enlargement or cataracts, may also cause seizures (Fiorelli et al. 1990).

Cerebral amyloid angiopathy, classically causing lobar hematomas and, in some cases, a dementia, may also manifest with simple partial seizures, which may occur before any lobar hemorrhages and either before or concurrent with a dementia (Greenberg et al. 1993).

Creutzfeldt–Jakob disease, typically characterized by dementia or delirium with myoclonus, may also, albeit uncommonly and late in the course of the disease, cause partial or grand mal seizures (Brown et al. 1986).

Granulomatous angiitis, or isolated angiitis of the central nervous system, presents subacutely with headache, which is quite prominent, and delirium, and may, in a minority, be accompanied by seizures (Vollmer et al. 1993).

Certain degenerative disorders of relatively early onset, from childhood to early adult years, may also cause partial or grand mal seizures, including metachromatic leukodystrophy (Alves et al. 1986; Betts et al. 1968a; Hageman et al. 1995; Haltia et al. 1980; Lima et al. 2006; Rauschka et al. 2006), adrenoleukodystrophy (Moser et al. 1984), pantothenate kinase-associated neurodegeneration (Rozdilsky et al. 1968), juvenile Huntington's disease (Campbell et al. 1961; Siesling et al. 1997), and, especially, subacute sclerosing panencephalitis (Koehler and Jakumeit 1976; Kornberg et al. 1991; Prashanth et al. 2006).

CONGENITAL DISORDERS

Mental retardation, of severe or profound degree, is commonly associated with seizures (Steffenburg et al. 1996), and over one-third of patients with autism will also have seizures, which may be seen both in those with and without retardation (Danielsson et al. 2005; Gillberg 1991; Olsson et al. 1988).

Various specific congenital disorders, most associated with mental retardation, also cause seizures, with each one being marked by various distinctive features.

Down's syndrome, typified by a variable degree of mental retardation and a characteristic dysmorphism with narrowed palpebral fissures, epicanthal folds, and a small mouth, often with a large protruding tongue, may be accompanied by partial or grand mal seizures in adults (Pueschel et al. 1991), the proportion affected rising from about one-tenth of young adults, to about one-half of those over 50 years old (McVicker et al. 1994), and to over three-quarters of those who go on to develop a dementia (Lai and Williams 1989).

Fragile X syndrome, seen generally, but not always, in males, is typified by a variable degree of mental retardation, macro-orchidism, and a characteristic dysmorphism, with a long, narrow face, prominent forehead, and large ears. A minority of these patients will also have either partial or grand mal seizures (Finelli et al. 1985; Wisniewski et al. 1985).

Klinefelter's syndrome, characterized by tall stature and eunuchoidism in post-pubertal males, may, albeit rarely, be accompanied by complex partial or grand mal seizures (Tatum et al. 1998).

Sturge–Weber syndrome is classically characterized by a unilateral facial port-wine stain, hemiplegia contralateral to the port-wine stain, mental retardation, and seizures (Bebin and Gomez 1988; Pascual-Castroviejo *et al.* 1993). Importantly, there is an association between frequent seizures and dementia in this disorder (Lichenstein 1954; Petermann *et al.* 1958), an association that underlines the importance of seizure control.

Von Recklinghausen's disease (neurofibromatosis type I) is characterized by neurofibromas and café au lait spots: seizures may occur in 4–5 percent of sufferers (Korf *et al.* 1993; Kulkantrakorn and Geller 1998).

Rett's syndrome (Hagberg *et al.* 1983), seen virtually only in females, is suggested by a typical evolution of symptoms in childhood, resulting in microcephaly and mental retardation. In a minority of adults either partial or grand mal seizures may be seen.

Tuberous sclerosis classically presents in childhood with the triad of seizures, adenoma sebaceum, and mental retardation (Critchley and Early 1932). Seizures generally, but not always, precede the appearance of adenoma sebaceum (Alsen *et al.* 1994; Ross and Dickerson 1943), and although generally of the 'salaam' type in infancy, manifest with typical grand mal or partial seizures by early or mid-childhood (Pampiglione and Moynahan 1976). Tuberous sclerosis may rarely present in the adult years: in one case, a 26-year-old developed adenoma sebaceum, followed, at the age of 31, by partial seizures (Kofman and Hyland 1959).

Prader–Willi syndrome is characterized by extreme obesity secondary to a ravenous hunger. Dysmorphic features are common, with a narrow head, almond-shaped eyes, a thin upper lip, thin arms, and, in males, micropenis and cryptorchidism. Perhaps one-half will also have mental retardation, generally of a mild degree. Seizures may occur in about one-fifth of these patients (Bray *et al.* 1983).

MISCELLANEOUS CAUSES

The miscellaneous causes may be divided into various groups; these include: *systemic or autoimmune disorders,* such as hypertensive encephalopathy or Hashimoto's encephalopathy; the *autosomal dominant partial epilepsies; multiple sclerosis*; certain *disorders typically presenting in childhood or adolescence,* such as Rasmussen's syndrome; and, finally, a group characterized by obvious *precipitating events,* such as cerebral anoxia.

Systemic or autoimmune disorders

Various systemic or autoimmune disorders may cause partial or grand mal seizures. Hypertensive encephalopathy (Chester *et al.* 1978; Healton *et al.* 1982) and the reversible posterior leukoencephalopathy syndrome (Hinchey *et al.* 1996) both present with headache, delirium, and seizures, and should be suspected in cases of severe hypertension or treatment with immunosuppressants. Hashimoto's encephalopathy (Henchey *et al.* 1995; Shaw *et al.* 1991) and limbic encephalitis (Alamowitch *et al.* 1997) may both

present with delirium and either partial or grand mal seizures; in the case of limbic encephalitis, seizures may constitute either the presentation (Brennan and Craddock 1983; Corsellis *et al.* 1968), or, rarely, the primary clinical expression of the disease (Shavit *et al.* 1999; Tsukamoto *et al.* 1993). Systemic lupus erythematosus may likewise cause partial or grand mal seizures (Devinsky *et al.* 1988a) in well over 10 percent of patients (Appenzeller *et al.* 2004). Thrombotic thrombocytopenic purpura should be suspected in cases of seizures occurring in the context of delirium and thrombocytopenia (Blum and Drislane 1996). Hyperthyroidism, rarely, may directly cause seizures, and is suggested by the accompanying autonomic symptoms (Korczyn and Bechar 1976; Jabbari and Huott 1980). Central pontine myelinolysis, suggested by the occurrence of quadriplegia or abnormal movements in the setting of rapid correction of hyponatremia, may also, rarely, cause seizures (Karp and Laureno 1993). Hepatic porphyria may be suspected when seizures occur in the context of abdominal pain and delirium (Byelsjo *et al.* 1996). Wernicke's encephalopathy, presenting with variable combinations of nystagmus, ataxia, and delirium in the setting of nutritional deficiency (as in chronic alcoholism), may, rarely, also cause seizures (Harrison *et al.* 2006). Marchiafava–Bignami disease, a very rare disorder also associated with chronic alcoholism, may present with delirium and seizures (Ironside *et al.* 1961; Koeppen and Barron 1978). Sarcoidosis is immediately suggested by typical findings on chest radiograph (Ferriby *et al.* 2001; Krumholz *et al.* 1991; Oksanen 1986). Other, rare, causes include: Behçet's syndrome, suggested by delirium accompanied by oral or genital aphthous ulcers (Aykutlu *et al.* 2002); Wegener's granulomatosus (Nishino *et al.* 1993), suggested by a combination of upper respiratory and renal disease; Whipple's disease, suggested by abdominal pain and arthralgia (Louis *et al.* 1996; Romanul *et al.* 1977); and celiac disease, also known as gluten enteropathy, suggested by abdominal pain or bloating (Chapman *et al.* 1978) or by the finding of occipital calcification (Gobbi *et al.* 1992; Tinuper *et al.* 1996b).

Autosomal dominant partial epilepsies

Autosomal dominant partial epilepsy should be suspected in cases of partial seizures, with or without grand mal seizures, which exhibit a family history consistent with autosomal dominant inheritance, and wherein the MR scan is normal. Three, more or less distinct, types have been recognized, including autosomal dominant lateral temporal lobe epilepsy (also known as autosomal dominant partial epilepsy with auditory features), autosomal dominant nocturnal frontal lobe seizures, and familial partial epilepsy with variable foci. Autosomal dominant lateral temporal lobe epilepsy is suggested clinically by complex partial seizures occurring with an auditory aura, which may range from simple buzzing to, at times, complex auditory hallucinations, such as music or voices (Berkovic *et al.* 2004a; Brodtkorb *et al.* 2005; Hedera *et al.* 2004; Michelucci *et al.* 2003; Ottman *et al.* 1995; Poza *et al.* 1999;

Winawer *et al.* 2000). Autosomal dominant nocturnal frontal lobe seizures is a syndrome distinguished by complex partial seizures that arise from sleep (Combi *et al.* 2005; Gambardella *et al.* 2000; Hayman *et al.* 1997; Hirose *et al.* 1999; Oldani *et al.* 1998; Phillips *et al.* 2000; Saenz *et al.* 1999; Scheffer *et al.* 1994, 1995; Willoughby *et al.* 2003). In both these types, the seizure type generally 'runs true' among family members; in familial partial epilepsy with variable foci, however, there is a marked heterogeneity in seizure types among family members (Berkovic *et al.* 2004b), and it is this heterogeneity which distinguishes this disorder. In addition to these three well-recognized type, there are also reports of other, less clear-cut autosomal dominant types of partial epilepsy (Brodtkorb *et al.* 2002; Depondt *et al.* 2002; Picard *et al.* 2000; Provini *et al.* 1999), and many researchers believe that what has been discovered so far represents merely the tip of the iceberg.

Multiple sclerosis

Multiple sclerosis, rarely, may cause seizures (Nicoletti *et al.* 2003; Thompson *et al.* 1993; Trouillas and Courjon 1972) and in one very rare case, multiple sclerosis presented with simple partial status epilepticus with motor signs secondary to a plaque in the precentral gyrus (Spatt 1995).

Disorders typically presenting in childhood or adolescence

Certain disorders typically presenting in childhood or adolescence may also be considered, including Rasmussen's encephalitis, the Landau–Kleffner syndrome, and Sydenham's chorea. Rasmussen's encephalitis typically presents with partial seizures, with or without secondary generalization; over time seizures are joined by a progressive hemiparesis, and, in some cases, a dementia (Aguilar and Rasmussen 1960; Bien *et al.* 2002; Granata *et al.* 2003; Rasmussen and Andermann 1989; Rasmussen *et al.* 1958); motor simple partial status epilepticus is not uncommon. Although pathologic studies have revealed an underlying encephalitic process consistent with an autoimmune etiology (Pardo *et al.* 2004); the nature of this autoimmune disorder remains, as yet, unknown. Although the onset is generally in childhood under the age of 10 years, adult onsets, albeit rare, may also be seen (McLachlan *et al.* 1993). Landau–Kleffner syndrome is characterized by a childhood onset of aphasia with seizures, which may be either partial or grand mal in type (Hirsch *et al.* 1990; Landau and Kleffner 1957; Mantovani and Landau 1980; Paquier *et al.* 1992). Sydenham's chorea is suggested by the onset of chorea in childhood or adolescence, and may also, albeit rarely, cause seizures (Nausieda *et al.* 1980). Interestingly, and again, very rarely, epilepsy may occur as a sequela to Sydenham's chorea (Aron *et al.* 1965).

Precipitating events

Seizures may also occur after certain, obvious, precipitating events, such as in the context of either post-anoxic encephalopathy (Krumholz *et al.* 1988) or post-radiation encephalopathy (Shewmon and Masdeu 1980), during the dialysis dysequilibrium syndrome or as part of the now vanishingly rare dialysis dementia (Burks *et al.* 1976; Garrett *et al.* 1988; Lederman and Henry 1978; O'Hare *et al.* 1983), or during eclampsia (Manfredi *et al.* 1997) or, very rarely, as a sequela to electroconvulsive therapy (ECT) (Devinsky and Duchowny 1983; Varma and Lee 1992).

DIAGNOSTIC WORK-UP

The diagnostic work-up, in part, is determined by the kinds of seizures the patient has. Cases characterized by an onset in childhood or adolescence of petit mal and/or non-focal grand mal seizures probably represent one of the idiopathic generalized epilepsies, and in such cases generally an interictal EEG is indicated: if it shows the typical findings discussed below, no further work-up may be required. In cases of non-focal grand mal seizures of later onset, and in all cases of focal seizures (i.e., grand mal seizures with focal features and all cases of either simple partial, complex partial seizures, atonic, or amnestic seizures) one should assume that a lesion is present and take steps to determine its location and nature (King *et al.* 1999). These steps, discussed below, include an *EEG*, *neuroimaging* (preferably using MRI), and a specifically focused history and examination, looking for certain distinctive *lateralizing and localizing symptoms and signs*. Lumbar puncture is reserved for cases of suspected meningitis or encephalitis. Additionally, one should always be alert to toxic or metabolic factors or substance withdrawal, which may cause grand mal seizures in otherwise normal individuals and may precipitate seizures in patients with epilepsy of any cause. If, after a thorough work-up, the cause of the patient's epilepsy remains obscure it is customary to make a diagnosis of 'cryptogenic' epilepsy. Such a diagnosis, however, should not be taken for more than it is, a mere confession of our ignorance, and the clinician should remain alert to the emergence of new clinical features that may ultimately reveal the underlying cause.

Electroencephalogram

An EEG (discussed in detail in Section 1.5) should be obtained in all cases. An interictal EEG is, in the vast majority of cases, sufficient, and should include hyperventilation, photic stimulation, and a sleep recording. Ictal EEGs, although helpful, are generally not required except for presurgical work-ups; however, in cases of reflex seizures, consideration may be given to inducing a seizure with the appropriate reflexive stimulus (Fariello *et al.* 1983).

Idiopathic generalized epilepsies are associated with generalized, bilaterally symmetric, and synchronous interictal epileptiform discharges. Patients with petit mal seizures will have classic spike and dome discharges, and patients with non-focal grand mal seizures will generally have spike and wave, polyspike, or polyspike and wave discharges.

Focal epilepsies typically display focal or multifocal interictal epileptiform discharges; however, it may require up to four routine EEGs to capture them, and even this strategy, as noted below, may fail. In cases where a focus is suspected in one of the temporal lobes, consideration should be given to the use of supplemental leads: 'true' anterior temporal leads are routinely appropriate in these cases, while invasive sphenoidal or nasopharyngeal leads are typically held in reserve for particularly difficult cases.

As important as the finding of interictal or ictal activity is, its absence does not rule out the diagnosis of focal epilepsy. In the case of simple partial seizures, both interictal (Devinsky et al. 1989b; Mauguire and Courjon 1978) and ictal (Bare et al. 1994; Devinsky et al. 1988b, 1989b) EEGs are often normal. In the case of complex partial seizures, interictal EEGs may likewise be normal (Goodin et al. 1990); furthermore, although ictal EEGs are more likely to be abnormal, even here the EEG may be normal during a seizure, especially when the seizure focus is on the medial surface of the frontal (Williamson and Spencer 1986; Williamson et al. 1985c) or temporal (Lieb et al. 1976) lobe. In these limiting cases when routine EEGs remain unrevealing, consideration may be given to admission to an epilepsy monitoring unit, or, more simply, to the utilization of a computer-assisted 24-hour ambulatory EEG.

Neuroimaging

Neuroimaging should, whenever possible, be performed using MRI rather than computed tomography (CT) scanning, as MR scanning is far more sensitive (Franceschi et al. 1989; Swartz et al. 1992). When MR scanning is utilized, it is important to obtain coronal images as these are superior to axial or sagittal images for the detection of mesial temporal sclerosis (Berkovic et al. 1991). Furthermore, it must be borne in mind that in some cases of mesial temporal sclerosis the temporal lobes and their contents may appear quite symmetric, and the only abnormality may be increased signal intensity on the T2-weighted scan (Jackson et al. 1994). Although MRI is more sensitive, a normal MRI examination certainly does not rule out a focal lesion, such as a small area of focal cortical dysplasia (Devinsky et al. 1988; Williamson et al. 1993).

In evaluating the MRI, it must be kept in mind that, albeit rarely, seizures themselves may induce reversible changes. For example, after complex status epilepticus the mesial aspect of the temporal lobe may demonstrate increased signal intensity on diffusion weighted imaging (Parmar et al. 2006; Szabo et al. 2005) and T2-weighted imaging (Henry et al. 1994; Kramer et al. 1987). CT scanning may also be misleading in the same situation, revealing a transient radiolucency (Kramer et al. 1987; Sammaritano et al. 1985).

Lateralizing and localizing symptoms and signs

Certain aspects of simple partial, complex partial or focal grand mal seizures may be helpful in both lateralizing and localizing the responsible lesion, and consequently a good grasp of the clinical symptomatology of the patient's seizure is very helpful. In the case of simple partial seizures, patients

may be able to provide a sufficiently clear history, however in the case of complex partial and grand mal seizures, this is not possible, and one must rely on a history provided by other observers. When this is not reliable, consideration may be given to asking family members to videotape seizures (Newmark 1981; Samuel and Duncan 1994) or, if this is unsuccessful, to admission for video–EEG monitoring.

Before discussing the lateralizing and localizing features peculiar to each seizure type, mention should be made of two post-ictal features, either of which can be seen with any of these three seizure types and which both have strong lateralizing value. The first of these is a post-ictal unilateral Babinski sign. Although it is well recognized that this may be found after a grand mal seizure, it also occurs post-ictally after approximately 20 percent of complex partial seizures (Walczak and Rubinsky 1994). The second is Todd's paralysis. This phenomenon, first described by Todd in 1855, is characterized by a unilateral post-ictal paresis, usually of the upper extremity, which may range in severity from a total paralysis to a mere drift of the upper extremity and which lasts for from seconds up to almost half an hour. It may be found after simple partial seizures with motor symptomatology, complex partial or grand mal seizures (Gallmetzer et al. 2004; Kellinghaus and Kotagal 2004). Both of these features reliably lateralize the lesion to the contralateral hemisphere.

Simple partial seizures often display both lateralizing and localizing signs. In the case of simple partial seizures with either motor or somatosensory signs, the focus is typically, but not always (Herskowitz and Swerdlow 1972), lateralized to the hemisphere contralateral to the side on which the patient is experiencing the symptoms (Mauguire and Courjon 1978). With regard to localization to a particular lobe, in most cases motor signs suggest the frontal lobe, somatosensory symptoms the parietal lobe, simple visual hallucinations or hemianopia the occipital lobe, structured visual hallucinations the occipitoparietal or occipitotemporal region, and most 'psychic' symptoms the temporal lobe (Acharya et al. 1998; Bien et al. 2000; Mauguire and Courjon 1978; Morris et al. 1988; Nystrom 1966; Russell and Whitty 1955; Salanova et al. 1995). In cases in which more than one sort of symptom is seen, careful attention must be paid to which occurred first as this is the one with most localizing value: for example, a simple partial seizure that began with a crude visual hallucination and was immediately followed by a motor sign would indicate a focus in the occipital rather than the frontal lobe (Salanova et al. 1992; Williamson et al. 1992a).

Complex partial seizures, like simple partial seizures, may also display both lateralizing and localizing signs. Lateralizing features include: speech; unilateral ictal clonic, tonic, or dystonic movements or paresis; unilateral automatisms; possibly ictal head version; and, finally, interictal emotional facial palsy. Speech may occur either during an aura, during the seizure itself, or post-ictally, and may be either coherent or aphasic. Ictal speech that is coherent suggests a focus in the non-dominant hemisphere (Fakhoury et al.

1994; Gabr *et al.* 1989; Koerner and Laxer 1988; Marks and Laxer 1998; Yen *et al.* 1996); however, exceptions to this rule do occur (Kaiboriboon *et al.* 2006). Aphasic speech occurring either as an aura (Kanemoto and Janz 1989) or post-ictally (Ajmone-Marsan and Ralston 1957; Devinsky *et al.* 1994a; Fakhoury *et al.* 1994; Gabr *et al.* 1989; Koerner and Laxer 1988; Marks and Laxer 1998; Privitera *et al.* 1991; Serafetinides and Falconer 1963) suggests a focus in the dominant hemisphere. Unilateral ictal clonic, tonic or dystonic movement (Kotagal *et al.* 1989; Marks and Laxer 1998; Rusu *et al.* 2005) and unilateral paresis (Oestreich *et al.* 1995) all suggest a focus on the contralateral side. Unilateral automatisms (Janszky *et al.* 2006; Marks and Laxer 1998) or unilateral ictal eye-blinking (Benbadis *et al.* 1996) both generally indicate an ipsilateral focus. Head version at the start of a seizure is of controversial lateralizing significance: some studies (e.g., Quesney *et al.* 1990; Salanova *et al.* 1995) report that the head turns away from the side with the focus, whereas others (e.g., Geier *et al.* 1977; Ochs *et al.* 1984) have not found such a relationship. With regard to this controversy over the lateralizing significance of head version, one study offered a potential solution by noting first that there are two types of head version: in one the head turning is casual, whereas in the other it is forced and unnatural and often accompanied by hemifacial clonic movements on the side toward which the head is turning. Cases with forced head version lateralized to the hemisphere away from which the head turned (Rheims *et al.* 2005). Interictal emotional facial palsy suggests that the focus is contralateral to the side with the palsy (Cascino *et al.* 1993b; Jacob *et al.* 2003; Remillard *et al.* 1977).

Localization of the focus of a complex partial seizure may not be as straightforward as was once thought. In the not-too-distant past, the assumption that complex partial seizures all originated from foci in the temporal lobe was so unquestioned that some authors used the terms 'complex partial epilepsy' and 'temporal lobe epilepsy' synonymously. It has become clear, however, that even though most complex partial seizures do arise from foci in the temporal lobe (Nystrom 1966), they may also occur secondary to foci in the frontal (Geier *et al.* 1977; Rasmussen 1983; Salanova *et al.* 1995; Sutherling *et al.* 1990; Williamson *et al.* 1985c), occipital (Ludwig and Marsan 1975; Salanova *et al.* 1992; Williamson *et al.* 1992a), or parietal (Cascino *et al.* 1993c; Ho *et al.* 1994; Williamson *et al.* 1992b) lobes. In cases where the focus is in a site other than the temporal lobe, electrical activity spreads rapidly from the originating lobe to the temporal lobes, thus producing the symptomatology of the complex partial seizure itself. As suggested by Jackson (1894), it stands to reason that, in such cases, the aura to the complex partial seizure may indicate the lobe of origin, and this does in fact appear to be the case (Boon *et al.* 1991; Palmini and Gloor 1992), the various aurae having the same localizing value as discussed for simple partial seizures, above. Finally, before leaving the subject of localization in complex partial seizures, note should be made of the significance of ictal bilateral

'bicycling' movements. Some have held that these indicate a frontal lobe onset (Williamson *et al.* 1985c), but such movements have also been noted in complex partial seizures of temporal lobe origin (Sussman *et al.* 1989; Swartz 1994).

Grand mal seizures may also display lateralizing and localizing features. A post-ictal Babinski sign or Todd's paralysis, as described above, may lateralize to the contralateral hemisphere, and any aurae may localize, as described for simple partial seizures, above.

DIFFERENTIAL DIAGNOSIS

In differentiating between seizures and other disorders capable of producing a more or less similar clinical picture, two features are generally helpful. The first feature to consider is the exquisitely paroxysmal onset of all seizure types, occurring over seconds: such an onset is rare in other disorders. Second, one should always, in obtaining a history, search for other seizure types, as their occurrence strongly suggests that the event in differential question is likewise a seizure. Additional differential considerations specific for each of the seizure types are discussed in turn, below, followed by a discussion of pseudoseizures.

Simple partial seizures

A transient ischemic attack or a migrainous aura may mimic most of the symptoms seen in simple partial seizures. Transient ischemic attacks (TIAs), of course, are unlikely in the young; however, when the clinical event in question occurs in an elderly patient with various vascular risk factors, the differential becomes quite problematic. A prototypical case involves patients with episodes of paralysis of a limb, which could represent either a TIA or an inhibitory motor simple partial seizure. The EEG, if productive of an interictal epileptiform discharge, is helpful, but a negative EEG still leaves the differential open, for, as noted earlier, EEGs are typically normal in patients with simple partial seizures. In doubtful cases, consideration may be given to empirical treatment with either an antiplatelet agent or an AED. In the case of migraine, the differential is much simpler: most migrainous aurae are followed by a typical migraine headache, and in those cases of migrainous aura without headache, the history will reveal typical events, with headache, in the past.

Some further considerations come into play in cases of hallucinations or anxiety. Simple partial seizures constitute but one of many disorders capable of causing isolated hallucinations, and the differential for these events, as discussed in Section 4.30, should be pursued. In a similar vein, simple partial seizures, likewise, are but one cause of anxiety attacks, and the differential for these, as outlined in Section 6.5, should also be consulted.

Complex partial seizures

Relatively brief episodes of confusion may be caused not only by complex partial seizures, but also by TIAs when the ischemia is found in one of the temporal lobes or in the thalamus. The differential here proceeds much as discussed immediately above for simple partial seizures; however, here the EEG may be more useful, as interictal epileptiform discharges are more common in cases of complex partial seizures.

Brief episodes of confusion arising from sleep may represent either a nocturnal complex partial seizure or a parasomnia such as REM sleep behavior disorder, night terrors, or somnambulism. REM sleep behavior disorder may be readily identified, as patients with this disorder will, upon 'coming to', report a vivid dream that explains their behavior during the event. Night terrors and somnambulism, however, lack such distinctive clues, and may be closely mimicked by nocturnal complex seizures (Boller *et al.* 1975; Pedley and Guilleminault 1977; Plazzi *et al.* 1995); consequently, polysomnography may be required.

Brief episodes of unprovoked and uncharacteristic violence may suggest either a complex partial seizure or an entity known as *intermittent explosive disorder*. This is a controversial entity putatively characterized by episodes wherein patients, either without any precipitants or with only trivial ones, experience a growing sense of tension and irritability, culminating in an explosion of violence, after which they have only a spotty memory of the event; importantly, at other times in the patients' lives, there are no significant abnormalities (e.g., no chronic irritability). As demonstrated by the examples provided earlier regarding violence during complex partial seizures, it is clear that the similarities between the putative intermittent explosive disorder and a complex partial seizure with reactive automatisms may be compelling. In fact, some believe that intermittent explosive disorder is in fact a species of complex partial epilepsy. Resolving this nosologic question will require further research; in the meantime, one should, when evaluating patients with sporadic, seemingly unmotivated episodes of violence, enquire closely regarding the all-important history of other seizure types.

Prolonged episodes of confusion may represent complex partial status epilepticus; however, in such cases the differential becomes quite large as it encompasses the syndrome of delirium, and in such cases that differential, as discussed in Section 5.3, should be considered.

Petit mal seizures

Apart from complex partial seizures, there is little else that can even come close to mimicking typical petit mal seizures. The presence of an aura or a duration longer than 10 or 15 seconds points toward a diagnosis of a complex partial seizure; in doubtful cases, an interictal EEG will resolve the issue.

Grand mal seizures

Apart from pseudoseizures, discussed below, there is very little that can reduplicate the tonic–clonic activity of a typical grand mal seizure.

Amnestic seizures

Amnestic seizures must be distinguished from transient global amnesia and alcoholic blackouts, a differential discussed in Section 5.4.

Atonic seizures

Atonic seizures may be mimicked by cataplexy or by syncope. In this differential, a good history is essential as in almost all cases of atonic seizures one will find a long history of other seizure types.

Cataplectic attacks are always preceded by some strong emotion and are accompanied by preservation of consciousness, and although atonic seizures, as discussed above, may share the same characteristics, this is very rare.

Syncope may be difficult to distinguish from an atonic seizure (Lempert *et al.* 1994). A 'swoon', in contrast with the 'stricken' fall of an atonic seizure, suggests a vasovagal syncopal episode, and syncope upon standing suggests hypotension. Cardiac syncope may be very similar to an atonic seizure, and Holter monitoring may be required. Furthermore, as noted earlier, some cases of complex partial seizures are accompanied by sinus arrest, and in such cases an AED, rather than anti-arrhythmic, drug, is in order.

Pseudoseizures

Pseudoseizures are paroxysmal events that, rather than occurring on the basis of an electrical paroxysm in the brain, represent a simulation of a seizure, and may be seen in conversion disorder, malingering, and factitious disorder (including 'epileptic Munchausen's syndrome' [Savard *et al.* 1988]). In practice, this differential possibility comes to mind when patients present with episodes that, although resembling either grand mal or complex partial seizures, have some atypical features. After discussing some of these atypical features, consideration will be given to an appropriate work up.

Pseudo-grand mal seizures may begin with a cry, but unlike the inarticulate brief cry of a 'true' grand mal seizure, this cry may involve words and may persist long into the event. The movements seen in a pseudo-grand mal seizure may be thrashing rather than rhythmic, and if attempts are made to restrain these movements the patient with a pseudoseizure may show active resistance. Patients with pseudoseizures may bite their lips, but the tongue is usually spared; furthermore, urinary incontinence is rare during a pseudoseizure.

Pseudo-complex partial seizures often come into the differential when the behavior during the event is quite complex. Although this indeed is suggestive, as most 'true' complex partial seizures are characterized by simple stereotyped automatisms, it is not definitive: as indicated by the examples cited earlier in the chapter, some of the reactive automatisms seen in complex partial seizures are quite complex indeed.

The work up in such cases proceeds in a fashion similar to that described earlier, and should include the following: testing for a post-event Babinski sign; appropriately timed testing for prolactin, neuron-specific enolase and, when grand mal seizures are in question, creatine phosphokinase (CPK) levels; EEG; neuroimaging; consideration of placebo induction, and, in selected cases, single photon emission computed tomography (SPECT) or positron emission tomography (PET) imaging.

A temporary Babinski sign may, as noted earlier, be seen after both grand mal and complex partial seizures As this phenomenon will generally lie outside the knowledge of most pseudoseizure patients, even medically sophisticated ones, its presence is a reliable sign of epileptic activity. Its absence, of course, is of little diagnostic import.

The serum prolactin level rises with depth-electrode stimulation of either the hippocampus or the amygdala (Gallagher *et al.* 1987; Parra *et al.* 1980; Sperling and Wilson 1986), thus serving as a marker for paroxysmal activity in these or related structures and as an indicator that the clinical event in question is a 'true' rather than a 'pseudo' seizure (Laxer *et al.* 1985; Pritchard *et al.* 1985a). Prolactin elevation is, however, not entirely specific to epileptic events, as such elevations may also be seen after hypotensive syncope (Oribe *et al.* 1996). A twofold or greater rise in serum prolactin level is found about 15 minutes post-ictally in most cases of complex partial seizures with temporal lobe onset (Bauer *et al.* 1994; Sperling *et al.* 1986) and in grand mal seizures (Wyllie *et al.* 1984). However, with seizures arising from foci outside the temporal lobe, whether complex partial (Meierkord *et al.* 1992) or simple partial (Dana-Haeri *et al.* 1983; Laxer *et al.* 1985; Sperling *et al.* 1986), prolactin elevation is less likely to occur. Furthermore, after frequent seizures (Jackel *et al.* 1987; Malkowitz *et al.* 1995) or after status epilepticus (Tomson *et al.* 1989) one may find a normal prolactin level, presumably reflecting an exhaustion of the pituitary prolactin stores secondary to prolonged stimulation.

Neuron-specific enolase is a marker of neuronal injury, and, in contrast with the prolactin level, which tends to be normal after status epilepticus, the level of enolase is elevated in such situations (DeGiorgio *et al.* 1999), peaking at one (DeGiorgio *et al.* 1995) to two days (Rabinowicz *et al.* 1995). Neuron-specific enolase may at times also be elevated after single complex partial or grand mal seizures (Rabinowicz *et al.* 1996).

CPK levels rise with muscle injury, and in cases when the differential is between a 'true' grand mal seizure and a pseudoseizure, this should be determined. Rises occur within 3 hours and tend to peak at a day and a half (Chesson *et al.* 1983; Libman *et al.* 1991).

An EEG, if possible, should be obtained concurrent with a typical event, as the finding of ictal electrical activity is obviously very important. The absence of any electrical change, however, does not unequivocally argue against an epileptic etiology given that, albeit very rarely, the ictal EEG during a complex partial seizure may be normal despite clear paroxysmal activity on depth recordings (Lieb *et al.* 1976; Morris *et al.* 1988; Williamson *et al.* 1986).

Neuroimaging, preferably by MR scanning, should be considered to determine whether or not a lesion is present that could, with some probability, be expected to cause seizures. Interpretation here must proceed with some caution, however: in some cases, epileptogenic lesions (e.g., small areas of focal cortical dysplasia) may be very difficult to detect on MRI and, conversely, not all lesions, even although they are easily detected (e.g., a small convexity meningioma), are likely to cause seizures.

Placebo induction, for example with saline infusion (Cohen and Suter 1982; Devinsky *et al.* 1996; Walczak *et al.* 1994), has been used as a diagnostic test for pseudoseizures on the not-implausible assumption that placebos are unlikely to induce paroxysmal electrical activity. It must be borne in mind, however, that placebo may, albeit rarely, induce 'true' seizures (Lesser *et al.* 1983).

Cumulatively, the absence of a Babinski sign, normal prolactin and neuron-specific enolase levels (and CPK levels when grand mal seizures are in question), and a normal ictal EEG and MR scan, coupled with a reproduction of the event in question by placebo induction would, when present in combination, argue very strongly for the diagnosis of pseudoseizure. It must, however, be borne in mind that some 'true' seizures will, albeit very rarely, 'slip by' all these tests. Consequently, in doubtful cases, consideration may be given to ictal SPECT or PET recordings. Essentially, in the work up of a suspected pseudoseizure, one is attempting to 'prove a negative', that is, to 'prove' that the event in question is not accompanied by a paroxysmal electrical discharge. Given that one can never definitively prove a negative, however, the diagnosis of pseudoseizure should always remain somewhat tentative.

A further complication in the diagnostic work up of pseudoseizures is the fact that it is not uncommon for patients to have both pseudoseizures and 'true' seizures (Krumholz and Niedermeyer 1983). Thus, simply demonstrating that a patient has had a pseudoseizure does not mean that the patient does not also have epilepsy.

Treatment

This section will begin with a discussion of *non-emergent treatment*, followed by a consideration of *status epilepticus*.

NON-EMERGENT TREATMENT

In non-emergent cases, when treatment of the underlying cause is either not possible or ineffective, utilization of an AED is appropriate. The first step in choosing among the many AEDs available today is to determine the etiology, as seizures due to one of the idiopathic generalized epilepsies respond differently than do focal seizures.

Idiopathic generalized epilepsies generally respond to treatment with valproic acid, and this is a reasonable first choice for patients with petit mal seizures (Sato *et al.* 1982) and/or non-focal grand mal seizures (Marson *et al.* 2002) with onset from childhood to early adult years. Ethosuximide is also effective for petit mal seizures but is not for grand mal seizures and, given that most patients with childhood or juvenile onset absence epilepsy also, in addition to petit mal seizures, have grand mal seizures, valproic acid seems preferable. Importantly, certain other AEDs, such as phenytoin (Genton et al. 2000), carbamazepine (Genton et al. 2000; Thomas et al. 2006), and oxcarbazepine (Gelisse et al. 2004) may worsen seizure control in patients with idiopathic generalized epilepsies and therefore should be avoided. In cases where valproic acid is only partially effective, further improvement may be obtained by adding topiramate (Biton et al. 1999), lamotrigine (Biton et al. 2005), or levetiracetam (Grunewald 2005). In patients who get little benefit from valproic acid or in whom it is poorly tolerated, consideration may be given to utilizing one of these 'add-on' drugs as monotherapy; however, it should be borne in mind that as yet there are no double-blind studies supporting this practice.

Epilepsy characterized by focal seizures may respond to monotherapy with any of the following: phenytoin or carbamazepine (Heller et al. 1995; Mattson et al. 1985; Ramsey et al. 1983; Rowan et al. 2005; Simonsen et al. 1976; Troupin et al. 1977), oxcarbazepine (Beydoun et al. 2000; Schacter et al. 1999), valproic acid (Beydoun et al. 1997; Callaghan et al. 1985; Heller et al. 1995; Mattson et al. 1992), gabapentin (Rowan et al. 2005), topiramate, or lamotrigine (Brodie et al. 1995; Rowan et al. 2005) and levetiracetam (Brodie et al. 2007). The choice among these is guided by considerations of the patient's general medical condition, potential drug–drug interactions with other medications, anticipated side-effects, etc. In cases where patients fail to respond to monotherapy, one may choose either to try monotherapy with a different AED or to add on an AED to the one already in place. In cases where the first AED used as monotherapy was relatively ineffective or simply not tolerated, then a switch to another monotherapy agent is reasonable, however when the first AED had definite benefit and was well-tolerated, then it is reasonable to consider an 'add-on' strategy. Most of the 'add-on' studies have been performed with patients already on either phenytoin or carbamazepine, however, admittedly, there is no consistency over all these studies. Consideration may be given to the following as 'add-on' AEDs: valproic acid (Willmore et al. 1996), gabapentin (Fuerstein et al. 1994; Sivenius et al. 1991; US Gabapentin Study Group 1993), pregabalin (Beydoun et al. 2005; Elger et al. 2005), topiramate (Faught et al. 1996; Privitera et al. 1996), lamotrigine (Binnie et al. 1989; Boas et al. 1996; Jawad et al. 1989; Loiseau et al. 1990b; Matsuo et al. 1993; Messenheimer et al. 1994), and levetiracetam (Cereghino et al. 2000; Leppik et al. 2003; Tsai et al. 2006) (which appears to be at times very effective [Stefan et al. 2006]). In choosing among these, particular attention must be paid to potential drug–drug interactions. In cases when patients fail to respond to treatment with two AEDs, various options are open. First, one may try either monotherapy with a different agent or try a different combination of two agents. In some cases, patients have responded to treatment with a combination of three AEDs but this strategy is very problematic: the risk of both pharmacokinetic and, especially, pharmacodynamic drug–drug interactions becomes so high that side-effects are often unacceptable. Furthermore, with such 'triple therapy' regimens there may be an exacerbation of the epilepsy: not uncommonly, patients on triple therapy who carry a diagnosis of 'treatment-resistant epilepsy' enjoy a substantial decrease in seizure frequency after one or more of their AEDs are discontinued.

The mechanism or mechanisms underlying treatment resistance are not clear. Recent research has focused on the role of what are known as multidrug resistance proteins. These proteins are normally found on capillary endothelial cells and serve to maintain the blood–brain barrier by pumping out foreign substances (such as AEDs) from the interstitial fluid back into the blood: one theory holds that they are up-regulated in patients with treatment resistance (Aronica et al. 2004). Regardless of the cause of treatment resistance, several options are open. In some cases, epilepsy surgery is appropriate, as for example in those with mesial temporal sclerosis (Engel 1996; Wiebe et al. 2001) or certain cases of focal cortical dysplasia (Kral et al. 2003). Vagal nerve stimulation (Handforth et al. 1998; Salinsky et al. 1996) may also be considered, and there is also some very preliminary evidence for the efficacy of transcranial magnetic stimulation in patients with various cortical dysplasias (Fregni et al. 2006).

In cases where patients have been seizure free for two or more years, the possibility of tapering and discontinuing AEDs may be entertained. The decision to embark on this course, however, is complex. To begin with, consideration should be given to the consequences of a recurrence of seizures and to the burden imposed by ongoing treatment. In patients with only simple partial seizures, the consequences of another seizure may not be severe, and if side-effects from current AED treatment are bothersome then discontinuation may seem attractive; on the other hand a history of grand mal seizures and a lack of side-effects might give one pause. Another consideration, of course, is the likelihood of recurrence, and several factors may enable one to make a rough estimate in this regard (Callaghan et al. 1988; Cardoso et al. 2006; Spooner et al. 2006), including the presence or absence of a lesion, the frequency of seizures and the difficulty encountered in initially controlling them, the kinds of seizures experienced by the patient, and the presence of interictal epileptiform discharges (IEDs). Not unreasonably, the presence of a lesion, such as mesial temporal sclerosis, increases the risk; by contrast, patients with idiopathic generalized epilepsies appear to be at lower risk. A history of very frequent seizures coupled with great difficulty in controlling them (as evidenced by the number of trials of AEDs required to do so) suggests a more severe underlying process and this also increases the risk of recurrence. The kinds of seizures experienced by the patient also may serve as an indicator of the severity of the underlying process. Thus, a history of complex partial seizures with secondary generalization poses a higher risk than does a history of simple or complex partial seizures without secondary generalization or a history of non-focal grand mal seizures (as seen in the idiopathic generalized epilepsies). Finally, the presence of IEDs on an EEG obtained close to the end of the 2-year seizure-free period indicates ongoing activity of the underlying disorder and suggests an increased risk of recurrence. Although some patients may fall at the extremes of these risk factors, most fall in between and, consequently, much clinical judgment should be utilized in balancing these various risk factors. If a decision is made to taper and discontinue AEDs the process should be a slow one, generally extending over 3–6 months, and if more than one AED is in place, only one should be tapered at a time.

In addition to the foregoing, some general measures are appropriate in all cases. First, certain non-specific stresses may aggravate epilepsy and these should be avoided or treated. They include poor sleep, irregular dietary habits, dehydration, febrile illnesses, hyperventilation, and excessive alcohol use. Second, there are certain specific disorders which also aggravate epilepsy, including migraine, sleep apnea and, in some females, the menstrual cycle. Although, of itself, migraine probably does not cause seizures, there is evidence that migraine may be able to precipitate seizures in patients with epilepsy. In particular, it appears that a migraine aura may trigger either a partial or a grand mal seizure, the seizure being intercalated between the migraine aura and the migraine headache (Marks and Ehrenberg 1993): in such cases effective migraine prophylaxis is essential and either valproic acid or topiramate are logical choices as they are effective not only as AEDs, but also as prophylaxis against migraine. Obstructive sleep apnea may aggravate seizures and treatment of the apnea with continuous positive airway pressure may be very effective in reducing seizure frequency (Devinsky et al. 1994b). Finally, some women will experience an increase in seizure frequency either toward the end of the follicular phase or during menstrual flow (Backstrom 1976), and although oral contraceptives have been advocated in such situations (Mattson et al. 1986) this is controversial (Dana-Haeri and Richens 1983).

Reflex seizures, of course, constitute an invitation to the utilization of common-sense measures at avoiding the reflex stimulus itself. In cases where this is not feasible, it may be possible, in certain cases, to blunt the provocative effect of the stimulus by repeatedly exposing the patient to that stimulus, as has been demonstrated in cases of musicogenic (Forster et al. 1967) and reading (Forster et al. 1969a) epilepsies.

Remarkably, albeit rarely, some patients have found it possible to abort partial seizures. Thus, in some cases of simple partial seizures that undergo a Jacksonian march, the seizure may be aborted by vigorously rubbing the part of the body that lies just proximal to the advancing march, and this holds true not only for motor (Russell and Whitty 1953; Symonds 1959), but also for sensory (Efron 1961; Sutherling et al. 1990) marches. In the case of complex partial seizures, Penfield (Penfield and Jasper 1954) noted that, when the aura consisted of some 'change in the stream of thought', the patient might be able to prevent the development of the seizure by 'forcing his thoughts with 'might and main' into some other channel'. Other techniques have been reported: one patient, whose aura consisted of an olfactory hallucination, was able to prevent a complex partial seizure by the application of a 'strong odor' (Efron 1956, 1957), and another patient, whose aura consisted of an auditory hallucination of music, was able to abort the seizure by 'imagining himself fishing, his favorite leisure pursuit' (Pritchard et al. 1985b).

Status epilepticus

Status epilepticus is approached differently depending on the kind of seizure involved. Grand mal status epilepticus is an acutely life-threatening event that also, in those who survive, entails significant sequelae; thus it requires emergent treatment. Complex partial status epilepticus, in contrast, is not life-threatening and, although sequelae have been noted, they are uncommon and, consequently, emergency treatment may not be required. Simple partial status, petit mal status and amnestic status are, of themselves, benign events and may be approached non-emergently.

In all cases of status, regardless of the seizure type, a finger stick glucose level is determined and if the level is low then 50 mL of D50W is given. Thiamine, 100 mg i.v., should also be given if there is any suspicion of alcoholism or severe malnutrition. Blood is sent for determination of glucose, sodium, potassium, calcium, magnesium, blood urea nitrogen (BUN), and, if appropriate, AED levels.

In cases requiring emergent treatment, intravenous access is obtained and lorazepam is given in a total dose of ~0.07 mg/kg at a rate no faster than 2 mg/min; as a rule, fosphenytoin should then be administered in a total dose of 15–25 mg/kg at a rate of 100–150 mg/min (Browne et al. 1996; Lowenstein et al. 1998; Ramsey and DeToledo 1996; Treiman et al. 1998). Exceptions to this rule include the following: allergy; a history of non-response to adequate levels of phenytoin; current treatment with phenytoin with blood levels in the therapeutic range; and cases where the grand mal seizures are occurring as part of one of the idiopathic generalized epilepsy syndromes. In cases where one of these exceptions obtain, consideration should be given to intravenous valproate in a total dose of 15–25 mg/kg (Misra et al. 2006): although current recommendations suggest infusing this at a rate no faster than 20 mg/min (or over a total of 60 min, whichever is longer), recent work suggests that much faster infusions, at 3–10 mg/kg/min are effective and well tolerated (Boggs et al. 2000; Limdi et al. 2007; Wheless et al. 2004). Regardless of whether fosphenytoin or valproate is given, an AED blood level should be obtained approximately 2 hours after the infusion is completed, with subsequent doses based on levels and response. When all of these measures are under way the patient must be closely monitored, preferably in an intensive care unit (ICU). In cases when status persists despite these measures, consideration may be given to utilizing two AEDs: thus, if a patient had been given fosphenytoin and failed to respond, valproate could be added; alternatives include levetiracetam (Patel *et al.* 2006) or phenobarbital, in a total dose of 20 mg/kg, at a rate no faster than 100 mg/min. In cases resistant to these measures, coma may be induced with pentobarbital, midazolam, or propofol.

Non-emergent treatment may involve oral loading with phenytoin, or, in cases of petit mal status, valproic acid. Phenytoin may be loaded in a dose of 15–25 mg orally, and valproic acid likewise in a dose of 15–25 mg/kg (importantly, divalproex should not be used emergently given the long time required to obtain peak blood levels). Alternatively, if the current episode of status occurred secondary to non-compliance with an AED other than phenytoin or valproic acid, and the patient had a clear history of response to that AED, one might simply load the patient with this previously effective agent.

7.4 STROKE

Stroke is defined as the more or less sudden occurrence of a neuropsychiatric deficit occurring secondary to a vascular event, such as an ischemic infarction or an intracerebral hemorrhage, and the diagnosis should be suspected in any patient with the acute onset of virtually any of the signs, symptoms or syndromes described in the preceding chapters including, most especially, weakness (such as hemiparesis), sensory changes, aphasia, agnosia, neglect, or delirium. The evaluation and care of stroke patients has undergone revolutionary advances in the recent past and, especially in acute cases, patients should generally be referred to stroke specialists.

Clinical features

Given that the clinical features of stroke are determined, in large part, by the vessel involved, this discussion will begin with a review of the *arterial supply and venous drainage of the brain*. Once this is in mind, attention is then turned to the most common cause of stroke, namely *ischemic infarction*, followed by discussions of less common causes such as *intracerebral hemorrhage* and *subarachnoid hemorrhage* and, finally, of two rare causes, namely *intraventricular hemorrhage* and *cerebral venous thrombosis*. Finally, attention is directed to various *sequelae of stroke*, such as dementia and post-stroke depression.

ARTERIAL SUPPLY AND VENOUS DRAINAGE OF THE BRAIN

Arterial supply

In tracing the arterial supply to the brain (Tatu *et al.* 1996, 1998), one may begin at the aortic arch, from which arises first the innominate artery, which, in turn, bifurcates into the right common carotid artery and the right subclavian artery. Passing further along the aortic arch, the left common carotid artery arises and, a little after that, the aortic arch gives off the left subclavian artery. From both subclavian

arteries arise the vertebral arteries. Under normal circumstances, the entire blood supply to the brain is derived from the internal carotid arteries and the vertebral arteries, as described below: in clinical work, arteries derived from the internal carotid arteries are referred to as part of the 'anterior circulation', whereas those derived from the vertebral arteries are referred to as part of the 'posterior circulation'.

Both common carotid arteries bifurcate at the level of the thyroid cartilage into an external carotid artery and an internal carotid artery (ICA). The internal carotid artery may then be divided into four segments, namely cervical, intrapetrosal, intracavernous, and supraclinoid. The cervical segment rises from the bifurcation and passes up through the neck, without giving off any branches. Upon arriving at the skull, the internal carotid artery then enters the petrous portion of the temporal bone via the foramen lacerum and passes through the temporal bone as the intrapetrosal segment. The artery emerges from the temporal bone into the cavernous sinus, and passes horizontally through the sinus close to its medial wall. This intracavernous portion bears important relations to the other occupants of the cavernous sinus, namely the third, fourth and sixth cranial nerves, and the first and second divisions of the fifth cranial nerve. After passing through the cavernous sinus, the internal carotid artery then swings superiorly and emerges medial to the anterior clinoid process as the supraclinoid segment.

After emerging from the cavernous sinus, the internal carotid artery gives off several branches, including the ophthalmic, posterior communicating, and anterior choroidal arteries. The ophthalmic artery passes forward in relation to the optic nerve and enters the orbit via the optic foramen. The posterior communicating artery passes posteriorly, and forms part of the circle of Willis, described below. The anterior choroidal artery also passes posteriorly, giving off important central branches, also described below. After giving off these three branches, the internal carotid artery then bifurcates into the anterior cerebral artery (ACA) and the middle cerebral artery (MCA).

The anterior cerebral artery passes anteriorly and medially, crossing superior to the optic nerve, to reach the interhemispheric fissure. Before passing into the fissure, it is joined to its partner on the opposite side by the anterior communicating artery. After passing into the interhemispheric fissure, the ACA, traveling inferior to the rostrum and genu of the corpus callosum, gives off orbitofrontal branches and a frontopolar artery. After rising over the genu, the ACA then bifurcates into a callosomarginal artery and a pericallosal artery, which extends along the body of the corpus callosum all the way to the splenium. Although this overall description of the ACA holds true in most cases, important normal variations may occur. In a few percent of cases, the ICA on one side does not give rise to an ACA, and in this situation the ACA on that side arises from the anterior communicating artery, such that both ACAs draw their blood from one ICA. Another very important variation is the fact that in over one-third of individuals a given ACA will supply not only its own hemisphere, but also will send various branches to the opposite hemisphere. Finally, in perhaps 5 percent of individuals, there may be only one ACA: this azygous, or unpaired, ACA then supplies the medial aspect of both hemispheres.

The MCA passes laterally, inferior to the anterior perforated substance, to reach the lateral cerebral fissure, where it typically bifurcates into superior and inferior divisions. The superior division gives rise to the orbitofrontal artery, pre-Rolandic artery, Rolandic artery, anterior parietal artery, posterior parietal artery and, in about one-half of individuals, the angular artery. The inferior division in turn gives rise to the temporopolar artery, the anterior temporal artery, the middle temporal artery, the posterior temporal artery, and, in the other one-half of normal individuals, the angular artery. In a small percentage of individuals, rather than bifurcating, the MCA may undergo a trifurcation, or, in an even smaller percentage, may directly divide into the numerous branches just named.

Turning now to the vertebral arteries (which have arisen from the subclavian arteries in the neck): these rise to the level of the sixth cervical vertebra where they enter the transverse foramina; subsequently, they rise through the transverse foramina of the remaining cervical vertebrae to eventually enter the cranium through the foramen magnum. Once inside the cranium, they initially ascend on either side of the medulla, and eventually merge at the junction of the medulla and pons to form the basilar artery. Before merging, however, in addition to giving off numerous small penetrating branches to the medulla, they also give rise to several large branches, namely the posterior spinal artery, the posterior inferior cerebellar artery, and the anterior spinal artery. The posterior spinal arteries move posteriorly and descend along the posterior aspect of the spinal cord. The posterior inferior cerebellar artery courses along the lateral aspect of the medulla and then reaches the inferior aspect of the cerebellum. The anterior spinal artery is formed by two branches, arising from both vertebral arteries, which meet in the midline to form this artery; the artery then descends along the anterior midline of the medulla to the cord below.

The basilar artery, arising from the junction of the two vertebral arteries, ascends along the ventral surface of the pons and onto the ventral surface of the midbrain whereupon it bifurcates into the two posterior cerebral arteries. The basilar artery gives off numerous branches. The anterior inferior cerebellar artery arises first and supplies the inferior surface of the cerebellum. Penetrating branches are given off throughout the course of the basilar artery and include paramedian, short circumferential, and long circumferential arteries. Just before the basilar artery bifurcates into the posterior cerebral arteries (PCAs) it gives off the superior cerebellar arteries, which nourish the superior surface of the cerebellum.

The PCA courses around the surface of the midbrain and passes superiorly medial to the tentorium, after which it bifurcates into a temporo-occipital artery and an internal occipital artery. The temporo-occipital artery courses laterally to supply the inferior surface of the temporal lobe and adjacent occipital lobe, including the occipitotemporal gyrus and the lingual gyrus. The internal occipital artery bifurcates into the parieto-occipital artery and the calcarine artery. The parieto-occipital artery, in addition to supplying the medial aspect of the occipital and parietal lobes, also supplies the splenium of the corpus callosum. The calcarine artery supplies the medial aspect of the occipital lobe, including the critically important calcarine cortex. An important normal variant of the posterior cerebral artery, seen in about 10 percent of individuals, consists of a 'fetal' pattern of circulation wherein one of the PCAs, rather than arising from the basilar artery, originates from the internal carotid artery, as it were replacing the posterior communicating artery.

The anterior, middle, and posterior cerebral arteries supply most of the cerebral cortex. Subcortical structures, including the basal ganglia and the thalamus, are supplied by various central branches, most, but not all, of which arise from the circle of Willis. The first component of the circle of Willis to consider is the posterior communicating artery, which, as noted earlier, arises from the ICA. The posterior communicating artery courses posteriorly to anastamose with the PCA. Subsequent components of the circle include the ipsilateral PCA, the contralateral PCA, the contralateral posterior communicating artery, the contralateral ACA, the anterior communicating artery, and the ipsilateral ACA, which then brings us full circle. In addition to some central branches, discussed immediately below, the circle of Willis also gives off multiple very small penetrating branches that nourish, among other structures, the hypothalamus and portions of the midbrain.

The central branches to be considered now include the following: the thalamopolar artery, the thalamo-perforating artery, the thalamogeniculate artery, the posterior choroidal artery, the recurrent artery of Heubner, the lenticulostriate arteries, and the anterior choroidal artery.

The thalamopolar artery arises from the posterior communicating artery and supplies anterior and lateral portions of the thalamus, including the dorsomedial nucleus, ventral lateral nucleus, and portions of the mammillothalamic tract. In a small minority of cases, both thalamopolar arteries may arise from a common pedicle arising from one or the other posterior communicating artery.

The thalamoperforating artery arises from the PCA medial to its junction with the posterior communicating artery, and supplies the central portion of the thalamus, including the intralaminar nuclei and portions of the mammillothalamic tract. In a small minority of cases both thalamoperforating arteries may arise from a common pedicle.

The thalamogeniculate artery arises from the posterior cerebral artery lateral to the junction with the posterior communicating artery and supplies portions of the lateral geniculate body and both the ventral posterolateral and ventral posteromedial nuclei of the thalamus.

The posterior choroidal artery arises from the PCA lateral to the origin of the thalamogeniculate artery. The posterior choroidal artery bifurcates into a medial posterior choroidal artery and a lateral posterior choroidal artery. The medial posterior choroidal artery courses medially to gain the medial aspect of the thalamus, where it supplies the anterior thalamic nuclei and the choroid plexus of the third ventricle. The lateral posterior choroidal artery courses laterally and enters the choroidal fissure of the temporal lobe to supply portions of the choroid plexus of the inferior horn of the lateral ventricle and portions of the hippocampus.

The recurrent artery of Heubner arises from the ACA and gives off branches that, after arising through the anterior perforated substance, supply the ventral portion of the head of the caudate, the inferior portion of the anterior limb of the internal capsule, and the anterior portion of the putamen.

The lenticulostriate arteries arise from the stem of the MCA before it reaches the lateral cerebral fissure. These arteries rise up through the anterior perforated substance, after which they supply the superior portion of the posterior limb of the internal capsule, the lateral portion of the globus pallidus, and most of the putamen.

The anterior choroidal artery, as noted earlier, arises from the internal carotid artery. It courses posteriorly, lateral to the midbrain and then turns laterally to pierce the choroidal fissure of the temporal lobe and supply portions of the choroid plexus of the inferior horn of the lateral ventricle and portions of the hippocampus. Before turning laterally, however, the anterior choroidal artery also gives off branches that supply the inferior portion of the posterior limb of the internal capsule, the retrolenticular portion of the posterior limb of the internal capsule and portions of the lateral geniculate body. A branch also supplies a portion of the globus pallidus.

Venous drainage

Venous drainage of the brain is accomplished via the superficial and deep cerebral veins, which in turn drain into the dural venous sinuses.

Of the dural sinuses, the first to consider is the superior sagittal sinus, which extends posteriorly along the superior edge of the falx cerebri to reach the sinus confluens. The inferior sagittal sinus extends posteriorly along the free edge of the falx cerebri to the edge of the tentorium cerebelli, where it joins with the great vein of Galen to form the straight sinus. The straight sinus, in turn, runs posteriorly in the junction of the falx cerebri and tentorium cerebelli to eventually join the terminus of the superior sagittal sinus at the sinus confluens. The sinus confluens then gives rise to the transverse sinuses, each of which courses anteriorly along the outer edge of the tentorium cerebelli. In a majority of cases, the straight sinus enters directly into the left transverse sinus, whereas the superior sagittal sinus drains directly into the right transverse sinus. The transverse sinus, upon reaching the junction of the occipital and petrosal bones, empties into the sigmoid sinus, which curves downward to drain into the internal jugular vein.

The next dural sinus to consider is the cavernous sinus, which lies lateral to the sella turcica and its enclosed pituitary gland. The cavernous sinus, in turn, drains posteriorly by two other sinuses, the superior petrosal and inferior petrosal sinuses, which connect, respectively, with the transverse sinus and the internal jugular vein.

The superficial cerebral veins lie on the cortex and drain into the various nearby dural sinuses. Importantly, these superficial cerebral veins are interconnected by various anastamotic veins that, by providing alternative outflows, minimize the consequences of a single occlusion. The deep cerebral veins drain subcortical structures and the medial aspects of the temporal lobes: the two most important types of these veins are the internal cerebral veins and the basal vein of Rosenthal, which join to form the great vein of Galen – as noted earlier this vein drains into the straight sinus.

ISCHEMIC INFARCTION

Ischemic infarctions of the brain may be subdivided into the following groups: *large vessel syndromes*, occurring secondary to occlusion of one of the large pial vessels, such as the MCA; *low-flow (watershed) infarctions* located in the boundary zone between the areas of distribution of two large vessels, for example the MCAs and ACAs; and *lacunar syndromes* resulting from occlusion of central or penetrating arteries. Attention is then turned to *transient ischemic attacks (TIAs)*, which occur due to temporary occlusion of a vessel, and, finally, to so-called 'silent' infarctions.

Large vessel syndromes

In the following paragraphs, the typical syndromes seen with occlusion of the large cerebral vessels, namely the middle, anterior, and posterior cerebral arteries, the anterior choroidal artery, and the basilar and vertebral arteries, are discussed. It must be borne in mind, however, that more often than not only fragments of these syndromes are seen. This is particularly the case with embolic infarction, wherein, rather than occluding the large vessel at or close to its origin, the embolus travels up the artery to lodge in a smaller branch.

MCA infarction may be only partial, involving only the superior division or the inferior division, or may be complete, involving both divisions. Infarction in the area of distribution of the superior division typically produces a contralateral hemiparesis and hemisensory loss, with preferential involvement of the face and upper extremity. When the right hemisphere is affected, left neglect and anosognosia (Hier *et al.* 1983) are commonly seen; other signs that may appear include asomatagnosia, constructional and dressing apraxia, and aprosodia. With involvement of the left hemisphere a motor aphasia typically occurs: in cases of left-sided infarction where the angular artery arises from the superior division, the additional involvement of Wernicke's area will produce a global aphasia; other signs that may occur include ideomotor or ideational apraxia and Gerstmann's syndrome.

Infarction in the area of distribution of the inferior division generally causes a contralateral hemianopia or quadrantopia. With right-sided infarction, a delirium, often accompanied by agitation (Caplan *et al.* 1986) is common and prosopagnosia may also be seen. With left-sided infarction, in cases where the angular artery arises from the inferior division, one typically sees a sensory aphasia; delirium may also occur but is less common than with right-sided infarction. Complete infarction, involving both the upper and lower divisions, is often a catastrophic event (Heinsius *et al.* 1998) and, in addition to a profound hemiplegia, such a 'malignant MCA infarction' may also be accompanied by stupor and vasogenic edema developing over the following 2–5 days may cause uncal or tentorial herniation with coma and death (Hacke *et al.* 1996): in such cases, decompressive hemicraniectomy may be life-saving.

ACA infarction, classically, produces a contralateral hemiplegia and hemianesthesia preferentially affecting the lower extremity (Critchley 1930); when the left hemisphere is involved, a transcortical motor aphasia may also appear. When the corpus callosum is infarcted, one may also see a 'disconnection syndrome' with left-sided, but not right-sided, agraphia, tactile agnosia or apraxia, and, rarely, the alien hand syndrome. In cases of bilateral infarction (e.g., as may occur with an azygous ACA), paraplegia may occur, as may abulia, a frontal lobe syndrome, or akinetic mutism.

PCA infarction typically causes a contralateral hemianopia (Castaigne *et al.* 1973; Pessin *et al.* 1987). If the infarction is on the left, one may also see alexia with agraphia, visual agnosia, and, if the temporal lobe is involved, a delirium. Infarctions on the right side that also involve the temporal lobe may be accompanied by prosopagnosia, and, in some cases a delirium (Medina *et al.* 1974). Bilateral infarction is signaled by cortical blindness, which may or may not be accompanied by Anton's syndrome, with denial of the blindness. In cases of bilateral infarction when both temporal lobes are involved, patients may also be left with a Korsakoff's syndrome. As described earlier, central branches arise from the PCA (i.e., thalamoperforating, thalamogeniculate, and posterior choroidal) and if these are also occluded, the typical symptoms just described will be joined by the syndromes peculiar to occlusion of these central branches, as described below, under 'lacunar syndromes'. Furthermore, when some of the very small penetrating branches to the mesencephalon are involved, there may be hemiparesis, oculomotor disturbances, and abnormal movements.

Anterior choroidal artery infarction is marked by contralateral hemiplegia and hemianopia (Helgason *et al.* 1986). Importantly, however, there is no accompanying aphasia or neglect, and generally no, or only transient, hemianesthesia, and it is the absence of these symptoms that distinguishes these infarctions from those that occur secondary to occlusion of the MCA.

Basilar artery occlusion is often a catastrophic event (Caplan 1979; von Campe *et al.* 2003). Involvement of the basis pontis produces a quadriparesis, and involvement of the midbrain will add diplopia.

Vertebral artery occlusion or occlusion of a posterior inferior cerebellar artery (or occlusion of one of the perforating branches of either of these arteries) may give rise to the classic Wallenberg or 'lateral medullary' syndrome (Kim 2003; Sacco *et al.* 1993). Infarction of the lateral medulla typically involves the following structures: inferior cerebellar peduncle, spinothalamic tract, the spinal tract and nucleus of the fifth cranial nerve, the nucleus ambiguus, vestibular nuclei, and descending sympathetic fibers. Respectively, the corresponding symptoms are: ipsilateral ataxia; contralateral hemianesthesia of the extremities; ipsilateral anesthesia of the face (which may be accompanied by pain); hoarseness and dysphagia; nausea, vomiting, and vertigo; and an ipsilateral Horner's syndrome. Occlusion of one of the originating branches of the anterior spinal artery may produce the 'medial medullary' syndrome (Kim *et al.* 1995). Here, infarction of the pyramid and of the emerging fibers of the twelfth cranial nerve give rise to an ipsilateral paresis of the tongue and a contralateral hemiparesis.

Cerebellar artery occlusion, including the posterior inferior, anterior inferior, and superior cerebellar arteries, may cause vertigo, nausea, nystagmus, or ipsilateral ataxia. Large infarctions, with attendant vasogenic edema, may, by compressing the underlying brainstem, cause stupor or coma, and in such cases emergent neurosurgical intervention may be required (Jensen *et al.* 2005).

Low–flow (watershed) infarctions

Watershed infarctions typically present with more or less atypical fragments of some of the large vessel syndromes. Thus, ACA–MCA watershed infarcts involving the prefrontal cortex and subjacent white matter may present with brachial or crural paresis, and, when the left hemisphere is involved one may see mutism, initially, which resolves into a transcortical motor aphasia. MCA–PCA watershed infarcts may present with hemianesthesia, hemianopia, and, if the left hemisphere is involved, a transcortical sensory aphasia. ACA–MCA infarcts involving the centrum semiovale present with a variable mixture of either of the foregoing syndromes. 'Internal' watershed infarcts in the border zone between the MCA and lenticulostriate arteries may present with hemiparesis with or without hemianesthesia (Kumral *et al.* 2004).

Lacunar syndromes

Lacunes are small cavities, ranging in size from 1 to 20 mm, which typically represent infarctions in the area of distribution of one of the central or perforating branches described earlier (Fisher 1965, 1982; Mohr 1982). Although the clinical presentation of lacunar infarctions is quite varied, depending on the location of the lacune (Arboix *et al.* 2006), certain presentations are quite distinctive and highly suggestive of lacunar infarction. These 'classic' lacunar syndromes include 'pure motor stroke', 'ataxic hemiparesis', 'dysarthria-clumsy hand', and 'pure sensory stroke'.

Pure motor stroke, as the name suggests, is characterized by a hemiparesis in the absence of sensory changes or other symptoms such as aphasia or neglect. Typically, the upper and lower extremities are more or less equally involved (with or without involvement of the ipsilateral lower face) and this pattern helps distinguish hemiplegia due to lacunar infarction from hemiplegia due to middle or anterior cerebral artery infarction wherein either, respectively, the upper or lower extremity is preferentially involved. The responsible lacune in pure motor stroke may be found in the contralateral corona radiata, internal capsule, cerebral peduncle, basis pontis, or medullary pyramid. In cases where the lacune is in the brainstem, one may see contralateral cranial nerve palsies, helping to further localize it: a third nerve palsy suggests a midbrain location; a sixth nerve palsy, a pontine location; and a twelfth nerve palsy, a medullary one.

In cases when pure motor stroke is characterized by either a monoparesis (of either the upper or the lower extremity) or an isolated facial paresis, the responsible lacune may not only be due to infarction in the area of distribution of the central or perforating arteries and located in the areas just described, but may also occur secondary to infarction due to occlusion of terminal branches of the MCA (or, less commonly, the ACA), producing small infarctions in the motor cortex (Maeder-Ingvar et al. 2005; Paciaroni et al. 2005).

Ataxic hemiparesis manifests with a combination of ataxia and hemiparesis and the lacune is typically found in the corona radiata, internal capsule, or basis pontis.

Dysarthria clumsy hand presents not only with dysarthria and clumsiness of the hand but also with a lower facial paresis ipsilateral to the clumsy hand; the lacune is typically found in the corona radiata, internal capsule (near the genu), or the rostral basis pontis (Arboix et al. 2004).

Pure sensory stroke is characterized by hemianesthesia occurring in isolation, and in the absence of motor weakness or other symptomatology. In such cases, a lacune is typically found in the ventrolateral thalamus: occasionally, when the lacune is surrounded by a substantial amount of edema, involvement of the adjacent posterior limb of the internal capsule may cause a contralateral hemiplegia, which, however, is usually relatively mild and clears as the edema resolves. In the months following a pure sensory stroke, a minority of patients may begin to experience chronic painful dysesthesiae in the involved limbs.

Other, less 'classic' lacunar syndromes may occur with infarction of other portions of the thalamus or with lacunar infarction of the caudate nucleus.

Lacunes affecting the anterior or central portions of the thalamus (Bogousslavsky et al. 1988; Giannopoulos et al. 2006; Graff-Radford et al. 1985), as may occur with occlusion of the thalamopolar or thalamoperforating arteries, typically present acutely with delirium or somnolence. Over time, patients typically become alert but are left with memory deficits (reflecting involvement of the mammillothalamic tract) or a frontal lobe syndrome (with involvement of the dorsomedial nucleus); furthermore, when the lacune is on the left, aphasia may occur and, when on the right, neglect may be seen.

Caudate lacunes (Caplan et al. 1990; Mendez et al. 1989), as may occur with occlusion of the recurrent artery of Heubner, are typically characterized by frontal lobe symptoms, especially abulia, and, less commonly, by chorea. Early on there may also be a dysarthria or mild hemiparesis, both transient, and agitation or restlessness, especially when the lacune is in the right caudate nucleus.

Finally, and before leaving this discussion of lacunar syndromes, mention should be made of a condition known either as a 'giant lacune' or a 'striatocapsular infarction' (Weiller et al. 1990). Here, all, or almost all, of the lenticulostriate arteries on one side are occluded, resulting in a relatively large infarction involving the posterior limb of the internal capsule and the putamen. These infarctions are typically larger than 20 mm in diameter and thus, technically, do not qualify as 'lacunes'. Their discrete shape and subcortical location, however, tempt one to use the word 'lacune' in referring to them, and this linguistic tension has given rise to the compromise term 'giant lacune'. Symptomatically, as might be expected, such a giant lacune generally presents with a contralateral hemiplegia that may be accompanied, if the lesion is on the left, by a transcortical motor aphasia or, if the lesion is on the right, by left neglect. The mechanism underlying such a 'giant lacune' varies according to the anatomy of the lenticulostriate arteries in question. As noted earlier, in most cases the lenticulostriate arteries arise sequentially from along the stem of the middle cerebral artery, and in these cases the responsible lesion is generally an embolus that lodges in the MCA stem proximal to the origin of the first of the lenticulostriate arteries. In such a scenario, the lack of collateral supply to the area nourished by the lenticulostriate arteries leads to infarction, whereas the cerebral cortex, being supplied with rich collaterals, may escape infarction. In other cases, all the lenticulostriate arteries arise from one common pedicle arising from the MCA stem, and in these cases the occlusion of this one pedicle, either by lipohyalinosis or encroachment of an atherosclerotic plaque, may do the job.

Transient ischemic attacks

A TIA represents the results of fully reversible neuronal ischemia due to a transient reduction in blood supply. Clinically, patients may experience any of the symptoms of ischemic infarction just described, with one critical difference: after a brief period of time, the symptoms resolve completely, with a full restoration of prior functional ability. There has been some controversy regarding the duration of symptoms seen in a TIA. In the past, it was felt that symptoms could persist for up to 24 hours; however, more recent studies with diffusion-weighted imaging (DWI) MR scanning have revealed that in cases when symptoms last much longer than 30 minutes (Inanatomia et al. 2004), and certainly for an hour or more (Ay et al. 2005), that actual infarction has generally occurred. Thus, it is probably best to reserve this diagnosis for cases where symptoms last no longer than a half hour, and in no case for more than an hour, and, if MR scanning is performed, for cases in which DWI is negative.

The transient reduction in blood flow may be due to either an embolus that fragments and passes on in a few minutes, or to temporary low flow past a thrombus or through a stenosed artery, as may occur during an episode of systemic hypotension. One very important kind of TIA, not mentioned earlier, is amaurosis fugax ('fleeting blindness', also referred to as transient monocular blindness), wherein the patient experiences partial or complete blindness for a matter of minutes in one eye: such episodes are highly suggestive of a disease in the ipsilateral carotid artery proximal to the origin of the ophthalmic artery.

TIAs may herald either embolic or thrombotic infarctions, including lacunar infarctions. Indeed, in one study (Rothwell *et al.* 2005), approximately 20 percent of TIA patients went on to have a stroke: in 17 percent of those who did develop stroke, the stroke occurred on the *same day* as the TIA, in 9 percent on the next day, and in 43 percent over the following week. These are sobering figures and serve to stress that a TIA is not a benign event but rather constitutes a serious warning of impending stroke. Given this, it is appropriate, if one is not already done, to immediately institute a work up, as described below, just as if the patient had already had an ischemic infarction, and then to pursue appropriate treatment.

'Silent' infarctions

It is important to note that ischemic infarctions may be 'silent', that is to say they either, in and of themselves, produce no symptoms or produce symptoms of such mildness that no attention is brought to them. This may be a common occurrence; indeed in patients who have a clinical history of stroke, MR scanning with DWI reveals subsequent silent infarctions in approximately one-third of all cases within the first 5 days, with approximately one-fifth of all cases going on to have silent infarcts in the 30- to 90-day period (Kang *et al.* 2006).

Despite being individually 'silent', these infarctions should not be considered as benign, given that, with an accumulation of them, a multi-infarct or a lacunar dementia (as discussed in Sections 10.1 and 10.2, respectively) may eventually develop.

INTRACEREBRAL HEMORRHAGE

Clinically, intracerebral hemorrhage is typified by the gradual evolution, over from 30 minutes to many hours, of headache, nausea, and vomiting, and a focal deficit appropriate to the location of the enlarging hemorrhage; with large putaminal or thalamic hemorrhages, stupor may also occur. In a significant minority seizures may also occur during the initial presentation (Caplan 1988). Such hemorrhages are readily visualized on CT scanning and their location gives a strong clue to the underlying mechanism of the bleed.

In some cases, the hemorrhage will extend into one of the ventricles, generally producing a catastrophic worsening clinically, with increased headache, decreased level of consciousness, and stiff neck. Such ventricular extension is most common when the hemorrhage is close to a ventricle, as may be seen with a caudate hemorrhage secondary to rupture of the recurrent artery of Heubner or a thalamic hemorrhage secondary to rupture of the thalamoperforating artery; putaminal hemorrhages, secondary to rupture of a lenticulostriate artery, may also extend into the nearby lateral ventricle.

In cases of cerebellar hemorrhage, the proximity of the hemorrhage to the brainstem sets the stage for another mechanism of catastrophic worsening, namely compression of the underlying brainstem. When this occurs, coma and death may occur, and surgical decompression is mandatory.

SUBARACHNOID HEMORRHAGE

Most cases of subarachnoid hemorrhage present in a catastrophic fashion (Suarez *et al.* 2006): the eruption of blood at arterial pressure within the subarachnoid space causes a very rapid rise in intracranial pressure, with severe headache, nausea and vomiting, delirium, stupor, or coma. The headache may rise to its maximal intensity over seconds, and is often described by patients as the worst in their lives. Neck stiffness is common but may not appear immediately. In some cases when the arterial eruption is directed toward the parenchyma, a jet of blood may pierce into the brain, causing an intracerebral hemorrhage.

In 20–40 percent of cases, this full picture may be preceded by transient 'sentinel' headaches occurring secondary to minor 'warning leaks' that terminate spontaneously (Ostergaard 1990).

Seizures may complicate the clinical picture within the first 24 hours, and are seen in up to one-fifth of all patients.

Patients who survive the initial event are at risk for significant complications (Hijdra 1988) over the following weeks, including rebleeding, vasospasm with cerebral infarction, and the development of hydrocephalus. Rebleeding may occur in up to 20 percent of patients and, although it is most common within the first 24 hours, the risk extends for two or more weeks. Vasospasm of cerebral arteries passing through the subarachnoid blood may occur, leading to clinically evident ischemic infarction in approximately one-third of all patients (Hijdra *et al.* 1986): serial MR scans have demonstrated that approximately a further fifth of patients will have 'silent' ischemic infarcts (Shimoda *et al.* 2001). The risk for vasospasm appears within the first few days, peaks at 5–10 days and then subsides by 2 weeks. Acute hydrocephalus, with headache and lethargy, may be seen in up to 20 percent of patients within the first hours or days, and occurs secondary to blockage, by clotted blood, of the exit foramina of the fourth ventricle. Chronic hydrocephalus, secondary to restricted passage of cerebrospinal fluid (CSF) through the arachnoid villi, may occur in the weeks or months following the initial bleed, presenting with dementia, incontinence, and gait disturbance.

Other complications include arrhythmias and hyponatremia. The hyponatremia, in turn, may be secondary to either the syndrome of inappropriate ADH secretion (SIADH), or, more commonly, cerebral salt wasting (CSW) (Rabinstein and Wijdicks 2003). Differentiating SIADH from CSW is critical, as the treatments are radically different. In SIADH there is an increased release of ADH, with consequent increased renal reabsorption of water leading to hyponatremia in the setting of volume expansion. By contrast, in CSW a release of natriuertic factors leads to renal sodium and fluid loss and a hyponatremia in a setting of volume contraction. SIADH is treated by fluid restriction, whereas CSW is treated by the administration of saline.

INTRAVENTRICULAR HEMORRHAGE

Intraventricular hemorrhage presents in a fashion similar to subarachnoid hemorrhage. Chronic communicating hydrocephalus is a common sequela.

CEREBRAL VENOUS THROMBOSIS

Thrombosis of one of the dural sinuses (most commonly the superior sagittal or the transverse sinus) may or may not be followed by cerebral infarction, depending both on whether drainage of a cerebral vein is blocked by the thrombus and on whether or not the vein in question lacks the anastamotic connections that might ensure adequate venous drainage. When these unfavorable conditions are met, venous congestion of the subserved area occurs with the gradual appearance of a hemorrhagic infarction and the appearance, clinically (Bousser *et al.* 1985; Cantu and Barregarrementeria 1993; Gosk-Bierska *et al.* 2006), of the gradual onset of headache, focal deficits appropriate to the infarcted area, and, in a significant minority, seizures. Thrombosis of the vein of Galen, although uncommon, may be given special consideration here, given its clinical expression. In these cases, the thalami, which are drained by the internal cerebral veins, may undergo hemorrhagic infarction, and this may result in stupor or coma (van den Bergh *et al.* 2005) or, in milder cases, a subacute onset of dementia (Krolak-Salmon *et al.* 2006).

Thrombosis of the superior sagittal sinus, by causing an elevation of intracranial pressure, may cause symptoms even in the absence of venous infarction, and patients may present with the gradual evolution of headache and delirium.

Thrombosis of the cavernous sinuses produces a distinctive syndrome with proptosis secondary to impaired venous drainage from the eye, and ophthalmoplegia, secondary to compression of the third and fourth cranial nerves found in the wall of the sinus itself.

The evolution of symptoms seen with venous infarction is very gradual, spanning days or even weeks. This leisurely onset reflects the gradual propagation of the clot and the equally gradual failure of collateral drainage.

SEQUELAE OF STROKE

The sequelae of stroke include *dementia*, *depression*, *anxiety*, and *other sequelae*, such as emotional incontinence, the catastrophic reaction, the frontal lobe syndrome, and, much less commonly, mania or psychosis.

Dementia

With multiple ischemic infarctions or intracerebral hemorrhages, patients may be left demented. This may occur with either cortical or white matter infarcts, producing a multi-infarct dementia (discussed further in Section 10.1), or with lacunes, producing a lacunar dementia (discussed in Section 10.2). Typically, in such cases, one finds a history of repeated stroke; however, occasionally, a 'strategically' placed single infarction or hemorrhage may leave the patient with a dementia, as for example with infarcts or hemorrhages within either temporal lobe or a hemorrhage or lacune in the thalamus.

Subarachnoid hemorrhage may also be followed by a dementia, due either to chronic hydrocephalus or multiple infarctions due to vasospasm. When infarction is at fault, one may find either a relatively small number of large vessel infarcts or a myriad of 'microinfarcts' occurring secondary to spasm of small vessels. CT scanning, although quite capable of demonstrating the large infarcts, will miss the smaller ones, and hence MRI may be required.

Cerebral venous thrombosis, if accompanied by multiple venous infarctions, may also leave patients demented; in the absence of these, most patients, if they survive, do so without cognitive sequelae.

Post-stroke depression

In the weeks or months following stroke, close to one-half of all patients will develop a depression of variable severity. The location of the infarct or hemorrhage plays a part here, with lesions in the anterior portions of the frontal lobes being more likely to cause depression. Of interest, in cases where the depression appears relatively early on, within the first week or two, left frontal lesions are more likely, whereas in cases where the onset is delayed for months, lesions are found with approximately equal frequency in either the left or the right frontal area. Depression has also been noted with lesions of the left basal ganglia.

In evaluating a patient for possible post-stroke depression, toxic and metabolic factors must also be considered. Medications (e.g., metoclopramide or nifedipine) may cause depression, and fatigue and loss of appetite are very common with infections and certain metabolic disorders, including hyponatremia and uremia.

Treatment with either citalopram (Anderson *et al.* 1994) or nortriptyline (Lipsey *et al.* 1984; Robinson *et al.* 2000) is effective; fluoxetine was found effective in one study (Wiart *et al.* 2000) but not in another (Robinson *et al.* 2000)

Of interest, given the frequency with which post-stroke depression occurs, efforts have been made to determine if antidepressants can prevent the appearance of depression. In this regard, both nortriptyline and fluoxetine were found effective; notably, however, when these medicines were discontinued after approximately 2 years of continuous treatment, whereas the fluoxetine-treated patients did well, the nortriptyline-treated patients were more likely to subsequently develop a depression (Narushima *et a*. 2002). Sertraline has also been studied, with one study (Rasmussen *et al.* 2003) demonstrating prophylactic efficacy and another not (Almeida *et al.* 2006).

Anxiety

Chronic anxiety is seen in a small minority of stroke patients and appears to be more common with right hemisphere infarctions.

In most cases of anxiety seen after stroke, the anxiety, rather than occurring in an isolated fashion, rather is part of a post-stroke depression and in such cases an additional diagnosis should not be made. Other differential possibilities include alcohol or benzodiazepine withdrawal, and general medical conditions such as chronic obstructive pulmonary disease or hypocalcemia.

Benzodiazepines are often prescribed: caution should be exercised here, however, as post-stroke patients may be more likely to develop cognitive deficits or lethargy secondary to these medications.

Other sequelae

Emotional incontinence, discussed further in Section 4.7, is characterized by displays of uncontrollable laughter or crying without any corresponding emotion and occurs secondary to bilateral interruption of the corticobulbar tracts. Nortriptyline (Robinson *et al.* 1993) and citalopram in doses of 10–20 mg/day (Andersen *et al.* 1993) are both effective.

A catastrophic reaction, as discussed further in Section 4.24, may be seen in close to 20 percent of patients and appears to be particularly common with infarction of the anterior left hemisphere or the left basal ganglia.

The frontal lobe syndrome, discussed in Section 7.2, may be seen with infarction or hemorrhage of the frontal lobes, caudate nucleus, or thalamus. Patients may present with varying combinations of disinhibition, perseveration, and affective changes.

Mania is a rare sequela to stroke and, as discussed in Section 6.3, may be seen after infarction of the midbrain, thalamus, anterior limb of the internal capsule, and adjacent head of the caudate nucleus, or the frontal or temporal lobes.

Psychosis, likewise, is a rare sequela, and, as discussed in Section 7.1, may occur with infarction of the frontal or temporal cortex, or the thalamus.

Etiology

The etiology of stroke varies according to whether it is due to *ischemic infarction, intracerebral hemorrhage, subarachnoid hemorrhage, intraventricular hemorrhage,* or *cerebral venous thrombosis*, and each of these is discussed in turn. Certain rare or unusual *other causes of stroke*, such as cerebral autosomal dominant arteriopathy with subcortical infarcts and leukoencephalopathy (CADASIL), are then discussed, followed by a *suggested work up* for the new stroke patient.

ISCHEMIC INFARCTION

Ischemic infarction occurs when arterial blood supply is reduced below that required for tissue viability and such reductions may occur via a variety of mechanisms. First, *embolic infarctions* occur when an embolus, say from the heart, lodges in an artery, thus occluding it. Second, *thrombotic infarctions* occur when a thrombus forms inside an artery, typically on top of an ulcerated atherosclerotic plaque, causing occlusion. These two mechanisms account for most large vessel syndromes, and may also underlie certain of the lacunar syndromes. Third, *low-flow (watershed) infarctions* occur secondary, not to occlusion, but to a critical reduction in perfusion pressure. Fourth, and finally, small penetrating arteries may be subject to *lipohyalinosis*, leading to their gradual occlusion and producing a lacunar syndrome.

Embolic infarctions

Emboli may be either cardiogenic (Caplan *et al.* 1983), arising from the heart, or 'artery-to-artery' wherein they arise from a thrombus on an arterial wall and travel downstream to eventually plug a smaller caliber artery. The most common cause of cardiogenic embolic infarction is atrial fibrillation, wherein thrombi form within either the left atrium or atrial appendage. Emboli are also seen in the sick sinus syndrome; however, here the increased risk is probably due to the associated atrial fibrillation. Atrial myxomas, although rare, are very prone to fragment and undergo embolization. Valvular disease is also associated with emboli. In the case of mitral stenosis, this increased risk may be related simply to the commonly associated atrial fibrillation; however, in both infective endocarditis (Anderson *et al.* 2003) and Libman–Sacks endocarditis, actual embolization from the affected valves does occur. Prosthetic valves may be complicated by thrombus formation with embolization, and this is much more likely with mechanical than with bioprosthetic valves. Myocardial infarction is associated with thrombus formation and embolization, both acutely and in the chronic phase. Acutely, thrombi may form on the damaged endocardium, and the period of risk here extends up through the first month or so post myocardial infarction. Chronically, thrombi may form in cases characterized by ventricular aneurysm or large areas of reduced cardiac contractility. Another cardiac condition favoring thrombus formation is dilated cardiomyopathy. In all the foregoing cardiac conditions, emboli arise from the left side of the heart: there is another condition, known as 'paradoxical embolization' wherein emboli travel first through the right heart. In these cases, one most commonly finds a patent foramen ovale; other defects allowing for such paradoxical embolization include atrial septal defect, ventricular septal defect, and pulmonary arteriovenous fistulae.

Artery-to-artery emboli typically have their origin in a thrombus atop an atherosclerotic plaque. Typical scenarios include emboli arising from the origin of the ICA and traveling downstream to occlude a branch of the MCA, or arising from the basilar artery, then traveling downstream to eventually occlude a branch of the PCA.

Emboli may also occur in association with cardiac surgery, especially valve replacement and coronary bypass grafting. Such cases are often associated with significant arteriosclerosis of the aorta, and when the aorta is clamped and unclamped, showers of embolic material may be dislodged. Mere cardiac catheterization may also cause embolic infarction, either secondary to dislodgment of a portion of an aortic plaque or secondary to thrombus formation on the tip of the catheter (Khatri and Kasner 2006).

Carotid artery dissection, although occurring across the lifespan, should be especially considered in any patient under the age of 45 years who has had an embolic infarction (Ahl *et al.* 2004). With dissection of the carotid artery and rupture of the intima, a thrombus forms, which may serve as a source for emboli (Fisher *et al.* 1978). Suggestive clinical evidence includes headache, neck pain, and, due to compression of ascending sympathetic fibers, Horner's syndrome, all occurring ipsilaterally to the infarction (Lee *et al.* 2006).

Regardless of the source of the embolus, whether it is cardiac or from an upstream artery, the sequence of events in embolic infarction is essentially the same. In all cases, the embolus is borne downstream, through arteries of progressively smaller caliber, until finally it lodges in an artery, causing its occlusion. Clinically, such plugging of an artery gives rise to a rapid onset of symptoms, over from seconds to minutes. In some cases, the embolic plug remains in place; however, in many cases the embolic thrombus fragments, dislodges, and passes further downstream, either to plug yet a smaller artery or, if the fragments are sufficiently small, to pass through the capillary bed into the venous circulation. In cases when such dislodgement occurs early, before tissue infarction occurs, one may see clinical improvement, which in some cases is dramatic: the so-called 'spectacular shrinking deficit' (Minematsu *et al.* 1992), wherein the clinical symptomatology undergoes a dramatic improvement as the embolus dislodges and travels downstream. However, in cases when infarction has already occurred, the passage of the embolus downstream, rather than leading to clinical improvement, is followed by 'hemorrhagic transformation' of the infarct (Okada *et al.* 1989). Here, with the renewed presence of blood flow in the infarcted area at arterial pressure, multiple petechial hemorrhages form within the area of infarction. Such hemorrhagic transformation occurs in about one-third of cases, and although it generally takes places within the first 2 days, transformation may occur for up to 10 days post-stroke. Importantly, there is usually little clinical change during hemorrhagic transformation: it is clinically 'silent'.

Thrombotic infarctions

Atherosclerotic occlusion of an artery, after embolus, is the next most common cause of cerebral infarction. Atherosclerosis is most likely to occur at areas of turbulent blood flow (Moosey 1966). In the anterior circulation, this includes the origin of the common carotid artery, its bifurcation into the internal and external carotid arteries, the intracavernous portion of the internal carotid artery, and the proximal portions of the middle cerebral and anterior cerebral arteries. In the posterior circulation, the likely areas include the origins of the subclavian arteries, the origin of the vertebral arteries, the proximal portion of the intracranial vertebral artery, the distal portion of the intracranial vertebral artery, the basilar artery, and the proximal portion of the PCA. The formation and enlargement of the atherosclerotic plaques is a slow process, extending over from months to years, and as this gradual encroachment of the arterial lumen occurs, collateral circulation forms to supply the downstream cerebral tissues that are being gradually deprived of their blood supply. The development of such collateral circulation explains why atherosclerotic occlusion of an artery may, even if complete, cause no symptoms at all. When, however, a thrombus forms on top of a cracked or ulcerated atherosclerotic plaque, the stage is set for infarction. One mechanism, as noted above, is embolization of a portion of the thrombus downstream to plug a smaller caliber artery. Another mechanism involves occlusion of the artery by the developing thrombus itself. Such thrombotic occlusion generally occurs over hours or a day or more, and thus most strokes due to thrombotic occlusion, as compared with embolic infarctions, have a relatively leisurely onset. An exception to this rule is when hemorrhage occurs inside an atherosclerotic plaque: here, enlargement of the plaque into the lumen may occur rapidly, with occlusion occurring within minutes.

In cases of thrombotic infarction when traditional risk factors, such as hypertension, hyperlipidemia, and diabetes mellitus are absent, or when the patient is under 45 years old, it is appropriate to look for other causes of thrombus formation. These include deficiencies of the naturally occurring antithrombotic agents protein S, protein C, and anti-thrombin III, and mutations in factor V Leiden (Bertina *et al.* 1994; Nedeltchev *et al.* 2005). The anti-phospholipid syndrome should also be tested for. This syndrome (Bailey *et al.* 1989), when fully developed, is characterized by a history of thrombophlebitis, miscarriage, stroke and heart attack, and by the presence of Libman–Sacks endocarditis, thrombocytopenia, and a false-positive VDRL test: laboratory testing reveals elevations of anti-cardiolipin antibodies (both IgG and IgM) and lupus anticoagulant. Consideration should also be given to carotid artery dissection. As noted above, such dissection may be followed by thrombus formation with embolization but, in some cases, rather than embolization, the thrombus may proceed to occlude the carotid artery itself.

Low-flow (watershed) infarctions

'Low-flow' infarctions differ from embolic and thrombotic infarctions in that the arteries serving the infarcted area are not, in fact, occluded. Certain portions of the cerebral cortex lie at the very periphery of the areas of distribution of major cerebral arteries and these areas are quite vulnerable. Perfusion pressure falls as one travels further down the arterial tree and at these peripheries pressure is relatively quite low. Consequently, whenever there is a substantial reduction of pressure upstream, the pressure at the periphery may fall below that required for tissue viability and infarction may occur. Such upstream reductions may occur with gradual artherosclerotic narrowing, with systemic hypotension (as may occur with cardiac arrest or as a side-effect of numerous drugs), or a combination of these mechanisms. Such 'low-flow' infarctions are generally referred to as either 'watershed' or 'border zone' infarctions and have a characteristic location. Watershed infarctions at the border zone of the anterior and middle cerebral arteries (ACA–MCA) occur either at the dorsolateral prefrontal cortex or extend through the central portion of the centrum semiovale. Those occurring at the border zone of the middle cerebral and posterior cerebral arteries (MCA–PCA) are typically found in the parieto-occipital cortex. Finally, there is an 'internal' border zone, lying between the lenticulostriate arteries and pial branches of the MCA: infarctions in this border zone are typically found in the periventricular white matter. In cases of unilateral watershed infarction, there is generally an associated tight stenosis of the internal carotid artery; simultaneous bilateral watershed infarcts generally only occur with dramatic systemic hypotension, for example with cardiac arrest.

Lipohyalinosis

Lipohyalinosis is generally considered to occur secondary to hypertension and affects the central branches, described above, and the penetrating branches arising from the vertebral and basilar arteries. With occlusion of one of these small arteries, a correspondingly small infarction, known as a 'lacune' typically occurs. Occlusion of central and penetrating arteries, while most commonly due to lipohyalinosis, may also occur secondary to atherosclerosis (Caplan 1989) and, rarely, to embolic occlusion. Atherosclerosis, as noted earlier, often involves the basilar artery, and in such a case an atherosclerotic plaque may, as it gradually enlarges, slowly lap over the ostium of the penetrating artery, thus occluding this innocent bystander. A similar sequence of events may occur in the stem of the MCA, leading to occlusion of one or all of the lenticulostriate arteries. Embolic occlusion of a small central or penetrating artery is unusual given that most emboli are borne along in the mainstream of the large parent artery and simply do not make the midstream turn required to enter central or penetrating arteries, which generally arise at a more or less right angle to their parent artery.

INTRACEREBRAL HEMORRHAGE

When the hemorrhage involves subcortical structures (e.g., putamen, caudate, or thalamus), brainstem (typically the pons) or cerebellum, the bleeding has usually occurred secondary to rupture of a microaneurysm on one of the central or penetrating arteries (Cole and Yates 1967), which, in turn has usually developed on the basis of longstanding uncontrolled hypertension.

By contrast, when the hemorrhage is 'lobar', that is to say situated in one of the lobes of the cerebrum, a variety of causes may be at fault, including cerebral amyloid angiopathy, hemorrhage into a tumor, rupture of a vascular malformation (e.g., an arteriovenous malformation, a cavernous angioma, or a venous angioma), vasculitis, or in the setting of anticoagulant or thrombolytic treatment: patients treated with warfarin may experience lobar hemorrhages secondary to minor trauma and intracerebral hemorrhage is a feared complication of treatment with tissue plasminogen activator. Other possible causes include vasculitis or use of sympathomimetic agents, such as cocaine.

SUBARACHNOID HEMORRHAGE

Subarachnoid hemorrhage (van Gijn and Rinkel 2001) is most often due to rupture of a berry aneurysm. Other causes include mycotic aneurysms, trauma, rupture of an arteriovenous malformation into the subarachnoid space, vasculitidies, and a condition known as perimesencephalic hemorrhage (van Gijn et al. 1985). This last entity is characterized by hemorrhage surrounding the midbrain and pons; symptoms are typically mild and it is suspected that the bleeding in this case, unlike all the other causes, is venous.

INTRAVENTRICULAR HEMORRHAGE

Hemorrhage into a ventricle may, as noted earlier, occur secondary to extension of an intracerebral hemorrhage. 'Primary' intraventricular hemorrhage may also occur: this is rare, and generally due to bleeding from a vascular malformation adjacent to the ventricle.

CEREBRAL VENOUS THROMBOSIS

Cerebral venous thrombosis, as noted earlier, generally is seen as a complication of thrombosis of one of the dural sinuses. Such thrombosis, in turn, may be due to a number of causes (Gosk-Bierska et al. 2006), such as Behçet's syndrome, the anti-phospholipid syndrome, deficiencies of anti-thrombin III or of proteins S or C, systemic lupus erythematosus, the puerperium, paroxysmal nocturnal hemoglobinuria, in association with certain malignancies, during treatment with oral contraceptives, and in association with certain infections: otitis or mastoiditis may lead to thrombosis of the transverse sinus, and facial or sinus infection to thrombosis of the cavernous sinus.

OTHER CAUSES OF STROKE

Other rare or relatively uncommon causes of stroke include CADASIL, moyamoya disease, vasculitidies (e.g., cranial arteritis and systemic lupus erythematosus), complicated migraine, and subclavian steal. CADASIL is suggested by a history of migraine and by the presence of leukaraiosis in the external capsule and temporal lobe. Moyamoya disease (Chiu *et al.* 1998; Mineharu *et al.* 2006) is characterized by stenosis of the terminal portions of both internal carotid arteries with development of a large number of collateral vessels from the circle of Willis: the name of this disorder is Japanese for 'puff of smoke', which is the appearance generated by these numerous collaterals as seen on arteriography. Clinically, patients present with both subcortical infarctions and subcortical hemorrhages. Moyamoya disease may be either primary or secondary to such conditions as Down's syndrome, von Recklinghausen's disease, or irradiation. Cranial arteritis is suggested by concurrent headache and an elevated erythrocyte sedimentation rate (ESR), and systemic lupus erythematosus by associated symptoms such as arthralgia and rash. Other vasculitidies to consider include Sjögren's syndrome, suggested by dryness of the eyes and mouth, and Sneddon's syndrome, heralded by livedo reticularis. Complicated migraine is suggested by the appearance of stroke in the setting of a migraine headache. The subclavian steal syndrome (Hennerici *et al.* 1988) occurs secondary to stenosis of the subclavian artery proximal to the origin of the vertebral artery on either the left, or, less commonly, the right side. With flow through the subclavian artery reduced, any exercise of the ipsilateral arm, with its concomitant increased blood demand, will 'steal' blood from the vertebral artery and thus reduce flow to the brainstem. Symptoms include 'claudication' of the ipsilateral arm with exercise-induced aching, and symptoms suggestive of brainstem TIA, such as vertigo, ataxia, or diplopia: actual brainstem infarction is rare. The clue to the diagnosis is found by taking the radial pulse on both arms simultaneously: on the affected side the pulse will be delayed and reduced.

SUGGESTED WORK UP

In the initial evaluation of a patient with acute stroke, one of the primary goals is to determine the cause of the stroke and to do this rapidly. Most strokes are secondary to ischemic infarction: ischemic infarction in the area of distribution of one of the large pial vessels (either embolic, or, less commonly, thrombotic in nature) is most common, followed by lacunar infarctions and watershed infarctions. Intracerebral hemorrhage is the next most common cause of stroke, followed by subarachnoid hemorrhage, intraventricular hemorrhage, and cerebral venous thrombosis.

Both the mode of onset and the presence or absence of severe headache help to differentiate the various causes of stroke. Strokes due to ischemic infarction may be either acute or gradual in onset but are generally not accompanied by severe headache. Embolic infarctions are generally of acute onset, with the maximal clinical deficit being reached rapidly, over minutes; by contrast thrombotic infarctions are typically of gradual or 'stuttering' onset, over hours or longer. Strokes due to intracerebral hemorrhage are relatively gradual in onset and are generally accompanied by significant headache. Strokes due to subarachnoid hemorrhage are of very acute onset, sometimes over seconds, and are typified by very severe headache; intraventricular hemorrhage shares these characteristics. Stroke due to cerebral venous thrombosis is generally of leisurely onset, over days or longer, and is generally accompanied by a more or less severe headache.

Although these clinical features are helpful, exceptions are not uncommon to these guidelines, and hence imaging is indispensable. Although MR scanning with DWI is far more sensitive than CT scanning (Chalela *et al.* 2007; Lansberg *et al.* 2000), CT scanning is generally utilized first, not only because of its speed and ready availability but also because it is at least as sensitive as is MRI for the detection of the blood characteristic of hemorrhage transformation of an ischemic infarction, intracerebral hemorrhage, subarachnoid hemorrhage, intraventricular hemorrhage, or cerebral venous thrombosis.

In ischemic infarction, the CT scan is generally normal early on. By 1 hour, some indistinctness of the gray-white boundary may occur, and in patients with occlusion of the MCA a 'hyperdense MCA sign' may be seen in about one-half of cases. Beginning 6 hours after onset, an increasing proportion of cases will demonstrate radiolucency in the area of the infarction, and up to 50 percent of cases will demonstrate this by 12 hours. If hemorrhagic transformation occurs one may see either stippled areas of radiodensity in the area of infarction, representing petechial hemorrhages, or, if the infarction is large, an actual hematoma.

If MR scanning is performed, at a minimum T2, fluid-attenuated inversion recovery (FLAIR) and DWI sequences with apparent diffusion coefficient (ADC) mapping should be obtained. Diffusion-weighted imaging may indicate an area of ischemic infarction within minutes of the event (Hjort *et al.* 2005) and tends to remain positive for 7–14 days; T2 and FLAIR images gradually become positive and then remain so chronically. If cerebral venous thrombosis is suspected, MR venography should be ordered.

Many hospitals also offer either perfusion CT or perfusion MRI, and these procedures may be very useful in cases of ischemic infarction. In such cases, the ischemic tissue may be divided into an ischemic 'core', which is destined to undergo necrosis no matter what treatment is offered, and an ischemic 'penumbra', consisting of 'stunned' tissue, which, although not functional, is capable of recovery. Identifying such a penumbra is of great import, for it invites therapies designed to restore circulation and thus salvage the stunned tissue, and such an identification is enabled by the use of either perfusion CT or perfusion MRI (Schramm *et al.* 2004; Wintermark *et al.* 2002a,b). In this regard, perfusion CT may have an advantage as it takes only about 15 minutes and can be performed in the emergency room.

Once imaging has been accomplished, and a decision has been made as to whether treatment with tissue plasminogen activator (discussed below) should be offered, further laboratory evaluation is undertaken to determine the mechanism of the stroke.

In cases of ischemic infarction, the following tests should be considered: Holter monitoring, echocardiography, duplex doppler studies of the carotid arteries, and either MR angiography or CT angiography. Holter monitoring is required to detect intermittent atrial fibrillation. Echocardiography may be either trans-thoracic (TTE) or trans-esophageal (TEE): although TEE is invasive, it is superior to TTE for imaging the left atrium, left atrial appendage, any atrial septal defects, and the aortic arch (Daniel and Mugge 1995; Sen *et al.* 2004). Duplex doppler studies identify plaques and stenotic lesions of the carotid arteries; MRA, and CTA, are likewise useful in this regard and also allow imaging of the larger intracranial vessels. If an embolic source is present, it is usually demonstrated by one or more of these tests. There are, however, exceptions. In some cases, the entire emboligenic lesion, for example a small atrial thrombus, may undergo embolization, leaving nothing behind to detect. Hence, some clinical judgment is required in interpreting these tests. For example, as noted earlier, a stroke which is 'maximal' at the onset is likely embolic in nature. Furthermore, ischemic infarction in one of the distal branches of the cerebral arteries is also likely embolic: thrombotic infarctions usually occur at areas of atherosclerotic plaque formation, which, as noted earlier, are generally in the more proximal portions of the arterial tree; by contrast, smaller emboli may readily pass distally to occlude an artery further downstream. Finally, if there is more than one acute infarction, and these infarctions are in different arterial territories then an embolic mechanism is a more likely explanation (Baird *et al.* 2000): multiple emboli, say, from a cardiac source, may course up different arteries, whereas it is unlikely that multiple different stenotic arteries would simultaneously give off emboli.

In thrombotic infarction, the underlying etiology is usually atherosclerosis, and one typically finds evidence of hyperlipidemia, diabetes mellitus, hypertension, or smoking. When these are absent, or the patient is under 45 years old, other causes must be considered, as discussed earlier, and consideration should be given to the following tests: protein S, protein C, anti-thrombin III, factor V Leiden, anti-cardiolipin antibodies (IgG and IgM), and lupus anticoagulant. The antiphospholipid syndrome may occur on an idiopathic basis or be secondary to systemic lupus erythematosus and, consequently, in the presence of anti-cardiolipin antibodies or lupus anticoagulant, an ANA test should also be ordered.

In patients with intracerebral hemorrhage, re-imaging with MRI (including a T2* sequence to detect evidence of old petechial hemorrhages in cases of suspected cerebral amyloid angiopathy) should be undertaken after a few weeks have passed, by which time enough blood will have been resorbed to allow the detection of most of the possible underlying causes.

Patients with spontaneous subarachnoid hemorrhage require arteriography to demonstrate the source of the arterial bleeding.

Differential diagnosis

Ischemic infarction may be mimicked by multiple sclerosis or a Bell's palsy. Multiple sclerosis is distinguished by imaging and CSF findings. Bell's palsy may suggest a 'pure motor' lacunar syndrome but only until recognition that the forehead is involved declares the lesion to be in the facial nerve.

Intracerebral hemorrhage may be mimicked by complicated migraine; however, in complicated migraine the headache is usually delayed for from 30 to 60 minutes after the onset of focal signs, whereas in intracerebral hemorrhage, the headache evolves more or less simultaneously with focal signs. Epidural or acute subdural hematomas may likewise mimic an intracerebral hemorrhage, and in the absence of a history of trauma the diagnosis may depend on imaging. Hypertensive encephalopathy may closely mimic intracerebral hemorrhage, with headache, nausea and vomiting, and seizures. Finding a grossly elevated blood pressure may or may not be helpful here, as this may be common to both conditions. Delirium and visual loss favor hypertensive encephalopathy; however, here the diagnosis often depends on imaging: although there may be petechial hemorrhages in hypertensive encephalopathy, one does not see the large, well-circumscribed collection of blood characteristic of intracerebral hemorrhage.

Subarachnoid and primary intraventricular hemorrhage, with the associated hyperacute onset of 'worst-ever' headache, are rarely imitated by any other disorder. Both meningitis and severe migraine might be considered, but imaging will quickly resolve the issue.

Cerebral venous thrombosis may be mimicked by subacute subdural hematoma, a brain tumor (e.g., glioblastoma multiforme) or a cerebral abscess, with, again, imaging resolving the question.

TIAs may be mimicked, with varying degrees of faithfulness, by partial seizures, 'transient tumor attacks', multiple sclerosis, transient global amnesia, and either hyper- or hypoglycemia. Inhibitory motor simple partial seizures are suggested by their exquisitely paroxysmal onset, over seconds, and by their association with other seizure types. A post-ictal Todd's paralysis may also enter the differential but this is immediately suggested by the history of the preceding seizure. 'Transient tumor attacks' occur in association with cerebral tumors, which are immediately apparent on imaging. Multiple sclerosis is suggested by the early adult onset, and may be confirmed by imaging and CSF analysis. Transient global amnesia (TGA) is, relative to a TIA, long-lasting; furthermore, there is no hemianopia or blindness in TGA, findings that would be expected in a TIA occurring secondary to ischemia in the area of distribution of the PCAs. Finally, hyperglycemia (as may be seen in hyperosmolar non-ketotic hyperglycemia) and hypo-glycemia may both present with focal signs, which resolve promptly with restoration of euglycemia.

Treatment

This section will focus first on certain aspects of the *acute treatment* of *ischemic infarction, intracerebral hemorrhage, subarachnoid hemorrhage, intraventricular hemorrhage,* and *cerebral venous thrombosis,* followed by certain recommended *routine measures* appropriate in most cases of stroke. It should be emphasized that the acute treatment of stroke typically requires admission to a specialized unit.

ACUTE TREATMENT

Ischemic infarction

The acute treatment of patients with ischemic infarction may involve the use of tissue-type plasminogen activator (t-PA). Normally, plasminogen is converted by endogenous tissue plasminogen activator to plasmin, which in turn is a fibrinolytic enzyme. The administration of t-PA, by increasing fibrinolysis, may dissolve a clot (whether part of an embolus or occurring on an atherosclerotic plaque in a large vessel), thus restoring flow to cerebral tissue, which, although 'stunned' by ischemia, has not as yet undergone necrosis. Acute ischemic infarctions, as noted earlier, consist of a 'core' of tissue that has been irreversibly damaged and a surrounding 'ischemic penumbra' of tissue, which, although 'stunned' and not functioning, may still survive if blood flow is promptly restored. The window of opportunity for restoration of blood flow is narrow, measured in hours, and thus decisions must be made rapidly. Current guidelines set the outside limit for treatment with t-PA at 3 hours post onset; however, this may not be appropriate in all cases: as noted earlier, both perfusion CT and perfusion MRI studies allow for a demonstration of the ischemic penumbra, and this may persist well past 3 hours (Albers *et al.* 2006; Parsons *et al.* 2002).

Even in cases of ischemic infarction when an ischemic penumbra is present not all patients should receive t-PA, given the risk of causing an intracerebral hemorrhage. Contraindications to t-PA include: stroke, head trauma, or myocardial infarction within 3 months; major surgery within 2 weeks; a history of gastrointestinal or genitourinary bleeding within 3 weeks; a history of intracerebral hemorrhage at any time; thrombocytopenia (with a platelet count below 100 000), anticoagulation (with an INR >1.7), or use of heparin within 48 hours (and a prolonged aPTT); grossly elevated blood pressure (systolic over 180 mmHg or diastolic over 110 mmHg); and, finally, evidence of a large infarct: large infarcts, for example infarcts encompassing the entire area of distribution of the MCA, are more likely to undergo hemorrhagic transformation and thus treatment may do more harm than good.

In cases of embolic infarction when systemic t-PA fails, consideration may be given to local, intra-arterial thrombolysis or to mechanical embolectomy (Gobin *et al.* 2004).

Patients should also be given aspirin in a dose of 325 mg for the first 2 weeks, as this reduces the risk of recurrent stroke within that timeframe (Chen *et al.* 2000): if t-PA is not given, aspirin should be given immediately; in cases where t-PA is utilized, aspirin may be started after 24 hours.

Some authors advocate the use of heparin in cases of thrombotic infarction, in the hope of preventing propagation of the offending thrombus. As yet, however, there is no convincing evidence for the effectiveness of heparin and the risks attendant on its use argue against this practice.

Most patients with ischemic infarction will also have hypertension, and it cannot be stressed enough that rigid control of blood pressure is *not* indicated in the acute phase of stroke treatment (Caplan 1976). The risks of neuronal ischemia secondary to systemic hypotension are simply too great; indeed, in cases of watershed infarction, a case may be made for allowing the pressure to run a little high. Recent work has also indicated that in acute patients, lying flat in bed, as compared to sitting up, not only improves flow within the MCA territory, but may also be followed, in some cases, by prompt clinical improvement (Wojner-Alexandrov *et al.* 2005).

Obstructive sleep apnea is a common condition, and recent work indicates that obstructive apneas are associated with early clinical worsening (Iranzo *et al.* 2002). Given this, it appears appropriate to ensure, if possible, that all patients with obstructive sleep apnea receive appropriate treatment.

Once acute treatment is accomplished, preventive treatment should be instituted: in addition to control of risk factors such as diabetes mellitus, hypertension, hyperlipidemia, and smoking cessation, consideration may be given to secondary stroke prevention with either warfarin or antiplatelet agents. Warfarin is indicated in cases of embolic infarction secondary to atrial fibrillation, atrial or ventricular thrombi, cardiomyopathy, and mechanical prosthetic valves. In other cases, or when warfarin is contraindicated, antiplatelet agents are indicated. A time-release combination of aspirin and dipyridamole (Aggrenox) is superior to aspirin alone (Halkes *et al.* 2006; Sacco *et al.* 2005), and clopidogrel (Plavix) is equal in efficacy to aspirin: the combination of clopidogrel and aspirin should probably not be used, as it carries an increased risk of hemorrhage. If aspirin is used alone, the best dose, whether 81 mg or 325 mg is uncertain; whichever dose is used, an enteric-coated preparation should be utilized. In patients on aspirin, it is important to avoid treatment with ibuprofen, which inhibits aspirin's antiplatelet effect (Catella-Lawson *et al.* 2001).

In cases when carotid artery stenosis is present at greater that 70 percent, consideration may be given to carotid endarterectomy (Barnett *et al.* 1998; Chaturvedi *et al.* 2005) or carotid stenting (Yadav *et al.* 2004).

Intracerebral hemorrhage

As yet there are no specific treatments for intracerebral hemorrhage: recent work suggests a role for recombinant activated factor VII to reduce the growth of the hemorrhage (Mayer et al. 2005); however, this has not as yet been approved for clinical use. In cases when the hemorrhage is causing significant herniation or compressing critical structures, treatment with dexamethasone, mannitol, or furosemide may be indicated. In emergent situations, surgery may be required to remove the clot. There is debate as to whether surgery is safe in cases of cerebral amyloid angiopathy, given the widespread vascular fragility; however, on balance, even here surgery may be worth the risk. In cases where there is doubt as to the etiology of the bleed, as for example may occur with lobar hemorrhages, follow-up MRI is indicated to detect underlying neoplasms or vascular malformations.

Subarachnoid hemorrhage

Patients with subarachnoid hemorrhage should be treated in an ICU. Various measures are undertaken (Naidech et al. 2005; Suarez et al. 2006): benzodiazepines (e.g., lorazepam), are given for agitation, nimodipine to reduce vasospasm, and either phenytoin or valproate for seizure prophylaxis; serial transcranial doppler studies are made to monitor the development of vasospasm, and should this appear, consideration is given both to 'triple-H' therapy (hypertension, hypervolemia, hemodilution) to facilitate flow through constricted arteries, and to angioplasty. Serial CT scans are also indicated to monitor for the development of hydrocephalus and external ventricular drainage may be required. Arteriography is generally performed to identify the bleeding source, and when, as is usually the case, an aneurysm is identified, patients should be considered for endovascular coiling (International Subarachnoid Aneurysm Trial [ISAT] Collaborative Group 2002) or neurosurgical clipping.

Intraventricular hemorrhage

In the case of intraventricular hemorrhage, treatment in an ICU is generally required, as is external ventricular drainage.

Cerebral venous thrombosis

For cerebral venous thrombosis, there is debate as to whether patients should be treated with heparin. Although increased hemorrhage is a risk, it appears that, in this case, the benefits obtained by preventing thrombus propagation may outweigh it. Increased intracranial pressure, as is often seen with thrombosis of the superior sagittal sinus, may require treatment with dexamethasone and mannitol.

ROUTINE MEASURES

Routine measures include proper nutrition (utilizing, if necessary, nasogastric tube feedings or percutaneous endoscopic gastrostomy tube placement), physical therapy, prevention or treatment of aspiration, decubiti, urinary tract infections, and deep venous thrombosis. A close watch should be kept early on for a worsening neurologic deficit. In ischemic infarction, recurrent emboli may lead to new infarctions, as may propagation of a thrombus. In intracerebral hemorrhage renewed bleeding may occur (Kazui et al. 1996), and in subarachnoid hemorrhage either ischemic infarction secondary to vasospasm or renewed bleeding may occur. Vasogenic edema typically appears within the first few days, and, if substantial, this too may cause a clinical downturn; typically the edema resolves within a week or two. A deterioration in the patient's general medical condition, by compromising the functioning of 'stunned' neuronal structures, may also cause a worsening of the initial deficit, and a close watch should be kept for hypoglycemia, hyponatremia, infections (e.g., pneumonia or urinary tract infections) and for any toxicity from such commonly administered medications as opioids, benzodiazepines, or antipsychotics.

Treatment with anti-epileptic drugs (e.g., phenytoin), may or may not be required. Seizures may be immediate, early (within the first 2 weeks) or late (from 2 weeks to 2 years). Early and immediate seizures occur in about 5 percent of patients with ischemic infarction, and up to 25 percent of patients with intracerebral hemorrhage: they generally occur only in those with cortical involvement and are rare in those with lacunar infarctions or hemorrhages confined to subcortical structures. In the case of subarachnoid hemorrhage, early and immediate seizures may be seen in up to 25 percent of patients, and in cerebral venous thrombosis, about 15 percent. The EEG may help in predicting seizures: periodic lateralized epileptiform discharges (PLEDs) and focal spikes are strongly associated with their development (Gupta et al. 1988; Holmes 1980). In the case of ischemic infarction, treatment with an AED is generally withheld until a seizure occurs, but in cases of intracerebral hemorrhage with cortical involvement or subarachnoid hemorrhage or venous thrombosis the risk is so high that prophylactic treatment with phenytoin is generally given for the first 2 weeks. Should a seizure occur after stroke, it is not clear how long treatment should continue: a prudent course would be to continue prophylactic treatment until 2 years had passed without seizure.

Once the patient is medically stable, consideration should also be given to transfer to a rehabilitation facility.

7.5 TRAUMATIC BRAIN INJURY

Traumatic brain injury (also known as closed head injury) occurs in the United States with a yearly incidence of approximately 120/100 000. Two age peaks are found, between 15 and 24 years of age, wherein motor vehicle accidents are the most common cause, and over the age of 64 years, wherein falls are most common. Males are more commonly affected than females at all ages, and alcohol intoxication is a very common factor, being found in from one-third to one-half of all cases (Corrigan 1995). Although multiple forms of brain injury may occur, this syndrome refers primarily to cases occurring with sudden 'acceleration–deceleration', as during a motor vehicle accident or a fall or blow to the head; trauma due to gunshot wounds and crush injuries are not considered here. This chapter will discuss the clinical features and treatment of the various aspects of traumatic brain injury, the etiology of these clinical features, and the differential diagnosis between traumatic brain injury and concussion.

Clinical features and treatments

In considering the clinical features (and their treatments) of traumatic brain injury, it is convenient to divide them into two groups, namely an *acute phase* and a *chronic phase*. The acute phase, from a neuropsychiatric point of view, is often dominated by a delirium; as the confusion clears, patients gradually enter into the chronic phase, which in turn may be characterized by numerous sequelae, including cognitive deficits that may, at times, be severe enough to constitute a dementia.

ACUTE PHASE

Almost all patients with significant traumatic brain injury will sustain a loss of consciousness, of variable duration, immediately after the injury. Those who do survive will typically emerge into a delirium. This delirium, in addition to such characteristic symptoms as confusion, disorientation, and decreased short-term memory, is also often marked by hallucinations, delusions, and, especially, agitation, which is seen in the majority of cases (Rao and Lyketsos 2000; van der Naalt *et al.* 2000).

It must be borne in mind that although the delirium in such cases is generally due to the intracranial injuries directly caused by the trauma, that other factors, as discussed in Section 5.3, may also be involved as the hospitalization proceeds. Toxicity from such medications as opioids, baclofen, anticholinergics, metoclopramide, and even amantadine must be considered, along with metabolic factors, such as hyponatremia, hypoglycemia, hypomagnesemia, and systemic effects of infections, such as pneumonia. Other metabolic factors to consider relate to the frequency with which alcoholism is involved, and include Wernicke's encephalopathy due to thiamine deficiency and delirium tremens. Consideration may also be given to the effects of global cerebral ischemia secondary to severe hypotension and, in those with fractures of long bones, to the fat embolism syndrome.

Treatment of patients during the acute phase is, at least initially, generally undertaken in either a trauma unit or an ICU. Neurosurgical treatment may be required for evacuation of epidural or subdural hematomas or large contusions or intracerebral hemorrhages, and serial CT scans are obtained. In comatose patients, intracranial pressure monitoring is often indicated, and treatment with intravenous sedation, mannitol, and other agents may be required to reduce pressure. Intubation is often required, and pneumonia is a frequent occurrence.

Treatment of delirium, in all cases, involves simple environmental measures designed to reduce confusion. These include, whenever possible, having the patient in a quiet room, with a window. Large calendars and digital clocks should be in full view, and the nurse's call button should be readily available. Sleep is essential and consequently the room should be darkened and very quiet at night, and all non-emergency procedures (e.g., vital signs, weights, baths, laboratory testing) should be forbidden during the sleeping hours. Restraints may occasionally be required and can be life-saving. For patients prone to get out of bed unsupervised, keeping the bedrails up may be sufficient; if not, or if these are impractical, utilizing a 'low-boy' bed, surrounded by mats, may help prevent injury. In some cases, round-the-clock sitters may be required.

In cases where these environmental measures are ineffective, pharmacologic treatment may be considered with either an antipsychotic or, in certain emergent cases, lorazepam. Antipsychotics are indicated for treatment of hallucinations or delusions, and are also effective for agitation. A second-generation agent, such as risperidone, is often used, and, in practice quetiapine and olanzapine are also utilized. Initial doses should generally be low, for example 0.5–1 mg of risperidone, 12.5–25 mg of quetiapine, and 2.5–5 mg of olanzapine. The first-generation agent haloperidol is also often used, with initial doses of 2–5 mg. Repeat doses, in approximately similar milligram amounts, may then be given every hour or so until the patient is calm, limiting side-effects occur, or a maximum dose is reached: rough guidelines for dose maxima are 5 mg for risperidone, 150 mg for quetiapine, 20 mg for olanzapine, and 20 mg for haloperidol. In cases when the patient responds satisfactorily, a regular daily dose is ordered for the next day (with the total daily dose approximately equivalent to the total required initially), divided into two or three doses. Provision is also made for further as-needed doses, with the total daily dose being adjusted according to the amount needed in p.r.n. doses. The eventual maintenance dose is then continued until the patient has been stable for a significant period of time, at which point it may be gradually tapered. Lorazepam is very commonly used, and given the rapidity of its effectiveness when given intravenously, has a place in emergent situations; however, given that lorazepam may also worsen confusion, it is appropriate to substitute another agent as soon as this is practical. If lorazepam is used, one may give anywhere from 0.5 to 2 mg i.v. every hour as needed until the patient is calm, limiting side-effects (such as sedation) occur, or a maximum of approximately 12 mg is reached.

Once patients have been stabilized, general rehabilitation efforts may be started, including physical, speech, and occupational therapy. Eventually, most patients are transferred to a specialized rehabilitation facility, where these general efforts are continued.

Two rating scales have come into widespread use in the evaluation of patients with traumatic brain injury: the Glasgow Coma Scale and the Rancho Los Amigos Cognitive Scale. The Glasgow Coma Scale (Teasdale and Jennett 1974) is designed for evaluating patients in the acute phase, and involves assessing three clinical features: eye opening, motor response, and verbal response, with, as noted in Table 7.8 a numerical score described for the various responses. Patients with total scores of ≤8 are said to have a severe injury, those with scores from 9 to 12, a moderate injury, and those with scores of from 13 to 15, a mild injury. The Rancho Los Amigos scale, described in Table 7.9 may also be utilized early on; however, it is often also employed as an instrument for following patients during the chronic phase. Although these scales are useful as a 'shorthand' they cannot and should not take the place of a detailed narrative description of the patient's clinical condition.

Post-traumatic seizures may occur during the acute phase, and these are discussed further, below.

Chronic phase

As the delirium gradually clears, almost all patients will be left with one or more chronic sequelae (Rao and Lyketos 2000), and these are discussed below, beginning with cognitive deficits, which are almost universal.

Cognitive deficits

Cognitive deficits typically remain after the confusion of delirium clears, and generally include inattentiveness, poor short-term memory (or simple 'forgetfulness'), poor concentration, and decreased abstracting ability (Levin et al. 1979; van Zomeren and van den Burg 1985). In some cases these may be quite mild and not terribly limiting; however, in others they amount to a clear, and disabling, dementia. Most patients show improvement over the first 6 months, with some further, but not as impressive, gains over the next 6 months: however, after 12 months, little further spontaneous recovery can be expected. Importantly, in assessing patients with cognitive deficits it is critical to check for the presence of depression, which, in and of itself, may cause cognitive impairment. Pharmacologic treatment may include donepezil, amantadine, bromocriptine, or methylphenidate. Donepezil, in doses of 10 mg/day, improves memory and attention (Morey et al. 2003; Zhang et al. 2004) (rivastigmine does not appear to be effective [Silver et al. 2006]). Amantadine, in doses of 100 mg in the morning and 100 mg in the early afternoon, may likewise improve cognitive performance (Meythaler et al. 2002), but not all studies support this (Schneider et al. 1999). Bromocriptine, in one double-blind study (McDowell et al. 1998) had some positive effect on executive functioning. Methylphenidate, titrated to a dose

Table 7.8　The Glasgow Coma Scale

Eye opening	
Spontaneous	4
To speech	3
To pain	2
Nil	1
Best motor response	
Obeys commands	6
Localizes	5
Withdraws	4
Abnormal flexion	3
Extensor response	2
Nil	1
Verbal response	
Oriented	5
Confused conversation	4
Inappropriate words	3
Incomprehensible sounds	2
Nil	1

Table 7.9　The Ranchos Los Amigos Scale*

I	*No response*: unresponsive to any stimulus
II	*Generalized response*: limited, inconsistent, and non-purposeful responses – often to pain only
III	*Localized response*: purposeful responses; may follow simple commands; may focus on presented object
IV	*Confused, agitated*: heightened state of activity; confusion and disorientation; aggressive behavior; unable to perform self care; unaware of present events; agitation appears related to internal confusion
V	*Confused, inappropriate*: non-agitated, appears alert; responds to commands; distractible; does not concentrate on task; agitated responses to external stimuli; verbally inappropriate; does not learn new information
VI	*Confused, appropriate*: goal-directed behavior, needs cueing; can relearn old skills as activities of daily living; serious memory problems, some awareness of self and others
VII	*Automatic, appropriate*: appears appropriately oriented; frequently robot-like in daily routine; minimal or absent confusion; shallow recall; increased awareness of self and interaction with environment; lacks insight into condition; decreased judgment and problem solving; lacks realistic planning for future
VIII	*Purposeful, appropriate*: alert and oriented; recalls and integrates past events; learns new activities and can continue without supervision; independent in home and living skills; capable of driving; defects in stress tolerance, judgment and abstract reasoning persist; may function at reduced levels in society

*Reprinted with permission from the Adult Brain Injury Service of the Rancho Los Amigos Medical Center, Downey, California

of 0.3 mg/kg b.i.d., may improve attention and speed of information processing (Whyte *et al.* 2004), but, as with amantadine, not all studies support this (Speech *et al.* 1993). Overall, it may be prudent to begin with either donepezil or amantadine, holding methylphenidate as a distant reserve.

Post-traumatic amnesia

'Post-traumatic amnesia' is defined differently by different authors. Some include under this rubric the decreased short-term memory seen during delirium, whereas others restrict the definition to cases wherein a short-term memory loss persists after resolution of delirium and, importantly, persists in relative 'isolation', being generally unaccompanied by other cognitive deficits. Utilizing the latter definition, Levin *et al.* (1988) found such a residual amnestic disturbance in approximately one-quarter of patients.

Anosognosia

Anosognosia is characterized by a failure to appreciate the severity of a deficit, or even its existence. Clinically significant anosognosia is found as a persistent symptom in almost one-half of patients (Flashman and McAllister 2002). Interestingly, the anosognosia appears selective, in that although patients tend to acknowledge such deficits as hemiplegia, they are much less likely to appreciate their cognitive deficits (Sbordone *et al.* 1998) or the existence of mood changes or a personality change (Fahy *et al.* 1967). Distinguishing anosognosia from denial may be difficult. One helpful point is the affect accompanying the patient's response to questions about deficits: in anosognosia the affect is often bland or matter of fact, whereas in denial there may be a degree of indignation or angry protest.

Importantly, given the high prevalence of anosognosia, it is critical, in the long-term treatment of these patients, to always question others, such as family members or friends, regarding the patient's condition. Relying on the anosognosic patient's report could lead to disastrous underdiagnosing.

Focal signs and symptoms

Focal signs and symptoms that persist after resolution of the delirium may include not only hemiplegia and various movement disorders, but also 'cortical' signs and symptoms such as neglect and aphasia. Aphasia is particularly common, and, to a variable degree, is found in the vast majority of cases (Levin *et al.* 1976; Sarno *et al.* 1986).

Agitation

Agitation is common and tends to fluctuate in severity, and may occur in up to two-thirds of all patients in the first few months (Nott *et al.* 2006). Up to one-third of patients may also exhibit aggressiveness, which may be either verbal or physical (Tateno *et al.* 2004). In evaluating agitated patients, consideration must be given to the possibility that the agitation in question is not directly due to the head injury but is rather secondary to other causes, such as pain, delusions of persecution, akathisia or disinhibition secondary to alcohol or benzodiazepines.

Pharmacologic treatment of agitation may include AEDs, amantadine, antipsychotics, propranolol, lithium, and antidepressants. In non-blind studies or case reports, carbamazepine (Azouvi *et al.* 1999; Chatham-Showalter 1996), valproic acid (Chatham-Showalter and Kimmel 2000; Wroblewski *et al.* 1997), and lamotrigene (Pachet *et al.* 2003) all appear effective. Amantadine, in a case report, was also effective (Chandler *et al.* 1988). Antipsychotics, such as the second-generation agents risperidone, quetiapine, or olanzapine, may be utilized. Although first-generation agents (e.g., haloperidol) have been associated with cognitive decrement (Stanislav 1997), and the same may be true with second-generation agents, the benefits of treatment with antipsychotics typically outweigh these cognitive side-effects. Propranolol also appears effective (Brooke *et al.* 1992): treatment is commenced at low doses, perhaps 20 mg/day, and increased gradually, in increments of perhaps 60 mg every few days, to clinical effectiveness, tolerance, or a maximum dose of 800 mg/day. Lithium has also been used (Glenn *et al.* 1989). Amitriptyline, in a large case series, has also been effective (Mysiw *et al.* 1988), and in the author's experience, mirtazapine has been remarkably effective; however, high doses of 60–90 mg may be required.

Given the lack of head-to-head studies, choosing among these agents is not straightforward. In my opinion, AEDs are a good first choice, and among these, preference may be given to either valproic acid or carbamazepine. Antipsychotics are probably a second choice, and among these, quetiapine is generally very well tolerated. Propranolol, given the high doses often required, should probably be held in reserve, and the same may be said of lithium, which is often poorly tolerated by patients with brain injuries. Amitriptyline, given its anticholinergic effects and possible negative effects on cognition, might also be held in reserve; as noted, the author has found mirtazapine quite effective, and with no significant adverse effects.

Sympathetic storms

Sympathetic storms, as described in Section 4.23, consist of episodes characterized by profuse diaphoresis, tachycardia, tachypnea, pupillary dilation, and, in some, rigid extensor posturing. The diaphoresis is indeed impressive, with beads of sweat dripping from the head. During the episode, patients may grimace as if in pain, and family members and other observers may become quite alarmed. The episodes themselves last from minutes to hours, and terminate slowly.

The distinction of these 'storms' from agitation is generally based on their course: the 'storms' come in discrete episodes, whereas agitation, although perhaps waxing and waning in intensity, usually does not assume an episodic course. In addition, sympathetic symptoms, such as impressive diaphoresis, although typical of sympathetic storms, are generally absent, or relatively minimal, during agitation.

Treatment with propranolol or bromocriptine usually prevents further attacks; alternatives include gabapentin and morphine.

Personality change

Personality change is very common, and over the long term may constitute one of the most disabling of residual symptoms (Thomsen 1984). A full or partial frontal lobe syndrome is typical, with disinhibition being the most common symptom; affective changes and perseveration may also occur. Before making this diagnosis, due regard must be paid to the patient's premorbid personality, with special attention to the presence of either an antisocial or borderline personality disorder. Pharmacologic treatment of the frontal lobe syndrome may include treatment with carbamazepine or an antipsychotic, such as quetiapine.

Depression

Depression appears during the first 2 years in up to one-half of patients, and may either remit spontaneously or persist (Jorge et al. 1993, 2004); of the typical symptoms of depression (i.e., depressed mood, fatigue, loss of interest, loss of appetite, difficulty with concentration, and insomnia), fatigue and poor concentration are often especially problematic (Kreutzer et al. 2001).

Importantly, in considering a diagnosis of depression, in this population one must keep in mind that transient displays of depressed mood or affect, as may be seen in emotionalism or emotional incontinence, simply do not qualify. Furthermore, both apathy and abulia must be kept in mind as other possibilities: in both cases, the requisite depressed mood is not present. Other differential possibilities to keep in mind include medications (e.g., steroids or metoclopramide) and a premorbid major depressive disorder.

Treatment generally includes an antidepressant, such as sertraline (Fann et al. 2000) or some other SSRI. Tricyclic antidepressants, although effective (e.g., desipramine [Wroblewski et al. 1996]) should be used with caution, given that they lower the seizure threshold (Wroblewski et al. 1990). Methylphenidate may also be considered, and in one double-blind study was similar to sertraline (Lee et al. 2005).

Emotionalism

Emotionalism is relatively common after head injury (Sloan et al. 1992). Typically, patients find themselves uncharacteristically prone to sadness and tearfulness. Importantly, although patients, especially males, may complain of their lack of emotional restraint, they do not complain that the sadness is unmotivated or out of place. Antidepressants, especially SSRIs, such as fluoxetine (Sloan et al. 1992), may be effective in this regard.

Emotional incontinence

Emotional incontinence (Muller et al. 1999) is characterized by the involuntary appearance of a sad or happy affect in the absence of any corresponding sense of sadness or mirth, and as such differs from emotionalism. Such 'empty' displays of affect may be seen as a late sequela in from 5 to 10 percent of patients (Tateno et al. 2004; Zeilig et al. 1996). Citalopram is effective here, sometimes in as little as 2 or 3 days (Muller et al. 1999).

Apathy

Apathy may occur (Kant et al.1998) and is distinct from either abulia or depression. Patients with abulia, if supervised, may complete tasks at a normal rate, whereas patients with apathy do not. Patients with depression may also complete tasks slowly; however, here, in contrast with apathy, there is a depressed mood. Apathy may respond to bromocriptine (Powell et al. 1996), amantadine (Van Reekum et al. 1995), or selegeline (Newburn and Newburn 2005).

Fatigue

Fatigue may be present in up to one-third of patients (Hillier et al. 1997). When severe, consideration may be given to treatment with methylphenidate or amphetamines; however, these agents should be given cautiously, if at all, in cases where they might be abused.

Mania

Mania may occur in the year following injury, but is relatively uncommon (Nizamie et al. 1988; Starkstein et al. 1990); it appears to be more likely when the polar regions of the temporal lobes have been involved, as for example by contusions. The episodes themselves tend to be relatively short, lasting on average 2 months (Jorge et al. 1993), and may occur soon after the injury or after a latent interval lasting months. In evaluating a patient suspected of having post-traumatic mania, it is important to differentiate manic exuberance from the disinhibition that is seen in the frontal lobe syndrome: the main differential point here is that whereas mood is heightened in mania, it is not in the frontal lobe syndrome. Furthermore, before attributing mania to head injury, a careful history is required to exclude a premorbid bipolar disorder. Treatment should generally include a mood stabilizer, such as divalproex or carbamazepine; lithium may also be considered, however, as noted earlier, patients with head injury may be especially prone to develop side-effects to this agent.

Sleep disturbances

Sleep disturbances occur in the majority of patients and may include hypersomnia, excessive daytime sleepiness or insomnia (Baumann et al. 2007).

Hypersomnia may be directly related to the head injury but consideration must also be given to the use of any sedating medications.

Excessive daytime sleepiness may be likewise be directly related to the head injury or may be due to sleep apnea, which in turn may be either central or obstructive (Castriotta and Lai 2001; Masel et al. 2001); periodic limb movements of sleep may also occur and, rarely, there may be post-traumatic narcolepsy (Lankford et al. 1994). Given that these latter disorders have specific treatments, it is reasonable to request polysomnography in any brain injury patient who complains of excessive daytime sleepiness. In cases of excessive daytime sleepiness occurring directly secondary to head injury, a case may be made for a trial of either methylphenidate or modafinil.

Insomnia may occur secondary to pain, or as part of depression, or exist independently (Beetar *et al.* 1996; Fichtenberg *et al.* 2000); treatment generally involves medications such as zolpidem or trazodone (typically effective in low doses of from 25 to 50 mg).

Psychosis

Psychosis, that is to say a condition characterized by delusions and/or hallucinations in the absence of delirium or dementia, is reported, albeit rarely, as a long-term sequela to traumatic brain injury (Fujii and Ahmed 2002; Sachdev *et al.* 2001); however, this assertion must be viewed with some caution. In the reported cases, latencies of 1–5 or more years are reported between the head injury and the gradual onset of the psychosis, and a family history of schizophrenia was found to be a significant risk factor (Sachdev *et al.* 2001). Given these findings, the argument may be made that the psychosis represents merely the coincidental occurrence of schizophrenia in a patient with a history of traumatic brain injury. Treatment involves use of an antipsychotic, preferably one of the better-tolerated second-generation agents, such as risperidone or quetiapine.

Post-traumatic seizures

Post-traumatic seizures may be defined as occurring early, during the first 7 days post-injury, or late, occurring at any time thereafter. Early seizures are reported in anywhere from 2 to 15 percent of cases, and are most likely to occur within the first 24 hours. Late seizures are seen in from 5 to 10 percent of cases, and in those destined to have a late seizure, the first one usually occurs within the first year post-injury (Mazzini *et al.* 2003): the range here, however, is wide, from weeks to up to 15 years. Several features increase the risk of occurrence of a late seizure, including the following: having an early seizure; the presence of contusions or intracerebral hemorrhages; intracranial operations; and dural penetration with bone or metal fragments (Englander *et al.* 2003; Mazzini *et al.* 2003; McQueen *et al.* 1983; Messori *et al.* 2005). Importantly, although the vast majority of seizures occurring post-traumatically are due to the intracranial pathology itself, other possibilities must also be kept in mind: in the case of early seizures, metabolic causes, such as hyponatremia, hypocalcemia, or hypomagnesemia are not uncommon. Simple partial, complex partial, and grand mal seizures may all occur.

With regard to treatment, two aspects exist: prophylaxis against an early seizure, and treatment after a seizure, whether early or late, has occurred.

With regard to prophylaxis of early seizures during the first week, both phenytoin (Temkin *et al.* 1990) and valproate (Temkin *et al.* 1999) are effective; however, there was an apparent trend toward increased mortality with valproate.

Consequently, phenytoin may be preferable for early prophylaxis. Importantly, neither of these agents provides prophylaxis after the first week: consequently, if the patient has gone through the first week without a seizure, the AED may generally be discontinued.

In cases where a seizure has occurred, whether early or late, treatment recommendations are not as clearly worked out. If a patient had an early seizure despite prophylactic treatment with phenytoin at therapeutic levels, some clinicians would continue phenytoin, on the assumption that it will decrease the frequency of later-occurring seizures, whereas others would opt for a different AED. In cases where there were no seizures during the first week, but one occurred later, perhaps much later, there are no firm guidelines regarding treatment, and consideration could be given not only to phenytoin or valproate, but also to other agents, such as levetiracetam, carbamazepine, oxcarbazepine, gabapentin, etc.

Endocrinologic changes

Endocrinologic changes appear in a majority of traumatic brain injury patients, and may occur secondary to either hypothalamic (Crompton 1971) or pituitary damage (Edwards and Clark 1986; Salehi *et al.* 2007). Diabetes insipidus, with hypernatremia, may occur early on; other endocrinologic changes, such as hypothyroidism or gonadal failure, may not become evident for months to years after the injury. In this regard, it is prudent to check a thyroid profile in any patient who develops depression, apathy or fatigue, and a testosterone level in patients who develop decreased libido.

Post-traumatic stress disorder

Post-traumatic stress disorder may occur after any major trauma, and traumatic brain injury is no exception. Indeed, anywhere from 6 percent (Bombardier *et al.* 2006) to 20 percent (Hibbard *et al.* 1998) of these patients will develop this disorder at some point.

Before making a diagnosis of post-traumatic stress disorder, however, careful consideration must be given to the fact that certain symptoms suggestive of this disorder may also occur as direct sequela of the brain injury itself, including poor concentration, insomnia, and fatigue.

Etiology

In traumatic brain injury, a variety of lesions may be seen (Freytag 1963; Jenkins *et al.* 1986), including diffuse axonal injury, contusions, intracerebral hemorrhage, subarachnoid hemorrhage, epidural or subdural hematomas, or infarctions. Cerebral edema accompanies most of these, and, in combination with space-occupying lesions, may cause uncal or subfalcine herniation. In some cases, hydrocephalus may appear. Fractures may or may not accompany these lesions.

Diffuse axonal injury (Adams *et al.* 1982), occurring secondary to the tremendous shearing and rotational forces occurring during acceleration/deceleration, is characterized by axonal rupture or damage. Although these effects are widespread throughout the cerebrum, certain areas are most vulnerable, including the junction between the cortex and white matter, the corpus callosum, and dorsolateral quadrants of the midbrain. In almost all cases, this diffuse axonal injury is also accompanied by diffuse vascular injury, wherein small penetrating arterioles, subjected to the same shearing and rotational forces, undergo rupture, producing widespread petechial hemorrhages.

Contusions occurring in acceleration–deceleration injuries typically occur along the inferior surfaces of the frontal and temporal lobes, as they slide along the bony protuberances at the base of the skull. In cases where there has been a blow to the head, a contusion may form under the point of impact (the 'coup' contusion) and also contralaterally, at the area where the brain is flung up against the inner surface of the skull (the 'contre-coup' contusion).

Intracerebral hemorrhages occur with rupture of relatively large penetrating arteries, and although these hemorrhages may be lobar in location they are most commonly seen in the basal ganglia (Katz et al. 1989; Macpherson et al. 1986). Rarely, intracerebral hemorrhages may be delayed in appearance for up to 2 days post-injury.

Subarachnoid hemorrhage may occur secondary to shearing of vessels traversing the subarachnoid space or due to leakage of blood from an area of contused or hemorrhagic cortex. In such cases, vasospasm of arteries traversing the bloody subarachnoid space may lead to ischemic infarction of subserved tissue.

Subdural hematomas occur in about one-fifth of patients, and may range in size from thin, inconsequential crescents to large, life-threatening lesions. Epidural hematomas may also occur, but are far less common.

Infarctions may occur secondary to herniations, vasospasm arterial dissection, or, if severe hypotension occurred, via a 'watershed' phenomenon (Marino et al. 2006).

Cerebral edema is common, and adds considerably to the clinical expression of diffuse axonal injury, contusions and intracerebral hemorrhages. Herniation may occur, with, as just noted, possible infarction secondary to vascular compression: with uncal herniation, such infarction may occur in the area of distribution of the posterior cerebral artery, whereas with subfalcine herniation, infarction may occur in the area of distribution of the anterior cerebral artery.

Hydrocephalus may occur via a number of mechanisms. Acute hydrocephalus may occur secondary to compression of the foramen of Monro by an expanding lesion, such as a contusion, or, when subarachnoid hemorrhage has occurred, secondary to a clot obstructing outflow from the exit foramina of the fourth ventricle. Chronic hydrocephalus, presenting weeks or months after the injury, may occur secondary to outflow obstruction at the arachnoid villi of the superior sagittal sinus.

Fractures may or may not occur, and it is important to keep in mind that there is not a good correlation between the presence of a fracture and the presence of brain damage; indeed in many cases of devastating traumatic brain injury, there is no fracture at all. Linear, depressed and compound fractures may all be seen, but of these linear fractures, typically at the base of the skull, are most common.

In addition to these direct effects of trauma, the occurrence of hypoxia and hypotension at the scene may lead, respectively, to global anoxic brain damage or, as noted earlier, watershed infarcts.

In determining which of these injuries have occurred, it must be borne in mind that MR scanning is more sensitive than CT scanning for diffuse axonal injury, contusions, subdural and epidural hematomas, infarcts, and global anoxic injury (Mittl et al. 1994; Orrison et al. 1994).

Differential diagnosis

Concussion is said to occur when, after an acceleration–deceleration injury or a blow to the head, there is either a very brief loss of consciousness or merely a sense of being dazed; there may also be an associated amnesia for the event. The post-concussion syndrome (discussed in Section 11.5), seen in a minority of patients after concussion, is characterized by minor cognitive deficits.

7.6 ACUTE ENCEPHALITIS

Although, technically, the term 'encephalitis' refers to any inflammation of the brain parenchyma, whether focal or diffuse, of any cause, in common clinical practice to say that a patient has an encephalitis is to imply that they are suffering from an acute and generalized infection. Most cases are due to viruses; bacterial and protozoal encephalitidies are much less common (Chaudhuri and Kennedy 2002).

Acute encephalitis constitutes a medical emergency, and hence recognizing the cardinal signs of encephalitis, namely fever, headache and delirium, is critically important.

Clinical features

In most cases, the encephalitis is preceded by a non-specific prodrome, lasting perhaps a few days, of fatigue, malaise, and fever. The encephalitis itself generally presents acutely, over hours, or at the most a day, with headache and delirium. In addition to confusion and variable disorientation, the delirium may also be accompanied by agitation, hallucinations (typically visual), and delusions. Focal findings, such as hemiparesis, aphasia, or hemianesthesia, may or may not be present, and there may also be partial or grand mal seizures. In most, but certainly not all, cases, signs of meningeal inflammation may also be present, with stiff neck or photophobia. With progression, stupor or coma may supervene.

Lumbar puncture is indicated in virtually every case (Steiner et al. 2005). Glucose is normal in viral infections, and decreased in bacterial and other causes. The total protein is increased. Essentially all cases will have a pleocytosis, ranging from 5 to 10 up to a 1000 white cells or more. In viral cases the pleocytosis is generally lymphocytic, whereas bacterial encephalitidies are generally marked by the presence of polymorphonuclear cells: an exception to this occurs with certain arbovirus infections wherein there may be a substantial number of polymorphonuclear cells for the first day or two; a persistent polymorphonuclear predominance after this time, however, is much more characteristic of bacterial infections. Gram stain and culture are performed routinely. Polymerase chain reactions (PCR) assay has revolutionized the identification of responsible organisms, and is useful in detecting herpes simplex, varicella-zoster, Epstein–Barr, cytomegalovirus, enterovirus, and various bacteria.

MRI, with contrast, should be performed; if this is not possible then CT scanning represents an alternative. Given the emergent nature of encephalitis, imaging should be promptly performed so as not to delay lumbar puncture. Importantly, early on, in the first day or two, imaging may not be impressive in the case of viral encephalitidies.

Electroencephalography typically shows generalized slowing, with or without interictal epileptiform discharges. Focal slowing in the temporal areas, with or without periodic complexes, is highly suggestive of herpes simplex encephalitis.

Etiology

As noted earlier, most cases of acute encephalitis are due to viral infection (Koskiniemi et al. 2001). Herpes simplex virus encephalitis (Section 14.5) is the most common cause of sporadic viral encephalitis, and, given its treatability, it should be high on the differential. Arboviral encephalitidies (Section 14.4) occur in both an epidemic and endemic fashion. Zoster encephalitis (Section 14.9) is suggested by a concurrent, generally widespread, zosteriform eruption; mumps encephalitis (Section 14.8) by an associated parotitis, and infectious mononucelosis (Section 14.7) by its occurrence in the setting of typical 'mono' with sore throat and cervical adenopathy. Rabies (Section 14.10) is suggested by the presence of parasthesiae near the site of the fateful bite (which may have occurred weeks or months earlier) and hypersalivation with hydrophobia. Other viral causes include influenza, enteroviruses, and adenoviruses. In the immunoincompetent patient, for example those with AIDS or those under treatment with steroids or immunosuppressants, one must also consider cytomegalovirus (Section 14.2). Furthermore, early on during human immunodeficiency virus (HIV) infection, a brief encephalitis may accompany seroconversion.

Bacterial causes include Rocky Mountain spotted fever (Section 14.19) and typhus, suggested by a concurrent rash, stage II Lyme disease (Section 14.16), suggested by a concurrent cranial or peripheral neuropathy, anthrax (Lanska 2002), mycoplasma pneumoniae infection, leptospirosis, listerosis, and cat scratch fever.

Protozoal causes include toxoplasmosis (Section 14.21), generally seen only in the severely immunocompromised, and cerebral malaria (Section 14.20).

Differential diagnosis

Acute disseminated encephalomyelitis, as discussed in Section 14.11, represents an autoimmune encephalitis triggered by a preceding viral or bacterial infection. Clinically, this syndrome may be indistinguishable from acute infectious encephalitis, and the differential may hinge on demonstrating the characteristic latent interval between a preceding infectious illness and the onset of the delirium.

Toxic and metabolic deliria are very common, and often occur in patients who have headache and fever due to a general medical illness, such as pneumonia or sepsis. Considerable clinical judgment is required here in deciding whether to perform a lumbar puncture; however, if the metabolic abnormalities are relatively mild, and the toxicity of current medications generally low, and the patient is not septic, one might lean toward obtaining CSF.

Subdural empyema, cerebritis or cerebral abscess, and cerebral thrombophlebitis are each apparent on magnetic resonance imaging.

The neuroleptic malignant syndrome (Section 22.1) is suggested by the presence of rigidity and coarse tremor in the proper pharmacologic setting: initiation or increased dose of an antipsychotic, or discontinuation or substantial dose decrease of a dopaminergic preparation, such as levodopa.

Treatment

Most patients should be admitted to an ICU, with strict attention to fluid and electrolyte balance: both diabetes insipidus and the syndrome of inappropriate antidiuretic hormone (ADH) secretion may occur. Intracranial pressure monitoring may be required. Seizures may be treated with fosphenytoin, and the general treatment of delirium is as discussed in Section 5.3.

Some encephalitidies have specific treatments, as discussed in the respective chapters. Given the devastating nature of herpes simplex encephalitis and its eminent treatability, it is customary to administer acyclovir pending the results of PCR testing.

Patients who survive may or may not be left with sequelae (Arciniegas and Anderson 2004), depending on the causative organism, the severity of the infection, and the age of the patient: both the very young and the elderly are more likely to have sequelae. Focal deficits may persist, and epilepsy may ensue. There may also be personality change, dementia, and various movement disorders. Specifics are discussed in the respective chapters.

7.7 SOMATOFORM DISORDERS

Somatoform disorders are characterized by complaints that either, as in the case of conversion disorder or somatization disorder, have no basis in the anatomic or physiologic facts of the matter, or, as in hypochondriasis, although having some basis in anatomy or physiology, yet are exaggerated far beyond what would be expected. Each of these is considered in turn.

Conversion disorder

Conversion disorder is characterized by symptoms that meet two criteria: first, they suggest a specific lesion of the central or peripheral nervous system; and, second, further investigation either reveals symptomatology that 'violates' the laws of anatomy or physiology, or demonstrates conclusively that the suspected lesion does not, in fact exist. Furthermore, and again despite thorough investigation, no motive can be discovered for the conversion symptom in question. This last point is critical, as it distinguishes conversion disorder from malingering, when the motive for the symptomatology, whether it be financial gain or avoidance of some unpleasant task, is fairly obvious.

A synonym for conversion disorder is hysteria (or, 'hysterical neurosis'): both terms, to a degree, are unfortunate, as both indicate etiologic theories that have not been substantiated. 'Conversion' implies a mechanism whereby emotionally charged ideas are in some unconscious way 'converted' into 'physical' symptoms. 'Hysteria', an ancient term, suggests that the disorder is in some way related to having a *hystera* (Greek for 'womb'), which is clearly not the case; although females are more likely to have this disorder than males (by a factor of from 2:1 up to 10:1), it clearly also occurs in males.

The lifetime prevalence of conversion disorder is not known with certainty: reported figures range from 0.01 to 0.5 percent of the general population.

CLINICAL FEATURES

Although conversion disorder may first appear anywhere from childhood to old age, most patients first experience symptoms in either adolescence or early adult years. In most cases, the onset is abrupt and typically follows closely upon a stressful life event.

Although a large number of conversion symptoms are possible, most patients have only one at a time. Common conversion symptoms include paralysis, anesthesia, ataxia, tremor, deafness, blindness, parkinsonism, syncope, coma, and seizures. As noted above, one of the distinctive features of conversion symptoms is that, in some way or other, they 'violate' the laws of anatomy or physiology, and it is this 'violation' that often alerts the examiner to the conversion nature of the symptom in question (Stone *et al.* 2002). An example would be a patient who complained of an area of anesthesia that involves the entire hand, extends up to the

middle of the forearm, and ends abruptly at a boundary that describes a perfect circle around the forearm. There simply is no lesion of either the central or peripheral nervous system that could conceivably produce such a pattern of anesthesia. In the following paragraphs, each of these common conversion symptoms is discussed in turn, with special attention to the associated 'violations' that one may find.

Conversion paralysis may mimic *monoplegia, hemiplegia,* or *paraplegia.* In conversion *monoplegia* involving, for example, the upper limb, one may find a non-physiologic pattern of weakness, involving perhaps the forearm and hand with complete strength maintained in the shoulder and arm. In conversion *hemiplegia,* one may find a positive Hoover test (Hoover 1908). The Hoover test may be performed by having the patient lie supine on the bed, positioning yourself at the foot of the bed and placing one hand under the heel of the 'bad' leg and the other on top of the ankle of the 'good' leg. At this point ask the patient to lift the 'good' leg up in the air against the resistance of your hand. As the patient attempts to lift the 'good' leg, you will feel the normal compensatory downward pressure of the contralateral leg on your hand as it lies under the heel of the 'bad' leg. Once this maneuver has been accomplished, ask the patient to rest the 'good' leg down and then switch the position of your hands, now placing one hand under the heel of the 'good' leg and placing the other hand on top of the 'bad' leg. At this point, encourage the patient to exert the greatest effort possible in raising the 'bad' leg up against the resistance of your hand. In a positive Hoover test one finds two things: first, the 'bad' leg moves little, if at all; second, one fails to feel any of the normally expected downward pressure on the hand underneath the heel of the 'good' leg, indicating that, in fact, the patient is putting no effort into the task of lifting the 'bad' leg. Recently, a similar test, designed to elicit the 'abductor sign' has been described (Sonoo 2004). In this test, with the patient with conversion hemiplegia supine in bed, stand at the foot of the bed, facing the patient, and place your hands on the lateral aspects of both of the patient's legs, maintaining a light inward pressure. At this point, ask the patient to abduct the 'bad' leg as forcefully as possible against the light pressure of your hand. In conversion paralysis, there is no movement of the 'bad' leg, and, critically, there is also no abduction of the 'good' leg either. In patients with 'true' hemiplegia one would appreciate the expected synergistic abduction of the 'good' leg, and it is the absence of this in conversion that indicates that, in fact, the patient is not putting effort into the task. Observing the patient on attempted ambulation is also helpful: when asked to walk, patients with conversion hemiparesis tend to drag the affected leg, pulling it up behind them, rather than circumducting it. Furthermore, patients with conversion hemiplegia may also display the 'wrong-way' tongue, with deviation of the protruded tongue away from the weak side, rather than toward it, as one would expect with stroke (Keane 1986). In both conversion monoplegia and hemiplegia one typically also finds symmetric deep tendon reflexes and bilaterally down-going toes. One may also find 'give-way' or 'collapsing' weakness. Here, the patient may be asked to flex the forearm after which the examiner, grasping the patient's hand, attempts to extend the forearm. In 'collapsing' weakness, one finds that an initial resistance is followed by an abrupt giving away of any resistance, as if the arm had suddenly become flaccid. Although this sign is useful, it must be borne in mind that a degree of collapsing weakness may at times be found in patients with hemiparesis due to stroke. Conversion *paraplegia* is suggested by normal reflexes, muscle tone, sensation, and sphincter function (Baker and Silver 1987).

Conversion anesthesia is suggested by the non-physiologic boundaries of the 'anesthetic' area. Thus, patients with a 'glove and stocking' pattern may complain of a precise boundary, with the anesthesia ending abruptly at a circular boundary just above the ankles or hands, rather than displaying the gradual 'fade' seen in a peripheral polyneuropathy. Furthermore, in such cases one may find a negative Romberg test. In cases where the conversion anesthesia suggests a mononeuropathy, one finds that the anesthetic area simply does not match any known dermatomal pattern. Finally, in cases suggesting central sensory loss, one may see a hemianesthesia with a boundary that precisely and exactly bisects the midline (care must be taken in interpreting this finding, however, for there are rare cases of hemianesthesia secondary to thalamic lesions wherein such a precise bisection is actually seen).

Before moving on to the next conversion symptom, it is worth remarking that the oft-stated rule that conversion paralysis and anesthesia are more likely to occur on the left than the right side does not, in fact, appear to hold true.

Conversion ataxia is suggested by elaborate lurching movements of the legs, which may be accompanied by similarly exaggerated flinging of the arms. In severe cases of conversion ataxia one may find astasia–abasia, that is to say, an inability to both walk and to stand. In such cases, one typically finds that, when supine on the bed, patients can perform finger-to-nose and heel-to-knee-to-shin testing adequately. Care must be taken here, however, for in some cases of lesions of the anterior vermis such a discrepancy may be found.

Conversion tremors are typically of large amplitude, and most importantly, vary in amplitude and frequency over small periods of time or with distraction; furthermore, when a weight is applied to the tremulous extremity, one often finds an exacerbation, rather than the expected diminution. In cases of unilateral tremor, the tremor may diminish when the patient is asked to perform a complex action with the contralateral extremity, for example touching the third, first, and fourth fingers with the thumb. One may also attempt to elicit a phenomenon known as 'chasing the tremor'. In cases of 'true' tremor, say, of a hand, when one grasps the hand the tremor diminishes and does not appear elsewhere. In conversion tremor, however, after grasping the hand, the forearm may begin to tremble, then, if the forearm is grasped, the tremor may appear in the upper arm, as if one were 'chasing' it.

Conversion deafness, if bilateral and complete, is suggested by observing a blink reflex to an unexpected and loud sound, thus demonstrating intactness of the brainstem.

Conversion blindness may be either monocular or bilateral. In both cases, an intact direct and consensual pupillary response demonstrates that the visual pathways to the lateral geniculate bodies are intact. In cases of bilateral conversion blindness, one finds that the patient does not sustain injury while attempting to navigate around the office or hospital room. In doubtful cases, one may have to resort to visual evoked potentials to demonstrate that the post-geniculate visual pathways are intact.

Conversion parkinsonism (Lang *et al.* 1995) may present with tremor, loss of associated arm movements, and postural instability; however, all of these may be accompanied by atypical features. Tremor may persist or even increase with action, and the arms, upon ambulation, are often held tightly against the patient's sides. Postural instability may be tested, provided adequate help is available in the case of a fall, by standing in front of the patient and then administering an abrupt and forceful push against the patient's sternum. In such cases, if the patient does fall back, there may be a tell-tale and distinctive fluid upswing of the arms, a movement that does not appear in bradykinetic patients.

Conversion syncope is suggested by a lack of autonomic changes, such as pallor, and by a typical, dramatic swoon that does not result in any injury.

Conversion coma is suggested by a number of findings. First, eye movements, as observed under the closed lids, are, rather than roving, typically saccadic. Next, upon gently stroking the eyelashes, one may see a responsive fluttering of the eyelids, and if one attempts to open the eyes by pulling up the lids, there is typically some more or less forceful resistance; furthermore, one finds that the pupillary responses are normal. Finally, when the eyes are allowed to close, they do so abruptly or with a jerky motion, in contrast to the smooth lowering seen in coma. If doubt remains, one may raise the patient's flaccid arm, hold it over the head and then let it drop, observing carefully to see if the arm is pulled to the side to avoid injuring the face. One may also consider the ice cube test, wherein, without warning, one touches an ice cube to a sensitive area, perhaps the cheek, whereupon one typically sees an abrupt turning of the head away from the stimulus.

Conversion seizures, also referred to as 'pseudoseizures', 'psychogenic non-epileptic seizures', or simply 'psychogenic seizures', may mimic either *grand mal* or *complex partial* seizures. Conversion *grand mal* seizures, like true grand mal seizures, may begin with a cry, but, unlike the inarticulate cry of a grand mal seizure, this cry may be more of a scream, and may involve words; furthermore, the scream may persist well past the initial part of the episode. The movements seen in a conversion grand mal seizure, rather than being symmetric and rhythmic, are typically asymmetric and may involve wild thrashing and rocking from side to side; furthermore, if attempts are made to restrain the patient, these are generally met with some resistance. In a conversion grand mal seizure, some patients may bite their lips, but the tongue is generally spared; furthermore, it is very rare to see urinary incontinence during a conversion seizure. After the event one typically does not see any confusion, nor does one find a positive Babinski sign. Conversion *complex partial* seizures are more difficult to diagnose given, as discussed in Section 7.3, the extraordinary range of symptomatology seen in true complex partial seizures. In general, however, as the behavior becomes more complex and the episode lasts longer, well past 5 minutes, the greater the likelihood is that the event represents a conversion seizure. Laboratory testing, including video–EEG and serum prolactin, neuron-specific enolase and CPK levels, may be required to confirm the diagnostic impression, and these are discussed further in Section 7.3.

Other conversion symptoms, of course, are possible, and these include aphonia, anosmia, nystgmus, convergence spasm, and ageusia.

Demonstrating a 'violation' may at times require considerable ingenuity on the part of the examining physician, and in all cases requires a thorough and detailed neurologic examination coupled with a firm grasp of the anatomy and physiology of the nervous system. Whether or not investigation beyond the clinical examination is required, for example with MR scanning, evoked potentials or EEGs, is a question that should be decided on a case-by case basis. Certainly, if the 'violation' is questionable, such investigation should be considered.

Although conversion disorder may occur in isolation, most patients have other disorders (Binzer *et al.* 1997), most commonly either a depression or a personality disorder of the histrionic, passive–aggressive, borderline, or antisocial types. Another feature often said to occur in association with conversion symptoms is 'la belle indifference', that is to say a casual indifference to symptoms, such as blindness or hemianesthesia, which would normally provoke considerable alarm. Unfortunately, this is not a reliable symptom, as it may either be absent or seen in other disorders (Stone *et al.* 2006). Furthermore, it may be confused with anosognosia.

COURSE

Conversion disorder may pursue either an episodic or chronic course (Mace and Trimble 1996). In episodic cases, recovery is seen typically in a matter of weeks or months; this favorable turn of events is more likely in younger patients, those of good intelligence, and in cases wherein the onset is acute, and occurs shortly after a major emotional stress. In those who do recover, however, recurrences are common in the following years; when recurrences do occur, the symptoms may or may not be the same. Chronicity may be anticipated when initial symptoms persist much beyond 6 months.

ETIOLOGY

The experience of patients with conversion symptoms is quite remarkable. Although it may be clear to the examining physician that the symptoms are, in some sense or other, 'produced' by the patient, the patient is not aware of doing so: for the patient, the symptom simply appeared, and did so not on the basis of any motivation or intention that the patient was aware of. Various theories have been proposed to explain this. Some invoke the concept of dissociation or suggest an association with hypnotic phenomena, whereas others involve unconscious motivations. For example, in explaining of conversion paralysis, say, of the right arm, one might speculate that the patient experienced a number of events unconsciously, including anger and a desire to strike out, guilt at entertaining such a notion and a sense of shame at not acting decisively. Here, the 'paralysis' of the arm serves two purposes: it effectively prevents the patient from hurting anyone, thus avoiding guilt, but also provides a ready excuse why decisive action cannot be taken, thus avoiding shame. Although such theories have a strong intuitive appeal, there is not, as yet, compelling evidence in their support.

Imaging studies have provided some interesting results. SPECT scanning has revealed decreased activity in the striatum and thalamus contralateral to conversion paralysis, with this asymmetry resolving with remission of the paralysis (Vuilleumier *et al.* 2001). Positron emission tomography (PET) scanning has revealed underactivation of the motor cortex contralateral to conversion paralysis when patients are requested to move the limb, with associated increased activation of the orbitofrontal and anterior cingulate cortex (Marshall *et al.* 1997), and, in a similar vein, functional MR scanning revealed decreased activity in the sensory cortex contralateral to conversion anesthesia (Ghaffar *et al.* 2006). Finally, in one study, MR scanning revealed slight atrophy of both striata and the right thalamus in patients with conversion disorder (Atmaca *et al.* 2006).

Overall, it may be prudent to say that the appearance of conversion symptoms involves dysfunction of the cortico-striato-thalamic circuitry, which, in some as yet unknown fashion, is associated with behavior whose motivation is unknown to the patient.

DIFFERENTIAL DIAGNOSIS

The most important differential to make, of course, is between conversion symptoms and 'true' symptoms that are, in fact, occurring on the basis of central or peripheral nervous system disease. In this regard, it must be borne in mind that, despite thorough investigation, a small minority of patients who receive the diagnosis of conversion disorder will, on follow-up, be found to have lesions missed during the initial evaluation (Binzer and Kullgren 1998; Moene *et al.* 2000). Consequently, the importance of a detailed and thorough examination, coupled with appropriate imaging and laboratory testing, cannot be overemphasized.

Conversion symptoms may occur not only in conversion disorder, but also in Briquet's syndrome and schizophrenia.

Conversion disorder is characterized solely by conversion symptoms. By contrast, in these two other disorders one sees multiple other symptoms. In Briquet's syndrome there are multiple complaints referable to organ systems other than the central nervous system, and hence one typically hears of complaints regarding pulmonary, gastrointestinal, and musculoskeletal functioning. In schizophrenia, one sees a variable mixture of psychotic symptoms, such as delusions, hallucinations, loosened associations, and overall bizarreness.

Malingering is distinguished from conversion disorder in that, in the case of malingering, the patient does intentionally, and with full awareness, feign the symptom that, in turn, clearly answers to an obvious motivation. For example, a patient who had been in a minor motor vehicle accident might feign a paralysis, and maintain that weakness until a large legal settlement had been obtained. Factitious disorder must also be considered, and here the motivation is simply to be a patient in the hospital.

TREATMENT

After the diagnosis is made, one should inform the patient in a calm and quietly authoritative way that the investigation and testing indicate that the nervous system is intact and not damaged. One may then go on to add that although it is not known why these symptoms have appeared, it is known that, with time, most patients recover. In some cases, especially those with conversion symptoms involving motor function, such as paralysis, engaging the patient in a course of physical therapy may be followed by a rapid resolution of symptoms (Watanabe *et al.* 1998). Hypnosis and psychotherapy have both been utilized, and, anecdotally, with success.

Somatization disorder

Somatization disorder, also known as Briquet's syndrome (in honor of Pierre Briquet, who first described it in 1859), is characterized by multiple complaints, referable to multiple organ systems, all occurring in the absence of any disease entity that could reasonably account for them (Perley and Guze 1962). These complaints persist chronically, and typically occasion multiple evaluations, hospitalizations, and often-needless diagnostic procedures or surgeries. Conservative estimates indicate a lifetime prevalence in females of from 0.2 to 2 percent; although Briquet's syndrome may also occur in males, this is probably very uncommon, if not rare (Smith *et al.* 1985).

CLINICAL FEATURES

This syndrome generally first appears in teenage years; onset past the age of 30 is extremely rare.

Patients tend to be excessively vague or dramatic in relating their history, often moving restlessly from one symptom to another, never lingering long enough on one symptom to give an adequately detailed account. As noted earlier, multiple complaints are heard, implicating multiple organ systems, including the gastrointestinal tract, the genitourinary system, central and peripheral nervous systems, and the musculoskeletal system. There is debate as to how many symptoms and how many organ systems are required to make a diagnosis: a conservative approach requires at least one unexplained complaint from each system.

Gastrointestinal complaints often center on vague and poorly localized abdominal pain, often accompanied by nausea and bloating. Constipation is common, diarrhea somewhat less so, and patients often complain of multiple food intolerances. Rectal pain or burning may also be present.

Of genitourinary complaints, irregular, painful or heavy menstrual flow is prominent, and patients who have been pregnant may complain of having had severe, intractable vomiting throughout the entire pregnancy. Decreased libido is common; females may complain of decreased vaginal lubrication and dyspareunia, and males may complain of erectile dysfunction. Dysuria and partial urinary retention may also occur.

Musculoskeletal complaints include backache, arthralgia, and diffuse chest pain.

Central and peripheral nervous system complaints include paralysis, anesthesia, ataxia, deafness, blurry vision, diplopia, blindness, dizziness, fainting, pseudoseizures, globus hystericus, aphonia, and headache.

The large number of complaints, and the inability of the physician to pin the patient down as to details, often make the interview very frustrating for the physician, and it is typical to find chart entries indicating merely that the review of systems was 'diffusely positive'. Many physicians turn to the physical examination with some relief, hoping to determine some definite findings. Generally, however, if there are any findings, they are typically minor and not indicative of any disease or condition that could possibly account for the patient's multitudinous complaints.

When physicians attempt to reassure patients regarding the benign nature of the examination, they are often met with disbelief, if not hostility, and patients typically demand tests, and when basic tests are unremarkable, the demands persist. Some physicians may call it quits at this point, but others will proceed to invasive procedures or even to surgery. In some cases, patients have welcomed so many abdominal surgeries that they finally develop a 'battlefield abdomen'. 'Doctor shopping' is common, as exasperated physicians 'fire' their patients, or patients, dissatisfied with the diagnostic approach offered by their physicians, move on to find a more aggressive diagnostician.

In addition to these multiple complaints, depression and panic attacks are common, as is alcohol abuse or alcoholism. Personality disturbances of the borderline, histrionic, or antisocial type, are also common.

COURSE

Briquet's syndrome typically pursues a chronic course, with the intensity and variety of complaints fluctuating gradually over the lifespan of the patient; spontaneous remissions are very uncommon.

ETIOLOGY

Briquet's syndrome may have both environmental and genetic determinants. The prevalence in first-degree relatives of females with this syndrome is increased to as high as 20 percent, and adoption studies of females have demonstrated an increased prevalence of alcohol abuse and antisocial behavior in their biological fathers (Bohman et al. 1984; Golding et al. 1992; Guze et al. 1986). It has been suggested that Briquet's syndrome and antisocial personality disorder result from a common genetic background, with sex-mediated expression.

DIFFERENTIAL DIAGNOSIS

The most important differential consideration, of course, is one, or perhaps an unfortunate combination of diseases, that could produce a 'diffusely positive' review of systems with few informative findings on physical examination. Possibilities include multisystem diseases such as systemic lupus erythematosus and sarcoidosis. Consequently, it is necessary to evaluate each new complaint on its own merits, before deciding that it can be ascribed to Briquet's. In this regard, when complaints referable to the central or peripheral nervous system are present, the techniques suggested in the preceding section, on conversion disorder, may be helpful.

Conversion disorder may also be considered on the differential but is ruled out on two counts: first, rather than a multitude of symptoms, there are generally only one, or perhaps two; and, second, rather than a multitude of organ systems, only one is involved in conversion disorder, namely the nervous system.

Malingering and factitious disorder, like conversion disorder, generally are not associated with multiple complaints; furthermore, the complaints are intentionally feigned with a more or less obvious motive behind them.

Hypochondriasis may also be considered, as hypochondriacal patients often have multiple complaints referable to multiple organ systems. The difference here, however, relates to the patients' attitude toward the complaint. In hypochondriasis, rather than being concerned about any suffering associated with the complaint, patients are worried about what the symptom implies, namely the presence of a serious, but undiagnosed, disease. In Briquet's syndrome, however, the focus is more on the suffering associated with the symptom.

Depression may be associated with multiple unexplained complaints, and thus can present a picture similar to Briquet's syndrome. To complicate matters further, as noted above, patients with Briquet's syndrome often do have concurrent depression. The key to making the differential here lies in the time course: in cases where the complaints are secondary to depression, one finds the onset of depressed mood and associated vegetative symptoms well before the appearance of multiple complaints. In doubtful cases, it may be appropriate to attempt a 'diagnosis by treatment response' by prescribing an antidepressant and watching to see if the multiple complaints subside.

Schizophrenia may also be associated with multiple complaints, but these typically have a bizarre cast to them, and are associated with other typical psychotic symptoms, such as delusions, hallucination, etc.

TREATMENT

A conservative medical approach is appropriate, and, if at all possible, patients should remain under the care of one physician, either an internist or family practitioner; psychiatric consultation to the primary care physician has also been demonstrated to improve patient care (Smith et al. 1986). Preliminary work suggests that cognitive behavior therapy may also be beneficial (Allen et al. 2001).

Hypochondriasis

In hypochondriasis (Barsky 2001), patients, on the basis of minor symptoms or signs, come to believe, or, at the very least, strongly suspect, that they have a serious, perhaps even life-threatening, disease. Their concerns occasion multiple consultations, often with multiple physicians, and, importantly, despite negative examinations and earnest reassurances regarding their condition, these patients remain beset by their concerns. This condition probably has a lifetime prevalence of between 1 and 5 percent, and is equally common among males and females.

CLINICAL FEATURES

Although the onset of hypochondriasis may occur at any point between adolescence and old age, most patients first begin to experience their concerns in their twenties or thirties. Although in most cases there does not appear to be a precipitating event, occasionally the onset may be triggered either by observing a serious illness in an acquaintance or personally suffering one. A good example of the latter is the 'cardiac cripple' who remains an invalid, consumed by hypochondriacal concerns after recovering from a heart attack, despite reassurances from the cardiologist.

Patients come to the physician already convinced that their symptoms, no matter how mild or trivial, indicate the presence of a severe disease. A mild, non-productive cough means they have pneumonia, or perhaps lung cancer; a few palpitations indicate that the heart is about to fail; slight nausea is a sure sign that an ulcer has eaten through the stomach, and simple constipation can only mean that colon cancer has finally appeared.

Patients often present their complaints in minute and maddening detail. If they have been to other physicians, as is typically the case, they may present copies of prior evaluations coupled with accusations that the prior physicians did not take their complaints with sufficient seriousness: the often thinly-veiled hostility of such patients may put the current physician on guard, as if he or she is under attack. An appropriate history and examination is typically unrevealing, or, if findings are noted, they are usually indicative of an often trivial condition. Rather than being reassured, however, patients are often upset. They want more tests, and if the physician expresses some skepticism regarding this, they may become demanding. Predictably, 'doctor shopping' is common.

The expression of hypochondriacal concerns is not confined to hospital or doctor visits but permeates these patients' lives. They may share their worries about their health at the dinner table, the office, or at social gatherings, anxiously going from person to person until they find a sympathetic listener who will tolerate their complaints. In some cases, their complaints are so wearying that others begin to avoid these patients, who become isolated and even more miserable. Some, paralyzed by their concerns, will opt to enter a nursing home in order to be sure that medical care is immediately available.

Depression or panic disorder are present in a majority of cases (Noyes *et al.* 1994).

COURSE

Hypochondriasis, in the majority of cases, appears to be chronic, with symptoms waxing and waning in intensity over the years (Barsky *et al.* 1998). Although it appears that spontaneous full remissions do occur, the frequency with which this occurs is not clear.

ETIOLOGY

Hypochondriasis does not appear to run in families (Noyes *et al.* 1997), and the etiology is as yet unclear. Although these patients recall having more serious illnesses in childhood and going through more emotionally traumatic events (Barsky *et al.* 1994; Noyes *et al.* 2002), there have been no prospective studies, and hence these findings may well be due to recall bias.

Based on the similarity between the persistent recurring concerns seen in hypochondriasis and obsessions seen in obsessive–compulsive disorder, there has been speculation that hypochondriasis is but one example of the 'obsessive–compulsive spectrum' disorders but as yet proof of this is lacking.

DIFFERENTIAL DIAGNOSIS

Hypochondriasis must be distinguished from transient hypochondriacal concerns, which are very common in the general population: the notorious 'Doctor's diseases' suffered by medical students are a good example. The differential here rests on the duration of hypochondriacal concerns: most transient concerns resolve spontaneously in a matter of weeks, and in any case, persist no longer than 6 months.

Depression is perhaps the most important differential to consider. Especially in the elderly, depression may manifest with hypochondriacal concerns; indeed, such patients may limit their presentation to such complaints, and not spontaneously report the accompanying vegetative symptoms, such as anergia, anhedonia, anorexia, and insomnia. These 'masked depressions' may at times be difficult to diagnose, as in some cases patients may deny feeling depressed.

Briquet's syndrome is distinguished both by the nature of the patients' complaints and by the manner in which they are made. In Briquet's syndrome, patients typically have a multitude of complaints, and here, it is not so much a concern that the symptoms indicate a serious underlying disease as it is with the debilitating nature of the symptom itself. Thus, whereas a hypochondriacal patient complaining of constipation may admit that it is mild, and relieved with simple fiber laxatives, the patient with Briquet's syndrome may complain that it is painful, unbearable, and impossible to overcome. Further, whereas the hypochondriacal patient typically reports complaints in precise detail, the patient with Briquet's syndrome is for the most part vague, and difficult to pin down.

Conversion disorder is likewise suggested by the nature of the complaint. In conversion disorder, the complaint always refers to the nervous system: in hypochondriasis, such complaints may also be heard, but other organ systems are more commonly implicated. Furthermore, in conversion disorder the patients' concerns are not so much related to a fear of some undiagnosed and underlying disease, as is the case in hypochondriasis, as they are to the effects of the symptom itself, such as an inability to walk because of conversion paralysis.

Malingering and factitious disorder are both distinguished by the fact that these patients either intentionally lie about symptoms or intentionally inflict wounds, all in the service of an understandable goal, such as financial gain, or, in the case of factitious disorder, merely being a patient in the hospital.

Finally, one must remain alert to the possibility that new complaints, rather than being hypochondriacal, may signal a serious underlying disease: each new complaint must be evaluated on its own merits.

TREATMENT

Cognitive–behavioral therapy is effective (Barsky and Ahern 2004), and paroxetine is roughly equivalent to cognitive–behavioral therapy, with both being better than placebo (Greeven *et al.* 2007). In cases where such therapy is either not available or when patients refuse to enter treatment, it is appropriate to maintain a conservative medical approach and to see patients in regularly scheduled follow-up visits. Should depression or panic disorder be present, these must be treated.

7.8 MALINGERING AND FACTITIOUS ILLNESS

Both malingering (LoPiccolo *et al.* 1999) and factitious illness (Krahn *et al.* 2003) are characterized by the intentional feigning of illness; they are distinguished from one another by the motive underlying this behavior. In malingering the motive is readily understandable, as for example when someone complains of a 'bad back' to get out of work or to obtain narcotics. In factitious illness, however, the motive is a little more obscure, in that the goal of these individuals is merely to be a patient in the hospital, and to assume, as it were, the 'sick role'.

Before making a diagnosis of malingering or factitious illness, one must be reasonably certain that there is no true underlying illness that could reasonably account for the individual's complaints. Furthermore, one must also distinguish malingering and factitious illness from conversion disorder, Briquet's syndrome, and hypochondriasis; these differential possibilities are distinguished by the lack of any associated intentionality and by the lack of any recognizable 'goal'. Thus, in the case of 'paralysis', the malingerer and the individual with factitious illness both consciously and intentionally feign weakness, with the goal, respectively, of either an understandable gain (e.g., winning a lawsuit) or of simply being a patient on the neurologic ward. By contrast, in the case of, say, conversion disorder, the 'paralysis' simply appears, without any planning or intention on the part of the patient, and persists despite there being no advantage to the patient.

Malingering

Some malingerers may limit their dissimulation to simply voicing more or less convincing complaints. Others may take advantage of an actual illness, and embellish their symptoms out of all proportion to the actual underlying disease or condition. Some may go so far as to actually stage an accident or inflict a wound and then go on to exaggerate their effects. Falsification of medical records may also occur.

Neurologic, psychiatric, and rheumatologic illnesses are often chosen as models. Malingerers may complain of headaches, anesthesia, paralysis, 'whiplash', and pain, especially low back pain. Depression, post-traumatic stress disorder, and psychosis may also be feigned. A peculiar form of malingering may be seen in prisoners awaiting trial or sentencing, known as the 'Ganser syndrome' (Carney *et al.* 1987; Tsoi 1973). Also known as the 'nonsense syndrome', this is characterized by 'nonsense' responses to questions, which are always just off the mark or past the point. For example, if the individual is asked to add 5 plus 3, he may respond '7'; with coaching and encouragement he may give other responses, such as '6' or '9', but never the correct one. In a similar vein, if asked how many legs a horse has, the response may be '3'. Typically, although these individuals appear confused and dazed, they are generally able to find their way around the jail and to do those things that are necessary to maintain a certain degree of comfort and safety. All in all, these individuals are acting out the 'popular' conception of 'insanity', and once the trial is over, or the sentence imposed, this 'insanity' clears up quickly.

Several features may alert the physician to the possibility of malingering. First, look for obvious gains should the individual be certified as 'ill', such as obtaining insurance payments or narcotics, or winning a lawsuit. Second, be alert to inconsistencies in the clinical presentation. In this regard, when neurologic complaints are heard, the diagnostic tips discussed in the Section 7.7 for conversion disorder may be kept in mind. Third, be suspicious when patients are uncooperative with treatment, or when the offering of a good prognosis is met with thinly veiled hostility.

In doubtful cases, obtaining collateral history may be very helpful. For example, if, on interviewing the spouse of an individual who complains of incapacitating back pain, one gathers a history that the 'patient' spends his weekends playing volleyball, the diagnostic evaluation is essentially complete. Laboratory testing may be helpful, as for example neuroimaging in cases of feigned paralysis; however, most malingerers tend to feign illnesses that lack distinctive laboratory findings.

What the physician should do, once it becomes clear that malingering is present, is not clear. Some advocate a simple, but non-judgmental, discussion of the facts, and indeed some malingerers may respond favorably to this. Most, however, will not and indeed may become even more demanding or hostile. Regardless of what approach is taken, however, it is important to 'do no harm', and in this regard, one should not prescribe narcotics, certify nonexistent illnesses, or do anything else that reinforces the patient's deception.

Factitious illness

The illnesses feigned here tend to be severe, as might be expected, given that the goal of the dissimulation is admission to the hospital. Typically, the patient arrives at the emergency room with a very convincing presentation (Reich and Gottfried 1983). Some may complain of several episodes of severe chest pain, suggesting crescendo angina. Others may report having had a 'seizure', and even bite their tongue to make the picture more convincing. Others may swallow blood and then vomit, thus simulating hematemesis, whereas others may hold the blood in their mouths and then cough, producing a picture of hemoptysis. A urine specimen may be contaminated with feldspar to mimic renal calculi, or with feces to suggest a severe urinary tract infection. More malignantly, feces may be injected to create a septic picture. Laxatives may be taken to induce diarrhea, furosemide to create hypokalemia, myelosuppressants to mimic aplastic anemia, thyroid hormone to produce hyperthyroidism, and either insulin or oral antidiabetic agents to produce hypoglycemia and raise the question of an insulinoma; in this last case, determining simultaneous insulin and C-peptide levels is helpful to rule out surreptitious injection of insulin: in an insulinoma both are elevated, whereas when insulin is injected the C-peptide level will be normal (Grunberger et al. 1988).

Once admitted, these individuals may make frequent demands for narcotics, and staff are often split and played off, one against the other. Diagnostic tests are welcomed, even demanded, and as the tests become ever more invasive and dangerous, these individuals often become calmer, even content. As more and more tests come back negative or inconsistent (Wallach 1994), the complaints may change: chest pain may fail to recur, but now abdominal pain and diarrhea come to the forefront. Eventually, when told by the physician that there is 'nothing wrong', these individuals typically become angry, accuse the physician of incompetence, and leave the hospital abruptly, often against medical advice.

The majority of individuals with factitious illness are female; most are in their twenties or thirties, and most have some medical background, having worked as aides, nurses, or therapists of one sort or other. In these cases, the frequency with which hospitalization is sought varies over time, and is often related to stressful events. In most cases, the dissimulation eventually stops after a matter of years.

In a minority of cases, however, the course is chronic and severe, and in such cases one speaks of 'Munchausen's syndrome', named after the famous German baron who traveled from city to city telling elaborate tales about himself (Asher 1951). In contrast with the typical individual with factitious illness, these individuals tend to be male and middle-aged, and to have a history of traveling from city to city with, at times, literally hundreds of hospital admissions. Also known as 'hospital hoboes' (Clarke and Melnick 1958) or 'hospital addicts' (Barker 1962), these individuals have made being a patient into a way or life.

A particularly loathsome variant of factitious illness (or Munchausen's syndrome) is that which occurs 'by proxy' (Souid et al. 1998). Here, a parent, typically the mother, may induce illness in a young child by any of the means noted above, and use the result as a ticket for the child's admission. These parents may, at least initially, seem appropriately concerned; however, suspicions may be aroused when staff note a certain satisfaction, even contentment, on the parent's part as the child is subjected to ever more invasive diagnostic procedures. In some cases, laboratory results may clinch the diagnosis, whereas in others it may be necessary to resort to covert video surveillance to 'catch' the parent injecting or otherwise harming the child (Hall et al. 2000). Although such 'proxy' factitious illness most often involves a parent and child, there have also been cases where adults have induced illness, either in their spouses or, more commonly, their elderly parents.

Although most cases of factitious illness involve 'physical' signs and symptoms, cases may also occur where 'psychological' signs and symptoms are feigned (Gelenberg 1977; Pope et al. 1982; Popli et al. 1992). Individuals may report suicidal or homicidal ideation, or may complain of voices, visions, deep depression, or post-traumatic stress. Given that laboratory testing is generally irrelevant in such cases, unmasking the dissimulation may take a little longer; however, eventually inconsistencies become apparent. In such cases, when confronted by the physician's suspicions, these individuals may, like those with 'physical' symptoms, become indignant and demand discharge, or they may 'up the ante' by making a suicidal gesture.

As with malingering, it is not clear what the best approach is to factitious illness. Some advocate confrontation, whereas others will attempt to engage the individual in some form of psychotherapy. In cases of 'proxy' illness, legal authorities must be involved.

REFERENCES

Abd El Naby S, Hassanein M. Neuropsychiatric manifestations of chronic manganese poisoning. *J Neurol Neurosurg Psychiatry* 1965; **28**:282–8.

Abenson MH. Epileptic fits provoked by taste. *Br J Psychiatry* 1969; **115**:123.

Acharya V, Acharya J, Luders H. Olfactory epileptic auras. *Neurology* 1998; **51**:56–61.

Adachi N, Arima K, Kato M *et al.* Dentatorubral-pallidoluysian atrophy (DRPLA) presenting with psychosis. *J Neuropsychiatry Clin Neurosci* 2001; **13**:258–60.

Adachi N, Kato M, Sekimoto M *et al.* Recurrent postictal psychosis after remission of interictal psychosis: further evidence of bimodal psychosis. *Epilepsia* 2003; **44**:1218–22.

Adachi N, Kanemoto K, Muramatsu R *et al.* Intellectual prognosis of status epilepticus in adult epilepsy patients: analysis with Wechsler Adult Intelligence Scale-revised. *Epilepsia* 2005; **46**:1502–9.

Adair JC, Williamson DJG, Schwartz RL *et al.* Ventral tegmental area injury and frontal lobe disorder. *Neurology* 1996; **46**:442–3.

Adam C, Baulac M, Saint-Hilaire J-M *et al.* Value of magnetic resonance imaging-based measurements of hippocampal formation in patients with partial epilepsy. *Arch Neurol* 1994; **51**:130–8.

Adamec DE, Stark-Adamec C. Limbic kindling in animal behavior: implications for human psychopathology associated with complex partial seizures. *Biol Psychiatry* 1983; **18**:269–74.

Adams JH, Graham DI, Murray AI *et al.* Diffuse axonal injury due to nonmissile head injury in humans: an analysis of 45 cases. *Ann Neurol* 1982; **12**:557–63.

Agius MA, Chan JW, Chung S *et al.* Role of antiribosomal P protein antibodies in the diagnosis of lupus isolated to the central nervous system. *Arch Neurol* 1997; **54**:862–4.

Agnetti V, Carreras M, Pinna L *et al.* Ictal prosopagnosia and epileptogenic damage of the dominant hemisphere. *Cortex* 1978; **14**:50–7.

Aquilar MJ, Rasmussen T. Role of encephalitis in pathogenesis of epilepsy. *Arch Neurol* 1960; **2**:663–76.

Ahl B, Bokemeyer M, Ennen JC et al. Dissection of the brain supplying arteries over the life span. *J Neurol Neurosurg Psychiatry* 2004; **75**:1194–6.

Ahuja GK, Mohandas S, Narayanaswamy AS. Eating epilepsy. *Epilepsia* 1980; **21**:85–9.

Ajmone-Marsan C, Ralston BL. *The epileptic seizure: its functional morphology and diagnostic significance.* IL: Springfield, Charles C. Thomas, 1957.

Akelaitis AJ. Lead encephalopathy in children and adults. *J Nerv Ment Dis* 1941; **93**:313–32.

Alajouanine T, DeRobert L, Thieffry S. Etude clinique de 210 cas d'intoxication par les sels organiques d'etain. *Rev Neurol* 1958; **98**:85–96.

Alamowitch S, Graus F, Uchuya M et al. Limbic encephalitis and small cell lung cancer: clinical and immunological features. *Brain* 1997; **120**:923–8.

Al-Asmi A, Jansen AC, Badhwar AP et al. Familial temporal lobe epilepsy as a presenting feature of choreoacanthocytosis. *Epilepsia* 2005; **46**:1256–63.

Albers GW, Thijs VN, Wechsler L et al. Magnetic resonance imaging profile predict clinical response to early reperfusion: the diffusion and perfusion imaging evaluation for understanding stroke evolution (DEFUSE) study. *Ann Neurol* 2006; **60**:508–17.

Albert A, Mirza S, Mirza KAH et al. Morbid jealousy in alcoholics. *Br J Psychiatry* 1996; **167**:668–72.

Alemayehu S, Bergey GK, Barry E et al. Panic attacks as ictal manifestations of parietal lobe seizures. *Epilepsia* 1995; **36**:824–30.

Alexander MP, Freedman M. Amnesia after anterior communicating artery aneurysm rupture. *Neurology* 1984; **34**:752–7.

Alldredge BK, Lowenstein DH, Simon RP. Seizures associated with recreational drug abuse. *Neurology* 1989; **39**:1037–9.

Allen LA, Woolfoldk RL, Lehrer PM et al. Cognitive behavior therapy for somatization disorder: a preliminary investigation. *J Behav Ther Exp Psychiatry* 2001; **32**: 53–62.

Allen RM, Young SJ. Phencyclidine induced psychosis. *Am J Psychiatry* 1978; **135**:1081–4.

Almeida OP, Waterreus A, Hankey GJ. Preventing depression after stroke: results from a randomized, placebo-controlled trial. *J Clin Psychiatry* 2006; **67**:1104–9.

Almeida S, Ranjith G. Using pramipexole in neuropsychiatry: a cautionary tale. *J Neuropsychiatry Clin Neurosci* 2006; **18**:556–7.

Alpers BJ. Relation of the hypothalmus to disorders of personality: report of a case. *Arch Neurol Psychiatry* 1937; **38**:291–303.

Alpers BJ, Grant FC. The clinical syndrome of the corpus callosum. *Arch Neurol Psychiatry* 1931; **25**:67–86.

Alsen G, Gillberg IC, Lindblom R et al. Tuberous sclerosis in Western Sweden: a population study of cases with early childhood onset. *Arch Neurol* 1994; **51**:76–81.

Alves D, Pires MM, Guimaraes A et al. Four cases of late onset metachromatic leukodystrophy in a family: clinical, biochemical and neuropathological studies. *J Neurol Neurosurg Psychiatry* 1986; **49**:1417–22.

Amatniek JC, Hauser WA, DelCastillo-Castenada C et al. Incidence and predictors of seizures in patients with Alzheimer disease. *Epilepsia* 2006; **47**:867–72.

Ames FR, Enderstein O. Ictal laughter: a case report with clinical, cinefilm, and EEG observations. *J Neurol Neurosurg Psychiatry* 1975; **38**:11–17.

Ames FR, Enderstein O. Gelastic epilepsy and hypothalamic hamartoma. *S Afr Med J* 1980; **58**:163–5.

Aminoff MJ, Simon RP. Status epilepticus. Causes, clinical features and consequences in 98 patients. *Am J Med* 1980; **69**:657–66.

Andermann F, Robb JP. Absence status: a reappraisal following review of thirty-eight patients. *Epilepsia* 1972; **13**:177–87.

Andersen G, Vestergaard K, Riis J. Citalopram for poststroke pathological crying. *Lancet* 1993; **342**:837–9.

Andersen G, Vestergaard K, Lauritzen L. Effective treatment of poststroke depression with the selective serotonin reuptake inhibitor citalopram. *Stroke* 1994; **25**:1099–104.

Anderson DJ, Goldstein LB, Wilkinson WE et al. Stroke location, characterization, severity, and outcome in mitral vs aortic valve endocarditis. *Neurology* 2003; **61**:1334–6.

Anderson G, Vestergaard F, Lauritzen L. Effective treatment of poststroke depression with the selective serontonin reuptake inhibitor citalopram. *Stroke* 1994; **25**:1099–104.

Anderson J. On sensory epilepsy. A case of cerebral tumour, affecting the left temporo-sphenoidal lobe, and giving rise to a paroxysmal taste-sensation and dreamy state. *Brain* 1886; **8**:385–95.

Andrews E, Ballard J, Walter-Ryan WG. Monosymptomatic hypochondriacal psychosis manifesting as delusion of infestation: case studies of treatment with haloperidol. *J Clin Psychiatry* 1986; **47**:188–90.

Annegers JF, Grabow JD, Groover RD et al. Seizures after head trauma: a population study. *Neurology* 1980; **30**:683–9.

Annegers JF, Hauser WA, Beghi E et al. The risk of unprovoked seizures after encephalitis and meningitis. *Neurology* 1988; **38**:1407–10.

Annegers JF, Hauser A, Coan SP et al. A population-based study of seizures after traumatic brain injuries. *N Engl J Med* 1998; **383**:20–4.

Appenzeller S, Cendes F, Costallat LTL. Epileptic seizures in systemic lupus erythematosus. *Neurology* 2004; **63**:1808–12.

Appleton RE, Farrell K, Teal P et al. Complex partial status epilepticus associated with cyclosporin-A therapy. *J Neurol Neurosurg Psychiatry* 1989; **52**:1068–71.

Arboix A, Bell Y, Garcia-Eroles L et al. Clinical study of 35 patients with dysarthria-clumsy hand syndrome. *J Neurol Neurosurg Psychiatry* 2004; **75**:231–4.

Arboix A, Lopez-Grau M, Casanovas C et al. Clinical study of 39 patients with atypical lacunar syndromes. *J Neurol Neurosurg Psychiatry* 2006; **77**:381–4.

Arcineagas DB, Anderson CA. Viral encephalitis: neuropsychiatric and neurobehavioral aspects. *Curr Psychiatry Rep* 2004; **6**:372–9.

Armstrong DD. The neuropathology of temporal lobe epilepsy. *J Neuropathol Exp Neurol* 1993; **52**:499–506.

Aron AM, Freeman JM, Carter S. The natural history of Sydenham's chorea. *Am J Med* 1965; **38**:83–95.

Aronica E, Gorter JA, Ramkema M et al. Expression and cellular distribution of multidrug resistance-related proteins in the hippocampus of patients with mesial temporal lobe epilepsy. *Epilepsia* 2004; **45**:441–5.

Arroyo S, Lesser RP, Gordon B. Mirth, laughter and gelastic seizures. *Brain* 1993; **116**:757–80.

Ashcroft PB. Traumatic epilepsy after gunshot wounds in the head. *BMJ* 1941; **1**:739–44.

Asher R. Myxoedematous madness. *BMJ* 1949; **2**:555–62.

Asher R. Munchausen's syndrome. *Lancet* 1951; **1**:339–41.

Ashford JW, Schulz SC, Walsh GO. Violent automatism in a partial complex seizure: report of a case. *Arch Neurol* 1980; **37**:120–2.

Ashkenazi A, Kaufman Y, Ben-hur T. Bilateral focal motor status epilepticus with retained consciousness after stroke. *Neurology* 2000; **54**:976–8.

Atmaca M, Aydin A, Texcan E *et al.* Volumetric investigation of brain regions in patients with conversion disorder. *Prog Neuropsychopharmacol Biol Psychiatry* 2006; **30**:708–13.

Aurahami E, Weiss-Peretz J, Cohn AF. Focal epileptic activity following intravenous contrast material injection in patients with metastatic brain disease. *J Neurol Neurosurg Psychiatry* 1987; **50**:221–3.

Avery TL. Seven cases of frontal tumor with psychiatric presentation. *Br J Psychiatry* 1971; **119**:19–23.

Ay H, Koroshetz WJ, Benner T *et al.* Transient ischemic attack with infarction: a unique syndrome. *Ann Neurol* 2005; **57**:679–83.

Aykutlu E, Baykan B, Serdaroglu P *et al.* Epileptic seizures in Behcet's disease. *Epilepsia* 2002; **43**:832–5.

Azouvi P, Jokic C, Attal N *et al.* Carbamazepine in agitation and aggressive behavior following severe closed-head injury: results of an open trial. *Brain Inj* 1999; **13**:797–804.

Backstrom T. Epileptic seizures in women related to plasma estrogen and progesterone during the menstrual cycle. *Acta Neurol Scand* 1976; **54**:321–47.

Bagedahl-Strindlund M. Postpartum mental illness: timing of illness onset and its relation to symptoms and sociodemographic characteristics. *Acta Psychiatr Scand* 1986; **74**:490–6.

Bailey DP, Coull BM, Goodnight SH. Neurological disease associated with antiphospholipid antibodies. *Ann Neurol* 1989; **25**:221–7.

Baird AE, Lovblad KO, Schlaug G *et al.* Multiple acute stroke syndrome: marker of embolic disease? *Neurology* 2000; **54**:674–8.

Baker JH, Silver JR. Hysterical paraplegia. *J Neurol Neurosurg Psychiatry* 1987; **50**: 375–82.

Baker RW, Conley RR. Seizures during clozapine therapy. *Am J Psychiatry* 1991; **148**:1265–6.

Balkan S. Painful unilateral epileptic seizure. *Acta Neurol Scand* 1995; **91**:414–16.

Ballenger CE, King DW, Gallagher BB. Partial complex status epilepticus. *Neurology* 1983; **33**:1545–52.

Bare MA, Burnstine TH, Fisher RS *et al.* Electroencephalographic changes during simple partial seizures. *Epilepsia* 1994; **35**:715–20.

Barker JC. The syndrome of hospital addiction (Munchausen syndrome): a report on the investigation of seven cases. *J Ment Sci* 1962; **108**:167–82.

Barkovich AJ, Kjos BO. Gray matter heterotopias: MR characteristics and correlation with developmental and neurologic manifestations. *Radiology* 1992; **182**:493–9.

Barkovich AJ, Rowley HA, Andermann F. MR in partial epilepsy: value of high-resolution volumetric techniques. *AJNR* 1995; **16**:339–43.

Barnes J, David AS. Visual hallucinations in Parkinson's disease: a review and phenomenological survey. *J Neurology Neurosurg Psychiatry* 2001; **70**:727–33.

Barnett HJM, Taylor DW, Eliasziw M *et al.* Benefit of carotid endarterectomy in patients with symptomatic moderate or severe stenosis. *N Engl J Med* 1998; **339**:1415–25.

Barry E, Sussman NM, Bosley TM *et al.* Ictal blindness and status epilepticus amauroticus. *Epilepsia* 1985; **26**:577–84.

Barsky AJ. The patient with hypochondriasis. *N Engl J Med* 2001; **345**:1395–9.

Barsky AJ, Ahern DK. Cognitive behavior therapy for hypochondriasis: a randomized controlled trial. *JAMA* 2004; **291**:1464–70.

Barsky AJ, Wool C, Barnett MC *et al.* Histories of childhood trauma in adult hypochondriacal patients. *Am J Psychiatry* 1994; **151**:397–401.

Barsky AJ, Fama JM, Bailey ED *et al.* A prospective 4- to 5-year study of DSM-III-R hypochondriasis. *Arch Gen Psychiatry* 1998; **55**:737–44.

Battaglia G, Chiapparini L, Fransceschetti S *et al.* Periventricular nodular heterotopia: classification, epileptic history, and genesis of epileptic discharges. *Epilepsia* 2006; **47**:86–97.

Bauer J, Kaufmann P, Elger CE *et al.* Similar postictal serum prolactin response in complex partial seizures of temporal or frontal lobe onset. *Arch Neurol* 1994; **51**:645.

Baumann CR, Werth E, Stocker R *et al.* Sleep-wake disturbances 6 months after traumatic brain injury: a prospective study. *Brain* 2007;**130**:1873–83.

Bautista RE, Ciampetti MZ. Expressive aprosody andamuia as a manifestation of right hemisphere seizures. *Epilepsia* 2003; **44**:466–7.

Baykan B, Matur Z, Gurses C *et al.* Typical absence seizures triggered by photosensitivity. *Epilepsia* 2005; **46**:159–63.

Bear DM. Temporal lobe epilepsy: a syndrome of sensory-limbic hyperconnection. *Cortex* 1979; **15**:357–69.

Bear DM, Fedio P. Qualitative analysis of interictal behavior in temporal lobe epilepsy. *Arch Neurol* 1977; **34**:454–67.

Bear DM, Levin K, Blumer D *et al.* Interictal behavior in hospitalized temporal lobe epileptics: relationship to idiopathic psychiatric syndromes. *J Neurol Neurosurg Psychiatry* 1982; **45**:481–8.

Beard AW. The association of hepatolenticular degeneration with schizophrenia. *Acta Psychiatr Neurol Scand* 1959; **34**:411–28.

Bebin EM, Gomez ER. Prognosis in Sturge–Weber disease: comparison of unihemispheric and bihemispheric involvement. *J Child Neurology* 1988; **3**:181–4.

Beetar JT, Guilmette TJ, Sparadeo FR. Sleep and pain complaints in symptomatic traumatic brain injury and neurologic populations. *Arch Phys Med Rehabil* 1996; **77**:1288–302.

Belafsky MA, Carwille S, Miller P *et al.* Prolonged epileptic twilight states: continuous recordings with nasopharyngeal electrodes and videotape analysis. *Neurology* 1978; **28**:239–45.

Beling CC, Martland HS. A case of tumor of the corpus callosum and frontal lobes. *J Nerv Ment Dis* 1919; **50**:425–32.

Bell DS. The experimental reproduction of amphetamine psychosis. *Arch Gen Psychiatry* 1973; **29**:35–40.

Bell WL, Harmes J, Logue P *et al*. Neologistic speech automatisms during complex partial seizures. *Neurology* 1990; **40**:49–52.

Bell WL, Walczak TS, Shin C *et al*. Painful generalized clonic and tonic seizures with retained consciousness. *J Neurol Neurosurg Psychiatry* 1997; **63**:792–5.

Benbadis SR, Kotagal P, Klem GH. Unilateral blinking: a lateralizing sign in partial seizures. *Neurology* 1996; **46**:45–8.

Benton CS, de Silva R, Rutledge SL *et al*. Molecular and genetic studies in SCA-7 define a broad clinical spectrum and the infantile phenotype. *Neurology* 1998; **51**:1081–6.

Bercel NA, Travis LE, Olinger LB *et al*. Model psychoses induced by LSD-25 in normals. I. Psychophysiological investigations, with special reference to the mechanism of the paranoid reaction. *Arch Neurol Psychiatry* 1956; **75**:588–611.

Beresford OD, Graham AM. Chorea gravidarum. *J Obs Gynecol Br Emp* 1950; **57**:616–25.

Berger JR, Ros DB. Reversible Parkinson syndrome complicating postoperative hypoparathyroidism. *Neurology* 1981; **31**:81–2.

Bergeron C, Pollanen MS, Weyer L *et al*. Unusual clinical presentation of cortical-basal ganglionic degeneration. *Ann Neurol* 1996; **40**:893–900.

van den Bergh MW, van der Schaaf I, van Gijn J. The spectrum of presentations of venous infarction caused by deep cerebral vein thrombosis. *Neurology* 2005; **65**:192–6.

Berkovic SF. Andermann F, Melanson D *et al*. Hypothalamic hamartomas and associated ictal laughter: evolution of the characteristic epileptic syndrome and diagnostic value of magnetic resonance imaging. *Ann Neurol* 1988; **23**:429–39.

Berkovic SF, Andermann F, Olivier A *et al*. Hippocampal sclerosis in temporal lobe epilepsy demonstrated by magnetic resonance imaging. *Ann Neurol* 1991; **29**:175–82.

Berkovic SF, Izzillo P, McMahon JM *et al*. LGI1 mutations in temporal lobe epilepsy. *Neurology* 2004a; **62**:1115–19.

Berkovic SF, Serratosa JM, Phillips HA *et al*. Familial partial epilepsy with variable foci: clinical features and linkage to chromosome 22q12. *Epilepsia* 2004b; **45**:1054–60.

Bertina RM, Koelman BPC, Rosendall FR *et al*. Mutation in the blood coagulation factor factor V associated with resistance to protein C. *Nature* 1994; **369**:64–7.

Betting LE, Mory SB, Lopes-Cendes I *et al*. EEG features in idiopathic generalized epilepsy: clues to diagnosis. *Epilepsia* 2006; **47**:523–8.

Betts TA, Smith WT, Kelly RE. Adult metachromatic leukodystrophy (sulphatide lipidosis) simulating schizophrenia. *Neurology* 1968a; **18**:1140–2.

Betts TA, Kalra PL, Cooper R *et al*. Epileptic fits as a possible side-effect of amitriptyline. *Lancet* 1968b; **1**:390–2.

Beydoun A, Uthman BM, Kugler AR *et al*. Safety and efficacy of two pregabalin regimens for add-on treatment of epilepsy. *Neurology* 2005; **64**:475–80.

Beydoun A, Sackellares JC, Shu V *et al*. Safety and efficacy of divalproex sodium monotherapy in partial epilepsy: a double-blind, concentration–response design clinical trial. *Neurology* 1997; **48**:182–8.

Beydoun A, Sachdeo R, Rosenfeld WE *et al*. Oxcarbazepine monotherapy for partial-onset seizures: a multicenter, double-blind, clinical trial. *Neurology* 2000; **54**:2245–51.

Bicknell JN, Moore RA. Psychological meaning of disulfiram (Antabuse) therapy. *Arch Gen Psychiatry* 1960; **2**:661–8.

Bien CG, Benniger FO, Urbach H *et al*. Localizing value of epileptic visual auras. *Brain* 2000; **123**:244–53.

Bien CG, Widman G, Urbach H *et al*. The natural history of Rasmussen's encephalitis. *Brain* 2002; **125**:1751–9.

Binnie LD, Debets RMC, Engelsman M *et al*. Double-blind crossover trial of lamotrigene (Lamictal) as add-on therapy in intractable epilepsy. *Epilepsia Res* 1989; **4**:222–9.

Binzer M, Kullgren G. Motor conversion disorder. A prospective 2- to 5-year follow-up study. *Psychosomatics* 1998; **39**:519–27.

Binzer M, Andersen PM, Kullgren G. Clinical characteristics of patients with motor disability due to conversion disorder: a prospective control group study. *J Neurol Neurosurg Psychiatry* 1997; **63**: 83–8.

Biton V, Montouris GD, Ritter F *et al*. A randomized, placebo-controlled study of topiramate in primary generalized tonic-clonic seizures. *Neurology* 1999; **52**:1330–7.

Biton V, Sackellares JC, Vuong A *et al*. Double-blind, placebo-controlled study of lamotriginein primary generalized tonic-clonic seizures. *Neurology* 2005; **65**:1737–43.

Bleuler E. *Textbook of psychiatry*, 1924. New York: Arno Press, 1976.

Blinkenberg M, Rune K, Jonsson A *et al*. Cerebral metabolism in a case of multiple sclerosis with acute mental disorder. *Acta Neurol Scand* 1996; **94**:310–13.

Blum AS, Drislane FW. Nonconvulsive status epilepticus in thrombotic thrombocytopenic purpura. *Neurology* 1996; **47**:1079–81.

Blume WT, Jones DC, Young GB *et al*. Seizures involving secondary sensory and related areas. *Brain* 1992; **115**:1509–20.

Blumer D. Hypersexual episodes in temporal lobe epilepsy. *Am J Psychiatry* 1970; **126**:1099–106.

Blumer D, Walker AE. Sexual behavior in temporal lobe epilepsy. *Arch Neurol* 1967; **16**:37–43.

Boas J, Dam M, Friis ML *et al*. Controlled trial of lamotrigene (Lamictal) for treatment-resistant partial seizures. *Acta Neurol Scand* 1996; **54**:247–52.

Boggs J, Preis K. Successful initiation of combined therapy with valproate sodium injection and divalproex sodium extended-release tablets in the epilepsy monitoring unit. *Epilepsia* 2000; **46**:940–51.

Bogousslavsky J, Regli F, Uske A. Thalamic infarcts: clinical syndromes, etiology, and prognosis. *Neurology* 1988; **38**:837–48.

Bogousslavsky J, Martin R, Regli F *et al*. Persistent worsening of stroke sequelae after delayed seizures. *Arch Neurol Psychiatry* 1992; **49**:385–8.

Bohman M, Cloninger CR, von Knorring AL *et al*. An adoption study of somatoform disorders. III. Cross-fostering analysis and genetic relationship to alcoholism and criminality. *Arch Gen Psychiatry* 1984; **41**:872–8.

Boller F, Wright DG, Cavalieri R *et al.* Paroxysmal 'nightmares': sequel of a stroke responsive to diphenylhydantoin. *Neurology* 1975; **25**:1026–8.

Bolt JMW. Huntington's disease in the West of Scotland. *Br J Psychiatry* 1970; **116**:259–70.

Bombardier CH, Fann JR, Temkin N *et al.* Posttraumatic stress disorder symptoms during the first six months after traumatic brain injury. *J Neuropsychiatry Clin Neurosci* 2006; **18**:501–8.

Boon PA, Williamson PD, Fried I *et al.* Partial seizures: an anatomoclinical, neuropsychological, and surgical correlation. *Epilepsia* 1991; **32**:467–76.

Borchert CD, Labar DR. Permanent hemiparesis due to partial status epilepticus. *Neurology* 1995; **45**:187–8.

Bornstein M, Coddon D, Song S. Prolonged alterations in behavior associated with a continuous electroencephalographic (spike and dome) abnormality. *Neurology* 1956; **6**:444.

Boudreau EA, Liow K, Frattali CM *et al.* Hypothalamic hamartomas and seizures: distinct natural history of isolated and Pallister-Hall syndrome cases. *Epilepsia* 2005; **46**:42–7.

Bousser M-G, Chiras J, Bories J *et al.* Cerebral venous thrombosis: a review of 38 cases. *Stroke* 1985; **16**:199–213.

Bouton SM. Pick's disease. *J Nerv Ment Dis* 1940; **91**:9–30.

Brady KT, Lydiard RB, Malcolm R *et al.* Cocaine-induced psychosis. *J Clin Psychiatry* 1991; **52**:509–12.

Bray GA, Dahms WT, Swerdhoff RS *et al.* The Prader–Willi syndrome: a study of 40 patients and a review of the literature. *Medicine* 1983; **62**:59–88.

Breningstall GN. Gelastic seizures, precocious puberty, and hypothalamic hamartoma. *Neurology* 1985; **35**:1180–3.

Brennan LV, Craddock PR. Limbic encephalopathy as a non-metastatic complication of oat cell lung cancer: its reversal after treatment of the primary lung lesion. *Am J Med* 1983; **75**:518–20.

Brey RL, Holliday SL, Saklad AR *et al.* Neuropsychiatric syndromes in lupus. Prevalence using standardized definitions. *Neurology* 2002; **58**:1214–20.

Brick JF, Gutrecht JA, Ringel RA. Reflex epilepsy and non-ketotic hyperglycemia in the elderly. *Neurology* 1989; **39**:394–9.

Briellman RS, Kalnins RM, Hopwood MJ *et al.* TLE patients with postictal psychosis: mesial dysplasia and anterior hippocampal preservation. *Neurology* 2000; **55**:1027–30.

Briellmann RS, Berkovic SF, Syngeniotis A *et al.* Seizure-associated hippocampal volume loss: a longitudinal magnetic resonance study of temporal lobe epilepsy. *Ann Neurol* 2002; **51**:641–4.

Britton JW, Ghearing GR, Benarroch EE *et al.* The ictal bradycardia syndrome: localization and lateralization. *Epilepsia* 2006; **47**:374–84.

Bridgman O, Smyth FS. Progressive lenticular degeneration. *J Nerv Ment Dis* 1944; **99**:534–43.

Brodie MJ, Richens A, Yuen AW. Double-blind comparison of lamotrigene and carbamazepine in newly diagnosed epilepsy. *Lancet* 1995; **345**:476–9.

Brodie MJ, Perucca E, Ryvlin P *et al.* Comparison of levetiracetam and controlled-release carbamazepine in newly diagnosed epilepsy. *Neurology* 2007; **68**:402–8.

Brodtkorb E, Nilsn G, Smevik O *et al.* Epilepsy and anomalies of neuronal migration: MRI and clinical aspects. *Acta Neurol Scand* 1992; **86**:24–32.

Brodtkorb E, Gu W, Nakken KO *et al.* Familial temporal lobe epilepsy with aphasic seizures and linkage to chromosome 10q22–q24. *Epilepsia* 2002; **43**:228–35.

Brodtkorb E, Michler RP, Gu W *et al.* Speech-induced aphasic seizures in epilepsy caused by *LGI1* mutations. *Epilepsia* 2005; **46**:963–6.

Brooke MM, Patterson DR, Questad KA *et al.* The treatment of agitation during initial hospitalization after traumatic brain injury. *Arch Phys Med Rehabil* 1992; **73**:917–21.

Brooks N, Campsie L, Symington C *et al.* The five year outcome of severe blunt head injury: a relative's view. *J Neurol Neurosurg Psychiatry* 1986; **49**:764–70.

Brown P, Rodgers-Johnson P, Cathala F *et al.* Creutzfeldt–Jakob disease of long duration: clinicopathological characteristics, biotransmissability, and differential diagnosis. *Ann Neurol* 1984; **16**:295–304.

Brown P, Cathala F, Castaigne P *et al.* Creutzfeldt–Jakob disease: clinical analysis of a consecutive series of 230 neuropathologically verified cases. *Ann Neurol* 1986; **20**:597–602.

Brown P, Gibbs CJ, Rodgers-Johnson P *et al.* Human spongiform encephalopathy: the National Institutes of Health series of 300 cases of experimentally transmitted disease. *Ann Neurol* 1994; **35**:513–29.

Browne TR, Kugler AR, Eldon MA. Pharmacology and pharmacokinetics of fosphenytoin. *Neurology* 1996; **46**(suppl. 1):3–7.

Brugger P, Agosti R, Regard M *et al.* Heautoscopy, epilepsy and suicide. *J Neurol Neurosurg Psychiatry* 1994; **57**:838–9.

Brun A, Englund B, Gustafson L *et al.* Clinical and neuropathological criteria for frontotemporal dementia. *J Neurol Neurosurg Psychiatry* 1994; **57**:416–18.

Bruton CJ. *The neuropathology of temporal lobe epilepsy.* Oxford: Oxford University Press, 1988.

Buckley P, Stack JP, Madigan C *et al.* Magnetic resonance imaging of schizophrenia-like psychoses associated with cerebral trauma: clinicopathological correlates. *Am J Psychiatry* 1993; **150**:146–8.

Bulrich N, Cooper DA, Freed A. HIV infection associated with symptoms indistinguishable from functional psychosis. *Br J Psychiatry* 1988; **152**:649–53.

Burks JS, Alfrey AC, Huddlestone J *et al.* A fatal encephalopathy in chronic hemodialysis patients. *Lancet* 1976; **1**:764–8.

Bursten B. Psychoses associated with thyrotoxicosis. *Arch Gen Psychiatry* 1961; **4**:267–73.

Butler CR, Graham KS, Hodges JR *et al.* The syndrome of transient epileptic amnesia. *Ann Neurol* 2007; **61**:587–98.

Byelsjo I, Forsgren L, Lithner F *et al.* Epidemiology and clinical characteristics of seizures in patients with acute intermittent porphyria. *Epilepsia* 1996; **37**:230–5.

Caine ED, Shoulson I. Psychiatric syndromes in Huntington's disease. *Am J Psychiatry* 1983; **140**:728–33.

Callaghan N, Kenny RA, O'Neill B *et al.* A prospective study between carbamazepine, phenytoin and sodium valproate in previously untreated and recently diagnosed patients with epilepsy. *J Neurol Neurosurg Psychiatry* 1985; **48**:639–44.

Callaghan N, Garrett A, Goggin T. Withdrawal of anticonvulsant drugs in patients free of seizures for two years. A prospective study. *N Engl J Med* 1988; **318**:942–6.

Cameron MM. Chronic subdural hematoma: a review of 114 cases. *J Neurol Neurosurg Psychiatry* 1978; **41**:834–9.

von Campe G, Regli F, Bogousslavsky J. Heralding manifestations of vascular artery occlusion with lethal or severe stroke. *J Neurol Neurosurg Psychiatry* 2003; **74**:1621–6.

Campbell AMG, Corner B, Norman RM *et al.* The rigid form of Huntington's disease. *J Neurol Neurosurg Psychiatry* 1961; **24**:71–7.

Cantu C, Barinagarrementeria F. Cerebral venous thrombosis associated with pregnancy and puerperium. Review of 67 cases. *Stroke* 1993; **24**:1880–4.

Cape CA, Martinez AJ, Robertson JT *et al.* Adult onset of subacute sclerosing panencephalitis. *Arch Neurol* 1973; **28**:124–7.

Caplan LR. Positional cerebral ischemia. *J Neurol Neurosurg Psychiatry* 1976; **39**:385–91.

Caplan LR. Occlusion of the vertebral or basilar artery. *Stroke* 1979; **10**:272–82.

Caplan LR. Intracerebral hemorrhage revisited. *Neurology* 1988; **38**:624–7.

Caplan LR. Intracranial branch atheromatous disease. *Neurology* 1989; **39**:1246–50.

Caplan LR, Hier DB, D'Cruz I. Cerebral embolism in the Michael Reese Stroke Registry. *Stroke* 1983; **14**:530–6.

Caplan LR, Kelly M, Kase CS *et al.* Infarcts of the inferior division of the right middle cerebral artery. *Neurology* 1986; **36**:1015–20.

Caplan LR, Schmahmann JD, Kase CS *et al.* Caudate infarcts. *Arch Neurol* 1990; **47**:133–43.

Cardoso TAM, Coan AC, Kobayashi E *et al.* Hippocampal abnormalities and seizure recurrence after antiepileptic drug withdrawal. *Neurology* 2006; **67**:134–6.

Carlson C, St. Louis EK. Vacuum cleaner epilepsy. *Neurology* 2004; **63**:190–1.

Carney MW, Chary TK, Robotis P *et al.* Ganser syndrome and its management. *Br J Psychiatry* 1987; **151**:697–700.

Cascino GD, Andermann F, Berkovic SF *et al.* Gelastic seizures and hypothalamic hamartomas. *Neurology* 1993a; **43**:747–50.

Cascino GD, Luckstein RR, Sharbrough FW *et al.* Facial asymmetry, hippocampal pathology, and remote symptomatic seizures. *Neurology* 1993b; **43**:725–7.

Cascino GD, Hulihan JF, Sharbrough FW *et al.* Parietal lobe lesional epilepsy: electroclinical correlation and operative outcome. *Epilepsia* 1993c; **34**:522–7.

Castaigne P, Lhermitte F, Gautier J *et al.* Arterial occlusion in the vertebral-basilar system. *Brain* 1973; **96**:133–54.

Castriotta RJ, Lai JM. Sleep disorders associated with traumatic brain injury. *Arch Phys Med Rehabil* 2001; **82**:1403–6.

Castro LH, Ferreira LK, Teles LR *et al.* Epilepsy syndromes associated with hypothalamic hamartomas. *Seizure* 2007;**16**:505–8.

Catella-Lawson F, Reilly MP, Kapoor SC *et al.* Cyclooxygenase inhibitors and the antiplatelet effects of aspirin. *N Engl J Med* 2001; **345**:1809–17.

Cavalleri F, De Renzi E. Amyotrophic lateral sclerosis with dementia. *Acta Neurol Scand* 1994; **89**:391–4.

Caveness WF. Epilepsy, a product of trauma in our time. *Epilepsia* 1976; **17**:207–15.

Celesia GG, Barr AN. Psychosis and other psychiatric manifestations of levodopa therapy. *Arch Neurol* 1970; **23**:193–200.

Cendes F, Andermann F, Gloor P *et al.* Atrophy of medial structures in patients with temporal lobe epilepsy: cause or consequence of repeated seizures? *Ann Neurol* 1993a; **34**:795–801.

Cendes F, Andermann F, Dubeau F *et al.* Early childhood prolonged febrile convulsions, atrophy and sclerosis of medial structures, and temporal lobe epilepsy: an MRI volumetric study. *Neurology* 1993b; **43**:1083–7.

Cendes F, Andermann F, Carpenter S *et al.* Temporal lobe epilepsy caused by domoic acid intoxication: evidence for glutamate receptor-mediated excitotoxicity in humans. *Ann Neurol* 1995; **37**:123–6.

Cereghino JJ, Biton V, Abou-Khalil B *et al.* Levetiracetam for partial seizures: results of a double-blind, randomized clinical trial. *Neurology* 2000; **55**:236–42.

Chalela JA, Kidwell CS, Nentwich LM *et al.* Magnetic resonance imaging and computed tomography in emergency assessment of patients with suspected acute stroke: a prospective comparison. *Lancet* 2007; **369**:293–8.

Chandler JH, Bebin J. Hereditary cerebellar ataxia: olivopontocerebellar type. *Neurology* 1956; **6**:187–95.

Chandler MC, Barnhill JL, Gualtieri CT. Amantadine for the agitated head-injury patient. *Brain Inj* 1988; **2**:309–11.

Chapman RWG, Laidlow JM, Colin-Jones D *et al.* Increased prevalence of epilepsy in coeliac disease. *BMJ* 1978; **2**:250–1.

Charles JR. Manganese toxaemia, with special reference to the effects of liver feeding. *Brain* 1927; **50**:30–43.

Chassagnon S, Minotti L, Kremer S *et al.* Restricted frontomesial epileptogenic focus generates dyskinetic behavior and laughter. *Epilepsia* 2003; **44**:859–63.

Chatham-Showalter PE. Carbamazepine for combativeness in acute traumatic brain injury. *J Neuropsychiatry Clin Neurosci* 1996; **8**:96–9.

Chatham-Showalter PE, Kimmel DN. Agitated symptom response to divalproex following acute brain injury. *J Neuropsychiatry Clin Neurosci* 2000; **12**:395–7.

Chaturvedi S, Bruno A, Feasby T *et al.* Carotid endarterectomy – an evidence-based review. *Neurology* 2005; **65**:794–801.

Chaudhuri A, Kennedy PG. Diagnosis and treatment of viral encephalitis. *Postgrad Med J* 2002; **78**:575–83.

Chen R-C, Forster FM. Cursive epilepsy and gelastic epilepsy. *Neurology* 1973; **23**:1019–29.

Chen ZM, Sandercock P, Pan HC *et al.* Indications for early aspirin use in acute ischemic stroke: a combined analysis of 40 000 randomized patients from the Chinese acute stroke trial and the international stroke trial. *Stroke* 2000; **31**:1240–9.

Chesson AL, Kasarkis EJ, Small VW. Postictal elevation of serum creatine kinase level. *Arch Neurol* 1983; **40**:315–17.

Chester EM, Agamanolis DP, Banker BQ *et al.* Hypertensive encephalopathy: a clinicopathologic study of 20 cases. *Neurology* 1978; **28**:928–39.

Chopra HD, Beatson JA. Psychotic symptoms in borderline personality disorder. *Am J Psychiatry* 1986; **143**:1605-7.

Chouinard G, Jones BD. Neuroleptic-induced supersensitivity psychosis. *Am J Psychiatry* 1980; **137**:16-21.

Cittandi E, Goadsby PJ. Psychiatric side effects during methysergide treatment. *J Neurol Neurosurg Psychiatry* 2005; **76**:1037-8.

Chiu D, Shedden P, Bratina P *et al.* Clinical features of Moyamaya disease in the United States. *Stroke* 1998; **29**:1347-51.

Clarke DJ. Prader–Willi syndrome and psychoses. *Br J Psychiatry* 1993; **163**:680-4.

Clarke E, Melnick SC. The Munchausen syndrome or the problem of hospital hoboes. *Am J Med* 1958; **25**:6-12.

Classen J, Peery S, Kreiter KT *et al.* Predictors and clinical import of epilepsy after subarachnoid hemorrhage. *Neurology* 2003; **60**:208-14.

Cleghorn RA. Adrenal cortical insufficiency: psychological and neurological observations. *CMAJ* 1951; **65**:445-57.

Clomipramine Collaborative Study Group. Clomipramine in the treatment of patients with obsessive-compulsive disorder. *Arch Gen Psychiatry* 1991; **48**:730-8.

Coats J. A study of two illustrative cases of epilepsy. *BMJ* **1876**:647-9.

Cockerell OC, Walker MC, Sander JWAS *et al.* Complex partial status epilepticus: a recurrent problem. *J Neurol Neurosurg Psychiatry* 1994; **57**:835-7.

Cockerell OC, Tothwell J, Marsden CD *et al.* Clinical and physiological features of epilepsia partialis continua: cases ascertained in the UK. *Brain* 1996; **116**:393-407.

Cohen RJ, Suter C. Hysterical seizures: suggestion as a provocative EEG test. *Ann Neurol* 1982; **11**:391-5.

Cole AJ, Gloor P, Kaplan R. Transient global amnesia: the electroencephalogram at onset. *Ann Neurol* 1987; **22**:721-2.

Cole F, Yates, P. Intracerebral microaneurysms and small cerebrovascular lesions. *Brain* 1967; **90**:759-68.

Combi R, Dalpra L, Ferini-Strambi L *et al.* Frontal lobe epilepsy and mutations of the corticotropin-releasing hormone gene. *Ann Neurol* 2005; **58**:899-904.

Commission of Classification and Terminology of the International League Against Epilepsy. *Epilepsia* 1981; **22**:489-501.

Commission of Classification and Terminology of the International League Against Epilepsy. *Epilepsia* 1989; **30**:389-99.

Corrigan JD. Substance abuse as a mediating factor in outcome from traumatic brain injury. *Arch Phys Med Rehabil 1995*; **76**:302-9.

Corsellis JAN, Golberg GJ, Norton AR. 'Limbic encephalitis' and its association with carcinoma. *Brain* 1968; **91**:481-96.

Critchley M. The anterior cerebral artery, and its syndromes. *Brain* 1930; **53**:120-65.

Critchley M, Early CJC. Tuberose sclerosis and allied conditions. *Brain* 1932; **55**:311-46.

Critchley M. Musicogenic epilepsy. *Brain* 1937; **60**:13-27.

Critchley M. Two cases of musicogenic epilepsy. *J Royal Navy Med Serv* 1942; **27**:182-4.

Critchley M, Greenfield JG. Olivo-ponto-cerebellar atrophy. *Brain* 1948; **71**:343-64.

Critchley M, Cobb W, Sears TA. On reading epilepsy. *Epilepsia* 1959; **1**:403-17.

Crompton M. Hypothalamic lesions following closed head injury. *Brain* 1971; **94**:165-72.

Currie S, Heathfield KWG, Henson RA *et al.* Clinical course and prognosis of temporal lobe epilepsy: a survey. *Brain* 1971; **97**:173-90.

Currier RD, Little SC, Suess SJ *et al.* Sexual seizures. *Arch Neurol* 1971; **25**:260-4.

D'Agostino MD, Bernasconi A, Das S *et al.* Subcortical band heterotopia (SBH) in males: clinical, imaging and genetic findings in comparison with females. *Brain* 2002; **125**:2507-22.

Daly D. Ictal affect. *Am J Psychiatry* 1958; **115**:97-108.

Daly DD, Barry MJ. Musicogenic epilepsy: report of three cases. *Psychosom Med* 1957; **19**:399-408.

Dam AM, Fuglsang-Fredricksen A, Svarre-Olsen U *et al.* Late-onset epilepsy: etiologies, types of seizure, and value of clinical investigation, EEG and computerized tomography scan. *Epilepsia* 1985; **26**:227-31.

Dana-Haeri J, Richens A. Effect of norethisterone on seizures associated with menstruation. *Epilepsia* 1983; **24**:377-81.

Dana-Haeri J, Trimble MR, Oxley J. Prolactin and gonadotropin changes following generalized and partial seizures. *J Neurol Neurosurg Psychiatry* 1983; **46**:331.

Danek A, Rubio JP, Rampoldi L *et al.* McLeod neuroacanthocytosis: genotype and phenotype. *Ann Neurol* 2001; **50**:755-64.

Daniel WG, Mugge A. Transesophageal echocardiography. *N Engl J Med* 1995; **332**:1268-79.

Daniele O, Mattaliano A, Tassinari CA *et al.* Epileptic seizures and cerebrovascular disease. *Acta Neurol Scand* 1989; **80**:117-22.

Danielsson S, Gillberg C, Billstedt E *et al.* Epilepsy in young adults with autism: a prospective population-based follow-up study of 120 individuals diagnosed in childhood. *Epilepsia* 2005;**46**:918-23.

Davidson J. Seizures and bupropion: a review. *J Clin Psychiatry* 1989; **50**:256-61.

DeGiorgio CM, Tomiyasu U, Gott PS, *et al.* Hippocampal pyramidal cell loss in human status epilepticus. *Epilepsia* 1992;**33**:23-7.

DeGiorgio CM, Correale JD, Gott PS *et al.* Serum neuron-specific enolase in human status epilepticus. *Neurology* 1995; **45**:1134-7.

DeGiorgio CM, Heck CN, Rabinowicz AL *et al.* Serum neuron-specific enolase in the major subtypes of status epilepticus. *Neurology* 1999; **52**:746-9.

Degos J-D, da Fonseca N, Gray F *et al.* Severe frontal syndrome associated with infarcts of the left anterior cingulate gyrus and the head of the right caudate nucleus. *Brain* 1993; **116**:1541-8.

Deisenhammer E. Transient global amnesia as an epileptic manifestation. *J Neurol* 1981; **225**:289-92.

Delgado-Escueta AV. Epileptogenic paroxysms: modern approaches and clinical correlations. *Neurology* 1979; **29**:1014-22.

Delgado-Escueta AV, Mattson RH, King L *et al.* The nature of aggression during epileptic seizures. *N Engl J Med* 1981; **305**:711-16.

Delgado-Escueta AV, Bascal FE, Treiman DM. Complex partial seizures on closed-circuit television and EEG: a study of 691 attacks in 79 patients. *Ann Neurol* 1982; **11**:292–300.

Denier C, Orgibct A, Foffi F *et al.* Adult-onset vanishing white matter leukoencephalopathy presenting as psychosis. *Neurology* 2007; **68**:1538–9.

Dening TR, Berrios GE. Wilson's disease: psychiatric symptoms in 195 cases. *Arch Gen Psychiatry* 1989; **46**:1126–34.

Dening TR, Berrios GE, Walshe JM. Wilson's disease and epilepsy. *Brain* 1988; **111**:1139–55.

Depondt C, Van Paesschen W, Matthijs G *et al.* Familial temporal lobe epilepsy with febrile seizures. *Neurology* 2002; **58**:1429–33.

van Der Naalt J, van Zomeren AH, Sluiter WJ *et al.* Acute behavioral disturbances related to imaging studies and outcome in mild-to-moderate head injury. *Brain Inj* 2000; **14**:781–8.

Dervaux A, Laine H, Czermak M *et al.* Creutzfeldt-Jakob disease presenting as psychosis. *Am J Psychiatry* 2004; **161**:1307–8.

Desbiens R, Berkovic S, Dubeau F *et al.* Life-threatening focal status epilepticus due to occult cortical dysplasia. *Arch Neurol* 1993; **50**:695–700.

Devinsky O, Duchowny MS. Seizures after convulsive therapy: a retrospective case series. *Neurology* 1983; **33**:921–5.

Devinsky O, Petito CK, Alonso DR. Clinical and neuropathological findings in systemic lupus erythematosus: the role of vasculitis, heart emboli and thrombotic thrombocytopenic purpura. *Ann Neurol* 1988a; **23**:380–4.

Devinsky O, Kelley K, Porter RJ *et al.* Clinical and electroencephalographic features of simple partial seizures. *Neurology* 1988b; **38**:1347–52.

Devinsky O, Felmann E, Burrowes K *et al.* Autoscopic phenomena with seizures. *Arch Neurol* 1989a; **46**:1080–8.

Devinsky O, Sato O, Kufta CV *et al.* Electroencephalographic studies of simple partial seizures with subdural electrode recordings. *Neurology* 1989b; **39**:527–33.

Devinsky O, Honigfield G, Patin J. Clozapine-related seizures. *Neurology* 1991; **41**:369–71.

Devinsky O, Kelley K, Yacubian EMT *et al.* Postictal behavior. *Arch Neurol* 1994a; **51**:254–9.

Devinsky O, Ehrenberg B, Barthlen GM *et al.* Epilepsy and sleep apnea syndrome. *Neurology* 1994b; **44**:2060–4.

Devinsky O, Sanchez-Villasenor F, Vazquez B *et al.* Clinical profile of patients with epileptic and nonepileptic seizures. *Neurology* 1996; **46**:1530–3.

Dewhurst K, Beard AW. Sudden religious conversions in temporal lobe epilepsy. *Br J Psychiatry* 1970; **117**:497–507.

Dewhurst K, Todd J. The psychosis of association – folie a deux. *J Nerv Ment Dis* 1956; **124**:451–9.

Dimitri D, Jehel L, Durr A *et al.* Fatal familial insomnia presenting as psychosis in an 18-year-old man. *Neurology* 2006; **67**:363–4.

Dixit S, Kurle P, Buyan-Dent L *et al.* Status epilepticus associated with cefipime. *Neurology* 2000; **54**:2153–5.

Donaire A, Carreno M, Gomez B *et al.* Cortical laminar necrosis related to prolonged focal status epilepticus. *J Neurol Neurosurg Psychiatry* 2006; **77**:104–6.

Drachman DA, Adams RD. Herpes simplex and acute inclusion-body encephalitis. *Arch Neurol* 1962; **7**:45–63.

Drury I, Klass DW, Westmoreland BF *et al.* An acute syndrome with psychiatric symptoms and EEG abnormalities. *Neurology* 1985; **35**:911–14.

D'Souza WJ, O'Brien TJ, Murphy M *et al.* Toothbrushing-induced epilepsy with structural lesions in the primary somatosensory area. *Neurology* 2007; **68**:769–71.

Dubeau F, Tampieri E, Carpenter S *et al.* Periventricular and subcortical nodular heterotopia: a study of 33 patients. *Brain* 1995; **118**:1273–87.

Duncalf CM, Kent JNG, Harbord M *et al.* Subacute sclerosing panencephalitis presenting as schizophreniform psychosis. *Br J Psychiatry* 1989; **155**:557–9.

Earnest MP, Feldman H, Marx JA *et al.* Intracranial lesions shown by CT scans in 259 cases of first alcohol-related seizures. *Neurology* 1988; **38**:1561–5.

Edwards OM, Clark JDA. Post-traumatic hypopituitarism: six cases and a review of the literature. *Medicine* 1986; **65**:281–90.

Efron R. The effect of olfactory stimuli in arresting uncinate fits. *Brain* 1956; **79**:267–81.

Efron R. The conditioned inhibition of uncinate fits. *Brain* 1957; **80**:251–62.

Efron R. Post-epileptic paralysis: theoretical critique and report of a case. *Brain* 1961; **84**:381–94.

Eisen JL, Rasmussen SA. Obsessive compulsive disorder with psychotic features. *J Clin Psychiatry* 1993; **54**:373–9.

Ellis JM, Lee SI. Acute prolonged confusion in later life as an ictal state. *Epilepsia* 1978; **19**:119–28.

Elger CE, Brodie MJ, Anhut H *et al.* Pregabalin add-on treatment in patients with partial seizures. A novel evaluation of flexible-dose and fixed-dose treatment in a double-blind, placebo-controlled study. *Epilepsia* 2005; **46**:1926–36.

Engel J. Surgery for seizures. *N Engl J Med* 1996; **334**:647–52.

Engel J, Driver MV, Falconer MA. Electrophysiological correlates of pathology and surgical results in temporal lobe epilepsy. *Brain* 1975; **98**:129–56.

Engel J, Ludwig BI, Fetele M. Prolonged partial complex status epilepticus: EEG and behavioral observations. *Neurology* 1978; **28**:863–9.

Englander J, Bushnik T, Duong TT *et al.* Analyzing risk factors for late posttraumatic seizures: a prospective, multicenter investigation. *Arch Phys Med Rehabil* 2003; **84**:365–73.

Eraut D. Idiopathic hypoparathyroidism presenting as dementia. *BMJ* 1974; **1**:429–30.

Erickson TC. Erotomania (nymphomania) as an expression of cortical epileptiform discharge. *Arch Neurol Psychiatry* 1945; **53**:226–31.

Espir ML, Rose FC. Alcohol, seizures and epilepsy. *J R Soc Med* 1987; **9**:542–3.

Escueta AV, Kunze U, Waddell G *et al.* Lapse of consciousness and automatisms in temporal lobe epilepsy: a videotape analysis. *Neurology* 1977; **27**:144–55.

Evans DL, Edelsohn GA, Golden RN. Organic psychosis without dementia or spinal cord symptoms in patients with vitamin B12 deficiency. *Am J Psychiatry* 1983; **140**:218–21.

Fahy TJ, Irving MJ, Millac P. Severe head injuries. A six-year follow-up. *Lancet* 1967; **2**:475–9.

Fairweather DS. Psychiatric aspects of the post-encephalitic syndrome. *J Ment Sci* 1947; **93**:201–54.

Fakhoury T, Abou-Khalil B, Peguero E. Differentiating clinical features of right and left temporal lobe seizures. *Epilepsia* 1994; **35**:1038–44.

Falconer MA. Clinical manifestations of temporal lobe epilepsy and their recognition in relation to surgical treatment. *BMJ* 1954; **2**:939–44.

Falconer MA. Genetic and related aetiological factors in temporal lobe epilepsy. *Epilepsia* 1971; **12**:13–31.

Falconer MA, Driver MV, Serafetinides EA. Seizures induced by movement: report of a case relieved by operation. *J Neurol Neurosurg Psychiatry* 1963; **26**:300–7.

Falconer MA, Serafetinides EA, Corsellis JAN. Etiology and pathogenesis of temporal lobe epilepsy. *Arch Neurol* 1964; **10**:233–48.

Fann JR, Uomoto JM, Katon WJ. Sertaline in the treatment of major depression following mild traumatic brain injury. *J Neuropsychiatry Clin Neurosci* 2000; **12**:226–32.

Fariello RG, Booker HE, Chun RWM *et al.* Reenactment of the triggering situation for the diagnosis of epilepsy. *Neurology* 1983; **33**:878–84.

Faught E, Wilder BJ, Famsay RE *et al.* Topiramate placebo-controlled dose-ranging trial in refractory partial epilepsy using 200-, 400-, and 600-mg daily dosages. *Neurology* 1996; **46**:1684–90.

Fauser S, Huppertz H-J, Bast T *et al.* Clinical characteristics in focal cortical dysplasia: a retrospective evaluation in a series of 120 patients. *Brain* 2006; **129**:1907–16.

Feinberg TE, Cianci CD, Morrow JS *et al.* Diagnostic tests for choreoacanthocytosis. *Neurology* 1991; **41**:1000–6.

Feinberg WM, Rapcsak SZ. 'Peduncular hallucinosis' following paramedian thalamic infarction. *Neurology* 1989; **39**:1535–6.

Feldman RG, White RF, Eriator II. Triethyltin encephalopathy. *Arch Neurol* 1993; **50**:1320–4.

Fenelon G, Mahieux F, Huon R *et al.* Hallucinations in Parkinson's disease: prevalence, phenomenology and risk factors. *Brain* 2000; **123**:733–45.

Fenton WS, McGlashen TH. Natural history of schizophrenia subtypes. I. Longitudinal study of paranoid, hebephrenic, and undifferentiated schizophrenia. *Arch Gen Psychiatry* 1991; **48**:969–77.

Fenwick PBC, Brown SW. Evoked and psychogenic seizures. *Acta Neurol Scand* 1989; **80**:535–40.

Fernandez-Torre JL, Martinez-Martinez M, Gonzalez-Rato J *et al.* Cephalosporin-induced nonconvulsive status epilepticus: clinical and electroencephalographic features. *Epilepsia* 2005; **46**:1550–2.

Ferriby D, de Seze J, Stojkovic T *et al.* Long-term follow-up of neurosarcoidosis. *Neurology* 2001; **57**:927–9.

Fichtenberg NL, Millis SR, Mann NR *et al.* Factors associated with insomnia among post-acute traumatic brain injury survivors. *Brain Inj* 2000; **14**:659–67.

Finelli PF. Metachromatic leukodystrophy manifesting as a schizophrenic disorder: computed tomographic correlation. *Ann Neurol* 1985; **18**:94–5.

Finelli PF, Pueschel SM, Padre-Mendoza T *et al.* Neurological findings in patients with the fragile-X syndrome. *J Neurol Neurosurg Psychiatry* 1985; **45**:150–63.

Fiol ME, Leppik IE, Pretzel K. Eating epilepsy: EEG and clinical study. *Epilepsia* 1986; **27**:441–5.

Fiorelli M, Di Piero V, Bastianello S *et al.* Cerebrotendinous xanthomatosis: clinical and MRI study (a case report). *J Neurol Neurosurg Psychiatry* 1990; **53**:76–8.

Fisher CM. Lacunes: small deep cerebral infarcts. *Neurology* 1965; **15**:774–84.

Fisher CM. Lacunar strokes and infarcts: a review. *Neurology* 1982; **32**:871–6.

Fisher CM, Ojemann R, Robertson G. Spontaneous dissection of cervico-cerebral arteries. *Can J Neurol Sci* 1978; **5**:9–19.

Flashman LA, McAllister TW. Lack of awareness and its impact in traumatic brain injury. *NeuroRehabilitation* 2002; **17**:285–96.

Flugel D, Cerlignani M, Symms MR *et al.* Diffusion tensor imaging findings and their correlation with neuropsychological deficits in patients with temporal lobe epilepsy and interictal psychosis. *Epilepsia* 2006; **47**:941–4.

Fontaine B, Seilhean D, Tourbah A *et al.* Dementia in two histologically confirmed cases of multiple sclerosis: one with isolated dementia and one case associated with psychiatric symptoms. *J Neurol Neurosurg Psychiatry* 1994; **57**:353–9.

Forster FM. Epilepsy associated with eating. *Trans Am Neurol Assn* 1971; **96**:106–7.

Forster FM. *Reflex epilepsy, behavioral therapy and conditioned reflexes.* IL: Springfield, Charles C. Thomas, 1977.

Forster FM, Liske E. Role of environmental clues in temporal lobe epilepsy. *Neurology* 1963; **13**:301–5.

Forster FM, Booker HE, Gascon G. Conditioning in musicogenic epilepsy. *Trans Am Neurol Assn* 1967; **92**:236–7.

Forster FM, Paulsen WA, Baughman FA. Clinical therapeutic conditioning in reading epilepsy. *Neurology* 1969a; **19**:717–23.

Forster FM, Hansotia P, Cleeland CS *et al.* A case of voice-induced epilepsy treated by conditioning. *Neurology* 1969b; **19**:325–31.

Fortemps E, Amand G, Bomboir A *et al.* Trimethyltin poisoning. Report of two cases. *Int Arch Occupat Environment Hlth* 1978; **41**:1–6.

Foster HG, Hillbrand M, Chi CC. Efficacy of carbamazepine in assaultive patients with frontal lobe dysfunction. *Prog Neuropsychopharmacol Biol Psychiatry* 1989; **13**:865–74.

Franceschi M, Triulzi F, Ferini-Strambi L *et al.* Focal cerebral lesions found by magnetic resonance imaging in cryptogenic nonrefractory temporal lobe epilepsy patients. *Epilepsia* 1989; **30**:540–6.

Francis A, Freeman H. Psychiatric abnormality and brain calcification over four generations. *J Nerv Ment Dis* 1984; **172**:166–70.

Frazier CH. Tumor involving the frontal lobe alone: a symptomatic survey of one hundred and five verified cases. *Arch Neurol Psychiatry* 1936; **35**:525–51.

Freemon FR, Nevis AH. Temporal lobe sexual seizures. *Neurology* 1969; **19**:87–90.

Fregni F, Otachi PTM, de Valle A *et al.* A randomized clinical trial of repetitive transcranial magnetic stimulation in patients with refractory epilepsy. *Ann Neurol* 2006; **60**:447–55.

French JA, Williamson PD, Thadani VM *et al.* Characteristics of medial temporal lobe epilepsy: I. Results of history and physical examination. *Ann Neurol* 1993; **34**:774–80.

Freytag E. Autopsy findings in head injuries from blunt forces: statistical evaluation of 1,367 cases. *Arch Pathol* 1963; **75**:402–13.

Friedlander WJ, Feinstein GH. Petit mal status: Epilepsia minoris continua. *Neurology* 1956; **6**:357–62.

Friedman A, Sienkiewicz J. Psychotic complications of long-term levodopa treatment of Parkinson's disease. *Acta Neurol Scand* 1991; **84**:111–13.

Friedman HM, Allen N. Chronic effects of complete limbic lobe destruction in man. *Neurology* 1969; **19**:679–90.

Fuerst D, Shah J, Shah A *et al.* Hippocampal sclerosis is a progressive disorder: a longitudinal volumetric MRI study. *Ann Neurol* 2003; **53**:413–16.

Fuerstein TJ, Sauerman W, Anhut H *et al.* Gabapentin (Neurontin) as add-on therapy in patients with partial seizures: a double-blind placebo-controlled study. *Epilepsia* 1994; **35**:795–801.

Fujii DE, Ahmed I. Risk factors in psychosis secondary to traumatic brain injury. *J Neuropsychiatry Clin Neurosci* 2001; **13**:61–9.

Fujii DE, Ahmed I. Characteristics of psychotic disorders due to traumatic brain injury: an analysis of case studies in the literature. *J Neuropsychiatry Clin Neurosci* 2002; **14**:130–40.

Fuster B, Castells C, Rodriguez B. Psychomotor attacks (primary automatisms) of subcortical origin. *Arch Neurol Psychiatry* 1954; **71**:455–72.

Gabr M, Luders H, Dinner D. Speech manifestations in lateralization of temporal lobe seizures. *Ann Neurol* 1989; **25**:82–7.

Gal P. Mental symptoms in cases of tumor of the temporal lobe. *Am J Psychiatry* 1958; **115**:157–60.

Gallagher BB, Flanigan HF, King DW *et al.* The effect of electrical stimulation of medial temporal lobe structures in epileptic patients upon ACTH, prolactin, and growth hormone. *Neurology* 1987; **37**:299–303.

Gallmetzer P, Leutezer F, Serles W *et al.* Postictal paresis in focal epilepsies: incidence, duration and causes. *Neurology* 2004; **62**:2160–4.

Gambardella A, Reutens DC, Andermann F *et al.* Late onset drop attacks in temporal lobe epilepsy. *Neurology* 1994; **44**:1074–8.

Gambardella A, Annesi G, De Fusco M *et al.* A new locus for autosomal dominant nocturnal frontal lobe epilepsy maps to chromosome 1. *Neurology* 2000; **55**:1467–71.

Garrett PJ, Mulcahy D, Carmody M *et al.* Aluminum encephalopathy: clinical and immunologic findings. *Q J Med* 1988; **69**:775–83.

Garron D. Huntington's chorea and schizophrenia. *Adv Neurol* 1973; **1**:729–34.

Gascon GG, Lombroso CT. Epileptic (gelastic) laughter. *Epilepsia* 1971; **12**:63–76.

Gastaut H. Clinical and electroencephalographic classification of epileptic seizures. *Epilepsia* 1970; **11**:102–13.

Gastaut H, Tassinari CA. Triggering mechanisms in epilepsy: the electroclinical point of view. *Epilepsia* 1966; **7**:85–138.

Gastaut H, Caveness WF, Landolt H *et al. Epilepsia* 1964; **5**:297–306.

Gastaut H, Gastaut JL, Goncalves E *et al.* Relative frequency of different types of epilepsy: a study employing the classification of the International League Against Epilepsy. *Epilepsia* 1975; **16**:457–61.

Gatzonis SD, Stamboulis E, Siafakis A. Acute psychosis and EEG normalization after vagus nerve stimulation. *J Neurol Neurosurg Psychiatry* 2000; **69**:278–9.

Gautier-Smith PC. Neurological complications of glandular fever (infectious mononucleosis). *Brain* 1965; **88**:323–34.

Geier S, Bancaud J, Talairach J *et al.* The seizures of frontal lobe epilepsy: a study of clinical manifestations. *Neurology* 1977; **27**:951–8.

Gelenberg AJ. Munchausen's syndrome with a psychiatric presentation. *Dis Nerv Syst* 1977; **38**:378–80.

Gelisse P, Genton P, Kuate C *et al.* Worsening of seizures by oxcarbazepine in juvenile idiopathic generalized epilepsies. *Epilepsia* 2004; **45**:1282–6.

Genton P, Gelisse P, Thomas P *et al.* Do carbamazepine and phenytoin aggravate juvenile myoclonic epilepsy? *Neurology* 2000; **55**:1106–9.

Geocaris K. Psychotic episodes heralding the diagnosis of multiple sclerosis. *Bull Men Clin* 1957; **21**:107–16.

Geyer JD, Payne TA, Drury I. The value of pelvic thrusting in the diagnosis of seizures and pseudoseizures. *Neurology* 2000; **54**:227–9.

Ghaffar O, Stains R, Feinstein A *et al.* Unexplained neurologic symptoms: an fMRI study of sensory conversion disorder. *Neurology* 2006; **67**:2036–8.

Giannopoulos S, Kostadima V, Selvi A, *et a.* Bilateral paramedian thalamic infarcts. *Arch Neurol* 2006; **63**:1652.

Gibbs FA, Gibbs EC. *Atlas of electroencephalography*, Vol. II. *Epilepsy.* London: Addison-Wesley, 1952.

van Gijn J, Rinkel GJ. Subarachnoid hemorrhage: diagnosis, causes and management. *Brain* 2001; **124**:249–78.

van Gijn J, van Dongen KJ, Vermeulen M *et al.* Perimesencephalic hemorrhage: a nonaneurysmal and benign form of subarachnoid hemorrhage. *Neurology* 1985; **35**:493–7.

Gillberg C. Outcome in autism and autistic-like conditions. *J Am Acad Child Adolesc Psychiatry* 1991; **30**:375–82.

Gillig P, Sackellares JC, Greenberg HS. Right hemisphere partial complex seizures: mania, hallucinations, and speech disturbances during ictal events. *Epilepsia* 1988; **29**:26–9.

Glaser GH, Levy LL. Seizures and idiopathic hypoparathyroidism. *Epilepsia* 1960; **4**:454–65.

Glass HC, Prieur B, Molnar C *et al.* Micturition and emotion-induced reflex epilepsy: case report and review of the literature. *Epilepsia* 2007; **47**:2180–2.

Glenn MB, Wroblewski B, Parziale J *et al.* Lithium carbonate for aggressive behavior or affective instability in ten brain-injured patients. *Am J Phys Med Rehabil* 1989; **68**:221–6.

Globus M, Lavi E, Fich E *et al*. Ictal hemiparesis. *Eur Neurol* 1982; **21**:165–8.

Gloor P. Electrophysiological studies of the amygdala (stimulation and recording): their possible contribution to the understanding of neural mechanisms of aggression. In: Fields WS, Sweet WH eds. *Neural bases of violence and aggression*. St Louis: C.V. Mosby, 1975.

Gobbi G, Bouquet F, Greco L *et al*. Coeliac disease, epilepsy, and cerebral calcification. *Lancet* 1992; **340**:439–43.

Gobin YP, Starkman S, Duckwiler GR *et al*. MERCI 1: a phase 1 study of Mechanical Embolus Removal in Cerebral Ischemia. *Stroke* 2004; **35**:2848–54.

Goetz CG, Fan W, Leurgans S *et al*. The malignant course of 'benign hallucinations' in Parkinson disease. *Arch Neurol* 2006; **63**:713–16.

Golden RN, James S, Sherer M *et al*. Psychoses associated with bupropion treatment. *Am J Psychiatry* 1985; **142**:1459–62.

Goldensohn ES, Gold AP. Prolonged behavioral disturbances as ictal phenomena. *Neurology* 1960; **10**:1–9.

Golding JM, Rost K, Kashner TM *et al*. Family psychiatric history of patients with somatization disorder. *Psychiatr Med* 1992; **10**:33–47.

Golub LM, Guhlman HV, Merlis JK. Seizure patterns in psychomotor epilepsy. *Dis Nerv Syst* 1951; **12**:73–6.

Goodin DS, Aminoff MJ, Laxer KD. Detection of epileptiform activity by different noninvasive EEG methods in complex partial epilepsy. *Ann Neurol* 1990; **27**:330–4.

Goodman L. Alzheimer's disease: a clinico-pathologic analysis of twenty-three cases with a theory on pathogenesis. *J Nerv Ment Dis* 1953; **118**:97–130.

Gordon A. Transition of obsessions into delusions. *Am J Psychiatry* 1950; **107**:455–8.

Gosk-Bierska I, Wysokinski W, Brown RD *et al*. Cerebral venous sinus thrombosis. Incidence of venous thrombosis recurrence and survival. *Neurology* 2006; **67**:814–19.

Gothelf D, Feinstein C, Thompson T *et al*. Risk factors for the emergence of psychotic disorders in adolescents with 22q11.2 deletion syndrome. *Am J Psychiatry* 2007; **164**:663–9.

Graff-Radford NR, Damasio H, Yamada T *et al*. Non-hemorrhagic thalamic infarction. *Brain* 1985; **108**:495–516.

Graham JM, Gruenwald RA, Sagar HJ. Hallucinosis in idiopathic Parkinson's disease. *J Neurol Neurosurg Psychiatry* 1997; **63**:434–40.

Granata T, Gobbi G, Spreafico R *et al*. Rasmussen's encephalitis. Early characteristics allow diagnosis. *Neurology* 2003; **60**:422–5.

Grant C, Warlow C. Focal epilepsy in diabetic non-ketotic hyperglycemia. *BMJ* 1985; **290**:1204–5.

Greenberg MK, Vance SC. Focal seizure disorder complicating iodophenylate myelography. *Lancet* 1980; **1**:312–13.

Greenberg SM, Vonsattel JPG, Stakes JW *et al*. The clinical spectrum of cerebral amyloid angiopathy: presentations without lobar hemorrhage. *Neurology* 1993; **43**:2073–9.

Greene KA, Marciano FF, Dickman CA *et al*. Anterior communicating aneurysm paraparesis syndrome: clinical manifestations and pathologic correlates. *Neurology* 1995; **45**:45–50.

Greer S, Parsons V. Schizophrenia-like psychosis in thyroid crisis. *Br J Psychiatry* 1968; **114**:1357–62.

Greeven A, van Balkom AJLM, Visser S *et al*. Cognitive behavioral therapy and paroxetin in the treatment of hypochodriasis: a randomized controlled trial. *Am J Psychiatry* 2007; **164**:91–9.

Grewal RP, Achari M, Matsuura T *et al*. Clinical features and ATTC repeat expansion in spinocerebellar ataxia type 10. *Arch Neurol* 2002; **59**:1285–90.

Griffith JD, Cavanaugh J, Held J *et al*. Dextroamphetamine: evaluation of psychotomimetic properties in man. *Arch Gen Psychiatry* 1972; **26**:97–100.

Grunberger G, Weiner JL, Silverman R *et al*. Factitious hypoglycemia due to surreptitious administration of insulin. Diagnosis, treatment, and long-term follow-up. *Ann Intern Med* 1988; **108**:252–7.

Grunewald R. Levetiracetam in the treatment of idiopathic generalized epilepsies. *Epilepsia* 2005; **46**(suppl. 9):154–60.

Guinena YH, Taher Y. Psychosensory seizures 'visual and auditory' of primary subcortical origin. *Electroencephalogr Clin Neurophysiol* 1955; **7**:425–8.

Gumpert J, Hansotia P, Upton A. Gelastic epilepsy. *J Neurol Neurosurg Psychiatry* 1970; **33**:479–83.

Gunderson JG, Kolb JE. Discriminating features of borderline patients. *Am J Psychiatry* 1978; **135**:792–6.

Gupta AK, Jeavons PM, Hughes RC *et al*. Aura in temporal lobe epilepsy: clinical and electroencephalographic correlation. *J Neurol Neurosurg Psychiatry* 1983; **46**:1079–83.

Gupta SR, Nasheedy MH, Elias D *et al*. Postinfarction seizures: a clinical study. *Stroke* 1988; **19**:1477–81.

Guze SB. Cloninger CR, Martin RL *et al*. A follow-up and family study of Briquet's syndrome. *Br J Psychiatry* 1986; **149**:17–23.

Gysin WM, Cooke ET. Unusual mental symptoms in a case of hepatolenticular degeneration. *Dis Nerv Syst* 1950; **28**:305–9.

Hacke W, Schwab S, Horn M *et al*. 'Malignant' middle cerebral artery territory infarction: clinical course and prognostic signs. *Arch Neurol* 1996; **53**:309–15.

Hagberg B, Aicardi J, Ramos O. A progressive syndrome of autism, ataxia, and loss of purposeful hand use in girls: Rett's syndrome: report of 35 cases. *Ann Neurol* 1983; **14**:471–9.

Hageman ATM, Gabreels FJM, de Jong JGN *et al*. Clinical symptoms of adult metachromatic leukodystrophy and arylsulfatase A pseudodeficiency. *Arch Neurol* 1995; **52**:408–13.

Hahn RD, Webster B, Weickhardt G *et al*. Penicillin treatment of general paresis (dementia paralytica). *Arch Neurol Psychiatry* 1959; **81**:557–90.

Halkes PH, van Gijn J, Kappelle LJ *et al*. Aspirin plus dipyridamole versus aspirin alone after cerebral ischaemia of arterial origin (ESPRIT): randomized controlled trial. *Lancet* 2006; **367**:1665–73.

Hall DE, Eubanks L, Meyyaxhagan LS *et al*. Evaluation of covert video surveillance in the diagnosis of Munchausen syndrome by proxy: lessons from 41 cases. *Pediatrics* 2000; **105**:1305–12.

Hall DP, Young SA. Frontal lobe cerebral aneurysm rupture presenting as psychosis. *J Neurol Neurosurg Psychiatry* 1992; **55**:1207–8.

Hall RCW, Joffe JR. Hypomagnesemia: physical and psychiatric symptoms. *JAMA* 1973; **224**:1749–51.

Haller E, Binder RL. Clozapine and seizures. *Am J Psychiatry* 1980; **147**:1069–71.

Haltia T, Palo J, Haltia M *et al.* Juvenile metachromatic dystrophy: clinical, biochemical, and neuropathologic studies in nine new cases. *Arch Neurol* 1980; **37**:42–5.

Hammes EM. Psychoses associated with Sydenham's chorea. *J Am Med Assoc* 1922; **79**:804–7.

Handforth A, DeGiorgio CM, Schacter SC *et al.* Vagus nerve stimulation therapy for partial-onset seizures: a randomized active-control trial. *Neurology* 1998; **51**:48–55.

Hanson PA, Chodos R. Hemiparetic seizures. *Neurology* 1978; **28**:920–3.

Hardie RJ, Pullon HWH, Harding AE *et al.* Neuroacanthocytosis: a clinical, haematological and pathological study of 19 cases. *Brain* 1991; **114**:13–49.

Harlow JM. Passage of an iron rod through the head. *Bost Med Surg J* 1848; **39**:389–93.

Harlow JM. Recovery from passage of an iron bar through the head. *J Mass Med Soc* 1868; **2**:327–47.

Harris MJ, Jeste DV, Gleghorn A *et al.* New-onset psychosis in HIV-infected patients. *J Clin Psychiatry* 1991; **52**:369–76.

Harrison RA, Vu T, Hunter AJ. Wernicke's encephalopathy in a patient with schizophrenia. *J Gen Int Med* 2006; **21**:1338.

Hauser WA, Morris ML, Hewston LL *et al.* Seizures and myoclonus in patients with Alzheimer's disease. *Neurology* 1986; **36**:1226–30.

Haymaker W. Herpes simplex encephalitis in man. *J Neuropathol Exp Neurol* 1949; **8**:132–54.

Hayman M, Scheffer IE, Chinvarun Y *et al.* Autosomal dominant nocturnal frontal lobe epilepsy: demonstration of focal frontal onset and intrafamilial variation. *Neurology* 1997; **49**:969–75.

Healton EB, Brust JC, Feinfeld DA *et al.* Hypertensive encephalopathy and the neurologic manifestations of malignant hypertension. *Neurology* 1982; **32**:127.

Heathfield KWG. Huntington's chorea. Investigation into the prevalence of this disease in the area covered by the North East Metropolitan Regional Hospital Board. *Brain* 1967; **90**:203–32.

Hedera P, Abou-Khalil B, Cronk AE *et al.* Autosomal dominant lateral temporal epilepsy: two families with novel mutations in the *LGI1* gene. *Epilepsia* 2004; **45**:218–22.

Heilman KM, Howell GJ. Seizure-induced neglect. *J Neurol Neurosurg Psychiatry* 1980; **43**:1035–40.

Heinsius T, Bogousslavsky J, van Melle G. Large infarcts in the middle cerebral artery territory. Etiology and outcome patterns. *Neurology* 1998; **50**:341–50.

Helgason C, Caplan LR, Goodwin J *et al.* Anterior choroidal artery territory infarction. *Arch Neurol* 1986; **43**:681–6.

Heller AJ, Chesterman P, Elwes RDC *et al.* Phenobarbitone, phenytoin, carbamazepine, or sodium valproate for newly diagnosed adult epilepsy: a randomized comparative monotherapy trial. *J Neurol Neurosurg Psychiatry* 1995; **58**:44–50.

Henchey R, Cibula J, Helveston W *et al.* Electroencephalographic findings in Hashimoto's encephalopathy. *Neurology* 1995; **45**:977–81.

Hennerici M, Klemm C, Rautenberg W. The subclavian steal phenomenon: a common vascular disorder with rare neurologic deficits. *Neurology* 1988; **38**:669–73.

Hennis A, Corbin D, Fraser H. Focal seizures and non-ketotic hyperglycemia. *J Neurol Neurosurg Psychiatry* 1992; **55**:195–7.

Henriksen GF. Status epilepticus partialis with fear as clinical expression: report of a case and EEG findings. *Epilepsia* 1973; **14**:39–46.

Henry TR, Drury I, Brunberg JA *et al.* Focal cerebral magnetic resonance changes associated with partial status epilepticus. *Epilepsia* 1994; **35**:35–41.

Hermann BP, Riel P. Interictal personality and behavioral traits in temporal lobe and generalized epilepsy. *Cortex* 1981; **17**:125–8.

Hermann BP, Whitman S, Wyler AR *et al.* The neurological, psychosocial and demographic correlates of hypergraphia in patients with epilepsy. *J Neurol Neurosurg Psychiatry* 1988; **51**:203–8.

Herskowitz A, Swerdlow M. Focal seizures – a false lateralizing sign. *Dis Nerv Syst* 1972; **33**:523–5.

Hertz PE, Nadas E, Wojtkowski H. Case report: Cushing's syndrome and its management. *Am J Psychiatry* 1955; **112**:144–5.

Heutink P, Stevens M, Rizzu P *et al.* Hereditary frontotemporal dementia is linked to chromosome 17q21–q22: a genetic and clinicopathological study of three Dutch families. *Ann Neurol* 1997; **41**:150–9.

Hibbard MR, Uysal S, Kepler K *et al.* Axis I psychopathology in individuals with traumatic brain injury. *J Head Trauma Rehabil* 1998; **13**:24–39.

Hier DB, Mondlock J, Caplan LR. Behavioral abnormalities after right hemisphere stroke. *Neurology* 1983; **33**:337–44.

Hijdra A, Van Gijn J, Stefanko S *et al.* Delayed cerebral ischemia after aneurysmal subarachnoid hemorrhage: clinico-anatomic correlations. *Neurology* 1986; **36**:329–33.

Hijdra A, van Gijn J, Nagelkerke NJD *et al.* Prediction of delayed cerebral ischemia, rebleeding and outcome after aneurismal subarachnoid hemorrhage. *Stroke* 1988; **19**:1250–6.

Hildebrand J, Lecaille C, Perennes J *et al.* Epileptic seizures during follow-up of patients treated for primary brain tumor. *Neurology* 2005; **65**:212–15.

Hillbom E. Schizophrenia-like psychoses after brain trauma. *Acta Psychiatr Neurol Scand* 1951(suppl. 60):36–47.

Hillier SL, Sharpe MH, Metzer J. Outcomes 5 years post-traumatic brain injury (with further reference to neurophysical impairment and disability). *Brain Inj* 1997; **11**:661–75.

Hinchey J, Chaves C, Appignani B *et al.* A reversible posterior leukoencephalopathy syndrome. *N Engl J Med* 1996; **334**:494–500.

Hirose S, Iwata H, Akiyoshi H *et al.* A novel mutation of *CHRNA4* responsible for autosomal dominant nocturnal frontal lobe epilepsy. *Neurology* 1999; **53**:1749–53.

Hirsch E, Marescaux C, Maquet P *et al.* Landau-Kleffner syndrome: a clinical and EEG study of five cases. *Epilepsia* 1990; **31**:756–67.

Hirsch S, Dunsworth FA. An interesting case of porphyria. *Am J Psychiatry* 1955; **111**:703.

Hjort N, Christensen S, Solling C et al. Ischemic injury detected by diffusion imaging in 11 minutes. Ann Neurol 2005; 58:462–5.

Ho SS, Berkovic SF, Newton MR et al. Parietal lobe epilepsy: clinical features and seizure localization by SPECT. Neurology 1994; 44:2277–84.

Hodgson RE, Murray D, Woods MR. Othello's syndrome and hyperthyroidism. J Nerv Ment Dis 1992; 180:663–4.

Hoefer PFA, Guttman SA, Sands IJ. Convulsive states and coma in cases of islet cell carcinoma of the pancreas. Am J Psychiatry 1946; 102:486–95.

Holmes G. Local epilepsy. Lancet 7 May 1927; 957–73.

Holmes GL. The electroencephalogram as a predictor of seizures following cerebral infarction. Clin Electroencephalogr 1980; 11:83–6.

Holmes GL. Partial complex seizures in children: an analysis of 69 seizures in 24 patients using EEG FM radiotelemetry and videotape recordings. Electroencephalogr Clin Neurophysiol 1984; 57:13–20.

Holmes GL, McKeever M, Adamson M. Absence seizures in children: clinical and electroencephalographic features. Ann Neurol 1987; 21:268–73.

Hoover CF. A new sign for detection of malingering and functional paresis of the lower extremities. J Am Med Assoc 1908; 51:1309–10.

Hopkins A, Shorvon S, Cascino G. Epilepsy, 2nd edn. London: Arnold 1995.

van der Horst L. Affective epilepsy. J Neurol Neurosurg Psychiatry 1953; 16:25–9.

Hudson EA, Munoz DG, Miller L et al. Amygdaloid sclerosis in temporal lobe epilepsy. Ann Neurol 1993; 33:622–31.

Hunter R, Blackwood W, Bull J. Three cases of frontal meningiomas presenting psychiatrically. BMJ 1968; 3:9–16.

Hyde TM, Ziegler JL, Weinberger DR. Psychiatric disturbances in metachromatic leukodystrophy: insights into the neurobiology of psychosis. Arch Neurol 1992; 49:401–6.

Inanatomia Y, Kimura K, Yonehara T et al. DWI abnormalities and clinical characteristics in TIA patients. Neurology 2004; 62:376–80.

Ingham SD, Nielsen JM. Thyroid psychosis: difficulties in diagnosis. J Nerv Ment Dis 1931; 74:271–7.

Insel TR, Akiskal HS. Obsessive-compulsive disorder with psychotic features: a phenomenologic analysis. Am J Psychiatry 1986; 143:1527–33.

International Subarachnoid Aneurysm Trial (ISAT) Collaborative Group. International subarachnoid aneurysm trial (ISAT) on neurosurgical clipping versus endovascular coiling in 2143 patients with ruptured intracranial aneurysm: a randomized trial. Lancet 2002; 360:1267–74.

Inzelberg R, Kipervasser S, Korczyn AD. Auditory hallucinations in Parkinson's disease. J Neurol Neurosurg Psychiatry 1998; 64:533–5.

Iranzo A, Santamaria J, Berenguer J et al. Prevalence and clinical importance of sleep apnea in the first night after cerebral infarction. Neurology 2002; 58:911–16.

Ironside R, Bosanquet FD, McMenemy WH. Central demyelination of the corpus callosum (Marchifava–Bignami disease): with report of a second case in Great Britian. Brain 1961; 84:212–30.

Isbell H, Fraser HF, Wickler A et al. An experimental study of etiology of 'rum fits' and delirium tremens. Q J Study Alcohol 1955; 16:1–33.

Ivanov D, Kirov G, Norton N et al. Chromosome 22q11 deletions, velo-cardio-facial syndrome and early onset psychosis. Br J Psychiatry 2003;183:409–13.

Iwanami A, Sugiyama A, Kuroki N et al. Patients with methamphetamine psychosis admitted to a psychiatric hospital in Japan. Acta Psychiatr Scand 1994; 89:428–32.

Jabbari B, Huott AD. Seizures in thyrotoxicosis. Epilepsia 1980; 21:91–6.

Jabbari B, Bryan GE, Marsh EE et al. Incidence of seizures with tricyclic and tetracyclic antidepressants. Arch Neurol 1985; 42:480–1.

Jackel RA, Malkowitz D, Trivedi R et al. Reduction of prolactin response with repetitive seizures. Epilepsia 1987; 28:588.

Jackson GD, Kuzniecky RI, Cascino GD. Hippocampal sclerosis without detectable hippocampal atrophy. Neurology 1994; 44:42–6.

Jackson JA, Zimmerman SL. A case of pseudosclerosis associated with a psychosis. J Nerv Ment Dis 1919; 49:5–13.

Jackson JH. On a particular variety of epilepsy ('intellectual aura'). One case with symptoms of organic brain disease. Brain 1889; 11:179–207.

Jackson JH. Neurological fragments. Lancet 1894; 2:182–3.

Jackson JH, Beevor CE. Case of tumour of the right temporo-sphenoidal lobe bearing on the localization of the sense of smell and on the interpretation of a particular variety of epilepsy. Brain 1890; 12:346–57.

Jackson JH, Colman WJ. Case of epilepsy with tasting movements and 'dreamy state' – very small patch of softening in the left uncinate gyrus. Brain 1898; 21:580–91.

Jackson JH, Stewart P. Epileptic attacks with a warning of a crude sensation of smell and with the intellectual aura (dreamy state) in a patient who had symptoms pointing to gross organic disease of the right temporo-sphenoidal lobe. Brain 1899; 22:534–49.

Jacob A, Cherian PJ, Radhakrishnan K et al. Emotional facial paresis in temporal lobe epilepsy: its prevalence and lateralizing value. Seizure 2003; 12:60–4.

Jacome DE, Risko M. Pseudocataplexy: gelastic–atonic seizures. Neurology 1984; 34:1381–3.

Jacome DE, McLain W, Fitzgerald R. Postural reflex gelastic seizures. Arch Neurol 1980; 37:249–51.

Jaffe R. Ictal behavior as the only manifestation of seizure disorder: case report. J Nerv Ment Dis 1962; 134:470–6.

James WE, Mefferd RB, Kimbell I. Early signs of Huntington's chorea. Dis Nerv Syst 1969; 30:550–9.

Janszky J, Fogarai A, Magalova V et al. Unilateral hand automatisms in temporal lobe epilepsy. Seizure 2005; 15:393–6.

Jawad S, Richens A, Goodwin G et al. Controlled trial of lamotrigene (Lamictal) for refractory partial seizures. Epilepsia 1989; 30:356–63.

Jenkins CD, Mellins RB. Lead poisoning in children: a study of forty-six cases. Arch Neurol Psychiatry 1957; 77:70–8.

Jenkins A, Teasdale G, Hadley MD *et al.* Brain lesions detected by magnetic resonance imaging in mild and severe head injuries. *Lancet* 1986; **2**:445–6.

Jennett B. Early traumatic epilepsy. *Arch Neurol* 1973; **30**:394–8.

Jennett B. Epilepsy and acute traumatic intracranial haematoma. *J Neurol Neurosurg Psychiatry* 1975; **38**:378–81.

Jennett B, Teather D, Bennie S. Epilepsy after head injury. *Lancet* 1973; **2**:652–3.

Jensen I, Klinken L. Temporal lobe epilepsy and neuropathology. *Acta Neurol Scand* 1976; **54**:391–414.

Jensen MB, St. Louis EK. Management of acute cerebellar stroke. *Arch Neurol* 2005; **62**:537–44.

Johnson KP, Rosenthal MS, Lerner PI. Herpes simplex encephalitis. *Arch Neurol* 1972; **27**:103–8.

Johnson RI, Richardson EP. The neurological manifestations of systemic lupus erythematosus. *Medicine* 1968; **47**:337–69.

Johnston JA, Lineberry CG, Archer JA *et al.* A 102–center prospective study of seizure in association with bupropion. *J Clin Psychiatry* 1991; **52**:450–6.

Jorge RE, Robinson RG, Arndt SV *et al.* Comparison between acute-and delayed-onset depression following traumatic brain injury. *J Neuropsychiatry Clin Neurosci* 1993; **5**:43–9.

Jorge RE, Robinson RG, Moser D *et al.* Major depression following traumatic brain injury. *Arch Gen Psychiatry* 2004; **61**:42–50.

Joynt J, Green D, Gren R. Musicogenic epilepsy. *JAMA* 1962; **179**:501–4.

Kaiboriboon K, Parent JM, Barbaro NM *et al.* Speech preservation during language-dominant, left temporal lobe seizures: report of a rare, potentially misleading finding. *Epilepsia* 2006; **47**:1343–6.

Kaiko RF, Foley KM, Grabinski PY *et al.* Central nervous system excitatory effects of meperidine in cancer patients. *Ann Neurol* 1983; **13**:180–5.

Kalinowsky LB. Convulsions in nonepileptic patients on withdrawal of barbiturates, alcohol and other drugs. *Arch Neurol Psychiatry* 1942; **48**:946–56.

Kanemoto K. Periictal Capgras syndrome after clustered ictal fear: depth-electroencephalogram study. *Epilepsia* 1997; **38**:847–50.

Kanemoto K, Janz D. The temporal sequence of aura-sensations in patients with complex partial focal seizures with particular attention to ictal aphasia. *J Neurol Neurosurg Psychiatry* 1989; **52**:52–6.

Kanemoto K, Watanabe Y, Tsuji T *et al.* Rub epilepsy: a somatosensory evoked reflex epilepsy induced by prolonged cutaneous stimulation. *J Neurol Neurosurg Psychiatry* 2001; **70**:541–3.

Kang D-W, Lattimore SU, Latour LL *et al.* Silent ischemic lesion recurrence on magnetic resonance imaging predicts subsequent clinical vascular events. *Arch Neurol* 2006; **63**:1730–3.

Kanner AM, Morris HH, Dinner DS *et al.* Supplementary motor seizures mimicking pseudoseizures: some clinical differences. *Neurology* 1990; **40**:1404–7.

Kanner AM, Stagno S, Kotagal P *et al.* Postictal psychiatric events during prolonged video-electroencephalographic monitoring studies. *Arch Neurol* 1996; **53**:258–63.

Kant R, Duffy JD, Pivovarnik A. Prevalence of apathy following head injury. *Brain Inj* 1998; **12**:87–92.

Karnosh LJ, Stout RE. Psychoses of myxedema. *Am J Psychiatry* 1935; **91**:1263–74.

Karp BI, Laureno R. Pontine and extrapontine myelinolysis: a neurologic disorder following rapid correction of hyponatremia. *Medicine* 1993; **72**:359–73.

Kashiwase H, Kato M. *Folie a deux* in Japan – analysis of 97 cases in the Japanese literature. *Acta Psychiatr Scand* 1997; **96**:231–4.

Katz DI, Alexander MP, Seliger GM *et al.* Traumatic basal ganglia hemorrhage: clinicopathologic features and outcome. *Neurology* 1989; **39**:862–3.

Kazui S, Naritomi H, Yamamoto H *et al.* Enlargement of spontaneous intracerebral hemorrhage: incidence and time course. *Stroke* 1996; **27**:1983–7.

Keane JR. Wrong-way deviation of the tongue with hysterical hemiparesis. *Neurology* 1986; **36**:1406–7.

Kellinghaus C, Kotagal P. Lateralizing value of Todd's palsy in patients with epilepsy. *Neurology* 2004; **62**:289–91.

Kendler KS. The nosological validity of paranoia (simple delusional disorder): a review. *Arch Gen Psychiatry* 1980; **37**:699–706.

Kendler KS, McGuire M, Gruenberg AM *et al.* Outcome and family study of the subtypes of schizophrenia in the West of Ireland. *Am J Psychiatry* 1994; **151**:849–56.

Kennedy F. The symptomatology of temporosphenoidal tumors. *Arch Int Med* 1911; **8**:317–50.

Kennedy PGE. A retrospective analysis of forty-six cases of herpes simplex encephalitis seen in Glasgow between1962 and 1985. *Q J Med* 1988; **68**:533–40.

Keschner M, Bender MB, Strauss I. Mental symptoms in cases of tumor of the temporal lobe. *Arch Neurol Psychiatry* 1936; **35**:572–96.

Khatri P, Kasner SE. Ischemic strokes after cardiac catheterization. Opportune thrombolysis candidates? *Arch Neurol* 2006; **63**:817–21.

Kilpatrick CJ, Davis SM, Tress BM *et al.* Epileptic seizures in acute stroke. *Arch Neurol* 1990; **47**:157–60.

Kilpatrick CJ, Davis SM, Hopper JL *et al.* Early seizures after acute stroke: risk of late seizures. *Arch Neurol* 1992; **49**:509–11.

Kim JS. Pure lateral medullary infarction: clinical-radiological correlation of 130 acute, consecutive patients. *Brain* 2003; **126**:1864–72.

Kim JS, Kim HG, Chung CS. Medial medullary syndrome: report of 18 new patients and a review of the literature. *Stroke* 1995; **26**:1548–52.

King DW, Marsan CA. Clinical features and ictal patterns in epileptic patients with EEG temporal lobe foci. *Ann Neurol* 1977; **2**:138–47.

King MA, Newton MR, Jackson GD *et al.* Epileptology of the first seizure presentation: a clinical, electroencephalographic, and magnetic resonance imaging study of 300 consecutive patients. *Lancet* 1999; **352**:1007–11.

Kiok MC, Terrence CF, Fromm GH *et al.* Sinus arrest in epilepsy. *Neurology* 1986; **36**:115–16.

Kirby GH, Davis TK. Psychiatric manifestations of epidemic encephalitis. *Arch Neurol Psychiatry* 1921; **5**:491–555.

Kirubakaren V, Mayfield D, Rengachary S. Dyskinesia and psychosis in a patient following Baclofen withdrawal. *Am J Psychiatry* 1984; **141**:692–3.

Kluge M, Beyenburg S, Fernandez G *et al.* Epileptic vertigo: evidence for vestibular representation in human frontal cortex. *Neurology* 2000; **55**:1906–8.

Knight RT, Cooper J. Status epilepticus manifesting as reversible Wernicke's aphasia. *Epilepsia* 1986; **27**:301–4.

Kobayashi E, Li LM, Lopes-Cendes I *et al.* Magnetic resonance imaging evidence of hippocampal sclerosis in asymptomatic, first-degree relatives of patients with familial mesial temporal lobe epilepsy. *Arch Neurol* 2002; **59**:1891–4.

Kobayashi E, D'Agostino MD, Lopes-Cendes I *et al.* Hippocampal atrophy an T2-weighted signal changes in familial mesial temporal lobe epilepsy. *Neurology* 2003; **60**:405–9.

Kober D, Gabbard GO. Topiramate-induced psychosis. *Am J Psychiatry* 2005; **162**:1542.

Koehler K, Jakumeit U. Subacute sclerosing panencephalitis presenting as Leonhard's speech-prompt catatonia. *Br J Psychiatry* 1976; **129**:29–31.

Koepp MJ, Edwards M, Collins J *et al.* Status epilepticus and tiagabine therapy revisited. *Epilepsia* 2005; **46**:1625–32.

Koeppen AH, Barron KD. Marchiafava-Bignami disease. *Neurology* 1978; **28**:290–4.

Koerner M, Laxer KD. Ictal speech, postictal language dysfunction, and seizure lateralization. *Neurology* 1988; **38**:634–6.

Kofman O, Hyland HH. Tuberous sclerosis in adults with normal intelligence. *Arch Neurol Psychiatry* 1959; **81**:557–90.

Korczyn AD, Bechar M. Convulsive fits in thyrotoxicosis. *Epilepsia* 1976; **17**:33–4.

Korf BR, Carrazana E, Holmes GL. Patterns of seizures observed in association with neurofibromatosis. I. *Epilepsia* 1993; **34**:616–20.

Kornberg AJ, Harvery AS, Shield LK. Subacute sclerosing panencephalitis presenting as simple partial seizures. *J Child Neurol* 1991; **6**:146–9.

Koskiniemi M, Rantalaiho T, Piiparinen H *et al.* Infections of the central nervous system of suspected viral origin: a collaborative study from Finland. *J Neurovirol* 2001; **7**:400–8.

Kossoff EH, Bergey GK, Freeman JM *et al.* Levetiracetam psychosis in children with epilepsy. *Epilepsia* 2001; **42**:1611–13.

Kotagal P, Luders H, Morris HH *et al.* Dystonic posturing in complex partial seizures of temporal lobe onset: a new lateralizing sign. *Neurology* 1989; **39**:196–204.

Kothare SV, VanLandingham K, Armon C *et al.* Seizure onset from periventricular nodular heterotopias: depth-electrode study. *Neurology* 1998; **51**:1723–7.

Kotsopoulos IAW, van Merode T, Kessels FGH *et al.* Systematic review and meta-analysis of incidence studies of epilepsy and unprovoked seizures. *Epilepsia* 2002; **43**:1402–9.

Koutroumaniois M, Koepp MJ, Richardson MP *et al.* The variants of reading epilepsy: a clinical and video-EEG study of 17 patients with reading-induced seizures. *Brain* 1998; **121**:1409–27.

Kraepelin E. *Clinical psychiatry* 1902. Delmar, NY: Scholar's Facsimiles and Reprints, 1981.

Krahn LE, Li H, O'Connor MK. Patients who strive to be ill: factitious disorder with physical symptoms. *Am J Psychiatry* 2003; **160**:1163–8.

Kral T, Clusman H, Blumcke I *et al.* Outcome of epilepsy surgery in focal cortical dysplasia. *J Neurol Neurosurg Psychiatry* 2003; **74**:183–8.

Kramer DL, Awad IA. Vascular malformations and epilepsy: clinical considerations and basic mechanisms. *Epilepsia* 1994; **35**(suppl. 6):30–43.

Kramer RE, Lesser RP, Weinstein MR *et al.* Transient focal abnormalities of neuroimaging studies during focal status epilepticus. *Epilepsia* 1987; **28**:528–32.

Kramer RE, Luders H, Goldstick LP *et al.* Ictus emeticus: an electroclinical study. *Neurology* 1988; **38**:1048–52.

Kreutzer JS, Seel RT, Gourley E. The prevalence and symptom rates of depression after traumatic brain injury: a comprehensive examination. *Brain Inj* 2001; **15**:561–2.

Kristensen O, Sindrup EH. Psychomotor epilepsy and psychosis. III: Social and psychological correlates. *Acta Neurol Scand* 1979; **59**:1–9.

Krolak-Salmon P, Montanont A, Hermier A *et al.* Thalamic venous infarction as a cause of subacute dementia. *Neurology* 2006; **58**:1689–91.

Kroll P. Psychoses associated with marijuana abuse in Thailand. *J Nerv Ment Dis* 1975; **161**:149–56.

Krumholz A, Niedermeyer E. Psychogenic seizures: a clinical study with follow-up data. *Neurology* 1983; **33**:498–502.

Krumholz A, Stern BJ, Weiss HD. Outcome from coma after cardiopulmonary resuscitation: relation to seizures and myoclonus. *Neurology* 1988; **38**:401–5.

Krumholz A, Stern BJ, Stern EG. Clinical implications of seizures in neurosarcoidosis. *Arch Neurol* 1991; **48**:842–4.

Krumholz A, Sung GY, Fisher RS *et al.* Complex partial status epilepticus accompanied by serious morbidity and mortality. *Neurology* 1995; **45**:1499–504.

Kulkantrakorn K, Geller TJ. Seizures in neurofibromatosis. 1. *Pediatr Neurology* 1998; **19**:347–50.

Kumral E, Ozdemirkiran T, Alper Y. Strokes in the subinsular territory. Clinical, topographical, and etiological patterns. *Neurology* 2004; **63**:2429–32.

Kuramochi H, Takahashi R. Psychopathology of LSD intoxication: study of experimental psychosis induced by LSD-25: description of LSD symptoms in normal Oriental subjects. *Arch Gen Psychiatry* 1964; **11**:151–61.

Kuzniecky R, Guthrei B, Mountz J *et al.* Intrinsic epileptogenesis of hypothalamic hamartomas in gelastic epilepsy. *Ann Neurol* 1997; **42**:60–7.

Labar DR, Solomon GR, Wells CR. Aphasia as the sole manifestation of simple partial status epilepticus. *Epilepsia* 1992; **33**:84–7.

Labovitz DL, Hauser WA, Sacco RL. Prevalence and predictors of early seizure and status epilepticus after first stroke. *Neurology* 2001; **57**:200–6.

Lai F, Williams RS. A prospective study of Alzheimer's disease in Down syndrome. *Arch Neurol* 1989; **46**:849–53.

Lambert MT. Paranoid psychoses after abuse of proprietary cold remedies. *Br J Psychiatry* 1987; **151**:548–50.

Lamy C, Domigo V, Semah F et al. Early and late seizures after cryptogenic stroke in young adults. Neurology 2003;60:400–4.

Lancman ME, Craven WJ, Asconape JJ et al. Clinical management of recurrent postictal psychosis. J Epilepsy 1994; 7:47–51.

Landau WM, Kleffner FR. Syndrome of acquired aphasia with convulsive disorder in children. Neurology 1957; 7:523–30.

Landolt H. Some clinical electroencephalographic correlations in epileptic psychoses (twilight states). Electroencephalogr Clin Neurophysiol 1953; 5:121.

Landolt H. Serial electroencephalographic investigations during psychotic episodes in epileptic patients and during schizophrenic attacks. In: de Haas AML ed. Lectures on epilepsy. London: Elsevier, 1958.

Lang AE, Koller WC, Fahn S. Psychogenic parkinsonism. Arch Neurol 1995; 52:802–10.

Langworthy OR, Kolb LC, Androp S. Disturbances of behavior in patients with disseminated sclerosis. Am J Psychiatry 1941; 98:243–9.

Lankford DA, Wellman JJ, O'Hara C. Posttraumatic narcolepsy in mild to moderate closed head injury. Sleep 1994; 17(suppl. 8):S25–S28.

Lansberg Mg, Albers GW, Beaulieu C et al. Comparison of diffusion-weighted MRI and CT in acute stroke. Neurology 2000; 54:1557–61.

Lanska DJ. Anthrax meningoencephalitis. Neurology 2002; 59:327–34.

Lawson JA, Birchansky S, Pacheo E et al. Distinct clinicopathologic subtypes of cortical dysplasia of Taylor. Neurology 2005; 64:55–61.

Laxer KD, Mullooly JP, Howell B. Prolactin changes after seizures classified by EEG monitoring. Neurology 1985; 35:31–5.

Leal AJR, Moreira A, Robalo C et al. Different electroclinical manifestations of the epilepsy associated with hamartomas connecting to the middle or posterior hypothalamus. Epilepsia 2003; 44:1191–5.

Lebensohn ZM. Self-inflicted bullet wound of frontal lobes in a depression with recovery. Am J Psychiatry 1941; 48:56–62.

Lechtenberg R, Worner TM. Total ethanol consumption as a seizure risk factor in alcoholics. Acta Neurol Scand 1992; 85:90–4.

Lederman RJ, Henry CE. Progressive dialysis encephalopathy. Ann Neurol 1978; 4:199–204.

Lee H, Lerner A. Transient inhibitory seizures mimicking crescendo transient ischemic attacks. Neurology 1990; 40:165–6.

Lee H, Kim SW, Kim JM et al. Comparing effects of methyphenidate, sertraline and placebo on neuropsychiatric sequelae in patients with traumatic brain injury. Hum Psychopharmacol 2005; 20:97–104.

Lee VH, Brown RD, Madrekar JN et al. Incidence and outcome of cervical artery dissection. Neurology 2006; 67:1809–12.

Legg NJ, Gupta PC, Scott DF. Epilepsy following cerebral abscess. A clinical and EEG study of 70 patients. Brain 1973; 96:259–68.

Lehtinen L, Kivalo A. Laughter epilepsy. Acta Neurol Scand 1965; 41:255–61.

Lempert T, Bauer M, Schmidt D. Syncope: a videometric analysis of 56 episodes of transient cerebral hypoxia. Ann Neurol 1994; 36:233–7.

Lende RA, Popp AJ. Sensory Jacksonian seizures. J Neurosurg 1976; 44:706–11.

Leone M, Bottacchi E, Beghi E et al. Alcohol use is a risk factor for a first generalized tonic-clonic seizure. Neurology 1997; 48:614–20.

Leppik IE, Biton V, Sander JWA et al. Levetiracetam and partial seizure subtypes: pooled data from three randomized, placebo-controlled trials. Epilepsia 2003; 44:1585–7.

Lesser RP, Lueders H, Conomy JP et al. Sensory seizure mimicking a psychogenic seizure. Neurology 1983; 33:800–2.

Leutmezer F, Serles W, Bacher J et al. Genital automatisms in complex partial seizures. Neurology 1999; 52:1188–91.

Leutmezer F, Podreka I, Asenbaum S et al. Postictal psychosis in temporal lobe epilepsy. Epilepsia 2003; 44:582–90.

Levin HS, Grossman RG, Kelly PJ. Aphasic disorder in patients with closed head injury. J Neurol Neurosurg Psychiatry 1976; 39:1062–70.

Levin HS, Grossman RG, Rose JE et al. Long-term neuropsychological outcome of closed head injury. J Neurosurg 1979; 50:412–22.

Levin HS, Goldstein FC, High WM et al. Disproportionately severe memory deficit in relation to normal intellectual functioning after closed head injury. J Neurol Neurosurg Psychiatry 1988; 51:1294–301.

Levy AB. Delirium and seizures due to abrupt alprazolam withdrawal: case report. J Clin Psychiatry 1984; 45:38–9.

Libman MD, Potvin L, Coupal L et al. Seizure v. syncope: measuring serum creatine kinase in the emergency department. J Gen Intern Med 1991; 6:408–12.

Lichenstein BW. Sturge–Weber–Dimitri syndrome: cephalic form of neurocutaneous hemangiomatosus. Arch Neurol Psychiatry 1954; 71:291–301.

Liddell DW. Observations on epileptic automatisms in a mental hospital population. J Ment Sci 1953; 99:732–48.

Lieb JP, Walsh JO, Babb TL et al. A comparison of EEG seizure patterns with surface and depth electrodes in patients with temporal lobe epilepsy. Epilepsia 1976; 17:137–60.

Lim J, Yagnik P, Schraeder P et al. Ictal catatonia as a manifestation of nonconvulsive status epilepticus. J Neurol Neurosurg Psychiatry 1986; 49:833–6.

Lim L, Ron MA, Omerod IEC et al. Psychiatric and neurological manifestations in systemic lupus erythematosus. Q J Med 1988; 66:27–38.

Lima MA, Drislane FW, Kuralnik IJ. Seizures and their outcome in progressive multifocal leukoencephalopathy. Neurology 2006; 66:262–4.

Limdi Na, Knowlton RK, Cofield SS et al. Safety of rapid intravenous loading of valproate. Epilepsia 2007; 48:478–83.

Lin J T-Y, Ziegler DK. Psychiatric symptoms with initiation of carbidopa-levodopa treatment. Neurology 1976; 26:699–700.

Lindenbaum J, Healton EB, Savage DG et al. Neuropsychiatric disorders caused by cobalamin deficiency in the absence of anemia or macrocytosis. N Engl J Med 1988; 318:1720–8.

Lipinski CG. Epilepsies with astatic seizures of late onset. Epilepsia 1977; 18:13–20.

Lipsey JD, Robinson RG, Pearlson GD et al. Nortriptyline treatment of post-stroke depression: a double-blind study. Lancet 1984; 1:297–300.

Lishman WA. Brain damage in relation to psychiatric disability after head injury. Br J Psychiatry 1968; 114:373–410.

Lishman WA. The psychiatric sequelae of head injury: a review. Psychol Med 1973; 3:304–18.

List CF, Dowman CE, Bagchi BK et al. Posterior hypothalamic hamartomas and gangliogliomas causing precocious puberty. Neurology 1958; 8:164–74.

Litovitz TL, Troutman WG. Amoxapine overdose: seizures and fatalities. JAMA 1983; 250:1069–71.

Litvan IL, Agid Y, Sastrj N et al. What are the obstacles to the accurate clinical diagnosis of Pick's disease? Neurology 1997; 49:62–9.

Liu RSN, Lemieux L, Bell GS et al. The structural consequences of newly diagnosed seizures. Ann Neurol 2002; 52:573–80.

Livingston S, Torres I, Pauli L et al. Petit mal epilepsy. Results of a prolonged follow-up of 117 patients. JAMA 1965; 194:227–32.

Locke J, Merrill JP, Tyler HR. Neurologic complications of uremia. Arch Int Med 1961; 108:519–30.

Logothetis J. Spontaneous epileptic seizures and electroencephalographic changes in the course of phenothiazine therapy. Neurology 1967; 17:869–77.

Logsdail SJ, Toone BK. Postictal psychoses: a clinical and phenomenological description. Br J Psychiatry 1988; 152:246–52.

Logue V, Durward M, Pratt RTC et al. The quality of survival after rupture of an anterior cerebral aneurysm. Br J Psychiatry 1968; 114:137–60.

Loiseau J, Loiseau P, Duche B et al. A survey of epileptic disorder in southwest France: seizures in elderly patients. Ann Neurol 1990a; 27:232–7.

Loiseau P, Yuen AWC, Duche B et al. A randomized double-blind, placebo-controlled crossover add-on trial of lamotrigene in patients with treatment-resistant partial seizures. Epilepsia Res 1990b; 7:136–45.

LoPiccolo CJ, Goodkin K, Baldewicz TT. Current issues in the diagnosis and management of malingering. Ann Med 1999; 31:166–74.

Lossius MI, Ronning OM, Slapo GD et al. Poststroke epilepsy: occurrence and predictors: a long-term prospective controlled study. Epilepsia 2005; 46:1246–51.

Lossos A, Dobson-Stone C, Monaco AP et al. Early clinical heterogeneity in choreoacanthocytosis. Ann Neurol 2005; 62:611–14.

Louis ED, Lynch T, Daufmann P et al. Diagnostic guidelines in central nervous system Whipple's disease. Ann Neurol 1996; 40:561–8.

Lowenstein DH, Alldredge BK. Status epilepticus. N Engl J Med 1998; 338:970–6.

Lowenstein DH, Aminoff MJ. Clinical and EEG features of status epilepticus in comatose patients. Neurology 1992; 42:100–4.

Luciano D, Devinsky O, Perrine K. Crying seizures. Neurology 1993; 43:2113–17.

Ludwig BI, Marsan CA. Clinical ictal patterns in epileptic patients with occipital electroencephalographic foci. Neurology 1975; 25:463–71.

Lundquist G. Delirium tremens: a comparative study of pathogenesis, course and prognosis with delirium tremens. Acta Psychiatr Neurol Scand 1961; 36:443–66.

Maccario M, Messis CP, Vastola EF. Focal seizures as a manifestation of hyperglycemia without ketoacidosis. A report of seven cases with review of the literature. Neurology 1965; 15:195–206.

Mace CJ, Trimble MR. Ten-year prognosis of conversion disorder. Br J Psychiatry 1996; 169:282–8.

Macpherson P, Teasdale E, Dhakar S et al. The significance of traumatic hematoma in the region of the basal ganglia. J Neurol Neurosurg Psychiatry 1986; 49:29–34.

Macrae D. Isolated fear: a temporal lobe aura. Neurology 1954a; 4:497–505.

Macrae D. On the nature of fear, with reference to its occurrence in epilepsy. J Nerv Ment Dis 1954b; 120:385–93.

McCarthy DJ. Epileptic ambulatory automatism. J Nerv Ment Dis 1900; 27:143–9.

McDowell S, Whyte J, D'Esposito M. Differential effect of a dopaminergic agent on prefrontal function in traumatic brain injury patients. Brain 1998; 121:1155–64.

McElroy SL, Phillips KA, Keck PE et al. Body dysmorphic disorder: does it have a psychotic subtype? J Clin Psychiatry 1993; 54:389–95.

McFarland HR. Addisons's disease and related psychoses. Compr Psychiatry 1963; 4:90–5.

McGrath N, Anderson NE, Croxson MC et al. Herpes simplex encephalitis treated with acyclovir: diagnosis and long term outcome. J Neurol Neurosurg Psychiatry 1997; 63:321–6.

McLachlan RS, Blume WT. Isolated fear in complex partial status epilepticus. Ann Neurol 1980; 8:639–41.

McLachlan RS, Girvin JP, Blume WT et al. Rasmussen's chronic encephalitis in adults. Arch Neurol 1993; 50:269–74.

McQueen JK, Blackwood DH, Harris P et al. Low risk of late post-traumatic seizures following severe head injury: implications for clinical trials of prophylaxis. J Neurol Neurosurg Psychiatry 1983; 46:899–904.

McVicker RW, Shanks OEP, McClelland RJ. Prevalence and associated features of epilepsy in adults with Down's syndrome. Br J Psychiatry 1994; 164:528–32.

Maeder-Ingvar M, van Melle G, Bogousslavsky J. Pure monoparesis. A particular stroke subgroup? Arch Neurol 2005; 62:1221–4.

Malamud N. Psychiatric disorder with intracranial tumors of limbic system. Arch Neurol 1967; 17:113–23.

Malkowitz DE, Legido A, Jackel RA et al. Prolactin secretion following repetitive seizures. Neurology 1995; 45:448–52.

Malouf R, Brust JCM. Hypoglycemia: causes, neurological manifestations and outcome. Ann Neurol 1985; 17:421–30.

Mandalos GE, Szarek BL. Dose-related paranoid reaction associated with fluoxetine. J Nerv Ment Dis 1990; 178:57–8.

Mandoki MW, Sumner GS. Psychiatric manifestations of hereditary coproporphyria in a child. J Nerv Ment Dis 1994; 182:117–18.

Manford MRA, Fish DR, Shorvon SD. Startle provoked epileptic seizures: features in 19 patients. J Neurol Neurosurg Psychiatry 1996; 61:151–6.

Manfredi M, Beltramello A, Bongiovanni LG et al. Eclamptic encephalopathy: imaging and pathogenetic considerations. Acta Neurol Scand 1997; 96:277-82.

Manowitz P, Kling A, Kohn H. Clinical course of adult metachromatic leukodystrophy presenting as schizophrenia: a report of two living cases in siblings. J Nerv Ment Dis 1978; 166:500-6.

Mantovani JF, Landau WM. Acquired aphasia with convulsive disorder: course and prognosis. Neurology 1980; 30:524-9.

Marchini C, Romito D, Lucci B et al. Fits of weeping as an unusual manifestation of speaking: case report. Acta Neurol Scand 1994; 90:218-21.

Margerison JH, Corsellis JAN. Epilepsy and the temporal lobes. Brain 1966; 89:499-530.

Marini C, Scheffer IE, Crossland KM et al. Genetic architecture of idiopathic generalized epilepsy: clinical genetic analysis of 55 multiplex families. Epilepsia 2004; 45:467-78.

Marino R, Gasparotti R, Pinelli L et al. Posttraumatic cerebral infarction in patients with moderate or severe head trauma. Neurology 2006; 67:1165-71.

Marks DA, Ehrenberg BC. Migraine-related seizures in adults with epilepsy, with EEG correlation. Neurology 1993; 43:2476-83.

Marks DA, Laxer KD. Semiology of temporal lobe seizures: value in lateralizing the seizure focus. Epilepsia 1998; 39:721-6.

Marks DA, Kim J, Spencer D et al. Characteristics of intractable seizures following meningitis and encephalitis. Neurology 1992; 42:1513-18.

Marsh GG. Neuropsychological syndrome in a patient with episodic howling and violent motor behavior. J Neurol Neurosurg Psychiatry 1978; 41:366-9.

Marshall JC, Halligan PW, Fink GR et al. The functional anatomy of a hysterical paralysis. Cognition 1997; 64:1-8.

Marson AG, Williamson PR, Clough H et al. Carbamazepine versus valproate monotherapy for epilepsy: a meta-analysis. Epilepsia 2002; 43:505-13.

Martinez O, Reisin R, Andermann F et al. Evidence for reflex activation of experiential complex seizures. Neurology 2001; 56:121-3.

Masel BE, Scheibel RS, Kimbark T et al. Excessive daytime sleepiness in adults with brain injuries. Arch Phys Med Rehabil 2001; 82:1526-32.

Massman PJ, Sims J, Cooke N et al. Prevalence and correlates of neuropsychological deficits in amytrophic lateral sclerosis. J Neurol Neurosurg Psychiatry 1996; 61:450-5.

Mathews WB. Multiple sclerosis presenting with acute remitting psychiatric symptoms. J Neurol Neurosurg Psychiatry 1979; 42:859-63.

Matsuo F, Beren D, Faught E et al. Placebo-controlled study of the efficacy and safety of lamotrigene in patients with partial seizures. Neurology 1993; 43:2284-91.

Mattson RH Cramer JA, Collins JF et al. Comparison of carbamazepine, phenobarbital, phenytoin, and primidone in partial and secondarily generalized tonic-clonic seizures. N Engl J Med 1985; 313:145-51.

Mattson RH, Cramer JA, Darney PD et al. Use of oral contraceptives by women with epilepsy. JAMA 1986; 255:238-40.

Mattson RH, Cramer JA, Collins JF et al. A comparison of valproate with carbamazepine for the treatment of complex partial seizures and secondarily generalized tonic-clonic seizures in adults. N Engl J Med 1992; 327:765-71.

Maudsley H. Responsibility in mental disease. New York: D. Appleton, 1874.

Mauguire F, Courjon J. Somatosensory epilepsy: a review of 127 cases. Brain 1978; 101:307-32.

Mayer SA, Brun SC, Begtrup K et al. Recombinant activated factor VII for acute intracerebral hemorhage. N Engl J Med 2005; 352:777-85.

Mayeux R, Lueders H. Complex partial status epilepticus: case report and proposal for diagnostic criteria. Neurology 1978; 28:957-61.

Mayeux R, Alexander MP, Benson DF et al. Poriomania. Neurology 1979; 29:1616-19.

Mazzini L, Cossa FM, Angelino E et al. Posttraumatic epilepsy: neuroradiologic and neuropsychological assessment of long-term outcome. Epilepsia 2003; 44:569-74.

Medina J, Rubino F, Ross E. Agitated delirium caused by infarctions of the hippocampal formation and fusiform and lingual gyri: a case report. Neurology 1974; 24:1181-3.

Meencke HJ, Janz D. Neuropathological findings in primary generalized epilepsy: a study of eight cases. Epilepsia 1984; 25:8-21.

Mega MS, Cummings JL, Fiorello T et al. The spectrum of behavioral changes in Alzheimer's disease. Neurology 1996; 46:130-5.

Meierkord H, Shorvon S, Lightman S et al. Comparison of the effects of frontal and temporal lobe partial seizures on prolactin levels. Arch Neurol 1992:49:225-30.

Mendez MF, Adams NL, Lewandowski KS. Neurobehavioral changes associated with caudate lesions. Neurology 1989; 39:349-54.

Mendez MF, Selwood A, Mastri AR et al. Pick's disease versus Alzheimer's disease: a comparison of clinical characteristics. Neurology 1993; 43:289-92.

Mendez MF, Chernier MM, Perryman KM. Epileptic forced thinking from left frontal lesions. Neurology 1996; 47:79-83.

Meninger KA. Influenza and schizophrenia. Am J Psychiatry 1926; 82:469-529.

Merriam AE, Medalia A, Levine B. Partial complex status epilepticus associated with cocaine abuse. Biol Psychiatry 1988; 23:515-18.

Merritt HH, Springlova M. Lissauer's dementia paralytica: a clinical and pathologic study. Arch Neurol Psychiatry 1932; 27:987-1030.

Messenheimer J, Ramsey RE, Willmore LJ et al. Lamotrigene therapy for partial seizures: a multicenter, placebo-controlled, double-blind, cross-over trial. Epilepsia 1994; 35:113-21.

Messing RO, Closson RG, Simon RP. Drug-induced seizures: a 10-year experience. Neurology 1984; 34:1582-6.

Messori A, Polonara G, Carle F et al. Predicting posttraumatic epilepsy with MRI; prospective longitudinal morphologic study in adults. Epilepsia 2005; 46:1472-81.

Mesulam M-M. Dissociative states with abnormal temporal lobe EEG. Arch Neurol 1981; 38:176-81.

Meythaler JM, Brunner RC, Johnson A et al. Amantadine to improve neurorecovery in traumatic brain injury-associated diffuse axonal injury: a pilot double-blind randomized trial. *J Head Trauma Rehabil* 2002; **17**:300–13.

Michelucchi R, Rubboli G, Passarelli D et al. Electroclinical features of idiopathic generalized epilepsy with persisting absences in adult life. *J Neurol Neurosurg Psychiatry* 1996; **61**:471–7.

Michelucchi R, Poza JJ, Sovia V et al. Autosomal dominant lateral temporal lobe epilepsy: clinical spectrum, new epitempin mutations, and genetic heterogeneity in seven European families. *Epilepsia* 2003; **44**:1289–97.

Michelucchi R, Gardella E, de Haan G-J et al. Telephone-induced seizures: a new type of reflex epilepsy. *Epilepsia* 2004; **45**:280–3.

Miguel EC, Rodriguez Pereira RM, de Braganca Pereira CA et al. Psychiatric manifestations of systemic lupus erythematosus: clinical features, symptoms and signs of central nervous system activity in 43 patients. *Medicine* 1994; **73**:224–32.

Mikati MA, Lee WL, DeLong GR. Epileptiform encephalopathy: an unusual form of partial complex status epilepticus. *Epilepsia* 1985; **26**:563–77.

Mineharu Y, Takenada K, Yamakawa H et al. Inheritance pattern of familial Moyamoya disease: autosomal dominant mode and genetic imprinting. *J Neurol Neurosurg Psychiatry* 2006; **77**:1025–9.

Minematsu K, Yamaguchi T, Omae T. Spectacular shrinking deficit: rapid recovery from a major hemispheric syndrome by migration of an embolus. *Neurology* 1992; **42**:157–62.

Misra UK, Kalita J, Patel R. Sodium valproate vs phenytoin in status epilepticus: a pilot study. *Neurology* 2006; **67**:340–2.

Mitchell C. Successful treatment of chronic delusional parasittosis. *Br J Psychiatry* 1989; **155**:556–7.

Mitchell W, Falconer MA, Hill D. Epilepsy with fetishism relieved by temporal lobectomy. *Lancet* 1954; **2**:626–30.

Mitchell WG, Messenheimer JA, Greenwood RS. Abdominal epilepsy. Cyclic vomiting as the major symptom of simple partial seizures. *Arch Neurol* 1983; **40**:251–2.

Mittle RL, Grossman RI, Hiehle JF et al. Prevalence of MR evidence of diffuse axonal injury in patients with mild head injury and normal head CT findings. *AJNR* 1994; **15**:1583–9.

Moder KG, Hurley DL. Fatal hypernatremia from exogenous salt intake: report of a case and review of the literature. *Mayo Clin Proc* 1990; **65**:187–94.

Moene FC, Landberg EH, Hoogduin KA et al. Organic syndromes diagnosed as conversion disorder: identification and frequency in a study of 85 patients. *J Psychosom Res* 2000; **49**:7–12.

Moersch FP. Psychic manifestations in cases of brain tumors. *Am J Psychiatry* 1925; **81**:707–24.

Mohr JP. Lacunes. *Stroke* 1982; **13**:3–11.

Molina JA, Calandre L, Bermejo F. Myoclonic encephalopathy due to bismuth salts: treatment with dimercaprol and analysis of CSF transmitters. *Acta Neurol Scand* 1989; **79**:200–3.

Monteiro L, Nunes B, Mendonca D et al. Spectrum of epilepsy in neuroacanthocytosis: a long-term follow-up of 143 patients. *Acta Neurol Scand* 1995; **92**:33–40.

Moore DP. A case of petit mal epilepsy aggravated by lithium. *Am J Psychiatry* 1981; **138**:690–1.

Moore DP. *Partial seizures and interictal disorders.* Boston: Butterworth-Heinemann, 1997.

Moosey J, Morphology, sites and epidemiology of cerebral atherosclerosis. *Res Publ Assoc Res Nerv Ment Dis* 1966; **51**:1–22.

Morey CE, Cilo M, Berry J et al. The effect of Aricept in persons with persistent memory disorder following traumatic brain injury: a pilot study. *Brain Inj* 2003; **17**:809–15.

Morris CE, Heyman A, Pozefsky T. Lead encephalopathy caused by ingestion of illicitly distilled whiskey. *Neurology* 1964; **14**:493–9.

Morris HH, Dinner DS, Luders H et al. Supplementary motor seizures: clinical and electroencephalographic findings. *Neurology* 1988; **38**:1075–82.

Moser HW, Moser AE, Singh I et al. Adrenoleukodystrophy: survey of 303 cases: biochemistry, diagnosis and therapy. *Ann Neurol* 1984; **16**:628–41.

Moskovitz C, Moses H, Klawans HL. Levodopa-induced psychosis: a kindling phenomenon. *Am J Psychiatry* 1978; **135**:669–75.

Motamedi M, Nguyen DK, Zaatreh M et al. Levetiracetam efficacy in refractory partial-onset seizures, especially after failed epilepsy surgery. *Epilepsia* 2003; **44**:211–14.

Mula M, Trimble MR, Yuen A et al. Psychiatric adverse events during levetiracetam therapy. *Neurology* 2003; **61**:704–6.

Mulder DW, Daly D. Psychiatric symptoms associated with lesions of temporal lobe. *JAMA* 1952; **150**:173–6.

Mulder DW, Parrott M, Thaler M. Sequelae of western equine encephalitis. *Neurology* 1951; **1**:318–27.

Mullatti N, Selway R, Nashef L et al. The clinical spectrum of epilepsy in children and adults with hypothalamic hamartoma. *Epilepsia* 2003; **44**:1310–19.

Muller D, Pilz H, Ter Meulen V. Studies on adult metachromatic leukodystrophy. I. Clinical, morphological and histochemical observations in two cases. *J Neurol Sci* 1969; **9**:567–84.

Muller T, Buttner TH, Kuhn W et al. Palinopsia as sensory epileptic phenomenon. *Acta Neurol Scand* 1995; **91**:433–6.

Muller U, Murai T, Bauer-Wittmund T et al. Paroxetine versus citalopram treatment of pathological crying after brain injury. *Brain Inj* 1999; **13**:805–11.

Mungas D. Interictal behavior abnormality in temporal lobe epilepsy. *Arch Gen Psychiatry* 1982; **39**:108–11.

Murphy CP, Harden EA, Thompson JM. Generalized seizures secondary to high dose busulfan therapy. *Ann Pharmacother* 1992; **26**:30–1.

Murphy KC, Jones LA, Owen MJ. High rates of schizophrenia in adults with velo-cardio-facial syndrome. *Arch Gen Psychiatry* 1999; **56**:940–5.

Murthy P, Jayakumar PN, Sampat S. Of insects and eggs: a case report. *J Neurol Neurosurg Psychiatry* 1997; **63**:522–3.

Mysiw WJ, Jackson RD, Corrigan JD. Amitriptyline for post-traumatic agitation. *Am J Phys Med Rehabil* 1988; **67**:29–33.

Naidech AM, Janjua N, Kreiter KT et al. Predictors and impact of aneurysm rebleeding after subarachnoid hemorrhage. *Arch Neurol* 2005; **62**:410–16.

Nakada T, Lee H, Kwee IL et al. Epileptic Kluver–Bucy syndrome: case report. *J Clin Psychiatry* 1984; **45**:87–8.

Narushima K, Kosier JT, Robinson R. Preventing poststroke depression: a 12-week double-blind randomized treatment trial and 21-month follow-up. *J Nerv Ment Dis* 2002; **190**:296–303.

Nasrallah HA, Fowler RC, Judd LL. Schizophrenia-like illness following head injury. *Psychosomatics* 1981; **22**:359–61.

Nausieda PA, Grossman BJ, Koller WC *et al.* Sydenham chorea: an update. *Neurology* 1980; **30**:331–4.

Navia BA, Jordan BD, Price RW. The AIDS dementia complex. I. Clinical features. *Ann Neurol* 1986a; **19**:517–24.

Navia BA, Petito CK, Gold JWM *et al.* Cerebral toxoplasmosis complicating the acquired immune deficiency syndrome: clinical and neuropathological findings in 27 patients. *Ann Neurol* 1986b; **19**:224–38.

Neary D, Snowden JS, Mann DMA *et al.* Frontal lobe dementia and motor neuron disease. *J Neurol Neurosurg Psychiatry* 1990; **53**:23–32.

Neary D, Snowden JS, Mann DMA. Familial progressive atrophy: its relationship to other forms of lobar atrophy. *J Neurol Neurosurg Psychiatry* 1993; **56**:1122–5.

Nedeltchev K, der Maur TA, Georgiadis D *et al.* Ischemic stroke in young adults: predictors of outcome and recurrence. *J Neurol Neurosurg Psychiatry* 2005; **76**:191–5.

Newburn G, Newburn D. Selegeline in the management of apathy following traumatic brain injury. *Brain Inj* 2005; **19**:149–54.

Newman P, Saunders M. A unique case of musicogenic epilepsy. *Arch Neurol* 1980; **37**:244–5.

Newmark ME. Diagnosis of epilepsy with home video-cassette recorder. *N Engl J Med* 1981; **305**:769.

Neylan TC. Frontal lobe function: Mr. Phineas Gage's famous injury. *J Neuropsychiatry Clin Neurosci* 1999; **11**:281–3.

Nicoletti A, Sofia V, Biondi R *et al.* Epilepsy and multiple sclerosis in Italy: a population-based study. *Epilepsia* 2003; **44**:1445–8.

Nielsen H, Kristensen O. Personality correlates of sphenoidal EEG foci in temporal lobe epilepsy. *Acta Neurol Scand* 1981; **64**:289–300.

Nightingale S, Welch JL. Psychometric assessment in absence status. *Arch Neurol* 1982; **39**:516–19.

Nishida T, Kudo T, Inoue Y *et al.* Postictal mania versus postictal psychosis: differences in clinical features, epileptogenic zone, and brain functional changes during postictal period. *Epilepsia* 2006; **47**:2104–14.

Nishino H, Rubino FA, DeRemee RA *et al.* Neurological involvement in Wegener's granulomatosis: an analysis of 324 consecutive patients at the Mayo clinic. *Ann Neurol* 1993; **33**:4–9.

Nizamie SH, Nizamie A, Borde M *et al.* Mania following head injury: case reports and neuropsychological findings. *Acta Psychiatr Scand* 1988; **77**:637–9.

Noachtar S, Luders HO. Focal akinetic seizures as documented by electroencephalography and video recordings. *Neurology* 1999; **53**:427–9.

Nott MT, Chapparo C, Baguley IJ. Agitation following traumatic brain injury: an Australian sample. *Brain Inj* 2006; **20**:1175–82.

Novak J, Corke P, Fairley N. 'Petit mal status' in adults. *Dis Nerv Syst* 1971; **32**:245–8.

Noyes R, Kathol RG, Fisher MM *et al.* Psychiatric comorbidity among patients with hypochondriasis. *Gen Hosp Psychiatry* 1994; **16**:78–87.

Noyes R, Holt CS, Happel RL *et al.* A family study of hypochondriasis. *J Nerv Ment Dis* 1997; **185**:223–32.

Noyes R, Sturat S, Langbehn DR *et al.* Childhood antecedents of hypochondriasis. *Psychosomatics* 2002; **43**:282–9.

Nystrom HM. Relationship between location of cerebral lesion and epilepsy. A statistical study of 350 cases. *Acta Neurol Scand* 1966; **42**:191–206.

O'Carroll RE, Masterton G, Dougall N *et al.* The neuropsychiatric sequelae of mercury poisoning: the Mad Hatter's disease. *Br J Psychiatry* 1995; **167**:95–8.

Ochs R, Gloor P, Quesney F *et al.* Does head-turning during a seizure have lateralizing or localizing significance? *Neurology* 1984; **34**:884–90.

Oder W, Goldenberg G, Spatt J *et al.* Behavioral and psychosocial sequelae of severe closed head injury and regional cerebral blood flow: a SPECT study. *J Neurol Neurosurg Psychiatry* 1992; **55**:475–80.

Oestreich LJ, Berg MJ, Bachmann DL *et al.* Ictal contralateral paresis in complex partial seizures. *Epilepsia* 1995; **36**:671–5.

Ogunyemi AO, Locke GE, Kramer LD *et al.* Complex partial status epilepticus provoked by 'crack' cocaine. *Ann Neurol* 1989; **26**:785–6.

O'Hare JA, Callaghan NM, Murnaghan DJ. Dialysis encephalopathy. Clinical, electroencephalographic, and interventional aspects. *Medicine* 1983; **62**:129–41.

Okada Y, Yamaguchi T, Minematsu K *et al.* Hemorrhagic transformation in cerebral embolism. *Stroke* 1989; **20**:598–603.

Oksanen V. Neurosarcoidosis: clinical presentations and course in 50 patients. *Acta Neurol Scand* 1986; **73**:283–90.

Oldani A, Zucconi M, Asselta R *et al.* Autosomal dominant nocturnal frontal lobe epilepsy: a video-polysomnographic and genetic appraisal of 40 patients and delineation of the epileptic syndrome. *Brain* 1998; **121**:205–23.

Olivier AP, Luchins DJ, Wyatt RJ. Neuroleptic-induced seizures. *Arch Gen Psychiatry* 1982; **39**:206–9.

Olsson I, Steffenberg S, Gillberg C. Epilepsy in autism and autistic-like conditions. *Arch Neurol* 1988; **45**:666–8.

Ono J, Mano T, Andermann E *et al.* Band heterotopia or double cortex in a male: bridging structures suggest abnormality of the radial glial system. *Neurology* 1997; **48**:1701–3.

Opjordsmoen S, Rettersol N. Delusional disorder: the predictive validity of the concept. *Acta Psychiatr Scand* 1991; **84**:250–4.

Oribe E, Rohullah A, Nissenbaum E *et al.* Serum prolactin concentrations are elevated after syncope. *Neurology* 1996; **47**:60–2.

Orrison WW, Gentry LR, Stimae GK *et al.* Blinded comparison of cranial CT and MR in closed head injury evaluation. *AJNR* 1994; **15**:351–6.

d'Orsi G, Tinuper P, Bisulli F *et al.* Clinical features and long term outcome of epilepsy in periventricular nodular heterotopia. Simple compared with plus forms. *J Neurol Neurosurg Psychiatry* 2004; **75**:873–8.

Ostergarrd JRI Warning lead in subarachnoid hemorrhage. *BMJ* 1990; **301**:190–1.

Ottman R, Risch N, Hauser WA *et al.* Localization of a gene for partial epilepsy to chromosome 10q. *Nat Genet* 1995; **10**:56–60.

Oxbury JM, Whitty CWM. Causes and consequences of status epilepticus in adults: a study of 86 cases. *Brain* 1971; **94**:733–44.

Ozkara C, Ozdemir S, Yilmaz A *et al.* Orgasm-induced seizures: a study of six patients. *Epilepsia* 2006; **47**:2193–7.

Pachet A, Friesen S, Winkelaar D *et al.* Beneficial behavioral effects of lamotrigene in traumatic brain injury. *Brain Inj* 2003; **17**:715–22.

Pacia SV, Devinsky O. Clozapine-related seizures: experience with 5,629 patients. *Neurology* 1994; **44**:2247–9.

Paciaroni M, Caso V, Milia P *et al.* Isolated monoparesis following stroke. *J Neurol Neurosurg Psychiatry* 2005; **76**:805–7.

Pakainis A, Drake ME, John K *et al.* Forced normalization: acute psychosis after seizure control in seven patients. *Arch Neurol* 1987; **44**:289–92.

Palmini A, Gloor P. The localizing value of auras in partial seizures: a prospective and retrospective study. *Neurology* 1992; **42**:801–8.

Palmini A, Andermann F, Olivier A *et al.* Focal neuronal migration disorders and intractable partial epilepsy: a study of 30 patients. *Ann Neurol* 1991; **30**:741–9.

Palmini AL, Gloor P, Jones-Gotman M. Pure amnestic seizures in temporal lobe epilepsy. *Brain* 1992; **115**:749–69.

Pampiglione G, Moynahan EJ. The tuberous sclerosis syndrome: clinical and EEG studies in 100 children. *J Neurol Neurosurg Psychiatry* 1976; **39**:666–73.

Panayiotopoulus CP. Vomiting as an ictal manifestation of epileptic siezures and syndromes. *J Neurol Neurosurg Psychiatry* 1988; **51**:1448–51.

Paquier PF, Van Dongen HR, Loonen CB. The Landau–Kleffner syndrome or 'acquired aphasia with convulsive disorder': long-term follow-up of six children and a review of the recent literature. *Arch Neurol* 1992; **49**:354–9.

Pardo CA, Vining SPG, Guo L *et al.* The pathology of Rasmussen syndrome: stages of cortical involvement and neuropathological studies in 45 hemispherectomies. *Epilepsia* 2004; **45**:516–26.

Parker N. Disseminated sclerosis presenting as schizophrenia. *Med J Aust* 1956; **1**:405–7.

Parmar H, Lim S-H, Tan NCK *et al.* Acute symptomatic seizures and hippocampal damage: DWI and MRS findings. *Neurology* 2006; **66**:1732–5.

Parra A, Velasco M, Cervantes C *et al.* Plasma prolactin increase following electrical stimulation of the amygdala in humans. *Neuroendocrinology* 1980; **31**:60–5.

Parsons MW, Barber PA, Chalk J *et al.* Diffusion- and perfusion-weighted MRI response to thrombolysis in stroke. *Ann Neurol* 2002; **51**:28–37.

Partlow GD, del Carpio-ODonovan R, Melanson D *et al.* Bilateral thalamic glioma: review of eight cases with personality change and mental deterioration. *AJNR* 1992; **13**:1125–30.

Partridge M. One operation cures three people: effect of prefrontal leukotomy on a case of folie a deux et demie. *Arch Neurol Psychiatry* 1950; **54**:792–6.

Pascual-Castroviejo I, Diaz-Gonzalez G, Garcia-Melian RM *et al.* Sturge–Weber syndrome: study of 40 patients. *Pediatr Neurology* 1993; **9**:283–8.

Paskavitz JF, Anderson CA, Filley CM *et al.* Acute arcuate fiber demyelinating encephalopathy following Epstein–Barr virus infection. *Ann Neurol* 1995; **38**:127–31.

Passero S, Rocchi R, Rossi S *et al.* Seizures after spontaneous supratentorial intracerebral hemorrhage. *Epilepsia* 2002; **43**:1175–80.

Patel NC, Landan IR, Levin J *et al.* The use of levetiracetam in refractory status epilepticus. *Seizure* 2006; **15**:137–41.

Pazzaglia P, D'Alessandro R, Ambrosetto G *et al.* Drop attacks: an ominous change in the evolution of partial epilepsy. *Neurology* 1985; **35**:1725–30.

Peavy GM, Herzog AG, Rubin NP *et al.* Neuropsychological aspects of dementia of motor neuron disease: a report of two cases. *Neurology* 1992; **42**:1004–8.

Pedley TA, Guilleminault C. Episodic nocturnal wanderings responsive to anticonvulsant drug therapy. *Ann Neurol* 1977; **2**:30–5.

Penfield W, Jasper H. *Epilepsy and the functional anatomy of the human brain.* Boston: Little, Brown, 1954.

Penry JK, Dreifuss FE. Automatisms associated with the absence of petit mal epilepsy. *Arch Neurol* 1969; **21**:142–9.

Penry JK, Porter RJ, Dreifuss FE. Simultaneous recording of absence seizures with video tape and electroencephalography: a study of 374 seizures in 48 patients. *Brain* 1975; **98**:427–40.

Peppercorn MA, Herzog AG, Dichter MA *et al.* Abdominal epilepsy: a case of abdominal pain in adults. *JAMA* 1978; **240**:2450–1.

Perez NM, Trimble MR. Epileptic psychosis – diagnostic comparison with process schizophrenia. *Br J Psychiatry* 1980; **137**:245–9.

Perley M, Guze B. Hysteria: the stability and usefulness of clinical criteria: a quantitative study based on a 6–8 year follow-up of 39 patients. *N Engl J Med* 1962; **266**:421–6.

Peroutka SJ, Sohmer BH, Kumer AJ *et al.* Hallucinations and delusions following a right temporo-parietal-occipital infarction. *Johns Hopkins Med J* 1982; **151**:181–5.

Pessin MS, Lathi E, Cohen M *et al.* Clinical features and mechanism of occipital infarction. *Ann Neurol* 1987; **21**:290–9.

Petermann AF, Hayles AB, Dockerty MB *et al.* Encephalotrigeminal angiomatosis (Sturge–Weber disease). Clinical study of thirty-five cases. *J Am Med Assoc* 1958; **167**:2169–76.

Petry S, Cummings JL, Hill MA *et al.* Personality alterations in dementia of the Alzheimer type. *Arch Neurol* 1988; **45**:1187–90.

Petti TA, Campbell M. Imipramine and seizures. *Am J Psychiatry* 1975; **132**:538–40.

Petty RG, Bonner D, Mouratoglou V *et al.* Acute frontal lobe syndrome and dyscontrol associated with bilateral caudate infarctions. *Br J Psychiatry* 1996; **168**:237–40.

Pflanz S, Besson JAO, Ebmeier KP *et al.* The clinical manifestations of mental disorder in Huntington's disease: a retrospective case record study of disease progression. *Acta Psychiatr Scand* 1991; **83**:53–60.

Phillips HA, Marini C, Scheffer IE *et al.* A de novo mutation in sporadic nocturnal frontal lobe epilepsy. *Ann Neurol* 2000; **48**:264–7.

Picard F, Baulac S, Kahane P *et al.* Dominant partial epilepsies: a clinical, electrophysiological and genetic study of 19 European families. *Brain* 2000; **123**:1247–62.

Placidi F, Floris R, Bozzao A et al. Ketotic hyperglycemia and epilepsia partialis continua. *Neurology* 2001; **57**:534–7.

Plazzi G, Tinuper P, Montagna P et al. Epileptic nocturnal wanderings. *Sleep* 1995; **18**:749.

Pomeroy SL, Holmes SJ, Dodge PR et al. Seizures and other neurologic sequelae of bacterial meningitis in children. *N Engl J Med* 1990; **323**:1651–7.

Pope HG, Katz DL. Affective and psychotic symptoms associated with anabolic steroid use. *Am J Psychiatry* 1988; **145**:487–90.

Pope HG, Jonas JM, Jones B. Factitious psychosis: phenomenology, family history and long-term outcome of nine patients. *Am J Psychiatry* 1982; **139**:1480–3.

Popli AP, Masand PS, Dewan MJ. Factitious disorders with psychological symptoms. *J Clin Psychiatry* 1992; **53**:315–18.

Porter NT, Meyer MA, Zimmerman AW et al. Molecular and clinical findings in a family with dentatorubral-pallidoluysian atrophy. *Ann Neurol* 1995; **37**:273–7.

Porter SB, Sande MA. Toxoplasmosis of the central nervous system in the acquired immunodeficiency syndrome. *N Engl J Med* 1992; **327**:1643–8.

Poskanzer DC, Brown AE, Miller H. Musicogenic epilepsy caused only by a discrete frequency band of church bells. *Brain* 1962; **85**:7–92.

Powell JH, al-Adawi S, Morgan J et al. Motivational deficits after brain injury: effects of bromocriptine in 11 patients. *J Neurol Neurosurg Psychiatry* 1996; **60**:416–21.

Poza JJ, Saenz A, Martinez-Gil A et al. Autosomal dominant lateral temporal lobe epilepsy: clinical and genetic study of a large Basque pedigree linked to chromosome 10q. *Ann Neurol* 1999; **45**:182–8.

Prashanth LK, Taly AB, Ravi V et al. Adult subacute sclerosing panencephalitis: clinical profile of 39 patients from a tertiary care center. *J Neurol Neurosurg Psychiatry* 2006; **77**:630–3.

Pritchard PB, Wannamaker BB, Sagel J et al. Serum prolactin and cortisol levels in evaluation of pseudoepileptic seizures. *Ann Neurol* 1985a; **18**:87–9.

Pritchard PB, Holmstrom VL, Giacinto J. Self-abatement of complex partial seizures. *Ann Neurol* 1985b; **18**:265–7.

Privitera MD, Morris GL, Gilliam F. Postictal language assessment and lateralization of complex partial seizures. *Ann Neurol* 1991; **30**:391–6.

Privitera MD, Fincham R, Penry J et al. Topiramate placebo-controlled dose-ranging trial in refractory partial epilepsy using 600-, 800-, and 1,000-mg daily dosages. *Neurology* 1996; **46**:1678–83.

Provini F, Plazzi G, Tinuper P et al. Nocturnal frontal lobe epilepsy: a clinical and polygraphic overview of 100 consecutive cases. *Brain* 1999; **122**:1017–31.

Pueschel SM, Louis S, McKnight P. Seizure disorders in Down syndrome. *Arch Neurol* 1991; **48**:318–20.

Putzel L. Cerebral complications of chorea. *New York Medical Record* 1879; (6 Sept):220–2.

Quesney LF, Constain M, Fish DR et al. The clinical differentiation of seizures in the parasaggital and anterolateral frontal convexities. *Arch Neurol* 1990; **47**:677–9.

Quirk JA, Fish DR, Smith SJM et al. First seizures associated with playing electronic screen games: a community-based study in Great Britian. *Ann Neurol* 1995; **37**:733–7.

Rabinowicz AL, Correale JD, Bracht KA et al. Neuron specific enolase is increased after nonconvulsive status epilepticus. *Epilepsia* 1995; **36**:475–9.

Rabinowicz AL, Correale J, Boutros RB. Neuron-specific enolase is increased after single seizures during inpatient video/EEG monitoring. *Epilepsia* 1996; **37**:122–5.

Rabinstein AA, Wijdicks EF. Hyponatremia in critically ill neurological patients. *Neurologist* 2003; **9**:290–300.

Ramsey RE, DeToledo J. Intravenous administration of fosphenytoin: options for the management of seizures. *Neurology* 1996; **46**(suppl. 1):17–19.

Ramsey RE, Wilder BJ, Berger JR et al. A double-blind study comparing carbamazepine with phenytoin as initial seizure therapy in adults. *Neurology* 1983; **33**:904–10.

Rao V, Lyketsos C. Neuropsychiatric sequelae of traumatic brain injury. *Psychosomatics* 2000; **41**:95–103.

Rasmussen A, Matsuura T, Ruano L et al. Clinical and genetic analysis of four Mexican families with spinocerebellar ataxia type 10. *Ann Neurol* 2001; **50**:234–9.

Rasmussen A, Lunde M, Poulsen DL et al. A double-blind, placebo-controlled study of sertraline in the prevention of depression in stroke patients. *Psychosomatics* 2003; **44**:216–21.

Rasmussen T, Olszewski J, Lloyd-Smith D. Focal seizures due to chronic localized encephalitis. *Neurology* 1958; **8**:435–45.

Rasmussen T. Surgical therapy of frontal lobe epilepsy. *Epilepsia* 1963; **4**:181–98.

Rasmussen T. Characteristics of a pure culture of frontal lobe epilepsy. *Epilepsia* 1983; **24**:482–93.

Rasmussen T, Andermann F. Update on the syndrome of 'chronic encephalitis' and epilepsy. *Cleve Clin J Med* 1989; **56**(suppl. 2):181–4.

Rauschka H, Colsch B, Baumann N et al. Late-onset metachromatic leukodystrophy. Genotype strongly influences phenotype. *Neurology* 2006; **67**:859–63.

Raymond AA, Fish DR, Sisodiya SM et al. Abnormalities of gyration, heterotopias, tuberous sclerosis, focal cortical dysplasia, microdysgenesis, dysembroplastic neuroepithelial tumor and dysgenesis of the archicortex in epilepsy. Clinical, EEG and neuroimaging findings. *Brain* 1995; **118**:629–60.

Raymond RW, Williams RL. Infectious mononucleosis with psychosis. *N Engl J Med* 1948; **239**:542–4.

Reading PJ, Will RG. Unwelcome orgasms. *Lancet* 1997; **350**:1747.

Reami DO, Silva DF, Albuquerque M et al. Dreams and epilepsy. *Epilepsia* 1991; **32**:51–3.

Reed K, Bland RL. Masked 'myxedema madness'. *Acta Psychiatr Scand* 1977; **56**:421–6.

van Reekum R, Bayley M, Garner S et al. N of 1 study: amantadine for the amotivational syndrome in a patient with traumatic brain injury. *Brain Inj* 1995; **9**:49–53.

Reich P, Gottfried LA. Factitious disorders in a teaching hospital. *Ann Intern Med* 1983; **99**:240–7.

Remillard GM, Andermann F, Rhi-Sausa A et al. Facial assymetry in patients with temporal lobe epilepsy. *Neurology* 1977; **27**:109–14.

Remillard GM, Andermann F, Testa GF et al. Sexual ictal manifestations predominate in women with temporal lobe epilepsy: a finding suggesting sexual dimorphism in the human brain. Neurology 1983; 33:323–30.

Rennick PM, Perez-Borja C, Rodin EA. Transient mental deficits associated with recurrent prolonged epileptic clouded state. Epilepsia 1969; 10:397–405.

Rennick PM, Noland DC, Bauer RB et al. Neuropsychologic and neurologic follow-up after herpes hominis encephalitis. Neurology 1973; 23:42–7.

Rheims S, Demarquay G, Isnard J et al. Ipsilateral head deviation in frontal lobe seizures. Epilepsia 2005; 46:1750–3.

Rice E, Gendelman S. Psychiatric aspects of normal pressure hydrocephalus. JAMA 1973; 223:409–12.

Richardson EP, Dodge PR. Epilepsy in cerebral vascular disease. Epilepsia 1954; 3:49–74.

Richfield EK, Twyman R, Berent S. Neurological syndrome following bilateral damage to the head of the caudate nuclei. Ann Neurol 1987; 22:768–71.

Roberts AH. Sequelae of closed head injuries. Proc R Soc Med 1976; 69:137–41.

Roberts JKA, Trimble MR, Robertson M. Schizophrenic psychosis associated with aqueductal stenosis in adults. J Neurol Neurosurg Psychiatry 1983; 46:892–8.

Roberts MA, Humphrey PRD. Prolonged complex partial status epilepticus: a case report. J Neurol Neurosurg Psychiatry 1988; 51:586–8.

Robinson RG, Parikh RM, Lipsey JR et al. Pathological laughing and crying after stroke: validation of a measurement scale and a double-blind treatment study. Am J Psychiatry 1993; 150:286–93.

Robinson RG, Schultz SK, Castillo C et al. Nortriptyline versus fluoxetine in the treatment of depression and in short-term recovery after stroke: a placebo-controlled, double-blind study. Am J Psychiatry 2000; 157:658–60.

Rocamora R, Kurthen M, Lickfett L et al. Cardiac asystole in epilepsy: clinical and neurophysiologic features. Epilepsia 2003; 44:179–85.

Rodin E, Schmaltz S. The Bear–Fedio personality inventory and temporal lobe epilepsy. Neurology 1984; 34:591–6.

Rodin EA. Psychomotor epilepsy and aggressive behavior. Arch Gen Psychiatry 1973; 28:210–13.

Romanelli MF, Morris JC, Ashkin K et al. Advanced Alzheimer's disease is a risk factor for late-onset seizures. Arch Neurol 1990; 47:847–50.

Romanul FCA, Radvany J, Rosales RK. Whipple's disease confined to the brain: a case confirmed clinically and pathologically. J Neurol Neurosurg Psychiatry 1977; 40:901–9.

Roos R, Cajdusek DC, Gibbs CJ. The clinical characteristics of transmissible Creutzfeldt–Jakob disease. Brain 1973; 96:1–20.

Rosenbaum M, Lewis M, Piker P et al. Convulsive seizures in delirium tremens. Arch Neurol Psychiatry 1941; 45:486–93.

Rosenberg GA, Kornfeld M, Stovring J et al. Subcortical arteriosclerotic encephalopathy (Binswanger's): computerized tomography. Neurology 1979; 29:1102–6.

Ross AT, Dickerson WW. Tuberous sclerosis. Arch Neurol Psychiatry 1943; 50:233–57.

Rothschild D. Dementia paralytica accompanied by manic-depressive and schizophrenic psychoses. Am J Psychiatry 1940; 96:1043–60.

Rothwell PM, Warlow CP. Timing of TIAs preceding stroke. Time window for prevention is very short. Neurology 2005; 64:817–20.

Rowan AJ, Scott DF. Major status epilepticus: a series of 42 patients. Acta Neurol Scand 1970; 46:573–84.

Rowan AJ, Ramsey RE, Collins JF et al. New onset geriatric epilepsy. A randomized study of gabapentin, lamotrigine, and carbamazepine. Neurology 2005; 64:1868–73.

Rozdilsky B, Cummings JN, Huston AF. Hallervorden–Spatz disease: late infantile and adult type, report of two cases. Acta Neuropathologica 1968; 10:1–16.

Ruff RL. Orgasmic epilepsy. Neurology 1980; 30:1252.

Rugg-Gunn FJ, Duncan JS, Smith SJM. Epileptic cardiac asystole. J Neurol Neurosurg Psychiatry 2000; 68:108–10.

Rush JL, Everett BA, Adams AH et al. Paroxysmal atrial tachycardia and frontal lobe tumor. Arch Neurol 1977; 34:578–80.

Russell WR, Whitty CWM. Studies in traumatic epilepsy. 1. Factors influencing the incidence of epilepsy after brain wounds. J Neurol Neurosurg Psychiatry 1952; 15:93–8.

Russell WR, Whitty CWM. Studies in traumatic epilepsy. 2. Focal motor and somatic sensory fits: a study of 85 cases. J Neurol Neurosurg Psychiatry 1953; 16:73–97.

Russell WR, Whitty CWM. Studies in traumatic epilepsy. 3. Visual fits. J Neurol Neurosurg Psychiatry 1955; 18:79–96.

Russo LS, Beace G, Sandroni S et al. Aluminum intoxication in undialysed adults with chronic renal failure. J Neurol Neurosurg Psychiatry 1992; 55:697–700.

Rusu V, Chassoux F, Landre E et al. Dystonic posturing in seizures of mesial temporal origin. Electroclinical and metabolic pattern. Neurology 2005; 65:1612–19.

Sacco RL, Freddo L, Bello JA et al. Wallenberg's lateral medullary syndrome. Clinical-magnetic resonance imaging correlations. Arch Neurol 1993; 50:609–14.

Sacco RL, Sivenius J, Diener H-C. Efficacy of aspirin plus extended-release dipyridamole in preventing recurrent stroke in high-risk populations. Arch Neurol 2005; 62:403–8.

Sachdev P, Smith JS, Cathcart S. Schizophrenia-like psychosis following traumatic brain injury: a chart-based descriptive and case-control study. Psychol Med 2001; 31:231–9.

Sadleir LG, Farrell K, Smith S et al. Electroclinical features of absence seizures in childhood absence epilepsy. Neurology 2006; 67:413–18.

Sadler RM, Rahey S. Prescience as an aura of temporal lobe epilepsy. Epilepsia 2004; 45:982–4.

Saenz A, Galan J, Caloustian C et al. Autosomal dominant nocturnal frontal lobe epilepsy in a Spanish family with a SER252PHE mutation in the CHRNA4 gene. Arch Neurol 1999; 56:1004–9.

Salanova V, Andermann F, Olivier A et al. Occipital lobe epilepsy: electroclinical manifestations, electrocorticography, cortical stimulation and outcome in 42 patients treated between 1930 and 1991. Brain 1992; 115:1655–80.

Salanova V, Morris HH, Van Ness P et al. Frontal lobe seizures: electroclinical syndromes. Epilepsia 1995; 36:16–24.

Salazar AM, Jabbari B, Vance SC et al. Epilepsy after penetrating head injury. I. Clinical correlates: a report of the Viet Nam head injury study. Neurology 1985; 35:1406–14.

Salehi F, Kovacs K, Scheihauer BW et al. Histologic study of the human pituitary gland in acute traumatic injury. Brain Inj 2007; 21:651–6.

Salib EA. Subacute sclerosing panencephalitis (SSPE) presenting at the age of 21 as a schizophrenia-like state with bizarre dysmorphophobic features. Br J Psychiatry 1988; 152:709–10.

Salinsky MC, Uthman BM, Ristanovic RK et al. Vagus nerve stimulation for the treatment of medically intractable seizures: results of a 1–year open-extension trial. Arch Neurol 1996; 53:1176–80.

Salmenpara T, Kononen M, Roberts N et al. Hippocampal damage in newly diagnosed focal epilepsy: a prospective MRI study. Neurology 2005; 64:62–8.

Sammaritano M, Andermann F, Melanson D et al. Prolonged focal cerebral edema associated with partial status epilepticus. Epilepsia 1985; 26:334–9.

Samuel M, Duncan JS. Use of hand held video camcorder in the evaluation of seizures. J Neurol Neurosurg Psychiatry 1994; 57:1417–18.

Sander JWAS, Hart YM, Johnson AL et al. National General Practice Study of Epilepsy: newly diagnosed epileptic seizures in a general population. Lancet 1990; 336:1267–71.

Sander JWAS, Hart YM, Trimble MR et al. Vigabatrin and psychosis. J Neurol Neurosurg Psychiatry 1991; 54:435–9.

Sands IJ. The acute psychiatric type of epidemic encephalitis. Am J Psychiatry 1928; 84:975–87.

Sandson TA, Daffner KR, Carvalho PA et al. Frontal lobe dysfunction following infarction of the left-sided medial thalamus. Arch Neurol 1991; 48:1300–3.

Sano K, Malamud N. Clinical significance of sclerosis of cornu Ammonis. Arch Neurol Psychiatry 1953; 70:40–53.

Sarno MT, Buonaguro A, Levita E. Characteristics of verbal impairment in closed head injury patients. Arch Phys Med Rehabil 1986; 67:400–5.

Satel SL, Southwick SM, Gawin FH. Clinical features of cocaine-induced paranoia. Am J Psychiatry 1991; 148:495–8.

Sato S, Dreifuss FE, Penry JK. Prognostic factors in absence seizures. Neurology 1976; 26:788–96.

Sato S, White BG, Penry JK et al. Valproic acid versus ethosuximide in the treatment of absence seizures. Neurology 1982; 32:157–3.

Savard G, Andermann F, Teitelbaum J et al. Epileptic Munchausen's syndrome: a form of pseudoseizures distinct from hysteria and malingering. Neurology 1988; 38:1628–9.

Savard G, Andermann F, Olivier A et al. Postictal psychoses after partial complex seizures: a multiple case study. Epilepsia 1991; 32:225–31.

Saygi S, Spencer SS, Scheyer R et al. Differentiation of temporal lobe ictal behavior associated with hippocampal sclerosis and tumor of the temporal lobe. Epilepsia 1994; 35:737–42.

Sbordone RJ, Seyranian GD, Ruff RM. Are the subjective complaints of traumatically brain injured patients reliable? Brain Inj 1998; 12:505–15.

Schacter SC, Vazquez B, Fisher RS et al. Oxcarbazepine: double-blind, randomized, placebo-controlled monotherapy trial for partial seizures. Neurology 1999; 52:732–7.

Schaumburg HH, Powers JM, Raine CS et al. Adrenoleukodystrophy: a clinical and pathological study of 17 cases. Arch Neurol 1975; 32:577–91.

Scheffer IE, Bhatia KP, Lopes-Cendes I et al. Autosomal dominant nocturnal frontal epilepsy misdiagnosed as a sleep disorder. Lancet 1994; 343:515–17.

Scheffer IE, Bhatia KP, Lopes-Cendes I et al. Autosomal dominant nocturnal frontal lobe epilepsy: a distinctive clinical disorder. Brain 1995; 118:61–73.

Schneider WN, Drew-Cates J, Wong TM et al. Cognitive and behavioral efficacy of amantadine in acute traumatic brain injury: an initial double-blind placebo-controlled study. Brain Inj 1999; 13:863–72.

Scholtes FB, Renier WO, Meinardi H. Simple partial status epilepticus: causes, treatment, and outcome in 47 patients. J Neurol Neurosurg Psychiatry 1996a; 61:90–2.

Scholtes FB, Renier WO, Meinardi H. Non-convulsive status epilepticus: causes, treatment and outcome in 65 patients. J Neurol Neurosurg Psychiatry 1996b; 61:93–5.

Schramm P, Schelliger PD, Klotz E et al. Comparison of perfusion computed tomography and computed tomography angiography source images with perfusion-weighted imaging and diffusion-weighted imaging in patients with acute stroke of less than 6 hours' duration. Stroke 2004; 35:1652–8.

Schube PG. Emotional states of general paresis. Am J Psychiatry 1934; 91:625–38.

Schuckitt MA, Smith TL, Anthenelli R et al. Clinical course of alcoholism in 636 male inpatients. Am J Psychiatry 1993; 150:786–92.

Schufle SU, Bermeo AC, Alexopoulos AV et al. Video-electrographic and clinical features in patients with ictal asystole. Neurology 2007; 69:439–41.

Schulz R, Luders HO, Noachtar S et al. Amnesia of the epileptic aura. Neurology 1995; 45:231–5.

Schwab RS. A case of status epilepticus in petit mal. Electroencephalogr Clin Neurophysiol 1953; 5:441–2.

Scott GM, Gibberb FB. Epilepsy and other factors in the prognosis of gliomas. Acta Neurol Scand 1980; 61:227–39.

Scott JS, Masland RL. Occurrence of 'continuous symptoms' in epilepsy patients. Neurology 1953; 3:297–301.

Seeley WW, Bauer AM, Miller BL et al. The natural history of temporal variant frontotemporal dementia. Neurology 2005; 64:1384–90.

Semel JD. Complex partial status epilepticus presenting as fever of unknown origin. Arch Int Med 1987; 147:1571–2.

Sen S, Laowatana S, Lima J et al. Risk factors for intracardiac thrombus in patients with recent ischemic cerebrovascular events. J Neurol Neurosurg Psychiatry 2004; 75:1421–5.

Serafetinides EA, Falconer MA. Speech disturbance in temporal lobe seizures: a study in 100 epileptic patients submitted to anterior temporal lobectomy. Brain 1963; 86:333–46.

Serby M, Angrist B, Lieberman A. Mental disturbances during bromocriptine and lergotrile treatment of Parkinson's disease. *Am J Psychiatry* 1978; **135**:1227–9.

Seshia SS, McLachlan RS. Aura continua. *Epilepsia* 2005; **46**:454–5.

Sethi PK, Surya R. Gelastic, quiritarian, and cursive epilepsy. *J Neurol Neurosurg Psychiatry* 1976; **39**:823–8.

Shah P, Kaplan SL. Catatonic symptoms in a child with epilepsy. *Am J Psychiatry* 1980; **137**:738–9.

Shavit YB, Graus F, Probst A *et al.* Epilepsia partialis continua: a new manifestation of anti-Hu associated paraneoplastic encephalomyelitis. *Ann Neurol* 1999; **45**:255–8.

Shaw PJ, Walls TJ, Newman PK *et al.* Hashimoto's encephalopathy: a steroid-responsive disorder associated with high anti-thyroid antibody titers – report of 5 cases. *Neurology* 1991; **41**:228–33.

Sherer MA, Kumor KM, Cone EJ *et al.* Suspiciousness induced by four-hour intravenous infusion of cocaine. Preliminary findings. *Arch Gen Psychiatry* 1988; **45**:673–7.

Sheth RD, Drazkowski JF, Sirven JI. Protracted ictal confusion in elderly patients. *Arch Neurol* 2006; **63**:529–32.

Shewmon DA, Masdeu JC. Delayed radiation necrosis of the brain contralateral to original tumor. *Arch Neurol* 1980; **37**:592–4.

Shimoda M, Takeuchi M, Tominaga J *et al.* Asymptomatic versus symptomatic infarcts from vasospasm in patients with subarachnoid hemorrhage: serial magnetic resonance imaging. *Neurosurgery* 2001; **49**:1341–8.

Shiozawa Z, Sasaki H, Ozaki Y *et al.* Epilepsia partialis continua following metrizamide cisternography. *Ann Neurol* 1981; **10**:400–1.

Shukla GD, Mishra DN. Vomiting as sole manifestation of simple partial seizure. *Arch Neurol* 1985; **42**:626.

Siegel AM, Cascino GD, Elger CE *et al.* Adult-onset epilepsy in focal cortical dysplasia of Taylor type. *Neurology* 2005; **64**:1771–4.

Siegel RK. Cocaine hallucinations. *Am J Psychiatry* 1978; **135**:309–14.

Silver JM, Koumaras B, Chen M *et al.* Effects of rivastigmine on cognitive function in patients with traumatic brain injury. *Neurology* 2006; **67**:748–55.

Siesling S, Vegter-van der Vlis M, Roos RAC. Juvenile Huntington's disease in the Netherlands. *Pediatr Neurol* 1997; **17**:34–43.

Silverstein A, Steinberg G, Nathanson M. Nervous system involvement in infectious mononucleosis. *Arch Neurol* 1972; **26**:353–8.

Simonsen N, Olsen PZ, Kuhl V *et al.* A comparative controlled study between carbamazepine and diphenylhydantoin in psychomotor epilepsy. *Epilepsia* 1976; **17**:169–76.

Singh BM, Strobos RJ. Epilepsia partialis continua associated with nonketotic hyperglycemia: clinical and biochemical profile of 21 patients. *Ann Neurol* 1980; **8**:155–60.

Singh BM, Gupta DR, Strobos RJ. Nonketotic hyperglycemia and epilepsia partialis continua. *Arch Neurol* 1973; **29**:187–90.

Sisler GC, Levy LL, Roseman E. Epilepsia cursiva: syndrome of running fits. *Arch Neurol Psychiatry* 1953; **69**:73–9.

Sisodiya SM, Free SL, Stevens JM *et al.* Widespread cerebral structural changes in patients with cortical dysgenesis and epilepsy. *Brain* 1995; **118**:1039–50.

Sisodiya SM, Stevens JM, Fish DR *et al.* The demonstration of gyral abnormalities in patients with cryptogenic partial epilepsy using three-dimensional MRI. *Arch Neurol* 1996; **53**:28–34.

Sittig O. A clinical study of sensory Jacksonian fits. *Brain* 1925; **48**:233–54.

Sivenius J, Kalviainen R, Ylinen A *et al.* Double-blind study of gabapentin in the treatment of partial seizures. *Epilepsia* 1991; **32**:539–42.

Slater E, Beard AW. The schizophrenia-like psychoses of epilepsy. I. Psychiatric aspects. *Br J Psychiatry* 1963a; **109**:95–112.

Slater E, Beard AW. The schizophrenia-like psychoses of epilepsy. V. Discussion and conclusion. *Br J Psychiatry* 1963b; **109**:143–50.

Sloan RL, Brown KW, Pentland B. Fluoxetine as a treatment for emotional lability after brain injury. *Brain Inj* 1992; **6**:315–19.

Smaje JC, Davidson C, Teasdale GM. Sino-atrial arrest due to temporal lobe epilepsy. *J Neurol Neurosurg Psychiatry* 1987; **50**:112–13.

Smith GR, Monson RA, Livingston RL. Somatization disorder in men. *Gen Hosp Psychiatry* 1985; **7**:4–8.

Smith GR, Monson RA, Ray DC. Psychiatric consultation in somatization disorder. A randomized controlled study. *N Engl J Med* 1986; **314**:1407–13.

Smith LH. Mental and neurologic changes in pernicious anemia. *Arch Neurol Psychiatry* 1929; **22**:551–7.

Smith RF, Devinsky O, Luciano D. Inhibitory motor status: two new cases and a review of inhibitory motor seizures. *J Epilepsy* 1997; **10**:15–21.

Smyth GE, Stern K. Tumours of the thalamus: a clinico-pathological study. *Brain* 1938; **61**:339–74.

Snavely SR, Hodges GR. The neurotoxicity of antibacterial agents. *Ann Int Med* 1984; **101**:92–104.

So EL, Schauble BS. Ictal asomatognosia as a cause of epileptic falls. Simultaneous video, EMG, and invasive EEG. *Neurology* 2004; **63**:2153–4.

So EL, King DL, Muruin AJ. Misdiagnosis of complex absence seizures. *Arch Neurol* 1984; **41**:640–1.

So EL, Annegers JF, Hauser WA *et al.* Population-based study of seizure disorders after cerebral infarction. *Neurology* 1996; **46**:350–1.

Sonoo M. Abductor sign: a reliable new sign to detect unilateral non-organic paresis of the lower limb. *J Neurol Neurosurg Psychiatry* 2004; **75**:121–5.

Souid AK, Keith DV, Cunningham AS. Munchausen syndrome by proxy. *Clin Pediatr* 1998; **37**:497–503.

Sowa MV, Pituck S. Prolonged spontaneous visual hallucinations and illusions as ictal phenomena. *Epilepsia* 1989; **30**:524–6.

Soyka M. Psychopathological characteristics in alcohol hallucinosis and paranoid schizophrenia. *Acta Psychiatr Scand* 1990; **81**:255–9.

Soyka M, Naber G, Volcker A. Prevalence of delusional jealousy in different psychiatric disorders. *Br J Psychiatry* 1991; **158**:549–53.

Spatt J. Epilepsia partialis continua in multiple sclerosis. *Lancet* 1995; **345**:658–9.

Speech TJ, Rao SM, Osmon DC et al. A double-blind controlled study of methylphenidate treatment in closed head injury. Brain Inj 1993; 7:333-8.

Spencer SS, Spencer DD, Williamson PD et al. Sexual automatisms in complex partial epilepsy. Neurology 1983; 33:527-33.

Sperling MR, Wilson CL. The effect of limbic and extralimbic electrical stimulations upon prolactin secretion in humans. Brain Res 1986; 371:293-7.

Sperling MR, Pritchard PB, Engel J et al. Prolactin in partial epilepsy: an indicator of limbic seizures. Ann Neurol 1986; 20:716-22.

Sperling MR, Lieb JP, Engel J et al. Prognostic significance of independent auras in temporal lobe seizures. Epilepsia 1989; 30:322-31.

Spooner CG, Berkovic SF, Mitchell LA et al. New-onset temporal lobe epilepsy in children. Lesion on MRI predicts poor seizure control. Neurology 2006; 67:2147-53.

Spratling WP. Epilepsy, its etiology, pathology and treatment briefly considered. JAMA 1902; 38:1126-30.

Stanislav SW. Cognitive effects of antipsychotic agents in persons with traumatic brain injury. Brain Inj 1997; 11:335-41.

Starkstein SE, Mayberg HS, Berthier ML et al. Mania after brain injury: neuroradiological and metabolic findings. Ann Neurol 1990; 27:652-9.

Starosta-Rubinstein S, Young AB, Kluin K et al. Clinical assessment of 31 patients with Wilson's disease: correlations with structural changes on magnetic resonance imaging. Arch Neurol 1987; 44:365-70.

Steegmann AT, Winer B. Temporal lobe epilepsy resulting from ganglioglioma. Neurology 1961; 11:406-12.

Stefan H, Wang-Tilz Y, Pauli E et al. Onset of action of levetiracetam; a RCT trial using therapeutic intensive seizure analysis. Epilepsia 2006; 47:516-22.

Steffenburg S, Gillberg C, Steffenburg U. Psychiatric disorders in children and adolescents with mental retardation and active epilepsy. Arch Neurol 1996; 53:904-12.

Steiner I, Budka H, Chaudhuri A et al. Viral encephalitis: a review of diagnostic methods and guidelines for management. Eur J Neurol 2005; 12:331-43.

Steiner W, Laporta M, Chouinard G. Neuroleptic-induced supersensitivity psychosis in patients with bipolar affective disorder. Acta Psychiatr Scand 1990; 81:437-40.

Stone J, Zeman A, Sharpe M. Functional weakness and sensory disturbance. J Neurol Neurosurg Psychiatry 2002; 73:241-5.

Stone J, Townend E, Kwan J et al. Personality change after stroke: some preliminary observations. J Neurol Neurosurg Psychiatry 2004; 75:1708-13.

Stone J, Smyth R, Carson A et al. La belle indifference in conversion symptoms and hysteria: systematic review. Br J Psychiatry 2006; 188:204-9.

Storm-Mathisen A. General paresis: a follow-up study of 203 patients. Acta Psychiatr Scand 1969; 45:118-32.

Stracciari A, Ciucci G, Bianchedi G et al. Epileptic transient amnesia. Eur Neurol 1990; 30:176-9.

Strauss H. Paroxysmal convulsive running and the concept of epilepsia cursiva. Neurology 1960; 10:341-4.

Strauss I, Keschner M. Mental symptoms in cases of tumor of the frontal lobe. Arch Neurol Psychiatry 1935; 33:986-1007.

Strobos RRJ. Tumors of the temporal lobe. Neurology 1953; 3:752-60.

Strub RL. Frontal lobe syndrome in a patient with bilateral globus pallidus lesions. Arch Neurol 1989; 46:1024-7.

Sturm JW, Andermann F, Berkovic SF. 'Pressure to laugh': an unusual epileptic symptom associated with small hypothalamic hamartomas. Neurology 2000; 54:971-3.

Sturm JW, Fedi M, Berkovic SF et al. Exercise induced temporal lobe epilepsy. Neurology 2002; 59:1246-8.

Suarez JI, Tarr RW, Selman WR. Aneurysmal subarachnoid hemorrahge. N Engl J Med 2006; 354:387-96.

Supino-Viterbo V, Sicard C, Risvegliato M et al. Toxic encephalopathy due to ingestion of bismuth salts: clinical and EEG studies of 45 patients. J Neurol Neurosurg Psychiatry 1977; 40:748-52.

Sussman NM, Jackel RA, Kaplan LR et al. Bicycling movements as a manifestation of complex partial seizures of temporal lobe origin. Epilepsia 1989; 30:527-31.

Sutherling WW, Risinger MW, Crandall PH et al. Focal functional anatomy of dorsolateral frontocentral seizures. Neurology 1990; 40:87-98.

Swanson AG, Iseri OA. Acute encephalopathy due to water intoxication. N Engl J Med 1958; 258:831-4.

Swartz BE. Electrophysiology of bimanual-bipedal automatisms. Epilepsia 1994; 35:264-74.

Swartz BE, Tomiyasu U, Delgado-Escueta AV et al. Neuroimaging in temporal lobe epilepsy: test sensitivity and relationships to pathology and postoperative outcome. Epilepsia 1992; 33:624-34.

Swigar ME, Bowers MB. Baclofen withdrawal and neuropsychiatric symptoms: a case report and review of other case literature. Compr Psychiatry 1986; 27:394-400.

Symonds C. Excitation and inhibition in epilepsy. Brain 1959; 82:133-46.

Szabo K, Poepel A, Pohlmann-Eden B et al. Diffusion-weighted and perfusion MRI demonstrates parenchymal changes in complex partial status epilepticus. Brain 2005; 128:1369-76.

Tachibana N, Shinde A, Ikede A et al. Supplementary motor area seizure resembling sleep disorder. Sleep 1996; 19:811-16.

Tanaka N, Sakurai K, Kamada K et al. Neuromagnetic source localization of epileptiform actitivity in patients with graphigenic epilepsy. Epilepsia 2006; 47;1963-7.

Tassi L, Colombo N, Cossu M et al. Electroclinical, MRI and neuropathological study of 10 patients with nodular heterotopia, with surgical outcomes. Brain 2005; 128:321-37.

Tassinari CA, Tassi L, Calandra-Buonaura G et al. Biting behavior, aggression, and seizures. Epilepsia 2005; 46:654-63.

Tateno A, Jorge RE, Robinson RG. Pathological laughing and crying after traumatic brain injury. J Neuropsychiatry Clin Neurosci 2004; 16:126-34.

Tatu L, Moulin T, Bogousslavsky J et al. Arterial territories of human brain: brainstem and cerebellum. Neurology 1996; 47:1125-35.

Tatu L, Moulin T, Bogousslavsky J et al. Arterial territories of human brain: cerebral hemispheres. Neurology 1998; 50:1699-708.

Tatum WO, Passaro EA, Elia M *et al.* Seizure in Klinefelter's syndrome. *Pediatr Neurology* 1998; **19**:275–82.

Tayah TF, Abou-KhalilB, Gilliam FG *et al.* Musicogenic seizures can arise from multiple temporal lobe foci: intracranial EEG analyses of three patients. *Epilepsia* 2006; **47**:1402–6.

Taylor DC, Marsh SM. Hughlings Jackson's Dr. Z: the paradigm of temporal lobe epilepsy revealed. *J Neurol Neurosurg Psychiatry* 1980; **43**:758–67.

Taylor DC, Falconer MA, Bruton CJ *et al.* Focal dysplasia of the cerebral cortex in epilepsy. *J Neurol Neurosurg Psychiatry* 1971; **34**:369–87.

Taylor J ed. *Selected writings of John Hughlings Jackson.* London: Hodder & Stoughton, 1931.

Teasdale G, Jennett B. Assessment of coma and impaired consciousness. A practical scale. *Lancet* 1974; **2**:81–4.

Temkin NR, Dikmen SS, Wilensky AJ *et al.* A randomized, double-blind study of phenytoin for the prevention of post-traumatic seizures. *N Engl J Med* 1990; **323**:497–502.

Temkin NR, Dikmen SS, Anderson GD *et al.* Valproate therapy for prevention of posttraumatic seizures: a randomized trial. *J Neurosurg* 1999; **91**:593–600.

Tenembaum S, Chamoles N, Fejerman N. Acute disseminated encephalomyelitis. A long-term follow-up study of 84 pediatric patients. *Neurology* 2002; **59**:1224–31.

Thacore VR, Shukla SRP. Cannabis psychosis and paranoid schizophrenia. *Arch Gen Psychiatry* 1976; **33**:383–6.

Theodore WH, Porter RJ, Penry JK. Complex partial seizures: clinical characteristics and differential diagnosis. *Neurology* 1983; **33**:1115–21.

Theodore WH, Porter RJ, Albert P *et al.* The secondarily generalized tonic-clonic seizure: a videotape analysis. *Neurology* 1994; **44**:1403–7.

Thomas CS, Szabadi E. Paranoid psychosis as the first presentation of a fulminating lethal case of AIDS. *Br J Psychiatry* 1987; **151**:693–5.

Thomas JE, Reagen TJ, Klass DW. Epilepsia partialis continua. A review of 32 cases. *Arch Neurol* 1977; **34**:266–75.

Thomas P, Valton L, Genton P. Absence and myoclonic status epilepticus precipitated by antiepileptic drugs in idiopathic generalized epilepsies. *Brain* 2006; **129**:1281–92.

Thompson AJ, Kermode AG, Moseley JF *et al.* Seizures due to multiple sclerosis: seven patients with MRI correlations. *J Neurol Neurosurg Psychiatry* 1993; **56**:1317–20.

Thompson GN, Nielsen JM. The organic paranoid syndrome. *J Nerv Ment Dis* 1949; **110**:478–96.

Thompson SW, Greenhouse HH. Petit mal status in adults. *Ann Intern Med* 1968; **68**:1271–9.

Thomsen IV. Late outcome of very severe blunt head trauma: a 10–15 year second follow-up. *J Neurol Neurosurg Psychiatry* 1984; **47**:260–8.

Tinuper P, Provini F, Marini C *et al.* Partial epilepsy of long duration: changing semiology with age. *Epilepsia* 1996a; **37**:162–4.

Tinuper P, Plazzi G, Provini F *et al.* Celiac disease, epilepsy, and occipital calcification: histopathological study and clinical outcome. *J Epilepsy* 1996b; **9**:206–9.

Tinuper P, Cerullo A, Marini C *et al.* Epileptic drop attacks in partial epilepsy: clinical features, evolution, and prognosis. *J Neurol Neurosurg Psychiatry* 1998; **64**:231–7.

Todd R. *Clinical lectures on paralysis, diseases of the brain, and other affections of the nervous system.* Philadelphia: Lindsay & Blakiston, 1855.

Tomson T, Svanborg E, Wedlund J-E. Nonconvulsive status epilepticus: high incidence of complex partial status. *Epilepsia* 1986; **27**:276–85.

Tomson T, Lindbom U, Nilsson BY *et al.* Serum prolactin during status epilepticus. *J Neurol Neurosurg Psychiatry* 1989; **52**:1435–7.

Tomson T, Lindbom U, Nilsson BY. Nonconvulsive status epilepticus in adults. Thirty-two consecutive patients from a general hospital population. *Epilepsia* 1992; **33**:829–35.

Towne AR, Waterhouse EJ, Boggs JG *et al.* Prevalence of nonconvulsive status epilepticus in comatose patients. *Neurology* 2000; **54**:340–5.

Treiman DM, Meyers PD, Walton NY *et al.* A comparison of four treatments for generalized convulsive status epilepticus. Veterans Affairs Status Epilepticus Cooperative Study Group. *N Engl J Med* 1998; **339**:792–8.

Trethowan WH, Cobb S. Neuropsychiatric aspects of Cushing's syndrome. *Arch Neurol Psychiatry* 1952; **67**:283–309.

Trouillas P, Courjon J. Epilepsy with multiple sclerosis. *Epilepsia* 1972; **13**:325–33.

Troupin A, Ojemann LM, Halpern L *et al.* Carbamazepine – a double-blind comparison with phenytoin. *Neurology* 1977; **27**:511–19.

Tsai JJ, Yen DJ, Hsih MS *et al.* Efficacy and safety of levetiracetam (up to 2000 mg/day) in Taiwanese patients with refractory partial seizures: a multicenter, randomized, double-blind, placebo-controlled study. *Epilepsia* 2006; **47**:72–81.

Tsoi WF. The Ganser syndrome in Singapore: a report on ten cases. *Br J Psychiatry* 1973; **123**:567–72.

Tsukamoto T, Mochizuki R, Mochizuki H *et al.* Paraneoplastic cerebellar degeneration and limbic encephalitis in a patient with adenocarcinoma of the colon. *J Neurol Neurosurg Psychiatry* 1993; **56**:713–16.

Tucker GJ, Price TRP, Johnson VB *et al.* Phenomenology of temporal lobe dysfunction: a link to atypical psychosis: a series of cases. *J Nerv Ment Dis* 1986; **174**:348–56.

Tucker WM, Forster FM. Petit mal epilepsy occurring in status. *Arch Neurol Psychiatry* 1958; **64**:823–7.

Tukel K, Jasper H. The electroencephalogram in parasaggital lesions. *Electroencephalogr Clin Neurophysiol* 1952; **4**:481–94.

Tyler RH. Neurologic disorders in renal failure. *Am J Med* 1968; **44**:734–48.

Umbricht D, Degreef G, Barr WB *et al.* Postictal and chronic psychoses in patients with temporal lobe epilepsy. *Am J Psychiatry* 1995; **152**:224–31.

US Gabapentin Study Group. Gabapentin as add-on therapy in refractory partial epilepsy: a double-blind, placebo-controlled, parallel-group study. *Neurology* 1993; **43**:2292–8.

Van Rossum J, Groeneveld-Ockhuysen AAW, Arts RJHM. Psychomotor status. *Arch Neurol* 1985; **42**:989–93.

Varma NK, Lee SI. Nonconvulsive status epilepticus following electroconvulsive therapy. *Neurology* 1992; **42**:263–4.

Venneri A, Caffarra P. Transient autobiographic amnesia: EEG and single-photon emission CT evidence of an organic etiology. *Neurology* 1998; **50**:186–91.

Verny M, Jellinger KA, Hauw J-J *et al.* Progressive supranuclear palsy: a clinicopathological study of 21 cases. *Acta Neuropathologica* 1996; **61**:427–31.

Vickrey BG, Bahls FH. Nonconvulsive status epilepticus following cerebral angiography. *Ann Neurol* 1989; **25**:199–201.

Victor M, Brausch J. The role of abstinence in the genesis of alcohol epilepsy. *Epilepsia* 1967; **8**:1–20.

Victor M, Hope JM. The phenomenon of auditory hallucinations in chronic alcoholism. *J Nerv Ment Dis* 1958; **126**:451–8.

Videbech T. Chronic olfactory paranoid syndrome. *Acta Psychiatr Scand* 1966; **42**:183–213.

Villani F, D'Amico D, Pincherle A *et al.* Prolonged focal negative motor seizures: a video-EEG study. *Epilepsia* 2006; **47**:1949–52.

Vizioli R, Magliocco EB. A case of prolonged petit mal seizures. *Electroencephalogr Clin Neurophysiol* 1953; **5**:439–40.

Vollmer TL, Guarnaccia J, Harrington W *et al.* Idiopathic granulomatous angiitis of the central nervous system: diagnostic challenges. *Arch Neurol* 1993; **50**:925–30.

Vroom FQ, Greer M. Mercury vapor intoxication. *Brain* 1972; **95**:305–18.

Vuilleumier P, Chicherio C, Assal F *et al.* Functional neuroanatomical correlates of hysterical sensorimotor loss. *Brain* 2001; **124**:1077–90.

Wallin WT, Kurtzke JF. Neurocysticercosis in the United States. Review of an important emerging infection. *Neurology* 2004; **63**:1559–64.

Walczak TS, Rubinsky M. Plantar responses after epileptic seizures. *Neurology* 1994; **44**:2191–3.

Walczak TS, Williams DT, Berten W. Utility and reliability of placebo infusion in the evaluation of patients with seizures. *Neurology* 1994; **44**:394–9.

Walshe FMR. On the mode of representation of movements in the motor cortex, with special reference to 'convulsions beginning unilaterally' (Jackson). *Brain* 1943; **66**:104–39.

Walshe JM, Yealland M. Wilson's disease: the problem of delayed diagnosis. *J Neurol Neurosurg Psychiatry* 1992; **55**:692–6.

Wallach J. Laboratory diagnosis of factitious disorders. *Arch Int Med* 1994; **154**:1690–6.

Walton RG. Seizure and mania after high intake of aspartame. *Psychosomatics* 1986; **27**:218–20.

Waltz G, Harik SI, Kaufman B. Adult metachromatic leukodystrophy: value of computed tomographic scanning and magnetic resonance imaging of the brain. *Arch Neurol* 1987; **44**:225–7.

Waltzer H. A psychotic family – folie a douze. *J Nerv Ment Dis* 1963; **137**:67–75.

Warner TT, Williams LD, Walker RWH *et al.* A clinical and molecular genetic study of dentatorubropallidoluysian atrophy in four European families. *Ann Neurol* 1995; **37**:452–9.

Watanabe TK, O'Dell MW, Togliatti TJ. Diagnosis and rehabilitation strategies for patients with hysterical

hemiparesis: a report of four cases. *Arch Phys Med Rehabil* 1998; **79**:1482–3.

Waxman SG, Geschwind M. Hypergraphia in temporal lobe epilepsy. *Neurology* 1974; **24**:629–36.

Waxman SG, Geschwind N. The interictal behavior syndrome of temporal lobe epilepsy. *Arch Gen Psychiatry* 1975; **32**:1580–6.

Weil AA. Depressive reactions associated with temporal lobe–uncinate seizures. *J Nerv Ment Dis* 1955; **121**:505–10.

Weil AA. Ictal depression and anxiety in temporal lobe disorders. *Am J Psychiatry* 1956; **113**:149–57.

Weil AA. Ictal emotions occurring in temporal lobe dysfunction. *Arch Neurol Psychiatry* 1959; **1**:101–11.

Weilburg JB, Bear DM, Sachs G. Three patients with concomitant panic attacks and seizure disorder: possible clues to the neurology of anxiety. *Am J Psychiatry* 1987; **144**:1053–6.

Weiller C, Ringelstein EB, Reiche W *et al.* The large striatocapsular infarct: a clinical and pathological entity. *Arch Neurol* 1990; **47**:1085–91.

Weinberger J. Simultaneous bilateral focal seizures without loss of consciousness. *Mt Sinai J Med* 1973; **40**:693–6.

Wells CE. Transient ictal psychosis. *Arch Gen Psychiatry* 1975; **32**:1201–3.

Wharton RM. Grand mal seizures with lithium treatment. *Am J Psychiatry* 1969; **125**:1446.

Wheless JW, Vazquez BR, Kanner AM *et al.* Rapid infusion with valproate sodium is well-tolerated in patients with epilepsy. *Neurology* 2004; **63**:1507–8.

Whitfield CL, Ch'ien LT, Whitehead JD. Lead encephalopathy in adults. *Am J Med* 1972; **52**:289–98.

Whyte J, Hart T, Vaccaro M *et al.* Effects of methylphenidate on attention deficits after traumatic brain injury: a multidimensional, randomized, controlled trial. *Am J Phys Med Rehabil* 2004; **83**:401–20.

Wiart L, Petit H, Joseph PA *et al.* Fluoxetine in early poststroke depression: a double-blind placebo-controlled study. *Stroke* 2000; **31**:1829–32.

Wiebe S, Blume WT, Girvin JP *et al.* A randomized, controlled trial of surgery for temporal-lobe epilepsy. *N Engl J Med* 2001; **345**:311–18.

Wieser HG. Temporal lobe or psychomotor status epilepticus. A case report. *Electroencephalogr Clin Neurophysiol* 1980; **48**:558–72.

Wieser HG, Hungerbuhler H, Siegel AM *et al.* Musicogenic epilepsy: review of the literature and case report with ictal single photon emission computed tomography. *Epilepsia* 1997; **38**:200–7.

Wijdicks EFM, Plevak DJ, Wiesner RH *et al.* Course and outcome of seizures in liver transplant patients. *Neurology* 1996; **47**:1523–5.

Wilder-Smith E. Complete atrio-ventricular block during complex partial seizure. *J Neurol Neurosurg Psychiatry* 1992; **55**:734–6.

Wilkinson HA. Epileptic pain. An uncommon manifestation with localizing value. *Neurology* 1973; **23**:518–20.

Williams BB, Lerner AM. Some previously unrecognized features of herpes simplex encephalitis. *Neurology* 1978; **28**:1193–6.

Williams D. The structure of emotions reflected in epileptic experiences. *Brain* 1956; **79**:29–67.

Williamson PD, Spencer SS. Clinical and EEG features of complex partial seizures of extratemporal origin. *Epilepsia* 1986; **27**(suppl. 2):46–63.

Williamson PD, Spencer DD, Spencer SS *et al.* Episodic aphemia and epileptic focus in the nondominant hemisphere: relieved by section of the corpus callosum. *Neurology* 1985a; **35**:1069–71.

Williamson PD, Spencer DD, Spencer SS *et al.* Complex partial status epilepticus: a depth-electrode study. *Ann Neurol* 1985b; **18**:647–54.

Williamson PD, Spencer DD, Spencer SS *et al.* Complex partial seizures of frontal lobe origin. *Ann Neurol* 1985c; **18**:497–504.

Williamson PD, Thadani VM, Darcey TM *et al.* Occipital lobe epilepsy: clinical characteristics, seizure spread patterns, and results of surgery. *Ann Neurol* 1992a; **31**:3–13.

Williamson PD, Boon PA, Thadani VM *et al.* Parietal lobe epilepsy: diagnostic considerations and results of surgery. *Ann Neurol* 1992b; **31**:193–201.

Williamson PD, French JA, Thadani VM *et al.* Characteristics of medial temporal lobe epilepsy. II. Interictal and ictal scalp electroencephalography, neuropsychological testing, neuroimaging, surgical results, and pathology. *Ann Neurol* 1993; **34**:781–7.

Williamson RT. On the symptomatology of gross lesions (tumours and abscesses) involving the pre-frontal regions of the brain. *Brain* 1896; **19**:346–65.

Willmore LJ, Shu V, Wallin B. Efficacy and safety of add-on divalproex sodium in the treatment of complex partial seizures. *Neurology* 1996; **46**:49–53.

Willoughby JO, Pope KJ, Eaton V. Nicotine as an antiepileptic agent in ADNFLE: an N-of-one study. *Epilepsia* 2003; **44**:1238–40.

Wilson LG. Viral encephalopathy mimicking functional psychosis. *Am J Psychiatry* 1976; **133**:165–70.

Wilson P, Preece AA. Chorea gravidarum. *Arch Intern Med* 1932; **49**:671–97.

Wilson SAK. Progressive lenticular degeneration: a familial nervous disease associated with cirrhosis of the liver. *Brain* 1912; **34**:295–509.

Wilson SAK. Nervous semiology, with special reference to epilepsy. *BMJ* 1930; **2**:50–4.

Wilson WH, Claussen AM. Seizures associated with clozapine treatment in a state hospital. *J Clin Psychiatry* 1994; **55**:184–8.

Winawer MR, Ottman R, Hauser A *et al.* Autosomal dominant partial epilepsy with auditory features: defining the phenotype. *Neurology* 2000; **54**:2173–6.

Winokur G. Delusional disorder (paranoia). *Compr Psychiatry* 1977; **18**:511–21.

Wintermark M, Reichart M, Cuisenaire O *et al.* Comparison of admission perfusion computed tomography and qualitative diffusion- and perfusion weighted magnetic resonance imaging in acute stroke patients. *Stroke* 2002a; **33**:2025–31.

Wintermark M, Reichart M, Thiran J-P *et al.* Prognostic accuracy of cerebral blood flow measurement by perfusion computed tomography, at the time of emergency room admission, in acute stroke patients. *Ann Neurol* 2002b; **51**:417–32.

Wisniewski KE, Frency JH, Fernando S *et al.* Fragile X syndrome: associated neurological abnormalities and developmental disabilities. *Ann Neurol* 1985; **18**:665–9.

Wojner-Alexandrov AW, Garami Z, Chernyshev OY *et al.* Heads down. Flat positioning improves blood flow velocity in acute ischemic stroke. *Neurology* 2005; **64**:1354–7.

Worrell GA, Sencakova D, Jack CR *et al.* Rapidly progressive hippocampal atrophy: evidence for a seizure-induced mechanism. *Neurology* 2002; **58**:1553–6.

Wroblewski BA, McColgan K, Smith K *et al.* The incidence of seizures during tricyclic antidepressant drug treatment in a brain-injured population. *J Clin Psychopharmacol* 1990; **10**:124–8.

Wroblewski BA, Joseph AB, Cornbatt RR. Antidepressant pharmacotherapy and the treatment of depression in patients with severe traumatic brain injury: a controlled, prospective study. *J Clin Psychiatry* 1996; **57**:582–7.

Wroblewski BA, Joseph AB, Kupfer J *et al.* Effectiveness of valproic acid on destructive and aggressive behaviors in patients with acquired brain injury. *Brain Inj* 1997; **11**:37–47.

Wyllie E, Luders H, MacMillan JP *et al.* Serum prolactin levels after epileptic seizures. *Neurology* 1984; **34**:1601–3.

Yadav JS, Wholex MH, Kuntz RF *et al.* Protected carotid artery stenting versus endarterectomy in high-risk patients. *N Engl J Med* 2004; **351**:1493–1501.

Yamada H, Yoshida H. Laughing attack: a review and report of nine cases. *Folia Psychiatr Neurol Japonica* 1977; **31**:129–37.

Yen D-J, Su M-S, Shih Y-H *et al.* Ictal speech manifestations in temporal lobe epilepsy: a video-EEG study. *Epilepsia* 1996; **37**:45–9.

Yenjun S, harvey AS, Marini C *et al.* EEG in adult-onset idiopathic generalized epilepsy. *Epilepsia* 2003; **44**:252–6.

York GK, Gabor AJ, Dreyfuss PM. Paroxysmal genital pain: an unusual manifestation of epilepsy. *Neurology* 1979; **29**:516–19.

Young GB, Blume WT. Painful epileptic seizures. *Brain* 1983; **106**:537–44.

Young GB, Blume WT. Painful epileptic seizures involving the secondary sensory area. *Ann Neurol* 1986; **19**:412.

Zak R, Solomon G, Petito F *et al.* Baclofen-induced generalized nonconvulsive status epilepticus. *Ann Neurol* 1994; **36**:113–14.

Zappoli R. Two cases of prolonged twilight state with almost continuous 'wave-spikes'. *Electroencephalogr Clin Neurophysiol* 1955; **7**:421–3.

Zarling EJ. Abdominal epilepsy: an unusual cause of recurrent abdominal pain. *Am J Gastroenterol* 1984; **79**:687–8.

Zeidler M, Johnstone EC, Bamber RWK *et al.* New variant Creutzfeldt–Jakob disease: psychiatric features. *Lancet* 1997a; **350**:908–10.

Zeidler M, Stewart GE, Barraclough CR *et al.* New variant Creutzfeldt–Jakob disease: neurological features and diagnostic tests. *Lancet* 1997b; **350**:903–7.

Zeilig G, Drubach DA, Katz-Zeilig M *et al.* Pathological laughter and crying in patients with closed traumatic brain injury. *Brain Inj* 1996; **10**:591–7.

Zeman A, Stone J, Porteous M *et al.* Spinocerebellar ataxia type 8 in Scotland: genetic and clinical features in seven unrelated cases and a review of published reports. *J Neurol Neurosurg Psychiatry* 2004; **75**:459–65.

Zeman AZJ, Boniface SJ, Hodges JR. Transient epileptic amnesia: a description of the clinical and neuropsychological features in 10 cases and a review of the literature. *J Neurol Neurosurg Psychiatry* 1998; **64**:435–43.

Zeng S, Kim CH, Rahman H. Psychotic symptoms presented in familial Creutzfeldt-Jakob disease, subtype E200K. *J Clin Psychiatry* 2001; **62**:735.

Zentner J, Hufnagel A, Wolf HK *et al.* Surgical treatment of temporal lobe epilepsy: clinical, radiological, and histopathological findings in 178 patients. *J Neurol Neurosurg Psychiatry* 1995; **58**:666–73.

Zhang L, Plotkin RC, Wang G *et al.* Cholinergic augmentation with donepezil enhances recovery in short-term memory and sustained attention after traumatic brain injury. *Arch Phys Med Rehabil* 2004; **85**:1050–5.

Zifko U, Lindner K, Wimberger D *et al.* Jarisch–Herxheimer reaction in a patient with neurosyphilis. *J Neurol Neurosurg Psychiatry* 1994; **57**:865–7.

van Zomeren AH, van den Berg W. Residual complaints of patients two years after severe head injury. *J Neurol Neurosurg Psychiatry* 1985; **48**:21–8.

PART III

SPECIFIC DISORDERS

8 Neurodegenerative and movement disorders

8.1 ALZHEIMER'S DISEASE

Alzheimer's disease is the most common cause of dementia in the elderly, accounting for about one-half of all cases in this age group. The prevalence of Alzheimer's disease increases with age: in those under 65 years approximately 1 percent will be affected, whereas in those aged 65 years some 5–10 percent will have the disease, and in those 85 years or older the prevalence rises to 20–40 percent. Women are slightly more likely to be affected than men.

The first known case of this disease occurred in a 51-year-old woman, Auguste D, who was initially seen by Alois Alzheimer in 1901 at the Frankfurt State Asylum. Alzheimer subsequently moved to Munich to work with Kraepelin and, after Auguste D died, he presented his findings on 3 November 1906 at the 37th annual meeting of the Southwest German Psychiatrists in Tubingen; these findings were published in 1907 (Alzheimer 1907). Alzheimer himself was diffident about lending his name to the disease, and it was only at the urging of Kraepelin that he agreed, thus giving us now the most famous of all medical eponyms (Amaducci et al. 1986; Maurer et al. 1997).

Clinical features

Although onsets in early adulthood may occur, the vast majority of cases present gradually and insidiously past the age of 50 years. In the vast majority of cases, the presentation is with a progressively worsening amnesia; in most of these cases, the amnesia is joined by a gradually progressive personality change.

With amnesia as the presenting feature, patients gradually become more and more forgetful (Bowler et al. 1997; Didic et al. 1998; Linn et al. 1995): the location of keys, wallets, or purses is forgotten, and patients may have difficulty recollecting what has happened earlier in the day; eventually, disorientation to time and place occur. Over time, as this anterograde component of the amnesia grows more profound, it is typically joined by a progressively worsening retrograde component: patients may forget where they have worked, the names of their children, the fact that they have been married, where they went to high school, etc. The fact that the amnesia is of the declarative or 'episodic' form, rather than the 'procedural' type, can make for some startling contrasts in the clinical picture. Thus, profoundly amnestic patients may still 'remember' how to play card games or musical instruments (Beatty *et al.* 1994). For example, one patient (Crystal *et al.* 1989), a professional musician, although unable to remember the names of various musical pieces or their composers, was nevertheless still able to play Beethoven's fifth symphony flawlessly on the piano.

Personality change may take various forms: apathy, indifference, and withdrawal are most common. Patients may also develop a frontal lobe syndrome, with coarseness, impulsivity, and disinhibition (Mega *et al.* 1996; Petry *et al.* 1988).

Rarely, Alzheimer's disease may present with an aphasia that may be expressive or, much less commonly, receptive, which gradually worsens as dementia supervenes (Clark *et al.* 2003; Galton *et al.* 2000; Green *et al.* 1990; Greene *et al.* 1996; Karbe *et al.* 1993; Knibb *et al.* 2006). Even more rarely, the presentation may be with a gradually worsening apraxia (Ross *et al.* 1996).

With gradual progression, further cognitive deficits accrue to eventually complete the clinical syndrome of dementia. Attempts have been made to subdivide the course of the dementia of Alzheimer's disease into various stages, such as 'mild', 'moderate', and 'severe' and, although this has some merit, it must be kept in mind that there is substantial overlap among these stages. The mild stage is characterized primarily by cognitive deficits: in addition to the amnesia, one also finds a decrease in abstracting and calculating abilities; there is also often a degree of anomia and apraxia. In the moderate stage, cognitive ability deteriorates further and speech may deteriorate into a fluent aphasia (Faber-Langendoen *et al.* 1988; Price *et al.* 1993). In the severe stage there is a profound cognitive deficit, and patients are often totally dependent on others for their care; mutism may occur, or there may be echolalia or palilalia.

In addition to cognitive deficits most patients will also develop mood changes and psychotic symptoms, generally during the moderate stage. Mood changes may include depression, apathy, anxiety and irritability, agitation, and euphoria (Mega *et al.* 1996). Depressive symptoms are fairly common, with prevalence figures noted of 14 percent (Klatka *et al.* 1996), 24 percent (Burns *et al.* 1990a) and 52 percent (Starkstein *et al.* 2005), and these symptoms tend to persist over a long follow-up period (Starkstein *et al.* 1997). The severity of the depression varies from mild to that encountered in the depressive episodes of a major depression (Migliorelli *et al.* 1995). Apathy may accompany depression, but it may also be seen in a pure form in roughly one-third of all patients (Starkstein *et al.* 2006). Anxiety and irritability are about as common as depression, being found in a little less than one-half of patients (Litvan *et al.* 1996a; Mega *et al.* 1996). Agitation is very common, found in over one-half of patients (Lopez *et al.* 2003). Euphoria, by contrast, is uncommon, being found in from 4 percent (Burns *et al.* 1990a) to 8 percent (Mega *et al.* 1996) of cases.

Psychotic symptoms include hallucinations, either visual or auditory, and delusions. Hallucinations are noted in from 10 percent (Mega *et al.* 1996) to 35 percent (Klatka *et al.* 1996) of patients and are more commonly visual than auditory (Burns *et al.* 1990b; Forstl *et al.* 1993; Ropacki and Jeste 2005). Delusions are found in from 16 percent (Burns *et al.* 1990c) to 53 percent (Klatka *et al.* 1996). Common delusional themes (Binetti *et al.* 1993; Burns *et al.* 1990c; Devanand *et al.* 1997; Forstl *et al.* 1993; Hirono *et al.* 1998) include misidentification, theft, the Capgras phenomenon, and the phantom boarder. Patients may misidentify other people and sometimes their own homes. They may insist that things have been stolen or taken from them, and they may be terrified that family members are actually imposters who have come to annoy or torment them; some may insist that someone, perhaps someone malevolent, is in fact hiding in the house, perhaps in the attic or the cellar. In some cases, misidentification may be quite remarkable, and patients may insist that their own reflection in the mirror is in fact not them (Forstl *et al.* 1993). Interestingly, although it is very rare for Alzheimer's disease to present with psychosis, this was in fact the presentation in Alzheimer's first patient, Auguste D, who presented, at the age of 51 years, with a delusion of jealousy regarding her husband (Maurer *et al.* 1997; Wilkins and Brody 1969a).

Other symptoms may appear as the dementia progresses, including 'frontal release' signs (such as snout and grasp reflexes), astereognosis, and agraphesthesia (Huff *et al.* 1987). Anosognosia is seen in a minority early on, but becomes common with disease progression (Starkstein *et al.* 1997). Parkinsonism may be seen late in the course in a minority of cases, being typically characterized by rigidity and bradykinesia, with tremor being relatively rare (Clark *et al.* 1997; Scarmeas *et al.* 2004). Seizures may also occur in a small minority (Amatniek *et al.* 2006; Goodman 1953); these tend to be grand mal and occur late in the course of the disease (Romanelli *et al.* 1990). Very late in the course, a minority may also have myoclonus (Benesch *et al.* 1993; Chen *et al.* 1991; Faden and Townsend 1976). Other possible symptoms include emotional incontinence (Starkstein *et al.* 1995), the Kluver–Bucy syndrome (Lilly *et al.* 1983), and, very rarely, hemiparesis (Jagust *et al.* 1990).

Magnetic resonance imaging (MRI) and computed tomography (CT) scanning reveal cortical atrophy and ventricular dilation. Early on in the course, the degree of this change may still be within the broadly defined limits of normal for the elderly population, but with progression, the changes become quite pronounced, as illustrated in Figures 8.1 and 8.2. The electroencephalogram is typically normal in mild disease; however, with progression generalized theta, and eventually delta, slowing appears. Although routine cerebrospinal fluid (CSF) studies are normal, measurement of CSF beta-amyloid and tau protein may be of diagnostic import. As noted below, Alzheimer's disease is characterized pathologically by neuritic plaques composed of an amyloid core, and by neurofibrillary tangles composed of hyperphosphorylated tau protein. CSF studies have demonstrated both a decreased level of beta-amyloid

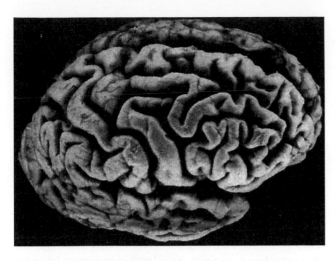

Figure 8.1 Note the relative sparing of the pre- and post-central gyri compared with the rest of the cortex in this case of Alzheimer's disease. (Reproduced from Rees *et al.* 1996.)

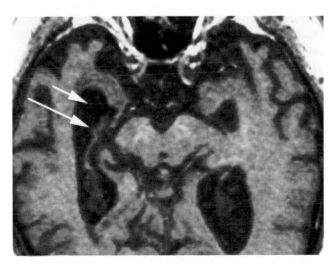

Figure 8.2 This T1-weighted magnetic resonance imaging scan demonstrates the cortical atrophy and ventricular dilation found in advanced Alzheimer's disease. Note in particular that the hippocampus, indicated by the arrows, has shrunk down to a thin remnant. (Reproduced from Gillespie and Jackson 2000.)

and an increased level of tau protein (Andreasen *et al.* 2001; Galasko *et al.* 1998; Hampel *et al.* 2004), and a recent autopsy study demonstrated a good correlation between CSF levels of tau protein and the burden of neurofibrillary tangles (Buerger *et al.* 2006).

Although single photon emission computed tomography (SPECT) scanning may show areas of decreased activity in association with neocortical areas, this technique is probably not appropriate for routine clinical work as in an autopsy control study (McNeill *et al.* 2007) it added little to diagnostic accuracy over and above a good history and examination.

Course

Although a small minority of patients may experience temporary plateaus, Alzheimer's disease, for the most part, is relentlessly and steadily progressive, death occurring for most within 5–15 years. At the end, patients are vegetative, bedfast, and incontinent. Although it is generally held that cases with an early onset, before the age of 65 years, tend to run a more rapid course (Koss *et al.* 1996), not all studies agree on this (Bracco *et al.* 1994).

Etiology

Macroscopically, as illustrated in Figure 8.1, there is widespread cortical atrophy affecting primarily the temporal, parietal, and frontal lobes, with prominent sparing of the pre- and post-central gyri; relative to the other lobes the occipital lobe is less affected. Within the temporal lobe, the hippocampus (as illustrated in Figure 8.2) and amygdala are also very prominently involved. Subcortical and brainstem nuclei, including the nucleus basalis of Meynert (especially its cholinergic neurons) (Whitehouse *et al.* 1981), the locus ceruleus (Mann *et al.* 1984), and the dorsal raphe nucleus (Yamamoto and Hirano 1985), also undergo significant damage.

Microscopically (Kidd 1964) there are widespread neurofibrillary tangles and neuritic plaques (also known as senile plaques) accompanied by neuronal loss (Terry *et al.* 1981). Neurofibrillary tangles are fibrillar structures found in the neuronal cytoplasm that, by electron microscopy, are seen to be composed of paired helical filaments. These paired helical filaments are composed of hyperphosphorylated tau proteins, which are one of the microtubule-associated proteins (MAP) that ensure the integrity and stability of the cellular microtubules. Neuritic plaques are spherical extracellular structures composed of an amyloid core surrounded by 'neurites', or swollen axonal fragments. The amyloid core of the neuritic plaque is composed primarily of beta-amyloid.

Interestingly, although the clinical severity of Alzheimer's disease correlates with the number of neurofibrillary tangles, there is little correlation with the number of neuritic plaques (Arriagada *et al.* 1992; Bierer *et al.* 1995). Furthermore, it appears that, in general, there is an orderly appearance of neurofibrillary tangles during the course of the disease, beginning first in the transentorhinal cortex and then progressing sequentially to the entorhinal cortex, hippocampus, temporal cortex, parietal and prefrontal cortex, and finally all neocortical areas (Braak and Braak 1991; Delacourte *et al.* 1999). This progression appears to supply a pathologic underpinning to the evolution of clinical features noted above, in that damage to medial temporal structures would be expected to cause an amnesia, whereas later damage to cortical areas would account for the appearance of further cognitive deficits.

In addition, there appears to be a correlation between the depth of the memory loss in Alzheimer's disease and the extent of damage in the cholinergic nucleus basalis of Meynert (Neary *et al.* 1986; Rasool *et al.* 1986; Whitehouse *et al.* 1982). There is also a correlation between depression and cell loss in the superior central nucleus (Zweig *et al.* 1988) and probably the locus ceruleus (Zubenko and Moosy 1988; Zweig *et al.* 1988), although not all have replicated this finding (Hoogendijk *et al.* 1999).

Much progress has been made in the search for the etiology of Alzheimer's disease, especially with regard to genetic factors. In a small minority of cases, probably less than 1 percent, especially those of early onset before the age of 50 years, Alzheimer's disease is clearly inherited in an autosomal dominant fashion. Mutations have been identified in three genes (Janssen *et al.* 2003): the APP (amyloid precursor protein) gene on chromosome 21 (Brouwers *et al.* 2006; Chartier-Harlin *et al.* 1991), the presenilin-1 gene on chromosome 14 (Bird *et al.* 1996; Wasco *et al.* 1995), and the presenilin-2 gene on chromosome 1 (Levy-Lahad *et al.* 1995). The role of genetic factors in the remaining vast majority of cases of apparently sporadic Alzheimer's disease is not clear. Some (Bergem *et al.* 1997; Breitner *et al.* 1995; Gatz *et al.* 1997), but not all (Cook *et al.* 1981), studies support a higher concordance among monozygotic than dizygotic twins. Likewise, whereas some studies indicate a higher prevalence of Alzheimer's disease among the first-degree relatives of probands than among the equivalent relatives of controls, others do not. One of the reasons for these discordant results might be that, although Alzheimer's disease may be inherited, there is such great intrafamily variability in the age of its expression that most cases among relatives are missed in cross-sectional studies. Life-table studies support this notion; indeed, studies using the life-table approach have found that the projected risk among first-degree relatives is approximately 50 percent (Mohs *et al.* 1987), just what would be expected if sporadic Alzheimer's disease was, in fact, an autosomal dominant disorder.

Another gene associated with Alzheimer's disease is that for apolipoprotein E on chromosome 19. Apolipoprotein E occurs in several forms, depending on which alleles are present – epsilon-2, epsilon-3, or epsilon-4 – and there is a correlation between which alleles are present and the risk of Alzheimer's disease. Thus, the risk for patients with one or two of the epsilon-4 alleles is substantially higher (Corder *et al.* 1993; Saunders *et al.* 1993) than that for patients who lack this allele. Importantly, the presence of the epsilon-4 allele is merely a 'risk factor': patients without this allele can and do get the disease and, conversely, those with it may never develop Alzheimer's.

In contrast to these positive results in genetic studies, efforts to identify environmental causes have generally been unsuccessful, with possibly one exception: it does appear that a history of significant head trauma may increase the risk of Alzheimer's disease (Schofield *et al.* 1997).

The actual mechanism or mechanisms responsible for the formation of neurofibrillary tangles and neuritic plaques remain unclear. One current hypothesis (the 'amyloid cascade hypothesis') focuses on the neurotoxicity of one form of beta-amyloid, the 42-amino acid form. APP is a transmembrane protein that is normally cleaved by several secretases, namely alpha, beta, and gamma secretase. Depending on which secretases are involved, different fragments are produced; when cleavage is via beta and then gamma secretase it appears that two forms of beta-amyloid are produced, a 40-amino acid form and a 42-amino acid form. The 42-amino acid form of beta-amyloid is relatively insoluble and undergoes fibrillization to form what are known as 'diffuse' plaques. These diffuse plaques prompt an inflammatory response and are neurotoxic; according to the theory, this neurotoxicity leads both to the breakdown of axons, thus creating neurites that surround the 'diffuse' plaques, thereby creating classic neuritic plaques, and to the formation of neurofibrillary proteins in surviving neurons. This amyloid cascade hypothesis gains support from several quarters. First, it is well known that patients with Down's syndrome, should they survive past the age of 40 years, almost always develop Alzheimer's disease (Evenhuius 1990; Jervis 1948; Lai and Williams 1989; Olson and Shaw 1969). Down's syndrome occurs secondary to an extra chromosome 21, with a consequent extra gene for APP; this leads in turn to an overproduction of APP, which would 'start' the amyloid cascade going from the top. Second, as noted earlier, there are rare inherited cases of Alzheimer's disease that are caused by mutations in the gene for APP, which, again, could start the cascade going. Third, it appears that presenilin interacts with gamma secretase and, as noted earlier, there are also rare inherited forms of Alzheimer's disease that occur secondary to mutations in the genes for presenilin-1 or -2; conceivably, if these mutations lead to an increased activity of gamma secretase, this would lead to an overproduction of beta-amyloid, specifically of the neurotoxic 42-amino acid form. Finally, it also appears that the epsilon-4 form of apolipoprotein E increases the rate of beta-amyloid production. Although taken together these considerations lend considerable weight to the 'amyloid cascade' hypothesis, it should be borne in mind that the hypothesis remains simply that, an hypothesis, and as yet has not been proven.

Differential diagnosis

As noted above, the typical presentation of Alzheimer's disease is characterized by the gradual onset of amnesia, with a subsequent accrual of other cognitive deficits; a personality change may occur, but usually only after cognitive deficits have become prominent, and, at least in the mild stage of the disease, there are few distinctive features. The differential diagnosis for such a dementia of gradual onset, lacking in distinctive features, as detailed in Section 5.1 and Table 5.1, is fairly wide, but certain considerations enable one to narrow it down.

Diffuse Lewy body disease may present in a similar fashion, but, within the first year, one sees several features that are not typical for early Alzheimer's disease, namely parkinsonism, visual hallucinations, and spontaneous confusional episodes.

Binswanger's disease and lacunar dementia may be suggested by a history of stroke; however, this may at times be absent, especially in the case of Binswanger's disease. Magnetic resonance scanning, however, will typically resolve the issue, revealing severe white matter disease in the case of Binswanger's disease, and a dozen or more subcortical infarcts in the case of lacunar dementia. Multi-infarct dementia is often listed in the differential at this point, but this entity is always characterized by a history of stroke, typically multiple strokes, and either CT or MRI will reveal appropriately placed lesions.

Pick's disease and frontotemporal dementia both typically present with a personality change, which dominates the clinical picture for a long time before cognitive deficits appear; as noted earlier, although a personality change may occur in Alzheimer's disease, this typically has an onset only after cognitive deficits are well established.

Tumors of the frontal lobes, corpus callosum, or diencephalon may be considered, but are immediately revealed by imaging.

Cerebral amyloid angiopathy, although typically presenting with lobar intracerebral hemorrhage, may, at times, present with a gradually progressive dementia due to miliary microbleeds. The differential in such cases may depend on performing MR scanning with gradient recall imaging to detect these lesions.

Vitamin B12 and folate deficiency may be clinically indistinguishable from Alzheimer's disease, and, although these are uncommon, they should always be tested for, given their eminent treatability.

Depression in the elderly may manifest with prominent cognitive deficits and thus enters the differential. Clinical features suggestive of this include the following: a history of typical depressive symptoms predating the onset of cognitive deficits; a history of prior episodes of depression; and, on mental status examination, a lack of effort on the patient's part in attempting cognitive tasks. As noted earlier, Alzheimer's disease itself may cause depression; however, in contrast to the dementia syndrome of depression, the depression seen in Alzheimer's disease occurs not before the onset of cognitive failure but only well after cognitive deficits have been thoroughly established. In cases in which a reliable history is lacking it is appropriate to attempt a 'diagnosis by treatment response' and to prescribe an antidepressant and then observe the course of both the depressive and cognitive symptoms.

Treatment

In addition to the routine environmental measures discussed in Section 5.1, certain medications may be considered that may reduce the risk of getting the disease or reduce symptoms.

Agents that may reduce the risk of the disease include non-steroidal anti-inflammatory drugs and, possibly, estrogen replacement therapy. With regard to the use of non-steroidal anti-inflammatory drugs (primarily ibuprofen), several epidemiologic studies have suggested a decreased risk with chronic use (Aisen and Davis 1994; in t' Veld et al. 2001; MacKenzie and Munoz 1998; McGeer et al. 1996; Stewart et al. 1997). With regard to estrogens, some (Scooter et al. 1999; Tang et al. 1996; Zandi et al. 2002), but not all (Roberts et al. 2006; Seshadri et al. 2001), studies suggest that, in post-menopasual women, estrogen replacement therapy may also reduce the risk. It is not clear whether, and to whom, these treatments should be recommended, if at all; certainly in the case of ibuprofen, the risks may well outweigh any putative benefits. Pending prospective studies it might, however, be reasonable to discuss them with patients who are at high risk, such as those with a family history of Alzheimer's disease or those with two epsilon-4 alleles of apolipoprotein E.

Agents capable of causing a modest symptomatic improvement include the acetylcholinesterase inhibitors donepezil (Feldman et al. 2001; Greenberg et al. 2000; Rogers and Friedhoff 1996; Rogers et al. 1998), rivastigmine (Rosler et al. 1999), and galantamine (Rockwood et al. 2001). As noted above, there is a correlation between the loss of cholinergic neurons in the nucleus basalis of Meynert and memory loss, and it is probably by partly restoring cholinergic tone that the acetylcholinesterase inhibitors exert their therapeutic effect. Another agent to consider is the N-methyl-D-aspartic acid (NMDA) antagonist memantine (Cummings et al. 2006), which may be used either alone or, more commonly, as an 'add-on' drug to one of the cholinesterase inhibitors, such as donepezil. Importantly, with treatment with a cholinesterase inhibitor or memantine, one sees not only some cognitive improvement but also some improvement in other clinical features, such as mood changes and, in some cases, delusions or hallucinations. Finally, some studies suggest benefit from D-cycloserine (Schwartz et al. 1996; Tsai et al. 1999), and some (Le et al. 1997; Mazza et al. 2006; Oken et al. 1998), but not all (Schneider et al. 2005), also suggest benefit from Ginkgo biloba. The optimum strategy with regard to these medications has not as yet been established. In my opinion it is reasonable to begin with a cholinesterase inhibitor, for example donepezil, and then monitor for a matter of months; if there has been some improvement but, as is usually the case, there is room for further improvement, memantine may then be added. The place of d-cycloserine and Gingko biloba has simply not been elucidated; however, during a time of relative clinical stability, one may consider adding one of these.

Other symptoms that may respond to pharmacologic treatment include depression, insomnia, apathy, agitation, and delusions and hallucinations. Depression may respond to treatment with an antidepressant, and a selective serotonin reuptake inhibitor (SSRI; e.g., escitalopram), given their tolerability, should receive consideration. Insomnia may, of course, be part of a depressive syndrome and, as such, may eventually respond to treatment with an antidepressant; in cases in which a hypnotic is required, consideration may be given to melatonin or zolpidem. Apathy in Alzheimer's disease, as discussed in Section 6.2, may respond to methylphenidate. Agitation, as discussed in Section 6.4, may respond to risperidone or olanzapine; in my opinion it is reasonable to begin with a low dose of risperidone (e.g., 0.25–0.5 mg/day) and to titrate it slowly and carefully. Although quetiapine has been associated with sedation, in my experience this agent, if started at a low dose (e.g., 6.25–12.5 mg) and titrated very carefully, may be extremely useful. With regard to the use of antipsychotics, concern has been raised that they may accelerate cognitive decline; however, at least in the case of risperidone, this does not appear to be the case (Livingston et al. 2007). Carbamazepine, as pointed out in Section 6.4, is also effective for agitation, although the side-effect burden of this agent may give one pause. Delusions and hallucinations, whether accompanied by agitation or not, may respond to the same antipsychotics as used for agitation; however, as with all symptoms, one must be sure that these delusions or hallucinations are sufficiently troubling to warrant the risk attendant on the use of antipsychotics.

8.2 PICK'S DISEASE

Pick's disease, first described by the neuropsychiatrist Arnold Pick in 1892 (Pick 1892), is a rare cause of dementia in which the dementia is distinguished by its presentation with a personality change of the frontal lobe type or by a more or less complete Kluver–Bucy syndrome; it is probably equally common in men and women.

Before proceeding with this discussion, it is necessary to mention nomenclature. Pick's disease has been well-described, both clinically and pathologically, for about a century. More recently it has become apparent that a fairly large number of different pathologic entities may cause a similar clinical picture, and some authors have recommended grouping all of these disorders together with Pick's disease, with different authors suggesting different names for the resulting collection: some have proposed the term 'Pick complex', whereas others favor 'frontotemporal dementia'. In this area of uncertain nomenclature, it is my opinion that we should preserve Pick's disease as an independent entity while leaving these newer disorders with similar clinical presentations provisionally grouped under the rubric of frontotemporal dementia until, with further work, they become clearly differentiated, both clinically and pathologically, at which time they may be regarded as independent entities on their own.

Clinical features

The onset is gradual and insidious, typically occurring in the fourth through the seventh decades; onsets as young as 21 (Lowenberg et al. 1939) or 25 (Coleman et al. 2002) years of age have, however, been noted. In most cases, the presentation is with a personality change, typically of the frontal lobe type, with disinhibition, coarsening of behavior, and perseveration (Bouton 1940; Ferraro and Jervis 1936; Litvan et al. 1997a; Mendez et al. 1993; Munoz et al. 1993; Munoz-Garcia and Ludwin 1984; Nichols and Weigner 1938); elements of the Kluver–Bucy syndrome, such as hyperorality and hypersexuality, are also common (Cummings and Duchen 1981; Mendez et al. 1993; Munoz et al. 1993; Munoz-Garcia and Ludwin 1984). Some patients may also be prone to restless wandering; however, in contrast to patients with Alzheimer's disease, who tend to wander off and get lost, patients with Pick's disease tend to get back to their starting point (Mendez et al. 1993; Munoz et al. 1993). Eventually, cognitive deficits appear, such as short-term memory loss, concreteness, and difficulty with calculations; in many cases an aphasia, typically of the expressive type, will supervene, and, in a small minority, seizures may occur.

Rarely, Pick's disease may present with a slowly progressive aphasia (Graff-Radford et al. 1990; Kertesz et al. 1994; Knibb et al. 2006; Wechsler et al. 1982), amnesia (Wisniewski et al. 1972), or apraxia (Fukui et al. 1996).

Computed tomography or MR scanning reveals lobar atrophy (Knopman et al. 1989; Wechsler et al. 1982), typically affecting the frontal and anterior temporal lobes; in some cases the atrophy is so severe as to present a 'knife-blade' appearance.

Course

Pick's disease is relentlessly progressive, leading to a profound dementia with death within 5–10 years (Robertson et al. 1958), generally from an intercurrent pneumonia.

Etiology

Pick's disease is an example of 'lobar' atrophy, with the frontal and temporal lobes bearing the brunt of the disease process. Interestingly, even when the temporal lobes are very hard hit, the posterior two-thirds of the superior temporal gyrus is generally spared, often to a remarkable degree, as illustrated in Figure 8.3. Although in most cases both the frontal and the temporal lobes are clearly affected, in a minority only one lobe will be macroscopically abnormal (Sjorgen et al. 1952). Microscopically one sees widespread neuronal loss and gliosis. Pick cells (large, ballooned neurons) and Pick bodies (rounded or oval argentophilic intracytoplasmic inclusions) may be seen in affected areas; the Pick bodies are composed of neurofilaments that are

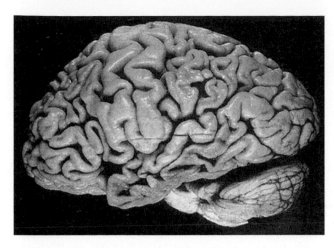

Figure 8.3 Sparing of the posterior two-thirds of the superior temporal gyrus relative to the frontal lobe and the rest of the temporal lobe in a case of Pick's disease. (Reproduced from Graham and Lantos 1996.)

straight or twisted (Murayama *et al.* 1990; Rewcastle and Ball 1968; Zhukareva *et al.* 2002).

Although most cases of Pick's disease are sporadic (Malamud and Waggoner 1943), hereditary cases do occur (Groen and Endtz 1982; Heston *et al.* 1987) and are usually consistent with dominant inheritance (Sjorgen *et al.* 1952). Most of these familial cases are associated with mutations in the tau gene (Bronner *et al.* 2005; Neumann *et al.* 2001; Pickering-Brown *et al.* 2000); however, a case has also been reported secondary to a mutation in presenilin-1 (Dermaut *et al.* 2004).

Differential diagnosis

Both Pick's disease (Litvan *et al.* 1997a) and fronto-temporal dementia are distinguished from most other dementing disorders by their presentation with a personality change; at present, a reliable differentiation of Pick's and frontotemporal dementia from each other on clinical grounds may not be possible. Tumors of the frontal or temporal lobes may mimic these disorders, but are immediately identified by imaging.

Treatment

The general treatment of dementia is discussed in Section 5.1, of the frontal lobe syndrome in Section 7.2, and of the Kluver–Bucy syndrome in Section 4.12. There is no specific treatment for Pick's disease itself.

8.3 FRONTOTEMPORAL DEMENTIA

At the outset it must be recognized that, with regard to frontotemporal dementia, there is considerable confusion regarding nomenclature. To begin with it must be emphasized that the term 'frontotemporal dementia' refers not to a discrete disease but rather to a syndrome that in turn results from multiple different diseases. The syndrome itself, as noted below, is characterized initially by a personality change, with, in most cases, the eventual development of a dementia. As noted in the discussion of Pick's disease, some authors would subsume Pick's disease under the rubric of frontotemporal dementia; however, in my opinion this represents inappropriate 'lumping' and in this text Pick's disease is treated as a disease in its own right (see Section 8.2). As noted in the section on etiology below, recent work has begun to identify some of the specific disease entities responsible for frontotemporal dementia, and it is hoped that, with further study, our understanding of these will mature to the point where they are as well-described as Pick's disease and thus eventually merit sections in their own right. Frontotemporal dementia, among the neurodegenerative disorders, is a relatively common cause of dementia.

Clinical features

The onset is insidious and generally in the sixth decade. Clinically (Heutink *et al.* 1997; Mann *et al.* 1993a; Neary *et al.* 1998), a personality change is usually the first sign of the disease, and, depending on the kind of personality change present, one may speak of a 'frontal variant' frontotemporal dementia or a 'temporal variant' frontotemporal dementia.

The frontal variant, as might be expected, is characterized by the frontal lobe syndrome, with varying mixtures of disinhibition, mood changes, perseveration, and overall coarsening of behavior; some patients may become quite gluttonous and some will show a pronounced taste for sweets. In some cases the environmental dependency syndrome may occur; as discussed in Section 4.11, such patients may compulsively utilize objects that come into view.

The temporal variant, in turn, is characterized by elements of the Kluver–Bucy syndrome (with hypersexuality and hyperorality, wherein patients will eat or drink almost anything, including, in one case, coffee grounds or banana peels [Edwards-Lee *et al.* 1997]) and by ritualistic and compulsive behaviors, which may include collecting or hoarding things. Patients with the temporal variant may also exhibit an anomia, and in such cases the term 'semantic dementia' is often used (Davies *et al.* 2005).

Over time, and well after the personality change has become established, a dementia supervenes, which, however, may remain relatively mild. Judgment and abstract thinking fail, and eventually there may be amnestic features. Over time, many patients will also develop an expressive aphasia (Neary *et al.* 1993; Snowden *et al.* 1992); gradually, this aphasia worsens, gathers receptive elements, and finally leads to mutism.

Subsequent to the onset of the personality change, some patients may also gradually develop parkinsonism or a syndrome similar to amyotrophic lateral sclerosis, with upper or lower motor neuron signs.

Uncommonly, frontotemporal dementia may present with an expressive aphasia (Bak *et al.* 2001; Turner *et al.* 1996) or with a progressive amnesia (Graham *et al.* 2005).

Computed tomography or MR scanning reveals atrophy of the frontal or temporal lobes, or both. This may be quite pronounced, to the point of a 'knife-blade' appearance of remaining gyri; in some cases the posterior portion of the superior temporal gyrus may be spared.

Course

Frontotemporal dementia is gradually progressive, with most patients dying within 5–10 years.

Etiology

Macroscopically (Heutink *et al.* 1997; Mann *et al.* 1993a) there is cortical atrophy in the frontal and temporal lobes; microscopically, neuronal loss, gliosis, and spongiform change are seen primarily in the superficial layers of the frontal and temporal cortices. Similar, although less severe, changes may be seen in the insula, cingulate cortex, hippocampus, basal ganglia, substantia nigra, and, in some, anterior horn cells. Importantly, there are no Pick cells and no Pick bodies. Appropriate staining, however, may reveal intracytoplasmic inclusions. In some cases these inclusions are tau positive, whereas in others they are tau negative but ubiquitin positive.

Both sporadic and familial, autosomal dominant cases occur. Autosomal dominant cases may be divided into those that have tau-positive inclusions and those that have inclusions which are tau negative but ubiquitin positive. Tau-positive inclusions are seen in frontotemporal dementia with parkinsonism linked to chromosome 17 (FTDP-17), a disorder secondary to mutations in the *MAPT* gene on chromosome 17 (Janssen *et al.* 2002; Lantos *et al.* 2002; Pickering-Brown *et al.* 2000; Yasuda *et al.* 2005). Tau-negative, ubiquitin-positive inclusions may be seen in several disorders, including frontotemporal lobar dementia with motor neuron disease (FTLD-MND) (Josephs *et al.* 2006) and frontotemporal lobar dementia-ubiquitinated (FTLD-U), due to mutations in the gene for progranulin, also on chromosome 17 (Bruni *et al.* 2007; Mackenzie *et al.* 2006; Mesulam *et al.* 2007; Snowden *et al.* 2006). As might be expected from the names of these disorders, FTDP-17 is associated with the later appearance of parkinsonism, and FTLD-MND with the later appearance of upper and lower motor neuron signs.

Differential diagnosis

When, as is typically the case, frontotemporal dementia presents with a personality change, it may not be possible, on clinical grounds, to differentiate it from Pick's disease. Tumors of the frontal or temporal lobes may cause a similar presentation but are immediately identified on imaging.

When frontotemporal dementia is accompanied by parkinsonism, the possibility of diffuse Lewy body disease may be raised. Clinical features preceding the development of parkinsonism, however, enable a differential: in frontotemporal dementia one sees a personality change, whereas in diffuse Lewy body disease one sees a dementia marked by visual hallucinations and confusional episodes.

Treatment

There are no well-established symptomatic treatments specific for frontotemporal dementia: one open study supported the use of rivastigmine (Moretti *et al.* 2004), whereas another open study reported no cognitive benefit from donepezil and a behavioral worsening (Mendez *et al.* 2007); one blind study reported behavioral improvement with low-dose trazodone (Lebert *et al.* 2004), whereas another blind study reported that with paroxetine there was no behavioral improvement but a cognitive decrement (Deakin *et al.* 2004).

Given that the personality change is generally the focus of treatment, consideration may be given to carbamazepine or a second-generation antipsychotic, as discussed in Section 7.2 on the frontal lobe syndrome and Section 4.12 on the Kluver–Bucy syndrome. Dementia, as noted, is often mild, and treatment considerations are discussed in Section 5.1.

8.4 AMYOTROPHIC LATERAL SCLEROSIS

Amyotrophic lateral sclerosis (ALS), first clearly delineated by the French neurologist Jean-Martin Charcot in 1874, is classically characterized by a combination of upper and lower motor neuron signs; recent work, however, has indicated additional involvement of the frontal and temporal cortices in this disease, with, in a substantial minority of patients, the development of a dementia. In Europe, ALS is often referred to as Charcot's disease or motor neuron disease, and in the United States it is, at times, colloquially referred to as Lou Gehrig's disease, after the famous baseball player who, in 1939, was forced to retire as the disease took its toll.

ALS has a lifetime prevalence of roughly 4–6 per 100 000 and is more common in men than women by a ratio of approximately 1.5:1.

Clinical features

Onset is gradual, most patients falling ill between the ages of 40 and 70 years. Classically, patients present with weakness in one of the upper extremities, often in the hand, and there may be difficulty buttoning clothes or using small tools; over time other limbs become involved. Eventually, with involvement of both upper and lower neurons, one finds the distinctive combination of brisk deep tendon reflexes with atrophic muscular weakness and fasciculations. With involvement of the upper motor neurons destined for the cranial nerve nuclei, a 'pseudobulbar palsy' may appear, with dysarthria, dysphagia, and 'emotional incontinence' with forced laughter and crying (Gallagher 1989; Ironside 1956); the jawjerk reflex tends also to be quite brisk. With involvement of the lower motor neurons in the cranial nerve nuclei, the tongue may become atrophic and demonstrate fasciculation. Sensory changes are generally absent.

Subsequent to the onset of the upper and lower motor neuron symptoms, a dementia may gradually appear in up to one-quarter of all patients, and in a significant minority of others there will be a cognitive decrement of less severe degree, characterized by poor short-term memory and judgment (Rippon et al. 2006).

Although most patients present with a combination of upper and lower motor neuron signs and symptoms, in a small minority of cases the presentation will be heavily weighted toward either the upper motor neuron (producing a syndrome known as primary lateral sclerosis) or the lower motor neuron (producing progressive muscular atrophy). Primary lateral sclerosis (Pringle et al. 1992) is characterized clinically by a progressive spastic paresis, accompanied in roughly one-half of patients by a pseudobulbar palsy (Kuipers-Upmeijer et al. 2001). Progressive muscular atrophy, in contrast, presents with progressive weakness, atrophy, and fasciculations. In most cases, patients with progressive lateral sclerosis or progressive muscular atrophy go on to develop clear clinical evidence of involvement of both upper and motor neurons (e.g., the eventual development of fasciculations in patients with progressive lateral sclerosis [La Forestier et al. 2001]), thus leaving no doubt as to the correct diagnosis. However, in a small minority of cases the clinical picture throughout life persistently demonstrates involvement of only the upper motor neuron or only the lower motor neuron, and these cases have raised the question as to whether primary lateral sclerosis and progressive muscular atrophy might each be a disease sui generis and distinct from ALS. Autopsy studies, however, have indicated subclinical involvement of both the upper and lower motor neurons in these cases, thereby justifying their inclusion under the overall rubric of ALS (Brownell et al. 1970; Lawyer and Netsky 1953).

Electromyography typically reveals evidence of denervation, and nerve condition velocity studies are typically normal.

T2-weighted or fluid-attenuated inversion recovery (FLAIR) MR imaging may reveal increased signal intensity bilaterally in the centrum semiovale, corresponding to the corticospinal tracts; rarely, atrophy may be noted in the prefrontal gyrus.

Course

ALS is almost invariably progressive, with death, often from respiratory failure or an intercurrent pneumonia, generally occurring within about 3 years; survival past 5 years is quite uncommon (del Aguila et al. 2003).

Etiology

As noted, the motor symptomatology of ALS reflects involvement of both the upper and lower motor neurons (Brownell et al. 1970): the upper motor neurons include those sending fibers into both the corticospinal and corticobulbar tracts, whereas the lower motor neurons include those found in certain lower brainstem cranial nerve nuclei (especially the hypoglossal nucleus and the nucleus ambiguus) and in the anterior horn of the spinal cord. Concurrent with the degeneration of the upper motor neurons, Wallerian degeneration leads to a thinning of both the corticospinal and corticobulbar tracts, and with degeneration of the anterior horn cells, there is subsequent atrophy of the ventral roots. Cognitive deficits reflect cell loss in the frontal and temporal cortices (Wilson et al. 2001). In remaining cells one typically finds tau-negative, ubiquitin-positive inclusions.

Ninety percent of all cases of ALS are sporadic; roughly 10 percent are inherited in an autosomal dominant fashion, secondary to mutations in the gene for superoxide dismutase on chromosome 21 (Rosen et al. 1993; Siddique et al. 1991), and there are very rare cases of inheritance on a recessive basis. Although the mechanism underlying cell loss in ALS is not known, excitotoxicity is strongly suspected.

Differential diagnosis

Diseases capable of causing diagnostic confusion are best grouped according to whether they mimic classic ALS, primary lateral sclerosis, progressive muscular atrophy, or the dementia seen in ALS.

Classic ALS, with evidence of both upper and lower motor neuron damage, may be mimicked by cervical spondylosis and syringomyelia; rarely, a similar picture may occur on a paraneoplastic basis or secondary to lymphoma (Younger et al. 1991). Finally, there is a rare disorder known as amyotrophic lateral sclerosis–parkinsonism dementia complex of Guam, found in Guam, parts of Japan, and other Pacific islands (Garruto et al. 1981; Hirano et al. 1967; Malamud et al. 1961).

Primary lateral sclerosis may be mimicked by multiple sclerosis, adrenoleukodystrophy, hereditary spastic paraplegia, and vitamin B12 deficiency.

Progressive muscular sclerosis is very closely mimicked by two rare, recessively inherited disorders, namely spinal muscular atrophy type III (or the Kugelberg–Welander syndrome [Kugelberg and Welander 1956]), which presents in adolescence or early adulthood with proximal muscle weakness, and X-linked spinal muscular atrophy (or Kennedy's disease [Harding *et al.* 1982; Kennedy *et al.* 1968]), which presents in the middle years with progressive weakness and fasciculations, often accompanied by a degree of gynecomastia. Consideration may also be given to various peripheral motor neuropathies; however, these are immediately identified on nerve conduction velocity studies.

As noted earlier, dementia occurring in ALS appears after the motor signs and symptoms are well-established, and this distinguishes this dementia from certain of the frontotemporal dementias. As noted in Section 8.3, certain of the frontotemporal dementias are accompanied by upper and lower motor neuron signs; however, these motor signs occur well after the personality change and dementia have appeared. However, this neat division, based on the evolution of signs and symptoms, has been brought into question by the discovery of certain families in which some members have ALS that is later complicated by a dementia, whereas others have developed a dementia first, followed by an ALS-like picture (Vance *et al.* 2006). Further research is clearly needed here.

Treatment

Meticulous general medical care goes far to ensure an optimum quality of life as the disease progresses. Physical therapy is helpful for spasticity and, when this is severe, a trial of baclofen may be considered. Emotional incontinence, as discussed in Section 4.7, may respond to a combination of 30 mg of dextromethorphan and 30 mg of quinidine, given twice daily; consideration may also be given to a trial of citalopram, nortriptyline, or amitriptyline. As respiratory insufficiency supervenes, bi-level positive airway pressure (BIPAP) is indicated. At some point the question of a feeding tube must be considered, and in most cases this is appropriate. Eventually one must also discuss tracheostomy, which is perhaps the most difficult decision of all. Tracheostomy clearly prolongs life but, as the disease progresses, patients may become completely 'locked in'. For some patients this amounts to a 'living death' and, rather than risk this, they may forego tracheostomy. Eventually, hospice care is appropriate.

Riluzole may also be considered. This agent both inhibits pre-synaptic release of glutamate and blocks post-synaptic glutamate receptors, and has been shown to retard the progression of the disease. At most, however, it generally adds only a few months to the patient's life.

8.5 PARKINSON'S DISEASE

Parkinson's disease, also known as idiopathic parkinsonism or paralysis agitans, presents with a classic parkinsonism; over time, however, the majority of patients will develop a dementia, and a significant minority will also develop depression. Furthermore, of patients treated with levodopa or direct-acting dopaminergics, a majority will develop significant neuropsychiatric side-effects, most notably visual hallucinations.

This is a common disease, with a prevalence of roughly 0.2 percent in the general population; it is slightly more common in men than women, by a ratio of roughly 1.5:1.

Clinical features

The onset of Parkinson's disease is gradual and insidious, with symptoms generally first appearing in the mid-50s; the range, however, is wide, from 20 to 80 years.

As just noted, the disease initially manifests with parkinsonism (Hoehn and Yahr 1967; Hughes *et al.* 1993; Martin *et al.* 1973): patients typically present with asymmetric tremor or rigidity affecting an upper or, less commonly, lower extremity. Over time, the opposite side becomes involved, and eventually all four limbs are affected.

Once fully established, Parkinson's disease leaves a stamp on patients that is, once recognized, almost unforgettable. Patients stand in a stooped, 'flexion' posture, with their arms and knees in flexion. A rhythmic, 3–7 cycles per second (cps) rest tremor is present, most noticeably in the hands but also evident, when seated, in the feet; the jaw is also often tremulous; of note, although the tremor typically resolves with sleep, in a minority it may persist (April 1966; Stern *et al.* 1968). The face is often 'masked' and expressionless, and there is a reduced frequency of blinking; there may also be copious drooling. Speech is hypophonic, soft, monotonous, and lacking in emotional inflection. Handwriting undergoes a 'micrographic' change, producing scratchy, small letters. Passive extension of the limbs reveals the rigidity, which, although often of the 'cogwheel' type, may at times be 'lead pipe' in character.

While walking there is reduced arm swing and patients often display 'marche a petit pas', wherein they take small, shuffling steps; furthermore, they often display 'festination' in which, as they walk, their steps become ever more rapid and closely spaced, to the point at which a catastrophic fall forward seems almost inevitable. Upon evaluating the station of these patients, one typically finds retropulsion, wherein a gentle push on the patient's chest will induce a gradual toppling backward that the patient cannot keep up with by backward steps. Another important symptom is bradykinesia, which manifests as a slowness in virtually any activity. For example, even in the absence of tremor or significant rigidity, it may take many minutes to fasten a button. A related phenomenon is bradyphrenia, in which thoughts, although coherent and logical, move very slowly, as if stuck in molasses.

Another curious phenomenon is 'freezing': in this, patients on the brink of an intentional act suddenly become 'frozen' and unable to move at all (Giladi *et al.* 1992). For example, a patient standing in a doorway and desirous of walking down the hall may be unable to lift a foot, take a step, or move at all. Amazingly, however, such 'freezing' may be prevented by providing appropriate visual 'cues'. For example, if the hallway is marked off with pieces of tape set about one footstep apart, the patient may well be able to begin and finish the walk down the hall without any difficulty; furthermore, in some cases, patients may be able to lyse their own frozen state by simply *imagining* such cues (Morris *et al.* 1996).

Finally, akathisia may occur in Parkinson's disease (Comella and Goetz 1994) and may appear early in the course of the disease, before any pharmacologic treatment (Lang and Johnson 1987).

Autonomic symptoms such as dysphagia, constipation, urinary frequency or incontinence, and nocturia are common, being seen in well over one-half of patients after 10 or more years of disease (Verbaan *et al.* 2007).

Dementia is more common in patients with Parkinson's disease than in age-matched controls (Biggins *et al.* 1992), with overall prevalence figures of 11 percent (Mayeux *et al.* 1988), 17 percent (Aarsland *et al.* 1996), 18 percent (Tison *et al.* 1995), 19 percent (Marder *et al.* 1995), 29 percent (Marttila and Rinne 1976), and 41 percent (Mayeux *et al.* 1992) being noted. The prevalence of dementia in Parkinson's disease rises with age: Mayeux *et al.* (1992) noted a prevalence of 0 percent for those under 50 years and 69 percent for those over 80 years. In a similar vein, over an 8-year follow-up, Aarsland *et al.* (2003) noted that 78 percent became demented. It also appears that dementia is more likely in those with more severe motor symptoms (Kuzis *et al.* 1997; Marder *et al.* 1995). Importantly, the dementia does not appear until after the motor symptoms have been well established: one study found that the onset of dementia occurred at a mean of 13 years after the appearance of motor symptoms, with a range of 6–21 years (Aarsland *et al.* 2005). It is of interest that James Parkinson, who described this disease in 1817 (Ostheimer 1922; Wilkins and Brody 1969b), maintained that dementia did not occur, an opinion that was echoed in textbooks for over one and one-half centuries. This mistake of his may be forgiven, based as it was on the observation of a mere six patients, two of whom were encountered only 'casually' and one of whom was 'seen only at a distance'. The dementia itself is fairly non-specific: patients may experience difficulty with memory and concentration, and, less commonly, such focal deficits as aphasia or apraxia may appear.

Depressive symptoms of sufficient severity to meet the criteria for a depressive episode as set out in DSM-III (American Psychiatric Association 1980) have been noted in 3 percent (Hantz *et al.* 1994), 5 percent (Tandberg *et al.* 1996), and, in two separate studies (Mayeux *et al.* 1984; Starkstein *et al.* 1990), 21 percent of patients; minor depressive symptomatology may be found in others (Tandberg *et al.* 1996), indeed up to 20 percent (Mayeux *et al.* 1986; Starkstein *et al.* 1990). As might be expected, the presence of depression worsens the cognitive deficits in those also demented (Kuzis *et al.* 1997). Of interest, it appears that in patients with primarily unilateral motor symptomatology,

depressive symptoms are more likely when the right side of the body is affected compared with the left, indicating an involvement of the left hemisphere in the genesis of depression (Starkstein *et al.* 1990).

Rapid eye movement (REM) sleep behavior disorder is fairly common in patients with Parkinson's disease, and may either precede or follow the onset of motor symptoms (Gagnon *et al.* 2002; Iranzo *et al.* 2005).

Course

Untreated, most patients become incapacitated within 8–10 years, with death often from pneumonia; with treatment, however, survival of 15 or more years may be expected.

Etiology

Macroscopically, there is depigmentation of the substantia nigra (as illustrated in Figure 8.4) and the locus ceruleus. Microscopically (Hughes *et al.* 1993), neuronal loss is present not only in these structures but also in the dorsal raphe

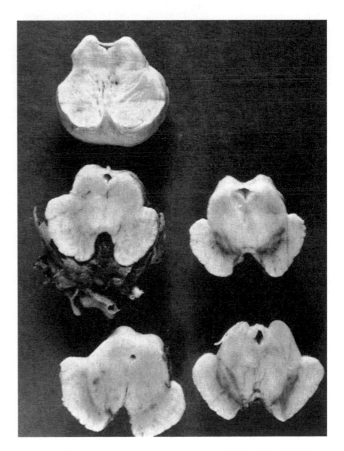

Figure 8.4 Note the depigmentation, especially evident in the substantia nigra, in the case of Parkinson's disease on the left compared with a normal control on the right. (Reproduced from Stern 1990.)

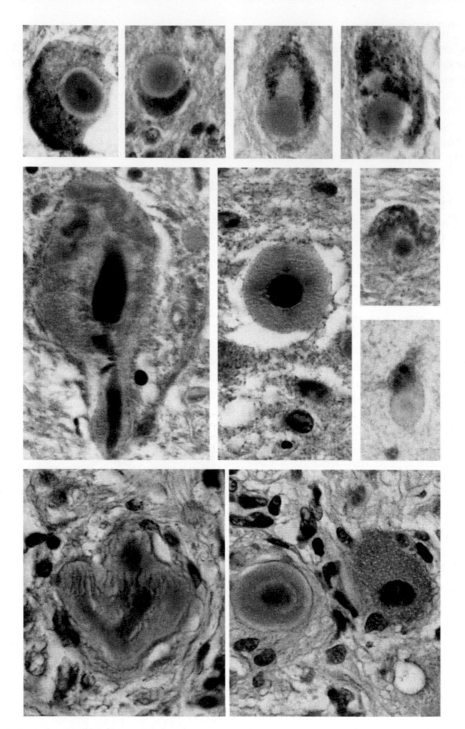

Figure 8.5   Lewy bodies in surviving neurons of the substantia nigra. (Reproduced from Stern 1990.)

nucleus, the pedunculopontine nucleus, the dorsal motor nucleus of the vagus, the thalamus, hypothalamus, nucleus basalis of Meynert, the amygdala, and in various areas of the cortex, including the temporal, insular, and cingulate cortices. Remaining neurons typically display the hallmark of Parkinson's disease, namely the Lewy body, which, as illustrated in Figure 8.5, is an intracytoplasmic inclusion, composed of alpha-synuclein, neurofilaments, and ubiquitin.

Motor symptoms correlate with cell loss in the substantia nigra, and generally do not appear until 60 percent or more of these cells have been lost. Dementia correlates

with cell loss and Lewy bodies in the cortex (Aarsland *et al.* 2005; Apaydin *et al.* 2002; Braak *et al.* 2005; Hurtig *et al.* 2000), and depression with similar changes in the locus ceruleus (Chan-Palay and Asan 1989) and the dorsal raphe nucleus (Becker *et al.* 1997); of note, the dorsal raphe nucleus serves as one of the main sources of serotonergic innervation to the cortex and a correlation has been found between CSF levels of 5-hydroxyindoleacetic acid, a metabolite of serotonin, and the presence of depression in patients with Parkinson's disease (Mayeux *et al.* 1984, 1986).

Table 8.1 Genetic forms related to Parkinson's disease

Inheritance pattern	Chromosome	Locus	Gene	Protein	Onset	Parkinsonism
AD	12p11–q13	PARK8	LRRK2	Leucine-rich repeat kinase 2	Late	Typical
AD	4q21	PARK1	SCNA	Alpha-synuclein	Early to late	Typical or atypical
AD	4q21	PARK4	SCNA	Alpha-synuclein	Early to late	Typical or atypical
AD	4p14	PARK5	UCH-L1	Ubiquitin C-terminal hydrolase	Late	Typical
AD	2p13	PARK3	?	?	Late	Typical
AD	1p	PARK11	?	?	Late	Typical
AR	6q25.2–27	PARK2	PRKN	Parkin	Early to late	Atypical
AR	1p36	PARK6	PINK1	PTEN-induced putative kinase 1	Early to late	Typical
AR	1p36	PARK7	DJ-1	DJ-1	Early	Typical
AR	1p36	PARK9	?	?	Early	Atypical
?	1p	PARK10	?	?	Late	Typical

AD, autosomal dominant; AR, autosomal recessive.

Although the mechanism or mechanisms underlying cell loss and Lewy body formation are not known, it is theorized that, perhaps related to mitochondrial respiratory chain dysfunction, there is an increased formation of free radicals with subsequent cell damage. Genetic factors and environmental factors may both be involved. Although idiopathic Parkinson's disease has long been thought to be sporadic, recent epidemiologic work strongly suggests familial factors (Sveinbjornsdottir et al. 2000). Furthermore, fluorodopa positron emission tomography has demonstrated not only reduced dopamine uptake in the striatum of patients but also a reduced uptake in their clinically unaffected co-twins, suggesting that the co-twins had asymptomatic disease (Piccini et al. 1999). Environmental toxins have long been suspected, and suspicion has focused on exposure to pesticides (Ascherio et al. 2006). Of interest, it also appears that cigarette smoking appears to reduce the risk of developing Parkinson's disease (Thacker et al. 2007).

Interest in genetic factors has recently been stimulated by the investigation of cases having a clear-cut, unequivocal familial basis (Feany 2004; Klein 2006; Tan and Jankovic 2006). These constitute only a small percentage of cases, no more than 10 percent, and the pattern of inheritance may be either autosomal dominant or autosomal recessive. Table 8.1 lists the various forms that have been discovered, grouping them according to whether they are dominantly or recessively inherited. As noted these cases may be either early (under 40 years) or late onset, and the parkinsonism may be typical or have atypical aspects. Two of the more common forms are PARK8, due to mutations in LRRK, and PARK2, due to mutations in PRKN. PARK8 cases may be clinically indistinguishable from idiopathic Parkinson's disease (Gaig et al. 2007; Papapetropoulos et al. 2006); PARK2 cases may also be indistinguishable or may present with a combination of parkinsonism and foot dystonia (Khan et al. 2003; Lucking et al. 2000). It is unclear at present how relevant these discoveries are to an understanding of the overwhelming majority of cases that do not exhibit a clear-cut familial basis, as they may not have the same pathology as that described above. For example, although Lewy bodies, the pathologic hallmark of Parkinson's disease, are found in some cases of PARK8 (Papapetropoulos et al. 2006) and PARK2 (Farrer et al. 2001; Pramstaller et al. 2005), they are not found in other cases, both of PARK8 (Funayama et al. 2002; Gaig et al. 2007) and PARK2 (Mori et al. 1998; Takahashi et al. 1994).

The place of genetic testing, at present, is uncertain. Where a strong family history exists, a case could be made for testing to allow for genetic counselling; otherwise, such testing is probably best reserved for research settings.

Differential diagnosis

Parkinson's disease constitutes only one of many different causes of parkinsonism, and the full differential for parkinsonism is discussed at length in Section 3.8. Of the disorders noted there, several should especially come to mind when considering a diagnosis of Parkinson's disease, including diffuse Lewy body disease, multiple system atrophy, progressive supranuclear palsy, corticobasal ganglionic degeneration, and vascular parkinsonism.

Diffuse Lewy body disease may present with a classic parkinsonism; however, within a year of onset of the movement disorder, this disease also causes a dementia marked by confusional episodes and visual hallucinations. Although most patients with Parkinson's disease will also develop a dementia, this, as noted above, is a late occurrence, appearing only many years after the onset of the movement disorder, and it is this disparity in time of onset of the dementia which is most helpful in distinguishing these two disorders.

Multiple system atrophy may cause a fairly classic parkinsonism; however, these patients will also typically have evidence of either cerebellar degeneration with ataxia, or autonomic failure with postural dizziness, erectile dysfunction and either urinary incontinence or retention.

Progressive supranuclear palsy may cause parkinsonism, but this is usually accompanied by certain atypical features, such as the early occurrence of frequent, unexplained falls, a symmetric onset, an extension (rather than flexion) posture, and, most importantly, the appearance within several years of a supranuclear ophthalmoplegia.

Corticobasal ganglionic degeneration, like Parkinson's disease, causes a parkinsonism of asymmetric onset. However, here the onset is markedly asymmetric and, furthermore, the rigidity often has a dystonic aspect to it and is typically accompanied by cortical sensory loss and apraxia.

Vascular parkinsonism, occurring in the setting of multiple lacunar infarctions, produces a somewhat atypical parkinsonism in that tremor is often absent and the rigidity and bradykinesia are accompanied by evidence of damage to the corticospinal tracts (e.g., hyper-reflexia and Babinski signs) and corticobulbar tracts (e.g., pseudobulbar palsy with emotional incontinence).

One very important clue in the differential of parkinsonism is the presence or absence of 'levodopa responsiveness'. The parkinsonism of Parkinson's disease is almost always robustly responsive to levodopa; although parkinsonism seen in other disorders may also respond, this is not as common and the response is typically not robust, hence a lack of a robust response to levodopa should prompt a reconsideration of the diagnosis.

Treatment

The treatment of Parkinson's disease begins with its *motor symptoms*; over time, as noted earlier, *dementia* and *depression* typically appear and require their own treatments. Each aspect of treatment is discussed in turn, beginning with motor symptoms.

MOTOR SYMPTOMS

Motor symptoms may be treated with a variety of agents, including monoamine oxidase inhibitors (e.g., selegiline and rasagiline), anticholinergics (e.g., benztropine and trihexyphenidyl), amantadine, levodopa/carbidopa (with or without entacapone), and direct-acting dopamine agonists (bromocriptine, cabergoline, pramipexole, and ropinirole). Each of these agents will be discussed in turn, followed by a discussion of an overall treatment strategy. Treatment with levodopa or dopamine agonists eventually causes significant neuropsychiatric side-effects (e.g., visual hallucinations) in most patients, and these are discussed further below.

The monoamine oxidase inhibitors selegiline (used in doses of 10 mg or less daily) (Myllyla *et al.* 1997; Palhagen *et al.* 1998) and rasagiline (Parkinson Study Group 2005) are both selective against monoamine oxidase type B and, as such, inhibit intracellular metabolism of levodopa, thus

increasing the amount available in the striatum and thereby exerting a modest therapeutic effect. Although perhaps controversial, there is also evidence that both selegiline (Palhagen *et al.* 2006) and rasagiline (Parkinson Study Group 2004) may have a 'neuroprotective' effect and may, to a modest degree, slow the progression of the disease. As there have been no 'head to head' comparisons of these two agents, it is not clear which one should be used.

Anticholinergics, although useful for tremor, have a limited effect on bradykinesia and rigidity, and in some patients may cause confusion or a memory deficit. In light of this, they are generally reserved for cases in which tremor is prominent, with due regard for any emerging cognitive deficits.

Amantadine, in a dose of 200–300 mg/day, may have a mild effect on motor symptoms, but the effect may be short-lived, with little benefit seen after a matter of months (Thomas *et al.* 2004; Timberlake and Vance 1978). Given this limited benefit, and the side-effects seen with amantadine, routine use is probably not justified. There may, however, be a place for amantadine in the treatment of levodopa-induced dyskinesias (Verhagen Metman *et al.* 1998).

Levodopa is the most effective treatment for the motor symptomatology of Parkinson's disease, and is generally given in combination with a peripheral aromatic amino acid decarboxylase inhibitor (carbidopa or benzaride) in order to prolong its effect: both regular and sustained-release preparations are available. The initial response to levodopa/carbidopa is generally quite gratifying, but as levodopa does not retard the progression of the disease, a dosage increase is necessary over time, and most patients eventually begin to show motor fluctuations: such fluctuations can be 'peak dose' with dyskinesias, 'end of dose' with an early wearing off of effectiveness, or unpredictable. When fluctuations appear, using lower and more closely spaced doses of levodopa may help, or one may add tolcapone. Tolcapone is a peripheral catechol-*O*-methyltransferase inhibitor that extends the duration of levodopa's effect and also allows for a lowering of the levodopa dose (Adler *et al.* 1998; Brooks and Sagar 2003; Kurth *et al.* 1997; Rajput *et al.* 1997; Waters *et al.* 1997); although hepatotoxicity is a concern (Baas *et al.* 1997), the medication may be used safely with appropriate monitoring (Olanow *et al.* 2000). Recently a 'triple combination' preparation, containing levodopa, carbidopa, and tolcapone, has become available. Attention should also be paid to the possibility of *Helicobacter pylori* infection; in patients with confirmed infection, successful treatment with omeprazole, amoxicillin, and clarithromycin was followed by increased absorption of levodopa and increased on-time (Pierantozzi *et al.* 2006).

As noted above, dopamine agonists include a number of different agents: although bromocriptine is the oldest member of this group, problematic side-effects, combined with the fact that newer agents (e.g. ropinirole [Korczyn *et al.* 1999]) may be more effective, have limited its use. Dopamine agonists have been used as monotherapy in early, mild Parkinson's disease, and include cabergoline (Rinne et al. 1997), pramipexole (Parkinson Study Group 1997; Shannon et al. 1997), ropinirole (Adler et al. 1997; Korczyn et al. 1999; Rascol et al. 2000), and, most recently, transdermal rotigotine (Jankovic et al. 2007). Dopamine agonists are also used as 'add-on' drugs to levodopa, both to smooth out levodopa fluctuations and to allow for a levodopa dose reduction, this effect having been shown for cabergoline (Hutton et al. 1996; Inzelberg et al. 1996), pramipexole (Guttman et al. 1997; Lieberman et al. 1997; Pinter et al. 1999), and ropinirole (Lieberman et al. 1998). Of these dopamine agonists, cabergoline has been strongly associated with cardiac valvular disease (Zanettini et al. 2007) and, hence, if an oral dopamine agonist is used, consideration is best given to either pramipexole or ropinirole. When dopamine agonists are used, patients should be cautioned that sleep attacks may occur (Avorn et al. 2005; Ferreira et al. 2000; Frucht et al. 1999; Hauser et al. 2000); they should generally avoid driving or using hazardous machinery until, with prolonged use, it has become apparent whether or not this side-effect will occur.

The optimum overall treatment strategy is still a matter of some debate, and although the strategy recommended here is intended as a middle of the road approach, not all authors will be in agreement.

In general, pharmacologic treatment should not be initiated until the motor symptomatology significantly interferes with the patient's ability to function. In mild cases one may begin with one of the monoamine oxidase inhibitors and, when tremor is prominent, some clinicians advocate the use of an anticholinergic. With disease progression, however, one must at some point add either levodopa or a dopamine agonist, and the question of which to use first has not been settled. Given the sometimes stunning effectiveness of levodopa, some advocate using this first, especially when a prompt response is required, for example when a patient is threatened with job loss. Others, however, with an eye towards delaying the emergence of levodopa-induced dyskinesias, advocate starting with dopamine agonist monotherapy and adding levodopa only as the disease progresses.

All other things being equal, it may be prudent to begin with a dopamine agonist, either pramipexole or ropinirole, increasing the dose as required until limiting side-effects occur or further dose increases are not effective, and then, with disease progression, to add levodopa. Between the regular and sustained-release preparations of levodopa, the sustained-release preparation may be preferable as it may allow for a longer duration of effect; given its slower onset of action, however, some patients may have to take a 'regular' release preparation first thing in the morning in order to 'jump start' themselves (Pahwa et al. 1996). When fluctuations in levodopa responsiveness begin to appear, the addition of tolcapone may be considered. If one begins with levodopa rather than with dopamine agonist monotherapy, at some point one will generally have to add a dopamine agonist to smooth out the effect of levodopa

and to allow a dose reduction and a reduction in levodopa-induced dyskinesias.

In treating patients with levodopa or dopaminergic agents, it is important to avoid suddenly stopping them as this may precipitate a neuroleptic malignant syndrome, as has been reported for levodopa (Sechi et al. 1984; Toru et al. 1981), the combination of levodopa and bromocriptine (Figa-Talamanca et al. 1985), and amantadine (Cunningham et al. 1991; Harsch 1987).

When motor symptoms become severe and resistant to pharmacologic treatment, consideration may be given to deep brain stimulation or to electroconvulsive therapy (ECT). Deep brain stimulation of the subthalamic nucleus is effective (Deep Brain Stimulation for Parkinson's Disease Study Group 2001; Rodriguez-Oroz et al. 2004), somewhat more so than stimulation of the pars interna of the globus pallidus (Deep Brain Stimulation for Parkinson's Disease Study Group 2001). In emergent situations, or in cases where neurosurgical intervention is not possible, consideration should be given to ECT. ECT has been shown in a double-blind study (Andersen et al. 1987) to improve motor symptoms regardless of whether patients are depressed or not, and the results are at times dramatic. As such, ECT may be life-saving, and although maintenance ECT may be required to prolong the benefit, this may, in selected cases, be a reasonable price to pay in light of the increased mobility.

Most patients treated with levodopa or dopamine agonists will eventually develop significant neuropsychiatric side-effects. The most common of these are visual hallucinations; others include psychosis, anxiety (during wearing off of levodopa), and certain other, much less common, phenomena, including impulsive behaviors, stereotypies, euphoria (with, rarely, mania), and delirium. Each of these is discussed in turn.

Visual hallucinations are very common with prolonged treatment with either levodopa or dopamine agonists: in one 6-year study, the percentage of patients with hallucinations gradually increased until, at the end of the study, fully 62 percent were experiencing them (Goetz et al. 2005). The hallucinations are typically complex, involving scenes, animals or people, and may last from minutes to hours or even days; importantly, early on, patients retain insight into the hallucinatory nature of these experiences and recognize that they are not 'real' (Barnes and David 2001; Fenelon et al. 2000; Friedman and Sienkiewicz 1991; Graham et al. 1997; Inzelberg et al. 1998). Auditory hallucinations, or even olfactory or gustatory hallucinations, may also occur, but these are much less common (Goetz et al. 2005; Holroyd et al. 2001). Of note, although it has traditionally been taught that visual hallucinations in patients with Parkinson's disease occur, as noted here, as side-effects, recent work suggests that, in a very small minority of patients, visual hallucinations may occur before any treatment is administered (Biousse et al. 2004). Furthermore, it appears that patients with greater cell loss and Lewy body pathology in the amygdala are more likely to develop hallucinations when treated with levodopa (Harding *et al.* 2002a). It may well be that amygdalar pathology not only renders patients more sensitive to the hallucinogenic effects of levodopa and dopamine agonists but may also, if severe enough, independently cause hallucinations.

Psychosis is said to be present when patients either experience hallucinations without insight or develop delusions. As just noted, visual hallucinations with preserved insight are very common; however, over a matter of several years, the majority of patients who do have hallucinations will lose insight and begin to react to the visual hallucinations as if they were real (Goetz *et al.* 2006). Delusions, often of persecution, may also occur, but are much less common (Holroyd *et al.* 2001).

Treatment of hallucinations or psychosis should generally involve an attempt at dose reduction of levodopa and/or dopamine agonists. These side-effects are generally dose-responsive and in some cases it may be possible to reduce the dose sufficiently to allow for a substantial resolution of them without sacrificing control of the parkinsonism. When dose reduction is either ineffective or impractical, consideration may be given to treatment with an antipsychotic. Various second-generation agents have been used. Quetiapine, in doses of 50–150 mg/day, in non-blind (Fernandez *et al.* 1999; Weiner *et al.* 2000) and single-blind (Merims *et al.* 2006) studies, appeared promising; however, a double-blind study failed to show any superiority to placebo (Rabey *et al.* 2006). Olanzapine, in doses of 2.5–15 mg in double-blind studies, was no better than placebo and less effective than clozapine, and tended to aggravate parkinsonism (Breier *et al.* 2002; Goetz *et al.* 2000). Risperidone, in a dose of 1–2 mg, was comparable to clozapine in a double-blind study but, in contrast to clozapine, worsened parkinsonism (Ellis *et al.* 2000). Clozapine, in doses of 6.25–50 mg, is clearly effective in double-blind studies (Parkinson Study Group 1999, Pollak *et al.* 2004) and, rather than worsening parkinsonism, may actually improve it (Durif *et al.* 2004; Parkinson Study Group 1999). On the basis of efficacy and motor effects, clozapine is clearly preferable; however, the risk of agranulocytosis and the need for regular blood counts make most clinicians pause before recommending it. A reasonable strategy might be to try another agent first, for example risperidone, keeping clozapine in reserve.

Anxiety may be seen during motor fluctuations of the 'wearing off' type, and full anxiety attacks may occur (Hillen and Sage 1996; Vazquez *et al.* 1993); other symptoms seen during the 'off' period include depressed mood, irritability, and various other symptoms, including sweating (Raudino 2001).

Impulsive behaviors, including pathologic gambling, compulsive shopping, and hypersexuality, may occur as side-effects of treatment in a few percent of patients, and appear more likely in those treated with dopamine agonists (Dodd *et al.* 2005; Pontone *et al.* 2006; Voon *et al.* 2006a,b); with discontinuation of treatment with the offending medication, symptoms resolve within days to months (Dodd *et al.* 2005).

Stereotypies seen with treatment may be complex and socially disabling. Known as 'punding', these may include repeatedly taking apart and putting together machinery or engaging in other purposeless behaviors (Evans *et al.* 2004).

Euphoria may occur, and some patients may escalate the dose in order to achieve this side-effect (Giovannoni *et al.* 2000); in some cases, albeit rarely, a manic episode may occur (Celesia and Barr 1970; O'Brien *et al.* 1971).

Delirium has been noted as a side-effect (Celesia and Barr 1970; Friedman and Sienkiewicz 1991; Serby *et al.* 1978), but this is rare.

DEMENTIA

Dementia may be treated with either donepezil (Emre *et al.* 2004; Ravina *et al.* 2005) or rivastigmine (Aarsland *et al.* 2002); donepezil may be preferred as there was no worsening of parkinsonism with donepezil, in contrast to rivastigmine, which did cause motor worsening, in particular an increase in tremor. The overall treatment of dementia is discussed in Section 5.1.

DEPRESSION

Depression may be treated with antidepressants such as sertraline (Antonini *et al.* 2006) or nortriptyline (Andersen *et al.* 1980); however, to date, there is no double-blind evidence to support their efficacy. Of interest, it appears that pramipexole may be more effective than sertraline in this regard; however, again this was an unblind study (Barone *et al.* 2006). Mirtazapine should be used only with caution, as it may precipitate REM sleep behavior disorder in these patients (Onofrj *et al.* 2003). In treatment-resistant cases, consideration may be given to either ECT or transcranial magnetic stimulation (TMS). In a naturalistic study (Douyon *et al.* 1989) ECT was effective, and, as noted earlier, ECT also improves motor symptoms. In a sham-controlled, double-blind study (Fregni *et al.* 2004), TMS was as effective as fluoxetine and did not aggravate motor symptomatology.

8.6 DIFFUSE LEWY BODY DISEASE

Diffuse Lewy body disease, also known as dementia with Lewy bodies, Lewy body dementia, cortical Lewy body disease, and senile dementia of the Lewy body type, is a relatively recently described (Okazaki *et al.* 1961) cause of dementia, now recognized in both autopsy (Barker *et al.* 2002) and clinical (Rahkonen *et al.* 2003) studies to be the second most common cause of dementia in the elderly, accounting for nearly 20 percent of all cases. Clinical studies have also indicated that, in the general population, diffuse Lewy body disease is the second most common cause of parkinsonism (Pineda *et al.* 2000).

Diffuse Lewy body disease is distinctive in that it may present in one of two ways, either with a dementia or with parkinsonism; eventually, all patients will display both features.

Clinical features

The onset is gradual, generally in the seventh decade, and, as noted, the presentation may be with either a dementia or parkinsonism (Byrne *et al.* 1989).

The dementia of diffuse Lewy body disease is characterized initially by difficulty in sustaining attention and by executive dysfunction, with deficits in judgment and decision-making; over time, these symptoms are joined by short-term memory loss. There are two other features of the dementia of diffuse Lewy body disease that deserve note, as they are helpful, as discussed later, in distinguishing diffuse Lewy body disease from other dementias: these two features are early-onset hallucinations or delusions and spontaneous episodes of confusion.

Hallucinations seen in diffuse Lewy body disease are typically visual, complex and well-formed, and are experienced without insight (Ala *et al.* 1997; Ballard *et al.* 1997, 1999, 2001; Crystal *et al.* 1990; Tiraboschi *et al.* 2006; Weiner *et al.* 1996). Auditory hallucinations may also occur, but are less common. Delusions are somewhat less common than hallucinations, and tend to be persecutory in nature (Marantz and Verghese 2002). As noted, these symptoms tend to appear early on, and indeed may occur at presentation.

Confusional episodes are common and occur early on (Ballard *et al.* 2001, McKeith *et al.* 1994a); they tend to last in the order of hours and, importantly, occur spontaneously, without any precipitating events (Bradshaw *et al.* 2004).

Depression may occur during the course of the dementia (Burkhardt *et al.* 1988) and indeed has been noted in up to one-half of all patients (Klatka *et al.* 1996).

The parkinsonism of diffuse Lewy body disease is very similar to the classic parkinsonian picture seen in Parkinson's disease, with bradykinesia, rigidity, and postural instability (Hely *et al.* 1996); tremor, however, is somewhat less commonly present (Louis *et al.* 1995, 1997). Like all parkinsonian patients, those with diffuse Lewy body disease are apt to experience a worsening of their parkinsonism upon exposure to antipsychotics; however, in diffuse Lewy body disease, the exacerbation tends to be quite severe, a phenomenon known as 'neuroleptic sensitivity' (McKeith *et al.* 1992a,b; Weiner *et al.* 1996). In some cases, the exacerbation may persist long after the antipsychotic has been discontinued, and fatalities have occurred.

In cases that present with dementia, parkinsonism typically appears within a matter of years. In cases that present with parkinsonism, a dementia supervenes relatively soon thereafter, typically within a year.

Other symptoms seen in diffuse Lewy body disease include myoclonus (seen in about one-fifth of patients [Louis *et al.* 1997]), autonomic dysfunction (with urinary incontinence, constipation, and orthostatic hypotension [Horimoto *et al.* 2003]) and REM sleep behavior disorder, which may actually constitute a very early presentation of the disorder, appearing long before any other symptoms (Boeve *et al.* 1998).

Magnetic resonance scanning may reveal cortical atrophy and atrophy of medial temporal structures; however, the degree of atrophy tends to be relatively mild (Tam *et al.* 2005). The EEG may reveal generalized slowing with temporal theta transients (Briel *et al.* 1999); frontal intermittent delta activity (FIRDA) (Calzetti *et al.* 2002) and periodic spike and slow-wave complexes (Doran and Larner 2004) have also been reported.

Course

The course is one of gradual progression, with death on average within 12–13 years.

Etiology

Microscopically (Gibb *et al.* 1987, Gomez-Tortosa *et al.* 1999, Hansen *et al.* 1990, Lennox *et al.* 1989, Lippa *et al.* 1994) there is cell loss and Lewy bodies in surviving neurons in the substantia nigra, nucleus basalis of Meynert, amygdala, and the cortex. Dementia correlates not only with cortical Lewy bodies but also with the presence of Lewy bodies in the nucleus basalis of Meynert. The nucleus basalis provides cholinergic innervation to the cortex, and there is a good correlation between loss of cortical choline acetyltransferase activity and the severity of the dementia (Tiraboschi *et al.* 2002). In turn, there is also a good correlation between the occurrence of visual hallucinations and the burden of Lewy bodies in the amygdala, parahippocampus, and inferior temporal cortex (Harding *et al.* 2002b).

It appears that most cases are sporadic, with only a few familial instances being reported (Galvin *et al.* 2002).

Differential diagnosis

The differential considerations vary depending on whether the presentation of diffuse Lewy body disease is with dementia or with parkinsonism.

In cases that present with dementia, consideration, as discussed in Section 5.1, must be given to certain other disorders capable of causing a dementia of gradual onset, including Alzheimer's disease, Binswanger's disease, and lacunar dementia. Several features of diffuse Lewy body disease facilitate this differential. The most important is the early appearance, within a year of the onset of the dementia, of parkinsonism. Other distinctive features are the early and prominent nature of visual hallucinations and the occurrence of confusional episodes. Although confusional episodes may occur, for example, in Alzheimer's disease, they generally appear later and typically occur only in stressful situations (e.g., when a patient is confronted with a cognitively demanding task), in contrast to the confusional episodes of diffuse Lewy body disease, which appear spontaneously. Neuroleptic sensitivity may also provide a clue: in some cases of diffuse Lewy body disease that present with dementia, there may be a subclinical parkinsonism, and in these patients treatment with an antipsychotic may be followed by a florid, and totally unexpected, parkinsonism (McKeith et al. 1992c, 1994b).

In cases that present with parkinsonism, other neurodegenerative disorders, as discussed in Section 3.8, must be considered, including Parkinson's disease, multiple system atrophy, progressive supranuclear palsy, and corticobasal ganglionic degeneration. With regard to Parkinson's disease, the most important distinguishing feature is what has come to be known as the '1-year rule'. As noted earlier, in cases of diffuse Lewy body disease that present with parkinsonism, there will generally be a dementia within 1 year; although Parkinson's disease may also cause dementia, the dementia typically 'breaks' the 1-year rule in that many years pass before cognitive features appear. Multiple system atrophy is suggested by concurrent ataxia; progressive supranuclear palsy by frequent falls, an extension posture, and supranuclear ophthalmoplegia; and corticobasal ganglionic degeneration by a strikingly asymmetric parkinsonism accompanied by dystonia and cortical sensory loss.

Treatment

The dementia may be treated with rivastigmine: doses of 6–12 mg not only improved cognition but also reduced the severity and frequency of hallucinations and delusions (McKeith et al. 2000, Wesnes et al. 2002); open-label studies also suggest benefit from donepezil (Thomas et al. 2005) and galantamine (Edwards et al. 2004). Memantine should probably be avoided, as it has been reported to worsen cognition (Sabbagh et al. 2005) and hallucinations and delusions (Ridha et al. 2005). In cases in which hallucinations and delusions persist despite treatment with rivastigmine, and which are clinically troubling, consideration may be given to using an antipsychotic. Given the neuroleptic sensitivity characteristic of diffuse Lewy body disease, first-generation agents, such as haloperidol, are best avoided, as they are more likely to cause parkinsonism than the second-generation agents. Second-generation agents used in diffuse Lewy body disease include olanzapine, quetiapine, and risperidone. Olanzapine, in a post hoc analysis of a larger study, was effective at doses from 5 to 10 mg, but not at doses of 15 mg (Cummings et al. 2002); an open study of olanzapine using doses from 2.5 to 7.5 mg reported either intolerable side-effects or minimal benefit (Walker et al. 1999). In two case series (Fernandez et al. 2002, Takahashi et al. 2003), quetiapine, in doses from 25 to 75 mg/day, was beneficial in the majority of cases but frequently caused sedation and orthostatic hypotension. Risperidone, at a dose of 1 mg/day, was beneficial in a case report (Kato et al. 2002). Interestingly, clozapine, at a dose of 6.25 mg/day, was not only ineffective but also actually worsened the hallucinations and delusions (Burke et al. 1998). Clearly, more work is needed here.

With regard to the treatment of depression, there are no controlled studies. Consideration may be given to an antidepressant, such as an SSRI (McKeith et al. 2005), or, in severe and treatment-resistant cases, ECT (Rasmussen et al. 2003). In case reports, patients with REM sleep behavior disorder have responded well to both clonazepam and donepezil (Massironi et al. 2003).

The parkinsonism of diffuse Lewy body disease may respond to combination treatment with levodopa/carbidopa (Byrne et al. 1989); however, the response is generally not as robust as that seen in Parkinson's disease (Molloy et al. 2005). There is little published experience regarding the use of dopamine agonists such as pramipexole or ropinirole.

8.7 PROGRESSIVE SUPRANUCLEAR PALSY

Progressive supranuclear palsy, also known as the Steele–Richardson–Olszewski syndrome, is characterized by an atypical parkinsonism, which is accompanied in most cases by a supranuclear ophthalmoplegia and, in about half of cases, by a dementia. This is an uncommon disorder, found somewhat more frequently in men than women.

Clinical features

The general clinical features have been described in several reports (Birdi et al. 2000; Collins et al. 1995; Litvan et al. 1996b; Maher and Lees 1986; Messert and Van Nuis 1966; Steele 1972; Steele et al. 1964). The onset is insidious, generally in the sixth decade, and the disease typically presents with frequent unexplained falls due to postural instability. An atypical parkinsonism then gradually appears, characterized by a more or less symmetric onset of rigidity, generally without tremor, and an abnormal gait typified by a wide-based stance with short, shuffling steps. Importantly, rather than the typical flexion posture seen in most cases of parkinsonism, patients with progressive supranuclear palsy typically display a dystonic axial rigidity, which may also affect the neck. Dystonic rigidity also affects the facial musculature, at times creating an 'astonished' appearance, as seen in Figure 8.6.

Classically, from 1 to 3 years after the parkinsonism is established, one also sees a supranuclear ophthalmoplegia for vertical gaze, wherein patients have difficulty voluntarily looking down, a difficulty that may make walking down stairs particularly treacherous. This feature, however, may

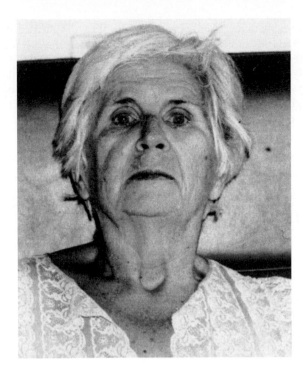

Figure 8.6 'Astonished' facial appearance in progressive supranuclear palsy. (Reproduced from Stern 1990.)

be delayed for many years, and in some cases may never appear (Birdi *et al.* 2002; Daniel *et al.* 1995).

Dementia occurs in about one-half of all patients, generally well after the parkinsonism has become established: patients have difficulty with concentration and memory, and there may be elements of a frontal lobe syndrome (Verny *et al.* 1996) with prominent apathy (Litvan *et al.* 1996a). Rarely, dementia may constitute the presenting symptom of progressive supranuclear palsy (Davis *et al.* 1985). Over time, pseudobulbar palsy with emotional incontinence (Menza *et al.* 1995) may occur, and seizures may occur in a small minority (Nygaard *et al.* 1989). Aphasia, agnosia, and apraxia are rare.

Magnetic resonance scanning may reveal atrophy of the midbrain and, in some cases, of the frontal and temporal cortices.

Course

Progressive supranuclear palsy is progressive, with death within 5–7 years (Golbe *et al.* 1988; Maher and Lees 1986).

Etiology

Macroscopically there is atrophy of the midbrain, globus pallidus and, in some cases, the frontotemporal cortex. Microscopically (Collins *et al.* 1995; Henderson *et al.* 2000; Litvan *et al.* 1996b; Steele *et al.* 1964), cell loss is noted in

the mesencephalic tectum, periaqueductal gray matter, locus ceruleus, substantia nigra, dentate nucleus, red nucleus, thalamus (especially in the caudal intralaminar nuclei), globus pallidus, subthalamic nucleus, and the temporal and inferior frontal cortices. This cell loss is accompanied by a gliosis and, in surviving neurons, one finds neurofibrillary tangles that are dissimilar to those found in Alzheimer's disease (Takahashi *et al.* 1989).

Although definite autosomal dominantly inherited cases have been identified (Brown *et al.* 1993; Rojo *et al.* 1999; Ros *et al.* 2005a,b; Stanford *et al.* 2000; de Yebenes *et al.* 1995), the vast majority of cases appear to be sporadic. There does, however, appear to be a 'susceptibility genotype', composed of normal variants in the gene for tau, which predisposes to classic progressive supranuclear palsy (Higgins *et al.* 1999; Morris *et al.* 2002).

Differential diagnosis

As discussed in detail in Section 3.8, progressive supranuclear palsy must be distinguished from certain other neurodegenerative disorders capable of causing a parkinsonism of gradual onset and slow progression, including Parkinson's disease, diffuse Lewy body disease, multiple system atrophy (of the striatonigral variant), and corticobasal ganglionic degeneration. Three clinical features of progressive supranuclear palsy, if present, generally allow for an accurate differentiation from all of these other disorders, namely postural instability, frequent unexplained falls, and supranuclear ophthalmoplegia; if all three of these are present during the first year of illness, the diagnosis of progressive supranuclear palsy is almost assured (Litvan *et al.* 1996c, 1997b). As noted above, however, supranuclear palsy may be delayed for years, and in some pathologically proven cases it may never have appeared. In such cases, one may look to other distinguishing features, namely the fact that Parkinson's disease, diffuse Lewy body disease, multiple system atrophy, and corticobasal ganglionic degeneration are all characterized by an asymmetric onset of parkinsonism with, if anything, a flexion posture, in marked contrast to progressive supranuclear palsy, in which one sees a symmetric onset with an extension posture.

Treatment

Levodopa or dopamine agonists may offer some benefit for the parkinsonism, but this is modest at best and any benefit is generally short-lived (Birdi *et al.* 2002). Interestingly, amitriptyline, in low doses from 25 to 50 mg, improves the parkinsonism, especially regarding gait (Kvale 1982; Newman 1985). Donepezil provided very modest benefit for dementia but worsened the parkinsonism, and on balance may not be beneficial (Litvan *et al.* 2001).

8.8 CORTICOBASAL GANGLIONIC DEGENERATION

Corticobasal ganglionic degeneration, also know as corticobasal degeneration, is a rare disorder, apparently equally common in men and women. It is characterized by an atypical parkinsonism, a dementia, or both.

Clinical features

The onset is gradual, usually in the sixth or seventh decade. Clinically (Litvan *et al.* 1997c; Riley *et al.* 1990; Rinne *et al.* 1994a; Wenning *et al.* 1998), most patients present with a strikingly asymmetric rigid akinetic parkinsonism affecting an upper limb; dystonic rigidity may also be present (Vanek and Jankovic 2001). Cortical sensory loss and apraxia are common, as is myoclonus. Dementia occurs in about one-half of patients and, although this usually follows the motor disturbance by years, it may at times be the presenting feature (Bergeron *et al.* 1996; Schneider *et al.* 1997); indeed, in two series (Grimes *et al.* 1999; Murray *et al.* 2007), the majority of patients presented with dementia. In patients who do develop dementia, depression is common; apathy and irritability may also occur (Litvan *et al.* 1998). Corticobasal ganglionic degeneration may rarely present with a primary progressive aphasia (Geda *et al.* 2007; Ikeda *et al.* 1996) or with a personality change with frontal lobe features (Geda *et al.* 2007). Many authors also comment on the presence of an alien hand sign in corticobasal ganglionic degeneration, but, as pointed out in Section 4.13, this sign is not in fact well described in this disorder: rather, patients display such purposeless movements as grasping, 'wandering' (Rinne *et al.* 1994a; Sawle *et al.* 1991), or levitation (Gibb *et al.* 1994; Riley *et al.* 1990).

MRI scanning may reveal asymmetric cortical atrophy affecting primarily the parietal and frontal cortices.

Course

Over a long period of time, the parkinsonism gradually becomes bilateral; in some cases cerebellar signs may appear and, rarely, a supranuclear ophthalmoplegia has been noted. Death typically occurs within 6–10 years, generally secondary to aspiration pneumonia.

Etiology

The pathology of corticobasal ganglionic degeneration has been described in a number of papers (Gibb *et al.* 1994; Rebeiz *et al.* 1968; Riley *et al.* 1990; Rinne *et al.* 1994a). Macroscopically there is asymmetric cortical atrophy, affecting primarily the parietal lobe and the posterior portion of the frontal lobe; over time, the atrophy may spread

to the contralateral side, and the temporal lobes and anterior portions of the frontal lobes may become involved. Microscopically, changes are seen in these areas and in the basal ganglia and substantia nigra, consisting of neuronal loss and astrocytosis; surviving neurons are large, ballooned, and achromatic and contain tau-positive filaments. The vast majority of cases are sporadic.

Differential diagnosis

When the presentation is with parkinsonism, consideration may be given to Parkinson's disease, diffuse Lewy body disease, multiple system atrophy, and progressive supranuclear palsy, as outlined in Section 3.8. Several features set corticobasal ganglionic degeneration apart from these disorders, including the striking asymmetry of the parkinsonism and the accompanying sensory loss and apraxia. When the presentation is with dementia, consideration, as discussed in Section 5.1, must be given to other disorders capable of causing a dementia of subacute or gradual onset, such as Alzheimer's disease, diffuse Lewy body disease, Binswanger's disease, etc. The correct diagnosis here may remain elusive until the asymmetric parkinsonism appears. In cases that present with aphasia, the differential diagnosis of primary progressive aphasia, as discussed in Section 2.1, should be considered.

Treatment

The general treatment of dementia is discussed in Section 5.1. Supportive measures, including physical and occupational therapy, may be beneficial for the movement disorder; the parkinsonism generally does not respond to levodopa (Rinne *et al.* 1994a).

8.9 MULTIPLE SYSTEM ATROPHY

Multiple system atrophy, as the name suggests, is characterized pathologically by involvement of multiple systems. This involvement, however, does not proceed evenly, and consequently the disease may present in different fashions, depending on which system is involved first (Papp and Lantos 1994; Quinn 1989). Three variants are generally recognized, namely the striatonigral variant, the olivopontocerebellar variant, and the Shy–Drager variant.

This is an uncommon disease and is somewhat more frequent in men than women.

Clinical features

The onset is gradual and typically occurs in the sixth decade. As noted, this disease may present in one of three fashions, each described below.

The striatonigral variant (Colosimo *et al.* 1995; Watanabe *et al.* 2002; Wenning *et al.* 1995), seen when the striatum and substantia nigra are most involved, is characterized by the gradual onset of parkinsonism. The parkinsonism is similar to that seen in Parkinson's disease, with the exceptions that the flexion posture is often extreme and tremor is seen in only a minority and is typically not of the classic pill-rolling type. Furthermore, patients with the striatonigral variant may have other signs not typical of Parkinson's disease, such as hyper-reflexia and extensor plantar responses, myoclonus, and, rarely, supranuclear ophthalmoplegia for downward gaze (Wenning *et al.* 1995).

The olivopontocerebellar variant (Watanabe *et al.* 2002), seen with involvement of the inferior olives, basis pontis, and cerebellar cortex, is characterized by the gradual onset of ataxia, intention tremor, dysarthria, and scanning speech; reflex myoclonus is also commonly seen (Rodriguez *et al.* 1994) and a recent study found emotional incontinence in roughly one-third of all cases (Parvizi *et al.* 2007).

The Shy–Drager variant (Shy and Drager 1960), seen when the intermediolateral gray matter of the spinal cord is heavily involved, is characterized by evidence of autonomic failure, such as urinary retention or incontinence, postural dizziness or syncope, erectile dysfunction, and, rarely, fecal incontinence (Wenning *et al.* 1994).

Dementia may occur in a minority of patients with multiple system atrophy and may be distinguished by elements of a frontal lobe syndrome (Robbins *et al.* 1992). Rarely, multiple system atrophy may present with a personality change and dementia, as has been noted in a case of the olivopontocerebellar variant (Critchley and Greenfield 1948).

Regardless of which variant the disease presents with, over a matter of years most patients will eventually display features of all three variants. Many patients also eventually develop laryngeal stridor.

Interestingly, there is a strong association between multiple system atrophy and REM sleep behavior disorder (Iranzo *et al.* 2005): one report (Plazzi *et al.* 1997) noted that the vast majority of patients with multiple system atrophy had this disorder, which could precede the development of typical symptomatology by years.

Magnetic resonance scanning may reveal atrophy of the striatum, pons, inferior olives, and cerebellum. In some cases, especially those with the striatonigral variant, the putamen displays decreased signal intensity on T2-weighted scanning but laterally has a surrounding rim of increased signal intensity. In other cases, especially those with the olivopontocerebellar variant, the basis pontis will display the 'hot cross bun sign' on axial T2-weighted images, wherein the base of the pons is marked by lines that give it the appearance of a hot cross bun seen from above.

Course

The disease is gradually progressive, with death, often from aspiration pneumonia, generally within 6–9 years.

Etiology

Macroscopically there is variable atrophy of the cerebral cortex (particularly the frontal area), striatum (more so the putamen than the caudate), pons, inferior olives, and cerebellum (Ozawa *et al.* 2004; Wenning *et al.* 1996). Microscopically, cell loss and astrocytosis are seen not only in these areas but also in the substantia nigra, locus ceruleus, ventrolateral medulla (Benarroch *et al.* 1998), and intermediolateral gray matter of the spinal cord. Cytoplasmic inclusions containing alpha-synuclein are seen in oligodendroglia and in surviving neurons.

Multiple system atrophy is a sporadic disorder of unknown cause.

Differential diagnosis

Differential considerations vary according to the variant with which multiple system atrophy presents. In cases of the striatonigral variant, consideration, as discussed in Section 3.8, must be given to certain other neurodegenerative disorders capable of causing parkinsonism, such as Parkinson's disease, diffuse Lewy body disease, progressive supranuclear palsy, and corticobasal ganglionic degeneration. Although a relatively pure case of the striatonigral variant might be difficult to distinguish from other causes of classic parkinsonism, especially Parkinson's disease or diffuse Lewy body disease, the eventual appearance of evidence of other system involvement, for example the appearance of ataxia, will secure the diagnosis. In cases of the olivopontocerebellar variant, consideration is given to alcoholic or paraneoplastic cerebellar degeneration, and to spinocerebellar ataxia, which is distinguished by its autosomal dominant inheritance; fragile X-associated tremor/ataxia syndrome (FXTAS) may be difficult to distinguish on clinical grounds, and genetic testing may be required.

Treatment

Parkinsonism may be treated with levodopa, but the response is neither prolonged nor robust and side-effects are common (Wenning *et al.* 1995). Interestingly, there is a double-blind study that demonstrated an improvement in parkinsonism after treatment with paroxetine, in doses of up to 60 mg/day (Freiss *et al.* 2006). There is no known treatment for the cerebellar symptoms. Postural dizziness may respond to fludrocortisone or midodrine. Erectile dysfunction has been treated with sildenafil; however, this was often not tolerated because of an aggravation of hypotension (Hussain *et al.* 2001). The general treatment of dementia is discussed in Section 5.1. Continuous positive airway pressure (CPAP) or BIPAP may be helpful in cases of laryngeal stridor; however, tracheostomy may eventually be required.

8.10 HUNTINGTON'S DISEASE

Huntington's disease, also known as Huntington's chorea or chorea major, is an autosomal dominantly inherited disorder that is characterized, in its full expression, by a combination of chorea and dementia. This disorder was first clearly characterized by George Huntington in 1872, who observed a number of affected families in East Hampton on Long Island (Brody and Wilkins 1967; Huntington 1872). Although the lifetime prevalence is not high (from 0.004 to 0.008 among white populations, and only one-third of that in black populations and one-tenth among Japanese populations), these patients are not uncommonly seen in hospital and clinic.

Clinical features

The onset is generally highly insidious and may occur anywhere from childhood to the eighth decade, with most patients falling ill in their 30s. The presentation may be with either chorea or a personality change; over time, in the vast majority of patients, both these syndromes will become present and be joined by the gradual development of a dementia (Pflanz et al. 1991). Exceptions to this rule do occur, especially in those with late onset in the sixth decade or beyond, when one may see primarily chorea, with little or no cognitive deficit (Britton et al. 1995).

Chorea may initially present as fidgetiness, clumsiness, or a tendency to drop things; obvious choreiform movements are generally first visible on the face (including the forehead), from where they spread to involve the trunk and extremities. There may be facial grimacing, brow wrinkling, and blinking; upper extremity involvement may lead to shoulder shrugging, abrupt flinging of the arms, or purposeless 'piano-playing' movements of the hands. In shaking the patient's hand, one may note the classic 'milkmaid' grip, wherein the patient's grasping of the examiner's hand feels as if the patient is attempting to milk a cow. Lower extremity involvement may lead to a lurching, staggering, or 'dancing and prancing' gait, which in some cases may so resemble the gait seen in alcohol intoxication that patients have been arrested for public intoxication (Lesse 1946). Importantly, these choreiform movements are quite brief, appearing and disappearing on a random basis from one location to another with lightning-like rapidity. Interestingly, although some patients seem fully aware of their chorea, it is not at all uncommon to find patients with obvious chorea denying that anything is amiss. The depth of this denial is at times extreme: I have seen patients with chorea of such severity as to preclude safe ambulation who nevertheless stoutly deny that anything at all is amiss.

Early on in the course of the disease, patients may attempt, with varying degrees of success, to disguise the choreic movements by merging them with purposeful movements: for example, a choreic fling of the arm up to the head may be purposefully extended to draw the fingers through the hair, as if the purpose had all along been to straighten the hair. Dysarthria often occurs, as does dysphagia, which may lead to aspiration (Leopold and Kagel 1985). The chorea eventually makes almost all purposeful activity, whether eating, dressing, or walking, almost impossible, and patients eventually become chairbound or bedridden. At the end, the chorea may gradually disappear, to be replaced by a rigid, akinetic state (Feigin et al. 1995). In advanced cases, seizures may also occur.

The personality change presents with poor judgment, impulsivity, irritability, and an overall coarsening of behavior. Over time, as noted earlier, a dementia develops, characterized by deficits in memory, concentration, calculation, and abstraction; focal signs, such as aphasia and apraxia, are generally not seen. Associated symptoms are found in the vast majority of patients (Caine and Shoulson 1983; Folstein et al. 1983; Paulsen et al. 2001). These include depression of variable severity in roughly half, agitation, irritability, apathy and anxiety, and, in a minority, euphoria or, rarely, mania. Delusions, generally of persecution, and, less commonly, hallucinations may be seen in a small minority, and, albeit rarely, Huntington's disease may present with a psychosis (Caine and Shoulson 1983). Suicidal ideation is common (Paulsen et al. 2005), and suicide itself occurs in a significant minority (Schoenfeld et al. 1984).

As noted earlier, Huntington's disease may present in childhood or adolescence, and when it does one often sees what is known as the Westphal variant of Huntington's disease, in which, rather than chorea, there is often a rigid, akinetic state that is generally accompanied by severe dementia, often with seizures, myoclonus, and ataxia (Bird and Paulson 1971; Campbell et al. 1965; Hansotia et al. 1968; Jervis 1979; Siesling et al. 1997); in other cases, rather than parkinsonism, the presentation may be with chorea, myoclonus, or dementia (Ribai et al. 2007).

Computed tomography or axial MR scanning may be normal early in the course of the disease; over time, however, because of atrophy of the caudate nuclei, there is a characteristic dilation of the frontal horns of the lateral ventricles, yielding a characteristic 'butterfly' configuration. Cortical atrophy, especially of the frontal lobes, may also be seen.

As noted below, Huntington's disease is a fully penetrant, autosomal dominant disease, and genetic testing is highly specific and sensitive (International Huntington Association 1994; Kremer et al. 1994). A positive family history is almost universally found, and in one American family it was possible to trace the disease back to an ancestor who arrived with the Puritans (Vessie 1932). Exceptions to this rule may occur secondary to rarely occurring spontaneous mutations or, more commonly, to uncertain parentage (Ramos-Arroyo et al. 2005).

Course

Huntington's disease is relentlessly progressive: most patients die within 10–30 years of onset, with an average life expectancy of about 15 years. Those with an earlier age of onset, for example those with the Westphal variant, experience a more rapid course, with death within about 10 years; conversely, those with a late onset, in the fifth decade or beyond, typically experience a more leisurely course.

Etiology

Huntington's disease is a fully penetrant autosomal dominant disorder: the affected gene codes for a protein known as huntingtin and is located on chromosome 4. The gene normally contains anywhere from 10 to 29 CAG trinucleotide repeats, whereas in Huntington's disease, anywhere from 36 to 121 repeats may be found (Kremer *et al.* 1994). Very rarely, sporadic cases may occur: in such cases, it appears that the patient's father, himself unaffected, harboured a number of CAG repeats that, although still within the bounds of normal, were unstable and underwent expansion (Myers *et al.* 1993). Although an inverse correlation has been found with the number of repeats and the age of onset (Marder *et al.* 2002), there is apparently no correlation with the appearance of mood changes or delusions or hallucinations (Tsuang *et al.* 2000; Zappacosta *et al.* 1996).

Macroscopically, atrophy is noted in the caudate (as illustrated in Figure 8.7), less so in the putamen, and to a degree in the frontal and parietal cortices. Neuronal loss and reactive astrocytosis is noted in these areas; in the caudate nucleus in particular, spiny neurons are lost first (Mann *et al.* 1993b; Myers *et al.* 1988). Surviving neurons may display intranuclear inclusions, which contain the huntingtin protein.

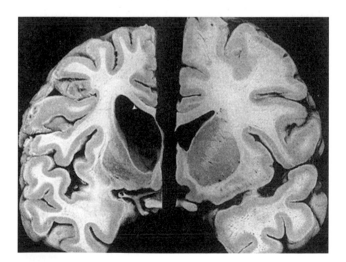

Figure 8.7 Marked atropy of the caudate, with compensatory ventricular dilation, in a case of Huntington's disease compared with a control brain on the right. (Reproduced from Graham and Lantos 1996.)

Differential diagnosis

Genetic testing has greatly simplified the differential diagnostic task, and should be considered in any patient with the gradual onset of chorea in late adolescence or early adult years. The other disorders to consider in the differential are discussed in Section 3.4, and certain clinical features, atypical for Huntington's disease, should suggest a close look. These include tics, dystonia or lip-biting (seen in choreoacanthocytosis), ataxia (in dentatorubropallidoluysian atrophy), dystonia or parkinsonism (in Fahr's syndrome), and dystonia or tremor (in Wilson's disease).

Another differential possibility to consider is schizophrenia, especially when this is complicated by tardive dyskinesia. As noted above, the dementia of Huntington's disease may be complicated by delusions or hallucinations, and in some cases these symptoms may be very prominent, thus creating a clinical syndrome of psychosis and chorea, which, at first glance, may appear similar to that seen when schizophrenia is complicated by tardive dyskinesia. Certain features of the chorea seen in these two situations, however, may enable a clinical differentiation. The chorea of tardive dyskinesia is generally stereotyped and repetitive, almost never involves the forehead, and generally leaves gait relatively unaffected. This is in contrast to the chorea of Huntington's disease, which is mercurial, flitting from one body part to another in an unpredictable fashion, and which typically affects the forehead and gait.

Treatment

The severity of chorea may be reduced by treatment with antipsychotics. Of the antipsychotics, the first-generation agent haloperidol is most often used, in doses from 1 to 10 mg/day (Barr *et al.* 1988). Akathisia may occur with haloperidol and, hence, second-generation agents, such as olanzapine (Bonelli *et al.* 2002; Dipple 1999; Paleacu *et al.* 2002), are also being used. Tetrabenazine, a dopamine depleter not available in the United States, is also beneficial (Huntington Study Group 2006). Amantadine may have a place here also. Although a double-blind study of amantadine, in a dose of 300 mg/day, found no benefit relative to placebo (O'Suilleabhain and Dewey 2003), another study (Verhagen Metman *et al.* 2002) did find a benefit, but only with a higher dose of 400 mg/day.

The general treatment of dementia is discussed in Section 5.1. In cases complicated by agitation or delusions or hallucinations, antipsychotics may also be useful. Depression may respond to an antidepressant, such as an SSRI. With progression of the disease, institutionalization becomes almost inevitable.

Ongoing research efforts are underway to find treatments that may retard the progression of the disease, and many patients are highly motivated to participate.

As noted earlier, genetic testing is now available, and should be offered to patients with a compatible clinical picture and to unaffected relatives. Extensive counselling resources should be available for instances when the test is positive.

8.11 CHOREOACANTHOCYTOSIS

Choreoacanthocytosis, also known as chorea-acanthocytosis, is a rare autosomal recessively inherited disorder that typically manifests with chorea, as well as dementia in roughly half of cases; in all cases one also finds an excessive percentage of acanthocytic red blood cells. This last characteristic, namely acanthocytosis, qualifies choreoacanthocytosis as one member of a larger group of disorders known as the neuroacanthocytoses, which, as noted below in the discussion on differential diagnosis, includes such conditions as the McLeod syndrome.

Clinical features

The onset is generally in the late twenties or early thirties but may occur anywhere from late childhood to the seventh decade. Clinically (Critchley *et al.* 1968; Feinberg *et al.* 1991; Hardie *et al.* 1991; Kartsounis and Hardie 1996; Lossos *et al.* 2005; Sakai *et al.* 1981), most cases present with a gradually progressive chorea, which, over time, is often joined by other abnormal movements, such as tics, dystonia, or a mild parkinsonism. A classic symptom, seen, however, in only a minority, is self-mutilating lip- or tongue-biting. Importantly, this self-mutilation is outside the patient's control: one patient (Medalia *et al.* 1989), despite attempting to 'restrain herself . . . by placing her fingers or a folded towel in her mouth . . . nevertheless had bleeding and scarred lesions of her oral mucosa and lips'. Most patients will also develop a sensorimotor peripheral poly-neuropathy, and, in a minority, seizures may occur. Roughly half of all patients will also develop a personality change, a dementia, or both.

Acanthocytosis to a degree of 10 percent or more is seen on peripheral smears; importantly, the smears must be fresh wet preparations and, given the chance of false negatives, at least three smears should be examined (Hardie *et al.* 1991). Genetic testing is available.

Creatinine kinase is elevated in most cases and MR scanning may reveal atrophy of the caudate nucleus.

Course

The disease is gradually progressive, with death, on average, after 14 years.

Etiology

Choreoacanthocytosis is an autosomal recessive condition occurring secondary to mutations in the *VPS13A* gene on chromosome 9q21 (formerly known as *CHAC*), which codes for a protein known as chorein. There may be considerable phenotypic heterogeneity in the same family.

Macroscopically, there is atrophy of the caudate, putamen, and, to a lesser degree, the globus pallidus. Microscopically, neuronal loss and gliosis are seen in these structure and in the substantia nigra (Rinne *et al.* 1994b). Axonal loss occurs in the peripheral nerves (Hardie *et al.* 1991; Ohnishi *et al.* 1981).

Differential diagnosis

The differential for chorea is discussed in Section 3.4; of the disorders considered there, several others, in addition to choreoacanthocytosis, present with chorea in early adult years and must be distinguished from choreoacanthocytosis. Huntington's disease is marked by autosomal dominant inheritance and an absence of a peripheral neuropathy and, critically, a lack of acanthocytosis. As noted earlier, other disorders, in addition to choreoacanthocytosis, may also present with chorea and acanthocytosis, and these include the McLeod syndrome and Huntington's disease-like 2 (Walker *et al.* 2002). The McLeod syndrome is distinguished by X-linked inheritance and Huntington's disease-like 2 by an autosomal dominant pattern of inheritance. Genetic testing is available for all of these disorders.

Treatment

As for Huntington's disease, chorea may be treated with antipsychotics; the general treatment of dementia is discussed in Section 5.1.

8.12 FXTAS

FXTAS, also known as the fragile X-associated tremor/ataxia syndrome, is a recently described inherited disorder characterized by the gradual development of tremor, ataxia, and, in a minority, dementia in middle-aged or older adults. This is not an uncommon disorder, and although cases have been reported in women (Hagerman *et al.* 2004), it is far more common in men.

Clinical features

Clinical features have been described in a number of papers (Greco *et al.* 2006; Hagerman *et al.* 2001; Hall *et al.* 2005). Although the age of onset ranges from the fourth to the ninth decade, most patients fall ill in the seventh decade with the gradual onset of ataxia and tremor. The tremor, although typically of the intention type, may also have a rest or postural component. Over time, a mild parkinsonism may also accrue, with rest tremor, rigidity, and bradykinesia. A peripheral neuropathy is common, and some patients may experience autonomic symptoms, such as erectile dysfunction.

Cognitive deficits eventually appear, and anywhere from one-quarter to one-half of all patients may eventually become demented: short-term memory loss, poor concentration, concreteness, and poor judgment are common. Frontal lobe symptomatology may also be seen, with disinhibition, perseveration, and inappropriate jocularity, and mood changes are common, with agitation, irritability, apathy, or depression (Bacalman *et al.* 2006; Bourgeois *et al.* 2007).

Magnetic resonance scanning may reveal both cerebral and cerebellar cortical atrophy. The most characteristic finding, however, is the 'middle cerebellar peduncle' sign: on T1-weighted scans these peduncles show decreased signal intensity, and on T2-weighted scans there is increased signal intensity (Brunberg *et al.* 2002). This sign, although not universally present, becomes more likely later in the course of the disease. Genetic testing is available.

Course

Symptoms progress very slowly.

Etiology

As might be gathered from the name of this syndrome, FXTAS bears a relationship to the fragile X syndrome: both occur as the result of a mutation in the fragile X mental retardation 1 (*FMR1*) gene, located on the long arm of the X chromosome.

Normally, the *FMR1* gene contains anywhere from 5 to 55 CGG trinucleotide repeats. The mutation in question involves an increase in the number of these repeats beyond the normal range. Increases into the range of 55 to 200 repeats have traditionally been termed a 'premutation' whereas increases above 200 repeats have been considered to constitute a 'full' mutation. Individuals with full mutations, especially men, typically develop the fragile X syndrome, with mental retardation. Until recently, it had been thought that those with a 'premutation' were merely carriers who remained free of any symptoms. The recognition of FXTAS, however, has now made it clear that this 'premutation', rather than being benign, may cause symptoms in its own right. Indeed, among men with the premutation, the penetrance progressively rises from roughly 20 percent in those from 50 to 59 years of age up to 75 percent in those aged 80 or above (Jacquemont *et al.* 2004).

Macroscopically, there is cerebral and cerebellar cortical atrophy. Microscopically (Greco *et al.* 2002, 2006), there is neuronal loss in these areas, and status spongiosus in the cerebellar white matter and the middle cerebellar peduncles. Intranuclear inclusions are found in both astrocytes and surviving neurons.

Differential diagnosis

Spinocerebellar ataxia is suggested by the autosomal dominant pattern of inheritance. Multiple system atrophy may be difficult to distinguish on clinical grounds, and the differential may rest on genetic testing.

One clue to the diagnosis rests in the family history. When the diagnosis is considered in a middle-aged or elderly man, one should inquire whether any of his grandchildren have mental retardation. If the middle-aged or elderly man in question does have FXTAS, then any daughters would also have the 'pre-mutation'. Increases in repeat length are likely during oogenesis and, consequently, a daughter may have passed on a 'full' mutation to one of her children, who, in turn, might express the fragile X syndrome with mental retardation. As noted above, FXTAS is much less likely in females and, when it does occur, it is less severe; this is probably due to the fact that females who do have the 'pre-mutation' also have a normal gene on the other X chromosome. In cases of middle-aged or elderly women suspected of having FXTAS, the family history may also help; however, here one looks only to the children and not the grandchildren for the telltale finding of mental retardation.

Treatment

The general treatment of dementia is described in Section 5.1; as yet there are no controlled studies focusing on FXTAS itself.

8.13 SENILE CHOREA

Senile chorea is a rare disorder characterized by the gradual onset of chorea late in life, in the absence of a family history.

Clinical features

The onset is insidious and generally in the seventh decade. Clinically, one sees the gradual progression of a mild chorea, generally involving the upper extremities or the face (Delwaide and Desseilles 1977; Klawans and Barr 1981; Shinotoh *et al.* 1994; Varga *et al.* 1982). There are no other abnormal movements and no dementia.

Course

The disorder is very gradually progressive.

Etiology

Microscopically, neuronal loss is noted in the caudate. The mechanism is not known.

Differential diagnosis

Of the disorders capable of causing chorea, discussed in Section 3.4, special consideration should be given to the following (Warren *et al.* 1998): late-onset Huntington's disease, the anti-phospholipid syndrome, tardive dyskinesia, and Fahr's syndrome; of these, Huntington's disease is the most likely and, hence, genetic testing is in order (Garcia Ruiz *et al.* 1997). Edentulousness should also be considered, as it may be accompanied by orofacial movements that resemble chorea (Koller 1983).

Treatment

In general, no treatment other than simple reassurance is required. In those rare cases in which the chorea becomes severe enough to interfere with functioning, consideration may be given to treatment with antipsychotics, as described for Huntington's disease.

8.14 BENIGN HEREDITARY CHOREA

This is a rare autosomal dominantly inherited disorder, characterized by a childhood-onset chorea that is generally non-progressive.

Clinical features

Onset may be anywhere from infancy to late childhood, and is characterized by a generalized chorea that may be accompanied by a subtle degree of ataxia (Breedveld *et al.* 2002; Fernandez *et al.* 2001); hypothyroidism may also occur (Asmus *et al.* 2005). There is no dementia (Behan and Bone 1977).

Course

After a period in which the chorea becomes established, although in most cases there is no change over time, one may see in a minority either a mild progression (Kleiner-Fisman *et al.* 2003) or, conversely, in adolescence or early adult years, a partial remission of symptoms (Fernandez *et al.* 2001).

Etiology

As noted, this is an autosomal dominant condition and mutations have been found in the thyroid transcription factor 1 gene (*TITF1*) (Asmus *et al.* 2005). Neuronal loss has been reported in the striatum (Kleiner-Fisman *et al.* 2005) and astrocytosis has been noted in the globus pallidus, thalamus, hypothalamus, and periaqueductal gray (Kleiner-Fisman *et al.* 2003).

Differential diagnosis

Other disorders capable of causing chorea in childhood, as discussed in Section 3.4, include Sydenham's chorea and cerebral palsy. The autosomal dominant pattern displayed, and the course, however, are quite distinctive.

Treatment

There are no established treatments; in case reports, levodopa was beneficial (Asmus *et al.* 2005). Consideration may also be given to treatment with antipsychotics, as discussed for Huntington's disease.

8.15 DENTATORUBROPALLIDOLUYSIAN ATROPHY

The unwieldy name of this disorder is derived from the main structures that show pathological changes, namely the dentate nucleus, the nucleus rubor (the red nucleus), the globus pallidus, and the corpus Luysii (the subthalamic nucleus). Dentatorubropallidoluysian atrophy, also known as dentatorubralpallidoluysian atrophy or simply DRPLA, is a rare autosomal dominantly inherited disorder, which may present early, in childhood or adolescence, or late, in adult years: among adult-onset cases, one typically sees a movement disorder, with chorea or ataxia, and a dementia. Some authorities consider DRPLA to be one of the spinocerebellar ataxias; however, in this author's opinion, given that DRPLA may be characterized by chorea rather than ataxia, this seems to be inappropriate nosologic 'lumping' and the disorders are considered separately in this text.

Clinical features

The onset is gradual, regardless of whether it is early or late, and the clinical features are strongly influenced by the age of onset. Early-onset cases (Becher *et al.* 1997) are characterized by ataxia, myoclonus, seizures, and a dementia. Late-onset cases (Becher *et al.* 1997; Iizuka *et al.* 1984; Nielsen *et al.* 1996; Villani *et al.* 1998; Warner *et al.* 1994, 1995; Yoshii *et al.* 1998) are typified by either chorea or ataxia (or a combination of these); in a minority of cases one may also see a mild degree of dystonia or parkinsonism. In adults one also sees the eventual development of a dementia, which may be accompanied by prominent hallucinations and delusions; rarely, DRPLA may present with a psychosis in adult years (Adachi *et al.* 2001). A small minority of adults may also have seizures. Magnetic resonance scanning may reveal atrophy of the superior cerebellar peduncle and, on T2-weighted scans, increased signal intensity in the globus pallidus.

Course

DRPLA is a gradually progressive disorder.

Etiology

As noted earlier, DRPLA is an autosomal dominantly inherited disorder: mutations exist in the gene for atrophin-1, found on chromosome 12, which consist of an expansion of a normally occurring CAG trinucleotide repeat (Nagafuchi et al. 1994). There is considerable phenotypic heterogeneity both within and between families (Potter et al. 1995). Neuronal loss is found not only in the namesakes of this disorder (the dentate nuclei, red nucleus, globus pallidus, and subthalamic nucleus) but also in the striatum, substantia nigra, inferior olives, thalamus, and cerebral cortex (Becher et al. 1997; Goto et al. 1982; Iizuka et al. 1984; Warner et al. 1994). In surviving neurons, intranuclear inclusions, formed of abnormal atrophin-1, may be found.

Differential diagnosis

In adults, the differential is influenced by the nature of the movement disorder: when chorea is prominent, consideration is given to Huntington's disease, and when ataxia is foremost, spinocerebellar ataxia enters the differential. Genetic testing is often required to make the differential.

Treatment

There is no specific treatment. The general treatment of dementia is discussed in Section 5.1; in cases in which chorea is problematic, treatment with antipsychotics, as for Huntington's disease, may be considered.

8.16 WILSON'S DISEASE

Wilson's disease, also known as hepatolenticular degeneration, is an autosomal recessively inherited disorder characterized pathologically by copper deposition in the liver and brain. Although relatively rare, occurring in perhaps 1–2/100 000 population, it is an important diagnosis given its eminent treatability.

Clinical features

The clinical features of Wilson's disease have been described in several large series (Dening and Berrios 1989; Machado et al. 2006; Starosta-Rubinstein et al. 1987; Taly et al. 2007; Walshe and Yealland 1992). The onset is typically between late childhood and early adulthood, although the range is wide, from early childhood to the sixth decade. The presentation may be with a movement disorder, psychosis, personality change, or dementia; over time, most patients eventually develop a combination of these features. Other symptoms include seizures, a Kayser–Fleischer ring, hepatitis, and anemia.

The movement disorder may consist of dystonia, chorea, tremor, or parkinsonism; dysarthria may also appear. Dystonia may present with torticollis, dystonia of the upper or lower extremity, oculogyric crisis (Lee et al. 1999), or facial dystonia; classically, there is a fixed, vacuous, wide-mouthed dystonic smile. Chorea may involve either the upper or the lower extremities. The tremor may be rhythmic or irregular; at times, one may see the classic 'wing-beating' tremor in which a rhythmic elevation and lowering of the upper extremities, combined with flexion at the elbows, gives an overall appearance of a frightened bird flapping its wings.

Personality change is generally characterized by lability, disinhibition, and, at times, bizarre behavior (Bridgman and Smyth 1944; Dening and Berrios 1989; Walshe and Yealland 1992).

Psychosis is characterized by hallucinations and delusions (Dening and Berrios 1989; Gysin and Cooke 1950) and may be quite bizarre, with Schneiderian first rank symptoms. Indeed, one of Wilson's (1912) patients heard 'God and the devil talking to him simultaneously' and said that he was 'influenced, willed or hypnotized to do certain things'. In one case (Davis and Borde 1993), stuporous catatonia dominated the presentation.

Seizures may occur but are rare, occurring in about 5 percent of patients (Dening et al. 1988).

The Kayser–Fleischer ring is a golden-brown discoloration of the corneal limbus, visible either on slit-lamp examination or to the naked eye. Although this Kayser–Fleischer ring is present in the overwhelming majority of cases, cases of unequivocal Wilson's disease (with a movement disorder) without a Kayser–Fleischer ring do occur (Demirkiran et al. 1996).

Hepatic damage may lead to clinical hepatitis, with fever, malaise, abdominal pain, and elevated transaminase levels. With significant hepatic dysfunction, hepatic encephalopathy may occur (Starosta-Rubinstein et al. 1987).

A Coombs-negative hemolytic anemia may occur.

The ceruloplasmin and total serum copper levels are both low, but the serum free copper is elevated, as is the 24-hour urinary copper; in a small minority, the ceruloplasmin level may be normal. Liver biopsy reveals an elevated copper level.

Magnetic resonance scanning may reveal characteristic findings (Sinha et al. 2006). On T2-weighted scans, increased signal intensity may be seen in the head of the caudate and lateral aspect of the putamen, with decreased signal intensity in the globus pallidus; in the midbrain, T2-weighted scanning may reveal the 'face of the giant panda' sign, with increased signal intensity in the tegmentum and decreased signal intensity in the red nuclei. On T1-weighted scans, increased signal intensity may be seen in the caudate and the putamen.

Given the large number of possible mutations, genetic testing is not practical.

Course

Although there may be partial, temporary remissions, the overall course is one of progression, with death within 5–10 years.

Etiology

Wilson's disease is essentially a disease of copper metabolism. Normally, after copper is absorbed from the intestine, it is bound to hepatic ceruloplasmin and then for the most part undergoes biliary excretion. In Wilson's disease biliary excretion is deficient and copper accumulates, first in the liver, where it causes hepatitis, and then, once it spills over into the systemic circulation, in the brain, where copper deposition occurs primarily in a pericapillary distribution. Macroscopically (Howard and Royce 1919), there is atrophy and a brownish discoloration of the striatum, with, in advanced cases, cavitation (Wilson 1912) and a mild degree of cortical atrophy. Microscopically, there is neuronal loss and astrocytosis in the striatum (more so the putamen than the caudate) and to a lesser degree in the globus pallidus; other affected structures include the cerebral cortex (especially the frontal lobes [Barnes and Hurst 1926]), thalamus, red nucleus, substantia nigra, dentate nucleus, and cerebellar cortex. Copper deposition in Descemet's membrane gives rise to the classic Kayser–Fleischer ring.

As noted earlier, Wilson's disease is an autosomal recessive disease, and it results from mutations in the *ATP7B* gene on chromosome 13 that codes for the copper-binding ATPase (Bull *et al.* 1993; Chelly and Monaco 1993); multiple different mutations have been identified (Thomas *et al.* 1995).

Differential diagnosis

Given the pleomorphic symptomatology of Wilson's disease, the differential diagnosis is large. In practice, given the availability of treatment, and the consequent importance of not missing the diagnosis, it is appropriate to test for Wilson's disease in any young person with a clinical presentation consistent with Wilson's disease that cannot be readily and fully accounted for by another disease process. One disorder in particular deserves mention as it may mimic Wilson's disease not only clinically but also with respect to laboratory values. Hereditary ceruloplasmin deficiency, like Wilson's disease, is characterized by low ceruloplasmin and total serum copper levels, but, unlike Wilson's disease, it is characterized by a low 24-hour urinary copper level (Kawanami *et al.* 1996).

Treatment

Treatment is aimed at reducing the total copper burden. Several methods are available, including chelation with penicillamine, trientine, or tetrathiomolybdate; treatment with zinc; and limiting copper intake.

Chelation has traditionally been accomplished with penicillamine; however, this agent has multiple, severe side-effects and also, in a significant minority of patients, will either exacerbate pre-existing symptoms (Starosta-Rubinstein *et al.* 1987) or, in pre-symptomatic patients, cause them (Brewer *et al.* 1994; Glass *et al.* 1990). Consequently, attention has shifted to two other chelating agents, namely trientine and tetrathiomolybdate; of these, tetrathiomolybdate is more effective than trientine (Brewer *et al.* 2006), and is generally well-tolerated (Brewer *et al.* 1996).

Zinc induces intestinal metallothionein, which in turn binds copper and prevents its absorption; it is less effective than chelating agents. Zinc is given in a dose of 50 mg three times daily, before meals (Hoogenraad *et al.* 1987).

Dietary restriction of copper is the least effective of the treatment measures and requires an avoidance of shellfish, legumes, nuts, grains, coffee, chocolate, and organ meats.

On balance, symptomatic patients should probably be treated with tetrathiomolybdate and zinc. Asymptomatic patients, with no evidence of liver or brain involvement, might be treated with zinc, with careful monitoring. With chelation treatment of symptomatic patients, recovery is slow, and up to a year or more may be required to see full improvement. The degree of recovery varies with the severity of symptoms before treatment; in mild cases there may be complete recovery, whereas in severe cases, some degree of residual symptomatology is to be expected.

A final alternative is liver transplantation, which, as it restores the body's ability to handle copper, is curative. This should be considered in either treatment-resistant or fulminant cases (Bax *et al.* 1998; Stracciari *et al.* 2000).

Symptomatic treatment of dementia is discussed in Section 5.1, of personality change in Section 7.2, and of psychosis in Section 7.1. Given that almost all patients with Wilson's disease will have some degree of hepatic failure, doses of hepatically metabolized medications must be adjusted accordingly.

All of the patient's siblings should be offered testing for copper and ceruloplasmin levels and, in doubtful cases, consideration should be given to liver biopsy.

8.17 SPINOCEREBELLAR ATAXIA

Spinocerebellar ataxia (SCA), also known as autosomal dominant cerebellar ataxia, is an uncommon, dominantly inherited disorder characterized, in most cases, by a slowly progressive ataxia, joined, over time, by various other features, which may include dementia, personality change, or delusions or hallucinations.

Some words are required regarding the synonym for this disorder, namely autosomal dominant cerebellar ataxia or ADCA. This name was initially utilized by Harding (1982, 1984), who went on to divide ADCA into three different subtypes, namely types III, II, and I. Type III was described as being characterized solely by cerebellar signs, without any associated features. Types II and I, by contrast, did encompass associated features, the difference between type II and type I being that type II could be accompanied by pigmentary retinopathy, whereas type I cases were specifically free of this sign. The nosologic status of this proposed subdivision is, however, in doubt, on both clinical and etiologic grounds. From a clinical point of view, it appears that type III cases are exceedingly rare, perhaps (with a sufficiently long follow-up) non-existent, and that, when comparing types II and I, type I patients (that is to say, those with associated features but without pigmentary retinopathy) comprise the overwhelming majority. Furthermore, from an etiologic point of view, it appears that this subdivision does not 'cleave' nature at the genetic 'joints', in that mutations at the same gene locus may cause two different clinical types (e.g., spinocerebellar ataxia type 6 [SCA6] is associated with both type III [Ishikawa et al. 1999] and type I [Schols et al. 1998]). Given this nosologic uncertainty, it may be prudent, for the time being, to refrain from subtyping cases as III, II, or I, but rather to concentrate on making sure that one has a case of ADCA and then proceeding to identify the responsible genetic locus.

Clinical features

The clinical hallmark of SCA is the appearance of a gradually progressive cerebellar ataxia, which is generally accompanied by dysarthria and nystagmus. The onset, although generally in the early to mid-adult years, may occur anywhere from childhood to senescence. With disease progression, almost all patients will also develop one or more of the following associated features: hyper-reflexia and extensor plantar responses; decreased vibratory sense, atrophy, and fasciculations; supranuclear ophthalmoplegia; tremor (including titubation), dystonia, chorea, myoclonus or parkinsonism; or pigmentary retinopathy. Seizures may also occur; however, they are uncommon and may be grand mal, simple, or complex partial in type.

Dementia may occur in a minority as may a personality change (often of the frontal lobe type), and some patients may develop delusions and hallucinations. Rarely, SCA may present with dementia, a personality change, or a psychosis.

The plenitude of these associated features should not, however, distract attention from the central feature of this syndrome, namely a progressive cerebellar ataxia; the associated features, usually few in number in any given case, generally play only a minor part in the overall clinical picture.

Genetic testing is available. Interestingly, given the wide phenotypic heterogeneity, it does not appear possible to reliably predict which SCA type is present based on the clinical picture (Giunti et al. 1998; Schols et al. 1998; Tang et al. 2000).

Magnetic resonance scanning may reveal atrophy of the cerebellum, pons, and inferior olives (Arpa et al. 1999; Ueyama et al. 1998).

Etiology

As noted, SCA is an autosomal dominantly inherited syndrome, and 26 different loci have been identified (Duenas et al. 2006): SCA1 on chromosome 6 (Goldfarb et al. 1989, 1996; Sasaki et al. 1996; Schols et al. 1997a; Tang et al. 2000), SCA2 on chromosome 12 (Adams et al. 1997; Burk et al. 1999; Giunti et al. 1998; Hsieh et al. 1999; Schols et al. 1997a,b; Tang et al. 2000; Ueyama et al. 1998; Zhou et al. 1998), SCA3 (also known as Machado–Joseph disease) on chromosome 14 (Durr et al. 1996; Lopes-Cendes et al. 1996; Schols et al. 1996, 1997b; Takiyama et al. 1994; Tang et al. 2000; Zhou et al. 1997), SCA4 on chromosome 16 (Nagaoka et al. 2000), SCA5 on chromosome 11 (Stevanin et al. 1999), SCA6 on chromosome 19 (Arpa et al. 1999; Ikeuchi et al. 1997; Ishikawa et al. 1999; Kaseda et al. 1999; Matsumara et al. 1997; Schols et al. 1998; Stevanin et al. 1997), SCA7 on chromosome 3 (Benton et al. 1998; Jobsis et al. 1997; Modi et al. 2000), SCA8 on chromosome 13 (Ikeda et al. 2000), SCA10 on chromosome 22 (Grewal et al. 2002; Matsuura et al. 1999), SCA11 on chromosome 15 (Worth et al. 1999), SCA12 on chromosome 5 (Seltzer et al. 1999), SCA13 on chromosome 19, SCA14 on chromosome 19 (Yamashita et al. 2000), SCA 15 on chromosome 3, SCA16 on chromosome 8, SCA17 on chromosome 6 (Lasek et al. 2006; Maltecca et al. 2003; O'Hearn et al. 2001), SCA18 on chromosome 7, SCA19 on chromosome 1, SCA20 on chromosome 11, SCA21 on chromosome 7, SCA23 on chromosome 20, SCA24 on chromosome 1, SCA25 on chromosome 2, SCA26 on chromosome 19, SCA27 on chromosome 13, and SCA28 on chromosome 18. Some authors also include dentatorubropallidoluysian atrophy among the SCAs (specifying it as 'SCA9'), but given that patients with dentatorubropallidoluysian atrophy may have little or no ataxia, and often have prominent chorea, this inclusion may not be warranted, and, in this text, dentatorubropallidoluysian atrophy is discussed separately, in its own section.

Most of the known mutations involve trinucleotide repeat expansions, as has been found for SCA1, -2, -3, -6, -7, -12, and -17; a CTG trinucleotide repeat expansion has been noted for SCA8, a pentanucleotide repeat expansion for SCA10, and missense mutations for SCA5, -23, -14, and -27.

The pathologic hallmark of this syndrome is atrophy of the cerebellum, pons, and inferior olives; in addition to these findings, associated atrophy may also be found in one or more of the following structures: the spinocerebellar tracts, Clarke's column, the globus pallidus, the subthalamic nucleus, the substantia nigra, and the cerebral cortex (Durr *et al.* 1996; Ikeuchi *et al.* 1997; Ishikawa *et al.* 1999; Jobsis *et al.* 1997; Takiyama *et al.* 1994).

Differential diagnosis

Two autosomal dominant disorders to consider include dentatorubropallidoluysian atrophy and Gerstmann–Straussler–Scheinker disease. Dentatorubropallidoluysan atrophy is marked, in many cases, by prominent chorea, and this may be a clue, but genetic testing is typically required to rule out both these disorders. Friedrich's ataxia is suggested by an autosomal recessive mode of inheritance and a typically early age of onset. Multiple system atrophy of the olivopontocerebellar type is suggested by concurrent autonomic signs and by its sporadic nature. Other sporadic disorders to consider include vitamin B12 deficiency, hypothyroidism, paraneoplastic cerebellar degeneration, and alcoholic cerebellar degeneration.

Treatment

In one double-blind study (Botez *et al.* 1996), amantadine reduced ataxia in patients with SCA1 and SCA2. The general treatment of dementia is discussed in Section 5.1, of personality change in Section 7.2, and of psychosis in Section 7.1.

Genetic testing should be offered to at-risk relatives.

8.18 PANTOTHENATE KINASE–ASSOCIATED NEURODEGENERATION

Pantothenate kinase-associated neurodegeneration is a rare autosomal recessively inherited disease due to mutations in the gene for panthothenate kinase. It typically presents in childhood or adolescence with a movement disorder, generally dystonia, followed, in most, by a dementia.

The original name for this disease was Hallervorden–Spatz disease; however, the use of this eponym is now discouraged on ethical grounds (Shevell 2003). Although there is no dispute that Drs Hallervorden and Spatz originally described this disease, concerns have been raised about honoring them with an eponym, given their participation in the extraordinarily unethical euthanasia programs practiced in Germany during the Third Reich.

Clinical features

The onset is typically gradual and, although most patients fall ill in childhood or adolescence, adult-onset cases may occur. The clinical symptomatology is heavily influenced by the age of onset.

Childhood-onset cases (Dooling *et al.* 1974, 1980; Hayflick *et al.* 2003; Pellecchia *et al.* 2005; Swaiman 1991)

are generally characterized by a slowly progressive dystonic rigidity, prominent in both the extremities and the face; although this dystonia may be unilateral initially, bilateral involvement eventually occurs. Over time, other abnormal movements may appear, including tremor or choreoathetosis; tics have also been noted in a small minority, as have obsessions and compulsions. Over time, a dementia gradually appears.

Adult-onset cases (Alberca *et al.* 1987; Jankovic *et al.* 1985; Rozdilsky *et al.* 1968) may present with parkinsonism, dystonia, or athetosis. Over time, and with progression of the abnormal movements, a dementia may occur. Rarely the presentation may be with dementia, followed years later by a movement disorder (Cooper *et al.* 2000; Dooling *et al.* 1974; Murphy *et al.* 1989; Rozdilsky *et al.* 1968). In some cases depressive symptomatology may occur or, rarely, delusions and hallucinations.

In addition to the abnormal movements, many patients may also develop signs of spasticity, with hyper-reflexia and the Babinski sign; in a minority pigmentary retinopathy may occur.

Magnetic resonance scanning generally reveals the distinctive 'eye of the tiger' sign (Angelini *et al.* 1992). On T2-weighted scans, increased signal intensity is seen in the lateral aspect of the globus pallidus, whereas on the inner aspect there is a gross loss of signal intensity: the overall effect, seen on axial imaging, is of looking a tiger in the eye.

Course

Childhood-onset cases show gradual progression, with death occurring within 10–15 years; adult-onset cases tend to pursue a much more leisurely course, and some patients may remain ambulatory for decades.

Etiology

As noted earlier, this is a recessively inherited disorder, and mutations are found in the gene for pantothenate kinase, *PANK2*, found on chromosome 20 (Zhou *et al.* 2001). Macroscopically, the globus pallidus is atrophic and exhibits a rust-brown discoloration. Microscopically, iron deposition and axonal spheroids are seen not only in the globus pallidus but also in the pars reticulata of the substantia nigra and in the cerebral cortex (Dooling *et al.* 1974).

Differential diagnosis

In childhood- or adolescent-onset cases, consideration must be given to Wilson's disease, idiopathic torsion dystonia, and dopa-responsive dystonia. In adult-onset cases, given the variety of abnormal movements seen, the differential is very wide and the reader is directed to Sections 3.5,

3.7, and 3.8 for athetosis, dystonia, and parkinsonism respectively.

One finding that is very helpful in the differential diagnosis is the 'eye of the tiger' sign. This is seen in almost all cases and indeed may be found before the onset of symptoms (Hayflick *et al.* 2001). Consequently, the sensitivity of this sign is very high. The specificity is also fairly high, although there are some cases that are clinically similar to pantothenate kinase-associated neurodegeneration, even to the point of demonstrating the 'eye of the tiger' sign, but which are not apparently associated with mutations in the pantothenate kinase gene (Hartig *et al.* 2006). The nosologic status of these cases is not clear.

Treatment

Pharmacologic treatment of the abnormal movements may be attempted as described in Sections 3.5, 3.7, and 3.8; however, the responses are generally not robust. In severe cases, success has been reported with deep brain stimulation of the globus pallidus (Castelnau *et al.* 2005). The general treatment of dementia is discussed in Section 5.1.

8.19 DOPA-RESPONSIVE DYSTONIA

Dopa-responsive dystonia is an uncommon inherited syndrome that classically presents in childhood with a dystonia which, as the name indicates, is quite responsive to levodopa. Given its eminent treatability, it is a diagnosis that must not be missed.

Clinical features

Although the classic onset is in childhood, later onsets in adolescence or adult years have also been reported. Regardless of the age of onset, symptoms generally both appear and accrue gradually.

Childhood-onset cases (Deonna 1986; Harwood *et al.* 1994; Nygaard and Duvoisin 1986; Nygaard *et al.* 1990, 1991) generally present with an intermittent dystonia of one foot; over time the dystonia spreads, eventually involving the other lower extremity and then the upper extremities; truncal and cervical dystonia may also eventually appear. A characteristic feature of the dystonia has been termed 'sleep benefit': after a good night's sleep, the dystonia may be very mild, or even absent, only to gradually reappear and worsen as the day wears on. In some cases, a mild parkinsonism may appear; myoclonus has also been noted. The movement disorder may, in some cases, be accompanied by depression or obsessions and compulsions.

Later-onset cases, although at times presenting similarly to childhood-onset cases, may also be marked by a more prominent parkinsonism (Harwood *et al.* 1994); in some cases the syndrome may present with depression or obsessions and compulsions without any abnormal movements (Hahn *et al.* 2001; Van Hove *et al.* 2006).

Course

In childhood-onset cases the dystonia eventually generalizes over about 3 or 4 years, after which it remains static.

Etiology

Dopa-responsive dystonia is a genetically heterogenous syndrome and, at present, three different diseases have been described, namely DYT5a, DYT5b, and DYT14.

DYT5a, also known as the Segawa syndrome, is an autosomal dominant disorder and constitutes the most common cause of dopa-responsive dystonia. In DYT5a there is a mutation in the gene for guanosine triphosphate cyclohydrolase 1 (GCH1) on chromosome 14 (Bandmann *et al.* 1998; Illarioshkin *et al.* 1998; Ohye *et al.* 1994; Steinberger *et al.* 2000). GCH1 is the rate-limiting enzyme for the synthesis of tetrahydrobiopterin, which in turn is an essential co-factor for tyrosine hydroxylase, the rate-limiting enzyme in the production of dopamine. The net result of this mutation is a reduction in the production of dopamine.

DYT5b is an autosomal recessive disorder caused by a mutation in the gene for tyrosine hydroxylase on chromosome 11 (Furukawa *et al.* 2001; Schiller *et al.* 2004).

DYT14 is an autosomal dominant disorder linked to a site on chromosome 14 (Grotzch *et al.* 2002); the gene has not as yet been identified.

Pathologic studies have demonstrated a reduction in melanin pigment in the substantia nigra, without cell loss, in both DYT5a (Rajput *et al.* 1994) and DYT14 (Grotzch *et al.* 2002).

Differential diagnosis

The full differential diagnosis for dystonia is discussed in Section 3.7: of the disorders noted there, primary torsion dystonia is highest on the differential. A key feature in making the diagnosis is the responsiveness to levodopa, and an attempt at a 'diagnosis by treatment response' is warranted in most cases of childhood-onset dystonia.

Treatment

As indicated earlier, the dystonia of dopa-responsive dystonia responds well to levodopa, and generally only low doses are required; of note, and in contrast to other conditions treated with levodopa, such as Parkinson's disease, the response to levodopa is sustained over long periods, with little need for dosage increases (Nygaard *et al.* 1991).

8.20 PRIMARY TORSION DYSTONIA

Primary torsion dystonia, also known as dystonia musculorum deformans, is a syndrome characterized classically by the onset of a focal dystonia in childhood or adolescence that eventually generalizes. As noted below, however, atypical presentations may also occur.

Clinical features

Classic cases (Johnson *et al.* 1962; Marsden and Harrison 1974) are characterized by an onset of dystonia between the ages of 5 and 15 years, appearing first in one of the lower extremities. Typically, and only intermittently, the young patient may experience some dystonic inversion and plantar flexion of the foot while walking. Curiously, this dystonia is not present at rest, and it may also be absent when walking backwards or dancing. Over time, however, the dystonia becomes more frequent and begins to involve more proximal portions of the lower extremities, often with flexion at the knees and hips. With progression of the disease, the dystonia becomes more and more constant and spreads not only to the upper extremities but also to the trunk, producing lordosis and tortipelvis. In a small minority, the face may be involved, with dystonic grimacing.

Atypical presentations (Bressman *et al.* 1989; Fletcher *et al.* 1990; Gasser *et al.* 1998; Johnson *et al.* 1962) are more common with later onset in adolescence or early adult years; patients may present with focal dystonias, such as writer's cramp or a cervical dystonia. Although such cases may show some spread, generalization of the sort seen in classic cases is not common.

Genetic testing is available for the most common cause of this syndrome, namely DYT1, and should be considered in any patient with an early-onset dystonia that has generalized (Brassat *et al.* 2000; Bressman *et al.* 2000).

Course

When progression does occur it typically reaches a maximum after some 5–10 years, after which the course is more or less static. In a very small minority partial remissions may occur, but these are generally only temporary.

Etiology

Three different autosomal dominant diseases have been identified that can cause the syndrome of primary torsion dystonia, namely DYT1, DYT6, and DYT13; the remaining cases, as yet, are considered idiopathic. Of the known causes, DYT1 was the first to be recognized and is by far the most common and the most likely to cause a classic presentation (Kramer *et al.* 1990; Ozelius *et al.* 1992).

DYT1, also known as Oppenheim disease, occurs secondary to a mutation in the gene for torsin A on chromosome 9 (Ozelius *et al.* 1997); penetrance is low, of the order of 30–40 percent. Although the underlying pathology is not known, one study found neuronal inclusion bodies in the pedunculopontine nucleus, the cuneiform nucleus, and the periaqueductal gray (McNaught *et al.* 2004).

DYT6 has been linked to chromosome 8 and tends to have an atypical presentation, often with a cervical dystonia (Almasy *et al.* 1997).

DYT13 is linked to chromosome 1 and also has an atypical presentation, with dystonia of an upper limb or a cervical dystonia (Bentivoglio *et al.* 1997; Valente *et al.* 2001).

Differential diagnosis

The full differential diagnosis of dystonia is discussed in Section 3.7. Of the disorders noted there, the most important for the differential diagnosis is dopa-responsive dystonia; given that this disorder may be clinically indistinguishable from primary torsion disorder, a 'diagnosis by treatment response', as discussed above (Section 8.19), should be attempted by giving levodopa.

Treatment

Perhaps the best-established pharmacologic treatment is trihexyphenidyl: children and adolescents may do well with this and, in contrast to adults, may tolerate high doses of 30 mg or more per day (Burke *et al.* 1986). In severe cases, consideration may be given to intrathecal baclofen or to deep brain stimulation of the globus pallidus (Vidhailet *et al.* 2005).

8.21 IDIOPATHIC CERVICAL DYSTONIA

Idiopathic cervical dystonia, also known as spasmodic torticollis or 'wry neck', is the most common of the primary focal dystonias and is somewhat more frequent in women.

Clinical features

Clinically (Chan *et al.* 1991; Jankovic *et al.* 1991; Rondot *et al.* 1991; Sorensen and Hamby 1966), the onset is generally between the ages of 20 and 60 years, with most patients falling ill in their forties. The presentation is generally with some intermittent dystonia of the neck musculature, pulling the head into a dystonic posture. The most common position is torticollis, the head being rotated to one side or the other; other positions, in order of decreasing frequency, include lateralcollis, with the head tilted to one side, retrocollis, with the head bent back, or anterocollis, with the head pulled down toward the chest. Isolated positions are the exception: most patients exhibit a combination, such as torticollis and lateralcollis. Pain is a common accompaniment.

In most cases patients are able to use a *geste antagoniste* to temporarily relieve the dystonia (Jahanshahi 2000; Muller *et al.* 2001a). These 'tricks' consist of lightly touching a specific body part, such as the chin, face, or occiput, resulting in a prompt, but temporary, relief of the dystonic stiffness.

Over time, the dystonia becomes more constant and sustained, and will, in a minority, undergo segmental spread to an adjacent part such as the arm.

A tremor of the head, similar to that seen in essential tremor, is present in a substantial minority of patients.

Course

In most cases there is a gradual progression with, as noted, some segmental spread in a minority; generalization, however, does not occur. There may be remissions in some 10–20 percent of patients during the first few years (Chan *et al.* 1991; Friedman and Fahn 1986; Jayne *et al.* 1984); however, most of these patients eventually relapse within 5 years (Dauer *et al.* 1998).

Etiology

Both familial (Bressman *et al.* 1996; Chan *et al.* 1991; Jankovic *et al.* 1991) and sporadic cases occur. In some familial cases, a genetic cause has been identified, for example the *DYT7* locus, mapped to chromosome 18 (Leube *et al.* 1997). The neuropathology is unknown.

Differential diagnosis

The full differential for dystonia is discussed in Section 3.7. Of the disorders noted there, special consideration should be given to an atypical presentation of primary torsion dystonia.

Treatment

Local injection of botulinum toxin (Greene *et al.* 1990) is effective; although some patients may benefit from treatment with trihexyphenidyl, botulinum toxin is more effective (Brans *et al.* 1996). In severe, treatment-resistant cases, consideration may be given to deep brain stimulation of the globus pallidus (Hung *et al.* 2007).

8.22 TASK–SPECIFIC DYSTONIA

Task-specific dystonia, one of the primary dystonias, is characterized by the occurrence of a dystonia upon attempting to perform a learned task. Also known as occupational dystonia, this movement disorder is typically divided into several subtypes depending on the task that occasions the dystonia; thus we have writer's cramp, typist's cramp, musician's cramp, etc.

Clinical features

Task-specific dystonias generally appear in adulthood between the ages of 20 and 50 years, and typically only after the patient has been engaging in the task in question for at least a number of years.

Writer's cramp (Cohen and Hallett 1988; Jedynak *et al.* 2001; Sheehy and Marsden 1982) is perhaps the most common of the task-specific dystonias and manifests as a dystonic cramping of the hand upon using a pen or pencil. Although early on in the course the dystonia may appear only after the patient has been writing for a while, with time the dystonia appears earlier and earlier until it may manifest as soon as the patient picks up the pen; furthermore, and again with time, the dystonia may spread to involve the forearm. Some patients may try and evade the cramping by writing with their non-dominant hand; however, in a minority, the dystonia will reappear on this opposite side. Musician's cramp may appear in the hands of violinists or pianists, and it may also appear in the orofacial musculature in wind-instrument players. This latter type of musician's cramp is referred to as embouchure dystonia or, colloquially, as 'loss of lip', and manifests variously with lip dystonia or dystonic jaw movements (Frucht *et al.* 2001).

Course

The dystonia gradually worsens over perhaps years and then typically remains static; remissions are unusual.

Etiology

Most cases are sporadic. Familial cases are generally consistent with an autosomal dominant mode of inheritance. Of interest, in some familial cases different family members may manifest different subtypes of task-specific dystonia (Schmidt *et al.* 2006). In one family, writer's cramp occurred as part of DYT7 with linkage to chromosome 18 (Bhidayasiri *et al.* 2005). The neuropathologic basis of this disorder is not known.

Differential diagnosis

Writer's cramp has been noted as an atypical presentation of both primary torsion dystonia (Gasser *et al.* 1998) and dopa-responsive dystonia (Deonna *et al.* 1997), and these disorders should be considered whenever task-specific dystonic movements occur in children or adolescents.

Treatment

Writer's cramp has been treated with botulinum toxin injections (Kruisdijk *et al.* 2007; Rivest *et al.* 1991), biofeedback, retraining, splint immobilization for 4–5 weeks (Priori *et al.* 2001), and placement of a transcutaneous electrical nerve stimulation (TENS) unit (Tinazzi *et al.* 2005). Similar strategies may be considered for musician's cramp involving the hand (Jabusch *et al.* 2005).

8.23 MEIGE'S SYNDROME

Meige's syndrome (also known as essential blepharospasm or primary blepharospasm), first described by the French neurologist Henri Meige in 1910 (Tolosa and Klawans 1979), is one of the primary dystonias and is characterized, as the synonyms indicate, by blepharospasm.

Clinical features

Clinical features have been described in a number of series (Grandas *et al.* 1988; Paulson 1972; Tolosa 1981). Onset is usually in middle years, and the primary symptom is bilateral blepharospasm. Initially the blepharospasm is neither prolonged nor frequent, but over time it becomes persistent, forceful, and at times almost constant. Over a year or two, the adjacent musculature, especially the jaw and mouth, may also become involved and, in a small minority, the neck musculature may likewise be affected (Defazio *et al.* 1999). The blepharospasm may be worsened by bright light or sometimes by walking, and may be lessened by yawning, talking, or singing (Weiner and Nora 1984). *Gestes antagonistes*, such as touching the eyebrow or the temple, may relieve the blepharospasm.

Course

Symptoms tend to worsen over the first few years and then remain static. Spontaneous remissions may occur in roughly 10 percent of patients, usually within the first 5 years (Castelbuono and Miller 1998).

Etiology

A positive family history is found in only a small minority (Defazio *et al.* 2006), and the remaining cases appear sporadic. Several cases have come to autopsy, however, it is not clear how representative they are. In three patients no clear abnormalities were found (Gibb *et al.* 1988); in one case neuronal loss and gliosis were found in the striatum (Altrocchi and Forno 1983); and in two cases neuronal loss and Lewy bodies were found in brainstem nuclei (Kulisevsky *et al.* 1988; Mark *et al.* 1994). It may well be

that these last two cases represented atypical presentations of diffuse Lewy body disease or some variant thereof.

Differential diagnosis

The full diagnosis of dystonia is discussed in Section 3.7, and several of the disorders discussed there deserve consideration. Brueghel's syndrome, another primary dystonia, is distinguished by the fact that it presents with oromandibular dystonia in the absence of blepharospasm (Gilbert 1996). Atypical presentations of primary torsion dystonia may be characterized by blepharospasm (Bressman *et al.* 1994; Ozelius *et al.* 1989). Tardive dyskinesia may present with blepharospasm, but the diagnosis is immediately suggested by the appearance of symptoms in the context of long-term treatment with antipsychotics (Weiner *et al.* 1981). Blepharospasm has also been reported secondary to lesions in the basal ganglia (Jankovic 1986) or brainstem (Jankovic and Patel 1983).

Non-dystonic disorders to consider include hemifacial spasm, distinguished by its strictly unilateral occurrence, and facial tics, distinguished by their fleeting, unsustained nature. Ocular pathology must also be considered, as inflammation of the lid, conjunctiva or iris may all be associated with blepharospasm.

Treatment

Botulinum toxin represents standard treatment; when this fails, case reports and case series suggest a usefulness for anticholinergics (Tanner *et al.* 1982) (e.g., trihexyphenidyl or benztropine), clonazepam (Hipola *et al.* 1984), levetiracetam (Yardimci *et al.* 2006), and, interestingly, quetiapine (Reeves and Liberto 2003). In severe, treatment-resistant cases, consideration may be given to deep brain stimulation of the globus pallidus (Houser and Waltz 2005).

8.24 SPASMODIC DYSPHONIA

Spasmodic dysphonia, also at times referred to as spastic dysphonia, represents a focal dystonia of the laryngeal musculature that renders speech dysphonic.

Clinical features

Clinical features have been described in a number of reports (Aminoff *et al.* 1978; Bicknell *et al.* 1968; Pool *et al.* 1991). The onset is typically in middle or later years, and may be subacute or gradual. Dystonic spasm of the laryngeal musculature may occur either in adduction or abduction, and the quality of the dysphonia differs in these two forms. Adductor spasm, which is by far more common, renders the voice high-pitched, strained, and strangulated; with abductor spasm, the voice is more breathy and whispering. Some patients may find improvement with singing, or even with shouting.

Course

After a period of progression of variable duration, the dysphonia generally remains chronic.

Etiology

Spasmodic dysphonia is considered one of the primary dystonias; the etiology is not known.

Differential diagnosis

Dysphonia may result from lesions in the central or peripheral nervous system or in the larynx itself. Dysphonia has been noted with a putaminal lesion (Lee *et al.* 1996), lesions of the nucleus ambiguus or the vagus or recurrent laryngeal nerves, and with various intrinsic laryngeal lesions. Dysphonia has also been reported as a side-effect of valproic acid (Oh *et al.* 2004) and gabapentin (Reeves *et al.* 1996), and has also occurred as part of tardive dyskinesia (Lieberman and Reife 1989).

Treatment

Botulinum injection of the laryngeal musculature generally provides relief. In treatment-resistant cases, consideration may be given to lesioning the recurrent laryngeal nerve.

8.25 TOURETTE'S SYNDROME

Tourette's syndrome, first describe by the French neurologist Georges Gilles de la Tourette in 1885 (de la Tourette 1885), is the classic cause of chronic tics; this is a not uncommon disorder, with a lifetime prevalence of about 0.05 percent, and is about three times more common in males than females. Synonyms for this disorder include maladie des tics and tic convulsiv.

Clinical features

The onset of Tourette's syndrome is typically with a simple tic, more often motor than verbal, and more often on the head or face than elsewhere. Although the age of onset may be anywhere from infancy to the early adult years (Marneros 1983), most patients fall ill in childhood, around the age of 7 years.

In its fully developed form, both motor and verbal tics are present, and these may be either simple or complex (Cardoso *et al.* 1996; Lang *et al.* 1993; Lees *et al.* 1984;

Nee *et al.* 1980; Regeur *et al.* 1986); it has also become apparent that sensory tics, once thought to be unusual, are also present in most patients.

Motor tics are usually the first to appear. Simple motor tics include blinking, brow wrinkling, grimacing, and shoulder shrugging; complex motor tics may include touching, smelling, hopping, throwing, clapping, bending over, squatting, or even such very complex acts as echopraxia or copropraxia (wherein patients make obscene gestures). Motor tics usually appear first in the face or head and then spread in a caudal direction. In most cases, before having a tic, patients first experience an urge to tic (Lang 1991), an urge that may at times be resisted, albeit with difficulty. Furthermore, some patients are able to abort a motor tic with a *geste antagoniste*, such as placing a hand under the chin to prevent the emergence of a tic of the head (Wojcieszek and Lang 1995).

Vocal tics, like motor tics, may also be simple or complex. Simple vocal tics include snorting, hissing, coughing, throat-clearing, grunting, and, classically, barking. Complex vocal tics include the utterance of words, simple phrases, or entire sentences. Echolalia or palilalia may occur and, in a minority, classic coprolalia, or involuntary swearing, may be seen.

Sensory tics occur in the majority of patients and appear to exist in two forms. In one there is simply the experience of an itch or a tingle (Chee and Sachdev 1997), and this is seen in perhaps one-quarter of patients. In the other the sensory tic appears more as a premonitory urge to a motor tic (Cohen and Leckman 1992; Leckman *et al.* 1993), and this has been reported in over 90 percent of cases (Leckman *et al.* 1993). Remarkably, in one case a premonitory urge to itch was experienced by a patient as residing in another person, whom the patient then proceeded to scratch (Karp and Hallett 1996).

Rarely, dystonic movements, especially cervical or facial dystonias, may appear in the course of Tourette's syndrome, but not until 10–38 years have passed (Stone and Jankovic 1991).

Obsessions and compulsions are common in Tourette's syndrome, eventually appearing in nearly one-half of all patients (Frankel *et al.* 1986; Robertson *et al.* 1988); they typically begin to appear about 5 years into the course. Interestingly, compulsions experienced by patients with Tourette's syndrome often center on getting things 'just right' (Leckman *et al.* 1994).

Attention deficit/hyperactivity disorder (ADHD) very commonly accompanies Tourette's syndrome and, in those cases of Tourette's syndrome in which it does occur, the hyperactivity usually precedes the tics by a little over a year (Cardoso *et al.* 1996).

Course

In most cases, symptoms gradually worsen over a matter of a few years, peaking in severity around the age of 10 years;

subsequently there is a gradual and progressive remission of symptoms, such that by the age of 18 years roughly one-half of patients are left with either no, or only trivial, tics (Leckman *et al.* 1998; Pappert *et al.* 2003). In those cases where full remissions do occur, relapses may appear, sometimes decades later (Chouinard and Ford 2000; Klawans and Barr 1985).

Etiology

Tourette's syndrome is clearly familial, with concordance rates rising from about 5 percent in siblings to approximately 10 percent in dizygotic twins and 50 percent in monozygotic twins; indeed if one accepts the presence of simple tics as evidence of the disorder, the monozygotic concordance rises to over 75 percent (Price *et al.* 1985). Although earlier studies supported an autosomal dominant mode of inheritance (Eapen *et al.* 1993; Pauls and Leckman 1986; Pauls *et al.* 1990), more recent work has indicated that Tourette's syndrome is a complex genetic disorder.

Imaging and neuropathologic studies have focused on the basal ganglia. MRI studies strongly suggest a reduced size of the basal ganglia (Bloch *et al.* 2005; Hyde *et al.* 1995; Peterson *et al.* 1993; Singer *et al.* 1993). Although neuropathologic studies have not revealed distinctive microscopic findings, immunologic studies have revealed a decreased number of dopamine reuptake sites in the striatum (Singer *et al.* 1991) and a decrease in dynorphin staining in fibers coursing from the striatum to the globus pallidus (Haber *et al.* 1986).

Although the mechanism or mechanisms underlying these changes in the basal ganglia are not clear, some research suggests that, at least in a certain minority of cases, Tourette's syndrome may be an autoimmune disease, triggered, in turn, by a preceding beta-hemolytic streptococcal infection. Swedo *et al.*, in 1998, considered Tourette's to be part of a syndrome that they named PANDAS (pediatric autoimmune neuropsychiatric disorders associated with streptococcal infections). In this condition, similar to Sydenham's chorea, a preceding group A beta-hemolytic streptococcal pharyngitis triggers an immune response that cross-reacts with the basal ganglia, leading to, among other symptomatologies, tics; increased levels of anti-streptococcal antibodies in patients with Tourette's syndrome support this notion (Church *et al.* 2003; Muller *et al.* 2001b; Rizzo *et al.* 2006). Furthermore, most (Church *et al.* 2003; Rizzo *et al.* 2006; Singer *et al.* 1998), but not all (Singer *et al.* 2005), studies have also found an increased incidence of serum anti-basal ganglia antibodies in patients with Tourette's compared with controls. Although speculative, it is tempting to suggest that in Tourette's syndrome what is inherited is either a susceptibility to streptococcal infections or to the development of a particular immune response to such infections, with symptoms then appearing secondary to autoimmune damage to the basal ganglia.

Differential diagnosis

The full differential for tics is provided in Section 3.3, and of the causes noted there, several deserve special consideration. Autism may be complicated by tics, and this diagnosis is suggested by the other features seen in autism, such as the machine-like relationships patients have with others. Sydenham's chorea may occur in children, but is suggested by concurrent chorea; Huntington's disease and choreoacanthocytosis may also cause tics, but these too are associated with chorea and generally have an onset in adult years.

Technically, a diagnosis of Tourette's syndrome should not be made until the patient has both motor tics and vocal tics. Patients with only motor or only vocal tics are said to have 'transient tic disorder' if the tics last no longer than a year, or 'chronic motor or vocal tic disorder' if they last longer than a year. This distinction may be unwarranted, however, as it appears that these 'disorders' merely represent formes frustes of the full Tourette's syndrome (Golden 1978; Kurlan *et al.* 1988).

Treatment

Various medications are effective, including second-generation antipsychotics (olanzapine [Onofrj *et al.* 2000], ziprasidone [Sallee *et al.* 2000], risperidone [Bruggeman *et al.* 2001; Dion *et al.* 2002; Scahill *et al.* 2003]), first-generation antipsychotics (haloperidol and pimozide [Sallee *et al.* 1997; Shapiro *et al.* 1989]), alpha-2 autoreceptor agonists (clonidine [Cohen *et al.* 1980; Leckman *et al.* 1991] and guanfacine [Scahill *et al.* 2001]), desipramine (Spencer *et al.* 2002), and pergolide (Gilbert *et al.* 2003). Each is discussed in turn, followed by a discussion of overall pharmacologic strategy.

Of the antipsychotics, olanzapine is begun at a dose of 5 mg/day and increased, if necessary, 2 weeks later to a dose of 10 mg/day. The starting dose for ziprasidone is 5 mg, for risperidone 0.5 mg, for haloperidol 0.25–0.5 mg, and for pimozide 1 mg, and each agent may be increased in similar increments every week or two until a satisfactory response, limiting side-effects, or a maximum dose is reached. Dosage ranges (and average effective doses) are as follows: ziprasidone, 5–40 mg (30 mg); risperidone, 1–6 mg (3 mg); haloperidol, 1–10 mg (4 mg); pimozide, 1–10 mg (4 mg). Choosing between the various antipsychotics is not entirely straightforward. Although the second-generation agents olanzapine, ziprasidone, and risperidone are, overall, better tolerated than the first-generation agents, both olanzapine and risperidone are associated with weight gain, hyperlipidemia, and even diabetes mellitus, and risperidone may cause dysphoria (Margolese *et al.* 2002). Haloperidol and pimozide are less likely to cause weight gain but carry the liabilities of akathisia (which may manifest with an increase in the frequency of tics [Weiden and Bruun 1987]), tardive dyskinesia, dysphoria (Bruun 1988), and, in children, the capacity to cause severe separation anxiety to the point where 'school phobia' sets in (Linet 1985; Mikkelsen *et al.* 1981). Furthermore, pimozide carries the further risk of prolonging the corrected QT interval, with the possibility of torsades de pointe. All other things being equal, it may be prudent to begin with a second-generation agent; if the initial choice fails then another might be tried, or one could switch to a first-generation agent such as haloperidol.

Of the two alpha-2 autoreceptor agonists, clonidine is the best studied. The total daily starting dose for clonidine is 0.1 mg and for guanfacine is 1 mg. Dosage increases may be made in similar increments every week or so until one begins to see an initial response, limiting side-effects, or a maximum dose is reached of 1 mg for clonidine and 4 mg for guanfacine. In all cases the total daily dose should be divided into two or three doses. Importantly, in contrast to antipsychotics, where the response is fairly prompt, with the alpha-2 autoreceptor agonists the full response may take weeks or months to develop. Consequently, in titrating the dose it makes sense, as soon as an initial response is seen, to pause and see how things develop before increasing the dose further. It must also be borne in mind that these agents must not be abruptly discontinued, as this may be followed by a prolonged and severe 'rebound' of tics (Leckman *et al.* 1986): a gradual tapering, over weeks, is required. In making the choice between clonidine and guanfacine, although there is more experience with the use of clonidine, guanfacine may be better tolerated.

Desipramine, a tricyclic antidepressant, may be started at a dose of 25 mg and increased every few days to 100 mg, after which the patient should be observed for a few weeks to see what sort of response emerges. Importantly, as desipramine has been associated with lethal arrhythmias in children, its use should be restricted to adults.

Pergolide has recently been shown to be effective. Given the association between pergolide and cardiac valvulopathy, however, its use cannot be recommended. If ropinirole or pramipexole are found to be effective, this will open up an exciting new therapeutic option.

Overall, in children one should begin with either an antipsychotic or an alpha-2 autoreceptor agonist. Although the antipsychotics are by and large more effective, the burden of long-term side-effects is significant, and, based on that, some clinicians prefer to begin with an alpha-2 autoreceptor agonist, holding the antipsychotics in reserve. Furthermore, if the patient also has ADHD that requires treatment, special consideration should be given to an alpha-2 autoreceptor agonist, as these agents, unlike the antipsychotics, are also effective in ADHD. In adults, similar considerations apply; however, here one may also consider desipramine, which, like the alpha-2 autoreceptor agonists, is effective not only for Tourette's but also for ADHD. It must be emphasized that the foregoing constitute suggestions only: there simply are not enough comparative studies to allow for definitive recommendations. In many cases, a methodical approach, giving one agent a good trial (at an adequate dose and for an adequate duration),

followed, if necessary, by another, and perhaps another, is most appropriate.

In considering treatment of Tourette's, one should also keep in mind the possibility that some cases do occur as part of PANDAS, that is to say, on an autoimmune basis after a beta-hemolytic streptococcal pharyngitis. This should be suspected in cases in which there is a temporal relationship between either the onset of tics (or their exacerbation) and a preceding 'sore throat', keeping in mind that weeks or months may be required for the mounting of the autoimmune response. When suspicion is high, it is appropriate to determine ASO (anti-streptolysin O) and anti-DNAase B levels to confirm a preceding streptococcal infection. In cases in which it appears likely that the Tourette's is occurring as part of PANDAS, consideration may be given to chronic penicillin treatment to prevent future exacerbations, and, in severe cases, to plasmapheresis to acutely reduce symptoms (Perlmutter *et al.* 1999).

Finally, in severe and treatment-resistant cases, neurosurgical intervention, for example deep brain stimulation of the globus pallidus, may be considered (Shahed *et al.* 2007).

As noted earlier, ADHD is commonly seen in patients with Tourette's and, should an alpha-2 autoreceptor agonist (or desipramine in adults) not prove effective, consideration may then be given to utilizing a stimulant, such as methylphenidate. Despite the fact that stimulants may cause tics (Denckla *et al.* 1976), it appears that, in practice, the risk is negligible (Gadow *et al.* 1992, 1999); indeed, in one study tics actually decreased with methylphenidate treatment (Tourette's Syndrome Study Group 2002). Furthermore, given that in patients with combined Tourette's and ADHD it is the symptomatology of the ADHD that is often most problematic, it is critical to not withhold effective treatment.

8.26 MYOTONIC MUSCULAR DYSTROPHY

Of the several disorders capable of causing myotonia and muscular dystrophy, the classic example, described by Batten and Gibb in 1909, has had several names over the past century. The original name, bestowed by Batten and Gibb (1909), was myotonia atrophica; a similar one is myotonia dystrophica. Subsequently, this disease was referred to as myotonic muscular dystrophy or, simply, myotonic dystrophy. Recently it became apparent that some other disorders (as discussed below under differential diagnosis) could produce a similar clinical picture and, in an effort to standardize terminology, a recent conference proposed renaming myotonic muscular dystrophy as myotonic dystrophy type 1 (or DM1), with similar disorders named myotonic dystrophy type 2 (DM2), etc. (International Myotonic Dystrophy Consortium 2000). Ongoing use of the name 'myotonic muscular dystrophy' for DM1 was not forbidden, however, and it is retained in this text.

Myotonic muscular dystrophy is a not uncommon disorder, with a lifetime prevalence of about 5 per 100 000; it is equally common in males and females.

Clinical features

The onset is gradual and insidious and, although most patients fall ill in their late teens or early twenties, the range of age of onset is wide, from childhood up to the sixth decade.

The cardinal symptoms of the disease are myotonia and weakness. Myotonia may go unnoticed by the patient, or may manifest in difficulty in letting go of, for example, a doorknob, or in disengaging from a handshake. On physical examination, myotonia may be elicited by tapping the thenar eminence with a percussion hammer and observing for the characteristic muscle dimpling. Weakness is eventually accompanied by atrophy and, importantly, this is more prominent distally, being seen first in the upper extremities. Other signs may also accrue. Many patients have a distinctive 'myopathic facies', with frontal balding, ptosis, and wasting of the face and neck musculature; the voice often also becomes nasal and monotone. Cataracts are seen in over 90 percent of patients, and there may be deafness (Wright et al. 1988) and gonadal failure, with erectile dysfunction or menstrual irregularity. Cardiac conduction abnormalities and arrhythmias may occur, including atrioventricular block, fascicular block, intraventricular conduction block, atrial fibrillation, and ventricular premature contractions; a cardiomyopathy with congestive heart failure may also occur, but is less common. Alveolar hypoventilation may also occur.

Cognitive impairment is eventually seen in a majority of patients (Modoni et al. 2004; Perini et al. 1989) and, although this is generally quite mild, it may progress to a dementia (Huber et al. 1989). Personality change may also occur and, although it tends to be mixed in type, avoidant traits may be predominant (Delaporte et al. 1998; Winblad et al. 2005). Apathy appears to be more common than among comparable controls (Rubinsztein et al. 1998). Although depression may occur, it appears, in contrast to apathy, to be no more common among these patients than comparable controls: in considering the diagnosis of depression, one must guard against misinterpreting the expressionless 'myopathic facies' as a depressed affect (Adie and Greenfield 1924; Billings and Ravin 1941; Bungener et al. 1998).

Hypersomnia is not uncommon (Manni et al. 1991) and indeed may be the presenting complaint (Hansotia and Frens 1981): some patients may literally sleep for days (Phemister and Small 1961). Although some of these hypersomnic patients demonstrate sleep apnea (of either the central or obstructive type), the number of apneic episodes is not high enough to account for the degree of hypersomnolence (van der Meche et al. 1994).

As noted below, 'anticipation' may occur in this disease (Harper et al. 1992; Howeler et al. 1989), and some children may be born with 'congenital' myotonic muscular dystrophy, characterized, among other symptoms, by mental retardation (Koch et al. 1991).

Both CT (Avrahami et al. 1987) and MRI (Antonini et al. 2004) scanning may reveal a mild degree of cortical atrophy. On MR scanning patchy areas of increased signal intensity on T2-weighed scans may be seen in the white matter (Di Costanzo et al. 2002). Genetic testing is available.

Course

The disease is gradually progressive and, although those with later onsets and milder symptoms may experience a normal lifespan, cases of early onset and severe symptoms are often associated with premature death in early or middle-adult years, often from cardiac or respiratory causes.

Etiology

Myotonic muscular dystrophy is inherited in an autosomal dominant fashion with almost 100 percent penetrance but a quite variable expressivity, even within the same family (Pryse-Phillips et al. 1982). Mutations consist of an expansion of a normally occurring CTG triplet in the DMPK gene on chromosome 19, which codes for the myotonic dystrophy protein kinase (Brook et al. 1992). As in many inherited disorders due to triplet expansions, 'anticipation' may occur, in which in succeeding generations, and with expansion of the triplet repeat, the disease becomes more severe and has an earlier onset. Although anticipation is more likely with maternal transmission, it has been noted in paternal cases (Nakagawa et al. 1994).

Neuropathologic studies are few. Neuronal heterotopias have been noted in the cerebral cortex (Rosman and Kakulas 1966) and neurofibrillary tangles in the hippocampus (Maurage et al. 2005). In cases characterized by hypersomnolence, cell loss was noted in the superior central nucleus of the midbrain (Ono et al. 1998), and, in cases marked by alveolar hyperventilation, cell loss was seen in the medullary reticular formation (Ono et al. 1996).

Differential diagnosis

As noted earlier, myotonic muscular dystrophy, or DM1, is but one of several causes of myotonia and weakness. DM2, also known as the PROMM syndrome (or proximal myotonic myopathy), although similar to myotonic muscular dystrophy, may be distinguished clinically by the pattern of weakness, which is proximal rather than distal, and by the presence of myalgia, which is not seen in myotonic muscular dystrophy (Day et al. 2003; Ricker et al. 1994, 1995, 1999). Recently a third disorder, namely DM3, was described, which, like the PROMM syndrome, is also characterized by proximal weakness; it also apparently is notable for a prominent dementia (Le Ber et al. 2004).

Another disorder to consider is myotonia congenita. This is an inherited, non-progressive condition characterized by myotonia and, rather than weakness and atrophy, by a degree of muscular hypertrophy: autosomal dominant cases are referred to as Thomsen's disease and recessive cases as the Becker variant. Because the phenomenon of myotonia may be the only symptom of myotonic muscular dystrophy for many years, the clinical differential between myotonic muscular dystrophy and myotonia congenita may depend on long-term follow-up, watching closely for other symptoms to appear (Maas and Paterson 1950).

Treatment

There is no specific treatment for the disease. Hypersomnolence, which, in some cases, may be the most distressing feature of the disease, responds to modafinil (MacDonald et al. 2002; Wintzen et al. 2007); open work also suggests a usefulness for methylphenidate (van der Meche et al. 1994). Myotonia may respond to various medications, including phenytoin, disopyramide, procainamide, and nifedipine, but given that myotonia rarely causes distress or disability, these agents are typically not required. The general treatment of dementia is discussed in Section 5.1. Yearly electrocardiograms (ECGs) are required and, if there is suspicion of significant arrhythmia, a 24-hour Holter monitor is appropriate; some patients may require a pacemaker. As noted earlier, alveolar hypoventilation may occur; these patients do not appear to tolerate general anesthesia well, hence surgery, if possible, should be avoided. Hearing aids and cataract surgery may be required.

Genetic counseling is appropriate and, given the variable expression of the disease, it may be appropriate to offer testing to apparently unaffected relatives.

8.27 CEREBROTENDINOUS XANTHOMATOSIS

Cerebrotendinous xanthomatosis is a rare, recessively inherited lipid storage disease that may, in some cases, cause a dementia. Also known as cholestanolosis, cholestanol storage disease or Van Bogaert's disease, the current name is a felicitous one, given that it draws attention to the hallmarks of the disease, namely xanthomatous deposits in the cerebrum and tendons, most particularly the Achilles tendon.

Clinical features

The onset is very gradual and, although most patients begin to have symptoms in late childhood or early adolescence, the range in age of onset is wide, from infancy to middle years (Swanson and Cromwell 1986).

Fully developed, classic cerebrotendinous xanthomatosis (Bencze et al. 1990; Canelas et al. 1983; Farpour and

Mahloudji 1975; Soffer et al. 1995; Verrips et al. 2000a,b; Watts et al. 1996) is characterized by dementia, seizures, long-tract signs, ataxia, a peripheral sensorimotor polyneuropathy, gross tendon enlargement, especially evident in the Achilles tendon, cataracts, and chronic diarrhea. Although the disease may present with any one of these various features, in most cases the presentation will be with juvenile cataracts or with chronic, intractable diarrhea.

T2-weighted or, especially, FLAIR MR scanning will reveal increased signal intensity in the cerebral and cerebellar white matter; increased signal intensity may also be seen in the cerebellar dentate nuclei (De Stefano et al. 2001; Swanson and Cromwell 1986).

Serum cholestanol levels are grossly increased; cholesterol levels are either normal or decreased (Salen 1971).

Genetic testing is available (Meiner et al. 1994).

Course

This is a very slowly progressive disorder. In those with an early age of onset and severe symptoms, death typically occurs within 10 to 20 years, whereas those with later onsets and milder symptoms may experience a normal lifespan.

Etiology

Cerebrotendinous xanthomatosis occurs secondary to mutations in CYP27, a gene on chromosome 2 that codes for an enzyme known as sterol 27-hydroxylase (Verrips et al. 2000a). With defective activity of this enzyme, cholestanol accumulation occurs in the cerebral and cerebellar white matter, the cerebellar dentate nuclei, and peripheral nerves, tendons, and corneae (Menkes et al. 1968). Within the brain, widespread demyelinization occurs and, in some cases, actual xanthomas may form (Schimschock et al. 1968).

Differential diagnosis

Whenever dementia occurs in the setting of juvenile cataracts, chronic diarrhea, or, classically, Achilles tendon enlargement, the diagnosis of cerebrotendinous xanthomatosis is very likely. When these are not present, or are overlooked, consideration may be given to metachromatic leukodystrophy in children, and to spinocerebellar ataxia in adults.

Treatment

Chenodeoxycholic acid, at a dose of 750 mg/day, taken chronically, dramatically reduces serum cholestanol levels and leads to a either a stabilization of symptoms or to a degree of remission (Berginer et al. 1984). Pravastatin and simvastatin, although ineffective by themselves, enhance the effect of chenodeoxycholic acid.

At-risk relatives should be offered genetic testing.

8.28 THALAMIC DEGENERATION

Thalamic degeneration is a very rare syndrome characterized clinically by dementia and pathologically by relatively selective degeneration of the thalamus, in the absence of known causes such as Creutzfeldt–Jakob disease. In all likelihood, this syndrome subsumes several or more different disease processes, which, to date, have not been isolated.

Clinical features

As might be expected, there is considerable variability in the clinical features of this syndrome (Martin *et al.* 1983). The age of onset may range from adolescence to the seventh decade, and the mode of onset from subacute to insidious. Dementia is a common denominator in all cases, and this may be accompanied by apathy and somnolence (Janssen *et al.* 2000; Stern 1939), emaciation (Martin *et al.* 1983), or myoclonus (Little *et al.* 1986). In one case (Deymeer *et al.* 1989), a 46-year-old woman presented with 'bizarre behavior and paranoid ideas', eventually followed by a dementia accompanied by fasciculations.

Course

Survival ranges from a matter of several months (Stern 1939) to up to 20 years (Martin *et al.* 1983).

Etiology

Both familial (Little *et al.* 1986) and sporadic cases have been reported. Autopsy studies reveal neuronal loss and gliosis in the thalamus, especially the dorsomedial (Janssen *et al.* 2000; Moosey *et al.* 1987) and anterior (Martin *et al.* 1983) nuclei. Other structures may also be affected, including the cerebral cortex, cerebral white matter, and inferior olives (Stern 1939), as well as the basal ganglia and nucleus basalis of Meynert (Moosey *et al.* 1987).

Differential diagnosis

Creutzfeldt–Jakob disease and fatal familia insomnia are often included in the differential.

Treatment

The general treatment of dementia is discussed in Section 5.1.

8.29 METACHROMATIC LEUKODYSTROPHY

Metachromatic leukodystrophy is a rare, recessively inherited disorder that occurs secondary to mutations in the gene for arylsulfatase A, with a resulting accumulation of sulfatides in the brain, peripheral nerves, kidneys, and gallbladder. It is of particular interest in that, when appearing in adolescents or adults, it may present with a psychosis, personality change, or a dementia.

Clinical features

Three forms are recognized based on the age of onset: the late infantile form presents in infants up to the age of 4 years, the juvenile form from the age of 4 to 16 years, and the adult form from the age of 16 years onwards. In the adult form, although most cases present before the age of 30 years, cases presenting as late as the seventh decade have been noted (Bosch and Hart 1978). Each of these forms differs in their typical clinical symptomatology.

The late infantile form is characterized by hypotonia, weakness, and seizures (Brain and Greenfield 1950).

The juvenile form (Haltia *et al.* 1980) may present with a dementia or with a personality change that merges into a dementia. Ataxia, spasticity, and a peripheral neuropathy may also constitute the presentation, or, in cases that present with a dementia or personality change, any one or all of these features may emerge later in the course of the disease.

The adult-onset form may present with psychosis, personality change, or dementia: in those cases that present with a psychosis or a personality change, a dementia generally ensues (Hageman *et al.* 1995; Rauschka *et al.* 2006). Other symptoms and signs may also constitute presenting features, or may emerge in the context of psychosis, personality change or dementia, including ataxia, spasticity, seizures, or a peripheral neuropathy (Rauschka *et al.* 2006). It must be emphasized that in cases which do present with psychosis, personality change, or dementia, these other symptoms and signs may not appear for years.

The psychosis seen in the adult form is very similar to that seen in schizophrenia. One patient developed bizarre delusions, auditory hallucinations, loosening of associations, and flat affect at the age of 19 years, and the diagnosis became apparent only 12 years later when a peripheral polyneuropathy was noted (Manowitz *et al.* 1978). Another, at the age of 28 years, developed 'bizarre elation, true auditory hallucinations, and poorly formulated paranoid ideas', followed by a gradually progressive dementia over the next 4 years (Betts *et al.* 1968). In a third example (Waltz *et al.* 1987), a 31-year-old man began to talk to himself and pace the floor; he was eventually fired from his job and his wife left him. By the age of 38 years he had 'poor concentration, inappropriate smiling and laughing, . . . irrelevant remarks . . . with non sequiturs, restlessness and occasional auditory hallucinations'. The diagnosis was eventually suggested when nerve conduction velocity studies showed mild slowing. In some cases, the psychosis may have a distinct manic flair: one patient (Besson 1980) was 'grandiose . . . and called out the fire brigade', and another (Van Bogaert and Dewulf 1939) 'had ideas of grandeur, thought he was going to become an ambassador and gave himself honorary titles'. In both these cases, the patients eventually became demented.

The personality change may be non-specific; however, a frontal lobe syndrome may be prominent (Austin *et al.* 1968; Finelli 1985; Wulff and Trojaborg 1985) with disinhibition, perseveration, irritability, and socially inappropriate behavior.

As might be suspected, in addition to cognitive deficits, the dementia seen in metachromatic leukodystrophy is also often marked by delusions, hallucinations, and frontal lobe symptomatology (Alves *et al.* 1986; Bosch and Hart 1978; Hirose and Bass 1972; Hyde *et al.* 1992; Reider-Grosswasser and Bornstein 1987; Shapiro *et al.* 1994).

T2-weighted MR scanning reveals ventricular dilation and widespread increased signal intensity in the white matter (Reider-Grosswasser and Bornstein 1987; Rauschka *et al.* 2006). Nerve conduction velocity studies may reveal slowing in patients who lack clinical evidence of a peripheral neuropthy; however, it must be kept in mind that such studies may be normal. Lumbar puncture may reveal normal CSF or, especially in those with late infantile or juvenile forms, an increased total protein.

An often mentioned, but rarely seen, finding in metachromatic leukodystrophy is non-filling of the gallbladder on cholecystography, which occurs secondary to infiltration of the gallbladder by sulfatides.

Assays of leukocytes reveal decreased aryl sulfatase A activity, and assays of peripheral nerve tissue (obtained at sural nerve biopsy) or of urinary sediment will reveal increased sulfatide content. The phenomenon of metachromasia, from which this disorder derives its name, may also be observed in peripheral nervous tissue or urinary sediment. Both cresyl violet and toluidine blue undergo a chromatic metamorphosis, turning from violet or blue to brown or golden-brown, respectively, when applied to affected cells in the peripheral nerve or urinary sediment.

Course

The disease is gradually progressive, with death within 2–10 years in the late infantile or juvenile forms; in the adult form, death may be delayed for up to 15 years.

Etiology

As noted, metachromatic leukodystrophy is a recessively inherited disorder, and occurs secondary to any of a large number of mutations in the gene for arylsulfatase A, found on chromosome 22 (Barth *et al.* 1993). Arylsulfatase A

normally converts sulfatides into cerebroside, which is a normal constituent of myelin; with decreased activity of arylsulfatase A, there is an increase in sulfatide levels and a decrease in cerebroside levels, with resulting demyelinization. Of interest, the increased sulfatide content in peripheral nervous tissue and renal epithelial cells accounts for the metachromasia. Sulfatides are positively charged, and their excessive presence reorients the negatively charged molecules of cresyl violet or toluidine blue, thereby changing their color.

Within the central nervous system, widespread demyelinzation is seen, and this is especially evident in the centrum semiovale. In severe cases, the white matter of the centrum semiovale may be shrunken down to a thin gliotic remnant, with only relative sparing of the U-fibers, such that there is very little intervening tissue between the depths of the sulci and the lateral ventricles. The cerebellar white matter is affected in a similar fashion, and there is also peripheral demyelinization.

Rarely, rather than occurring secondary to a mutation in the gene for arylsulfatase A, metachromatic leukodystrophy may occur secondary to a mutation in a gene on chromosome 10 coding for a sulfatide activator protein (Schlote *et al.* 1991). This protein acts as an essential cofactor for arylsulfatase A and, in its absence, all of the biochemical defects seen with mutations in the gene for arylsulfatase A also accrue.

Differential diagnosis

Differential diagnostic considerations vary according to the age of the patient.

Juvenile-onset cases may be confused with adrenoleukodystrophy; however, in adrenoleukodystrophy one also sees either a hemianopia or cortical blindness, findings not seen in metachromatic leukodystrophy.

Adult-onset cases may, depending on their presentation, raise several differential considerations. Presentations with psychosis may be indistinguishable from schizophrenia until other signs and symptoms, such as ataxia or peripheral neuropathy, emerge, or until a dementia supervenes. Presentations with a personality change of the frontal lobe type or with a dementia may raise the possibility of frontotemporal dementia, and the differential here may also rest on the emergence of a peripheral neuropathy or ataxia.

As noted earlier, diagnosis rests on demonstrating decreased aryl sulfatase A activity in leukocytes and in finding increased sulfatide content in peripheral tissues, and it must be stressed that both tests must be positive. Finding a decreased aryl sulfatase A activity by itself is not diagnostic, because in about 10 percent of the general population there is a 'pseudodeficiency' of arylsulfatase A activity that is not associated with sulfatide accumulation or with any symptomatology (Hageman *et al.* 1995).

Treatment

Bone marrow transplantation may retard or halt the progression of the disease (Kidd *et al.* 1998; Krivit *et al.* 1987; Navarro *et al.* 1996). The general treatment of psychosis is discussed in Section 7.1, of personality change in Section 7.2, and of dementia in Section 5.1.

8.30 ADRENOLEUKODYSTROPHY

Adrenoleukodystrophy is a rare, X-linked disorder characterized pathologically by the accumulation of very-long-chain fatty acids in the brain, spinal cord, peripheral nerves, and adrenal glands, and clinically by a variable combination of dementia, spasticity, and adrenal failure.

Clinical features

Clinically (Moser *et al.* 1984), adrenoleukodystrophy may be characterized according to either the age of onset or the primary site of pathology. Thus, onset may be in childhood (at an average age of 8 years), adolescence, or adult years, and the primary site may be cerebral, spinal, or adrenal.

Childhood-onset adrenoleukodystrophy usually presents with cerebral symptomatology, often with a personality change and visual symptoms. These patients may become withdrawn and irritable, and school performance declines. Varying degrees of hemianopia or cortical blindness may occur, followed by a dementia accompanied by spasticity (Moser *et al.* 1984; Schaumburg *et al.* 1975). Adolescent-onset adrenoleukodystrophy tends to present in a fashion similar to that of the childhood-onset form.

Adult-onset adrenoleukodystrophy tends to present with spinal cord involvement, adrenal failure or, less commonly, with cerebral involvement; in cases that present with cord involvement or adrenal failure, long-term follow-up reveals the development of cerebral involvement in a significant minority (van Geel *et al.* 2001). Cord involvement yields a syndrome known as adrenomyeloneuropathy (Griffin *et al.* 1977), wherein gait becomes clumsy and stiff, and a spastic paraplegia eventually appears. Cerebral involvement produces a dementia that may be nonspecific in character, or which may be marked by manic symptoms (Weller *et al.* 1992) or a Kluver–Bucy syndrome (Powers *et al.* 1980).

Peripheral nerve involvement tends to be mild and may in some cases only be apparent with nerve conduction velocity studies.

Seizures occur in about one-fifth of all patients, usually late in the course of the disease.

Adrenal involvement may occur at any age and may indeed be the sole presentation of adrenoleukodystrophy (O'Neill *et al.* 1982). In some cases, the only evidence of adrenal cortical involvement may be a decreased cortisol level or an increased adrenocorticotrophic hormone level, whereas in others there may be melanoderma, nausea, vomiting, abdominal pain, diarrhea, and hyperkalemia. It must be kept in mind that, in some cases with cerebral or cord involvement, adrenal function may be normal.

Phenotypic variability is the rule in adrenoleukodystrophy, and even members of the same family may have different presentations (Erlington *et al.* 1989). Indeed, even monozygotic twins may exhibit phenotypic heterogeneity (Sobue *et al.* 1994), to the point of one twin being affected while the other is not (Korenke *et al.* 1996).

Female heterozygotes may occasionally have mild symptoms.

Computed tomography scanning in patients with cerebral involvement may reveal areas of radiolucency in the white matter: typically these first appear in the occipital lobes and then spread anteriorly into the parietal and temporal lobes. With contrast administration, enhancement is seen at the boundary between the areas of radiolucency and normal tissue. T2-weighted MR scanning reveals increased signal intensity in the white matter, following the same pattern as seen on CT scans, with the same pattern of enhancement upon administration of gadolinium. Cerebrospinal fluid analysis may reveal a mild lymphocytic pleocytosis and an elevated total protein. In patients with adrenal involvement, there may be hyperkalemia and decreased cortisol and increased adrenocorticotropic hormone (ACTH) levels. The diagnosis is confirmed by finding elevated levels of very-long-chain fatty acids in plasma or cultured skin fibroblasts. Given the very large number of mutations, genetic testing is not practical.

Course

Childhood-onset cases generally progress fairly rapidly, death supervening within 3–5 years; adolescent- and adult-onset cases, especially those with the adrenomyeloneuropathy syndrome, may progress very slowly. There may rarely be periods of partial remission, only to be followed eventually by relapse (Walsh 1980).

Etiology

Adrenoleukodystrophy is an X-linked disorder (Mosser *et al.* 1994) that occurs secondary to any of a large number of different mutations in the *ALD* gene on the X chromosome. These mutations cause defective functioning of a peroxisome membrane-associated protein, which in turn leads to an accumulation of very-long-chain fatty acids in the white matter of the brain or spinal cord, in the peripheral nerves, and in the adrenal cortex.

Within the brain (Schaumburg *et al.* 1975), one typically finds an advancing wave of demyelinization that begins in the occipital lobe and then moves forward into the parietal and temporal lobes; the frontal lobes are broached in only a minority. An inflammatory response is seen at the border between the demyelinization and the normal tissue, behind which much of the white matter is replaced by gliotic tissue. Importantly, the subcortical U-fibers are generally spared, as is the gray matter. Demyelinization also occurs in the spinal cord, especially in the corticospinal tracts, and the peripheral nerves may also be involved, albeit generally to a much lesser extent.

Differential diagnosis

In children or adolescents, a diagnosis of metachromatic leukodystrophy may be considered; however, the presence of visual symptoms and adrenal insufficiency favor adrenoleukodystrophy. In adults, multiple sclerosis is often considered. Adrenal insufficiency suggests adrenoleukodystrophy; however, in its absence the differential may rest on the determination of very-long-chain fatty acid levels.

Treatment

There was much hope that reducing very-long-chain fatty acid levels by means of 'Lorenzo's oil' would be curative; however, this hope does not seem to have been borne out. Although Lorenzo's oil does indeed reduce plasma very-long-chain fatty acid levels, and uncontrolled studies suggest that it may delay expression of the disease in asymptomatic boys (Moser et al. 2005), a controlled study in symptomatic patients failed to display any benefit (van Geel et al. 1999). Bone marrow transplantation, if undertaken very early in the course of the disease, may halt its progression or even lead to improvement (Shapiro et al. 2000). The general treatment of dementia is discussed in Section 5.1. Adrenal insufficiency is treated in the usual fashion.

Female relatives should be offered testing for very-long-chain fatty acid levels.

8.31 KUFS' DISEASE

Kufs' disease, also known as the adult form of neuronal ceroid lipofuscinosis, is a very rare disorder that typically presents in early adult years with either seizures or dementia.

Clinical features

Kufs' disease typically presents in early adult years in one of two fashions (Berkovic et al. 1988; Callagy et al. 2000). In one, referred to as 'type A', patients present with grand mal and myoclonic seizures and a dementia, which is often accompanied by ataxia or abnormal movements, such as athetosis or parkinsonism. In the other, 'type B', the presentation is typically with a personality change or dementia, which may also be accompanied by ataxia and other abnormal movements.

Magnetic resonance scanning may be normal or may reveal cortical atrophy.

In those with dementia, generalized slowing is seen on the EEG; when seizures are present, the EEG typically reveals generalized spike-and-wave discharges, and there may be a pronounced photosensitivity (Vadlamudi et al. 2003).

Diagnosis is confirmed by rectal, muscle, or skin biopsy, which reveals characteristic fingerprint or granular osmiophilic deposits on electron microscopy (Berkovic et al. 1988).

Course

The disease is relentlessly progressive, with death occurring on average after 12 years.

Etiology

The neuronal ceroid lipofuscinoses occur in four forms, namely infantile (CLN1), late infantile (CLN2), juvenile (CLN3), and the adult form, Kufs' disease (CLN4). Kufs' disease may occur on a sporadic or an inherited basis. Although most heritable cases occur on an autosomal recessive basis (Berkovic et al. 1988), families with dominant inheritance have been reported (Burneo et al. 2003; Nijssen et al. 2002). Although the genetic defect for most cases of Kufs' disease is not known, there is one case report of adult-onset neuronal ceroid lipofuscinosis occurring secondary to a mutation typically associated with the infantile form (van Diggelen et al. 2001).

Neuronal loss occurs, and in surviving neurons ceroid and lipofuscin deposits are seen within lysosomes, creating a typical fingerprint or granular pattern on electron microscopy.

Differential diagnosis

Kufs' disease is typically suspected in adults with a combination of myoclonus and dementia, and in such cases one must consider Creutzfeldt–Jakob disease and Hashimoto's encephalopathy. The EEG may be very helpful in making the differential here in cases with seizures, as the pattern seen in Kufs' disease is not present in these other disorders.

Treatment

The symptomatic treatment of dementia is discussed in Section 5.1; divalproex may be considered for seizures.

8.32 ESSENTIAL TREMOR

Essential tremor is a common condition characterized primarily by a postural tremor of the hands.

Clinical features

Although the range in age of onset is wide, from the first to the ninth decades of life, most patients experience the onset of tremor during the fifth decade.

Clinically speaking (Bain *et al.* 1994; Critchley 1949; Koller *et al.* 1994; Lou and Jankovic 1991; Martinelli *et al.* 1987), in the vast majority of cases, the tremor first becomes evident in the hand, generally bilaterally; only in a small minority is the onset unilateral. The tremor, at least initially, is fine, ranging in frequency from 4 to 8cps, and postural, being most evident when the hands are held outstretched with the fingers spread. In most cases, over time, the tremor also becomes apparent elsewhere, including, in decreasing order of frequency, the head, the voice, the chin, and, in a small minority, the feet. Head tremor is generally of the 'no-no' type (Bain *et al.* 1994) with a trembling oscillation of the head from side to side. Involvement of the voice may impart a quavering quality to the patients' speech (Ardran *et al.* 1966). Recent work (Benito-Leon *et al.* 2006) indicates that patients may also display some cognitive deficits, but these are quite mild and of questionable clinical importance.

Course

In most cases the course is characterized by progressive worsening to a certain plateau, which may persist for years or decades, after which there may be further progression. As the tremor worsens, it characteristically becomes of greater amplitude and slower frequency.

Etiology

Although sporadic cases do occur, both family and twin studies (Bain *et al.* 1994; Lorenz *et al.* 2004; Tanner *et al.* 2001) indicate that essential tremor is, in most cases, inherited, most likely on an autosomal dominant basis. Although the genetic basis remains obscure, in some families linkage has been found to sites on chromosomes 2, 3, and 6 (Shatunov *et al.* 2006).

Although routine pathologic studies have been unremarkable (Rajput *et al.* 2004), recent work has demonstrated some interesting findings (Louis *et al.* 2005, 2006a,b). Lewy bodies have been found in brainstem nuclei, most especially the locus ceruleus; furthermore, within the cerebellum, Purkinje cell loss has been noted, with, in surviving Purkinje cells, torpedoes, or massive collections of disoriented neurofilaments. Although speculative, these seemingly disparate findings may be reconciled as contributing to a final common pathway of reduced inhibitory output of the Purkinje cell layer. The locus ceruleus has massive stimulatory projections to the Purkinje cell layer, and with dysfunction of the locus ceruleus, and loss of this stimulation, Purkinje cell output would fall. A similar loss of output from the Purkinje cell layer would also, of course, occur with loss or damage to the Purkinje cells themselves. If these findings are replicated, and if this speculation is correct, then it may well be that essential tremor represents a syndrome composed of two or more inherited disorders causing pathology either in brainstem nuclei or in the cerebellum.

Differential diagnosis

Essential tremor is a postural tremor and, as discussed in Section 3.1, this must be distinguished from rest and intention tremors. Once it is clear that the patient does have a postural tremor, the differential may be pursued as outlined in Section 3.1, with special attention given to medication-induced tremors (e.g., sympathomimetics or caffeine), alcohol or sedative/hypnotic withdrawal, and hyperthyroidism.

Treatment

A large number of medications are effective in essential tremor. Primidone (Koller and Royse 1986) and propranolol (Winkler and Young 1974) are the mainstays; propranolol may be given in doses from 80 to 240 mg/day, and primidone from 25 to 750 mg/day. Alternatives include gabapentin (Gironell *et al.* 1999; Ondo *et al.* 2000), in doses from 1200 to 3600 mg/day, and topiramate (Connor 2002; Ondo *et al.* 2006), from 100 to 400 mg/day. Alprazolam is also effective (Gunal *et al.* 2000), but given the high risk of physiologic dependence, this should probably be held in reserve. Regardless of which medication is used, one should start at a low dose and increase gradually, looking for the lowest effective dose. Another 'medication', which many patients will already have discovered on their own, is alcohol (Growdon *et al.* 1975), which, for obvious reasons, cannot be recommended. In severe, treatment-resistant cases, consideration may be given to deep brain stimulation of the thalamus (Sydow *et al.* 2003).

8.33 HYPEREKPLEXIA

Hyperekplexia, also known as hyperexplexia or 'startle disease', is a rare disorder characterized by a pathologic startle response.

Clinical features

Hyperekplexia occurs in two varieties, namely the major form and the minor form, and these differ both in age of onset and in clinical symptomatology (Andermann *et al.* 1980; Kirsten and Silfverskiold 1958; Ryan *et al.* 1992; Suhren *et al.* 1966; Tijssen *et al.* 1995).

The major form of hyperekplexia becomes apparent in earliest infancy with episodes of hypertonus. By the time that the child is able to walk, or shortly thereafter, the response typical of hyperekplexia becomes apparent: to an appropriate stimulus, often a loud, unexpected noise, patients experience an exaggerated startle response (Brown et al. 1991) characterized by grimacing, flexion of the neck, arms and trunk, abduction of the arms, and generalized stiffness; many fall 'like a log' and injuries are common. Consciousness is maintained throughout and the stiffness resolves immediately, allowing the patient to stand again.

The minor form of hyperexplexia typically does not become apparent until childhood or later and consists simply of the exaggerated startle response without any associated stiffness.

Course

Although some partial reduction in severity of the startle response may occur in the adult years, the course is overall chronic and unremitting. Symptoms are typically worse during fatigue or stress.

Etiology

The etiology of the two forms of hyperekplexia probably differ.

Regarding the major form, although sporadic cases do occur (Saenz-Lope et al. 1984), most cases are inherited, and most are due to mutations in the gene for the alpha-1 subunit of the inhibitory glycine receptor (GLRA1) on chromosome 5; depending on the mutation, both autosomal dominant (Andrew and Owen 1997; Shiang et al. 1993) and recessive (Rees et al. 1994; Siren et al. 2006; Tsai et al. 2004) patterns of inheritance may occur.

The etiology of the minor form is not clear. The fact that both major and minor forms may occur in the same family (Andermann et al. 1980; Suhren et al. 1966) suggests that the minor form may merely be a forme fruste of the major form; however, genetic analysis of these cases, although revealing a mutation in the alpha subunit in those with the major form, failed to find mutations in those with the minor form (Tijssen et al. 1995).

Differential diagnosis

The reader is directed to Section 3.14, where the differential for pathologic startle is discussed.

Treatment

Clonazepam is generally effective in reducing the severity of the startle response (Ryan et al. 1992); divalproex has also been successfully used (Dooley and Andermann 1989).

REFERENCES

Aarsland D, Tandberg E, Larsen JP et al. Frequency of dementia in Parkinson disease. Arch Neurol 1996; 53:538–42.

Aarsland D, Laake K, Larsen JP et al. Donepezil for cognitive impairment in Parkinson's disease: a randomized controlled study. J Neurol Neurosurg Psychiatry 2002; 72:708–12.

Aarsland D, Andersen K, Larson JP et al. Prevalence and characteristics of dementia in Parkinson disease: an 8-year prospective study. Arch Neurol 2003; 60:387–92.

Aarsland D, Perry R, Brown A et al. Neuropathology of dementia in Parkinson's disease: a prospective, community-based study. Ann Neurol 2005; 58:773–6.

Adachi N, Arima K, Asada T et al. Dentatorubral-pallidoluysia atrophy (DRPLA) presenting with psychosis. J Neuropsychiatry Clin Neurosci 2001; 13:258–60.

Adams C, Starkman S, Pulst S-M. Clinical and molecular analysis of a pedigree of southern Italian ancestry with spinocerebellar ataxia type 2. Neurology 1997; 49:1163–6.

Adie WJ, Greenfield JG. Dystrophia myotonica (myotonia atrophica). Brain 1924; 47:73–127.

Adler CH, Sethi KD, Hauser RA et al. Ropinirole for the treatment of early Parkinson's disease. Neurology 1997; 49:393–9.

Adler CH, Singer C, O'Brien C et al. Randomized placebo-controlled study of tolcapone in patients with fluctuating Parkinson's disease treated with levodopa–carbidopa. Arch Neurol 1998; 55:1089–95.

del Aguila MA, Longstreth WT, McGuire V et al. Prognosis in amyotrophic lateral sclerosis. A population-based study. Neurology 2003; 60:813–19.

Aisen PS, Davis KL. Inflammatory mechanisms in Alzheimer's disease: implications for therapy. Am J Psychiatry 1994; 151:1105–13.

Ala TA, Yang KH, Sung JH et al. Hallucinations and signs of parkinsonism help distinguish patients with dementia and cortical Lewy bodies from patients with Alzheimer's disease at presentation: a clinicopathological study. J Neurol Neurosurg Psychiatry 1997; 62:16–21.

Alberca RA, Chinchon I, Vadillo J et al. Late onset parkinsonian syndrome in Hallervorden–Spatz disease. J Neurol Neurosurg Psychiatry 1987; 50:1665–8.

Almasy L, Bressman SB, Raymond D et al. Idiopathic torsion dystonia linked to chromosome 8 in two Mennonite families. Ann Neurol 1997; 42:670–3.

Altrocchi PH, Forno LS. Spontaneous oral-facial dyskinesia: neuropathology of a case. Neurology 1983; 33:802–5.

Alves D, Pires MM, Guimaraes A et al. Four cases of late onset metachromatic leukodystrophy in a family: clinical, biochemical and neuropathological studies. J Neurol Neurosurg Psychiatry 1986; 49:1417–22.

Alzheimer A. Ubr eine eigenartige erkrankung der hirnrinde. Allermeine Zeitschrift fur Psychiatrie 1907; 64:146–8.

Amaducci LA, Rocca WA, Schoenberg BS. Origin of the distinction between Alzheimer's disease and senile dementia: how history can clarify nosology. Neurology 1986; 36:1497–9.

Amatniek JC, Hauser WA, DelCastillo-Castenada C et al. Incidence and predictors of seizures in patients with Alzheimer's disease. Epilepsia 2006; 47:867–72.

American Psychiatric Association. *Diagnostic and statistical manual of mental disorders*, 3rd edn. Washington, DC: American Psychiatric Press, 1980.

Aminoff MJ, Dedo HH, Idebski K. Clinical aspects of spasmodic dysphonia. *J Neurol Neurosurg Psychiatry* 1978; **41**:361–5.

Andersen J, Asbo E, Gulmann N et al. Anti-depressive treatment in Parkinson's disease. A controlled trial of the effect of nortriptyline in patients with Parkinson's disease treated with L-DOPA. *Acta Neurol Scand* 1980; **62**:210–19.

Andersen K, Baldin J, Gottfries CG et al. A double-blind evaluation of electroconvulsive therapy in Parkinson's disease with 'on-off' phenomenon. *Acta Neurol Scand* 1987; **76**:191–9.

Andermann F, Keene DL, Andermann E et al. Startle disease or hyperekplexia: further delineation of the syndrome. *Brain* 1980; **103**:985–97.

Andreasen N, Minthon L, Davidsson P et al. Evaluation of CSF-tau and CSF-Abeta42 as diagnostic markers for Alzheimer disease in clinical practice. *Arch Neurol* 2001; **58**:349–50.

Andrew M, Owen MJ. Hyperekplexia: abnormal startle response due to glycine receptor mutations. *Br J Psychiatry* 1997; **170**:106–8.

Angelini L, Nardocci N, Rumi V et al. Hallervorden–Spatz disease: clinical and MRI study of 11 cases diagnosed in life. *J Neurol* 1992; **239**:417–25.

Antonini A, Mainero C, Romano A et al. Cerebral atrophy in myotonic dystrophy: a voxel-based morphometric study. *J Neurol Neurosurg Psychiatry* 2004; **75**:1611–13.

Antonini A, Tesel S, Zechinelli A et al. Randomized study of sertraline and low-dose amitriptyline in patients with Parkinson's disease and depression: effect on quality of life. *Mov Disord* 2006; **21**:1119–22.

Apaydin H, Ahlskog JE, Parisi JE et al. Parkinson disease neuropathology. *Arch Neurol* 2002; **59**:102–12.

April RS. Observations on parkinsonian tremor in all-night sleep. *Neurology* 1966; **16**:720–4.

Ardran G, Kinsbourne M, Rushworth G. Dysphonia due to tremor. *J Neurol Neurosurg Psychiatry* 1966; **29**:219–23.

Arpa J, Cuesta A, Cruz-Martinez A et al. Clinical features and genetic analysis of a Spanish family with spinocerebellar ataxia 6. *Acta Neurol Scand* 1999; **99**:44–7.

Arriagada PV, Growdon JH, Hedley-Whyte ET et al. Neurofibrillary tangles but not senile plaques parallel duration and severity of Alzheimer's disease. *Neurology* 1992; **42**:631–9.

Ascherio A, Chen C, Weisskopf MG et al. Pesticide exposure and risk for Parkinson's disease. *Ann Neurol* 2006; **60**:197–203.

Asmus F, Horber V, Pohlenz J et al. A novel TITF-1 mutation causes benign hereditary chorea with response to levodopa. *Neurology* 2005; **64**:1952–4.

Austin J, Armstrong D, Fouch S et al. Metachromatic leukodystrophy (MLD). VIII. MLD in adults: diagnosis and pathogenesis. *Arch Neurol* 1968; **18**:225–40.

Avorn J, Scneeweis S, Sudarksy LR et al. Sudden uncontrollable somnolence and medication use in Parkinson disease. *Arch Neurol* 2005; **62**:1242–8.

Avrahami E, Katz A, Bornstein N et al. Computed tomographic findings of brain and skull in myotonic dystrophy. *J Neurol Neurosurg Psychiatry* 1987; **50**:435–8.

Baas H, Beiske AG, Ghika J et al. Catechol-O-methyltransferase inhibition with tolcapone reduces the 'wearing off' phenomenon and levodopa requirements in fluctuating parkinsonian patients. *J Neurol Neurosurg Psychiatry* 1997; **63**:421–8.

Bacalman S, Farzin F, Bourgeois JA et al. Psychiatric phenotype of the Fragile X-associated tremor/ataxia syndrome (FXTAS) in males: newly described fronto-subcortical dementia. *J Clin Psychiatry* 2006; **67**:87–94.

Bain PG, Findley LJ, Thompson PD et al. A study of hereditary essential tremor. *Brain* 1994; **117**:805–24.

Bak TH, O'Donovan DG, Xuereb JH et al. Selective impairment of verb processing associated with pathological changes in Brodmann areas 44 and 45 in the motor neurone disease-dementia-aphasia syndrome. *Brain* 2001; **124**:103–20.

Ballard C, McKeith I, Harrison R et al. A detailed phenomenological comparison of complex visual hallucinations in dementia with Lewy bodies and Alzheimer's disease. *Int Psychogeriatr* 1997; **9**:381–8.

Ballard C, Holmes C, McKeith I et al. Psychiatric morbidity in dementia with Lewy bodies: a prospective clinical and neuropathological comparative study with Alzheimer's disease. *Am J Psychiatry* 1999; **156**:1039–45.

Ballard C, O'Brien J, Gray A et al. Attention and fluctuating attention in patients with dementia with Lewy bodies and Alzheimer disease. *Arch Neurol* 2001; **58**:977–82.

Bandmann O, Valente EM, Holmans P et al. Dopa-responsive dystonia: a clinical and molecular genetic study. *Ann Neurol* 1998; **44**:649–56.

Barker WW, Luis CA, Kashuba A et al. Relative frequencies of Alzheimer disease, Lewy body, vascular and frontotemporal dementia, and hippocampal sclerosis in the State of Florida Brain Bank. *Alzheimer Dis Assoc Disord* 2002; **16**:203–12.

Barnes J, David AS. Visual hallucinations in Parkinson's disease: a review and phenomenological survey. *J Neurol Neurosurg Psychiatry* 2001; **70**:727–33.

Barnes S, Hurst W. A further note on hepatolenticular degeneration. *Brain* 1926; **49**:36–60.

Barone P, Scarzella L, Marconi R et al. Pramipexole versus sertaline in the treatment of depression in Parkinson's disease: a national multicenter parallel-group randomized study. *J Neurol* 2006; **253**:601–7.

Barr AN, Fischer JH, Koller WC et al. Serum haloperidol concentrations and choreiform movements in Huntington's disease. *Neurology* 1988; **38**:84–8.

Barth ML, Fensom A, Harris A. Prevalence of common mutations in the arylsulfatase A gene in metachromatic leukodystrophy patients diagnosed in Britain. *Hum Genet* 1993; **91**:73–7.

Batten FE, Gibb HP. Myotonia atrophica. *Brain* 1909; **32**:187–96.

Bax RT, Hassler A, Luck W et al. Cerebral manifestation of Wilson's disease successfully treated with liver transplantation. *Neurology* 1998; **51**:863–5.

Beatty WW, Winn P, Adams RL et al. Preserved cognitive skills in dementia of the Alzheimer type. *Arch Neurol* 1994; **51**:1040–6.

Becher MW, Rubinsztein DC, Leggo J et al. Dentatorubral and pallidoluysian atrophy (DRPLA): clinical and neuropathological findings in genetically conformed North American and European pedigrees. *Mov Disord* 1997; **12**:519–30.

Becker T, Becker G, Seufert J *et al.* Parkinson's disease and depression: evidence for an alteration of the basal limbic system detected by transcranial sonography. *J Neurol Neurosurg Psychiatry* 1997; **63**:590–6.

Behan PO, Bone I. Hereditary chorea without dementia. *J Neurol Neurosurg Psychiatry* 1977; **40**:687–91.

Benarroch EE, Smithson IL, Low PA *et al.* Depletion of catecholaminergic neurons of the rostral ventrolateral medulla in multiple systems atrophy with autonomic failure. *Ann Neurol* 1998; **43**:156–63.

Bencze KS, Vande Polder DR, Prockop LD. Magnetic resonance imaging of the brain and spinal cord in cerebrotendinous xanthomatosis. *J Neurol Neurosurg Psychiatry* 1990; **53**:166–7.

Benesch CG, McDaniel KD, Cox C *et al.* End-stage Alzheimer's disease: Glasgow coma scale and neurologic examination. *Arch Neurol* 1993; **50**:1309–15.

Benito-Leon J, Louis ED, Bermejo-Pareja F *et al.* Population-based case-control study of cognitive function in essential tremor. *Neurology* 2006; **66**:69–74.

Bentivoglio AR, DelGrosso N, Albenese A *et al.* Non-DYT1 dystonia in a large Italian family. *J Neurol Neurosurg Psychiatry* 1997; **62**:357–60.

Benton CS, de Silva R, Rutledge SL *et al.* Molecular and clinical studies in SCA-7 define a broad clinical spectrum and the infantile phenotype. *Neurology* 1998; **51**:1081–6.

Bergem AL, Engedal K, Kringlen E. The role of heredity in late-onset Alzheimer disease and vascular dementia. A twin study. *Arch Gen Psychiatry* 1997; **54**:264–70.

Bergeron C, Pollanen MS, Weyer L *et al.* Unusual clinical presentation of cortical-basal ganglionic degeneration. *Ann Neurol* 1996; **40**:893–900.

Berginer VM, Salen G, Shefer S. Long-term treatment of cerebrotendinous xanthomatosis with chenodeoxycholic acid. *N Engl J Med* 1984; **311**:1649–54.

Berkovic SF, Carpenter S, Andermann F *et al.* Kufs' disease: a critical reappraisal. *Brain* 1988; **111**:27–62.

Besson JAO. A diagnostic pointer to adult metachromatic leukodystrophy. *Br J Psychiatry* 1980; **137**:186–7.

Betts TA, Smith WT, Kelly RE. Adult metachromatic leukodystrophy (subacute lipidosis) simulating acute schizophrenia: report of a case. *Neurology* 1968; **18**:1140–2.

Bhidayasiri R, Jen JC, Baloh RW. Three brothers with a very-late-onset writer's cramp. *Mov Disord* 2005; **20**:1375–7.

Bicknell JM, Greenhouse AH, Pesch RN. Spastic dysphonia. *J Neurol Neurosurg Psychiatry* 1968; **31**:158–61.

Bierer L, Hof P, Purohit D *et al.* Neocortical neurofibrillary tangles correlate with dementia severity in Alzheimer's disease. *Arch Neurol* 1995; **52**:81–8.

Biggins CA, Boyd JL, Harrop FM *et al.* A controlled, longitudinal study of dementia in Parkinson's disease. *J Neurol Neurosurg Psychiatry* 1992; **55**:566–71.

Billings EG, Ravin A. A psychiatric study of patients manifesting dystrophica myotonica. *Am J Psychiatry* 1941; **97**:1116–34.

Binetti G, Bianchetti A, Padovani A *et al.* Delusions in Alzheimer's disease and multi-infarct dementia. *Acta Neurol Scand* 1993; **88**:5–9.

Biousse V, Skibell BC, Watts RL *et al.* Ophthalmologic features of Parkinson's disease. *Neurology* 2004; **62**:177–80.

Bird MT, Paulson GW. The rigid form of Huntington's chorea. *Neurology* 1971; **21**:271–6.

Bird TD, Levy-Lahad E, Poorkaj P *et al.* Wide range in age of onset for chromosome 1-related familial Alzheimer's disease. *Ann Neurol* 1996; **40**:932–6.

Birdi S, Rajput AH, Fenton M *et al.* Progressive supranuclear palsy diagnosis and confounding features: report on 16 autopsied cases. *Mov Disord* 2002; **17**:1255–64.

Bloch MH, Leckman JF, Zhu HS *et al.* Caudate volumes in childhood predict symptom severity in adults with Tourette syndrome. *Neurology* 2005; **65**:1253–8.

Boeve BF, Silber MH, Ferman TJ *et al.* REM sleep behavior disorder and degenerative dementia: an association likely reflecting Lewy body disease. *Neurology* 1998; **51**:363–70.

Bonelli RM, Niederwieser G, Tribl GG *et al.* High-dose olanzapine in Huntington's disease. *Int Clin Psychopharmacol* 2002; **17**:91–3.

Bosch EP, Hart MN. Late adult-onset metachromatic leukodystrophy: dementia and polyneuropathy in a 63-year-old man. *Arch Neurol* 1978; **35**:475–7.

Botez MI, Botez-Marquard T, Elie R *et al.* Amantadine hydrochloride treatment in heredodegenerative ataxia: a double blind study. *J Neurol Neurosurg Psychiatry* 1996; **61**:259–64.

Bourgeois JA, Cogswell JB, Hessl D *et al.* Cognitive, anxiety and mood disorders in the fragile X-associated tremor/ataxia syndrome. *Gen Hosp Psychiatry* 2007; **29**:349–56.

Bouton SM. Pick's disease. *J Nerv Ment Dis* 1940; **91**:9–30.

Bowler JV, Eliaszaw M, Steenhuis R *et al.* Comparative evolution of Alzheimer disease, vascular dementia, and mixed dementia. *Arch Neurol* 1997; **54**:697–703.

Braak H, Braak E. Neuropathological staging of Alzheimer-related changes. *Acta Neuropathol* 1991; **82**:239–59.

Braak H, Rub U, Jansen Steur ENH *et al.* Cognitive status correlates with neuropathologic stage in Parkinson disease. *Neurology* 2005; **64**:1404–10.

Bracco L, Gallato R, Grigoletto F *et al.* Factors affecting course and survival in Alzheimer's disease. *Arch Neurol* 1994; **51**:1213–19.

Bradshaw J, Saling M, Hopwood M *et al.* Fluctuating cognition in dementia with Lewy bodies and Alzheimer's disease is qualitatively distinct. *J Neurol Neurosurg Psychiatry* 2004; **75**:382–7.

Brain WR, Greenfield JG. Late infantile metachromatic leukodystrophy with primary degeneration of the interfascicular oligodendroglia. *Brain* 1950; **73**:291–317.

Brans JWM, Lindeboom R, Snoek JW *et al.* Botulinum toxin versus trihexyphenidyl in cervical dystonia: a prospective, randomized, double-blind controlled trial. *Neurology* 1996; **46**:1066–72.

Brassat D, Camuzat A, Vidailhet M *et al.* Frequency of the *DYT1* mutation in primary torsion dystonia without family history. *Arch Neurol* 2000; **57**:333–5.

Breedveld GJ, Percy AK, MacDonald ME et al. Clinical and genetic heterogeneity in benign hereditary chorea. *Neurology* 2002; **59**:579–84.

Breier A, Sutton VK, Feldman PD et al. Olanzapine in the treatment of dopamimetic-induced psychosis in patients with Parkinson's disease. *Biol Psychiatry* 2002; **52**:438–45.

Breitner JCS, Walsh KA, Gau BA et al. Alzheimer's disease in the National Academy of Sciences – National Research Council of Aging Twin Veterans. III: Detection of cases, longitudinal results, and observations on twin concordance. *Arch Neurol* 1995; **52**:763–71.

Bressman SB, de Leon D, Brin MF et al. Idiopathic torsion dystonia among Ashkenazi Jews: evidence for autosomal dominant inheritance. *Ann Neurol* 1989; **26**:612–20.

Bressman SB, de Leon D, Kramer PL et al. Dystonia in Ashkenazi Jews: clinical characterization of a founder mutation. *Ann Neurol* 1994; **36**:771–7.

Bressman SB, Warner TT, Almasy L et al. Exclusion of the DYT1 locus in familial torticollis. *Ann Neurol* 1996; **40**:681–4.

Bressman SB, Sabatti C, Raymond D et al. The *DYT1* phenotype and guidelines for diagnostic testing. *Neurology* 2000; **54**:1746–52.

Brewer GJ, Turkay A, Yuzbasiyan-Gurkan V. Development of neurologic symptoms in a patient with asymptomatic Wilson's disease treated with penicillamine. *Arch Neurol* 1994; **51**:304–5.

Brewer GJ, Johnson V, Dick RD et al. Treatment of Wilson's disease with ammonium tetrathiomolybdate. II. Initial therapy in 33 neurologically affected patients and follow-up with zinc therapy. *Arch Neurol* 1996; **53**:1017–26.

Brewer GJ, Askari F, Lorincz MT et al. Treatment of Wilson disease with ammonium tetrathiomolybdate. IV. Comparison of tetrathiomolybdate and trientene in a double blind study of treatment of the neurologic presentation of Wilson disease. *Arch Neurol* 2006; **63**:521–7.

Bridgman O, Smyth FS. Progressive lenticular degeneration. *J Nerv Ment Dis* 1944; **99**:534–43.

Briel RC, McKeith IG, Barker WA et al. EEG findings in dementia with Lewy bodies and Alzheimer's disease. *J Neurol Neurosurg Psychiatry* 1999; **66**:401–3.

Britton JW, Uitti RJ, Ahlskog JE et al. Hereditary late-onset chorea without significant dementia: genetic evidence for substantial phenotypic variation in Huntington's disease. *Neurology* 1995; **45**:443–7.

Brody IA, Wilkins RH. Huntington's chorea. *Arch Neurol* 1967; **17**:331–3.

Bronner IF, ter Meulen BC, Azmani A et al. Hereditary Pick's disease with the G272V tau mutation showing predominant three-repeat tau pathology. *Brain* 2005; **128**:2645–53.

Brook JD, McCurrach ME, Harley HG et al. Molecular basis of myotonic dystrophy: expansion of a trinucleotide (CTG) repeat at the 3' end of a transcript encoding a protein kinase family member. *Cell* 1992; **68**:799–808.

Brooks DJ, Sagar H. Entacapone is beneficial in both fluctuating and non-fluctuating patients with Parkinson's disease: a randomized, placebo controlled, double blind, six month study. *J Neurol Neurosurg Psychiatry* 2003; **74**:1071–9.

Brouwers N, Sleegers K, Engelborghs S et al. Genetic risk and transcriptional variability of amyloid precursor protein in Alzheimer's disease. *Brain* 2006; **129**:2984–91.

Brown J, Lantos P, Stratton M et al. Familial progressive supranuclear palsy. *J Neurol Neurosurg Psychiatry* 1993; **56**:473–6.

Brown P, Rothwell JC, Thompson PD et al. The hyperekplexias and their relationship to the normal startle reflex. *Brain* 1991; **114**:1903–28.

Brownell B, Oppenheimer DR, Hughes JT. The central nervous system in motor neuron disease. *J Neurol Neurosurg Psychiatry* 1970; **33**:338–57.

Bruggeman R, van der Linden C, Butelaar JK et al. Risperidone versus pimozide in Tourette's disorder: a comparative double-blind parallel-group study. *J Clin Psychiatry* 2001; **62**:50–6.

Brunberg JA, Jacquemont S, Hagerman RJ et al. Fragile X premutation carriers: characteristic MR imaging findings of adult male patients with progressive cerebellar and cognitive dysfunction. *AJNR* 2002; **23**:1757–66.

Bruni AC, Momeni P, Bernardi L et al. Heterogeneity within a large kindred with frontotemporal dementia. *Neurology* 2007; **69**:140–7.

Bruun RD. Subtle and unrecognized side effects of neuroleptic treatment in children with Tourette's disorder. *Am J Psychiatry* 1988; **145**:621–4.

Buerger K, Ewers M, Pirtilla T et al. CSF phosphorylated tau protein correlates with neocortical neurofibrillary pathology in Alzheimer's disease. *Brain* 2006; **129**:3035–41.

Bull PC, Thomas GR, Rommens JM et al. The Wilson disease gene is a putative copper transporting P-type ATPase similar to Menkes gene. *Nature Gen* 1993; **5**:327–37.

Bungener C, Jouvent R, Delaporte C. Psychopathological and emotional deficits in myotonic dystrophy. *J Neurol Neurosurg Psychiatry* 1998; **65**:353–6.

Burk K, Globas C, Bosch S et al. Cognitive deficits in spinocerebellar ataxia 2. *Brain* 1999; **122**:769–77.

Burke RE, Fahn S, Marsden CD. Torsion dystonia: a double-blind, prospective trial of high-dosage trihexyphenidyl. *Neurology* 1986; **36**:160–4.

Burke WJ, Pfeiffer RF, McComb RD. Neuroleptic sensitivity to clozapine in dementia with Lewy bodies. *J Neuropsychiatry Clin Neurosci* 1998; **10**:227–9.

Burkhardt CR, Filley CM, Kleineschmidt-DeMasters BK et al. Diffuse Lewy body disease and progressive dementia. *Neurology* 1988; **38**:1520–8.

Burneo JG, Arnold T, Palmer CA et al. Adult-onset neuronal ceroid lipofuscinosis (Kufs' disease) with autosomal dominant inheritance in Alabama. *Epilepsia* 2003; **44**:841–6.

Burns A, Jacoby R, Levy R. Psychiatric phenomena in Alzheimer's disease. III. Disorders of mood. *Br J Psychiatry* 1990a; **157**:81–6.

Burns A, Jacoby R, Levy R. Psychiatric phenomena in Alzheimer's disease. II. Disorders of perception. *Br J Psychiatry* 1990b; **157**:76–81.

Burns A, Jacoby R, Levy R. Psychiatric phenomena in Alzheimer's disease. I. Disorders of thought content. *Br J Psychiatry* 1990c; **157**:72–6.

Byrne EJ, Lennox G, Lowe J et al. Diffuse Lewy body disease: clinical features in 15 cases. J Neurol Neurosurg Psychiatry 1989; 57:709-17.

Caine ED, Shoulson I. Psychiatric symptoms in Huntington's disease. Am J Psychiatry 1983; 140:728-33.

Callagy C, O'Neill G, Murphy SF et al. Adult neuronal ceroid lipofuscinosis (Kufs' disease) in two siblings in an Irish family. Clin Neuropathol 2000; 19:109-18.

Calzetti S, Bortone E, Negrotti A et al. Frontal intermittent rhythmic delta activity (FIRDA) in patients with dementia with Lewy bodies: a diagnostic tool? Neurol Sci 2002; 23(suppl. 2):S65-6.

Campbell AMG, Corner B, Norman RM et al. The rigid form of Huntington's disease. J Neurol Neurosurg Psychiatry 1965; 24:71-7.

Canelas HM, Quintao ECR, Scaff M et al. Cerebrotendinous xanthomatosis: clinical and laboratory study of 2 cases. Acta Neurol Scand 1983; 67:305-11.

Cardoso F, Veado CCM, de Oliveira JT. A Brazilian cohort of patients with Tourette's syndrome. J Neurol Neurosurg Psychiatry 1996; 60:209-12.

Castelbuono A, Miller NR. Spontaneous remission in patients with essential blepharospasm and Meige syndrome. Am J Ophthalmol 1998; 126:432-5.

Castelnau P, Cif L, Valente EM et al. Pallidal stimulation improves pantothenate kinase-associated neurodegeneration. Ann Neurol 2005; 57:738-41.

Celesia GG, Barr AN. Psychosis and other psychiatric manifestations of levodopa therapy. Arch Neurol 1970; 23:193-200.

Chan DB, Lang MF, Fahn S. Idiopathic cervical dystonia. Mov Disord 1991; 6:119-26.

Chan-Palay V, Asan E. Alterations in catecholamine neurons of the locus coeruleus in senile dementia of the Alzheimer type and in Parkinson's disease with and without dementia and depression. Comp Neurol 1989; 287:373-92.

Chartier-Harlin M, Crawford F, Houlden H et al. Early-onset Alzheimer's disease caused by mutations at codon 717 of the beta-amyloid precursor protein gene. Nature 1991; 353:844-6.

Chee KY, Sachdev P. A controlled study of sensory tics in Gilles de la Tourette syndrome and obsessive-compulsive disorder using a structured interview. J Neurol Neurosurg Psychiatry 1997; 62:188-92.

Chelly J, Monaco AP. Cloning the Wilson disease gene. Nature Gen 1993; 5:317-18.

Chen J-Y, Stern Y, Sano M et al. Cumulative risk of developing extrapyramidal signs, psychosis or myoclonus in the course of Alzheimer's disease. Arch Neurol 1991; 48:1141-3.

Chouinard S, Ford B. Adult onset tic disorder. J Neurol Neurosurg Psychiatry 2000; 68:738-43.

Church AJ, Dale RC, Lees AJ et al. Tourette's syndrome: a cross-sectional study to examine the PANDAS hypothesis. J Neurol Neurosurg Psychiatry 2003; 74:602-7.

Clark CM, Ewbank D, Lerner A et al. The relationship between extrapyramidal signs and cognitive performance in patients with Alzheimer's disease enrolled in the CERAD study. Neurology 1997; 49:70-5.

Clark DG, Mendez MF, Farag E et al. Clinicopathologic report: progressive aphasia in a 77-year old man. J Neuropsychiatry Clin Neurosci 2003; 15:231-8.

Cohen AJ, Leckman JF. Sensory phenomena associated with Gilles de la Tourette's syndrome. J Clin Psychiatry 1992; 23: 319-23.

Cohen DJ, Detlor RN, Young G et al. Clonidine ameliorates Gilles de la Tourette's syndrome. Arch Gen Psychiatry 1980; 37:1350-7.

Cohen LG, Hallett M. Hand cramps: clinical features and electromyographic patterns in a focal dystonia. Neurology 1988; 38:1005-12.

Coleman LW, Digre KB, Stephenson GM et al. Autopsy-proven, sporadic Pick disease with onset at age 25 years. Arch Neurol 2002; 59:856-9.

Collins SJ, Ahlskog JE, Parisi JE et al. Progressive supranuclear palsy: neuropathologically based diagnostic clinical criteria. J Neurol Neurosurg Psychiatry 1995; 58:167-73.

Colosimo C, Albanese A, Hughes AJ et al. Some specific clinical features differentiate multiple system atrophy (striatonigral variety) from Parkinson's disease. Arch Neurol 1995; 52:294-8.

Comella CL, Goetz CG. Akathisia in Parkinson's disease. Mov Disord 1994; 9:545-9.

Connor GS. A double-blind placebo-controlled trial of topiramate treatment of essential tremor. Neurology 2002; 59:132-4.

Cook RH, Schenck SA, Clark DB. Twins with Alzheimer's disease. Arch Neurol 1981; 38:300-1.

Cooper GE, Rizzo M, Jones RD. Adult-onset Hallervorden-Spatz syndrome presenting as cortical dementia. Alzheimer Dis Assoc Disord 2000; 14:120-6.

Corder EH, Saunders EM, Strittmatter WJ et al. Gene dose of apolipoprotein II type 4 allele and the risk of Alzheimer's disease in late onset families. Science 1993; 261:921-3.

Critchley EMR, Clark DB, Wikler A. Acanthocytosis and neurological disorder without abetalipoproteinemia. Arch Neurol 1968; 18:134-40.

Critchley M. Observation on essential (heredofamilial) tremor. Brain 1949; 72:113-39.

Critchley M, Greenfield JG. Olivo-ponto-cerebellar atrophy. Brain 1948; 71:343-64.

Crystal HA, Grober E, Masur D. Preservation of musical memory in Alzheimer's disease. J Neurol Neurosurg Psychiatry 1989; 52:1415-16.

Crystal HA, Dixon DW, Lizardi JE et al. Antemortem diagnosis of diffuse Lewy body disease. Neurology 1990; 40:1523-8.

Cummings JL, Duchen LW. Kluver-Bucy syndrome in Pick disease: Clinical and pathologic correlations. Neurology 1981; 31:1415-22.

Cummings JL, Street J, Masterman D et al. Efficacy of olanzapine in the treatment of psychosis in dementia with Lewy bodies. Dement Geriatr Cogn Disord 2002; 13:67-73.

Cummings JL, Schneider E, Tariot PN et al. Behavioral effects of memantine in Alzheimer disease patients receiving donepezil treatment. Neurology 2006; 67:57-63.

Cunningham MA, Darby DG, Donnan GA. Controlled-release delivery of L-dopa associated with nonfatal hyperthermia, rigidity and autonomic dysfunction. *Neurology* 1991; **41**:942–3.

Daniel SE, de Bruin VMS, Lees AJ. The clinical and pathological spectrum of Steele–Richardson–Olszewski syndrome (progressive supranuclear palsy): a reappraisal. *Brain* 1995; **118**:759–70.

Dauer WT, Burke RE, Greene P *et al.* Current concepts on the clinical features, aetiology and management of idiopathic cervical dystonia. *Brain* 1998; **121**:547–60.

Davies RR, Hodges JR, Kril JJ *et al.* The pathological basis of semantic dementia. *Brain* 2005; **128**:1984–95.

Davis EJB, Borde M. Wilson's disease and catatonia. *Br J Psychiatry* 1993; **162**:256–9.

Davis PH, Bergeron C, McLachlan DR. Atypical presentation of progressive supranuclear palsy. *Ann Neurol* 1985; **17**: 337–43.

Day JW, Ricker K, Jacobsen JF *et al.* Myotonic dystrophy type 2. Molecular diagnostic and clinical spectrum. *Neurology* 2003; **60**:657–64.

Deakin JB, Rahman S, Nestor PJ *et al.* Paroxetine does not improve symptoms and impairs cognition in frontotemporal dementia: a double-blind randomized controlled trial. *Psychopharmacology* 2004; **172**:400–8.

Deep Brain Stimulation for Parkinson's Disease Study Group. Deep brain stimulation of the subthalamic nucleus or the pars interna of the globus pallidus in Parkinson's disease. *N Engl J Med* 2001; **345**:956–63.

Defazio G, Berardelli A, Abbruzzese G *et al.* Risk factors for spread of primary adult onset blepharospasm: a multicentre investigation of the Italian movement disorders study group. *J Neurol Neurosurg Psychiatry* 1999; **67**:613–19.

Defazio G, Martino D, Aniello MS *et al.* A family study on primary blepharospasm. *J Neurol Neurosurg Psychiatry* 2006; **77**:252–4.

Delacourte A, David JP, Sergeant N *et al.* The biochemical pathway of neurofibrillary degeneration in aging and Alzheimer's disease. *Neurology* 1999; **52**:1158–65.

Delaporte C. Personality patterns in patients with myotonic dystrophy. *Arch Neurol* 1998; **55**:635–40.

Delwaide PJ, Desseilles M. Spontaneous buccolinguofacial dyskinesia in the elderly. *Acta Neurol Scand* 1977; **56**:256–62.

Demirkiran M, Jankovic J, Lewis RA *et al.* Neurologic presentation of Wilson disease without Kayser–Fleischer rings. *Neurology* 1996; **46**:1040–3.

Denckla MB, Bemporad JR, MacKay MC. Tics following methylphenidate administration: a report of 20 cases. *JAMA* 1976; **235**:1349–51.

Dening TR, Berrios GE, Walshe JM. Wilson's disease and epilepsy. *Brain* 1988; **111**:1139–55.

Dening TR, Berrios GE. Wilson's disease: psychiatric symptoms in 195 cases. *Arch Gen Psychiatry* 1989; **46**:1126–34.

Deonna T. DOPA-sensitive progressive dystonia of childhood with fluctuations of symptoms – Segawa's syndrome and possible variants. *Neuropediatrics* 1986; **17**:81–6.

Deonna T, Roulet E, Ghika J *et al.* Dopa-responsive childhood dystonia: a forme fruste with writer's cramp, triggered by exercise. *Dev Med Child Neurol* 1997; **39**:49–53.

Dermaut B, Kumar-Singh S, Engelborghs S *et al.* A novel presenilin 1 mutation associated with Pick's disease but not beta-amyloid plaques. *Ann Neurol* 2004; **55**:617–26.

De Stefano N, Dotti MT, Mortilla M *et al.* Magnetic resonance imaging and spectroscopic changes in brains of patients with cerebrotendinous xanthomatosis. *Brain* 2001; **124**:121–3.

Devanand DP, Jacobs DM, Tang M-X *et al.* The course of psychopathologic features in mild to moderate Alzheimer's disease. *Arch Gen Psychiatry* 1997; **54**:257–63.

Deymeer F, Smith TW, DeGirolami U *et al.* Thalamic dementia and motor neuron disease. *Neurology* 1989; **39**:58–61.

Di Costanzo A, De Salle F, Santoro L *et al.* Pattern and significance of white matter abnormalities in myotonic dystrophy type 1: an MRI study. *J Neurol* 2002; **249**:1175–82.

Didic M, Cherif AA, Gambarelli D *et al.* A permanent pure amnestic syndrome of insidious onset related to Alzheimer's disease. *Ann Neurol* 1998; **43**:526–30.

van Diggelen OP, Thobois S, Tilikete C *et al.* Adult neuronal ceroid lipofuscinosis with palmitoyl-protein thioesterase deficiency: first adult-onset patients of a childhood disease. *Ann Neurol* 2001; **50**:269–72.

Dion Y, Annable L, Stat D *et al.* Risperidone in the treatment of Tourette syndrome: a double-blind, placebo-controlled trial. *J Clin Psychopharmacol* 2002; **22**:31–9.

Dipple HC. The use of olanzapine for movement disorder in Huntington's disease: a first case report. *J Neurol Neurosurg Psychiatry* 1999; **67**:123–4.

Dodd CM, Klos KS, Bower JH *et al.* Pathological gambling caused by drugs used to treat Parkinson disease. *Arch Neurol* 2005; **62**:1377–81.

Dooley JM, Andermann F. Startle disease or hyperekplexia: adolescent onset and response to valproate. *Ped Neurology* 1989; **5**:126–7.

Dooling EC, Schoene WC, Richardson EP. Hallervorden–Spatz syndrome. *Arch Neurol* 1974; **30**:70–83.

Dooling EC, Richardson EP, Davis KR. Computed tomography in Hallervorden–Spatz disease. *Neurology* 1980; **30**: 1128–30.

Doran M, Larner AJ. EEG findings in dementia with Lewy bodies causing diagnostic confusion with sporadic Creutzfeldt-Jakob disease. *Eur J Neurol* 2004; **11**:838–41.

Douyon R, Serby M, Klutchbo B *et al.* ECT and Parkinson's disease revisited: a 'naturalistic' study *Am J Psychiatry* 1989; **146**:1451–5.

Duenas AM, Goold R, Giunti P. Molecular pathogenesis of spinocerebellar ataxias. *Brain* 2006; **129**:1357–70.

Durif F, Debilly B, Galitzky M *et al.* Clozapine improves dyskinesias in Parkinson disease. A double-blind, placebo-controlled study. *Neurology* 2004; **62**:381–8.

Durr A, Stevanin G, Cancel G *et al.* Spinocerebellar ataxia 3 and Machado–Joseph disease: clinical, molecular, and neuropathological features. *Ann Neurol* 1996; **39**:490–9.

Eapen V, Pauls DL, Robertson MM. Evidence for autosomal dominant transmission in Tourette's syndrome – United Kingdom cohort study. *Br J Psychiatry* 1993; **162**:593–6.

Edwards KR, Hershel L, Wray L *et al.* Efficacy and safety of galantamine in patients with dementia with Lewy bodies: a

12-week interim analysis. *Dement Geriatr Cogn Disord* 2004; **17**(suppl. 1):40–8.

Edwards-Lee T, Miller BL, Benson DF *et al*. The temporal variant of frontotemporal dementia. *Brain* 1997; **120**:1027–40.

Ellis T, Cudkowicz ME, Sexton PM *et al*. Clozapine and risperidone treatment of psychosis in Parkinson's disease. *J Neuropsychiatry Clin Neurosci* 2000; **12**:364–9.

Emre M, Aarsland D, Albanese A *et al*. Rivastigmine for dementia associated with Parkinson's disease. *N Engl J Med* 2004; **351**:2509–18.

Erlington GM, Bateman DE, Jeffrey MJ *et al*. Adrenoleukodystrophy: heterogeneity in two brothers. *J Neurol Neurosurg Psychiatry* 1989; **52**:310–14.

Evans AH, Katzenshlager R, Paviour D *et al*. Punding in Parkinson's disease: its relation to the dopamine dysregulation syndrome. *Mov Disord* 2004; **19**:367–70.

Evenhuius HM. The natural history of dementia in Down's syndrome. *Arch Neurol* 1990; **47**:263–7.

Faber-Langendoen K, Morris JC, Knesvich JW *et al*. Aphasia in senile dementia of the Alzheimer type. *Ann Neurol* 1988; **23**:365–70.

Faden AI, Townsend JJ. Myoclonus in Alzheimer's disease: a confusing sign. *Arch Neurol* 1976; **33**:278–80.

Farpour H, Mahloudji M. Familial cerebrotendinous xanthomatosis: report of a new family and review of the literature. *Arch Neurol* 1975; **32**:223–5.

Farrer M, Chan P, Chen R *et al*. Lewy bodies and parkinsonism in families with parkin mutation. *Ann Neurol* 2001; **50**:293–300.

Feany MB. New genetic insights in Parkinson's disease. *N Engl J Med* 2004; **351**:1937–40.

Feigin A, Kieburtz K, Bordwell K *et al*. Functional decline in Huntington's disease. *Mov Disord* 1995; **10**:211–14.

Feinberg TE, Cianci CD, Morrow JS *et al*. Diagnostic tests for choreoacanthocytosis. *Neurology* 1991; **41**:1000–6.

Feldman H, Gauthier S, Heker J *et al*. A 24-week, randomized, double-blind study of donepezil in moderate to severe Alzheimer's disease. *Neurology* 2001; **57**:613–20.

Fenelon G, Mahieux F, Huon R *et al*. Hallucinations in Parkinson's disease: prevalence, phenomenology and risk factors. *Brain* 2000; **123**:733–45.

Fernandez HH, Friedman JH, Jacques C *et al*. Quetiapine for the treatment of drug-induced psychosis in Parkinson's disease. *Mov Disord* 1999; **14**:484–7.

Fernandez HH, Trieschmann ME, Burke MA *et al*. Quetiapine for psychosis in Parkinson's disease versus dementia with Lewy bodies. *J Clin Psychiatry* 2002; **63**:513–15.

Fernandez M, Raskind W, Matsushita M *et al*. Hereditary benign chorea: clinical and genetic features of a distinct disease. *Neurology* 2001; **57**:106–10.

Ferraro A, Jervis GA. Pick's disease: clinicopathologic study with report of two cases. *Arch Neurol Psychiatry* 1936; **36**:738–67.

Ferreira JJ, Galitzky M, Montrastruc JL *et al*. Sleep attacks and Parkinson's disease treatment. *Lancet* 2000; **355**:1333–4.

Figa-Talamanca L, Gualandi C, Di Meo L *et al*. Hyperthermia after discontinuance of levodopa and bromocriptine therapy: impaired dopamine receptors a possible cause. *Neurology* 1985; **35**:258–61.

Finelli PF. Metachromatic leukodystrophy manifesting as a schizophrenic disorder: computed tomographic correlation. *Ann Neurol* 1985; **18**:94–5.

Fletcher NA, Harding AE, Marsden CD. A genetic study of idiopathic torsion dystonia in the United Kingdom. *Brain* 1990; **113**:379–95.

Folstein SE, Abbott MH, Chase GA *et al*. The association of affective disorder with Huntington's disease in a case series and in families. *Psychol Med* 1983; **13**:537–42.

Forstl H, Besthorn C, Geiger-Kabisch C *et al*. Psychotic features and the course of Alzheimer's disease: relationship to cognitive, electroencephalographic and computerized tomography findings. *Acta Psychiatr Scand* 1993; **87**:395–9.

Frankel M, Cummings JL, Robertson MM *et al*. Obsessions and compulsions in Gilles de la Tourette's syndrome. *Neurology* 1986; **36**:378–82.

Fregni F, Santos CM, Myczkowski ML *et al*. Repetitive transcranial magnetic stimulation is as effective as fluoxetine in the treatment of depression in patients with Parkinson's disease. *J Neurol Neurosurg Psychiatry* 2004; **75**:1171–4.

Friedman A, Fahn S. Spontaneous remissions in spasmodic torticollis. *Neurology* 1986; **36**:398–400.

Friedman A, Sienkiewicz J. Psychotic complications of long-term levodopa treatment of Parkinson's disease. *Acta Neurol Scand* 1991; **84**:111–13.

Freiss E, Kuempfel T, Modell S *et al*. Paroxetine treatment improves motor symptoms in patients with multiple system atrophy. *Parkinsonism Relat Disord* 2006; **12**:432–7.

Frucht S, Rogers JD, Greene PE *et al*. Falling asleep at the wheel: motor vehicle mishaps in persons taking pramipexole and ropinirole. *Neurology* 1999; **52**:1908–10.

Frucht SJ, Fahn S, Greene PE *et al*. The natural history of embouchure dystonia. *Mov Disord* 2001; **16**:899–906.

Fukui T, Sugita K, Kawamura M *et al*. Primary progressive apraxia in Pick's disease: a clinicopathologic report. *Neurology* 1996; **47**:467–73.

Funayama M, Hasegawa K, Kowa H *et al*. A new locus for Parkinson's disease (*PARK8*) maps to chromosome 12p11.2-q13.1. *Ann Neurol* 2002; **51**:296–301.

Furukawa Y, Graf WD, Wong H *et al*. Dopa-responsive dystonia simulating spastic paraplegia due to tyrosine hydroxylase (TH) gene mutation *Neurology* 2001; **56**:260–3.

Gadow KD, Nolan EE, Sverd J. Methylphenidate in hyperactive boys with comorbid tic disorder. II: Short-term behavioral effects in school settings. *J Am Acad Child Adolesc Psychiatry* 1992; **31**:462–71.

Gadow KD, Sverd J, Sprafkin J *et al*. Long-term methylphenidate therapy in children with comorbid attention-deficit hyperactivity disorder and chronic multiple tic disorder. *Arch Gen Psychiatry* 1999; **56**:330–6.

Gagnon J-F, Bedard M-A, Fantini MC *et al*. REM sleep behavior disorder and REM sleep without atonia in Parkinson's disease. *Neurology* 2002; **59**:585–9.

Gaig C, Marti MJ, Ezquerra M *et al*. G2019S *LRRK2* mutation causing Parkinson's disease without Lewy bodies. *J Neurol Neurosurg Psychiatry* 2007; **78**:626–8.

Galasko D, Chang I, Motter I et al. High cerebrospinal fluid tau and low amyloid beta-42 levels in the clinical diagnosis of Alzheimer disease and relation to apolipoprotein E genotype. Arch Neurol 1998; 55:937–45.

Gallagher JP. Pathologic laughter and crying in ALS: a search for their origin. Acta Neurol Scand 1989; 80:114–17.

Galton CJ, Patterson K, Xuereb JH et al. Atypical and typical presentations of Alzheimer's disease: a clinical, neuropsychological, neuroimaging and pathological study of 13 cases. Brain 2000; 123:484–98.

Galvin JE, Lee SL, Perry A et al. Familial dementia with Lewy bodies: clinicopathologic analysis of two kindreds. Neurology 2002; 59:1079–82.

Garcia Ruiz PJ, Gomez-Tortosa E, del Barrio A et al. Senile chorea: a multicenter prospective study. Acta Neurol Scand 1997; 95:180–3.

Garruto RM, Gajdusek DC, Chen KM. Amyotrophic lateral sclerosis and parkinsonism-dementia among Filipino immigrants to Guam. Ann Neurol 1981; 10:341–50.

Gasser T, Windgassen K, Bereznai B et al. Phenotypic expression of the DYT1 mutation: a family with writer's cramp of juvenile onset. Ann Neurol 1998; 44:126–8.

Gatz M, Pedersen NL, Berg S et al. Heritability for Alzheimer's disease: the study of dementia in Swedish twins. J Gerontol A Biol Sci Med Sci 1997; 52:17–25.

Geda YE, Boeve BF, Negash S et al. Neuropsychiatric features in 36 pathologically confirmed cases of corticobasal degeneration. J Neuropsychiatry Clin Neurosci 2007; 19:77–80.

van Geel BM, Assies J, Haverkort EB et al. Progression of abnormalities in adrenomyeloneuropathy and neurologically asymptomatic X-linked adrenoleukodystrophy despite treatment with 'Lorenzo's oil'. J Neurol Neurosurg Psychiatry 1999; 67:290–9.

van Geel BM, Bezman L, Loes DJ et al. Evolution of phenotypes in adult male patients with X-linked adrenoleukodystrophy. Ann Neurol 2001; 49:186–94.

Gibb WRG, Esiri MM, Lees AJ. Clinical and pathological features of diffuse cortical Lewy body disease (Lewy body dementia). Brain 1987; 110:1131–53.

Gibb WR, Lees AJ, Marsden CD. Pathological report of four patients presenting with cranial dystonia. Mov Disord 1988; 3:211–21.

Gibb WR, Luthert PJ, Marsden CD. Corticobasal degeneration. A clinical study of 36 cases. Brain 1994; 117:1183–96.

Giladi N, McMahon D, Przedborski S et al. Motor blocks in Parkinson's disease. Neurology 1992; 42:333–9.

Gilbert DL, Dure L, Sethuraman G et al. Tic reduction with pergolide in a randomized controlled trial in children. Neurology 2003; 60:606–11.

Gilbert GJ. Brueghel syndrome: its distinction from Meige syndrome. Neurology 1996; 46:1767–9.

Gillespie J, Jackson A. MRI and CT of the brain. London: Arnold, 2000.

Giovannoni G, O'Sullivan JD, Turner K et al. Hedonistic homeostatic dysregulation in patients with Parkinson's disease on dopamine replacement therapies. J Neurol Neurosurg Psychiatry 2000; 68:423–8.

Gironell A, Kulisevsky J, Barbanoj M et al. A randomized, placebo-controlled comparative trial of gabapentin and propranolol in essential tremor. Arch Neurol 1999; 56:475–80.

Giunti P, Sabbadini G, Sweeney MG et al. The role of the SCA2 trinucleotide repeat expansion in 89 autosomal dominant cerebellar ataxia families: frequency, clinical and genetic correlates. Brain 1998; 121:459–67.

Glass JD, Reich SG, DeLong MR. Wilson's disease: development of neurological disease after beginning penicillamine therapy. Arch Neurol 1990; 47:595–6.

Goetz CG, Blasucci LM, Leurgans S et al. Olanzapine and clozapine. Comparative effects on motor function in hallucinating PD patients. Neurology 2000; 55:789–94.

Goetz CG, Wuu J, Curgian LM et al. Hallucinations and sleep disorders in PD. Six-year prospective longitudinal study. Neurology 2005; 64:81–6.

Goetz CG, Fan W, Leurgans S et al. The malignant course of 'benign hallucinations' in Parkinson disease. Arch Neurol 2006; 63:713–6.

Golbe L, Davis P, Schoenberg B et al. Prevalence and natural history of progressive supranuclear palsy. Neurology 1988; 38:1031–4.

Golden GS. Tics and Tourette's: a continuum of symptoms? Ann Neurol 1978; 4:145–8.

Goldfarb LG, Chumakov MP, Petrov PA et al. Olivopontocerebellar atrophy in a large Iakut kinship in Eastern Siberia. Neurology 1989; 39:1527–30.

Goldfarb LG, Vasconcelos O, Platonov FA et al. Unstable triplet repeat and phenotypic variability of spinocerebellar ataxia type I. Ann Neurol 1996; 39:500–16.

Gomez-Tortosa E, Newell K, Irizarry MC et al. Clinical and quantitative pathologic correlates of dementia with Lewy bodies. Neurology 1999; 53:1284–91.

Goodman L. Alzheimer's disease: a clinico-pathologic analysis of twenty-three cases with a theory on pathogenesis. J Nerv Ment Dis 1953; 118:97–130.

Goto I, Tobimatsu S, Ohta M et al. Dentatorubropallidoluysian degeneration: clinical, neuro-ophthalmologic, biochemical and pathologic studies on autosomal dominant form. Neurology 1982; 32:1395–9.

Graff-Radford NR, Damasio AR, Hyman BT et al. Progressive aphasia in a patient with Pick's disease: a neuropsychological, radiologic, and anatomic study. Neurology 1990; 40:620–6.

Graham A, Davies R, Xuereb J et al. Pathologically proven frontotemporal dementia presenting with severe amnesia. Brain 2005; 128:597–605.

Graham DI, Lantos PL. Greenfield's neuropathology, 6th edn. London: Arnold, 1996.

Graham JM, Grunewald RA, Sagar HJ. Hallucinosis in idiopathic Parkinson's disease. J Neurol Neurosurg Psychiatry 1997; 63:434–40.

Grandas F, Elston J, Quinn N et al. Blepharospasm: a review of 264 patients. J Neurol Neurosurg Psychiatry 1988; 51:767–72.

Greco CM, Hagerman RJ, Tassone F et al. Neuronal intranuclear inclusions in a new cerebellar tremor/ataxia syndrome among fragile X carriers. Brain 2002; 125:1760–71.

Greco CM, Berman RF, Martin RM et al. Neuropathology of fragile X-associated tremor/ataxia syndrome. Brain 2006; 129:243–55.

Green J, Morris JC, Sandson J et al. Progressive aphasia: a precursor of global dementia? Neurology 1990; 48:423–9.

Greenberg SM, Tennis MK, Brown LB et al. Donepezil therapy in clinical practice. A randomized crossover study. Arch Neurol 2000; 57:94–9.

Greene JDW, Patterson K, Xuereb J et al. Alzheimer disease and nonfluent progressive aphasia. Arch Neurol 1996; 53: 1072–8.

Greene P, Kang U, Fahn S et al. Double-blind, placebo controlled trial of botulinum toxin injection for the treatment of spasmodic torticollis. Neurology 1990; 40:1213–18.

Grewal RP, Achari M, Matsura T et al. Clinical features and ATTCT repeat expansion in spinocerebellar ataxia type 10. Arch Neurol 2002; 59:1285–90.

Griffin JW, Goren E, Schaumburg H et al. Adrenomyeloneuropathy: a probable variant of adrenoleukodystrophy. Neurology 1977; 27:1107–10.

Grimes DA, Lang AE, Bergeron CB. Dementia as the most common presentation of cortical-basal ganglionic degeneration. Neurology 1999; 53:1969–74.

Groen JJ, Endtz LJ. Hereditary Pick's disease: second re-examination of a large family and discussion of other hereditary cases with particular reference to electroencephalography and computerized tomography. Brain 1982; 105:443–59.

Grotzch H, Pizzolato G-P, Ghika J et al. Neuropathology of a case of dopa-responsive dystonia associated with a new genetic locus, DYT14. Neurology 2002; 58:1839–42.

Growdon JH, Shahani BT, Young RR. The effect of alcohol on essential tremor. Neurology 1975; 25:259–62.

Gunal DI, Afsar N, Bekiroglu N et al. New alternative agents in essential tremor therapy: double-blind placebo-controlled study of alprazolam and acetazolamide. Neurol Sci 2000; 21:315–17.

Guttman M, International Pramipexole–Bromocriptine Study Group. Double-blind comparison of pramipexole and bromocriptine treatment with placebo in advanced Parkinson's disease. Neurology 1997; 49:1060–5.

Gysin WM, Cooke ET. Unusual mental symptoms in a case of hepatolenticular degeneration. Dis Nerv Syst 1950; 11: 305–9.

Haber SN, Kowall NW, Vonsattel JP et al. Gilles de la Tourette's syndrome. A postmortem neuropathological and immunohistochemical study. J Neurol Sci 1986; 75:225–41.

Hageman ATM, Gabreels FJM, de Jong JGN et al. Clinical symptoms of adult metachromatic leukodystrophy and arylsulfatase A pseudodeficiency. Arch Neurol 1995; 52:408–13.

Hagerman RJ, Leehey M, Heinrichs W et al. Intention tremor, parkinsonism, and generalized brain atrophy in male carriers of fragile X. Neurology 2001; 57:127–30.

Hagerman RJ, Leavitt BR, Farzin F et al. Fragile X-associated tremor/ataxia syndrome (FXTAS) in females with the FMR1 premutation. Am J Hum Genet 2004; 74:1051–6.

Hahn H, Trant MR, Brownstein MJ et al. Neurologic and psychiatric manifestations in a family with a mutation in exon 2 of the guanosine triphosphate-cyclohydrolase gene. Arch Neurol 2001; 58:749–55.

Hall DA, Berry-Kravis E, Jacquemont S et al. Initial diagnosis given to persons with the fragile X associated tremor/ataxia syndrome (FXTAS). Neurology 2005; 65:294–301.

Haltia T, Palo J, Haltia M et al. Juvenile metachromatic leukodystrophy: clinical, biochemical, and neuropathologic studies in nine new cases. Arch Neurol 1980; 37:42–6.

Hampel H, Buerger K, Zinkowski R et al. Measurement of phosphorylated tau epitopes in the differential diagnosis of Alzheimer disease: a comparative cerebrospinal fluid study. Arch Gen Psychiatry 2004; 61:95–102.

Hansen L, Salmon D, Galasko D et al. The Lewy body variant of Alzheimer's disease: a clinical and pathologic entity. Neurology 1990; 40:1–8.

Hansotia P, Frens D. Hypersomnia associated with alveolar hypo-ventilation in myotonic dystrophy. Neurology 1981; 31:1336–7.

Hansotia P, Cleeland CS, Chun RWM. Juvenile Huntington's chorea. Neurology 1968; 18:217–24.

Hantz P, Caradoc-Davies G, Caradoc-Davies T et al. Depression in Parkinson's disease. Am J Psychiatry 1994; 151:1010–14.

Hardie RJ, Pullon HWH, Harding AE et al. Neuroacanthocytosis: a clinical, haematological and pathological study of 19 cases. Brain 1991; 114:13–49.

Harding A. The clinical features and classification of the late onset autosomal dominant cerebellar ataxias: a study of eleven families including descendants of the 'Drew family of Walworth'. Brain 1982; 105:1–28.

Harding AE. The hereditary ataxias and related disorders. London: Churchill Livingstone, 1984.

Harding AE, Thomas PK, Baraitser M et al. X-linked recessive bulbo-spinal neuropathy: a report of ten cases. J Neurol Neurosurg Psychiatry 1982; 45:1012–19.

Harding AJ, Stimson E, Hernderson JM et al. Clinical correlates of selective pathology in the amygdala of patients with Parkinson's disease. Brain 2002a; 125:2431–45.

Harding AJ, Broe GA, Halliday GM. Visual hallucinations in Lewy body disease related to Lewy bodies in the temporal lobe. Brain 2002b; 125:391–403.

Harper PS, Harley HG, Reardon W et al. Anticipation in myotonic dystrophy: new light on an old problem. Am J Human Genet 1992; 51:10–16.

Harsch HH. Neuroleptic malignant syndrome: physiological and laboratory findings in a series of nine cases. J Clin Psychiatry 1987; 48:328–33.

Hartig MB, Hortnagel K, Garavaglia B et al. Genotypic and phenotypic spectrum of PANK2 mutations in patients with neurodegeneration with brain iron accumulation. Ann Neurol 2006; 59:248–56.

Harwood G, Hierons R, Fletcher NA et al. Lessons from a remarkable family with dopa-responsive dystonia. J Neurol Neurosurg Psychiatry 1994; 57:460–3.

Hauser RA, Gauger L, McDowell Anderson W et al. Pramipexole-induced somnolence and episodes of daytime sleep. Mov Disord 2000; 15:658–63.

Hayflick SJ, Penzien JM, Michl W et al. Cranial MRI changes may preceded symptoms in Hallervorden-Spatz syndrome. Pediatr Neurol 2001; 25:166-9.

Hayflick SJ, Westaway SK, Levinson B et al. Genetic, clinical, and radiographic delineation of Hallervorden-Spatz syndrome. N Engl J Med 2003; 348:33-40.

Hely MA, Reid WGJ, Halliday GM et al. Diffuse Lewy body disease: clinical features in nine cases without coexistent Alzheimer's disease. J Neurol Neurosurg Psychiatry 1996; 60:531-8.

Henderson JM, Carpenter K, Cartwright H et al. Loss of thalamic and intralaminar nuclei in progressive supranuclear palsy and Parkinson's disease: clinical and therapeutic implications. Brain 2000; 123:1410-21.

Heston LL, White JA, Mastri AR. Pick's disease. Clinical genetics and natural history. Arch Gen Psychiatry 1987; 44:409-11.

Heutink P, Stevens M, Rizzu P et al. Hereditary frontotemporal dementia is linked to chromosome 17q21-q22: a genetic and clinicopathological study of three Dutch families. Ann Neurol 1997; 41:150-9.

Higgins JJ, Adler RI, Loveless JM. Mutational analysis of the tau gene in progressive supranuclear palsy. Neurology 1999; 53:1421-4.

Hillen ME, Sage JI. Nonmotor fluctuations in patients with Parkinson's disease. Neurology 1996; 47:1180-3.

Hipola D, Mateo D, Gimenez-Roldan S. Meige's syndrome: acute and chronic responses to clonazepam and anticholinergics. Eur Neurol 1984; 23:474-8.

Hirano A, Arumugasamy N, Zimmerman HM. Amyotrophic lateral sclerosis: a comparison of Guam and classical cases. Arch Neurol 1967; 16:357-63.

Hirono N, Mori E, Yasuda M et al. Factors associated with psychotic symptoms in Alzheimer's disease. J Neurol Neurosurg Psychiatry 1998; 64:648-52.

Hirose G, Bass NH. Metachromatic leukodystrophy in the adult: a biochemical study. Neurology 1972; 22:312-20.

Hoehn MM, Yahr MD. Parkinsonism: onset, progression and mortality. Neurology 1967; 17:427-42.

Holroyd S, Currie L, Wooten GF. Prospective study of hallucinations and delusions in Parkinson's disease. J Neurol Neurosurg Psychiatry 2001; 70:734-8.

Hoogendijk WJG, Sommer IEC, Pool C et al. Lack of association between depression and loss of neurons in the locus coeruleus in Alzheimer disease. Arch Gen Psychiatry 1999; 56:45-51.

Hoogenraad TU, Van Hattum J, Van den Hamer CJA. Management of Wilson's disease with zinc sulphate: experience in a series of 27 patients. J Neurol Sci 1987; 77:137-46.

Horimoto Y, Matsumoto M, Akatsu H et al. Autonomic dysfunction in dementia with Lewy bodies. J Neurol 2003; 250:530-3.

Houser M, Waltz T. Meige syndrome and pallidal deep brain stimulation. Mov Disord 2005; 20:1203-5.

Howard CP, Royce CE. Progressive lenticular degeneration associated with cirrhosis of the liver (Wilson's disease). Arch Int Med 1919; 24:497-508.

Howeler CJ, Busch HF, Geraedts JP et al. Anticipation in myotonic dystrophy: fact or fiction? Brain 1989; 112:779-97.

Hsieh M, Li S-Y, Tsai C-J et al. Identification of five spinocerebellar ataxia type 2 pedigrees in patients with autosomal dominant cerebellar ataxia in Taiwan. Acta Neurol Scand 1999; 100:189-98.

Huber SJ, Kissel JT, Shuttleworth EC et al. Magnetic resonance imaging and clinical correlates of intellectual impairment in myotonic dystrophy. Arch Neurol 1989; 46:536-40.

Huff FJ, Boller J, Luchelli F et al. The neurologic examination in patients with probable Alzheimer's disease. Arch Neurol 1987; 44:929-32.

Hughes AJ, Daniel SE, Blankson S et al. A clinicopathologic study of 100 cases of Parkinson's disease. Arch Neurol 1993; 50:140-8.

Hung SW, Hamani C, Lozano AM et al. Long-term outcome of bilateral pallidal deep brain stimulation for primary cervical dystonia. Neurology 2007; 68:4579-9.

Huntington G. On chorea. Med Surg Reporter Philadelphia 1872; 26:317-21.

Huntington Study Group. Tetrabenazine as antichorea therapy in Huntington disease: a randomized controlled trial. Neurology 2006; 66:366-72.

Hurtig HI, Trojanowski JQ, Galvin J et al. Alpha-synuclein cortical Lewy bodies correlate with dementia in Parkinson's disease. Neurology 2000; 54:1916-21.

Hussain IF, Brady CM, Swinn MJ et al. Treatment of erectile dysfunction with sildenafil citrate (Viagra) in parkinsonism due to Parkinson's disease or multiple system atrophy. J Neurol Neurosurg Psychiatry 2001; 71:371-4.

Hutton JT, Koller WC, Ahlskog JE et al. Multicenter, placebo-controlled trial of cabergoline taken once daily in the treatment of Parkinson's disease. Neurology 1996; 46:1062-5.

Hyde TM, Ziegler JC, Weinberger DR. Psychiatric disturbances in metachromatic leukodystrophy: insights into the neurobiology of psychosis. Arch Neurol 1992; 49:401-6.

Hyde TM, Stacey ME, Coppoa R et al. Cerebral morphometric abnormalities in Tourette's syndrome: a quantitative MRI study of monozygotic twins. Neurology 1995; 45:1176-82.

Iizuka R, Hirayama K, Maehara KA. Dentato-rubro-pallido-luysian atrophy: a clinico-pathological study. J Neurol Neurosurg Psychiatry 1984; 47:1288-98.

Ikeda K, Akiyama H, Iritani S et al. Corticobasal degeneration with primary progressive aphasia and accentuated cortical lesion in superior temporal gyrus: case report and review. Acta Neuropath 1996; 92:534-9.

Ikeda Y, Shizuka M, Watanabe M et al. Molecular and clinical analysis of spinocerebellar ataxia type 8 in Japan. Neurology 2000; 54:950-5.

Ikeuchi T, Takano H, Koide R et al. Spinocerebellar ataxia type 6: CAG repeat expansion in alpha1a voltage-dependent calcium channel gene and clinical variations in Japanese population. Ann Neurol 1997; 42:879-84.

Illarioshkin SN, Markova ED, Slominsky PA et al. The GTP cyclohydrolase I gene in Russian families with dopa-responsive dystonia. Arch Neurol 1998; 55:789-92.

in t' Veld BA, Ruitenberg A, Hofman A et al. Nonsteroidal antiinflammatory drugs and the risk of Alzheimer's disease. N Engl J Med 2001; 345:1515-21.

International Huntington Association, World Federation of Neurology Research Group on Huntington's Chorea. Guidelines for the molecular genetics predictive test in Huntington's disease. *Neurology* 1994; **44**:1533–6.

International Myotonic Dystrophy Consortium. New nomenclature and DNA testing guidelines for myotonic dystrophy type 1 (DM1). *Neurology* 2000; **54**:1218–21.

Inzelberg R, Nisipeanu P, Rabey JM *et al.* Double-blind comparison of cabergoline and bromocriptine in Parkinson's disease patients with motor fluctuations. *Neurology* 1996; **47**:785–8.

Inzelberg R, Kipervasser S, Korczyn AD. Auditory hallucinations in Parkinson's disease. *J Neurol Neurosurg Psychiatry* 1998; **64**:533–5.

Iranzo A, Santamaria J, Rye DB *et al.* Characteristics of idiopathic REM sleep behavior disorder and that associated with MSA and PD. *Neurology* 2005; **65**:247–52.

Ironside R. Disorders of laughter due to brain lesions. *Brain* 1956; **79**:589–609.

Ishikawa K, Watanabe M, Yoshizawa K *et al.* Clinical, neuropathological, and molecular study in two families with spinocerebellar ataxia type 6 (SCA6). *J Neurol Neurosurg Psychiatry* 1999; **67**:86–9.

Jabusch HC, Zschucke D, Schmidt A *et al.* Focal dystonia in musicians: treatment strategies and long-term outcome in 144 patients. *Mov Disord* 2005; **20**:1623–6.

Jacquemont S, Hagerman RJ, Leehey MA *et al.* Penetrance of fragile X-associated tremor/ataxia syndrome in a premutation carrier population. *JAMA* 2004; **291**:460–9.

Jagust WJ, Davies P, Tiller-Borcich JK *et al.* Focal Alzheimer's disease. *Neurology* 1990; **90**:14–19.

Jahanshahi M. Factors that ameliorate or aggravate spasmodic torticollis. *J Neurol Neurosurg Psychiatry* 2000; **68**:227–9.

Jankovic J. Blepharospasm with basal ganglia lesions. *Arch Neurol* 1986; **43**:866–8.

Jankovic J, Patel S. Blepharospasm associated with brainstem lesions. *Neurology* 1983; **33**:1237–40.

Jankovic J, Kirkpatrick JB, Blomquist KA *et al.* Late-onset Hallervorden–Spatz disease presenting as familial parkinsonism. *Neurology* 1985; **35**:227–34.

Jankovic J, Leder S, Warner D *et al.* Cervical dystonia: clinical findings and associated movement disorders. *Neurology* 1991; **41**:1088–91.

Jankovic J, Watts RL, Martin W *et al.* Transdermal rotigotine. Double-blind, placebo-controlled trial in Parkinson's disease. *Arch Neurol* 2007; **64**:676–82.

Janssen JC, Lantos PL, Al-Sarraj S *et al.* Thalamic degeneration with negative prion protein immunostaining. *J Neurol* 2000; **247**:48–51.

Janssen JC, Warrington EK, Morris HR *et al.* Clinical features of frontotemporal dementia due to the intronic *tau* 10 + 16 mutation. *Neurology* 2002; **58**:1161–8.

Janssen JC, Beck JA, Campbell TA *et al.* Early onset familial Alzheimer's disease. Mutation frequency in 31 families. *Neurology* 2003; **60**:235–9.

Jayne D, Lees AJ, Stern GM. Remission in spasmodic torticollis. *J Neurol Neurosurg Psychiatry* 1984; **47**:1236–7.

Jedynak PC, Trenchant C, de Beyl DZ. Prospective clinical study of writer's cramp. *Mov Disord* 2001; **16**:494–9.

Jervis GA. Early senile dementia in mongoloid idiocy. *Am J Psychiatry* 1948; **105**:102–6.

Jervis GA. Huntington's chorea in childhood. *Arch Neurol* 1979; **23**:83–93.

Jobsis GJ, Weber JW, Barth PG *et al.* Autosomal dominant cerebellar ataxia with retinal degeneration (ADCA II): clinical and neuropathological findings in two pedigrees and genetic linkage to 3p12–p21.1. *J Neurol Neurosurg Psychiatry* 1997; **62**:367–71.

Johnson W, Schwartz G, Barbeau A. Studies on dystonia musculorum deformans. *Arch Neurol* 1962; **7**:301–13.

Josephs KA, Parisi JE, Knopman DS *et al.* Clinically undetected motor neuron disease in pathologically proven frontotemporal lobar degeneration with motor neuron disease. *Arch Neurol* 2006; **63**:506–12.

Karbe H, Kertesz A, Polk M. Profiles of language impairment in primary progressive aphasia. *Arch Neurol* 1993; **50**:192–201.

Karp BI, Hallett M. Extracorporeal 'phantom' tics in Tourette's syndrome. *Neurology* 1996; **46**:38–40.

Kartsounis LD, Hardie RJ. The pattern of cognitive impairments in neuroacanthocytosis: a frontosubcortical dementia. *Arch Neurol* 1996; **53**:77–80.

Kaseda Y, Kawakami H, Matsuyama Z *et al.* Spinocerebellar ataxia type 6 in relation to CAG repeat length. *Acta Neurol Scand* 1999; **99**:209–12.

Kato K, Wada T, Kawakatsu S *et al.* Improvement of both psychotic symptoms and parkinsonism in a case of dementia with Lewy bodies by the combination therapy of risperidone and L-dopa. *Prog Neuropsychopharmacol Biol Psychiatry* 2002; **26**:201–3.

Kawanami T, Kato T, Daimon M *et al.* Hereditary ceruloplasmin deficiency: clinicopathological study of a patient. *J Neurol Neurosurg Psychiatry* 1996; **61**:506–9.

Kennedy WR, Alter M, Sung JH. Progressive proximal spinal and bulbar muscular atrophy of late onset: a sex-linked recessive trait. *Neurology* 1968; **18**:671–80.

Kertesz A, Hudson L, Mackenzie IRA *et al.* The pathology and nosology of primary progressive aphasia. *Neurology* 1994; **44**:2065–72.

Khan NL, Graham E, Critchley P *et al.* Parkin disease: a phenotypic study of a large case series. *Brain* 2003; **126**:1279–92.

Kidd D, Nelson J, Jones F *et al.* Long-term stabilization after bone marrow transplantation in juvenile metachromatic leukodystrophy. *Arch Neurol* 1998; **51**:98–9.

Kidd M. Alzheimer's disease: an electron microscopic study. *Brain* 1964; **87**:307–20.

Kirsten L, Silfverskiold B. A family with emotionally precipitated drop seizures. *Lancet* 1958; **2**:471–6.

Klatka LA, Louis ED, Schiffer RB. Psychiatric features in diffuse Lewy body disease: a clinicopathologic study using Alzheimer's disease and Parkinson's disease comparison groups. *Neurology* 1996; **47**:1148–52.

Klawans HL, Barr A. Prevalence of spontaneous lingual-facial-buccal dyskinesias in the elderly. *Neurology* 1981; **31**:558–9.

Klawans HL, Barr A. Recurrence of childhood multiple tics in late adult life. *Arch Neurol* 1985; **42**:1079–80.

Klein C. Implications of genetics on the diagnosis and care of patients with Parkinson disease. *Arch Neurol* 2006; **63**:328–34.

Kleiner-Fisman G, Rogaeva E, Halliday W *et al*. Benign hereditary chorea: clinical, genetic, and pathological findings. *Neurology* 2003; **54**:244–7.

Kleiner-Fisman G, Calingasan NY, Putt M *et al*. Alterations of striatal neurons in benign hereditary chorea. *Mov Disord* 2005; **20**:1353–7.

Knibb J, Xuereb JH, Patterson K *et al*. Clinical and pathological characteristics of progressive aphasia. *Ann Neurol* 2006; **59**:156–65.

Knopman DS, Christensen KJ, Schut LJ *et al*. The spectrum of imaging and neuropsychological findings in Pick's disease. *Neurology* 1989; **39**:362–8.

Koch MC, Grimm T, Harley HG *et al*. Genetic risks for children of women with myotonic dystrophy. *Am J Human Genet* 1991; **48**:1084–91.

Koller WC. Edentulous orodyskinesia. *Neurology* 1983; **13**:97–9.

Koller WC, Royse VL. Efficacy of primidone in essential tremor. *Neurology* 1986; **36**:121–4.

Koller WC, Busenbark K, Miner K *et al*. The relationship of essential tremor to other movement disorders: report on 678 patients. *Ann Neurol* 1994; **35**:717–23.

Korczyn AD, Brunt ER, Larsen JP *et al*. A 3-year randomized trial of ropinirole and bromocriptine in early Parkinson's disease. *Neurology* 1999; **53**:364–70.

Korenke GC, Fuchs S, Kraseman E *et al*. Cerebral adreno-leukodystrophy in only one of monozygotic twins with an identical ALD genotype. *Ann Neurol* 1996; **40**:254–7.

Koss E, Edland S, Fillenbaum G *et al*. Clinical and neuropsychological differences between patients with earlier and later onset of Alzheimer's disease: a CERAD analysis, Part XII. *Neurology* 1996; **46**:136–41.

Kramer PL, de Leon D, Oselius L *et al*. Dystonia gene in Ashkenazi Jewish population is located on chromosome 9q32–34. *Ann Neurol* 1990; **27**:114–20.

Kremer B, Goldberg P, Andrew SE *et al*. A world-wide study of the Huntington's disease mutation: the sensitivity and specificity of measuring CAG repeats. *N Engl J Med* 1994; **330**:1401–6.

Krivit W, Lipton ME, Tsai M *et al*. Prevention of deterioration in metachromatic leukodystrophy by bone marrow transplantation. *Am J Med Sci* 1987; **249**:80–5.

Kruisdijk JJM, Koelman JHTM, Ongerboer BW *et al*. Botulinum toxin for writer's cramp: a randomized, placebo-controlled trial and 1-year follow-up. *J Neurol Neurosurg Psychiatry* 2007; **7 8**:264–70.

Kugelberg E, Welander L. Heredofamilial juvenile muscular atrophy simulating muscular dystrophy. *Arch Neurol Psychiatry* 1956; **75**:500–9.

Kuipers-Upmeijer J, de Jager AEJ, Hew JM *et al*. Primary lateral sclerosis: clinical, neurophysiological, and magnetic resonance findings. *J Neurol Neurosurg Psychiatry* 2001; **71**:615–20.

Kulisevsky J, Marti MJ, Ferrer I *et al*. Meige syndrome: neuropathology of a case. *Mov Disord* 1988; **3**:170–5.

Kurlan R, Behr J, Medved L *et al*. Transient tic disorder and the spectrum of Tourette's syndrome. *Arch Neurol* 1988; **45**:1200–1.

Kurth MC, Adler CH, St Hilaire M *et al*. Tolcapone improves motor function and reduces levodopa requirement in patients with Parkinson's disease experiencing motor fluctuations: a multicenter, double-blind, randomized, placebo-controlled trial. *Neurology* 1997; **48**:81–7.

Kuzis G, Sabe L, Tiberti C *et al*. Cognitive functions in major depression and Parkinson disease. *Arch Neurol* 1997; **54**:982–6.

Kvale JN. Amitriptyline in the management of progressive supranuclear palsy. *Arch Neurol* 1982; **39**:387–8.

La Forestier N, Maisonobe T, Piquard A *et al*. Does primary lateral sclerosis exist? A study of 20 patients and a review of the literature. *Brain* 2001; **124**:1989–99.

Lai F, Williams RS. A prospective study of Alzheimer's disease in Down syndrome. *Arch Neurol* 1989; **46**:849–53.

Lang AE. Patient perception of tics and other movement disorders. *Neurology* 1991; **41**:223–8.

Lang AE, Johnson K. Akathisia in idiopathic Parkinson's disease. *Neurology* 1987; **37**:477–81.

Lang AE, Consky E, Sandor P. 'Signing tics' – insights into the pathophysiology of symptoms in Tourette's syndrome. *Ann Neurol* 1993; **33**:212–15.

Lantos PL, Cairns NJ, Khan MN *et al*. Neuropathologic variations in frontotemporal dementia due to the intronic *tau* 10 + 16 mutation. *Neurology* 2002; **58**:1169–75.

Lasek K, Lencer R, Gaser C *et al*. Morphological basis for the spectrum of clinical deficits in spinocerebellar ataxia 17 (SCA17). *Brain* 2006; **129**:2341–52.

Lawyer T, Netsky MG. Amyotrophic lateral sclerosis: clinico-anatomic study of 53 cases. *Arch Neurol Psychiatry* 1953; **69**:171–92.

Le Bars PL, Katz MM, Berman N *et al*. A placebo-controlled, double-blind, randomized trial of *Ginkgo biloba* for dementia: North American EGb Study Group. *JAMA* 1997; **278**: 1327–32.

Le Ber I, Martinez M, Campion D *et al*. A non-DM1, non DM2 multisystem myotonic disorder with frontotemporal dementia: phenotype and suggestive mapping of the DM3 locus to chromosome 15q21-24. *Brain* 2004; **127**:1979–92.

Lebert F, Stekke W, Hasenbroek C *et al*. Frontotemporal dementia: a randomized, controlled trial with trazodone. *Geriatr Cogn Disord* 2004; **17**:355–9.

Leckman JF, Ort S, Caruso KA *et al*. Rebound phenomena in Tourette's syndrome after abrupt withdrawal of clonidine. Behavioral, cardiovascular, and neurochemical effects. *Arch Gen Psychiatry* 1986; **43**:1168–76.

Leckman JF, Hardin MT, Riddle MA *et al*. Clonidine treatment of Gilles de la Tourette's syndrome. *Arch Gen Psychiatry* 1991; **48**:324–8.

Leckman JF, Walker DE, Cohen DJ. Premonitory urges in Tourette's syndrome. *Am J Psychiatry* 1993; **150**:98–102.

Leckman JF, Walker DE, Goodman WK *et al*. 'Just right' perceptions associated with compulsive behavior in Tourette's syndrome. *Am J Psychiatry* 1994; **151**:675–80.

Leckman JF, Zhang H, Vitale A et al. Course of tic severity in Tourette syndrome: the first two decades. *Pediatrics* 1998; **102**:14–19.

Lee MS, Lee SB, Kim WC. Spasmodic dysphonia associated with a left ventrolateral putaminal lesion. *Neurology* 1996; **47**:827–8.

Lee MS, Kim YD, Lyoo CH. Oculogyric crisis as an initial manifestation of Wilson's disease. *Neurology* 1999; **52**:1714–15.

Lees AJ, Robertson M, Trimble MR et al. A clinical study of Gilles de la Tourette syndrome in the United Kingdom. *J Neurol Neurosurg Psychiatry* 1984; **47**:1–9.

Lennox G, Lowe J, Landon M et al. Diffuse Lewy body disease: correlative neuropathology using anti-ubiquitin immunocytochemistry. *J Neurol Neurosurg Psychiatry* 1989; **52**:1236–47.

Leopold NA, Kagel MC. Dysphagia in Huntington's disease. *Arch Neurol* 1985; **42**:57–60.

Lesse SM. Huntington's chorea: report of a case. *J Nerv Ment Dis* 1946; **104**:84–7.

Leube B, Hendgen J, Kessler KR et al. Sporadic focal dystonia in Northwest Germany: molecular basis on chromosome 18p. *Ann Neurol* 1997; **42**:111–14.

Levy-Lahad E, Wasco W, Poorkaj P et al. Candidate gene for the chromosome 1 familial Alzheimer's disease locus. *Science* 1995; **269**:973–7.

Lieberman A, Ranhosky A, Korts D. Clinical evaluation of pramipexole in advanced Parkinson's disease: results of a double-blind, placebo-controlled, parallel-group study. *Neurology* 1997; **49**:162–8.

Lieberman A, Olanow CW, Sethi K et al. A multicenter trial of ropinirole as adjunct treatment for Parkinson's disease. *Neurology* 1998; **51**:1057–62.

Lieberman JA, Reife R. Spastic dysphonia and denervation signs in a young man with tardive dyskinesia. *Br J Psychiatry* 1989; **154**:105–9.

Lilly R, Cummings JL, Benson DF et al. The human Kluver–Bucy syndrome. *Neurology* 1983; **33**:1141–5.

Linet LS. Tourette syndrome, pimozide, and school phobia: the neuroleptic separation anxiety syndrome. *Am J Psychiatry* 1985; **12**:613–15.

Linn RT, Wolf PA, Bachman DL et al. The 'preclinical phase' of probable Alzheimer's disease. *Arch Neurol* 1995; **52**:485–90.

Lippa CF, Smith TW, Swearer JM. Alzheimer's disease and Lewy body disease: a comparative clinicopathological study. *Ann Neurol* 1994; **35**:81–8.

Little BW, Brown PW, Rodgers-Johnson P et al. Familial myoclonic dementia masquerading as Creutzfeldt–Jakob disease. *Ann Neurol* 1986; **20**:231.

Litvan I, Mega MS, Cummings JL et al. Neuropsychiatric aspects of progressive supranuclear palsy. *Neurology* 1996a; **47**: 1184–9.

Litvan I, Mangone CA, McKee A et al. Natural history of progressive supranuclear palsy (Steele–Richardson–Olszewski syndrome) and clinical predictors of survival: a clinicopathologic study. *J Neurol Neurosurg Psychiatry* 1996b; **61**:615–20.

Litvan I, Agid Y, Jankovic J et al. Accuracy of clinical criteria for the diagnosis of progressive supranuclear palsy (Steele–Richardson Olszewski syndrome). *Neurology* 1996c; **46**:922–30.

Litvan I, Agid Y, Sastrj N et al. What are the obstacles for accurate clinical diagnosis of Pick's disease? *Neurology* 1997a; **49**:62–9.

Litvan I, Campbell G, Mangone CA et al. Which clinical features differentiate progressive supranuclear palsy (Steele–Richardson–Olszewski syndrome) from related disorders? A clinicopathological study. *Brain* 1997b; **120**:65–74.

Litvan I, Agid Y, Goetz C et al. Accuracy of the clinical diagnosis of corticobasal degeneration: a clinicopathologic study. *Neurology* 1997c; **48**:119–25.

Litvan I, Cummings JL, Mega M. Neuropsychiatric features of corticobasal degeneration. *J Neurol Neurosurg Psychiatry* 1998; **65**:717–21.

Litvan I, Phipps M, Pharr VL et al. Randomized placebo-controlled trial of donepezil in patients with progressive supranuclear palsy. *Neurology* 2001; **57**:467–73.

Livingston G, Walker AE, Katona CLE et al. Antipsychotics and cognitive decline in Alzheimer's disease: the LASER-Alzheimer's disease longitudinal study. *J Neurol Neurosurg Psychiatry* 2007; **78**:25–9.

Lopes-Cendes I, Silveira I, Maciel P et al. Limits of clinical assessment as the accurate diagnosis of Machado–Joseph disease. *Arch Neurol* 1996; **53**:1168–74.

Lopez OL, Becker JT, Sweet RA et al. Psychiatric symptoms vary with the severity of dementia in probable Alzheimer's disease. *J Neuropsychiatry Clin Neurosci* 2003; **15**:346–53.

Lorenz D, Frederiksen H, Moises H et al. High concordance for essential tremor in monozygotic twins of old age. *Neurology* 2004; **62**:208–11.

Lossos A, Dobson-Stone C, Monaco AP et al. Early clinical heterogeneity in choreoacanthocytosis. *Ann Neurol* 2005; **62**:611–14.

Lou J-S, Jankovic J. Essential tremor: clinical correlates in 350 patients. *Neurology* 1991; **41**:234–8.

Louis ED, Goldman JE, Powers JM et al. Parkinsonian features of eight pathologically diagnosed cases of diffuse Lewy body disease. *Mov Disord* 1995; **10**:188–94.

Louis ED, Klatka LA, Liu Y et al. Comparison of extrapyramidal features in 31 pathologically confirmed cases of diffuse Lewy body disease and 34 pathologically confirmed cases of Parkinson's disease. *Neurology* 1997; **48**:376–80.

Louis ED, Honig LS, Vonsattel JPG et al. Essential tremor associated with focal nonnigral Lewy bodies. *Arch Neurol* 2005; **62**:1004–7.

Louis ED, Vonsattel JPG, Honig LS et al. Neuropathologic findings in essential tremor. *Neurology* 2006a; **66**:1756–9.

Louis ED, Vonsattel JPG, Honig LS et al. Essential tremor associated with pathologic change in the cerebellum. *Arch Neurol* 2006b; **63**:1189–93.

Lowenberg K, Boyd DA, Salon DD. Occurrence of Pick's disease in early adult years. *Arch Neurol Psychiatry* 1939; **41**:1004–20.

Lucking CB, Durr A, Bonifati V et al. Association between early-onset Parkinson's disease and mutations in the Parkin gene. N Engl J Med 2000; 342:1560-7.

Maas O, Paterson AS. Myotonia congenita, dystrophia myotonica, and paramyotonia. Brain 1950; 73:318-32.

MacDonald JR, Hill JD, Tarnopolsky MA. Modafinil reduces excessive somnolence and enhances mood in patients with myotonic dystrophy. Neurology 2002; 59:1876-80.

Machado A, Chien HF, Deguti MM et al. Neurological manifestations of Wilson's disease: report of 119 cases. Mov Disord 2006; 21:2192-6.

MacKenzie IR, Munoz DG. Nonsteroidal anti-inflammatory drug use and Alzheimer-type pathology in aging. Neurology 1998; 50:986-90.

Mackenzie IRA, Baker M, Pickering-Brown S et al. The neuropathology of frontotemporal lobar degeneration caused by mutations in the progranulin gene. Brain 2006; 129:3081-90.

Maher ER, Lees AJ. The clinical features of the Steele-Richardson-Olszewski syndrome (progressive supranuclear palsy). Neurology 1986; 36:1005-8.

Malamud N, Waggoner RW. Genealogic and clinicopathologic study of Pick's disease. Arch Neurol Psychiatry 1943; 50:288-303.

Malamud N, Hirano A, Kurland LT. Pathoanatomic changes in amyotrophic lateral sclerosis on Guam. Neurology 1961; 5:401-14.

Maltecca F, Filla A, Castaldo I et al. Intergenerational instability and marked anticipation in SCA-17. Neurology 2003; 61:1441-3.

Mann D, Yates P, Marcyniuk B. A comparison of changes in the nucleus basalis and the locus coeruleus in Alzheimer's disease. J Neurol Neurosurg Psychiatry 1984; 47:201-3.

Mann D, South PW, Snowden JS et al. Dementia of frontal lobe type: neuropathology and immunohistochemistry. J Neurol Neurosurg Psychiatry 1993a; 56:605-14.

Mann D, Oliver R, Snowden JS. The topographic distribution of brain atrophy in Huntington's disease and progressive supranuclear palsy. Acta Neuropathol 1993b; 85:553-9.

Manni R, Zucca C, Martinetti M et al. Hypersomnia in dystrophica myotonica: a neurophysiological and immunogenetic study. Acta Neurol Scand 1991; 84:498-502.

Manowitz P, Kling A, Kohn H. Clinical course of adult metachromatic leukodystrophy presenting as schizophrenia: a report of two living cases in siblings. J Nerv Ment Dis 1978; 166:500-6.

Marantz AG, Verghese J. Capgras' syndrome in dementia with Lewy bodies. J Geriatr Psychiatry Neurol 2002; 15:239-41.

Marder K, Ming-Xin T, Cote L et al. The frequency and associated risk factors for dementia in patients with Parkinson's disease. Arch Neurol 1995; 52:695-701.

Marder K, Sandler S, Lechich A et al. Relationship between CAG repeat length and late-stage outcomes in Huntington's disease. Neurology 2002; 59:1622-4.

Margolese HC, Annable L, Dion Y. Depression and dysphoria in adult and adolescent patients with Tourette's disorder treated with risperidone. J Clin Psychiatry 2002; 63:1040-4.

Mark MH, Sage JI, Dickson DW et al. Meige syndrome in the spectrum of Lewy body disease. Neurology 1994; 44:1432-6.

Marneros A. Adult onset of Tourette's syndrome. Am J Psychiatry 1983; 140:924-5.

Marsden CD, Harrison MJG. Idiopathic torsion dystonia (dystonia musculorum deformans): a review of forty-two patients. Brain 1974; 97:793-810.

Martin JJ, Yap M, Nei LP et al. Selective thalamic degeneration – report of a case with memory and mental disturbances. Clin Neuropathol 1983; 2:156-62.

Martin WE, Loewenson RB, Resch JA et al. Parkinson's disease: clinical analysis of 100 patients. Neurology 1973; 23:783-90.

Martinelli P, Gabellini AS, Gulli MR et al. Different clinical features of essential tremor: a 200-patient study. Acta Neurol Scand 1987; 75:106-11.

Marttila RJ, Rinne UK. Dementia in Parkinson's disease. Acta Neurol Scand 1976; 54:431-44.

Massironi G, Galuzzi S, Frisoni GB. Drug treatment of REM sleep behavior disorders in dementia with Lewy bodies. Int Psychogeriatr 2003; 15:377-83.

Matsumara R, Futamura N, Fujimoto Y et al. Spinocerebellar ataxia type 6. Molecular and genetic features of 35 Japanese patients including one homozygous for the CAG repeat expansion. Neurology 1997; 49:1238-43.

Matsuura T, Achari M, Khajavi M et al. Mapping of the gene for a novel spinocerebellar ataxia with pure cerebellar signs and epilepsy. Ann Neurol 1999; 45:407-11.

Maurage CA, Udd B, Ruchoux MM et al. Similar brain tau pathology in DM2/PROMM and DM1/Steinert disease. Neurology 2005; 65:1636-8.

Maurer K, Volk S, Gerbaldo H. Auguste D and Alzheimer's disease. Lancet 1997; 349:1546-9.

Mayeux R, Stern Y, Cote L et al. Altered serotonin metabolism in depressed patients with Parkinson's disease. Neurology 1984; 34:642-6.

Mayeux R, Stern Y, Williams JBW et al. Clinical and biochemical features of depression in Parkinson's disease. Am J Psychiatry 1986; 143:756-9.

Mayeux R, Stern Y, Rosenstein R et al. An estimate of the prevalence of dementia in idiopathic Parkinson's disease. Arch Neurol 1988; 45:260-2.

Mayeux R, Denaro J, Hemenegildo N et al. A population-based investigation of Parkinson's disease with and without dementia: relationship to age and gender. Arch Neurol 1992; 49:492-7.

Mazza M, Capuano A, Bria P et al. Ginkgo biloba and donepezil: a comparison in the treatment of Alzheimer's disease in a randomized placebo-controlled double-blind study. Eur J Neurol 2006; 13:981-5.

McGeer PL, Schulzer M, McGeer EG. Arthritis and anti-inflammatory agents as possible protective factors for Alzheimer's disease: a review of 17 epidemiologic studies. Neurology 1996; 47:425-32.

McKeith I, Fairbarin A, Perry R et al. Neuroleptic sensitivity in patients with senile dementia of Lewy body type. BMJ 1992a; 305:1158-9.

McKeith IG, Perry RH, Fairbarin AF et al. Operational criteria for senile dementia of Lewy body type (SDLT). Psychol Med 1992b; 22:911–22.

McKeith IG, Fairbairn A, Perry RH et al. Neuroleptic sensitivity in patients with senile dementia of Lewy body type. BMJ 1992c; 305:673–8.

McKeith I, Fairbairn AF, Perry RH et al. The clinical diagnosis and a misdiagnosis of senile dementia of Lewy body type (SDLT). Br J Psychiatry 1994a; 165:324–32.

McKeith IG, Fairbairn AF, Bothwell RA et al. An evaluation of the predictive validity and inter-rater reliability of clinical diagnostic criteria for senile dementia of Lewy body type. Neurology 1994b; 44:872–7.

McKeith I, Del Ser T, Spano P et al. Efficacy of rivastigmine in dementia with Lewy bodies: a randomized, double-blind, placebo-controlled international study. Lancet 2000; 356:2031–6.

McKeith IG, Dickson DW, Lowe J et al. Diagnosis and management of dementia with Lewy bodies: third report of the DLB consortium. Neurology 2005; 65:1863–72.

McNaught KSP, Kaspussin A, Jackson T et al. Brainstem pathology in DYT1 primary torsion dystonia. Ann Neurol 2004; 56:540–7.

McNeill R, Sare GM, Manoharan M et al. Accuracy of single-photon emission computed tomography in differentiating frontotemporal dementia from Alzheimer's disease. J Neurol Neurosurg Psychiatry 2007; 78:350–5.

van der Meche FGA, Bogaard JM, van der Sluys JCM et al. Daytime sleep in myotonic dystrophy is not caused by sleep apnoea. J Neurol Neurosurg Psychiatry 1994; 57:626–8.

Medalia A, Merriam A, Sandberg M et al. Neuropsychological deficits in choreoacanthocytosis. Arch Neurol 1989; 46:573–83.

Mega MS, Cummings JL, Fiorello T et al. The spectrum of behavioral changes in Alzheimer's disease. Neurology 1996; 46:130–5.

Meiner V, Meiner Z, Reshef A et al. Cerebrotendinous xanthomatosis: molecular diagnosis enables presymptomatic detection of a treatable disease. Neurology 1994; 44:288–90.

Mendez MF, Selwood A, Mastr AR et al. Pick's disease versus Alzheimer's disease: a comparison of clinical characteristics. Neurology 1993; 43:289–92.

Mendez MF, Shapira JS, McMurtay A et al. Preliminary findings: behavioral worsening on donepezil in patients with frontotemporal dementia. Am J Geriatr Psychiatry 2007; 15:84–7.

Menkes JH, Schimschock JR, Swanson PD. Cerebrotendinous xanthomatosis: the storage of cholestanol within the nervous system. Arch Neurol 1968; 19:47–53.

Menza MA, Cocchiola J, Golbe LI. Psychiatric symptoms in progressive supranuclear palsy. Psychosomatics 1995; 36:550–4.

Merims D, Balas M, Peretz C et al. Rater-blinded, prospective comparison: quetiapine versus clozapine for Parkinson's disease psychosis. Clin Neuropharmacol 2006; 29:331–7.

Messert B, Van Nuis C. A syndrome of paralysis of downward gaze, dysarthria, pseudobulbar palsy, axial rigidity of neck and trunk and dementia. J Nerv Ment Dis 1966; 143:47–54.

Mesulam M, Johnson N, Kreftt TA et al. Progranulin mutations in primary progressive aphasia. The PPA1 and PPA3 families. Arch Neurol 2007; 64:43–7.

Migliorelli R, Teson A, Sabe L et al. Prevalence and correlates of dysthymia and major depression among patients with Alzheimer's disease. Am J Psychiatry 1995; 152:37–44.

Mikkelsen EJ, Detlor J, Cohen DJ. School avoidance and social phobia triggered by haloperidol in patients with Tourette's disorder. Am J Psychiatry 1981; 138:1572–6.

Modi G, Modi M, Martinus I et al. The clinical and genetic characteristics of spinocerebellar ataxia type 7 (SCA7) in three black South African families. Acta Neurol Scand 2000; 101:177–82.

Modoni A, Silvestri G, Pomponi MG et al. Characterization of the pattern of cognitive impairment in myotonic dystrophy type 1. Arch Neurol 2004; 61:1943–7.

Mohs RC, Breitner JCS, Silverman JM et al. Alzheimer's disease: morbid risk among first-degree relatives approximates 50% by 90 years of age. Arch Gen Psychiatry 1987; 44:405–8.

Molloy S, McKeith IG, O'Brien JT et al. The role of levodopa in the management of dementia with Lewy bodies. J Neurol Neurosurg Psychiatry 2005; 76:1200–3.

Moosey J, Martinez AJ, Hanin I et al. Thalamic and subcortical gliosis with dementia. Arch Neurol 1987; 44:510–13.

Moretti R, Torre P, Antonello RM et al. Rivastigmine in frontotemporal dementia: an open-label study. Drugs Aging 2004; 21:931–7.

Mori H, Kondo T, Yokochi M et al. Pathologic and biochemical studies of juvenile parkinsonism linked to chromosome 6q. Neurology 1998; 51:890–2.

Morris HR, Gibb G, Katzenschlager R et al. Pathological, clinical and genetic heterogeneity in progressive supranuclear palsy. Brain 2002; 125:969–75.

Morris ME, Iansek R, Matyas TA et al. Stride length regulation in Parkinson's disease: normalization strategies and underlying mechanisms. Brain 1996; 119:551–68.

Moser HW, Moser AE, Singh I et al. Adrenoleukodystrophy: survey of 303 cases: biochemistry, diagnosis and therapy. Ann Neurol 1984; 16:628–41.

Moser HW, Raymond GV, Lu S-E et al. Follow-up of 89 asymptomatic patients with adrenoleukodystrophy treated with Lorenzo's oil. Arch Neurol 2005; 62:1073–80.

Mosser J, Lutz Y, Stoeckel ME et al. The gene responsible for adrenoleukodystrophy encodes a peroxisomal membrane protein. Hum Mol Genet 1994; 3:265–71.

Muller J, Wissel J, Masuhr F et al. Clinical characteristics of the geste antagoniste in cervical dystonia. J Neurol 2001a; 248:478–82.

Muller N, Kroll B, Schwarz MJ et al. Increased titers of antibodies against streptococcal M12 and M19 proteins in patients with Tourette's syndrome. Psychiatry Res 2001b; 101:187–93.

Munoz MF, Selwood A, Mastri AR et al. Pick's disease versus Alzheimer's disease: a comparison of clinical abnormalities. Neurology 1993; 43:289–95.

Munoz-Garcia D, Ludwin SK. Classic and generalized variants of Pick's disease: a clinico-pathological, ultrastructural, and immunocytochemical comparative study. *Ann Neurol* 1984; **16**:467–80.

Murayama S, Mori H, Ihara Y *et al*. Immunocytochemical and ultrastructural studies of Pick's disease. *Ann Neurol* 1990; **27**:394–405.

Murphy MA, Feldman JA, Kilburn G. Hallervorden–Spatz disease in a psychiatric setting. *J Clin Psychiatry* 1989; **50**:100–3.

Murray R, Neumann M, Forman MS *et al*. Cognitive and motor assessment in autopsy-proven corticobasal degeneration. *Neurology* 2007; **68**:1274–83.

Myers RH, Vonsattel JP, Stevens TJ *et al*. Clinical and neuropathologic assessment of severity in Huntington's disease. *Neurology* 1988; **38**:341–7.

Myers RH, Mac DM, Koroshetz WJ *et al*. De novo expansion of a (CAG) repeat in sporadic Huntington's disease. *Nat Genet* 1993; **5**:174–9.

Myllyla VV, Sotaniemi KA, Hakulinen P *et al*. Selegeline as the primary treatment of Parkinson's disease – a long-term double-blind study. *Acta Neurol Scand* 1997; **95**:211–18.

Nagafuchi S, Yanagisawa H, Sato K *et al*. Dentatorubral and pallidoluysian atrophy expansion of an unstable CAG repeat on chromosome 12p. *Nat Genet* 1994; **6**:14–18.

Nagaoka U, Takashima M, Ishikawa K *et al*. A gene on SCA4 locus causes dominantly inherited pure cerebellar ataxia. *Neurology* 2000; **54**:1971–5.

Nakagawa M, Yamada H, Higucki I *et al*. A case of paternally inherited congenital myotonic dystrophy. *J Med Genet* 1994; **31**:397–400.

Navarro C, Fernandez JM, Dominguez C *et al*. Late juvenile metachromatic leukodystrophy treated with bone marrow transplantation: a 4-year follow-up study. *Neurology* 1996; **46**:254–6.

Neary D, Snowden J, Mann D *et al*. Alzheimer's disease – a correlative study. *J Neurol Neurosurg Psychiatry* 1986; **49**:229–34.

Neary D, Snowden JS, Mann DMA. Familial progressive atrophy: its relationship to other forms of lobar atrophy. *J Neurol Neurosurg Psychiatry* 1993; **56**:1122–5.

Neary D, Snowden JS, Gustafson L *et al*. Frontotemporal lobar degeneration: a consensus on clinical diagnostic criteria. *Neurology* 1998; **51**:1546–54.

Nee LE, Caine ED, Polinsky RJ *et al*. Gilles de la Tourette's syndrome: clinical and family study of 50 cases. *Ann Neurol* 1980; **7**:41–9.

Neumann M, Schulz-Schaeffer W, Crowther A *et al*. Pick's disease associated with the novel tau gene mutation K369I. *Ann Neurol* 2001; **50**:503–13.

Newman GC. Treatment of progressive supranuclear palsy with tricyclic antidepressants. *Neurology* 1985; **35**:1189–93.

Nichols IC, Weigner WC. Pick's disease – a specific type of dementia. *Brain* 1938; **61**:237–49.

Nielsen JE, Sorensen SA, Hasholt L *et al*. Dentatorubral-pallidoluysian atrophy. Clinical features of a five-generation Danish family. *Mov Disord* 1996; **11**:533–41.

Nijssen PC, Brusse E, Leyten AC *et al*. Autosomal dominant adult cerebral neuronal ceroid lipofuscinosis: parkinsonism due to

both striatal and nigral dysfunction. *Mov Disord* 2002; **17**:482–7.

Nygaard TG, Duvoisin RC. Hereditary dystonia–parkinsonism syndrome of juvenile onset. *Neurology* 1986; **36**:1424–8.

Nygaard TG, Duvoisin RC, Manocha M *et al*. Seizures in progressive supranuclear palsy. *Neurology* 1989; **39**:138–40.

Nygaard TG, Trugman JM, de Yebenes JG *et al*. Dopa-responsive dystonia: the spectrum of clinical manifestations in a large North American family. *Neurology* 1990; **40**:66–9.

Nygaard TG, Marsden CD, Fahn S. Dopa-responsive dystonia: long-term treatment response and prognosis. *Neurology* 1991; **41**:174–81.

O'Brien CP, DiGiacomo JN, Fahn S *et al*. Mental effects of high-dosage levodopa. *Arch Gen Psychiatry* 1971; **24**:61–4.

Oh J, Park KD, Cho HJ. Spasmodic dysphonia induced by valproic acid. *Epilepsia* 2004; **45**:880–1.

O'Hearn E, Holmes SE, Calvert PC *et al*. SCA-12: tremor with cerebellar and cortical trophy is associated with a CAG repeat expansion. *Neurology* 2001; **56**:299–303.

Ohnishi A, Sato Y, Nagara H *et al*. Neurogenic muscular atrophy and low density of large myelinated fibres of sural nerve in chorea–acanthocytosis. *J Neurol Neurosurg Psychiatry* 1981; **44**:645–8.

Ohye T, Takahashi E, Seki N *et al*. Hereditary progressive dystonia with marked diurnal fluctuation caused by mutations in the GTP cyclohydrolase I gene. *Nat Genet* 1994; **8**:236–42.

Okazaki H, Lipkin LE, Aronson SM. Diffuse intracytoplasmic ganglionic inclusions (Lewy type) associated with progressive dementia and quadriparesis in flexion. *J Neuropathol Exp Neurol* 1961; **20**:237–44.

Oken BS, Storzbach DM, Kaye JA. The efficacy of *Gingko biloba* on cognitive function in Alzheimer's disease. *Arch Neurol* 1998; **55**:1409–15.

Olanow CW, Tasmar Advisory Panel. Tolcapone and hepatotoxic effects. *Arch Neurol* 2000; **57**:263–7.

Olson MI, Shaw CM. Presenile dementia and Alzheimer's disease in mongolism. *Brain* 1969; **92**:147–56.

Ondo W, Hunter C, Dat Vuong K *et al*. Gabapentin for essential tremor: a multiple-dose, double-blind, placebo-controlled trial. *Mov Disord* 2000; **15**:678–82.

Ondo W, Jankovic J, Connor GS *et al*. Topiramate in essential tremor. A double-blind, placebo-controlled trial. *Neurology* 2006; **66**:672–7.

O'Neill BP, Moser HW, Saxena KM. Familial X-linked Addison disease as an expression of adrenoleukodystrophy (ALD): elevated C26 fatty acids in cultured skin fibroblasts. *Neurology* 1982; **32**:543–9.

Ono S, Kanda F, Takahashi K *et al*. Neuronal loss in the medullary reticular formation in myotonic dystrophy: a clinicopathological study. *Neurology* 1996; **46**:228–31.

Ono S, Takahashi K, Jinnai K *et al*. Loss of serotonin-containing neurons in the raphe of patients with myotonic dystrophy: a quantitative immunohistochemical study and relation to hypersomnia. *Neurology* 1998; **50**:535–8.

Onofrj M, Paci C, D'Andreamatteo G *et al*. Olanzapine in severe Gilles de la Tourette syndrome: a 5-week double-blind cross-over study vs. low-dose pimozide. *J Neurol* 2000; **247**:443–6.

Onofrj M, Luciano AL, Thomas A et al. Mirtazapine induces REM sleep behavior disorder in parkinsonism. Neurology 2003; **60**:113–15.

Ostheimer AJ. An essay on the shaking palsy, by James Parkinson, M.D., member of the Royal College of Surgeons. Arch Neurol Psychiatry 1922; **7**:681–710.

O'Suilleabhain P, Dewey RB. A randomized trial of amantadine in Huntington disease. Arch Neurol 2003; **60**:996–8.

Ozawa T, Pavious D, Quinn NP et al. The spectrum of pathological involvement of the striatonigral and olivopontocerebellar system in multiple system atrophy: clinicopathological correlations. Brain 2004; **127**:2657–71.

Ozelius L, Kramer PL, MosKowitz CB et al. Human gene for torsion dystonia located on chromosome 9q32–q34. Neuron 1989; **2**:1427–34.

Ozelius LJ, Kramer PL, de Leon D et al. Strong allelic association between the torsion dystonia gene (DYT 1) and loci on chromosome 9q34 in Ashkenazi Jews. Am J Hum Genet 1992; **50**:619–28.

Ozelius LJ, Hewett JW, Page CE et al. The early-onset torsion dystonia gene (DYT1) encodes an ATP-binding protein. Nat Genet 1997; **17**:40–8.

Pahwa R, Lyons K, McGuire D et al. Early morning akinesia in Parkinson's disease: effect of standard levodopa/carbidopa and sustained-release levodopa/carbidopa. Neurology 1996; **46**:1059–62.

Paleacu D, Anca M, Giladi N. Olanzapine in Huntington's disease. Acta Neurol Scand 2002; **105**:441–4.

Palhagen S, Heinonen EH, Hagglund J et al. Selegeline delays the onset of disability in de novo parkinsonian patients. Neurology 1998; **51**:520–5.

Palhagen S, Heinonen E, Hagglund J et al. Selegeline slows the progression of the symptoms of Parkinson's disease. Neurology 2006; **66**:1200–6.

Papapetropoulos S, Singer C, Ross OA et al. Clinical heterogeneity of the LRRK2 G2019S mutation. Arch Neurol 2006; **63**:1242–6.

Papp MI, Lantos PI. The distribution of oligodendroglial inclusions in multiple system atrophy and its relevance to clinical symptomatology. Brain 1994; **117**:235–43.

Pappert EJ, Goetz CG, Louis ED et al. Objective assessment of longitudinal outcome in Gilles de la Tourette's syndrome. Neurology 2003; **61**:936–40.

Parkinson Study Group. Safety and efficacy of pramipexole in early Parkinson's disease: a randomized dose-ranging study. JAMA 1997; **278**:125–30.

Parkinson Study Group. Low-dose clozapine for the treatment of drug-induced psychosis in Parkinson's disease. N Engl J Med 1999; **340**:757–63.

Parkinson Study Group. A controlled, randomized, delayed-start study of rasagaline in early Parkinson disease. Arch Neurol 2004; **61**:561–6.

Parkinson Study Group. A randomized placebo-controlled trial of rasagaline in levodopa-treated patients with Parkinson disease and motor fluctuations. Arch Neurol 2005; **62**:241–8.

Parvizi J, Joseph J, Press DZ et al. Pathological laughter and crying in patients with multiple system atrophy – cerebellar type. Mov Disord 2007; **22**:798–803.

Pauls DL, Leckman JF. The inheritance of Gilles de la Tourette's syndrome and associated behaviors. N Engl J Med 1986; **315**:993–7.

Pauls DL, Pakstis AJ, Kurlan R et al. Segregation and linkage analysis of Tourette's syndrome and related disorders. J Am Acad Child Adolesc Psychiatry 1990; **29**:195–203.

Paulson GW. Meige's syndrome. Dyskinesia of the eyelids and facial muscles. Geriatrics 1972; **27**:69–73.

Paulsen JS, Ready RE, Hamilton JN et al. Neuropsychiatric aspects of Huntington's disease. J Neurol Neurosurg Psychiatry 2001; **71**:31–4.

Paulsen JS, Hoth KF, Nehl C et al. Critical periods of suicide risk in Huntington's disease. Am J Psychiatry 2005; **162**:725–31.

Pellecchia MT, Valente EM, Cif L et al. The diverse phenotype and genotype of pantothenate kinase-associated neurodegeneration. Neurology 2005; **64**:1810–12.

Perini GI, Colombo G, Armani M et al. Intellectual impairment and cognitive evoked potentials in myotonic dystrophy. J Nerv Ment Dis 1989; **177**:750–4.

Perlmutter SJ, Leitman SF, Garvey MA et al. Therapeutic plasma exchange and intravenous immunoglobulin for obsessive-compulsive disorder and tic disorders in childhood. Lancet 1999; **354**:1153–8.

Peterson B, Riddle MA, Cohen DJ et al. Reduced basal ganglia volumes in Tourette's syndrome using 3-dimensional reconstruction techniques from magnetic resonance images. Neurology 1993; **43**:941–9.

Petry S, Cummings JL, Hill MA et al. Personality alterations in dementia of the Alzheimer type. Arch Neurol 1988; **45**:1187–90.

Pflanz S, Besson JAO, Ebmeier KP et al. The clinical manifestation of mental disorder in Huntington's disease: a retrospective case record study of disease progression. Acta Psychiatr Scand 1991; **83**:53–60.

Phemister JC, Small JM. Hypersomnia in dystrophia myotonica. J Neurol Neurosurg Psychiatry 1961; **24**:173–5.

Piccini P, Burn DJ, Ceravolo R et al. The role of inheritance in sporadic Parkinson's disease: evidence from a longitudinal study of dopaminergic function in twins. Ann Neurol 1999; **45**:577–82.

Pick A. Uber die beziehungen der senilin hirnatrophie zur aphasie. Prager Med Wochenschur 1892; **17**:165–7.

Pickering-Brown S, Baker M, Yen SH et al. Pick's disease is associated with mutations in the tau gene. Ann Neurol 2000; **48**:859–67.

Pierantozzi M, Pietrousti A, Brusa L et al. Helicobacter pylori eradication and L-dopa absorption in patients with PD and motor fluctuations. Neurology 2006; **66**:1824–9.

Pineda DA, Buritica O, Sanchez JL et al. Parkinsonian syndromes in Medellin (Colombia). Rev Neurol 2000; **31**:936–43.

Pinter MM, Pogarell O, Oertel WH. Efficacy, safety, and tolerance of the non-ergoline dopamine agonist pramipexole in the treatment of advanced Parkinson's disease: a double blind, placebo controlled, randomized, multicentre study. J Neurol Neurosurg Psychiatry 1999; **66**:436–41.

Plazzi G, Corsini R, Provini F et al. REM sleep behavior disorder in multiple system atrophy. Neurology 1997; **48**:1094–7.

Pollak P, Tison F, Rascol O *et al.* Clozapine in drug-induced psychosis in Parkinson's disease. A randomized, placebo controlled study with open follow up. *J Neurol Neurosurg Psychiatry* 2004; **75**:689–95.

Pontone G, Williams JR, Bassett SS *et al.* Clinical features associated with impulse control disorders in Parkinson disease. *Neurology* 2006; **67**:1258–61.

Pool KD, Freeman FJ, Finitzo T *et al.* Heterogeneity in spasmodic dysphonia. Neurologic and voice findings. *Arch Neurol* 1991; **48**:305–9.

Potter NT, Meyer MA, Zimmerman AW *et al.* Molecular and clinical findings in a family with dentatorubral-pallidoluysian atrophy. *Ann Neurol* 1995; **37**:273–7.

Powers JM, Schaumburg HH, Gaffney CL *et al.* Kluver–Bucy syndrome caused by adreno-leukodystrophy. *Neurology* 1980; **30**:1131–2.

Pramstaller PP, Schlossmacher MG, Jacques TS *et al.* Lewy body Parkinson's disease in a large pedigree with 77 *Parkin* mutation carriers. *Ann Neurol* 2005; **58**:411–22.

Price BH, Gurvit H, Weintraud S *et al.* Neuropsychological patterns and language deficits in 20 consecutive cases of autopsy-confirmed Alzheimer's disease. *Arch Neurol* 1993; **50**:931–7.

Price RA, Kidd KK, Cohen DJ *et al.* A twin study of Tourette syndrome. *Arch Gen Psychiatry* 1985; **42**:815–20.

Pringle CE, Hudson AJ, Munoz DJ *et al.* Primary lateral sclerosis. Clinical features, neuropathology and diagnostic criteria. *Brain* 1992; **115**:495–520.

Priori A, Pesenti A, Cappellari A *et al.* Limb immobilization for the treatment of focal occupational dystonia. *Neurology* 2001; **57**:405–9.

Pryse-Phillips W, Johnson GJ, Larsen B. Incomplete manifestations of myotonic dystrophy in a large kinship in Labrador. *Ann Neurol* 1982; **11**:582–4.

Quinn N. Multiple system atrophy – the nature of the beast. *J Neurol Neurosurg Psychiatry* 1989; **52**:78–85.

Rabey JM, Prokhorov T, Minlovitz A *et al.* Effect of quetiapine in psychotic Parkinson's disease patients: a double-blind labeled study of 3 month's duration. *Mov Disord* 2007; **22**:313–8.

Rajput AH, Gibb WRG, Zhong XH *et al.* Dopa-responsive dystonia: pathological and biochemical observations in a case. *Ann Neurol* 1994; **35**:396–402.

Rajput AH, Martin W, Saint-Hilaire M-H *et al.* Tolcapone improves motor function in Parkinsonian patients with the 'wearing-off' phenomenon: a double-blind, placebo-controlled, multicenter trial. *Neurology* 1997; **49**:1066–71.

Rajput A, Robinson CA, Rajput AH. Essential tremor course and disability. *Neurology* 2004; **62**:932–6.

Rahkonen T, Eloniemi-Sulkava U, Rissanen S *et al.* Dementia with Lewy bodies according to the consensus criteria in a general population aged 75 or older. *J Neurol Neurosurg Psychiatry* 2003; **74**:720–4.

Ramos-Arroyo MA, Moreno S, Valiente A. Incidence and mutation rates of Huntington's disease in Spain: experience of 9 years of direct genetic testing. *J Neurol Neurosurg Psychiatry* 2005; **76**:337–42.

Rascol O, Brooks DJ, Corczyn AD *et al.* A five-year study of the incidence of dyskinesia in patients with early Parkinson's disease who were treated with ropinirole or levodopa. *N Engl J Med* 2000; **342**:1484–91.

Rasool C, Svendsen CN, Selkoe DJ. Neurofibrillary degeneration of cholinergic and noncholinergic neurons of the basal forebrain in Alzheimer's disease. *Ann Neurol* 1986; **20**:482–8.

Rasmussen KG, Russell JC, Kung S *et al.* Electroconvulsive therapy for patients with major depression and probably Lewy body dementia. *J ECT* 2003; **19**:103–9.

Raudino F. Non motor off in Parkinson's disease. *Acta Neurol Scand* 2001; **104**:312–15.

Rauschka H, Colsch B, Bamann N *et al.* Late-onset metachromatic leukodystrophy. Genotype strongly influences phenotype. *Neurology* 2006; **67**:859–63.

Ravina B, Pott M, Siderowf A *et al.* Donepezil for dementia in Parkinson's disease: a randomized double-blind, placebo controlled crossover study. *J Neurol Neurosurg Psychiatry* 2005; **76**:934–9.

Rebeiz J, Kolodney E, Richardson EJ. Corticodentatonigral degeneration with neuronal achromasia. *Arch Neurol* 1968; **18**:20–33.

Rees L, Lipsedge M, Ball C. *Textbook of psychiatry*. London: Arnold, 1996.

Rees MI Andrew M, Jawad S *et al.* Evidence for recessive as well as dominant forms of startle disease (hyperekplexia) caused by mutations in the alpha 1 subunit of the inhibitory glycine receptor. *Hum Mol Genet* 1994; **3**:2175–9.

Reeves AL, So EL, Sharbrough FW *et al.* Movement disorders associated with the use of gabapentin. *Epilepsia* 1996; **37**:988–90.

Reeves RR, Liberto V. Treatment of essential blepharospasm with quetiapine. *Mov Disord* 2003; **18**:1072–3.

Regeur L, Pakkenberg B, Fog R *et al.* Clinical features and long-term treatment with pimozide in 65 patients with Gilles de la Tourette's syndrome. *J Neurol Neurosurg Psychiatry* 1986; **49**:791–5.

Reider-Grosswasser I, Bornstein N. CT and MRI in late-onset metachromatic leukodystrophy. *Acta Neurol Scand* 1987; **75**:64–9.

Rewcastle NB, Ball MJ. Electron microscopic structure of the 'inclusion bodies' in Pick's disease. *Neurology* 1968; **18**:1205–13.

Ribai P, Nguyen K, Hanhn-Barma V *et al.* Psychiatric and cognitive difficulties as indicators of juvenile Huntington's disease onset in 29 patients. *Arch Neurol* 2007; **64**:813–19.

Ricker K, Koch MC, Lehmann-Horn F *et al.* Proximal myotonic myopathy: a new dominant disorder with myotonia, muscle weakness and cataracts. *Neurology* 1994; **4**:1448–52.

Ricker K, Koch MC, Lehmann-Horn F *et al.* Proximal myotonic myopathy: clinical features of a multisystem disorder similar to myotonic dystrophy. *Arch Neurol* 1995; **52**:25–31.

Ricker K, Grimm T, Koch MC *et al.* Linkage of proximal myotonic myopathy to chromosome 3q. *Neurology* 1999; **52**:170–1.

Ridha BH, Josephs KA, Rossor MN. Delusions and hallucinations in dementia with Lewy bodies: worsening with memantine. *Neurology* 2005; **65**:481–2.

Riley DE, Lang AE, Lewis A *et al.* Cortical-basal ganglionic degeneration. *Neurology* 1990; **40**:1203–12.

Rinne J, Lee MS, Thompson PD *et al.* Corticobasal degeneration: a clinical study of 36 cases. *Brain* 1994a; **117**:1183–96.

Rinne J, Daniel SE, Scaravilli F *et al.* The neuropathological features of acanthocytosis. *Mov Disord* 1994b; **9**:297–304.

Rinne UK, Bracco F, Chouza C *et al.* Cabergoline in the treatment of early Parkinson's disease: results of the first year of treatment in a double-blind comparison of cabergoline and levodopa. *Neurology* 1997; **48**:363–8.

Rippon GA, Scarmeas N, Gordon PH *et al.* An observational study of cognitive impairment in amyotrophic lateral sclerosis. *Arch Neurol* 2006; **63**:345–52.

Rivest L, Lees AJ, Marsden CED. Writer's cramp: treatment with botulinum toxin injections. *Mov Disord* 1991; **6**:55–9.

Rizzo R, Gulisano M, Pavone P *et al.* Increased antistreptococcal antibody titers and anti-basal ganglia antibodies in patients with Tourette's syndrome: controlled cross-sectional study. *J Child Neurol* 2006; **21**:747–53.

Robbins TW, James M, Lange KW *et al.* Cognitive performance in multiple system atrophy. *Brain* 1992; **115**:271–91.

Roberts RO, Cha RH, Knopman DS *et al.* Postmenopausal estrogen therapy and Alzheimer disease: overall negative findings. *Alzheimer Dis Assoc Disord* 2006; **20**:141–6.

Robertson EE, Le Roux A, Brown JH. The clinical differentiation of Pick's disease. *J Ment Sci* 1958; **104**:1000–24.

Robertson MM, Trimble MR, Lees AJ. The psychopathology of Gilles de la Tourette's syndrome: a phenomenological analysis. *Br J Psychiatry* 1988; **152**:388–90.

Rockwood K, Mintzer J, Truyen L *et al.* Effects of a flexible galantamine dose in Alzheimer's disease: a randomized, controlled trial. *J Neurol Neurosurg Psychiatry* 2001; **71**:589–95.

Rodriguez MC, Articda O, Zubieta JL *et al.* Reflex myoclonus in olivopontocerebellar atrophy. *J Neurol Neurosurg Psychiatry* 1994; **57**:316–19.

Rodriguez-Oroz MC, Zamarbide I, Guridi J *et al.* Efficacy of deep brain stimulation of the subthalamic nucleus in Parkinson's disease 4 years after surgery: double-blind and open label evaluation. *J Neurol Neurosurg Psychiatry* 2004; **75**:1382–5.

Rogers SL, Friedhoff LT. The efficacy and safety of donepezil in patients with Alzheimer's disease: results of a US multicentre randomized, double-blind, placebo-controlled study. *Dementia* 1996; **7**:293–303.

Rogers SL, Farlow MR, Doody RS *et al.* A 24-week, double-blind, placebo-controlled trial of donepezil in patients with Alzheimer's disease. *Neurology* 1998; **50**:136–45.

Rojo A, Pernaute RS, Fontan A *et al.* Clinical genetics of familial progressive supranuclear palsy. *Brain* 1999; **122**:1233–45.

Romanelli MF, Morris JC, Ashkin K *et al.* Advanced Alzheimer's disease is a risk factor for late-onset seizures. *Arch Neurol* 1990; **47**:847–50.

Rondot P, Marchand MP, Dellatolas G. Spasmodic torticollis – review of 220 patients. *Can J Neurol Sci* 1991; **18**:143–51.

Ropacki SA, Jeste DV. Epidemiology of and risk factors for psychosis of Alzheimer's disease: a review of 55 studies published from 1990 to 2003. *Am J Psychiatry* 2005; **162**:2022–30.

Ros R, Garre P, Hirano M *et al.* Genetic linkage of autosomal dominant progressive supranuclear palsy to 1q31.1. *Ann Neurol* 2005a; **57**:634–1.

Ros R, Thobois S, Streichenberger N *et al.* A new mutation in the tau gene, G303V, in early-onset familial progressive supranuclear palsy. *Arch Neurol* 2005b; **62**:1444–50.

Rosen DR, Siddique T, Patterson D *et al.* Mutations in Cu/Zn superoxide dismutase gene are associated with familial amyotrophic lateral sclerosis. *Nature* 1993; **362**:59–62.

Rosler M, Anand R, Cicin-Sain A *et al.* Efficacy and safety of rivastigmine in patients with Alzheimer's disease: international randomized controlled trial. *BMJ* 1999; **318**:633–40.

Rosman NP, Kakulas BA. Mental deficiency associated with muscular dystrophy: a neuropathological study. *Brain* 1966; **89**:769–87.

Ross SJM, Graham N, Stuart-Green L *et al.* Progressive biparietal atrophy: an atypical presentation of Alzheimer's disease. *J Neurol Neurosurg Psychiatry* 1996; **61**:388–95.

Rozdilsky B, Cummings JN, Huston AF. Hallervorden–Spatz disease: late infantile and adult types: report of two cases. *Acta Neuropatholog* 1968; **10**:1–16.

Rubinsztein JS, Rubinsztein DC, Goodburn S *et al.* Apathy and hypersomnia are common features of myotonic dystrophy. *J Neurol Neurosurg Psychiatry* 1998; **64**:510–15.

Ryan SG, Sherman SL, Terry JC *et al.* Startle disease, or hyperekplexia: response to clonazepam and assignment of the gene (STHE) to chromosome 5q by linkage analysis. *Ann Neurol* 1992; **31**:663–8.

Sabbagh MN, Hake AM, Ahmed S *et al.* The use of memantine in dementia with Lewy bodies. *J Alzheimer's Dis* 2005; **7**:285–9.

Saenz-Lope E, Herranz-Tanarro FJ, Masdeu JC *et al.* Hyperekplexia: a syndrome of pathological startle responses. *Ann Neurol* 1984; **15**:36–41.

Sakai T, Mawatari S, Hiroshi I *et al.* Choreoacanthocytosis: clues to the clinical diagnosis. *Arch Neurol* 1981; **38**:333–8.

Salen G. Cholesterol deposition in cerebrotendinous xanthomatosis. *Ann Intern Med* 1971; **75**:843–51.

Sallee FR, Nesbitt L, Jackson C *et al.* Relative efficacy of haloperidol and pimozide in children and adolescents with Tourette's disorder. *Am J Psychiatry* 1997; **154**:1057–62.

Sallee FR, Kurlan R, Goetz CG *et al.* Ziprasidone treatment of children and adolescents with Tourette's syndrome: a pilot study. *J Am Acad Child Adolesc Psychiatry* 2000; **39**:292–9.

Sasaki H, Fukazawa T, Yanagihara T *et al.* Clinical features and natural history of spinocerebellar ataxia type 1. *Acta Neurol Scand* 1996; **93**:64–71.

Saunders AM, Strittmatter WJ, Schmechel D *et al.* Association of apolipoprotein E allele epsilon 4 with late-onset and sporadic Alzheimer's disease. *Neurology* 1993; **43**:1467–72.

Sawle GV, Leenders KL, Brooks DJ *et al.* Dopa-responsive dystonia: [18F]dopa positron emission tomography. *Ann Neurol* 1991; **30**:24–30.

Scahill L, Chappell PB, Kim YS *et al.* A placebo-controlled study of guanfacine in the treatment of children with tic disorders and attention deficit hyperactivity disorder. *Am J Psychiatry* 2001; **158**:1067–74.

Scahill L, Leckman JF, Schultz RT *et al.* A placebo-controlled trial of risperidone in Tourette's syndrome. *Neurology* 2003; **60**:1130–5.

Scarmeas N, Hadjigeorgiou GM, Papadimitrou A *et al.* Motor signs during the course of Alzheimer disease. *Neurology* 2004; **63**:95–82.

Schaumburg HH, Powers JM, Raine CS *et al.* Adrenoleukodystrophy. A clinical and pathological study of 17 cases. *Arch Neurol* 1975; **32**:577–91.

Schiller A, Wevers RA, Steenbergen GCH *et al.* Long-term course of L-dopa responsive dystonia caused by tyrosine hydroxylase deficiency. *Neurology* 2004; **63**:1524–6.

Schimschock JR, Alvord EC, Swanson PD. Cerebrotendinous xanthomatosis: clinical and pathological studies. *Arch Neurol* 1968; **18**:688–98.

Schlote W, Harzer K, Christomanou H *et al.* Sphingolipid activator protein 1 deficiency in metachromatic leukodystrophy with normal arylsulfatase A activity. A clinical, morphological, biochemical and immunological study. *Eur J Pediatr* 1991; **150**:584–91.

Schmidt A, Jabusch H-C, Altenmuller E *et al.* Dominantly transmitted focal dystonia in families of patients with musician's cramp. *Neurology* 2006; **67**:691–3.

Schneider JA, Watts RL, Gearing M *et al.* Corticobasal degeneration: neuropathologic and clinical heterogeneity. *Neurology* 1997; **48**:959–69.

Schneider LS, DeKosky ST, Farlow MR *et al.* A randomized, double-blind, placebo-controlled trial of two doses of *Ginkgo biloba* extract in dementia of the Alzheimer's type. *Curr Alzheimer Res* 2005; **2**:541–51.

Schoenfeld M, Myers RH, Cupples LA *et al.* Increased rate of suicide among patients with Huntington's disease. *J Neurol Neurosurg Psychiatry* 1984; **47**:1283–7.

Schofield PW, Tang M, Marder K *et al.* Alzheimer's disease after remote head injury: an incidence study. *J Neurol Neurosurg Psychiatry* 1997; **62**:119–24.

Schols L, Amoiridis G, Epplen JT *et al.* Relations between genotype and phenotype in German patients with the Machado–Joseph disease mutation. *J Neurol Neurosurg Psychiatry* 1996; **61**:466–70.

Schols L, Amoiridis G, Buttner T *et al.* Autosomal dominant cerebellar ataxia: phenotypic differences in genetically defined subtypes? *Ann Neurol* 1997a; **42**:924–32.

Schols L, Gispert S, Vorgero M *et al.* Spinocerebellar ataxia type 2. Genotype and phenotype in German kindreds. *Arch Neurol* 1997b; **54**:1073–80.

Schols L, Kruger R, Amoiridis G *et al.* Spinocerebellar ataxia type 6: genotype and phenotype in German kindreds. *J Neurol Neurosurg Psychiatry* 1998; **54**:67–73.

Schwartz BL, Hashtroudi S, Herting RL *et al.* d-Cycloserine enhances implicit memory in Alzheimer patients. *Neurology* 1996; **46**:420–4.

Scooter AJC, Bronzoua J, Witteman JCM *et al.* Estrogen use and early onset Alzheimer's disease: a population-based study. *J Neurol Neurosurg Psychiatry* 1999; **67**:779–81.

Sechi GP, Tanda F, Mutani R. Fatal hyperpyrexia after withdrawal of levodopa. *Neurology* 1984; **34**:249–51.

Seltzer WK, Boss MA, Vieria-Saecker A-M *et al.* Expansion of a novel CAG trinucleotide repeat in the 5' region of PPP2R2B is associated with SCA 12. *Nat Genet* 1999; **23**:391–2.

Serby M, Angrist B, Lieberman A. Mental disturbances during bromocriptine and lergotrile treatment of Parkinson's disease. *Am J Psychiatry* 1978; **135**:1227–9.

Seshadri S, Zornberg GL, Derby LE *et al.* Postmenopausal estrogen replacement therapy and the risk of Alzheimer disease. *Arch Neurol* 2001; **58**:435–40.

Shahed J, Poysky J, Kenney C *et al.* GPi deep brain stimulation for Tourette syndrome improves tics and psychiatric comorbidities. *Neuroelogy* 2007; **68**:159–60.

Shannon KM, Bennett JP, Friedman JH *et al.* Efficacy of pramipexole, a novel dopamine agonist, as monotherapy in mild to moderate Parkinson's disease. *Neurology* 1997; **49**:724–8.

Shapiro E, Shapiro A, Fulop G *et al.* Controlled study of haloperidol, pimozide, and placebo for the treatment of Gilles de la Tourette's syndrome. *Arch Gen Psychiatry* 1989; **46**:722–30.

Shapiro EG, Lockman LA, Knopman D *et al.* Characteristics of the dementia in late-onset metachromatic leukodystrophy. *Neurology* 1994; **44**:662–5.

Shapiro E, Krivit W, Lockman L *et al.* Long-term effect of bone-marrow transplant for childhood-onset X-linked adrenoleukodystrophy. *Lancet* 2000; **356**:713–18.

Shatunov A, Sambuughin N, Jankovic J *et al.* Genomewide scans in North American families reveal genetic linkage of essential tremor to a region on chromosome 6p23. *Brain* 2006; **129**:2318–31.

Sheehy MP, Marsden CD. Writer's cramp – a focal dystonia. *Brain* 1982; **105**:461–80.

Shevell M. Hallervorden and history. *N Engl J Med* 2003; **348**:3–4.

Shiang R, Ryan SG, Zhu YZ *et al.* Mutations in the alpha-1 subunit of the glycine receptor cause the dominant neurologic disorder, hyperekplexia. *Nat Genet* 1993; **5**:351–8.

Shinotoh H, Calne DB, Snow B *et al.* Normal CAG repeat length in the Huntington's disease gene in senile chorea. *Neurology* 1994; **44**:2183–4.

Shy GM, Drager GA. A neurological syndrome associated with orthostatic hypotension: a clinico-pathologic study. *Arch Neurol* 1960; **2**:511–27.

Siddique T, Figlewicz DA, Pericak-Vance MA *et al.* Linkage of a gene causing familial amyotrophic lateral sclerosis to chromosome 21 and evidence of genetic-locus heterogeneity. *N Engl J Med* 1991; **324**:1381–4.

Siesling S, Vegter-van der Vlis M, Roos RAC. Juvenile Huntington's disease in the Netherlands. *Pediatr Neurol* 1997; **17**:34–43.

Singer HS, Hahn L-S, Moran TH. Abnormal dopamine uptake sites in postmortem striatum from patients with Tourette's syndrome. *Ann Neurol* 1991; **30**:558–62.

Singer HS, Reiss AL, Brown JE *et al.* Volumetric MRI changes in basal ganglia of children with Tourette's syndrome. *Neurology* 1993; **43**:950–6.

Singer HS, Giuliano JD, Hansen BH *et al.* Antibodies against human putamen in children with Tourette syndrome. *Neurology* 1998; **50**:1618–24.

Singer HS, Hong JJ, Yoo DY et al. Serum autoantibodies do not differentiate PANDAS and Tourette syndrome from controls. Neurology 2005; 65:1701-7.

Sinha S, Taly AB, Ravishankar S et al. Wilson's disease: cranial MRI observations and clinical correlation. Neuroradiology 2006; 48:613-21.

Siren A, Legros B, Crahine L et al. Hyperekplexia in Kurdish families: a possible GLRA1 founder mutation. Neurology 2006; 67:137-9.

Sjorgen T, Sjorgen H, Lindgren AGH. Morbus Alzheimer and Morbus Pick. Acta Psychiatr Neurol Scand 1952; 82(suppl.):1-152.

Snowden JS, Neary D, Mann DMA et al. Progressive language disorder due to lobar atrophy. Ann Neurol 1992; 31:174-83.

Snowden JS, Pickering-Brown SM, Mackenzie IR et al. Progranulin gene mutations associated with frontotemporal dementia and progressive non-fluent aphasia. Brain 2006; 129:3091-102.

Sobue G, Ueno-Natsukari I, Okamoto H et al. Phenotypic heterogeneity of an adult form of adrenoleukodystrophy in monozygotic twins. Ann Neurol 1994; 36:912-15.

Soffer D, Benharroch D, Berginer V. The neuropathology of cerebrotendinous xanthomatosis: a case report and a review of the literature. Acta Neuropathol 1995; 90:213-20.

Sorensen BF, Hamby WB. Spasmodic torticollis: results in 71 surgically treated patients. Neurology 1966; 16:867-78.

Spencer T, Biederman J, Coffey B et al. A double-blind comparison or desipramine and placebo in children and adolescents with chronic tic disorder and comorbid attention-deficit/hyperactivity disorder. Arch Gen Psychiatry 2002; 59: 649-56.

Stanford PM, Halliday GM, Brooks WS et al. Progressive supranuclear palsy pathology caused by a novel silent mutation in exon 10 of the tau gene: expansion of the disease phenotype caused by tau gene mutations. Brain 2000; 123:880-93.

Starkstein SE, Preziosi TJ, Bolduc PL et al. Depression in Parkinson's disease. J Nerv Ment Dis 1990; 178:27-31.

Starkstein SE, Migliorelli R, Teson A et al. Prevalence and clinical correlates of pathological affective display in Alzheimer's disease. J Neurol Neurosurg Psychiatry 1995; 59:55-60.

Starkstein SE, Chemerinski E, Sabe L et al. Prospective longitudinal study of depression and anosognosia in Alzheimer's disease. Br J Psychiatry 1997; 171:47-52.

Starkstein SE, Jorge R, Mizrahi R et al. The construct of minor and major depression in Alzheimer's disease. Am J Psychiatry 2005; 162:2086-93.

Starkstein WE, Jorge R, Mizrahi R et al. A prospective longitudinal study of apathy in Alzheimer's disease. J Neurol Neurosurg Psychiatry 2006; 77:8-11.

Starosta-Rubinstein S, Young AB, Kluin K et al. Clinical assessment of 31 patients with Wilson's disease: correlations with structural changes on magnetic resonance imaging. Arch Neurol 1987; 44:365-70.

Steele JC. Progressive supranuclear palsy. Brain 1972; 95:693-704.

Steele JC, Richardson JC, Olszewski J. Progressive supranuclear palsy: a heterogenous degeneration involving the brain stem, basal ganglia and cerebellum, with vertical gaze and pseudobulbar palsy, vertical dystonia and dementia. Arch Neurol 1964; 10:333-59.

Steinberger D, Korinthenberg R, Topka H et al. Dopa-responsive dystonia: mutation analysis of GCH1 and analysis of therapeutic doses of L-dopa. Neurology 2000; 55:1735-7.

Stern G. Parkinson's disease. London: Arnold, 1990.

Stern K. Severe dementia associated with bilateral symmetric degeneration of the thalamus. Brain 1939; 62:157-71.

Stern M, Roffwarg H, Duvoisin R. The parkinsonian tremor in sleep. J Nerv Ment Dis 1968; 147:202-10.

Stevanin G, Durr A, David G et al. Clinical and molecular features of spinocerebellar ataxia type 6. Neurology 1997; 49:1243-6.

Stevanin G, Herman A, Brice A et al. Clinical and MRI findings in spinocerebellar ataxia type 5. Neurology 1999; 53:1355-7.

Stewart WF, Kawas C, Corrada A et al. Risk of Alzheimer's disease and duration of NSAID use. Neurology 1997; 48:626-32.

Stone LA, Jankovic J. The coexistence of tics and dystonia. Arch Neurol 1991; 48:862-5.

Stracciari A, Tempestini A, Borghi A et al. Effect of liver transplantation on neurological manifestations in Wilson's disease. Arch Neurol 2000; 57:384-6.

Suhren AL, Bruyn GW, Tuyman JA. Hyperekplexia: a hereditary startle syndrome. J Neurol Sci 1966; 3:577-86.

Sveinbjornsdottir S, Hicks AA, Jonsson T et al. Familial aggregation of Parkinson's disease in Iceland. N Engl J Med 2000; 343:1765-70.

Swaiman KF. Hallervorden-Spatz syndrome and brain iron metabolism. Arch Neurol 1991; 48:1285-93.

Swanson PD, Cromwell LD. Magnetic resonance imaging in cerebrotendinous xanthomatosis. Neurology 1986; 36:124-6.

Swedo SE, Leonhard HL, Garvey M et al. Pediatric autoimmune neuropsychiatric disorders associated with streptococcal infections: clinical description of the first 50 cases. Am J Psychiatry 1998; 154:264-71.

Sydow O, Thobois S, Alesch F et al. Multicentre European study of thalamic stimulation in essential tremor: a six year follow up. J Neurol Neurosurg Psychiatry 2003; 74:1387-91.

Takahashi H, Oyanagi K, Takeda S et al. Occurrence of 15-nm wide straight tubules in neocortical neurons in progressive supranuclear palsy. Acta Neuropathol 1989; 79:233-9.

Takahashi H, Ohama E, Suzuki S et al. Familial juvenile parkinsonism: clinical and pathologic study in a family. Neurology 1994; 44:437-41.

Takahashi H, Yoshida K, Sugita T et al. Quetiapine treatment of psychotic symptoms and aggressive behavior in patients with dementia with Lewy bodies: a case series. Prog Neuropsychopharmacol Biol Psychiatry 2003; 27:549-53.

Takiyama T, Oyanagi S, Kawashima S et al. A clinical and pathologic study of a large Japanese family with Machado-Joseph disease tightly linked to the DNA markers on chromosome 14q. Neurology 1994; 44:1302-8.

Taly AB, Meenakshi-Sundaram S, Sinha S et al. Wilson disease: description of 282 patients evaluated over 3 decades. Medicine 2007; 86:112-21.

Tam CW, Burton EJ, McKeith IG et al. Temporal lobe atrophy on MRI in Parkinson disease with dementia: a comparison with

Alzheimer disease and dementia with Lewy bodies. *Neurology* 2005; **64**:861-5.

Tan E-K, Jankovic J. Genetic testing in Parkinson's disease. *Arch Neurol* 2006; **63**:1232-7.

Tandberg E, Larsen JP, Aarsland D *et al.* The occurrence of depression in Parkinson's disease: a community-based study. *Arch Neurol* 1996; **53**:175-9.

Tang B, Liu C, Shen L *et al.* Frequency of SCA1, SCA2, SCA3/MJD, SCA6, SCA7, and DRPLA CAG trinucleotide repeat expansion in patients with hereditary spinocerebellar ataxia from Chinese kindreds. *Arch Neurol* 2000; **57**:540-4.

Tang MX, Jacobs D, Stern Y *et al.* Effect of oestrogen during menopause on risk and age at onset of Alzheimer's disease. *Lancet* 1996; **348**:429-32.

Tanner CM, Glantz RH, Klawans HL. Meige disease: acute and chronic anticholinergic effects. *Neurology* 1982; **32**:783-5.

Tanner CM, Goldman SM, Lyons KE *et al.* Essential tremor in twins: an assessment of genetic vs environmental determinants of etiology. *Neurology* 2001; **57**:1389-91.

Terry RD, Peck A, DeTeresa R *et al.* Some morphometric aspects of the brain in senile dementia of the Alzheimer type. *Ann Neurol* 1981; **10**:184-92.

Thacker EL, O'Reilly EJ, Weisskopf MG *et al.* Temporal relationship between cigarette smoking and risk of Parkinson disease. *Neurology* 2007; **68**:764-8.

Thomas A, Iacono D, Luciano AL *et al.* Duration of amantadine benefit on dyskinesia of severe Parkinson's disease. *J Neurol Neurosurg Psychiatry* 2004; **75**:141-3.

Thomas AJ, Burn DJ, Rowan EN *et al.* A comparison of the efficacy of donepezil in Parkinson's disease with dementia and dementia with Lewy bodies. *Int J Geriatr Psychiatry* 2005; **20**:938-44.

Thomas GR, Forbes JR, Roberts EA *et al.* The Wilson disease gene: spectrum of mutations and their consequences. *Nat Genet* 1995; **9**:210-17.

Tijssen MA, Shiang R, van Deutekom J *et al.* Molecular genetic reevaluation of the Dutch hyperekplexia family. *Arch Neurol* 1995; **52**:578-82.

Timberlake WH, Vance MA. Four-year treatment of patients with parkinsonism using amantadine alone or with levodopa. *Ann Neurol* 1978; **3**:119-28.

Tinazzi M, Farina S, Bhatia K *et al.* TENS for the treatment of writer's cramp dystonia: a randomized, placebo-controlled study. *Neurology* 2005; **64**:1946-8.

Tiraboschi P, Hansen LA, Alford M *et al.* Early and widespread cholinergic losses differentiate dementia with Lewy bodies from Alzheimer disease. *Arch Gen Psychiatry* 2002; **59**:946-51.

Tiraboschi P, Salmon DP, Hansen LA *et al.* What best differentiates Lewy body from Alzheimer's disease in early-stage dementia? *Brain* 2006; **129**:729-35.

Tison F, Dartigues JF, Auriacombe S *et al.* Dementia in Parkinson's disease: population-based study in ambulatory and institutionalized individuals. *Neurology* 1995; **45**:705-8.

Tolosa ES. Clinical features of Meige's disease (idiopathic orofacial dystonia): a report of 17 cases. *Arch Neurol* 1981; **38**:147-51.

Tolosa ES, Klawans HC. Meige's disease: a clinical form of facial convulsion, bilateral and medial. *Arch Neurol* 1979; **36**:635-7.

Toru M, Matsuda O, Makiguchi K *et al.* Single case study: neuroleptic malignant syndrome-like state following a withdrawal of antiparkinsonian drugs. *J Nerv Ment Dis* 1981; **169**:324-7.

de la Tourette G. Etude sur une affection nerveuse, characterisee par de 'incoordination motrice, accompagne d'cholalie et de coprolalie. *Arch Neurol* (Paris) 1885; **9**:158-200.

Tourette's Syndrome Study Group. Treatment of ADHD in children with tics: a randomized controlled trial. *Neurology* 2002; **58**:527-36.

Tsai CH, Chang FC, Su YC *et al.* Two novel mutations of the glycine receptor gene in a Taiwanese hyperekplexia family. *Neurology* 2004; **63**:893-6.

Tsai G, Falk W, Gunther J *et al.* Improved cognition in Alzheimer's disease with short-term D-cycloserine treatment. *Am J Psychiatry* 1999; **1567**:467-9.

Tsuang D, Almquist EW, Lipe H *et al.* Familial aggregation of psychotic symptoms in Huntington's disease. *Am J Psychiatry* 2000; **157**:1955-9.

Turner RS, Kenyon LC, Trojanowski JQ *et al.* Clinical, neuroimaging, and pathologic features of progressive nonfluent aphasia. *Ann Neurol* 1996; **39**:166-73.

Ueyama H, Kumanoto T, Nagao S *et al.* Clinical and genetic studies of spinocerebellar ataxia type 2 in Japanese kindreds. *Acta Neurol Scand* 1998; **98**:427-32.

Vadlamudi L, Westmoreland BF, Klass DW *et al.* Electroencephalographic findings in Kufs disease. *Clin Neurophysiol* 2003; **114**:1738-43.

Valente EM, Bentivoglio AR, Cassetta E *et al.* DYT13, a novel primary torsion dystonia locus, maps to chromosome 1p36.13-36.32 in an Italian family with cranial-cervical or upper limb onset. *Ann Neurol* 2001; **49**:362-6.

Van Bogaert L, Dewulf A. Diffuse progressive leukodystrophy in the adult with production of metachromatic degenerative products. *Arch Neurol Psychiatry* 1939; **42**:1083-97.

Vance C, Al-Chalabi A, Ruddy D *et al.* Familial amyotrophic lateral sclerosis with frontotemporal dementia is linked to a locus on chromosome 9p13.2-21.3. *Brain* 2006; **129**:868-76.

Vanek Z, Jankovic J. Dystonia in corticobasal degeneration. *Mov Disord* 2001; **16**:252-7.

Van Hove JLK, Steyaert J, Matthijs G *et al.* Expanded motor and psychiatric phenotype in autosomal dominant Segawa syndrome due to GTP cyclohydrolase deficiency. *J Neurol Neurosurg Psychiatry* 2006; **77**:18-23.

Varga E, Sugerman AA, Varga V *et al.* Prevalence of spontaneous oral dyskinesia in the elderly. *Am J Psychiatry* 1982; **139**:329-31.

Vazquez A, Jimenez-Jimenez FJ, Garcia-Ruiz P *et al.* 'Panic attacks' in Parkinson's disease. A long-term complication of levodopa therapy. *Acta Neurol Scand* 1993; **87**:14-18.

Verbaan D, Marinus J, Visser M *et al.* Patient-reported autonomic symptoms in Parkinson disease. *Neurology* 2007; **69**: 333-41.

Verhagen Metman L, Del Dotto P, van den Munckhof P *et al.* Amantadine as treatment for dyskinesias and motor fluctuations in Parkinson's disease. *Neurology* 1998; **50**:1323–6.

Verhagen Metman L, Morris MJ, Farmer C *et al*. Huntington's disease: a randomized, controlled trial using the NMDA-antagonist amantadine. *Neurology* 2002; **59**:694–9.

Verny M, Jellinger KA, Hauw J-J *et al*. Progressive supranuclear palsy: a clinicopathological study of 21 cases. *Acta Neuropathol* 1996; **91**:427–31.

Verrips A, Hofsloot LH, Steenbergen GCH *et al*. Clinical and molecular genetic characteristics of patients with cerebrotendinous xanthomatosis. *Brain* 2000a; **123**: 908–19.

Verrips A, van Engelen BGM, Wevers RA *et al*. Presence of diarrhea and absence of tendon xanthomas in patients with cerebrotendinous xanthomatosis. *Arch Neurol* 2000b; **57**:520–4.

Vessie PR. On the transmission of Huntington's chorea for 300 years – the Bures family group. *J Nerv Ment Dis* 1932; **76**:553–73.

Vidhailet M, Vercueil L, Houeto J-L *et al*. Bilateral deep-brain stimulation of the globus pallidus in primary generalized dystonia. *N Engl J Med* 2005; **352**:459–67.

Villani F, Gellera C, Spreafilo R *et al*. Clinical and molecular findings in the first identified Italian family with dentatorubral-pallidoluysian atrophy. *Acta Neurol Scand* 1998; **98**:324–7.

Voon V, Hassan K, Zurowski M *et al*. Prevalence of repetitive and reward-seeking behaviors in Parkinson disease. *Neurology* 2006a; **67**:1254–7.

Voon V, Hassan K, Zurowski M *et al*. Prospective prevalence of pathologic gambling and medication association in Parkinson disease. *Neurology* 2006b; **66**:1750–2.

Walker RH, Rasmussen A, Rudnicki D *et al*. Huntington's disease-like 2 can present as chorea-acanthocytosis. *Neurology* 2002; **61**:1002–4.

Walker Z, Grace J, Overshot N *et al*. Olanzapine in dementia with Lewy bodies: a clinical study. *Int J Geriatr Psychiatry* 1999; **14**:459–66.

Walsh PJ. Adrenoleukodystrophy: report of two cases with relapsing and remitting courses. *Arch Neurol* 1980; **37**:448–50.

Walshe JM, Yealland M. Wilson's disease: the problem of delayed diagnosis. *J Neurol Neurosurg Psychiatry* 1992; **55**:692–6.

Waltz G, Harik SI, Kaufman B. Adult metachromatic leukodystrophy: value of computed tomographic scanning and magnetic resonance imaging of the brain. *Arch Neurol* 1987; **44**:225–7.

Warner TT, Lennox GG, Janota I *et al*. Autosomal-dominant dentatorubropallidoluysian atrophy. *Mov Disord* 1994; **9**:289–96.

Warner TT, Williams LD, Walker RWH *et al*. A clinical and molecular genetic study of dentatorubropallidoluysian atrophy in four European families. *Ann Neurol* 1995; **37**:452–9.

Warren JD, Firgaira F, Thompson EM *et al*. The causes of sporadic and 'senile' chorea. *Aust N Z J Med* 1998; **28**:429–31.

Wasco W, Pettingell WP, Jondro PD *et al*. Familial Alzheimer's chromosome 14 mutations. *Nat Med* 1995; **1**:848.

Watanabe H, Saito Y, Terao S *et al*. Progression and prognosis in multiple system atrophy. An analysis of 230 Japanese patients. *Brain* 2002; **125**:1070–83.

Waters CH, Kurth M, Bailey P *et al*. Tolcapone in stable Parkinson's disease: efficacy and safety of long-term treatment. *Neurology* 1997; **49**:665–71.

Watts GF, Mitchell WD, Bending JJ *et al*. Cerebrotendinous xanthomatosis: a family study and pharmacotherapy. *Q J Med* 1996; **89**:55–63.

Wechsler AF, Verity A, Rosenschein S *et al*. Pick's disease: a clinical computed tomographic and histologic study with Golgi impregnation observation. *Arch Neurol* 1982; **39**:287–90.

Weiden P, Bruun R. Worsening of Tourette's syndrome due to neuroleptic-induced akathisia. *Am J Psychiatry* 1987; **144**:504–5.

Weiner MF, Risser RC, Cullum CM *et al*. Alzheimer's disease and its Lewy body variant: a clinical analysis of postmortem verified cases. *Am J Psychiatry* 1996; **153**:1269–73.

Weiner WJ, Nora LM. 'Trick' movements in facial dystonia. *J Clin Psychiatry* 1984; **45**:519–21.

Weiner WJ, Nausieda PA, Glantz RH. Meige syndrome (blepharospasm-oromandibulardysonia) after long-term neuroleptic therapy. *Neurology* 1981; **31**:1555–6.

Weiner WJ, Minagar A, Shulman LM. Quetiapine for L-dopa-induced psychosis in PD. *Neurology* 2000; **54**:1538.

Weller M, Liedtke W, Petersen D *et al*. Very-late-onset adrenoleukodystrophy: possible precipitation of demyelination by cerebral contusion. *Neurology* 1992; **42**:367–70.

Wenning GK, Shlomo YB, Megalhaes M *et al*. Clinical features and natural history of multiple system atrophy: an analysis of 100 cases. *Brain* 1994; **117**:835–45.

Wenning GK, Ben-Shlomo Y, Magalhaes M *et al*. Clinicopathological study of 35 cases of multiple system atrophy. *J Neurol Neurosurg Psychiatry* 1995; **58**:160–6.

Wenning GK, Tison F, Elliott L *et al*. Olivopontocerebellar pathology in multiple system atrophy. *Mov Disord* 1996; **11**:157–62.

Wenning GK, Litvan I, Jankovic J *et al*. Natural history and survival of 14 patients with corticobasal degeneration confirmed at postmortem examination. *J Neurol Neurosurg Psychiatry* 1998; **64**:184–9.

Wesnes KA, McKeith IG, Ferrara R *et al*. Effects of rivastigmine on cognitive function in dementia with Lewy bodies: a randomized, placebo-controlled international study using the cognitive drug research computerized assessment system. *Dement Geriatr Cogn Disord* 2002; **13**:183–92.

Whitehouse P, Price D, Clark A *et al*. Alzheimer's disease: evidence for a selective loss of cholinergic cells in the nucleus basalis. *Ann Neurol* 1981; **10**:122–6.

Whitehouse PJ, Price DL, Struble RG *et al*. Alzheimer's disease and senile dementia: loss of neurons in the basal forebrain. *Science* 1982; **215**:1237–9.

Wilkins RH, Brody IA. Alzheimer's disease. *Arch Neurol* 1969a; **21**:109–10.

Wilkins RH, Brody IA. Parkinson's syndrome. *Arch Neurol* 1969b; **20**:440–5.

Wilson CM, Grace GM, Munoz DG *et al.* Cognitive impairment in sporadic ALS. A pathologic continuum underlying a multisystem disorder. *Neurology* 2001; **57**:651–7.

Wilson SAK. Progressive lenticular degeneration: a familial nervous disease associated with cirrhosis of the liver. *Brain* 1912; **34**:295–509.

Winblad S, Lindberg C, Hansen S. Temperament and character in patients with classical myotonic dystrophy type 1 (DM-1). *Neuromuscul Disord* 2005; **15**:287–92.

Winkler GF, Young RR. Efficacy of chronic propranolol therapy in action tremors of the familial, senile or essential varieties. *N Engl J Med* 1974; **290**:984–8.

Wintzen AR, Lammers GJ, van Dijk JG. Does modafinil enhance activity of patients with myotonic dystrophy? A double-blind placebo-controlled crossover study. *J Neurol* 2007; **254**: 26–8.

Wisniewski HM, Coblentz JM, Terry RD. Pick's disease: a clinical and ultrastructural study. *Arch Neurol* 1972; **26**:97–108.

Wojcieszek JM, Lang AE. Gestes antagonistes in the suppression of tics: 'tricks for tics'. *Mov Disord* 1995; **10**:226–8.

Worth PF, Giunti P, Gardner-Thorpe C *et al.* Autosomal dominant cerebellar ataxia type III: linkage in a large British family to a 7.6cM region on chromosome 15q14–21.3. *Am J Hum Genet* 1999; **65**:420–6.

Wright RB, Glantz RH, Butcher J. Hearing loss in myotonic dystrophy. *Ann Neurol* 1988; **23**:202–3.

Wulff CH, Trojaborg W. Adult metachromatic leukodystrophy: neurophysiologic findings. *Neurology* 1985; **35**:1776–8.

Yamamoto T, Hirano A. Nucleus raphe dorsalis in Alzheimer's disease: neurofibrillary tangles and loss of large neurons. *Ann Neurol* 1985; **17**:573–7.

Yamashita I, Sasaki H, Yabe I *et al.* A novel locus for dominant cerebellar ataxia (SCA 14) maps to a 10.2–cM interval flanked by D19S206 and D19S605 on chromosome 19q13.4–qter. *Ann Neurol* 2000; **48**:156–63.

Yardimci N, Karatas M, Kilinc M *et al.* Levetiracetam in Meige's syndrome. *Acta Neurol Scand* 2006; **114**:63–6.

Yasuda M, Nakamura Y, Kawamata T *et al.* Phenotypic heterogeneity within a new family with the *MAPT* P301S mutation. *Ann Neurol* 2005; **58**:920–8.

de Yebenes JG, Sarasa JL, Daniel SE *et al.* Familial progressive supranuclear palsy: description of a pedigree and review of the literature. *Brain* 1995; **118**:1095–103.

Yoshii F, Tomiyasu H, Shinohara Y. Fluid attenuation inversion recovery (FLAIR) images of dentatorubropallidoluysian atrophy: case report. *J Neurol Neurosurg Psychiatry* 1998; **65**:396–9.

Younger DS, Rowland LP, Latov N *et al.* Lymphoma, motor neuron disease, and amyotrophic lateral sclerosis. *Ann Neurol* 1991; **29**:78–86.

Zandi PP, Carlson MC, Plassman BL *et al.* Hormone replacement therapy and incidence of Alzheimer disease in older women: the Cache County study. *JAMA* 2002; **288**:2123–9.

Zanettini R, Antonini A, Gatto G *et al.* Valvular heart disease and the use of dopamine agonists for Parkinson's disease. *N Engl J Med* 2007; **356**:39–46.

Zappacosta B, Monza D, Meoni C *et al.* Psychiatric symptoms do not correlate with cognitive decline, motor symptoms, or CAG repeat length in Huntington's disease. *Arch Neurol* 1996; **53**:493–7.

Zhou B, Westaway SK, Levinson B *et al.* A novel pantothenate kinase gene (*PANK2*) is defective in Hallervorden-Sptaz syndrome. *Nat Genet* 2001; **28**:345–9.

Zhou YX, Takiyama Y, Igarashi S *et al.* Machado–Joseph disease in four Chinese pedigrees: molecular analysis of 15 patients including two juvenile cases and clinical correlations. *Neurology* 1997; **48**:482–5.

Zhou Y-X, Wang G-X, Tang B-S *et al.* Spinocerebellar ataxia type 2 in China: molecular analysis and genotype–phenotype correlation in nine families. *Neurology* 1998; **51**:595–8.

Zhukareva V, Mann D, Pickering-Brown S *et al.* Sporadic Pick's disease: a tauopathy characterized by a spectrum of pathological tau isoforms in gray and white matter. *Ann Neurol* 2002; **51**:730–9.

Zubenko GS, Moosy J. Major depression in primary dementia: clinical and neuropathologic correlates. *Arch Neurol* 1998; **45**:1182–6.

Zweig RM, Ross CA, Hedreen JC *et al.* The neuropathology of aminergic nuclei in Alzheimer's disease. *Ann Neurol* 1988; **24**:233–42.

9

Congenital, developmental, and other childhood-onset disorders

9.1 STURGE–WEBER SYNDROME

The Sturge–Weber syndrome, also known as the Sturge–Weber–Dimitri syndrome or encephalotrigeminal angiomatosis, first described by William Sturge in 1879 (Sturge 1879), is a rare disorder, characterized, classically, by a unilateral facial port-wine stain, epilepsy, hemiplegia, and mental retardation, and, on appropriate imaging, cerebral cortical calcification in the hemisphere ipsilateral to the port-wine stain (Chao 1959; Lichtenstein 1954; Pascual-Castroviejo et al. 1993; Petermann et al. 1958; Sujansky and Conradi 1995a,b).

Clinical features

The port-wine stain, also known as a nevus flammeus, is present at birth, and, at a minimum, covers the area of distribution of the first division of the trigeminal nerve, including the upper eyelid; in some cases the stain may extend down the face to the second or even third division, and may even reach the side of the neck. Although in most cases the stain is unilateral, bilateral involvement may occur in a small minority; rarely there may be no port-wine stain (Aydin et al. 2000; Taly et al. 1987).

Seizures occur in the great majority of patients and, although they can first appear at any time from infancy to early adult years, the vast majority of patients will begin having seizures in the first year of life. Simple partial motor seizures are classic, and when these do occur the motor activity is seen contralateral to the hemisphere affected by calcification. Complex partial seizures may also occur, and secondary generalization to grand mal seizures is common.

Mental retardation occurs in the majority of patients, and, in those with frequent seizures, there may be a decrement in cognitive abilities (Lichtenstein 1954; Petermann et al. 1958).

Other symptoms that may occur include the following: hemiplegia and hemiatrophy, contralateral to the hemisphere with calcification; an enlarged eye, present in infancy, known as bupthalmos ('ox-eye'); and glaucoma, which may occur at any age. It is also becoming apparent that the majority of patients will also have stroke-like episodes (Maria et al. 1998).

Cortical calcification may not become evident on imaging until after the age of 2 years but becomes progressively more common with the passage of time, eventually appearing in approximately 90 percent of patients over the age of 20 years. On skull films, the calcification appears in a classic curvilinear 'trolly-track' pattern, and on computed tomography (CT) scanning, as illustrated in Figure 9.1, there is a 'serpiginous' pattern. Magnetic resonance (MR) scanning, in addition to revealing calcification, may also demonstrate leptomeningeal vascular malformations (Benedikt et al. 1993).

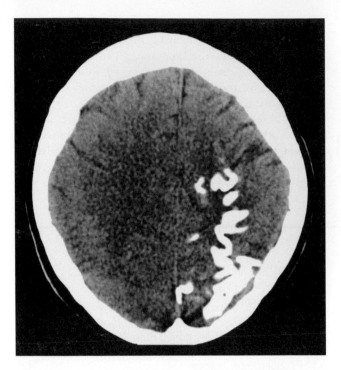

Figure 9.1 This unenhanced computed tomography scan demonstrates the serpiginous calcification seen in the Sturge–Weber syndrome. (Reproduced from Gillespie and Jackson 2000.)

Course

With the exception of intellectual decrement seen in some patients with frequent seizures, and of any decrements seen secondary to stroke-like episodes, the overall course is for the most part static.

Etiology

Neuropathologically (Roizen *et al.* 1972; Weber 1929; Wohlwill and Yakovlev 1957), the hallmark of the disorder is a unilateral leptomeningeal angiomatosis, primarily venular in type, which, though often confined to the occipitoparietal area, may extend forward to the frontal area and, in some cases, may be bilateral (Bebin and Gomez 1988). In the subjacent cortex there is calcification in the walls of small arteries, free calcium deposits within the brain parenchyma, and neuronal loss and gliosis.

The vast majority of cases are sporadic.

Differential diagnosis

The combination of a facial port-wine stain, seizures, and cortical calcification is pathognomonic for Sturge–Weber syndrome. In those rare cases in which the port-wine stain is absent, consideration is given to celiac disease, characterized by occipital calcification and seizures. It must also be borne in mind that isolated port-wine stains are not at all

uncommon, and that the diagnosis of Sturge–Weber syndrome should never be made on the basis of a port-wine stain alone.

Treatment

Given the association of seizures with intellectual decrement, vigorous treatment with anti-epilepsy drugs (AEDs) is imperative. In treatment-resistant cases, consideration should be given to neurosurgical intervention (Arzimanoglou *et al.* 2000). Given the possibility of stroke-like episodes, many physicians will also treat patients prophylactically with aspirin. The port-wine stain may be treated with laser surgery; glaucoma is treated in the usual way, and, in cases in which glaucoma is absent, yearly monitoring of intraocular pressure is indicated. The treatment of mental retardation is discussed in Section 5.5.

9.2 TUBEROUS SCLEROSIS

Tuberous sclerosis, also known as Bourneville's disease or epiloia, is a rare genetic disorder presenting, classically, with the triad of seizures, mental retardation, and a particular skin lesion known as adenoma sebaceum (Alsen *et al.* 1994; Critchley and Earl 1932; Devlin *et al.* 2006; Lagos and Gomez 1967; Monaghan *et al.* 1981; Pampiglione and Moynahan 1976; Ross and Dickerson 1943; Webb and Osborne 1995). Although brain lesions, known as tubers, figure most prominently in this disorder, it must be borne in mind that tuberous sclerosis is a systemic disease, with additional lesions in the skin, eye, kidneys, heart, and lungs.

Clinical features

In most cases, the first sign of tuberous sclerosis is the presence of hypomelanotic macules, evident in 90 percent or more of affected infants. These macules, which are best seen with Wood's light, range in size from a few millimeters to 2 or 3 cm, and are sometimes oval shaped, giving rise to the name 'ash leaf' spots. Additional skin lesions include adenoma sebaceum and what are known as 'shagreen patches'. Adenoma sebaceum typically appears gradually in early childhood and is present in over 90 percent of those over the age of 4 years; it consists of multiple minute facial nodules, generally arranged in a symmetrical butterfly shape over the nose, cheeks, and chin, with, typically, sparing of the upper lip. Shagreen patches are leathery-appearing areas, most frequently seen in the lumbar region.

Seizures may first appear at any point in childhood, adolescence, or even late adult years (Gutowski and Murphy 1992). Seizures appearing in the first 2 years of life are generally of the 'salaam' or infantile spasm type (Roth and Epstein 1971). Other seizure types, especially complex partial and grand mal seizures, may also appear, not only, as it were, to replace infantile spasms but also as the first seizure type in those patients whose seizures begin at a later age.

Mental retardation is seen in approximately two-thirds of patients. Furthermore, and especially in those with frequent seizures, there may be a progressive cognitive decline, thus constituting a dementia. Autism may occur in up to one-quarter of all patients (Alsen *et al.* 1994; Gutierrez *et al.* 1998; Lawlor and Maurer 1987), and is more likely in those both with tubers in the temporal lobe and frequent seizures of temporal lobe onset (Bolton and Griffiths 1997; Bolton *et al.* 2002). In a very small minority of patients, hydrocephalus may occur secondary to occlusion of the foramen of Monro by a tuber or astrocytoma, with the development of further cognitive decline accompanied by headache and gait disturbance.

Other lesions include subungual fibromas, retinal phakomas, renal angiomyolipomas and cysts, cardiac rhabdolipomas, and pulmonary cysts.

Neuroimaging reveals the distinctive tubers. Tubers typically undergo calcification and, when this occurs, they are immediately apparent on skull radiographs or CT scanning. Magnetic resonance scanning also reveals calcified tubers and may also identify uncalcified ones, which may be missed on CT scanning. The electroencephalogram (EEG) is marked by slowing and interictal epileptiform activity, which is often multifocal. Genetic testing is available.

Course

Tuberous sclerosis is a gradually progressive disease. Those with an early childhood onset, especially those with severe epilepsy, rarely survive for more than 15 years, eventually succumbing to status epilepticus or cardiac or renal complications. In adult-onset cases, the progression tends to be much slower, and the disease may be compatible with a normal lifespan.

Etiology

Tuberous sclerosis occurs secondary to mutations in either one of two genes: *TSC1* is located on chromosome 9 and codes for a protein known as hamartin; *TSC2* is on chromosome 16 and codes for tuberin (European Chromosome 16 Tuberous Sclerosis Consortium 1993; Fryer *et al.* 1987; Hyman and Whittemore 2000). Hamartin and tuberin function as tumor suppressor proteins, and it is presumably a lack of this normal 'suppression' that allows for the development of the tubers and other manifestations of the disease. Approximately two-thirds of cases represent spontaneous mutations, whereas in the remaining one-third the disease is inherited on an autosomal dominant basis.

Tubers are nodules of varying size, ranging from millimeters to 2 cm or more, and are composed of glia and enlarged, 'ballooned', neuronal elements. They are typically found both in the cerebral cortex and in the subependymal white matter: in some cases subependymal tubers may protrude into the ventricle and may be so numerous that they impart a 'candle guttering' appearance to the surface of the ventricle (Richardson 1991). Tubers, as noted, typically undergo calcification, and the calcification may be so pronounced as to produce 'brain stones' (Yakovlev and Corwin 1939). Some tubers may undergo malignant transformation into astrocytomas (Goh *et al.* 2004; Morimoto and Mogami 1986), and tubers (or astrocytomas) adjacent to the foramen of Monro may cause occlusion and noncommunicating hydrocephalus.

Differential diagnosis

The classic triad of seizures, mental retardation, and adenoma sebaceum is pathognomonic. As noted earlier, however, about one-third of patients will have normal intelligence, and such cases may present with seizures alone in adult years (Kofman and Hyland 1959). In these cases, diagnostic suspicion may be aroused by skin lesions, such as ash leaf spots or adenoma sebaceum, or by finding tubers on imaging.

Treatment

Seizure control is imperative. Infantile spasms may respond to adrenocorticotropic hormone (ACTH) or vigabatrin. Partial or grand mal seizures may be treated with the usual AEDs, with, however, some caveats. In some cases renal failure may occur, making the use of AEDs that undergo primary renal excretion problematic. Other AEDs, such as carbamazepine (Weig and Pollack 1993), may precipitate cardiac block in patients with cardiac lesions. In treatment-resistant cases in which there is a single, well-localized epileptogenic zone, surgical resection may be considered (Jarrar *et al.* 2004).

Obstructive hydrocephalus may respond to neurosurgical intervention. Tubers that have undergone transformation into astrocytomas may also respond to treatment with rapamycin (Franz *et al.* 2006).

Mental retardation and autism are treated in the usual fashion, as discussed in Sections 5.5 and 9.14 respectively. When severe, adenoma sebaceum may be surgically treated, but recurrences are the rule. Genetic counselling should be offered, not only to patients but also, given that some cases (perhaps manifest only by subtle skin lesions) may go undetected, to relatives.

9.3 VON RECKLINGHAUSEN'S DISEASE (NEUROFIBROMATOSIS TYPE 1)

Von Recklinghausen's disease, also known as neurofibromatosis type 1 or 'peripheral' neurofibromatosis, is a not uncommon genetic disorder characterized by skin lesions (such as café au lait spots), peripheral neurofibromas, and, in a minority, central nervous system tumors, such as optic nerve gliomas. Attention-deficit/hyperactivity disorder (ADHD), developmental disabilities, and, in a small minority, mental retardation may also occur.

Clinical features

The cardinal features of von Recklinghausen's disease are café au lait spots and neurofibromas (Huson *et al.* 1988). Café au lait spots are generally present in infancy and grow in number and size throughout adolescence. Neurofibromas appear around puberty, are generally either pedunculated or sessile, and may be as large as a walnut or no bigger than a grain of sand; they typically appear on the trunk or the extremities, generally sparing the face, and range in number from a few up to literally hundreds. Large plexiform neurofibromas may occasionally occur, and these may be extremely disfiguring. Neurofibromas may be painful to strong touch and at times spontaneous neuralgic pains may occur. In a small minority, neurofibromas may appear on the central portion of peripheral nerves, and in such cases compression of adjacent structures may occur.

Other features found in adults include Lisch nodules and axillary freckling. Lisch nodules (Lubs *et al.* 1991) are small, yellow-brown spots on the iris that are at times visible only by slit-lamp examination. Axillary freckling, although found only in a minority, is virtually pathognomonic of von Recklinghausen's disease. Seizures may occur in a very small minority (Kulkantrakorn and Geller 1998).

Central nervous system tumors, such as astrocytomas, meningiomas, and, most commonly, optic nerve gliomas, may occur (Creange *et al.* 1999; Guillamo *et al.* 2003; Listernick *et al.* 1989; Rodriguez and Barthrong 1966). Peripheral neurofibromas may undergo sarcomatous change, an event heralded both by an increase in size and by the occurrence or exacerbation of pain. Other malignancies seen in von Recklinghausen's disease include pheochromocytoma, Wilm's tumor, and various leukemias.

Attention-deficit/hyperactivity disorder occurs in roughly one-third of patients; various developmental disabilities, such as developmental dyslexia, also occur in about one-third of patients and appear more likely in males; and mental retardation is seen in a little over 5 percent (Hyman *et al.* 2005). Precocious puberty may occur in a small minority.

Magnetic resonance scanning will reveal central nervous system tumors. Of note, in children and adolescents there may also, on T2-weighted scans, be multiple areas of increased signal intensity in the brainstem, basal ganglia, thalamus, and cerebral and cerebellar white matter (Guillamo *et al.* 2003), which, in some (Feldmann *et al.* 2003; Hyman *et al.* 2003; North *et al.* 1994), but not all (Legius *et al.* 1995), studies, have been correlated with the occurrence of cognitive deficits. Of interest, the number of these areas within the gray matter structures actually decreases with age (DiMario *et al.* 1998; Hyman *et al.* 2003).

Course

Neurofibromas typically show a period of progression in early adolescence, whereas in adult years, although progression may still occur, there are typically long periods of quiescence. Pregnancy and the use of oral contraceptives may prompt renewed growth. Most patients live a normal lifespan; exceptions may occur in those who develop any of the various tumors noted earlier.

Etiology

Von Recklinghausen's disease occurs secondary to any of a large number of different mutations in a gene on chromosome 17 (Wallace *et al.* 1990) that codes for a protein known as neurofibromin (von Deimling *et al.* 1995). About half of cases represent spontaneous mutations, whereas the other half are inherited on an autosomal dominant basis. Of note, although penetrance is near 100 percent, expressivity is quite variable, and there is considerable inter- and intrafamilial phenotypic variability. Neurofibromin acts as a tumor suppressor protein, and it is apparently a deficiency of such suppression by the abnormal protein that allows for the clinical manifestations of the disease.

Neurofibromas constitute the neuropathologic hallmark of the disease, and these may occur peripherally, where they are composed of fibroblasts and Schwann cells, or centrally, in which case one finds fibroblasts and astrocytes. Within the central nervous system one also finds scattered glial nodules, neuronal heterotopias, and areas of cortical dysplasia (Rosman and Pearce 1967), and, in the white matter, areas of spongiosus (DiPaolo *et al.* 1995). Presumably these abnormalities account for the T2 hyperintensities seen on MR scanning and for the ADHD, developmental disabilities, and mental retardation. As noted earlier, various tumors, such as optic nerve gliomas, astrocytomas, and meningiomas, may also occur.

Differential diagnosis

The diagnosis is self-evident when numerous neurofibromas are present. When these are lacking, the diagnosis may depend on dermatologic findings, such as café au lait spots or axillary freckling. Importantly, isolated café au lait spots are not uncommon and, hence, to make the diagnosis it is necessary to find six or more of these measuring at least 0.5 cm in diameter in children and 1.5 cm in adults.

Von Recklinghausen's disease must be differentiated from neurofibromatosis type 2, also known as 'central' neurofibromatosis. Neurofibromatosis type 2 is a very rare disorder that is clinically and genetically distinct: clinically, it presents with intracranial tumors, classically bilateral acoustic neuromas, and genetically, it results from mutations in a gene on chromosome 22 (Rouleau *et al.* 1987); cutaneous manifestations in neurofibromatosis type 2 are either absent or very scant.

Treatment

Given that surgery to neurofibromas may predispose to sarcomatous change, excision should be reserved for disfiguring peripheral neurofibromas or for central neurofibromas that are causing compression injury. Other tumors are treated in the usual fashion; bilateral optic gliomas may also be subjected to radiation treatment. Attention-deficit/hyperactivity disorder, developmental disabilities, and mental retardation are treated in the usual fashion. Genetic counselling should be offered, and it should be stressed to patients with mild symptoms that, given the considerable intrafamilial phenotypic heterogeneity, should they have children then those children may be severely affected by the disease.

9.4 DOWN'S SYNDROME

Down's syndrome, first described by John Langdon Down in 1866 (Down 1866), is one of the most common causes of mental retardation in the United States. It is also known as trisomy 21; however, this synonym may not be appropriate because, although about 95 percent of cases are due to trisomy 21, the remainder, which are clinically indistinguishable, occur as a result of translocations.

Clinical features

The appearance of patients is so characteristic as to allow a diagnosis in infancy. The head is small with a flattened occiput. The palpebral fissures show a distinctive oblique slant, and epicanthal folds are present. The bridge of the nose is broad, the mouth is generally small, and the tongue, which is typically enlarged, often protrudes. The patients tend to be of short stature. The hands are broad and foreshortened, and the fifth finger is often curved inward; further, the palms often display a transverse or 'Simian' crease. The first and second toes are often separated by a wide gap. The external genitalia are often small; puberty may be delayed and fertility in males is often reduced.

Mental retardation ranges from mild to severe, but, in many cases, social skills are more advanced than cognitive ones, and patients with Down's syndrome tend to be affable, outgoing, and pleasant. A small minority will suffer from autism (Lund and Munk-Jorgensen 1988).

Dementia due to Alzheimer's disease occurs in adults with Down's syndrome (Collacott et al. 1992; Jervis 1948; Lai and Williams 1989; Lund and Munk-Jorgensen 1988), with an ever-increasing prevalence as patients pass the age of 20 years, rising to close to 50 percent in those who live to the fifth decade and beyond. In contrast to the stable level of reduced cognitive performance characteristic of the mental retardation, there is a gradual deterioration in functioning (Wisniewski et al. 1985a): those with severe retardation may become more apathetic and less sociable, whereas in those with only a mild or moderate degree of retardation, the dementia may present with decreased memory, disorientation to time, and reduced verbal output (Lai and Williams 1989).

Seizures are common in Down's syndrome and occur in a bimodal pattern: among infants and children, infantile spasms and grand mal seizures may be seen, whereas in adults, simple or complex partial seizures are more common, with a somewhat smaller percentage also having grand mal seizures (Prasher 1995; Pueschel et al. 1991). During the adult years, the prevalence of seizures increases dramatically with increasing age, and close to 50 percent of all patients over 50 years will experience them (McVicker et al. 1994): indeed, among those with dementia, the figure approaches 80 percent (Lai and Williams 1989).

Hypothyroidism may occur in both children and adults with Down's syndrome, and in adults this is often associated with the presence of anti-thyroid antibodies (Chinta 1988; Karlsson et al. 1998).

Depression may occur in a minority (Collacott et al. 1992), and in some cases this may be so severe as to cause a dementia (Warren et al. 1989).

Congenital heart disease, such as ventriculoseptal defect or patent ductus arteriosus, is found in up to 40 percent of patients. Emboli, some of which may be septic, may arise from the heart, and stroke may occur (Pearson et al. 1985); in cases with multiple strokes, a dementia may be seen (Collacott et al. 1994). Other abnormalities seen in Down's syndrome include duodenal obstruction, intestinal stenosis, megacolon, leukemia, and atlanto-axial instability. This last abnormality is very important to keep in mind, as it may lead to cord compression. Obstructive sleep apnea may also occur, and may cause daytime fatigue and irritability.

Although the diagnosis can usually be reliably made on clinical grounds alone, karyotyping is indicated, not only to confirm the diagnosis but also to identify the small proportion of cases that occur secondary to a translocation.

Course

The average age of death is 12 years, with most of those who die in childhood or adolescence succumbing to cardiac complications (Baird and Sadovnik 1987). Among those who survive into adult years, roughly half will live to the seventh decade (Baird and Sadovnik 1988) whereas the other half will succumb to Alzheimer's disease, usually within 5 years of its onset (Evenhuius 1990).

Etiology

Approximately 95 percent of cases of Down's syndrome are secondary to trisomy 21 due to non-disjunction during meiosis (Petersen and Luzzatti 1965; Stoll et al. 1998). In almost all cases this non-disjunction occurs in the mother, and the risk for this rises dramatically with age, from about 1 in 1000 in the early twenties to almost 1 in 100 at the age of 40 years and 1 in 50 at the age of 45 years. In a very small minority, mosaicism may occur, and cases secondary to

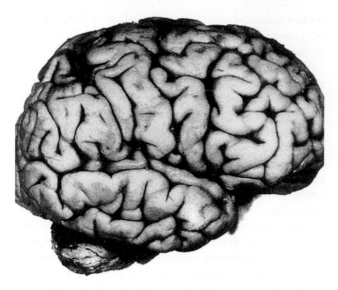

Figure 9.2   Note the marked hypoplasia of the superior temporal gyrus in this case of Down's syndrome. (Reproduced from Graham and Lantos 1996.)

this tend to be characterized by mild symptomatology. In the remaining 5 percent of cases not due to trisomy 21, there is a translocation, generally from chromosome 21 to 14: such translocations may occur sporadically or may be inherited from either parent.

The brain is small and rounded, with a flattened occiput. The overall sulcal pattern is often simple and undeveloped, and the superior temporal gyrus is often quite hypoplastic, as illustrated in Figure 9.2. The number of neurons in the cerebral cortex is reduced (Ross *et al.* 1984), and on the remaining neurons there is typically a reduced number of dendritic spines (Suetsugu and Mehraein 1980). As noted earlier, Alzheimer's disease is common in Down's syndrome and, among patients over 40 years, senile plaques and neurofibrillary tangles (Hyman *et al.* 1995; Schochet *et al.* 1973) are almost universal (Wisniewski *et al.* 1985b). Presumably, the appearance of Alzheimer's disease in this population is due to the fact that the gene for the amyloid precursor protein is on chromosome 21, and the extra gene leads to an overproduction of amyloid.

Differential diagnosis

The diagnosis of Down's syndrome is evident on inspection and difficult to confuse with other causes of mental retardation. In cases in which dementia supervenes in adult years, although the most common cause is Alzheimer's disease, consideration must also be given to dementia secondary to hypothyroidism, depression, and, rarely, a multi-infarct dementia.

Treatment

If karyotyping reveals a translocation, all first-degree relatives should be offered testing. Mothers of patients with

Down's syndrome due to trisomy 21 should be informed of the high risk of Down's syndrome in future children.

The treatment of mental retardation, seizures, dementia, and depression is discussed in Sections 5.5, 7.3, 5.1, and 6.1 respectively. When Alzheimer's disease occurs, a trial of donepezil is reasonable (Prasher *et al.* 2002). Given the frequency with which hypothyroidism occurs, it is appropriate to screen patients with a thyroid profile on a yearly basis. All patients should have a CT scan of the atlanto-axial junction, and if there is evidence of instability appropriate restrictions on contact and similar sports should be instituted.

9.5 KLINEFELTER'S SYNDROME

Klinefelter's syndrome, found only in males, occurs secondary to the presence of one or more extra X chromosomes and, when fully expressed, is characterized by a tall stature, hypogonadism, and infertility. Developmental disabilities may occur, and a very small minority may have mental retardation.

Clinical features

The classic clinical picture (Ratcliffe *et al.* 1982) of Klinefelter's syndrome becomes apparent in post-pubertal males and is characterized, as noted, by tall stature, hypogonadism, and infertility. Excessive height is primarily caused by a late closure of the epiphyseal plates and results from increased leg length. Hypogonadism manifests with gynecomastia, a female escutcheon, and a small penis and testes; although most patients have a heterosexual orientation, libido is often low and erectile dysfunction may occur (Pasqualini *et al.* 1957). Moderate to severe azoospermia is present, which accounts for the infertility. Importantly, in an unclear but probably significant proportion of patients, this classic picture is not present, and some patients may come to clinical attention only during a work-up for infertility or erectile dysfunction.

Although the vast majority of patients have an IQ within the normal range (Ratcliffe *et al.* 1982), mental retardation may be seen in a minority, and developmental disabilities, such as developmental dysphasia or developmental dyslexia, have been noted; rarely, seizures may occur (Graham *et al.* 1988; Khalifa and Struthers 2002; Pasqualini *et al.* 1957; Swanson and Stipes 1969; Tatum *et al.* 1998; Wakeling 1972). The presence of more than two X chromosomes is associated with more severe retardation (Forsman 1970). In those who are retarded, the personality may be characterized by a sullen sort of withdrawal, with a liability to hostile outbursts (Hunter 1969).

There is an uncertain association between Klinefelter's syndrome and various other disorders, such as alcoholism (Nielsen 1969), bipolar disorder (Everman and Stoudemire 1994), and schizophrenia (Nielsen 1969; Pomeroy 1980; Roy 1981).

Other associated disorders include Hashimoto's thyroiditis, acute myeloid leukemia, diabetes mellitus, chronic obstructive pulmonary disease, and breast cancer.

Pre-pubertally, hormone levels are generally within normal limits, but after puberty, abnormalities become apparent with a low testosterone level and an elevated follicle-stimulating hormone level.

Karyotyping will reveal one or more extra X chromosomes.

Course

The evolution of the clinical picture is usually complete by adult years.

Etiology

Klinefelter's syndrome occurs secondary to non-disjunction during either spermatogenesis or oogenesis, resulting in the presence of one or more extra X chromosomes. The most common karyotype is 47,XXY; in about 10 percent of cases, mosaicism is present, with a 46,XY/47,XXY karyotype. Rarely, more severe abnormalities may occur, yielding karyotypes such as 48,XXXY or 49,XXXXY.

Although much of the symptomatology of Klinefelter's syndrome can be explained on the basis of primary hypogonadism secondary to a progressive fibrosis of the testes, it is clear that hypogonadism alone is not sufficient to explain all of the neuropsychiatric features of the disorder, such as mental retardation (Pasqualini et al. 1957; Wakeling 1972). Recent MRI studies have indicated a mild global cerebral atrophy (Giedd et al. 2007; Itti et al. 2006); however, the mechanism underlying this is not certain.

Differential diagnosis

When fully expressed, the clinical picture in adults is distinctive. Diagnostic difficulties may arise in partial cases, and the correct diagnosis may be revealed only incidentally during a work-up for infertility or erectile dysfunction.

Treatment

Testosterone treatment improves libido and erectile function, and tends to help with energy and overall outlook (Nielsen et al. 1988); infertility, however, persists. Gynecomastia may require surgical correction. Developmental disabilities and mental retardation are treated in the usual fashion.

9.6 FRAGILE X SYNDROME

The fragile X syndrome is one of the most common causes of mental retardation in developed countries. Although the classic picture of mental retardation with a characteristic facial dysmorphism is far more common and severe in males, females may also be affected.

Clinical features

The classic syndrome (Baumgardner et al. 1995; Finelli et al. 1985; Wisniewski et al. 1985c), as noted, is most evident in males and is characterized by mental retardation, a characteristic dysmorphic facies, and macro-orchidism. Mental retardation ranges from mild to severe. Autistic features, such as gaze avoidance, are present in most cases, and a minority will have the full syndrome of autism; ADHD is also seen in a minority. Dysmorphic features include a long, narrow face, prognathism, a high forehead, and large ears (De Arce and Kearns 1984). Macro-orchidism is a constant feature in post-pubertal males and may also be seen in a minority during childhood (Chudley and Hagerman 1987; De Arce and Kearns 1984). Seizures, either complex partial or grand mal, occur in a significant minority (Finelli et al. 1985; Musumeci et al. 1999; Sabaratnam et al. 2001; Wisniewski et al. 1985c). Other features include hyperextensible joints and mitral valve prolapse (Chudley and Hagerman 1987), and in a minority there may also be hyperreflexia and Babinski signs (Finelli et al. 1985). Incomplete penetrance may occur in males, and some may be of normal intelligence; in these cases, however, elements of developmental dysphasia, with both receptive and expressive deficits, are common, and most post-pubertal males will also have macro-orchidism.

Females with the fragile X syndrome tend to have much milder cases. Mental retardation is seen in only about 50 percent and tends to be of mild degree; facial dysmorphism is seen in only a small minority.

Genetic testing is available.

Course

Although there is some evidence that, in males, intellectual functioning may undergo a decline in late childhood or early adolescence (Dykens et al. 1989), it appears that, for the most part, the clinical picture becomes set in adolescence and generally remains stable thereafter.

Etiology

The fragile X syndrome occurs secondary to mutations in the FMR1 gene on the long arm of the X chromosome (Verkerk et al. 1991), which codes for a protein known as the fragile X mental retardation-1 protein (FMRP). This gene normally contains a sequence of CGG trinucleotide repeats containing anywhere from 5 to 55 triplets. An expansion of this sequence to include from 55 to 200 repeats is known as a premutation, whereas expansions to over 200 triplets constitute full mutations. Patients with pre-mutations do not develop the fragile X syndrome; however, those with full mutations do. In those with full mutations, transcription of the gene fails and levels of functional FMRP are low or undetectable. The relatively minor symptomatology seen in females is due to random inactivation of the X chromosome, which allows for some production of FMRP. The fragile X syndrome derives its name from the fact that when the cells of patients are cultivated in a medium deficient in thymidine and folic acid, a fragile site will be found on the long arm of the X chromosome (Sutherland 1977), which, as might be expected, corresponds to the location of the expanded CGG repeat.

Interestingly, although both female and male parents with a premutation may pass a full mutation to their children, this is far more commonly the case with female parents. The reason for this is that expansion of a pre-mutation to a full mutation occurs readily during oogenesis but only rarely during spermatogenesis.

Magnetic resonance imaging studies have revealed hypertrophy of the hippocampus with atrophy of the superior temporal gyrus (Reiss et al. 1994) and atrophy of the cerebellar vermis (Mostofsky et al. 1998). Autopsy studies have demonstrated that, although neuronal cell counts are normal in the cortex, dendritic spines are long and tortuous in shape (Hinton et al. 1991; Rudelli et al. 1985).

Differential diagnosis

The full clinical syndrome of mental retardation, with or without autism, and the characteristic facial dysmorphism (with, in males, macro-orchidism) is distinctive.

Mention should also be made of a condition known as FXTAS, or fragile X-associated tremor/ataxia syndrome. As noted earlier, patients with pre-mutations do not develop the fragile X syndrome. This is not to say, however, that the pre-mutation is benign, given that those who carry this premutation are at high risk for developing FXTAS in middle or later years, with tremor, ataxia, and, in a minority, dementia.

Treatment

The general treatment of mental retardation, autism, and ADHD is discussed in Sections 5.5, 9.14, and 9.15 respectively. Importantly, fragile X patients with ADHD respond well to methylphenidate (Hagerman et al. 1988).

9.7 VELOCARDIOFACIAL SYNDROME

The velocardiofacial syndrome, also known as the 22q11.2 deletion syndrome, is an inherited disorder characterized by facial dysmorphism, intellectual deficits, and a number of neuropsychiatric syndromes, most notably a psychosis phenotypically similar to schizophrenia. First described in 1978 by Shprintzen et al., this disorder is now recognized as

the most common of the microdeletion syndromes, being found in up to 1 in 4000 live births.

Clinical features

The facial dysmorphism is characterized by hypertelorism, a large, bulbous nose with a squared-off nasal root, and micrognathia. Most patients have a degree of velopharyngeal insufficiency, leading to a hypernasal voice.

About 50 percent of patients suffer from either borderline intellectual functioning or mental retardation, which is generally of mild degree (Swillen et al. 1997); perhaps one-fifth of all patients will also have symptomatology similar to that seen in ADHD, with varying mixtures of hyperactivity, impulsiveness, and inattentiveness. Autism has been noted in a small minority (Fine et al. 2005).

As these patients pass through adolescence into adult years, up to one-third will develop a psychosis phenotypically similar to that seen in schizophrenia (Bassett et al. 2003; Gothelf et al. 2007; Murphy et al. 1999), with delusions and hallucinations. Mood disturbances may also occur and may be more frequent than psychosis: both manic or hypomanic episodes (Papolos et al. 1996) and depressive episodes (Murphy et al. 1999) may occur. Obsessions and compulsions have also been noted in roughly one-third of teenagers (Gothelf et al. 2004).

Other clinical features include cardiac defects, hypocalcemia secondary to hypoparathyroidism, and, in a small minority, seizures (Kao et al. 2004).

Course

The course is chronic; although some die of cardiac complications, most live a normal lifespan.

Etiology

This syndrome occurs secondary to a microdeletion at 22q11.2 and is inherited in an autosomal dominant fashion with variable penetrance (McDonald-McGinn et al. 2001). Magnetic resonance imaging studies (van Amelsvoort et al. 2004; Bish et al. 2004, Campbell et al. 2006, Eliez et al. 2000, Kates et al. 2006; Schaer et al. 2006) have revealed atrophy of the cerebral cortex and white matter, with reduced gyrification of the cortex; enlargement of the right caudate; enlargement of the amygdalae; and atrophy of the thalamus. In the cerebellum, atrophy of the cortex and white matter is also seen.

Differential diagnosis

In adults, velocardiofacial syndrome must be distinguished from schizophrenia, bipolar disorder, major depression, obsessive–compulsive disorder, and ADHD.

The distinctive facial dysmorphism, nasal voice, mental retardation, hypocalcemia, and cardiac defects may all suggest the correct diagnosis; however, at times these abnormalities may be absent or subclinical, and the diagnostic possibility may only be raised when the family history suggests the syndrome in a relative, thus prompting genetic testing.

Treatment

There are no blinded treatment studies for this disorder; the neuropsychiatric syndromes seen here are treated as described in the sections on mental retardation (Chapter 5), ADHD and autism (Chapter 9), psychosis (Chapter 7), mania and depression (Chapter 6), and obsessions and compulsions (Chapter 4).

9.8 LESCH–NYHAN SYNDROME

The Lesch–Nyhan syndrome, first described in 1964 (Lesch and Nyhan 1964), is a rare X-linked recessively inherited disorder, occurring almost exclusively in males, which is characterized, classically, by mental retardation, a movement disorder with both dystonic and choreoathetotic components, and, most notably, a striking degree of self-mutilative lip biting.

Clinical features

The overall clinical picture has been described in several studies (Christie et al. 1982; Jankovic et al. 1988; Jinnah et al. 2006; Lesch and Nyhan 1964; Nyhan 1972). Toward the end of the first year of life, dystonia and choreoathetosis gradually appear, and with time spasticity may also occur. Mental retardation eventually becomes apparent in early childhood, and may range from mild to severe; notably, in a very small minority the IQ may be in the normal range (Mathews et al. 1995).

The characteristic self-mutilation typically begins in early childhood, after teeth come in; later onsets, up to the age of 8 years, however, have been reported (Hatanaka et al. 1990). Despite being normally sensitive to pain, patients repeatedly bite at their lips, tongue, buccal mucosa, and fingers, to the point where the lips and fingers are literally bitten off in some cases. It must clearly be kept in mind that there is no anesthesia here and that the biting is involuntary: Lesch and Nyhan (1964) commented that one of their patients 'appeared terrified and screamed as if in pain during the process (of biting) and appeared happy only when restrained securely'.

A minority of patients may also have seizures.

Hyperuricemia is a constant feature of this disease, and tophaceous gout and gouty nephropathy may appear in adolescence. A megaloblastic anemia may also occur in some patients.

Genetic testing is available. As noted below, hypoxanthine-guanine phosphoribosyl transferase (HPRT) activity is grossly reduced or absent, and diagnosis may also be established by measuring this enzymatic activity in erythrocytes, hair roots or cultured skin fibroblasts.

Course

Self-mutilation may decrease, or even remit, in early adolescence (Mizuno 1986); most patients, however, die of infection or renal failure in their teenage or early adult years.

Etiology

The Lesch–Nyhan syndrome occurs secondary to any one of a large number of different mutations in the gene for HPRT, found on the X chromosome (Davidson et al. 1989; Edwards et al. 1990; Gibbs and Caskey 1987; Yang et al. 1984). Although cases in females have been reported (van Bogaert et al. 1992; Ogasawara et al. 1989), this disorder, as noted above, is seen almost exclusively in males. Hyperuricemia is a constant feature of this syndrome, and this occurs secondary to disturbances in purine metabolism due to the mutation in HPRT. The hyperuricemia, however, does not explain the mental retardation, movement disorder or self-mutilation.

Although routine neuropathologic examinations are unrevealing, MR scanning has demonstrated mild atrophy of both the cerebral cortex and of the caudate nucleus (Harris et al. 1998). Several studies have strongly suggested disturbances in dopaminergic functioning. Post-mortem work has demonstrated reduced dopamine content in the caudate (Saito et al. 1999), and cerebrospinal fluid (CSF) studies have demonstrated a reduction in the level of homovanillic acid (HVA), a metabolite of dopamine (Jankovic et al. 1988). Positron emission tomography (PET) studies have indicated a reduction in pre-synaptic dopamine stores (Ernst et al. 1996; Wong et al. 1996), and post-mortem work has demonstrated an increase in post-synaptic dopamine receptors (Saito et al. 1999). Taken together, these results are consistent with a reduction of dopamine in pre-synaptic neurons and an expected compensatory up-regulation of post-synaptic dopamine receptors.

Differential diagnosis

Although patients with other forms of mental retardation may bite themselves, the degree of self-biting rarely ever approaches that seen in the Lesch–Nyhan syndrome.

Treatment

Allopurinol, by forestalling gouty nephropathy, may prolong life; it has, however, no effect on the central nervous system manifestations.

Lip biting may be curtailed by lip or mouth guards or by face masks; however, in severe cases, teeth extraction may be required. In cases with finger biting, restraints may be helpful. Various medications have been reported in non-blind case reports or studies to be helpful in reducing the biting, including risperidone (Allen and Rice 1996), levodopa (Jankovic *et al.* 1988), gabapentin (McManaman and Tam 1999), and carbamazepine (Roach *et al.* 1996). In one case report, a patient with a severe movement disorder underwent deep brain stimulation of the globus pallidus that not only relieved the movement disorder but was also followed by a remission of the self-biting (Taira *et al.* 2003).

9.9 BARDET–BIEDL SYNDROME

The Bardet–Biedl syndrome is a rare autosomal recessively inherited disorder, characterized in its fully expressed form by obesity, polydactyly or syndactyly, retinal dystrophy, and mental retardation. Although this syndrome is well-characterized, there is some inconsistency in the literature regarding its name: in the past it was often referred to as the Laurence–Moon–Biedl syndrome; however, the currently preferred name is Bardet–Biedl syndrome.

Clinical features

Clinical features have been discussed in a number of papers (Beales *et al.* 1997; Green *et al.* 1989; Klein and Ammann 1969; Rathmell and Burns 1938; Roth 1947). Obesity is almost universal and tends to be of the central type. Syndactyly or polydactyly is also almost universal; when polydactyly is present, it typically manifests with an extra finger or toe, which may range from rudimentary to fully formed. Retinal dystrophy is also almost universal, but may not become symptomatic until later childhood or adolescence; by early adult years, however, a majority of patients will become blind. Mental retardation ranges from mild to severe, and is seen in the majority of cases. Other features include hypogenitalism in males, with a small penis and testes, menstrual irregularities in females, renal dysplasia (which may progress to renal failure in a minority), congenital heart disease, hypertension, and diabetes mellitus.

Course

Apart from retinal dystrophy and renal abnormalities, both of which are progressive, the overall clinical course remains static through adult life.

Etiology

As noted, this disorder is inherited on an autosomal recessive basis: 12 loci (*BBS1* through *BBS12*) have been identified. The neuropathology is not known.

Differential diagnosis

Both the Prader–Willi and Alstrom–Hallgren syndromes are characterized by obesity; however, neither of these disorders is associated with polydactyly or syndactyly. Further differentiating features include a ravenous hunger in the Prader–Willi syndrome and sensorineuronal deafness in the Alstron–Hallgren syndrome.

Treatment

The treatment of mental retardation is discussed in Section 5.5.

9.10 PRADER–WILLI SYNDROME

The Prader–Willi syndrome is a congenital disorder characterized by extreme hyperphagia, obesity, various dysmorphic features, and, in a majority, mild mental retardation; other neuropsychiatric features, as described below, may also be present. This is a not uncommon disorder, and is found with equal frequency in males and females.

Clinical features

The overall clinical features have been described in several papers (Bray *et al.* 1983; Burke *et al.* 1987; Butler *et al.* 1986; Dunn 1968; Greenswag 1987; Hall and Smith 1972; Robinson *et al.* 1992). This disorder presents in infancy with somnolence, hypotonia, and decreased oral intake. By the age of 2 years, however, a remarkable transformation occurs, in that these patients become alert and begin to display a remarkable hyperphagia.

The hyperphagia of the Prader–Willi syndrome is severe and leads to extreme obesity. It stems from a ravenous hunger: one patient literally 'took off running' and 'as soon as she could walk, she was constantly near the refrigerator, begging for food' (Zellweger and Schneider 1968). Patients often go to any lengths to satisfy this hunger and, if refrigerators and food cabinets are locked, may turn to other sources: one patient 'ate catfood, begged food from neighbors, and ate rotting chicken carcasses and other items removed from dustbins' (Clarke 1993).

Characteristic dysmorphic features include a narrow head, almond-shaped eyes, and a narrowed or tented upper lip. Micromelia is also often present, with slender arms and legs and small hands and feet. Hypogonadism is present, manifesting in males with micropenis and cryptorchidism, and in females with hypoplastic labia, a lack of breast development, and varying degrees of amenorrhea.

Mental retardation is present in the majority of patients, but is generally mild. Behavioral abnormalities include skin picking, which may be quite severe, temper tantrums, and stubbornness; ritualistic behaviors may also be present.

(Clarke *et al.* 2002). Depression occurs in a minority, and may be quite severe (Boer *et al.* 2002); psychosis has also been reported (Clarke 1993). Seizures may occur in a minority.

Hypersomnolence is common and appears to be multifactorial. With the extreme obesity, obstructive sleep apnea (Clift *et al.* 1994) and the Pickwickian syndrome (Bye *et al.* 1983) may occur; however, in some cases the degree of hypersomnolence seems more severe than can be accounted for by these disorders.

The diagnosis may be confirmed by DNA methylation analysis, as discussed below.

Course

The disorder is chronic and many die prematurely of the complications of obesity.

Etiology

The Prader–Willi syndrome occurs secondary to a lack of a critical portion of the paternally-derived chromosome 15, and this deficit may occur via any one of three mechanisms. The most common mechanism involves a microdeletion on the paternally derived chromosome 15; the next most common is uniparental disomy, with both chromosome 15s being derived maternally; finally, and rarely, mutations may occur on the paternally derived chromosome 15. The diagnosis, as indicated earlier, may be made via methylation analysis. The methylation pattern on chromosome 15 differs for paternally and maternally derived chromosomes, and hence analysis allows one to determine whether the patient has a normal, paternally-derived chromosome 15.

The neuropathology of the Prader–Willi syndrome is not clear. Magnetic resonance imaging (Miller *et al.* 2007) has indicated cortical atrophy and, in some cases, polymicrogyria. The remarkable hunger has suggested hypothalamic involvement, and one study found a reduction in the size and neuronal count of the hypothalamic paraventricular nucleus (Swaab *et al.* 1995).

Differential diagnosis

The Bardet–Biedl syndrome is distinguished by the presence of polydactyly or syndactyly.

Treatment

Growth hormone, given early in life, may improve both overall height and lean body mass (Myers *et al.* 2006).

Early dietary management is essential and in some cases institutionalization may be required to forestall the development of a lethal degree of obesity. In one double-blind study, fenfluramine was effective in reducing weight (Selikowitz *et al.* 1990); however, this agent is no longer available in the United States. An open study also suggested effectiveness of risperidone in this regard (Durst *et al.* 2000). Obstructive sleep apnea and the Pickwickian syndrome are treated as discussed in Sections 18.8 and 18.9 respectively.

Mental retardation is treated as outlined in Section 5.5. Of note, open work has found that topiramate, although ineffective for weight loss in this population, did reduce skin picking (Smathers *et al.* 2003); in cases with seizures, this would be a logical choice. Case reports also suggest that selective serotonin reuptake inhibitors (SSRIs) may reduce skin picking (Hellings and Warnock 1994).

9.11 CONGENITAL RUBELLA SYNDROME

The congenital rubella syndrome occurs secondary to fetal infection during the first trimester. In the past, this was an important cause of mental retardation; however, in developed countries, vaccination of females has made this a very rare disorder.

Clinical features

In its fully developed form (Forrest and Menser 1970; Forrest *et al.* 2002; Hardy 1973; Miller *et al.* 1982; Tartakow 1965), the syndrome is characterized by mental retardation, cataracts, deafness, and various cardiac abnormalities, such as patent ductus arteriosus and ventricular septal defect. A minority of patients may also have autism (Chess *et al.* 1978; Fombonne *et al.* 1997).

Course

In those who survive into late childhood or beyond, the course is static, except in the small minority who go on to develop the dementia of progressive rubella panencephalitis, as discussed in Section 14.14.

Etiology

Maternal rubella infection leads to fetal infection via transplacental spread and, if this occurs in the first trimester, various abnormalities may occur, including areas of focal necrosis, primarily in the basal ganglia, mesencephalon, and cord (Desmond *et al.* 1967; Plotkin *et al.* 1965; Rorke 1973; Rorke and Spiro 1967); microcephaly and spina bifida may also be present (Tartakow 1965).

Differential diagnosis

Fetal infection with toxoplasma, cytomegalovirus or herpes simplex virus can cause a similar syndrome.

Treatment

The treatment of mental retardation is discussed in Section 5.5, and of autism in Section 9.14. Hearing aids are generally required.

Prevention is critical, and females of child-bearing age should be vaccinated if they have not already had rubella. Contraception for the 3 months post-vaccination is critical, as, albeit rarely, congenital rubella has occurred in fetuses conceived during this time period.

9.12 FETAL ALCOHOL SYNDROME

The fetal alcohol syndrome, caused by *in utero* exposure to alcohol, consists, classically, of a characteristic facial dysmorphism, mental retardation, and behavioral problems, most notably hyperactivity (Clarren and Smith 1978; Jones and Smith 1973; Jones *et al.* 1974). This is a not uncommon disorder, being present in roughly 1 in 1000 live births, and represents one of the most common causes of mental retardation in the United States. Partial syndromes also occur, and such patients are often said to have 'fetal alcohol effect'.

Clinical features

The characteristic dysmorphism includes microcephaly, shortened palpebral fissures, epicanthal folds, maxillary hypoplasia, a thin upper lip, a flattened philtrum, and micrognathia. Mental retardation ranges from severe to mild, and some may be of normal intelligence: those with an IQ within the normal range, however, may have developmental disorders, such as developmental dyscalculia or developmental dysphasia (Larsson *et al.* 1985; Shaywitz *et al.* 1981). Behavioral problems are common, and patients may not only be irritable but also display hyperactivity and distractability reminiscent of ADHD. Cardiac abnormalities may also occur, such as atrial or ventricular septal defects.

Magnetic resonance scanning may be normal or, in severe cases, may disclose cortical atrophy, ventricular enlargement, and hypoplasia or agenesis of the corpus callosum.

Course

Although some improvement may occur during adolescence, especially with regard to the severity of the facial dysmorphism (Spohr *et al.* 1993; Streissguth *et al.* 1991), the overall course is one of a stable chronicity.

Etiology

Although the syndrome is clearly related to maternal alcohol ingestion, multiple uncertainties remain as to the details. For example, it is not clear whether it is the first or, rather, later trimesters that constitute the greatest period of risk.

Furthermore, it is also unclear whether it is the total amount of alcohol consumed that is important or whether relatively brief exposures to high levels, as may occur with binge drinking, are more toxic. Finally, there is also debate as to whether it is alcohol itself that is toxic, or its metabolite, acetaldehyde.

Neuropathologic studies (Clarren *et al.* 1978; Ferrer and Galofre 1987; Konovalov *et al.* 1997; Pfeiffer *et al.* 1979; Wisniewski *et al.* 1983) have revealed numerous abnormalities (which may be present in various combinations), including microcephaly, agenesis of the corpus callosum, and hypoplasia of the cerebellar vermis; microscopically, cortical dyslamination may be present, and glial and glial-neuronal nodules may be found in the white matter and also in the leptomeninges.

Differential diagnosis

The characteristic facial dysmorphism, coupled with a history of maternal alcohol use, strongly suggest the diagnosis. Difficulties may arise on two counts. First, it may not be possible to establish the degree of alcohol use during pregnancy. Second, as noted earlier, the facial dysmorphism tends to fade and hence may be very subtle, or even absent, in teenagers or adults: when the diagnosis is strongly suspected but the facial dysmorphism is absent, examining childhood photographs may be very helpful.

A similar syndrome may occur in cases of *in utero* exposure to various anti-epileptic drugs, most notably phenytoin and valproic acid.

Treatment

The treatment of mental retardation is discussed in Section 5.5; hyperactivity and distractability may be treated as described for ADHD in Section 9.15. Prevention, of course, is critical, and females of child-bearing age should be informed that binge drinking may be as dangerous as daily drinking and that there may indeed be no minimal 'threshold' of alcohol consumption below which a pregnant woman can drink without endangering the fetus.

9.13 RETT'S SYNDROME

Rett's syndrome, first described by Andreas Rett in 1966 (Rett 1966), is a rare disorder characterized by mental retardation, microcephaly, autistic features, and peculiar stereotypic hand movements. This is a rare disorder that occurs almost exclusively in females.

Clinical features

As described in a number of papers (Coleman *et al.* 1988; Hagberg 1989; Hagberg and Witt-Engerstrom 1986; Hagberg *et al.* 1983; Witt-Engerstrom 1990), the clinical features of Rett's syndrome in females may be roughly divided into four stages. It must be emphasized that the delineations between various stages are not precise, and that various features may overlap from one stage to another.

Stage I becomes apparent at around the age of 10 months and is characterized by a general stagnation of normal development. There may be a failure of normal weight gain, and, rather than beginning to crawl, patients may display a persistent 'bottom shuffling'. This stage persists for anywhere from a month up to a year and a half.

Stage II generally occurs around the age of 18 months and is characterized by a regression. Interestingly, although the onset of this stage is generally gradual, spanning weeks or months, it may at times occur relatively acutely, with an onset spanning days. The regression itself presents with autistic features, including a general withdrawal of contact with surroundings, and the appearance of characteristic stereotypies. Initially patients may suck their hands or grasp their tongues; however, with time, the classic hand stereotypies emerge, with hand-wringing, hand-clasping or washing movements. There may also be attacks of violent screaming, teeth gnashing, and nocturnal awakenings accompanied by peculiar laughter. Most patients also display episodes of irregular respiration while awake, with periods of hyperventilation followed by apneas. During this stage, head growth decelerates, and patients gradually develop microcephaly. Stage II generally lasts about a year and a half.

Stage III typically begins around the age of 3 years and is often referred to as the 'pseudostationary' stage, reflecting the fact that, for the most part, the regression seen in stage II ends and there is a period of relative stability. Patients are left with mental retardation, which is generally severe, and ambulation may or may not be possible. Seizures, if not already evident in stage II, now appear in most patients, and may be complex partial or grand mal. This stage lasts for many years, occasionally persisting into early adult years or even middle age.

Stage IV, also known as the stage of late motor deterioration, may appear at any point from late childhood to adult years, and is characterized by dystonia and lower motor neuron muscular atrophy, both most prominent in the lower extremities, and by scoliosis, which at times may be quite severe.

Although these clinical stages are the rule in females, exceptions do occur, and at times there may be mild or 'variant' cases in which speech is preserved.

As noted earlier, the vast majority of cases are seen in females. In those very rare instances in which Rett's syndrome occurs in males, it tends to be more severe (Dotti *et al.* 2002), with most patients dying in infancy (Kankirawatana *et al.* 2006)

Genetic testing is available.

Course

Stage IV may persist for decades and some patients may live into their 60s. Early death, however, is not uncommon and may occur secondary to infections or post-operative complications.

Etiology

Rett's syndrome is an X-linked dominant disorder due to any one of a large number of different mutations in the gene for methyl-CpG-binding protein 2 (*MECP2*) (Amir *et al.* 1999; Auranen *et al.* 2001). Phenotypic variation reflects not only the effects of different mutations (Dotti *et al.* 2002) but also non-random inactivation of the X chromosome (Amir *et al.* 2000). Almost all cases represent *de novo* mutations; in the few familial cases identified, it appears that the mother was a 'carrier' who was either unaffected (Dayer *et al.* 2007) or had a very mild phenotype (Huppke *et al.* 2006). The extreme rarity of this disorder in males probably reflects the lethal nature of most mutations when not 'balanced', as in females, by a normal X chromosome.

Neuropathologic studies have revealed microcephaly and hypopigmentation of the pars compacta of the substantia nigra (Jellinger and Seitelberger 1986; Jellinger *et al.* 1988). Microscopically, there is a loss of cortical pyramidal cells (Belichenko *et al.* 1997); remaining neurons are generally small and closely packed (Bauman *et al.* 1995), and dendrites show decreased branching (Armstrong *et al.* 1998). Cerebellar pathology is also present (Oldfors *et al.* 1990), with cerebellar cortical atrophy and a loss of Purkinje cells; of note, although gliosis may be present in those dying in adult years, it appears absent or scant in childhood.

Differential diagnosis

The overall differential diagnosis of mental retardation is discussed in Section 5.5; the combination of mental retardation, autistic features, and hand stereotypies in a female, although not specific for Rett's syndrome (Temudo *et al.* 2007), is very suggestive.

Treatment

The general treatment of mental retardation is discussed in Section 5.5. In one blind study, in a minority, bromocriptine was followed by some improvement in cognition and overall behavior (Zappella 1990). Non-blind work suggests that in some patients folinic acid treatment may be followed by overall improvement (Ramaekers *et al.* 2003). Naltrexone should not be used, as it may cause a distinct worsening of symptoms (Percy *et al.* 1994). With regard to seizures, although there are no blind studies, case series support the use of carbamazepine (Huppke *et al.* 2007), lamotrigine (Stenbom *et al.* 1998), or topiramate (Goyal *et al.* 2004).

9.14 AUTISM

Autism, first described by Leo Kanner in 1943 (Kanner 1943), is a chronic, lifelong disorder that is characterized by an inability on the patient's part to form normal relationships with others. The relationships that are formed exhibit a peculiar disturbance, in that patients act toward others as if those others were inanimate objects: there is a machine-like quality to the patient's overall behavior with others, as if the patient fails to sense the difference between the animate and inanimate. In severe cases patients may be almost totally inaccessible, whereas in milder ones an observer might note only a peculiar awkwardness and stiltedness in the patient's social behavior. Most, but certainly not all, patients also have mental retardation.

Autism is a relatively rare disorder, with a lifetime prevalence of about 0.05 percent; it is far more common in males than females, by a ratio of 3–4:1. Although some recent studies have indicated an increase in the rate with which the diagnosis of autism is made, it is unclear whether this represents an actual increase in prevalence or rather better case finding.

Clinical features

Autism has an insidious onset in infancy. Parents may recall that the child cried infrequently and seemed indifferent to being held or cuddled; some parents, as noted by Kanner (1943), were 'astonished at the children's *failure to assume at any time an anticipatory posture* to being picked up' (italics in original). Although symptoms are typically obvious by the age of 3 years, in mild cases they may escape notice, and children may not come to attention until they enter elementary school and their behavior is compared to that of their normal peers.

The full picture of autism is typically best seen in middle childhood. Autistic children prefer solitary play and, rather than playing with other children, occupy themselves with objects such as toys or machines of some sort. They seem, as noted by Kanner (1943), to be unable '*to relate themselves* in the ordinary way to people and situations' (italics in original); indeed, other people, whether adults or children, are often treated as if they were machines or perhaps mere props to be used during play. Attempts to make contact with such children generally fail. If one tries to catch their eyes, they will often exhibit 'gaze avoidance' (Richer and Coss 1976), staring fixedly at something else, perhaps something just to the side of the examiner's head. One gets the impression that a mannequin would be more satisfactory to the autistic child than an actual playmate.

The behavior of autistic children may, at times, seem bizarre. There are often what are known as 'fascinations', in which the child becomes intently interested in and fascinated with certain objects, such as a piece of cloth, jewelry, or, classically, spinning things such as tops. One of Kanner's patients (Kanner 1944) spun 'toys and lids of bottles and jars by the hour . . . He would watch them and get severely excited and jump up and down in ecstasy'. Stereotypies such as repetitive hand flapping or finger flicking may occur, and some patients may engage in posturing or, classically, toe walking. The persistence of stereotypies can be astonishing: one child (Ornitz and Ritvo 1968) sustained 'oscillatory hand-flapping throughout the entire day'. Some patients seem insensitive to pain, whereas others display an inordinate, often terrifying, sensitivity to innocuous stimuli: one of Kanner's (1943) patients 'was so afraid of the vacuum cleaner that she would not even go near the closet where it was kept, and when it was used, ran out into the garage, covering her ears with her hands'. Head banging and other self-injurious behaviors, such as self-biting, may also occur. An overall hyperactivity may also occur.

Another classic symptom of autism is an '*anxiously obsessive desire for the maintenance of sameness*' (Kanner 1943; italics in original). As noted further by Kanner (1951):

> the autistic child desires to live in a static world, a world in which no change is tolerated. The status quo must be maintained at all cost. Only the child himself may sometimes take it upon himself to modify existing combinations. But no one else may do so without arousing unhappiness and anger . . . The slightest change of arrangement, sometimes so minute that it is hardly perceived by others, may evoke a violent outburst of rage.

Not only arrangements but also routines and sequences must be maintained inviolate: the aisles in the grocery store must be traversed in exactly the same order and direction every time, and the exact same route must be taken to school every day.

Speech and language are also disturbed. Some patients are mute, and those who do speak often display a curious aprosody, wherein they not only seem insensitive to the emotional inflections of those speaking to them but also display a monotonous or 'sing-song' quality in their own speech. There may also be echolalia and, classically, pronomial reversals, wherein the patients refer to themselves in the third person.

Some patients (Kanner 1944) may display 'an astounding vocabulary . . . excellent memory for events of several years before . . . [and] phenomenal rote memory for poems and names'. Kanner (1944) was impressed with their 'strikingly intelligent physiognomies', believing that most, if not all, of his patients were of normal intelligence. It is now clear, however, that Kanner's original sample of 20 patients was not representative and that, in fact, about three-quarters of autistic patients have mental retardation, ranging in severity from mild to severe.

The mental retardation seen in autism is, however, peculiar in that, unlike most examples of mental retardation, the decrement in abilities is not even: indeed, in some cases one may find 'islets' of normal, or even superior, functioning in an otherwise retarded patient. For example, one autistic man with an IQ of 71, although unable to abstract on proverbs testing or do simple arithmetic, was nevertheless able to 'correctly give the day of the week of any day this century' (Hurst and Mulhall 1988). In the past, such patients have been referred to as '*idiots savants*' (Treffert 1988), and although this terminology is unfortunate, it does forcefully convey the sometimes astounding contrast between the 'islets' of superior functioning and the overall intellectual decrement.

Seizures occur in roughly one-third of patients and, although these are most common in those with mental retardation, they may also occur in those of normal intelligence. Infantile spasms may occur in younger children, whereas in older children and in adults, simple partial, complex partial, and grand mal seizures may be seen (Danielsson *et al.* 2005; Olsson *et al.* 1988).

Before leaving this discussion of the clinical features of autism, it is appropriate to comment on the putative entity known as Asperger's syndrome. As noted earlier, in some mild cases of autism, symptoms may not come to light until the child enters elementary school and, in very mild cases, recognition may be delayed until much later. Some authors believe that these cases represent a separate disorder, called Asperger's syndrome; myself and others, however, conceive of such patients as merely constituting the very 'high-functioning' end of the spectrum of clinical severity of autism.

Course

The overall outcome is strongly influenced by whether or not there is an associated mental retardation and, if so, its severity. With regard to autistic symptoms, there is typically some gradual improvement by adult years, and, from a prognostic point of view, the course during middle childhood is particularly important: those who attain some language and some social skills around this time have a much more favorable outcome than those who do not. No matter how great the spontaneous recovery, however, residual symptoms, such as aprosodia, social awkwardness, and a reduced awareness of social conventions, remain in adult years (Rumsey *et al.* 1985).

Etiology

Etiologic theories regarding autism have changed radically over the past few decades. This disorder was once believed to result from faulty child rearing by cold and distant parents. This theory has now been soundly discredited, and current research focuses primarily on genetics and neuropathology.

Family studies strongly support a genetic basis. As noted earlier, the lifetime prevalence is about 0.05 percent; however, the concordance among monozygotic twins is over 60 percent (Bailey *et al.* 1995; Folstein and Rutter 1977). Genetic heterogeneity is almost assured, and linkage studies have identified loci on various chromosomes, including chromosomes 2, 3, 7, 11, 15, 19, and X.

Although MRI studies overall have not been conclusive, with numerous contradictory results and failures of replication, two findings appear fairly solid, namely vermal hypoplasia and a degree of macroencephaly. Neuropathologic studies (as recently reviewed by Palmen *et al.* in 2004), although likewise not conclusive, do suggest cerebral cortical dysgenesis, abnormalities of neuronal cell packing and size within the limbic cortex, and a loss of Purkinje cells within the cerebellum.

It is unclear what role environmental factors play in the etiology of autism. Recent concerns regarding an etiologic role of the measles/mumps/rubella vaccine appear unfounded (Madsen *et al.* 2002).

Although the etiology of the vast majority of cases of autism thus remains unclear, it does appear that in a small minority, perhaps 10 percent, autism occurs secondary to certain other well-described disorders (Kielinen *et al.* 2004; Ritvo *et al.* 1990), including tuberous sclerosis (Alsen *et al.* 1994; Lawlor and Maurer 1987), the fragile X syndrome (Wisniewski *et al.* 1985c), Rett's syndrome (Percy *et al.* 1990), Down's syndrome (Lund and Munk-Jorgensen 1988), velocardiofacial syndrome (Fine *et al.* 2005), and the congenital rubella syndrome (Chess *et al.* 1978).

Differential diagnosis

As noted, mental retardation is seen in association with autism in about three-quarters of cases, and hence autism with mental retardation must be distinguished from mental retardation of other causes. At times this may be difficult, given that many patients with mental retardation of other causes will display repetitive, stereotyped behaviors, which at times may be similar to the 'fascinations' and stereotypies seen in autism. A cardinal differential feature, however, is the patient's social relatedness: upon approaching a child with mental retardation of other causes, one may be greeted by a smile and an expectant posture; by contrast, the child with autism may show no more interest in the approaching physician than might be evinced for a machine.

Developmental dysphasia, especially when both expressive and receptive components are present, may be confused with autism; however, here again the quality of the patient's social relatedness enables a differentiation. The child with developmental dysphasia, although unable to communicate verbally, will still, by gesture, tone of voice, and facial expression, clearly desire social contact, in stark contrast to the child with autism.

Schizophrenia may enter the differential, especially in cases characterized by significant inaccessibility and bizarre stereotypies. Here the age of onset is helpful. As noted earlier, most cases of autism become obvious by the age of 3 years; by contrast, schizophrenia only very rarely has an onset before the age of 8 years. Furthermore, in schizophrenia one finds hallucinations and delusions, symptoms that are absent in autism.

Treatment

Treatment of autism involves behavior modification, family counselling, special education, and medication. All components are important, and most patients generally receive a combination of these.

Behavior modification programs that target specific behaviors, such as head banging or aggressive behavior, are often quite effective. Unfortunately, however, there is often very little generalization: the learning of autistic patients is often quite state specific and, hence, although a program might eliminate, for example, head banging at school, the patient might continue to engage in this behavior at home, until a similar program is implemented at home.

Family counselling is aimed at helping parents adjust to their ill child, and to implementing and continuing behavior programs at home. In all cases it is also important to forcefully convey to the parents that they are in no way responsible for their child's illness.

Special education classes are generally appropriate. A class that is highly structured is more effective in fostering appropriate classroom behavior and learning than is a more permissive or 'open' classroom.

A variety of medications have been found useful in the treatment of autism. Stereotypies, repetitive behaviors, aggressiveness, hyperactivity, and, to a degree, overall social relatedness all improve with antipsychotics (risperidone [McCracken *et al.* 2002; McDougle *et al.* 1998, 2005; Research Units on Pediatric Psychopharmacology Autism Network 2002], olanzapine [Hollander *et al.* 2006a], and haloperidol [Anderson *et al.* 1984]), antidepressants (clomipramine [Gordon *et al.* 1993], fluvoxamine [McDougle *et al.* 1996], and fluoxetine [Hollander *et al.* 2005]), and divalproex (Hollander *et al.* 2006b). Hyperactivity also responds to clonidine (Frankhauser *et al.* 1992), methylphenidate (Research Units on Pediatric Psychopharmacology [RUPP] Autism Network 2005), atomoxetine (Arnold *et al.* 2006), and naltrexone (Felman *et al.* 1999).

Risperidone, in doses from 0.5 to 3 mg/day, is probably the best pharmacologic treatment overall, with haloperidol, in similar doses, coming a close second; olanzapine is associated with significant and problematic weight gain. Concerns regarding long-term side-effects of these antipsychotics often prompt clinicians to try an antidepressant first; however, at least in the case of clomipramine, haloperidol had fewer side-effects and was better tolerated in the short term (Remington *et al.* 2001); consequently fluvoxamine or fluoxetine might represent a better choice. The experience with divalproex is relatively limited.

Clonidine tends to cause sedation, and methylphenidate (and, to a lesser degree, atomoxetine) and naltrexone may cause irritability and increased social withdrawal.

All things being otherwise equal, it may be appropriate to begin with an antidepressant (or perhaps divalproex) and to hold an antipsychotic in reserve; of the antipsychotics, risperidone is preferable. Clonidine, methylphenidate, atomoxetine or naltrexone may occasionally constitute first-line treatment in cases in which hyperactivity far overshadows other symptoms; however, in most cases these are reserved as 'add-on' treatments in cases in which hyperactivity persists despite treatment with an antipsychotic or an antidepressant.

In planning the pharmacologic treatment of autism, it is important to adopt a methodical approach, using one agent at a time and giving each agent a 'good' trial before moving on to another: 'good' trials must involve not only adequate dosage but also adequate duration, keeping in mind that weeks or months may be required to see the effect of any given dose.

9.15 ATTENTION–DEFICIT/HYPERACTIVITY DISORDER

Attention-deficit/hyperactivity disorder (Biederman and Faraone 2005), often referred to simply as ADHD, is characterized by a variable mixture of hyperactivity, impulsivity, and inattentiveness. This is a common disorder, found in anywhere from 3 to 7 percent of school-age children, and occurs in males far more frequently than in females, with reported sex ratios varying from 2:1 to 10:1 depending on the diagnostic criteria utilized. Synonyms for ADHD include minimal brain dysfunction, hyperkinetic syndrome, or, simply, hyperactivity.

Clinical features

Although the onset of symptoms may occur as early as infancy, most patients do not come to clinical attention until kindergarten or early elementary school years. In infancy, one may see an unusual degree of fussiness and irritability, and during toddler years affected children may be constantly 'on the go' and forever 'into things', as if the 'motor' is never turned off. Preschoolers may be impulsive, and parents may find it almost impossible to impose discipline.

As these children enter kindergarten or elementary school, their behavior in the classroom generally brings them to attention. The clinical picture may be dominated by hyperactivity and impulsivity (in which case one speaks of ADHD 'predominantly hyperactive–impulsive type'), or inattentiveness (wherein the term ADHD 'predominantly inattentive type' is used), or a combination of all three symptoms (in which case one speaks of ADHD 'combined type').

Hyperactivity may first come to attention in the classroom as the children appear incapable of remaining seated. They may squirm in their seats, fidget constantly, get up abruptly, or walk to another desk or over to a shelf. Teachers may be able to get them seated again, but the success is generally only short-lived. These children may also be incessant talkers, and other students may be bothered by this. At home the hyperactivity persists, and children may restlessly go from room to room. Even favorite television shows may not be able to keep these children in one place, and asking about this point is often helpful in the attempt to make the diagnosis.

Impulsivity leads to multiple forms of 'thoughtless' behavior and may prompt teachers and parents to comment on an absence of any self-restraint. In the classroom, these children may blurt out answers even before the teacher has finished asking a question; in the lunch line, they may barge ahead to get a favorite dessert; and in the playground they may rush uninvited into the middle of other children's games. At home they may be in constant conflict with siblings and neighborhood children, commandeering their toys and generally bursting into otherwise quiet activities.

Inattentiveness is typically most apparent in the classroom. These children seem incapable of paying attention to their schoolwork, and this is particularly the case whenever attention to detail is required. At times, it may appear as if it's not so much a matter of inattentiveness as easy distractibility. A noise in the hallway, a car passing by outside, or simply something on another child's desk may pull their attention away from the task at hand, as if everything has the same degree of importance as the schoolwork in front of them. Thus, incapable of giving their work the required attention, these children predictably get very poor grades. At home, parents may complain about difficulties in getting the attention of these children: sometimes it may have been necessary for parents to literally hold a child's head still in order to 'get the message through', and even with this tactic the effort may fail.

As noted below, in the natural course of events there is a gradual and spontaneous diminution of symptoms as these young patients enter adolescence and then adult years, with a consequent change in the overall clinical presentation.

In adolescence, although the grosser manifestations of hyperactivity tend to diminish and patients may be able to stay seated in the classroom, there may still be an undue amount of fidgetiness. Impulsivity may result in merely a few too many 'larks', such as 'joyrides' or unplanned drinking bouts; in more severe cases, an otherwise easily resolved confrontation with another teenager, or with an authority figure, may rapidly escalate into violence. Inattentiveness, abetted by normal teenage restlessness, may lead to poor grades, despite normal intelligence.

Among adults, hyperactivity tends to fade into the clinical background, being manifest in these years merely by restlessness; impulsivity likewise recedes and may fade into a mere flightiness. Inattentiveness, however, tends to persist to a significant degree, and patients may find themselves unable to advance in work situations that require sustained attention.

Course

As just described, there is a gradual and spontaneous partial remission of symptoms as patients pass through adolescence into adulthood such that, by adult years, roughly two-thirds of patients, although perhaps not symptom free, have improved to the point where symptoms are no longer disabling.

Etiology

Attention deficit/hyperactivity disorder is clearly familial, however, genetic studies, although offering some promising leads regarding genes for dopamine receptors and dopamine transporters, have not as yet provided any conclusive results (Faraone et al. 2005). Magnetic resonance imaging studies have, however, demonstrated thinning of the cerebral cortex and atrophy of the cerebellar vermis (Berquin et al. 1998, Castellanos et al. 2002; Mackie et al. 2007; Shaw et al. 2006).

Attention deficit/hyperactivity disorder may also occur secondary to lead encephalopathy, a rare condition of inherited resistance to thyroid hormones (Hauser et al. 1993), or as a sequela of traumatic brain injury (Max et al. 2005).

Differential diagnosis

Autistic children may be quite hyperactive, impulsive, and distractible; however, here, in contrast with ADHD, one also sees the typical peculiar lack of relatedness with others, as if others were mere machines. This is an important differential to make, as a misdiagnosis here may lead to stimulant treatment, which may make some features of autism worse.

Childhood schizophrenia may also be characterized by hyperactivity and impulsivity; however, these children have additional symptoms not seen in ADHD, such as delusions, hallucinations, and loosened associations.

If accompanied by agitation, depression may make it impossible for a child to remain seated in class or attend to schoolwork; however, here one sees depressed mood, fatigue, and sleep disturbance, symptoms not typical of ADHD.

Mania is typified by hyperactivity, impulsivity, and distractibility, and, especially when mild, may be difficult to distinguish from ADHD. The age of onset here may help, as it is extremely rare for bipolar disorder to present at 10 years or earlier: in contrast, in most cases of ADHD the illness is well-established by this time. Symptomatology is also different: in mania the hyperactivity stems from an excess of energy, whereas in ADHD energy levels are generally not elevated.

Fetal alcohol syndrome may be characterized by the typical ADHD triad; however, here, one also sees a typical facial dysmorphism, with shortened palpebral fissures, epicanthal folds, a thin upper lip, and a smooth philtrum. Furthermore, most patients with the fetal alcohol syndrome also have either mental retardation or borderline intellectual functioning, in contrast to ADHD in which intelligence is normal.

Phenobarbital may cause hyperactivity as a side-effect.

Diagnosing ADHD in adults is a difficult task. First, one must rule out a host of other disorders that may be characterized by one or more of the ADHD triad. These include schizophrenia, agitated depression, mania, borderline personality disorder, antisocial personality disorder, and various substance use disorders, in particular dependence on alcohol or stimulants. In some cases, the differential task is relatively easy, as for example with cases of schizophrenia, depression or mania, in which other typical symptoms immediately suggest the correct diagnosis. In others, the only truly reliable way to make the differential involves documenting the onset of symptoms in early childhood (Mannuzza *et al.* 2002), an admittedly difficult task, involving, as it may, interviewing parents, siblings, and others.

Treatment

A large number of medications are useful in ADHD, including stimulants (and stimulant-like medications), certain antidepressants, lithium, and alpha-2 autoreceptor agonists.

Stimulant and stimulant-like medications include methylphenidate, mixed amphetamine salts, atomoxetine, modafinil, and dextroamphetamine. Methylphenidate and mixed amphetamine salts are roughly equivalent in efficacy (Pelham *et al.* 1999); methylphenidate appears superior to dextroamphetamine, and mixed amphetamine salts appear superior to atomoxetine (Wigal *et al.* 2005); modafinil appears roughly equivalent to dextroamphetamine (Taylor and Russo 2000). Methylphenidate is available in both immediate and time-release preparations; in general, the time-release preparation, given its convenience, should be used.

Antidepressants effective in ADHD include the tricyclic desipramine (Spencer *et al.* 2002), the monoamine oxidase inhibitors tranylcypromine (Zametkin *et al.* 1985) and selegiline (Mohammadi *et al.* 2004), and bupropion (Kuperman *et al.* 2001).

In adults, lithium appeared as effective as methylphenidate (Dorrego *et al.* 2002).

Alpha-2 autoreceptor agonists effective in ADHD include clonidine and guanfacine (Scahill *et al.* 2001, Taylor and Russo 2001).

Barring certain complicating factors, discussed below, it appears reasonable to start with a stimulant or stimulant-like medication and, of these, either methylphenidate or mixed amphetamine salts may be utilized. In cases in which these medications are either ineffective or poorly tolerated, consideration may be given to an antidepressant and, among the antidepressants, bupropion is a reasonable choice. Lithium may also be considered but the data supporting its effectiveness are not as robust as for the other agents. Alpha-2 autoreceptor agonists are less well-tolerated than the other agents and are generally held in reserve.

Certain complicating conditions may dictate a change in strategy, and these include substance abuse, depression, tic disorders, schizophrenia, and bipolar disorder. Substance abusers, in general, should not be given stimulants, and in this group it is reasonable to begin with bupropion. When depression is present, it also makes sense to use bupropion, in hopes of clearing both ADHD and depression with one medication. Tic disorders were once thought to constitute a relative contraindication to stimulants given the possibility that tics may be exacerbated by these agents. Recent research, however, suggests that, in fact, patients with tic disorders generally do well with stimulants. In those cases, however, in which tics are exacerbated by stimulants, consideration may be given to an alpha-2 autoreceptor agonist or, in adults, to desipramine, as both of these are effective not only for ADHD but also may ameliorate tics. Of the alpha-2 autoreceptor agonists, guanfacine is probably better tolerated; desipramine should be limited to adults, given the risk of arrhythmia in children. Schizophrenia does constitute a contraindication to stimulant use as these agents exacerbate psychotic symptoms: here, either bupropion or lithium may be considered. Bipolar disorder likewise constitutes a contraindication to stimulants given their propensity to precipitate mania, and here the obvious alternative is lithium.

Regardless of which medication is chosen for children or adolescents, it is also appropriate to offer psychosocial treatments, such as parent training classes and behavior modification programs for the classroom. It must be borne in mind, however, that medication, in particular stimulants, is more effective, sometimes far more effective, than psychosocial treatment.

9.16 DEVELOPMENTAL DYSPHASIA

Developmental dysphasia, also known as 'language disorder' or 'specific language impairment', is characterized by an incomplete acquisition of linguistic skills in children (Webster and Shevell 2004). In some cases, this results primarily in an expressive dysphasia, in which children, although capable of understanding what is said to them, have great difficulty in expressing their thoughts in speech. In other cases, in addition to this expressive deficit, there is also difficulty in understanding what others say, producing a clinical picture referred to as 'mixed receptive–expressive language disorder'.

Developmental dysphasia is seen in 2–4 percent of school age children, and is more common in boys than girls.

Clinical features

Depending on its severity, developmental dysphasia may come to clinical attention anywhere from the age of 2 years up to early school years.

In the expressive form of developmental dysphasia, children, although able generally to understand what is said to them, have a greater or lesser degree of difficulty in expressing their thoughts in speech (Sato and Dreifuss 1973). In severe cases vocabulary is restricted to simple words, and patients may be unable to speak in sentences. In milder cases, sentences may be possible, but are short, incomplete, and often telegraphic in form.

The mixed receptive–expressive form, when severe, may be characterized by muteness. In less severe cases, patients may be able to understand simple words, such as 'cat', or even simple sentences, such as 'sit down', but more complex vocabulary or sentences leave them baffled (Bartak *et al.* 1975; Cohen *et al.* 1989; Paul *et al.* 1983).

In addition to these linguistic problems, these children often have other difficulties, including anxiety, emotional lability, and, especially in boys, aggressiveness and hyperactivity.

Course

Although some degree of improvement may gradually occur during adolescence, for the most part this is a chronic disorder.

Etiology

Developmental dysphasia is familial and linkage has been found to loci on chromosomes 13, 16, and 19 (Bartlett *et al.* 2002, SLI Consortium 2004). In one well-studied family ('KE'), in which developmental dysphasia is inherited in a fully penetrant autosomal dominant fashion, a specific mutation was found on chromosome 7 (Lai *et al.* 2001).

Magnetic resonance imaging has demonstrated both a reversed asymmetry of linguistic cortex (De Fosse *et al.* 2004) and, in a substantial minority of cases, polymicrogyria in the peri sylvian region (Guerreiro *et al.* 2002).

Electroencephalogram studies have revealed an increased incidence of interictal epileptiform discharges (Nasr *et al.* 2001), especially evident in sleep studies (Picard *et al.* 1998).

One autopsy study demonstrated a dysplastic gyrus on the inferior surface of the left frontal cortex (Cohen *et al.* 1989).

Overall, it appears probable that developmental dysphasia occurs secondary to a genetically mediated disruption of normal neuronal migration to the peri-sylvian cortex, resulting in gyriform or dysplastic abnormalities. It is not clear whether the interictal epileptiform discharges are merely epiphenomenal, reflecting an unexpressed epileptogenic potential of dysplastic cortex, or are perhaps indicative of an epileptic process that, at least theoretically, could disturb normal development or function of the linguistic cortex.

Differential diagnosis

Deafness may simulate developmental dysphasia, and all children in whom this diagnosis is considered should have audiometry.

Severe deprivation may stunt language development; however, these children, in contrast to those with dysphasia, typically show rapid gains when placed in a linguistically stimulating environment.

Both autism and childhood-onset schizophrenia may be characterized by linguistic disturbances similar to those seen in the mixed form of developmental dysphasia; however, in these disorders other symptoms also occur (e.g., a lack of social relatedness in autism, or hallucinations and delusions in schizophrenia) that are not seen in dysphasia.

Acquired dysphasia is distinguished from developmental dysphasia by the course. In acquired dysphasia one sees a more or less normal acquisition of language followed by a 'regression' or loss of linguistic competence. By contrast, in developmental dysphasia, the gradual acquisition of language appears simply to 'stall out' and plateau at a level well below that expected for the child's age. Acquired dysphasia may be seen with head trauma, encephalitis, tumors, and the Landau–Kleffner syndrome, and has also been reported as a side-effect of topiramate (Gross-Tsur and Shalev 2004).

Finally, there is the question of the 'late talkers', that is children whose language development, although delayed, eventually results in normal linguistic competence. At present, there is no method whereby these children can be confidently distinguished from those whose development will eventually plateau at a lower than normal level, and consequently long-term clinical follow-up is required.

Treatment

Remedial education is critical and often helpful. Some practitioners recommend treatment with anti-epileptic drugs in cases with interictal epileptiform discharges; however, this is controversial and there are no controlled studies to support this practice.

9.17 DEVELOPMENTAL DYSLEXIA

In developmental dyslexia (Demonet *et al.* 2004), children, despite normal intelligence and adequate educational opportunity, have great difficulty in learning how to read. First described by Hinshelwood in 1896, this is a common disorder, seen in up to 4 percent of school age children. Although once thought to be far more common in boys, recent epidemiologic work suggests that the prevalence is roughly equal in boys and girls. Synonyms include reading disorder, specific reading disability, and congenital word blindness (Orton 1925).

Clinical features

Depending on its severity, developmental dyslexia may first come to light anywhere between the ages of 6 and 9 years as the child falls behind his or her peers in the acquisition of reading skills.

In attempting to read out loud, these young patients seem to stumble over certain words: they may skip words and go on to the next, or they may misread a word and say one that is different from that on the page. The errors in reading often involve omitting certain letters or supplying a different letter than the one printed; letter reversals often occur, such as 'd' for 'b'. In some cases, entire words are reversed, with the child saying 'pat' for the written word 'tap', for example. Reading comprehension is impaired and, after finally, and haltingly, reading a paragraph, the child may be unable to paraphrase it in his or her own words. In striking contrast, if the same paragraph is read out loud to the child, he or she may then be able to paraphrase it with little difficulty.

Writing is also impaired, and similar reversals may be seen. Thus, intending to write 'top', the child may write 'pot'. In some cases entire sentences may be reversed, with the written words reading from right to left on the page. Of note, if the child is asked to take a look at what he or she has written and then asked if there are any errors, the answer is often 'no'.

Course

Although there may be some spontaneous improvement over long periods of time, the overall natural course is marked by a chronic difficulty in reading.

Etiology

Developmental dyslexia is clearly familial; concordance among dizygotic twins is about 25 percent, and among monozygotic twins it rises to about 50 percent. Genetic heterogeneity exists (Williams and O'Donovan 2006), with loci identified on chromosomes 1, 3, 6, and 7. Autopsy studies in males reveal cortical dysgenesis, which, although widespread, is concentrated in the left peri-sylvian areas (Galaburda *et al.* 1985). In females, although similar findings were noted, there was, in addition, widespread glial scarring (Humphreys *et al.* 1990). Of note, and again in males, dysplastic changes have also been identified in the medial geniculate body and the posterior lateral nucleus of the thalamus (Galaburda and Eidelberg 1982). Magnetic resonance scanning has also suggested a lack of normal cerebral asymmetry of the planum temporale (Hynd *et al.* 1990); however, not all studies agree on this (Rumsey *et al.* 1997). Of interest, recent work has demonstrated that specific evoked potential abnormalities in infants predict the appearance of dyslexia (Molfese 2000).

Overall, it appears likely that developmental dyslexia occurs secondary to an inherited disturbance of neuronal migration, resulting in cortical microdysgenesis of the temporal cortex.

Differential diagnosis

Decreased visual acuity, severe anxiety, or a less than adequate educational setting may all impair a child's ability to learn to read.

Mental retardation is characterized by deficient reading, but here, in contrast to developmental dyslexia, one finds deficits in other academic skills.

Treatment

Remedial education is often strikingly effective. Piracetam, not available in the United States, may be helpful (Wilsher *et al.* 1987); however, not all studies agree on this (Ackerman *et al.* 1991).

9.18 DEVELOPMENTAL DYSGRAPHIA

Developmental dysgraphia (Deuel 1995; Gubbay and de Klerk 1995; Roeltgen and Tucker 1988), also known as developmental agraphia or 'disorder of written expression', is characterized by an impaired acquisition of the ability to write, despite normal intelligence and adequate educational opportunity. This is probably an uncommon disorder, and is probably more common in boys than girls.

Clinical features

Children with this disorder often misspell words; their sentences tend to be short and deficient in terms of grammar and syntax, and at times whole words may be missing, giving sentences a 'telegraphic' quality. Penmanship may or may not be poor; at times the penmanship far outshines what is actually written. Importantly, and in stark contrast to what they write, these children are often able to express themselves quite well when speaking.

Course

In the natural course of events, developmental dysgraphia appears to be chronic.

Etiology

Apart from the fact that dysgraphia tends to run in families (Schulte-Korne 2001), little is known about its etiology.

Differential diagnosis

Developmental dyslexia is distinguished by a concurrent difficulty with reading, and mental retardation by associated deficits in other academic abilities.

Treatment

Remedial education is effective.

9.19 DEVELOPMENTAL DYSCALCULIA

Developmental dyscalculia (Shalev 2004) is characterized by a more or less complete inability, despite otherwise normal intelligence and adequate educational opportunity, to acquire arithmetic skills. This is a relatively common disorder, occurring in 5–6 percent of school age children, and is seen with roughly equal frequency in boys and girls. Synonyms for this disorder include mathematics disorder and developmental arithmetic disorder.

Clinical features

In severe cases, patients are unable to perform the simplest of numerical operations, such as counting to 10. In other cases, children, although able to count, are unable to perform simple addition; those who progress to the mastery of simple addition may be unable to subtract, multiply, or divide.

Course

Roughly one-half of patients will experience considerable improvement by the early teenage years (Shalev et al. 2005).

Etiology

Although developmental dyscalculia is clearly familial (Shalev et al. 2001), the genetic basis for this is not clear. Autopsy studies are lacking; however, both magnetic resonance spectroscopy (Levy et al. 1999) and voxel-based morphometry (Issacs et al. 2001) indicate a lesion in the left parietal cortex.

Differential diagnosis

An inability to learn arithmetic has also been noted in children who were born prematurely with very low birth weight (Issacs et al. 2001) and in association with the fragile X syndrome or petit mal epilepsy (Shalev and Gross-Tsur 1993). Inability to learn arithmetic may also, of course, be seen in mental retardation of any cause; however, here it is associated with other cognitive disabilities, thus distinguishing it from developmental dyscalculia, in which the inability to learn arithmetic occurs in isolation.

New-onset dyscalculia in a child who has previously learned to do arithmetic is, of course, inconsistent with a diagnosis of developmental dyscalculia; such a scenario has been reported in a child with a left temporoparietal tumor (Martins et al. 1999).

Treatment

Remedial education is effective.

9.20 DEVELOPMENTAL STUTTERING

Developmental stuttering occurs in roughly 1 percent of school-age children, and is about four times as common in boys than girls.

Clinical features

Stuttering typically first appears between the ages of 2 and 10 years. The stuttering itself may occur with any word or, alternatively, only with certain syllables or letters. Typically, when stuttering occurs over syllables or letters, it is the first syllable or letter in a word that usually blocks speech; in this regard, 'b's, 'd's, 'k's, 'p's, and 't's are common precipitants. In attempting to speak, the patient feels 'blocked' and may appear to stumble over the word or sound, attempting to say it again and again, sometimes with increasingly explosive force. Often these attempts are accompanied by repetitive grimacing, blinking, hissing, or forceful thrusting of the head, arms, or even the trunk. After the sound or word is eventually spoken, there may be a veritable cascade of words, all correctly pronounced, until the next verbal stumbling block is encountered.

Stuttering is generally worse when patients are anxious, pressed for time, or speaking in front of a group. Interestingly, fluency may be improved or even restored if the patient reads a text, speaks in unison with others, or sings.

Course

Spontaneous remission occurs in about three-quarters of patients by early teenage years, and is more likely to occur in girls than boys.

Etiology

Developmental stuttering is clearly familial, and linkage studies suggest loci on chromosomes 7 and 12 (Suresh et al. 2006). Magnetic resonance imaging has indicated both reduced cerebral asymmetry of the plana temporalia and disruption of gyral architecture along the left peri-sylvian cortex (Foundas et al. 2001). PET scanning (Fox et al. 1996, Wu et al. 1995) has demonstrated reduced metabolic activity in the left frontal peri-sylvian cortex and increased activity in the homologous area on the right, which may, however, merely represent a compensatory change. Taken together, these findings are consistent with an inherited disorder of neuronal migration to the left superior perisylvian cortex.

Differential diagnosis

Acquired stuttering differs clinically from developmental stuttering in that acquired stuttering is likely to occur on any syllable, regardless of where it falls in a word, rather than on the first one, as is the case in developmental stuttering. Furthermore, those with acquired stuttering rarely demonstrate the kind of forceful effort to overcome a block as is seen with developmental stuttering. Acquired stuttering may be seen with lesions of the left frontal or parietal cortices or basal ganglia, and may also occur as a side-effect of various drugs, including methylphenidate, tricyclic antidepressants, monoamine oxidase inhibitors, SSRIs, certain antipsychotics, theophylline, and phenytoin.

Treatment

Speech therapy appears to be effective. In cases in which stuttering persists despite adequate speech therapy, consideration may be given to pharmacologic treatment. Various medications have been demonstrated to be effective in double-blind trials, including clomipramine (mean dose ~150 mg) (Gordon et al. 1995), haloperidol (mean dose ~3 mg) (Murray et al. 1977), olanzapine (2.5–5 mg/day) (Maguire et al. 2004), and risperidone (best results seen at 0.5 mg/day; in some cases, higher doses were associated with a loss of effect) (Maguire et al. 2000). As there have been no head-to-head comparative studies of these agents, choosing among them requires clinical judgment. In this regard, it should be borne in mind that haloperidol, although effective, was poorly tolerated. In addition to these blind studies, there is also a very intriguing case report of complete remission of developmental stuttering with chronic treatment with levetiracetam (Canevini et al. 2002).

REFERENCES

Ackerman PT, Dykman RA, Hooloway C et al. A trial of piracetam in two subgroups of students with dyslexia enrolled in summer tutoring. J Learn Disabil 1991; 24:542–9.

Allen SM, Rice SN. Risperidone antagonism of self-mutilation in a Lesch–Nyhan patient. Prog Neuropsychopharmacol Biol Psychiatry 1996; 20:793–800.

Alsen G, Gillberg IC, Lindblom R et al. Tuberous sclerosis in Western Sweden: a population study of cases with early childhood onset. Arch Neurol 1994; 51:76–81.

van Amelsvoort T, Daly E, Henry J et al. Brain anatomy in adults with velocardiofacial syndrome with and without schizophrenia: preliminary results of a structural magnetic resonance imaging study. Arch Gen Psychiatry 2004; 61:1085–96.

Amir RE, Van den Veyver IB, Wan M et al. Rett syndrome is caused by mutations in X-linked MECP2, encoding methyl-CpG-binding protein 2. Nat Genet 1999; 23:185–8.

Amir RE, Van den Veyver IB, Schultz R et al. Influence of mutation type and X chromosome inactivation on Rett syndrome phenotypes. Ann Neurol 2000; 47:670–9.

Anderson LT, Campbell M, Grega DM et al. Haloperidol in the treatment of infantile autism: effects on learning and behavioral symptoms. Am J Psychiatry 1984; 141:195–202.

Armstrong DD, Dunn K, Antalffy B. Decreased dendritic branching in frontal, motor and limbic cortex in Rett syndrome compared with trisomy 21. J Neuropathol Exp Neurol 1998; 57:1013–17.

Arnold LE, Aan MG, Cook AM et al. Atomoxetine for hyperactivity in autism spectrum disorders: placebo-controlled crossover pilot trial. J Am Acad Child Adolesc Psychiatry 2006; 45:1196–205.

Arzimanoglou AA, Andermann F, Aicardi J et al. Sturge–Weber syndrome. Indications and results of surgery in 20 patients. Neurology 2000; 55:1472–9.

Auranen M, Vanhala R, Vosman M et al. MECP2 gene analysis in classical Rett syndrome and in patients with Rett-like features. Neurology 2001; 56:611–17.

Aydin A, Cakmakci H, Kovanlikaya A et al. Sturge–Weber syndrome without facial nevus. Pediatr Neurol 2000; 22:400–2.

Bailey A, le Couteur A, Gottesmann I et al. Autism as a strongly genetic disorder: evidence from a British twin study. Psychol Med 1995; 25:63–77.

Baird PA, Sadovnik AD. Life expectancy in Down syndrome. J Pediatr 1987; 110:849–54.

Baird PA, Sadovnik AD. Life expectancy in Down syndrome adults. Lancet 1988; 2:1354–6.

Bartak L, Rutter M, Cox A. A comparative study of infantile autism and specific developmental receptive language disorder. I. The children. Br J Psychiatry 1975; 126:127–45.

Bartlett CW, Flax JF, Logue MW et al. A major susceptibility locus for specific language impairment is located on 13q21. Am J Hum Genet 2002; 71:45–55.

Bassett AS, Chow EWC, Abdelmalik P et al. The schizophrenia phenotype in 22q11 deletion syndrome. Am J Psychiatry 2003; 160:1580–6.

Bauman ML, Kemper TL, Arin DM. Pervasive neuroanatomic abnormalities of the brain in three cases of Rett's syndrome. Neurology 1995; 45:1581–6.

Baumgardner TL, Reiss AL, Freund LS et al. Specification of the neurobehavioral phenotype in males with fragile X syndrome. Pediatrics 1995; 95:744–52.

Beales PL, Warner AM, Hitman GA et al. Bardet-Biedl syndrome: a molecular and phenotypic study of 18 families. J Med Genet 1997; 34:92–8.

Bebin EM, Gomez MR. Prognosis in Sturge–Weber disease: comparison of unihemispheric and bihemispheric involvement. J Child Neurology 1988; 3:181–4.

Belichenko PV, Hagberg B, Dahlstrom A. Morphological study of neocortical areas in Rett syndrome. Acta Neuropathol 1997; 93:50–61.

Benedikt RA, Brown DC, Walker R et al. Sturge–Weber syndrome; cranial MR with Gd-DTPA. AJNR 1993; 14:409–15.

Berquin PC, Gledd JN, Jacobsen LK et al. Cerebellum in attention-deficit hyperactivity disorder: a morphometric MRI study. Neurology 1998; 50:1087–93.

Biederman J, Faraone SV. Attention-deficit hyperactivity disorder. Lancet 2005; 366:237–48.

Bish JP, Nguyen V, Ding L et al. Thalamic reductions in children with chromosome 22q11.2 deletion syndrome. Neuroreport 2004; 15:1413–15.

Boer H, Holland A, Whittington J et al. Psychotic illness in people with Prader Willi syndrome due to chromosome 15 maternal uniparental disomy. Lancet 2002; 359:135–6.

van Bogaert P, Ceballos I, Desguerre I et al. Lesch–Nyhan in a girl. J Inherit Metabol Dis 1992; 15:790–1.

Bolton PF, Griffiths PD. Association of tuberous sclerosis of temporal lobes with autism and atypical autism. Lancet 1997; 349:392–5.

Bolton PF, Park RJ, Higgins JN et al. Neuro-epileptic determinants of autism spectrum disorders in tuberous sclerosis complex. Brain 2002; 125:1247–55.

Bray GA, Dahms WT, Swerdloff RS et al. The Prader–Willi syndrome: a study of 40 patients and a review of the literature. Medicine 1983; 62:59–88.

Burke CM, Kousseff BG, Gleeson M et al. Familial Prader–Willi syndrome. Arch Int Med 1987; 147:673–5.

Butler MG, Meany FJ, Palmer CG. Clinical and cytogenetic survey of 39 individuals with Prader–Labhart–Willi syndrome. Am J Med Genet 1986; 23:793–809.

Bye AM, Vines R, Fronsek K. The obesity hypoventilation syndrome and the Prader–Willi syndrome. Aust Paediatr J 1983; 19:251–5.

Campbell LE, Daly E, Toal F et al. Brain and behavior in children with 22q11.2 deletion syndrome: a volumetric and voxel-based morphometry MRI study. Brain 2006; 129:1218–28.

Canevini MP, Chifari R, Piazzini A. Improvement of a patient with stuttering on levetiracetam. Neurology 2002; 59:1288.

Castellanos FS, Lee PP, Sharp W et al. Developmental trajectories of brain volume abnormalities in children and adolescents with attention-deficit/hyperactivity disorder. JAMA 2002; 288:1740–8.

Chao DHC. Congenital neurocutaneous syndromes of childhood. III. Sturge–Weber disease. J Pediatr 1959; 55:635–49.

Chess S, Fernandez P, Korn S. Behavioral consequences of congenital rubella. J Pediatr 1978; 93:699–703.

Chinta M. Hypothyroidism in Down's syndrome. Br J Psychiatry 1988; 153:102–4.

Christie R, Bay C, Kaufman IA et al. Lesch–Nyhan disease: clinical experience with nineteen patients. Dev Med Child Neurol 1982; 24:293–306.

Chudley AE, Hagerman RJ. Fragile X syndrome. J Pediatrics 1987; 110:821–31.

Clarke DJ. Prader–Willi syndrome and psychoses. Br J Psychiatry 1993; 163:680–4.

Clarke DJ, Baer H, Whittington J et al. Prader–Willi syndrome, compulsive and ritualistic behaviors: the first population-based survey. Br J Psychiatry 2002; 180:358–62.

Clarren SK, Smith DW. The fetal alcohol syndrome. N Engl J Med 1978; 298:1063–7.

Clarren SK, Alvord EC, Sumi SM et al. Brain malformations related to prenatal exposure to alcohol. J Pediatrics 1978; 92:64–7.

Clift S, Dahlitz M, Parkes JD. Sleep apnoea in the Prader–Willi syndrome. J Sleep Res 1994; 3:121–6.

Cohen M, Campbell R, Yaghmai F. Neuropathological abnormalities in developmental dysphasia. Ann Neurol 1989; 25:546–70.

Coleman M, Brubaker J, Hunter K et al. Rett syndrome: a survey of North American patients. J Ment Def Res 1988; 32:117–24.

Collacott RA, Cooper S-A, McGrother C. Differential rates of psychiatric disorder in adults with Down's syndrome compared with other mentally handicapped adults. Br J Psychiatry 1992; 161.671–4.

Collacott RA, Cooper SA, Ismail IA. Multi-infarct dementia in Down's syndrome. J Intellect Disabil Res 1994; 38:203–8.

Creange A, Zeller J, Rostaing-Rigattieri et al. Neurological complications of neurofibromatosis type 1 in adulthood. Brain 1999; 122:473–81.

Critchley M, Earl CJ. Tuberous sclerosis and allied conditions. Brain 1932; 55:311–46.

Danielsson S, Gillberg C, Billstedt E et al. Epilepsy in young adults with autism: a prospective population based follow-up study of 100 individuals diagnosed in childhood. Epilepsia 2005; 46:918–23.

Davidson BL, Tarle SA, Patella TD et al. Molecular basis of hypoxanthine-guanine phosphoribosyltransferase deficiency in ten subjects determined by direct sequencing of amplified transcripts. J Clin Invest 1989; 84:342–6.

Dayer AG, Bottani A, Bouchardy I et al. MECP2 mutant allele in a boy with Rett syndrome and his unaffected hemizygous mother. Brain Dev 2007; 29:47–50.

De Arce MA, Kearns A. The fragile X syndrome: the patients and their chromosomes. J Med Genet 1984; 21:84–91.

De Fosse L, Hodge SM, Makris N et al. Language-association cortex asymmetry in autism and specific language impairment. Ann Neurol 2004; 56:757–66.

von Deimling A, Krone W, Menon AG. Neurofibromatosis type 1: pathology, clinical features and molecular genetics. Brain Pathol 1995; 5:153–62.

Demonet JF, Taylor MJ, Chaix Y. Developmental dyslexia. Lancet 2004; 364:247–8.

Desmond M, Wilson G, Melnick J et al. Congenital rubella encephalitis. J Pediatrics 1967; 71:311–31.

Deuel RK. Developmental dysgraphia and motor skills disorders. J Child Neurol 1995; 10 (suppl. 1):6–8.

Devlin LA, Shepherd CH, Crawford H et al. Tuberous sclerosis complex: clinical features, diagnosis, and prevalence within Northern Ireland. Dev Med Child Neurol 2006; 48:495–9.

DiMario FJ, Ramsby G. Magnetic resonance imaging lesion analysis in neurofibromatosis type 1. Arch Neurol 1998; 55:500–5.

DiPaolo DP, Zimmerman RA, Rorke LB et al. Neurofibromatosis type 1: pathologic substrate of high-signal intensity in the brain. Radiology 1995; 195:721–4.

Dorrego MF, Canevaro L, Kuzia G et al. A randomized, double-blind, crossover study of methylphenidate and lithium in adults with attention-deficit/hyperactivity disorder: preliminary findings. J Neuropsychiatry Clin Neurosci 2002; 14:289–95.

Dotti MT, Orrico A, De Stefano N et al. A Rett syndrome MECP2 mutation that causes mental retardation in men. Neurology 2002; 58:226–30.

Down JLH. Observation on an ethnic classification of idiots. Clin Lect Rep Lond Hosp 1866; 3:259–62.

Dunn HG. The Prader–Labhart–Willi syndrome: a review of the literature and report of nine cases. Acta Paediatr Scand Suppl 1968; 186:1–38.

Durst R, Rubin-Jabotinsky K, Raskin S et al. Risperidone in treating behavioral disturbances of Prader–Willi syndrome. Acta Psychiatr Scand 2000; 102:461–5.

Dykens EM, Hodapp RM, Ort S *et al.* The trajectory of cognitive development in males with fragile X syndrome. *J Am Acad Child Adolesc Psychiatry* 1989; **28**:422–6.

Edwards A, Voss H, Rice P *et al.* Automated DNA sequencing of the human HPRT locus. *Genomics* 1990; **6**:593–608.

Eliez S, Schmitt JE, White CD *et al.* Children and adolescents with velocardiofacial syndrome: a volumetric MRI study. *Am J Psychiatry* 2000; **157**:409–15.

Ernst M, Zametkin AJ, Matochil JA *et al.* Presynaptic dopaminergic deficits in Lesch–Nyhan disease. *N Engl J Med* 1996; **334**:1568–72.

European Chromosome 16 Tuberous Sclerosis Consortium. Identification and characterization of the tuberous sclerosis gene on chromosome 16. *Cell* 1993; **75**:1305–15.

Evenhuius HM. The natural history in Down's syndrome. *Arch Neurol* 1990; **47**:263–7.

Everman DB, Stoudemire A. Bipolar disorder associated with Klinefelter's syndrome and other chromosomal abnormalities. *Psychosomatics* 1994; **35**:35–40.

Faraone SV, Perlis RH, Doyle AE *et al.* Molecular genetics of attention-deficit/hyperactivity disorder. *Biol Psychiatry* 2005; **57**:1313–23.

Feldmann R, Denecke J, Grenzebach M *et al.* Neurofibromatosis type 1. Motor and cognitive function and T2-weighted MRI hyperintensities. *Neurology* 2003; **61**:1725–8.

Felman HM, Kolmen BK, Gonzaga AM. Naltrexone and communication skills in young children with autism. *J Am Acad Child Adolesc Psychiatry* 1999; **38**:587–93.

Ferrer I, Galofre E. Dendritic spine abnormalities in fetal alcohol syndrome. *Neuropediatrics* 1987; **18**:161–3.

Fine SE, Weissman A, Gerdes M *et al.* Autism spectrum disorders and symptoms in children with molecularly confirmed 22q11.2 deletion syndrome. *Autism Dev Disord* 2005; **35**:461–70.

Finelli PF, Pueschel SM, Padre-Mendoza T *et al.* Neurological findings in patients with the fragile-X syndrome. *J Neurol Neurosurg Psychiatry* 1985; **48**:150–3.

Folstein S, Rutter M. Infantile autism: a genetic study of 21 twin pairs. *J Child Psychol Psychiatry* 1977; **18**:297–321.

Fombonne E, Du Mazuabrun C, Cans C *et al.* Autism and associated medical disorders in a French epidemiological study. *J Am Acad Child Adolesc Psychiatry* 1997; **36**:1561–9.

Foundas AL, Bollich AM, Corey DM *et al.* Anomalous anatomy of speech-language areas in adults with persistent developmental stuttering. *Neurology* 2001; **57**:207–15.

Forrest JM, Menser MA. Congenital rubella in school children and adolescents. *Arch Dis Child* 1970; **45**:63–9.

Forrest JM, Turnbull FM, Sholler GF *et al.* Gregg's congenital rubella patients 60 years later. *Med J Aust* 2002; **177**:664–7.

Forsman H. The mental implications of sex chromosome aberrations. The Blake Marsh lecture for 1970. *Br J Psychiatry* 1970; **117**:353–63.

Fox PT, Ingham RJ, Ingham JC *et al.* A PET study of the neural systems of stuttering. *Nature* 1996; **382**:158–61.

Frankhauser MP, Karumanchi VC, German ML *et al.* A double-blind placebo-controlled study of the efficacy of transdermal clonidine in autism. *J Clin Psychiatry* 1992; **53**:77–82.

Franz DN, Leonard J, Tudor C *et al.* Rapamycin causes regression of astrocytomas in tuberous sclerosis complex. *Ann Neurol* 2006; **59**:490–8.

Fryer AE, Chalmers A, Connor JM *et al.* Evidence that the gene for tuberous sclerosis is on chromosome 9. *Lancet* 1987; **1**:659–61.

Galaburda AM, Eidelberg D. Symmetry and asymmetry in the human posterior thalamus. II. Thalamic lesions in a case of developmental dyslexia. *Arch Neurol* 1982; **39**:333–6.

Galaburda AM, Sherman GF, Rosen GS *et al.* Developmental dyslexia: four consecutive patients with cortical abnormalities. *Ann Neurol* 1985; **18**:222–33.

Gibbs RA, Caskey CT. Identification and localization of mutations at the Lesch–Nyhan locus by ribonuclease A cleavage. *Science* 1987; **236**:303–5.

Giedd JN, Clasen LS, Wallace GL *et al.* XXY (Klinefelter syndrome): a pediatric quantitative brain magnetic resonance imaging case-control study. *Pediatrics* 2007; **119**:232–40.

Gillespie J, Jackson A. *MRI and CT of the brain.* London: Arnold, 2000.

Goh S, Butler W, Thiele EA. Subependymal giant cell tumors in tuberous sclerosis complex. *Neurology* 2004; **63**:1457–61.

Gordon CT, State RC, Nelson JE *et al.* A double-blind comparison of clomipramine, desipramine and placebo in the treatment of autistic disorder. *Arch Gen Psychiatry* 1993; **50**:441–7.

Gordon CT, Cotelingam GM, Stager S *et al.* A double-blind comparison of clomipramine and desipramine in the treatment of developmental stuttering. *J Clin Psychiatry* 1995; **56**:238–42.

Gothelf D, Presburger G, Zohar AH *et al.* Obsessive-compulsive disorder in patients with velocardiofacial (22q11 deletion) syndrome. *Am J Med Genet B Neuropsychiatr Genet* 2004; **126**:99–105.

Gothelf D, Feinstein C, Thompson T *et al.* Risk factors for the emergence of psychotic disorders in adolescents with 22q11.2 deletion syndrome. *Am J Psychiatry* 2007; **164**:663–9.

Goyal M, O'Riordan MA, Wiznetzer M. Effect of topiramate on seizures and respiratory dysrhythmia in Rett syndrome. *J Child Neurol* 2004; **19**:588–91.

Graham DI, Lantos PL. *Greenfield's neurology*, 6th edn. London: Arnold, 1996.

Graham JM, Bashir AS, Stark RE *et al.* Oral and written language abilities of XXY boys: implications for anticipatory guidance. *Pediatrics* 1988; **81**:795–806.

Green JS, Parfrey PS, Harnett JD *et al.* The cardinal features of Bardet-Biedl syndrome, a form of Laurence-Moon-Biedl syndrome. *N Engl J Med* 1989; **321**:1002–9.

Greenswag LR. Adults with Prader-Willi syndrome: a survey of 232 cases. *Dev Med Child Neurol* 1987; **29**:145–52.

Gross-Tsur V, Shalev RS. Reversible language regression as an adverse effect of topiramate treatment in children. *Neurology* 2004; **62**:299–300.

Gubbay SS, de Klerk NH. A study and review of developmental dysgraphia in relation to acquired dysgraphia. *Brain Dev* 1995; **17**:1–8.

Guerreiro MM, Hage SR, Guimaraes CA *et al.* Developmental language disorder associated with polymicrogyria. *Neurology* 2002; **59**:245–50.

Guillamo J-S, Creange A, Kalifa C et al. Prognostic features of CNS tumors in neurofibromatosis 1 (NF1): a retrospective study of 104 patients. *Brain* 2003; **126**:152–60.

Gutierrez GC, Smalley SL, Tanguey PE. Autism in tuberous sclerosis complex. *J Autism Dev Disord* 1998; **28**:97–103.

Gutowski NJ, Murphy RP. Late onset epilepsy in undiagnosed tuberous sclerosis. *Postgrad Med J* 1992; **68**:970–1.

Hagberg BA. Rett syndrome: clinical peculiarities, diagnostic approach, and possible cause. *Pediatr Neurol* 1989; **5**:75–83.

Hagberg BA, Witt-Engerstrom I. Rett's syndrome: a suggested staging system for describing the impairment profile with increasing age toward adolescence. *Am J Med Genet* 1986; **24**(suppl. 1):47–59.

Hagberg B, Aicardi J, Ramos O. A progressive syndrome of autism, ataxia and loss of purposeful hand use in girls: Rett's syndrome: report of 35 cases. *Ann Neurol* 1983; **14**:471–9.

Hagerman RJ, Murphy MA, Wittenberger MD. A controlled trial of stimulant medication in children with fragile X syndrome. *Am J Med Genet* 1988; **30**:377–92.

Hall BD, Smith DW. Prader–Willi syndrome. *J Pediatrics* 1972; **81**:286–93.

Hardy JB. Clinical and developmental aspects of congenital rubella. *Arch Otolaryngol* 1973; **98**:230–6.

Harris JC, Less RR, Jinnah HA et al. Craniocerebral magnetic resonance imaging measurement and findings in Lesch–Nyhan syndrome. *Arch Neurol* 1998; **55**:547–53.

Hatanaka T, Higashino H, Woo M et al. Lesch–Nyhan syndrome with delayed onset of self-mutilation: hyperactivity of interneurons at the brainstem and blink reflex. *Acta Neurol Scand* 1990; **81**:184–7.

Hauser P, Zametkin AJ, Martinez P et al. Attention deficit-hyperactivity disorder in people with generalized resistance to thyroid hormone. *N Engl J Med* 1993; **328**:997–1001.

Hellings JA, Warnock JK. Self-injurious behavior and serotonin in Prader-Willi syndrome. *Psychopharmacol Bull* 1994; **30**:245–50.

Hinshelwood J. A case of dyslexia – a peculiar form of word blindness. *Lancet* 1896; **2**:1454.

Hinton VJ, Brown WT, Wisniewski K et al. Analysis of neocortex in three males with the fragile X syndrome. *Am J Med Genet* 1991; **41**:289–94.

Hollander E, Phillips A, Chaplin W et al. A placebo controlled crossover trial of liquid fluoxetine on repetitive behaviors in childhood and adolescent autism. *Neuropsychopharmacology* 2005; **30**:582–9.

Hollander E, Wasserman S, Swanson EN et al. A double-blind placebo-controlled pilot study of olanzapine in childhood/adolescent pervasive developmental disorder. *J Child Adolesc Psychopharamcol* 2006a; **16**:541–8.

Hollander E, Soorya L, Wasserman S et al. Divalproex sodium vs. placebo in the treatment of repetitive behaviors in autism spectrum disorders. *Int J Neuropsychopharmacol* 2006b; **9**:209–13.

Humphreys P, Kaufmann WE, Galaburda AM. Developmental dyslexia in women: neuropathological findings in three patients. *Ann Neurol* 1990; **28**:727–38.

Hunter H. A controlled study of the psychopathology and physical measurements of Klinefelter's syndrome. *Br J Psychiatry* 1969; **115**:443–8.

Huppke P, Maier EM, Warnke A et al. Very mild cases of Rett syndrome with skewed X inactivation. *J Med Genet* 2006; **43**:814–16.

Huppke P, Kohler K, Brockmann K et al. Treatment of epilepsy in Rett syndrome. *Eur J Paediatr Neurol* 2007; **11**:10–16.

Hurst LC, Mulhall DJ. Another calendar savant. *Br J Psychiatry* 1988; **152**:274–7.

Huson SM, Harper PS, Compston DAS. Von Recklinghausen neurofibromatosis: a clinical and population study in south-east Wales. *Brain* 1988; **111**:1355–81.

Hyman BT, West HL, Rebeck GW et al. Neuropathological changes in Down's syndrome hippocampal formation. Effect of age and apolipoprotein E genotype. *Arch Neurol* 1995; **52**:373–8.

Hyman MH, Whittemore VH. National Institutes of Health consensus conference: tuberous sclerosis complex. *Arch Neurol* 2000; **57**:662–5.

Hyman SL, Gill DS, Shees EA et al. Natural history of cognitive deficits and their relationship to MRI T2-hyperintensities in NF1. *Neurology* 2003; **60**:1139–45.

Hyman SL, Shores A, North KN. The nature and frequency of cognitive deficits in children with neurofibromatosis type 1. *Neurology* 2005; **65**:1037–44.

Hynd GW, Semrud-Clikeman M, Lorys AR et al. Brain morphology in developmental dyslexia and attention deficit disorder/hyperactivity. *Arch Neurol* 1990; **47**:919–26.

Issacs EB, Edmonds CJ, Lucas A et al. Calculation difficulties in children of very low birthweight: a neural correlate. *Brain* 2001; **124**:1681–2.

Itti E, Gaw Gonsalo IT, Pawlikowska-Haddel A et al. The structural brain correlates of cognitive deficits in adults with Klinefelter's syndrome. *J Endocrinol Metabol* 2006; **91**:1423–7.

Jankovic J, Caskey TC, Stout T et al. Lesch–Nyhan syndrome: a study of motor behavior and cerebrospinal fluid neurotransmitters. *Ann Neurol* 1988; **33**:466–9.

Jarrar RG, Buchhalter JR, Raffel C. Long-term outcome of epilepsy surgery in patients with tuberous sclerosis. *Neurology* 2004; **62**:479–81.

Jellinger K, Seitelberger F. Neuropathology of Rett syndrome. *Am J Med Genet* 1986; **1**(suppl.):259–88.

Jellinger K, Armstrong D, Zoghbi HY et al. Neuropathology of Rett syndrome. *Acta Neuropath* 1988; **76**:142–58.

Jervis GA. Early senile dementia in mongoloid idiocy. *Am J Psychiatry* 1948; **105**:102–6.

Jinnah HA, Visser JE, Harris JC et al. Delineation of the motor disorder of Lesch–Nyhan disease. *Brain* 2006; **129**:1210–17.

Jones KL, Smith DW. Recognition of fetal alcohol syndrome in early infancy. *Lancet* 1973; **2**:999–1001.

Jones KL, Smith DW, Streissguth AP et al. Outcome in offspring of chronic alcoholic women. *Lancet* 1974; **1**:1076–8.

Kankirawatana P, Leonard H, Ellaway C et al. Early progressive encephalopathy in boys and *MECP2* mutation. *Neurology* 2006; **67**:164–6.

Kanner L. Autistic disturbances of affective contact. *Nervous Child* 1943; **2**:217–50.

Kanner L. Early infantile autism. *J Pediatrics* 1944; **25**:211–17.

Kanner L. The conception of wholes and parts in early infantile autism. *Am J Psychiatry* 1951; **108**:23–6.

Kao A, Mariani J, McDonald-McGinn DM *et al.* Increased prevalence of seizures in patients with a 22q11.2 deletion. *Am J Med Genet A* 2004; **129**:29–34.

Karlsson B, Gustafsson J, Hedov G *et al.* Thyroid dysfunction in Down's syndrome: relation to age and thyroid autoimmunity. *Arch Dis Child* 1998; **79**:242–5.

Kates WR, Miller AM, Abdulsabur N *et al.* Temporal lobe anatomy and psychiatric symptoms in velocardiofacial syndrome (22q11.2 deletion syndrome). *J Am Acad Child Adolesc Psychiatry* 2006; **45**:587–95.

Khalifa MM, Struthers JL. Klinefelter syndrome is a common cause for mental retardation of unknown etiology among prepubertal males. *Clin Genet* 2002; **61**:49–53.

Kielinen M, Rantala H, Timonen E *et al.* Associated medical disorders and disabilities in children with autistic disorder: a population-based study. *Autism* 2004; **8**:49–60.

Klein D, Ammann F. The syndrome of Laurence–Moon–Biedl–Bardet and allied diseases in Switzerland. *J Neurol Sci* 1969; **9**:479–513.

Kofman O, Hyland HH. Tuberous sclerosis in adults with normal intelligence. *Arch Neurol Psychiatry* 1959; **81**:557–90.

Konovalov HV, Kovetsky NS, Bobryshev YV *et al.* Disorders of brain development in the progeny of mothers who used alcohol during pregnancy. *Early Hum Dev* 1997; **25**:153–66.

Kulkantrakorn K, Geller TJ. Seizures in neurofibromatosis 1. *Pediatr Neurology* 1998; **19**:347–50.

Kuperman S, Perry PJ, Gaffney GR *et al.* Bupropion SR vs. methylphenidate vs. placebo for attention deficit hyperactivity disorder in adults. *Ann Clin Psychiatry* 2001; **13**:129–34.

Lagos JC, Gomez MR. Tuberos sclerosis: reappraisal of a clinical entity. *Mayo Clin Proc* 1967; **42**:26–49.

Lai CS, Fisher SE, Hurst JA *et al.* A forkhead-domain gene is mutated in severe speech and language disorder. *Nature* 2001; **413**:519–23.

Lai F, Williams RS. A prospective study of Alzheimer's disease in Down syndrome. *Arch Neurol* 1989; **46**:849–53.

Larsson G, Bohlin A-B, Tunell R. Prospective study of children exposed to variable amounts of alcohol in utero. *Arch Dis Child* 1985; **60**:316–21.

Lawlor BA, Maurer RG. Tuberous sclerosis and the autistic syndrome. *Br J Psychiatry* 1987; **150**:396–7.

Legius E, Descheemaeker MJ, Steyaert J *et al.* Neurofibromatosis type 1 in childhood: correlation of MRI findings with intelligence. *J Neurol Neurosurg Psychiatry* 1995; **59**:638–40.

Lesch M, Nyhan WL. A familial disorder of uric acid metabolism and central nervous system function. *Am J Med* 1964; **36**:561–70.

Levy AM, Reiss IL, Grafman J. Metabolic abnormalities detected by 1H-MRS in dyscalculia and dysgraphia. *Neurology* 1999; **53**:639–41.

Lichtenstein BW. Sturge–Weber–Dimitri syndrome: cephalic form of neurocutaneous hemangiomatosis. *Arch Neurol Psychiatry* 1954; **71**:291–301.

Listernick R, Charrow J, Greenwald MJ *et al.* Optic gliomas in children with neurofibromatosis type 1. *J Pediatr* 1989; **114**:788–92.

Lubs M-LE, Bauer MS, Formas ME *et al.* Lisch nodules in neurofibromatosis type 1. *N Engl J Med* 1991; **324**:1264–6.

Lund J, Munk-Jorgensen P. Psychiatric aspects of Down's syndrome. *Acta Psychiatr Scand* 1988; **78**:369–74.

Mackie S, Shaw P, Lenroot R *et al.* Cerebellar development and clinical outcome in attention deficit hyperactivity disorder. *Am J Psychiatry* 2007; **164**:645–55.

Madsen KM, Huiid A, Vestergaard M *et al.* A population-based study of measles, mumps, and rubella vaccination and autism. *N Engl J Med* 2002; **347**:1477–82.

Maguire GA, Riley GD, Franklin DL *et al.* Risperidone for the treatment of stuttering. *J Clin Psychopharmacol* 2000; **20**:479–82.

Maguire GA, Riley GD, Franklin DL *et al.* Olanzapine in the treatment of developmental stuttering: a double-blind, placebo-controlled trial. *Ann Clin Psychiatry* 2004; **16**:63–7.

Mannuzza S, Klein RG, Klein DF *et al.* Accuracy of adult recall of childhood attention deficit hyperactivity disorder. *Am J Psychiatry* 2002; **159**:1882–8.

Maria BL, Neufeld JA, Rosainz LC *et al.* Central nervous system structure and function in Sturge–Weber syndrome: evidence of neurologic and radiologic progression. *J Child Neurol* 1998; **13**:606–18.

Martins IP, Ferreira J, Borges L. Acquired procedural dyscalculia associated to a left parietal lesion in a child. *Child Neuropsychol* 1999; **5**:265–73.

Mathews WS, Solan A, Barabas G. Cognitive functioning in Lesch–Nyhan syndrome. *Dev Med Child Neurol* 1995; **37**:715–22.

Max JE, Schacher RJ, Levin HS *et al.* Predictors of secondary attention-deficit/hyperactivity disorder in children and adolescents 6 to 24 months after traumatic brain injury. *J Am Acad Child Adolesc Psychiatry* 2005; **44**:1041–9.

McCracken JT, McGough J, Shah H *et al.* Risperidone in children with autism and serious behavioral problems. *N Engl J Med* 2002; **347**:314–21.

McDonald-McGinn DM, Tonnesen MK, Laufer-Cahana A *et al.* Phenotype of the 22q11.2 deletion in individuals identified through an affected relative: cast a wide FISHing net! *Genet Med* 2001; **3**:23–9.

McDougle CJ, Naylor ST, Cohen DJ *et al.* A double-blind, placebo-controlled study of fluvoxamine in adults with autistic disorder. *Arch Gen Psychiatry* 1996; **53**:1001–8.

McDougle CJ, Holmes JP, Carlson DC *et al.* A double-blind, placebo-controlled study of risperidone in adults with autistic disorder and other pervasive developmental disorders. *Arch Gen Psychiatry* 1998; **55**:633–41.

McDougle CJ, Scahill L, Aman MG *et al.* Risperidone for the core symptom domains of autism: results from the study by the Autism Network of the Research Units on Pediatric Psychopharmacology. *Am J Psychiatry* 2005; **162**:1142–8.

McManaman J, Tam DA. Gabapentin for self-injurious behavior in Lesch–Nyhan syndrome. *Pediatr Neurology* 1999; **20**:381–2.

McVicker RW, Shanks OEP, McClelland RJ. Prevalence and associated features of epilepsy in adults with Down's syndrome. *Br J Psychiatry* 1994; **164**:528–32.

Miller E, Craddock-Watson JE, Pollock TM. Consequences of confirmed maternal rubella at successive stages of pregnancy. *Lancet* 1982; **2**:781–4.

Miller JL, Couch JA, Schmalfuss *et al.* Intracranial abnormalities detected by three-dimensional magnetic resonance imaging in Prader-Willi syndrome. *Am J Med Genet A* 2007; **143**:476–83.

Mizuno T. Long-term follow-up of ten patients with Lesch–Nyhan syndrome. *Neuropediatrics* 1986; **17**:158–61.

Mohammadi MR, Ghanizadeh A, Alaghband-Rad J *et al.* Selegeline in comparison with methylphenidate in attention deficit hyperactivity disorder children and adolescents in a double-blind, randomized trial. *J Child Adolesc Psychopharamcol* 2004; **14**:418–25.

Molfese DL. Predicting dyslexia at 8 years of age using neonatal brain responses. *Brain Lang* 2000; **72**:238–45.

Monaghan HP, Krafchik BR, Macgregor DL *et al.* Tuberous sclerosis complex in children. *Am J Dis Child* 1981; **135**:912–17.

Morimoto K, Mogami H. Sequential CT study of subependymal giant-cell astrocytoma associated with tuberous sclerosis. *J Neurosurg* 1986; **65**:874–7.

Mostofsky SH, Mazzocco MM, Aakalu G *et al.* Decreased cerebellar posterior vermis size in fragile X syndrome: correlation with neurocognitive performance. *Neurology* 1998; **50**:121–30.

Murphy KC, Jones LA, Owen MJ. High rates of schizophrenia in adults with velo-cardio-facial syndrome. *Arch Gen Psychiatry* 1999; **56**:940–5.

Murray TJ, Kelly P, Campbell L *et al.* Haloperidol in the treatment of stuttering. *Br J Psychiatry* 1977; **130**:370–3.

Musumeci SA, Hagerman RJ, Ferri R *et al.* Epilepsy and EEG findings in males with fragile X syndrome. *Epilepsia* 1999; **40**:1092–9.

Myers SE, Whitman BY, Carrel AL *et al.* Two years of growth hormone therapy in young children with Prader-Willi syndrome: physical and neurodevelopmental benefits. *Am J Med Genet A* 2006; **143**:443–8.

Nasr JT, Gabis L, Savatic M *et al.* The electroencephalogram in children with developmental dysphasia. *Epilepsy Beh* 2001; **2**:115–18.

Nielsen J. Klinefelter's syndrome and the XYY syndrome. *Acta Psychiatr Scand Suppl* 1969; **209**:1–353.

Nielsen J, Pelsen B, Sorensen K. Follow-up of 30 Klinefelter males treated with testosterone. *Clin Genet* 1988; **33**:262–9.

North K, Joy P, Yuille D *et al.* Specific learning disability in children with neurofibromatosis type 1: significance of MRI abnormalities. *Neurology* 1994; **44**:878–83.

Nyhan WL. Clinical features of the Lesch–Nyhan syndrome. *Arch Int Med* 1972; **130**:186–92.

Ogasawara N, Stout JT, Goto H *et al.* Molecular analysis of a female Lesch–Nyhan patient. *J Clin Invest* 1989; **84**:1024–7.

Oldfors A, Sourander P, Armstrong DL *et al.* Rett syndrome: cerebellar pathology. *Pediatr Neurol* 1990; **6**:310–14.

Olsson I, Steffenberg S, Billberg C. Epilepsy in autism and autistic-like conditions. *Arch Neurol* 1988; **45**:666–8.

Ornitz EM, Ritvo ER. Perceptual inconstancy in early infantile autism: the syndrome of early infant autism and its variants, including certain cases of childhood schizophrenia. *Arch Gen Psychiatry* 1968; **18**:76–8.

Orton ST. Word blindness in school children. *Arch Neurol Psychiatry* 1925; **14**:581–615.

Palmen SJ, von Engeland H, Hof PR *et al.* Neuropathological findings in autism. *Brain* 2004; **127**:2572–83.

Pampiglione G, Moynahan EJ. The tuberous sclerosis syndrome: clinical and EEG studies in 100 children. *J Neurol Neurosurg Psychiatry* 1976; **39**:666–73.

Papolos DF, Faedda GL, Veit S *et al.* Bipolar spectrum disorders in patients diagnosed with velo-cardio-facial syndrome: does a hemizygous deletion of chromosome 22q11 result in bipolar affective disorder? *Am J Psychiatry* 1996; **153**:1541–7.

Pascual-Castroviejo I, Diaz-Gonzales C, Garcia-Melian RM *et al.* Sturge–Weber syndrome: study of 40 patients. *Pediatr Neurology* 1993; **9**:283–8.

Pasqualini RQ, Vidal G, Bur GE. Psychopathology of Klinefelter's syndrome. Review of thirty-one cases. *Lancet* 1957; **2**:164–7.

Paul R, Cohen DJ, Caparulo BK. A longitudinal study of patients with severe developmental disorders of language learning. *J Am Acad Child Psychiatry* 1983; **22**:525–34.

Pearson E, Lenn NJ, Cail WS. Moymoya and other causes of stroke in patients with Down syndrome. *Pediatr Neurol* 1985; **1**:174–9.

Pelham WE, Gnagy EM, Chronis AM *et al.* A comparison of morning-only and morning/late afternoon Adderall to morning-only, twice-daily, and three times-daily methylphenidate in children with attention-deficit/hyperactivity disorder. *Pediatrics* 1999; **104**:1300–11.

Percy AK, Gillberg C, Hagberg B *et al.* Rett syndrome and the autistic disorders. *Neurol Clinics* 1990; **8**:659–76.

Percy AK, Glaze DG, Schultz RJ *et al.* Rett syndrome: controlled study of oral opiate antagonist naltrexone. *Ann Neurol* 1994; **35**:464–70.

Petermann AF, Hayles AB, Dockerty MB *et al.* Encephalotrigeminal angiomatosis (Sturge–Weber disease). Clinical study of 35 cases. *J Am Med Assoc* 1958; **167**:2169–76.

Petersen CD, Luzzatti K. The role of chromosome translocation in the recurrence risk of Down's syndrome. *Pediatrics* 1965; **35**:463–9.

Pfeiffer J, Majewski F, Fischbach H *et al.* Alcohol embryopathy and fetopathy: neuropathology of three children and three fetuses. *J Neurol Sci* 1979; **41**:125–37.

Picard A, Cheliout Heraut F, Bouskaoui M *et al.* Sleep EEG and developmental dysphasia. *Dev Med Child Neurol* 1998; **40**:595–9.

Plotkin SA, Oski SA, Hartnett EM *et al.* Some recently recognized manifestations of the rubella syndrome. *J Pediatrics* 1965; **67**:182–91.

Pomeroy JC. Klinefelter's syndrome and schizophrenia. *Br J Psychiatry* 1980; **136**:597–9.

Prasher VP. Epilepsy and associated effects on adaptive behavior in adults with Down syndrome. *Seizure* 1995; **4**:53–6.

Prasher VP, Huxley A, Haque MS *et al.* A 24-week, double-blind, placebo-controlled trial of donepezil in patients with Down syndrome and Alzheimer's disease – pilot study. *Int J Geriatr Psychiatry* 2002; **17**:270–8.

Pueschel SM, Louis S, McKnight P. Seizure disorders in Down syndrome. *Arch Neurol* 1991; **48**:318–20.

Ramaekers VT, Hansen SI, Holm J *et al.* Reduced folate transport to the CNS in female Rett patients. *Neurology* 2003; **61**:506–15.

Ratcliffe SG, Bancroft J, Axworthy D *et al.* Klinefelter's syndrome in adolescents. *Arch Dis Child* 1982; **57**:6–12.

Rathmell TK, Burns MA. The Laurence–Moon–Biedl syndrome occurring in a brother and a sister. *Arch Neurol Psychiatry* 1938; **39**:1022–42.

Reiss AL, Lee J, Freunc L. Neuroanatomy of fragile X syndrome: the temporal lobe. *Neurology* 1994; **44**:1317–24.

Remington G, Sloman L, Konstantareas M *et al.* Clomipramine versus haloperidol in the treatment of autistic disorder: a double-blind, placebo-controlled, crossover study. *J Clin Psychopharmacol* 2001; **21**:440–4.

Research Units on Pediatric Psychopharmacology Autism Network. Risperidone in children with autism and serious behavioral problems. *N Engl J Med* 2002; **347**:314–21.

Research Units on Pediatric Psychopharmacology (RUPP) Autism Network. Randomized, controlled, crossover trial of methylphenidate in pervasive developmental disorder with hyperactivity. *Arch Gen Psychiatry* 2005; **62**:1266–74.

Rett A. Uber ein eigenartiges hirnatrophisches syndrom bei hyperammonamie im kindersalter. *Wien Med Wochenschr* 1966; **116**:723–6.

Richardson EP. Pathology of tuberous sclerosis. Neuropathologic aspects. *Ann NY Acad Sci* 1991; **615**:128–39.

Richer JM, Coss RG. Gaze aversion in autistic and normal children. *Acta Psychiatr Scand* 1976; **53**:193–210.

Ritvo ER, Mason-Brothers A, Freeman BJ *et al.* The UCLA–University of Utah epidemiologic survey of autism: the etiological role of rare diseases. *Am J Psychiatry* 1990; **147**:1614–21.

Roach ES, Delgado M, Anderson L *et al.* Carbamazepine trial for Lesch-Nyhan self-mutilation. *J Child Neurol* 1996; **11**:476–8.

Robinson WP, Bottani A, Yagang X. Molecular, cytogenetic and clinical investigations of Prader–Willi syndrome patients. *Am J Hum Genet* 1992; **49**:1219–34.

Rodriguez HA, Barthrong M. Multiple primary intracranial tumors in von Recklinghausen's neurofibromatosis. *Arch Neurol* 1966; **14**:467–75.

Roeltgen DP, Tucker DM. Developmental phonological and lexical agraphia in adults. *Brain Lang* 1988; **35**:287–300.

Roizen L, Gold G, Berman HH *et al.* Congenital vascular anomalies and their histopathology in Sturge–Weber–Dimitri syndrome (nevus flammeus with angiomatosis and encephalosis calcificans). *J Neuropathol Exp Neurol* 1972; **14**:173–88.

Rorke LB. Nervous system lesions in the congenital rubella syndrome. *Arch Otolaryngol* 1973; **98**:249–51.

Rorke LB, Spiro AJ. Cerebral lesions in congenital rubella syndrome. *J Pediatrics* 1967; **70**:243–55.

Rosman NP, Pearce J. The brain in multiple neurofibromatosis (von Recklinghausen's disease): a suggested basis for the associated mental defect. *Brain* 1967; **90**:829–37.

Ross AT, Dickerson WW. Tuberous sclerosis. *Arch Neurol Psychiatry* 1943; **50**:233–57.

Ross MH, Galaburda AM, Kemper TL. Down's syndrome: is there a decreased population of neurons? *Neurology* 1984; **34**:909–16.

Roth AA. Familial eunuchoidism: the Laurence–Moon–Biedl syndrome. *J Urology* 1947; **57**:427–42.

Roth JC, Epstein CJ. Infantile spasms and hypopigmented macules: early manifestations of tuberous sclerosis. *Arch Neurol* 1971; **25**:547–51.

Rouleau GA, Wertelecki BR, Martuza RI *et al.* Genetic linkage of bilateral acoustic neurofibromatosis to a DNA marker on chromosome 22. *Nature* 1987; **329**:246–8.

Roy A. Schizophrenia and Klinefelter's syndrome. *Can J Psychiatry* 1981; **26**:262–4.

Rudelli RD, Brown WT, Wisniewski K *et al.* Adult fragile X syndrome: clinico-neuropathologic findings. *Acta Neuropathol* 1985; **67**:289–95.

Rumsey JM, Rapoport JL, Sceery WR. Autistic children as adults: psychiatric, social, and behavioral outcomes. *J Am Acad Child Psychiatry* 1985; **24**:465–73.

Rumsey JM, Donohue BC, Brady DR *et al.* A magnetic resonance imaging study of planum temporale asymmetry in men with developmental dyslexia. *Arch Neurol* 1997; **54**:1481–9.

Sabaratnam M, Vroegop PG, Gangadhran SK. Epilepsy and EEG findings in 18 males with fragile X syndrome. *Seizure* 2001; **10**:60–3.

Saito Y, Ito M, Hanaoka S *et al.* Dopamine receptor upregulation in Lesch-Nyhan syndrome: a postmortem study. *Neuropediatrics* 1999; **30**:66–71.

Sato S, Dreifuss FE. Electroencephalographic findings in a patient with developmental expressive aphasia. *Neurology* 1973; **23**:181–5.

Scahill L, Chappell PB, Kim YS *et al.* A placebo-controlled study of guanfacine in the treatment of children with tic disorders and attention deficit hyperactivity disorder. *Am J Psychiatry* 2001; **158**:1067–74.

Schaer M, Schmitt JE, Glaser B *et al.* Abnormal patterns of cortical gyrification in velo-cardio-facial syndrome (deletion 22q11.2): an MRI study. *Psychiatry Res* 2006; **146**:1–11.

Schochet SS, Lampert PW, McCormick WF. Neurofibrillary tangles in patients with Down's syndrome: a light and electron-microscopic study. *Acta Neuropathol* 1973; **23**:342–6.

Schulte-Korne G. Annotation: genetics of reading and spelling disorder. *J Child Psychol Psychiatry* 2001; **42**:985–97.

Selikowitz M, Sunman J, Pendergast A *et al.* Fenfluramine in Prader-Willi syndrome: a double blind, placebo controlled trial. *Arch Dis Child* 1990; **65**:112–14.

Shalev RS. Developmental dyscalculia. *J Child Neurol* 2004; **19**:765–71.

Shalev RS, Gross-Tsur V. Developmental dyscalculia and medical assessment. *J Learn Disabil* 1993; **26**:134–7.

Shalev RS, Manor O, Kerem B *et al.* Developmental dyscalculia is a familial learning disability. *J Learn Disabil* 2001; **34**:59–65.

Shalev RS, Manor O, Gross-Tsur V. Developmental dyscalculia: a prospective six-year follow-up. *Dev Med Child Neurol* 2005; **47**:121–5.

Shaw J, Lerch J, Greenstein D *et al.* Longitudinal mapping of cortical thickness and clinical outcome in children and adolescents with attention-deficit/hyperactivity disorder. *Arch Gen Psychiatry* 2006; **63**:540–9.

Shaywitz SE, Caparulo B, Hodgson ES. Developmental language disability as a result of prenatal exposure to ethanol. *Pediatrics* 1981; **68**:850–5.

Shprintzen RJ, Goldberg RB, Lewin ML *et al*. A new syndrome involving cleft palate, cardiac anomalies, typical facies, and learning disabilities: velo-cardio-facial syndrome. *Cleft Palate J* 1978; **15**:56–62.

SLI Consortium (SLIC). Highly significant linkage to the SLI1 locus in an expanded sample of individuals affected by specific language impairment. *Am J Hum Genet* 2004; **74**:1225–38.

Smathers SA, Wilson JG, Nigro MA. Topiramate effectiveness in Prader-Willi syndrome. *Pediatr Neurol* 2003; **28**:130–3.

Spencer T, Biederaman J, Coffey B *et al*. A double-blind comparison of desipramine and placebo in children and adolescents with chronic tic disorder and comorbid attention-deficit/hyperactivity disorder. *Arch Gen Psychiatry* 2002; **59**:649–56.

Spohr HL, Willms J, Steinhausen HC. Prenatal alcohol exposure and long-term developmental consequences. *Lancet* 1993; **341**:907–10.

Stenbom Y, Tonnby B, Hagberg B. Lamotrigine in Rett syndrome: treatment experience from a pilot study. *Eur Child Adolesc Psychiatry* 1998; **7**:49–52.

Stoll C, Alembik Y, Dott B *et al*. Study of Down syndrome in 238,942 consecutive births. *Ann Genet* 1998; **41**:44–51.

Streissguth AP, Aase JM, Clarren SK *et al*. Fetal alcohol syndrome in adolescents and adults. *J Am Med Assoc* 1991; **265**:1961–7.

Sturge WA. A case of partial epilepsy, apparently due to a lesion of one of the vaso-motor centres of the brain. *Trans Clin Soc London* 1879; **12**:162–7.

Suetsugu M, Mehraein P. Spine distribution along the apical dendrites of the pyramidal neurons in Down's syndrome. A quantitative Golgi study. *Acta Neuropathol* 1980; **50**:207–10.

Sujansky E, Conradi S. Sturge–Weber syndrome: age of onset of seizures and glaucoma and the prognosis for affected children. *J Child Neurol* 1995a; **10**:49–58.

Sujansky E, Conradi S. Outcome of Sturge–Weber syndrome in 52 adults. *Am J Med Genet* 1995b; **57**:35–45.

Suresh R, Ambrose N, Roe C *et al*. New complexities in the genetics of stuttering: significant sex-specific linkage signals. *Am J Hum Genet* 2006; **78**:554–63.

Sutherland GR. Heritable fragile sites on human chromosomes. Demonstration of their dependence on the type of tissue culture medium. *Science* 1977; **197**:265.

Swaab DJ, Purba JS, Hofman MA. Alterations in the hypothalamic paraventricular nucleus and its xytocin neurons (putative saticty cells) in Prader-Willi syndrome: a study of five cases. *J Clin Endocrinol Metab* 1995; **80**:573–9.

Swanson DW, Stipes AH. Psychiatric aspects of Klinefelter's syndrome. *Am J Psychiatry* 1969; **126**:814–22.

Swillen A, Devriendt K, Legius E *et al*. Intelligence and psychosocial adjustment in velocardiofacial syndrome: a study of 37 children and adolescents with VCFS. *J Med Genet* 1997; **34**:453–8.

Taira T, Kobayashi T, Hori T. Disappearance of self-mutilating behavior in a patient with Lesch-Nyhan syndrome after

bilateral chronic stimulation of the globus pallidus internus. *J Neurosurg* 2003; **98**:414–16.

Taly AB, Nagaraja D, Das S *et al*. Sturge–Weber–Dimitri disease without facial nevus. *Neurology* 1987; **37**:1063–4.

Tartakow IJ. The teratogenicity of maternal rubella. *J Pediatrics* 1965; **66**:380–91.

Tatum WO, Passaro EA, Elia M *et al*. Seizure in Klinefelter's syndrome. *Pediatr Neurology* 1998; **19**:275–82.

Taylor FB, Russo J. Efficacy of modafinil compared to dextroamphetamine for the treatment of attention deficit hyperactivity disorder in adults. *J Child Adolesc Psychopharmacol* 2000; **10**:311–20.

Taylor FB, Russo J. Comparing guanfacine and destroamphetamine for the treatment of adult attention-deficit/hyperactivity disorder. *J Clin Psychopharmacol* 2001; **21**:223–8.

Temudo T, Oliveira P, Santos M *et al*. Stereotypies in Rett syndrome. Analysis of 83 patients with and without detected MECP2 mutation. *Neurology* 2007; **68**:1183–7.

Treffert D. The idiot savant: a review of the syndrome. *Am J Psychiatry* 1988; **145**:563–72.

Verkerk AJ, Pieretti M, Sutcliffe JS *et al*. Identification of a gene (FMR1) containing a CGG repeat coincident with a breakage point cluster region exhibiting length variation in fragile X syndrome. *Cell* 1991; **65**:905–14.

Wakeling A. Comparative study of psychiatric patients with Klinefelter's syndrome and hypogonadism. *Psychol Med* 1972; **2**:139–54.

Wallace MR, Marchuk DA, Andersen LB *et al*. Type 1 neurofibromatosis gene: identification of a large transcript disrupted in three NF1 patients. *Science* 1990; **249**:181–6.

Warren AC, Holroyd S, Folstein MF. Major depression in Down's syndrome. *Br J Psychiatry* 1989; **155**:202–5.

Webb DW, Osborne JP. Tuberous sclerosis. *Arch Dis Child* 1995; **72**:471–4.

Weber FP. A note on the association of extensive haemangiomatous naevus of the skin with cerebral (meningeal) haemangioma especially cases of facial vascular naevus with contralateral hemiplegia. *Proc R Soc Med* 1929; **22**:431–42.

Webster RI, Shevell MI. Neurobiology of specific language impairment. *J Child Neurol* 2004; **19**:471–81.

Weig SG, Pollack P. Carbamazepine-induced heart block in a child with tuberous sclerosis and cardiac rhabdomyoma: implications for evaluation and follow-up. *Ann Neurol* 1993; **34**:617–19.

Wigal SB, McGough JJ, McCracken JT *et al*. A laboratory school comparison of mixed amphetamine salts extended release (Adderall XR) and atomoxatine (Strattera) in school-aged children with attention deficit/hyperactivity disorder. *J Attent Disord* 2005; **9**:275–89.

Williams J, O'Donovan MC. The genetics of developmental dyslexia. *Eur J Hum Genet* 2006; **14**:681–9.

Wilsher CR, Bennett D, Chase CH *et al*. Piracetam and dyslexia: effects on reading tests. *J Clin Psychopharmacol* 1987; **7**:230–7.

Wisniewski K, Dambska M, Sher JH *et al*. A clinical neuropathological study of the fetal alcohol syndrome. *Neuropediatrics* 1983; **14**:197–201.

Wisniewski KE, Dalton AJ, McLachlan DRC *et al.* Alzheimer's disease in Down's syndrome: clinicopathologic studies. *Neurology* 1985a; **35**:957–61.

Wisniewski KE, Wisniewski HM, Wen GY. Occurrence of neuropathological changes and dementia of Alzheimer's disease in Down's syndrome. *Ann Neurol* 1985b; **17**:278–82.

Wisniewski KE, Frency JH, Fernando S *et al.* Fragile X syndrome: associated neurological abnormalities and developmental disabilities. *Ann Neurol* 1985c; **18**:665–9.

Witt-Engerstrom I. Rett syndrome in Sweden. Neurodevelopment – disability – pathophysiology. *Acta Pediatr Scand Suppl* 1990; **369**:1–60.

Wohlwill FS, Yakovlev PI. Histopathology of meningo-facial angiomatosis (Sturge–Weber's disease). *J Neuropathol Exp Neurol* 1957; **16**:341–64.

Wong DF, Harris JC, Naidu S *et al.* Dopamine transporters are markedly reduced in Lesch-Nyhan disease in vivo. *Proc Natl Acad Sci* 1996; **93**:5539–43.

Wu JC, Maguire G, Riley G *et al.* A positron emission tomography (18F) deoxyglucose study of developmental stuttering. *Neuroreport* 1995; **15**:501–5.

Yakovlev PI, Corwin W. Roentgenographic sign in cases of tuberous sclerosis of the brain (multiple 'brain stones'). *Arch Neurol Psychiatry* 1939; **40**:1030–7.

Yang TP, Patel PI, Stout JT *et al.* Molecular evidence for new mutations in the HPRT locus in Lesch–Nyhan patients. *Nature* 1984; **310**:412–14.

Zametkin A, Rapoport JL, Murphy DL *et al.* Treatment of hyperactive children with monoamine oxidase inhibitors. I. Clinical efficacy. *Arch Gen Psychiatry* 1985; **42**:962–6.

Zappella M. A double blind trial of bromocriptine in the Rett syndrome. *Brain Dev* 1990; **12**:148–50.

Zellweger H, Schneider HJ. Syndrome of hypotonia–hypomentia–hypogonadism–obesity (HHHO) or Prader–Willi syndrome. *Am J Dis Child* 1968; **115**:588–98.

Vascular disorders

10.1 MULTI-INFARCT DEMENTIA

Multi-infarct dementia is the traditional name given to dementia occurring secondary to multiple, generally large, cortical infarctions; classically, in addition to the dementia, such patients also have focal signs, such as aphasia, and their history is characterized by a 'stepwise' course, with successive steps further down the cognitive ladder corresponding to successive large-vessel, territorial infarctions. As will be noted below, however, variations on this classic picture do occur. Thus conceived, multi-infarct dementia is, in all likelihood, a common cause of dementia in the elderly.

Before proceeding, some comments are in order regarding the term 'vascular dementia'. Vascular dementia is an umbrella term that includes not only multi-infarct dementia but also lacunar dementia (Section 10.2) and Binswanger's disease (Section 10.4). Lacunar dementia occurs secondary to multiple subcortical lacunar infarctions, whereas Binswanger's disease appears on the basis of a gradually progressive ischemic leukoencephalopathy. Unfortunately for those diagnosticians who yearn for precision, although 'pure' cases of each of these three types of vascular dementia do occur, it is common to find elements of two or even all three of these at the same time in any given patient.

Clinical features

The onset of multi-infarct dementia corresponds to the age of greatest risk for stroke, and hence most patients are in their sixties or older. In most cases, one finds a history of multiple strokes preceding the onset of cognitive decline. Although in some cases the dementia may be rather non-specific, with mere difficulties in memory, calculations, and abstractions, etc., in many cases multi-infarct dementia is marked by depression, agitation, and hallucinations or delusions (Cummings et al. 1987). Depression may be heavily tinged with irritability, and agitation may be extreme. Hallucinations are generally visual, and delusions tend to be either of persecution or misidentification. Focal signs, as noted, are common and may include aphasia, apraxia, neglect, and hemiparesis etc.; late in the course a pseudobulbar palsy may also appear, with, as discussed in Section 4.7, emotional incontinence. Seizures may also occur.

Neuroimaging, either with computed tomography (CT) or, preferably, magnetic resonance imaging (MRI), will reveal evidence of multiple old infarctions in, as discussed below, appropriately 'strategic' locations.

Course

As noted, the classic course of multi-infarct dementia is stepwise, with successive strokes bringing the patient down yet another step into further cognitive deterioration. Importantly, many of these steps are characterized by a delirium, which gradually resolves concurrent with the resolution of peri-lesional edema. Exceptions to this rule, however, do occur. In some cases, the course may be marked by one giant step down, as in cases of multiple simultaneous infarcts or with one infarct occurring in an exquisitely strategic location.

Etiology

In most cases, the dementia occurs secondary to bilateral, multiple, territorial large vessel infarctions involving the frontal, parietal, and temporal cortices (Erkinjunti *et al.* 1988; Jayakumar *et al.* 1989; Ladurna *et al.* 1982; Liu *et al.* 1992; Tomlinson *et al.* 1970); rarely, single infarctions, for example in the temporal or frontal lobes, may be responsible (Auchus *et al.* 2002; Yoshitake *et al.* 1995). Although most cases are due to infarction, as the name 'multi-infarct' suggests, a very similar clinical picture can emerge with multiple intracerebral hemorrhages, and it is probably appropriate to lump these cases under the rubric of multi-infarct dementia. A better name might be 'multi-stroke' dementia, but the term multi-infarct has great currency and probably will not change.

The multiple causes of these infarctions (and hemorrhages) are discussed in Section 7.4.

Differential diagnosis

The diagnosis of multi-infarct dementia should be considered in any patient with dementia and a history of stroke. In weighing this history, however, one must take into account the location of the lesion: whereas infarcts in such cognitively strategic locations as the frontal, parietal, or temporal cortices might be expected to cause dementia, one would be hard-pressed to attribute a dementia to infarctions occurring in the occipital lobes.

Lacunar dementia may also present with a history of stroke; however, here the strokes tend to be of the lacunar variety, such as pure motor stroke. Furthermore, and in contrast to multi-infarct dementia, lacunar dementia tends to be characterized by a frontal lobe syndrome.

As noted earlier, it is not uncommon to find patients with more than one vascular process underlying a dementia, and in such cases MR scanning is generally necessary to determine the various contributions of cortical infarctions, lacunar infarctions, and diffuse white matter disease. In some instances, it may not be possible to disentangle the effects of each of these separate processes, and in such cases, one may have to be content with merely making a diagnosis of vascular dementia.

Given the prevalence of Alzheimer's disease, it must also be borne in mind that it is not at all uncommon to find patients with a 'mixed' dementia, that is with a combination of multi-infarct dementia and Alzheimer's disease (Tomlinson *et al.* 1970). Such a diagnosis should be considered in cases in which the course is mixed, being composed of sequential downward steps occurring on a background of a steady, gradual decline.

Treatment

The general treatment of dementia is discussed in Section 5.1. Antidepressants, for example a selective serotonin reuptake inhibitor (SSRI), may be needed for depressive symptoms, and antipsychotics, such as risperidone, for hallucinations, delusions, and agitation. There is also evidence that both the cholinesterase inhibitors donepezil (Black *et al.* 2003; Wilkinson *et al.* 2003) and galantamine (Auchus *et al.* 2007), and memantine (Orgogozo *et al.* 2002; Wilcock *et al.* 2002) may improve overall cognitive function.

Concurrent with symptomatic treatment, steps should be taken to prevent future strokes if possible, as discussed in Section 7.4.

10.2 LACUNAR DEMENTIA

As discussed in Section 7.4, lacunes are small cavities that may be found in the thalamus, basal ganglia, and internal and external capsules, among other locations, and which occur as sequelae to infarctions in the areas of distribution of central or perforating arteries. Single lacunes may be clinically 'silent' or present with one of the classic lacunar syndromes, such as pure motor stroke. When multiple lacunes are present, one speaks of the 'lacunar state'; when significant cognitive impairment occurs on the basis of multiple lacunes (or, albeit uncommonly, on the basis of a single 'strategically' located lacune) it is customary to speak of subcortical vascular dementia or, more simply, lacunar dementia. Lacunar dementia, along with multi-infarct dementia and Binswanger's disease, is a vascular dementia, and although it may occur in a 'pure' state, it is not uncommonly accompanied by other evidence of vascular pathology, such as the large territorial infarcts seen in multi-infarct dementia or the ischemic leukoencephalopathy of Binswanger's disease.

Although the prevalence of lacunar dementia is not known with any precision, the clinical impression is that it is not uncommon.

Clinical features

In addition to cognitive deficits such as decreased short-term memory, slowed thinking, and disorientation (Mok *et al.* 2004), etc., one also classically sees elements of the frontal lobe syndrome such as disinhibition, affective change, perseveration or apathy (Ishii *et al.* 1986; Wolfe *et al.* 1990). In some cases, parkinsonism may occur, as discussed in Section 10.3. As might be expected, there is typically also a history of lacunar syndromes, such as pure motor stroke, ataxic hemiparesis, dysarthria–clumsy hand or pure sensory stroke. Furthermore, and in advanced cases of the lacunar state, it is common to see a psuedobulbar palsy with, as described in Section 4.7, emotional incontinence.

Although CT scanning may reveal some lacunes, MRI is far more sensitive and is strongly recommended.

Course

In most cases, lacunar dementia is a progressive condition, and the progression itself may be either 'stepwise' or more or less gradual (Ishii *et al.* 1986; Swartz and Black 2006; Yoshitake *et al.* 1995), depending on the size and location of subsequent lacunar infarctions. Larger or strategically placed lacunes may cause an obvious step down the cognitive ladder; conversely, small lacunes, although individually clinically 'silent', may, upon accumulation, cause a clinically noticeable, and more or less gradually appearing, cognitive deficit.

Etiology

In all likelihood, lacunes cause cognitive deficits by interrupting the circuit that runs from the frontal cortex to the basal ganglia, then to the thalamus and finally back to the frontal lobe, and this may account for the frequency with which the frontal lobe syndrome accompanies this dementia. A discussion of the mechanisms underlying the infarctions that create these lacunes is provided in Section 7.4.

Although in most cases multiple lacunes (generally a dozen or more [Ishii *et al.* 1986]) are found, in some instances single lacunes, if strategically located, for example in the anteromedial thalamus (Auchus *et al.* 2002; Katz *et al.* 1987; Mori *et al.* 1986; Sandson *et al.* 1991; Swartz and Black 2006), may cause a dementia.

Differential diagnosis

Lacunar dementia should be suspected in any demented patient with a history of lacunar syndromes or with multiple (or strategically placed) lacunes found on MR scanning. As noted earlier, it is not uncommon to find evidence of other vascular pathology and, in cases in which there are also large, territorial cortical infarcts or extensive white matter disease in addition to lacunes, clinical judgment must come into play in deciding how important the lacunes are in the development of the dementia. In this regard, one looks not only to the number of lacunes but also, as noted, to their location: whereas lacunes in the posterior limb of the internal capsule may not be that important, those situated in the thalamus, genu or anterior limb of the internal capsule or the head of the caudate are more likely to cause cognitive deficits.

Treatment

The overall treatment of dementia, the frontal lobe syndrome, and pseudobulbar palsy is discussed in Sections 5.1, 7.2, and 4.7 respectively. There is some evidence that donepezil (Black *et al.* 2003; Wilkinson *et al.* 2003), galantamine (Auchus *et al.* 2007), and memantine (Orgogozo *et al.* 2002; Wilcock *et al.* 2002) are helpful. Treatment aimed at preventing future lacunar infarctions is discussed in Section 7.4.

10.3 VASCULAR PARKINSONISM

Vascular parkinsonism, formerly known as arteriosclerotic parkinsonism, first described by Critchley in 1929, is characterized by an atypical parkinsonism occurring on the basis of lacunar infarctions either in the mesencephalon or basal ganglia. It is probably an uncommon disorder.

Clinical features

The onset is generally in the seventh or eighth decade. Clinically (Bruetsch and Williams 1954; Keschner and Sloane 1931; Murrow *et al.* 1990; Tolosa and Santamaria 1984; Winikates and Jankovic 1999; Zijlmans *et al.* 2004a), the parkinsonism is characterized by bradykinesia, lead-pipe rigidity, instability, and a tendency to fall. The posture of these patients may or may not be in flexion; the gait is either shuffling or 'magnetic' in that the feet seem 'stuck' to the floor. Overall, these parkinsonian features may be either symmetric or asymmetric. Notably, both tremor and cogwheeling are generally absent, and, as discussed below, the response to levodopa is generally poor. A lacunar dementia, as described in Section 10.2, may occur (Bruetsch and Williams 1954; Keschner and Sloane 1931), and typically one finds evidence of damage to corticospinal tracts (e.g., spasticity) and corticobulbar tracts, with pseudobulbar palsy.

Magnetic resonance scanning reveals multiple lacunes, with at least some of them involving either the basal ganglia or the mesencephalon (Zijlmans *et al.* 1995).

Course

The overall course is generally one of progression, and may be either 'stepwise' or more or less gradual.

Etiology

Case reports have clearly demonstrated that parkinsonism can occur secondary to solitary lacunar infarctions in such strategic locations as the basal ganglia (Lazzarino *et al.* 1990) or the substantia nigra (Akyol *et al.* 2006; Hunter *et al.* 1978). In most patients, however, vascular parkinsonism occurs in the setting of multiple lacunes (Bruetsch and Williams 1954; Keschner and Sloane 1931; Murrow *et al.* 1990; Zijlmans *et al.* 2004a) that affect not only the basal ganglia or substantia nigra but also the corticospinal and corticobulbar tracts as they course through the internal capsule, thus giving rise to the other symptoms described above.

Differential diagnosis

The full differential for parkinsonism is described in Section 3.8. Of the disorders considered there, the neurodegenerative causes of parkinsonism are most likely to be confused with vascular parkinsonism. Parkinson's disease is distinguished by the presence of tremor, cogwheel rigidity, and a good response to levodopa. Diffuse Lewy body disease is suggested by the early occurrence of a dementia marked by confusion and visual hallucinations, and multiple system atrophy by associated ataxia and autonomic failure. Progressive supranuclear palsy may appear very similar to vascular parkinsonism, and, in cases in which supranuclear ophthalmoplegia has not as yet appeared, the differential may rest on MR scanning, which reveals midbrain atrophy in progressive supranuclear palsy, in contrast to the multiple lacunes of vascular parkinsonism.

Treatment

Although the response to levodopa is generally not good (Winikates and Jankovic 1999), some patients may respond (Zijlmans *et al.* 2004b) and, hence, it is worth a try. Dementia may be treated as described for lacunar dementia in Section 10.2, and the treatment of pseudobulbar palsy is discussed in Section 4.7. Efforts should be undertaken to prevent further lacunar infarctions, as discussed in Section 7.4.

10.4 BINSWANGER'S DISEASE

Binswanger's disease, first described by Otto Binswanger in 1894 (Binswanger 1894), is characterized by a slowly progressive dementia occurring in the elderly on the basis of a diffuse microangiopathic ischemic leukoencephalopathy or leukoaraiosis. Thus conceived, Binswanger's disease is considered to be one of the vascular dementias, along with multi-infarct dementia and lacunar dementia. Traditional synonyms for this disease include subcortical arteriosclerotic encephalopathy, chronic progressive subcortical encephalopathy, and encephalitis subcorticalis chronica progressiva. Although precise figures regarding prevalence are not available, the clinical impression is that it is not uncommon.

Clinical features

The onset is generally gradual, occurring in the sixth or later decades. Clinically (Bogucki *et al.* 1991; Caplan and Schoene 1978), as described by Binswanger himself (Blass *et al.* 1991), there is a 'slow development of the deterioration of the intellectual capacities', and patients present with a non-specific dementia, with slowness of thought, decreased short-term memory, disorientation, and concreteness. In advanced cases, a pseudobulbar palsy may occur. Minor focal signs, such as asymmetric deep tendon reflexes or a Babinski sign, may be seen, but, in uncomplicated Binswanger's disease, major, clear-cut syndromes, such as aphasia or apraxia, do not occur.

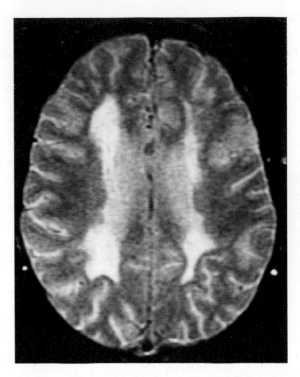

Figure 10.1 A T2-weighted magnetic resonance (MR) scan in a case of Binswanger's disease, with large confluent areas of increased signal intensity in the centrum semiovale. (Reproduced from Gillespie and Jackson 2000.)

Computed tomography scanning reveals widespread areas of radiolucency in the periventricular white matter and centrum semiovale. Magnetic resonance scanning is far more sensitive and on fluid-attenuated inversion recovery (FLAIR) or T2-weighted images one finds, as illustrated in Figure 10.1, multiple patchy and confluent areas of increased signal intensity in the periventricular region and the centrum semiovale, extending close to the cortex but sparing the U-fibers. In advanced cases, these patchy areas may coalesce to the point of creating a virtual 'white-out'.

Course

Although the course of Binswanger's disease has not been well-studied, it appears that the dementia undergoes a gradual progression over many years.

Etiology

The neuropathologic changes have been described in several reports (Akiguchi *et al.* 1997; Caplan and Schoene 1978; Lin *et al.* 2000; Revesz *et al.* 1989; Yamanouchi 1991). At autopsy, the small penetrating medullary vessels display lipohyalinosis and, in some cases, the lumens are obliterated. There is widespread demyelinization with some associated axonal loss and, in severe cases, cystic changes may occur. Although it is suspected that these microangiopathic changes occur on the basis of longstanding hypertension, other factors are probably also at work, as Binswanger's disease may occur in normotensive individuals.

Differential diagnosis

Binswanger's disease is one of the dementias of gradual onset that often lack distinctive features and, as discussed in Section 5.1, it must therefore be distinguished from several other disorders, including Alzheimer's disease, diffuse Lewy body disease, and normal pressure hydrocephalus. These disorders are immediately made doubtful by MR scanning, which fails to demonstrate the white matter pathology characteristic of Binswanger's disease. Clinical features may also help. Alzheimer's disease classically presents first with a slowly progressive short-term memory loss, in contrast to Binswanger's disease in which the memory loss occurs hand in hand with other cognitive changes. Diffuse Lewy body disease may present with a dementia, but here one finds visual hallucinations and spontaneous episodes of confusion early on, findings not seen in Binswanger's disease. Finally, in normal pressure hydrocephalus, one sees both a 'magnetic' gait and urinary urge incontinence, which are generally not seen in Binswanger's disease.

There are two disorders that present with dementia in the context of diffuse white matter changes, namely cerebral amyloid angiopathy and CADASIL (cerebral autosomal dominant arteriopathy with subcortical infarcts and leukoencephalopathy), and these may cause some diagnostic difficulty. In cerebral amyloid angiopathy, gradient echo recall MRI may reveal evidence of 'microbleeds'; furthermore, in most cases there will eventually also be lobar intracerebral hemorrhages, which clinch the diagnosis. CADASIL is suggested by a history of migraine headaches and also by the distinctive finding of a leukoencephalopathy that extends into the anterior temporal lobe.

As noted earlier, Binswanger's disease is one of the vascular dementias, and, given that patients may develop not only the microangiopathic changes of Binswanger's disease but also disease of the large pial vessels and the smaller penetrating central perforating vessels, it is not uncommon to find a mixture of vascular pathology; in such cases Binswanger's disease may be complicated by territorial infarctions and lacunar infarctions. There is often a history of multiple strokes in addition to the gradually progressive dementia, and clinical judgment is required in deciding what weight to give to each of the vascular pathologies with regard to the dementia. In cases characterized by a prominent amount of all three vascular pathologies, one may have to content oneself with an 'umbrella' diagnosis of 'vascular dementia'.

Finally, in evaluating a patient with a slowly progressive non-specific dementia, care must be taken not to place too much diagnostic weight on minor changes seen on MR scanning. Periventricular 'caps' and 'rims' are of no significance, and it is not at all uncommon to find multiple,

non-confluent, small patchy areas in the centrum semiovale or periventricular areas, which are, in fact, asymptomatic. The diagnosis of Binswanger's disease should not be made unless the white matter disease is severe and extensive, approaching, ideally, a 'white-out'.

Treatment

The general treatment of dementia is discussed in Section 5.1; there is some evidence that donepezil (Black et al. 2003; Wilkinson et al. 2003), galantamine (Auchus et al. 2007), and memantine (Orgogozo et al. 2002; Wilcock et al. 2002) may also be helpful. Control of blood pressure is important; however, one must not be overzealous here as given that other vascular pathology is common, creating hypotension runs the risk of watershed infarctions.

10.5 CRANIAL ARTERITIS

Cranial arteritis, also known as giant cell arteritis or temporal arteritis, is characterized pathologically by a segmental inflammation of various, primarily cranial, arteries, and clinically by symptoms related to ischemia in the areas of distribution of those arteries. Classically, this disorder presents with headache (due to inflammation of one of the branches of the external carotid artery, typically the superficial temporal artery) and either amaurosis fugax or blindness due to involvement of the ophthalmic artery.

In those over 50 years, this is a not uncommon disorder; it is seen primarily in Caucasians, especially those of Nordic descent.

Clinical features

The symptomatology of cranial arteritis varies according to which arteries are inflamed (Wilkinson and Russell 1972). Branches of the external carotid artery are commonly involved, and, as noted above, inflammation of the temporal artery is classic, causing a severe headache in the temporal region, which, although generally unilateral, can be bilateral. In some cases the occipital artery is involved and in these instances the headache may be localized to the neck. Involvement of the facial artery may lead to 'jaw claudication' with facial pain upon chewing, and involvement of the lingual artery may cause tongue necrosis. Of the branches of the internal carotid artery, the ophthalmic artery, as noted, is classically involved, and in such cases unilateral blindness may occur (Caselli et al. 1988), which may or may not be preceded by episodes of amaurosis fugax.

In about 10 percent of cases, strokes or transient ischemic attacks may occur (Caselli et al. 1988), and this may be seen with involvement of either the vertebral artery or the internal carotid artery. With vertebral artery involvement, clots may form that may then embolize further downstream, for example to the posterior cerebral artery. It also appears that small branches of the vertebral arteries may also be occluded, leading to medullary infarction. With involvement of the internal carotid artery, clots may also form, with embolization downstream to cause occlusion of the middle or anterior cerebral arteries or their branches. It is debated whether (or with what frequency) smaller arteries in the anterior circulation become inflamed; however, one report suggested that small penetrating arteries may be involved, causing multiple lacunes. In some cases, if the number and location of infarctions is appropriate, either a multi-infarct dementia (Caselli 1990) or a lacunar dementia (Nightingale et al. 1982) may ensue.

Most cases of cranial arteritis are further characterized by constitutional symptoms, such as malaise, fatigue, anorexia, and a low-grade fever, and most patients will also have an associated polymyalgia rheumatica, with muscle aching and stiffness, which, although diffuse, is most prominent in the neck and shoulders.

With rare exceptions (Kansu et al. 1977) the erythrocyte sedimentation rate (ESR) is elevated, generally above 50 mm/min (Westergen) and often above 100 mm/min. Mild anemia is common and the alkaline phosphatase may also be elevated. The diagnosis is confirmed by biopsy of an involved artery, such as the temporal artery; given the segmental nature of the inflammation, however, false negatives are possible and multiple biopsies may be required.

Course

The inflammatory process generally undergoes a gradual, spontaneous remission in anywhere from several months to several years.

Etiology

Involved arteries show a graulomatous inflammation characterized by the presence of giant cells. As noted, the inflammation is segmental, and between the involved segments the artery may be normal. Thrombi may form over the inflamed areas and, as noted earlier, emboli may be generated (Wilkinson and Russell 1972); in some cases the artery may become occluded. Although the mechanism underlying the inflammation is not known, an autoimmune process is suspected.

Differential diagnosis

The diagnosis should be suspected in cases of amaurosis fugax, blindness, or stroke, occurring in the setting of headache, constitutional symptoms, polymyalgia rheumatica, or an elevated ESR. Systemic lupus erythematosus may be considered in the differential, but here the anti-nuclear antibody (ANA) test is positive. Polyarteritis nodosa may also be suspected; however, here, renal or gastrointestinal involvement will indicate the correct diagnosis.

Treatment

Urgent treatment with steroids is essential to prevent stroke or blindness. Traditionally, prednisone is used, starting at doses of approximately 60 mg/day and, once symptoms are controlled and the ESR has dropped, tapering the dose gradually to the minimum required to keep the patient asymptomatic and the ESR down. Recent work suggests that aggressive treatment with methylprednisolone at 15 mg/kg (of ideal body weight) daily for the first 3 days, followed by prednisone, induces a more rapid remission and ensures a more favorable course (Mazlumzadeh et al. 2006). Uncontrolled work further suggests that use of low-dose aspirin concurrent with prednisone may also reduce the risk of stroke (Nesher et al. 2004).

10.6 CEREBRAL AMYLOID ANGIOPATHY

Cerebral amyloid angiopathy, also known as congophilic amyloid angiopathy, is a not uncommon disorder characterized by an amyloid angiopathy that may lead to spontaneous lobar intracerebral hemorrhages, a gradually progressive dementia secondary to a widespread leukoencephalopathy, or a combination of these findings; cerebral 'microhemorrhages' commonly accompany these findings.

Clinical findings

Cerebral amyloid angiopathy typically has an onset in the seventh or later decades, and may present with either spontaneous lobar intracerebral hemorrhages or with a gradually progressive dementia (Cosgrove et al. 1985; Gilles et al. 1984; Haan et al. 1990a; Nobuyoshi et al. 1984; Yoshimura et al. 1992).

The lobar intracerebral hemorrhages present with a gradual evolution, over perhaps a half-hour, of headache, nausea and vomiting, and a focal deficit appropriate to the location of the hemorrhage. Classically, the hemorrhage occurs spontaneously and recurrences are the rule. With multiple recurrences, a 'stepwise' accrual of cognitive deficits may occur, eventually leading to a picture of multi-infarct dementia.

Dementia, as noted, may also be of gradual onset and progression, and in this instance it is non-specific in character, with decreased short-term memory, variable disorientation, and deficits in abstracting and calculating ability.

Cerebral microhemorrhages may occur, and these may be silent or may present with relatively minor focal findings that, in most cases, resolve over time (Greenberg et al. 1993). Residual deposits of hemosiderin may serve as seizure foci, and partial seizures may also occur.

Magnetic resonance scanning will reveal evidence of any old intracerebral hemorrhages; in cases with a leukoencephalopathy, T2-weighted or FLAIR images reveal bilateral, more or less symmetric, patchy or confluent areas of increased signal intensity that spare the U-fibers. Gradient echo images may reveal punctate areas of decreased signal intensity, corresponding to old microhemorrhages (Greenberg *et al.* 1999). Recent work has also demonstrated that, in some cases, one will find large asymmetric areas of increased signal intensity on T2-weighted or FLAIR imaging in the subcortical white matter, which fail to enhance and which may represent vasogenic edema (Kinnecom *et al.* 2007).

Course

The course of cerebral amyloid angiopathy depends on the preponderance of the underlying pathology. With repeated intracerebral hemorrhages, a 'stepwise' course, as noted, may occur, whereas cases with leukoencephalopathy are characterized by a gradual progression of cognitive deficits. The combination of these two courses may also occur, and is quite distinctive for this disease (Nobuyoshi *et al.* 1984).

Etiology

Amyloid deposition occurs in the walls of small and medium-sized cortical arterioles, resulting in fibrinoid degeneration and the formation of microaneurysms (Okazaki *et al.* 1979). Affected vessels are 'congophilic', staining well with Congo red dye, thus accounting for the alternative name for this disorder, 'congophilic amyloid angiopathy'. The aneurysmal dilations of these vessels are quite fragile, and account for both spontaneous lobar intracerebral hemorrhages and microhemorrhages. Within the areas of distribution of the affected arteries, rarefaction of the white matter occurs (Gray *et al.* 1985), probably on an ischemic basis.

Although the vast majority of cases are sporadic, cerebral amyloid angiopathy may also occur on an autosomal dominant basis as 'hereditary cerebral hemorrhage with amyloidosis', either of the 'Dutch' (Haan *et al.* 1990a,b; Levy *et al.* 1990; Wattendorff *et al.* 1995) or 'Icelandic' (Gudmundsson *et al.* 1972; Palsdottir *et al.* 1988) type.

Differential diagnosis

Intracerebral hemorrhages of cerebral amyloid angiopathy must be distinguished from intracerebral hemorrhages of other causes. Hypertensive intracerebral hemorrhage is suggested by location: hypertensive hemorrhages tend to involve deep subcortical structures, such as the putamen, in contrast to the hemorrhages of cerebral amyloid angiopathy, which are lobar in location. Hemorrhage into tumors

or rupture of a vascular malformation when these are lobar are more difficult to distinguish and, in such cases, follow-up MRI scans, obtained after the hemorrhage has resolved, are often required. A helpful rule is that the occurrence of two or more spontaneous intracerebral hemorrhages that are lobar in location reliably indicates a diagnosis of cerebral amyloid angiopathy (Knudson *et al.* 2001).

Cerebral amyloid angiopathy may be very difficult to distinguish from Binswanger's disease, as both of these disorders present with a gradually progressive dementia associated with a diffuse, bilateral leukoencephalopathy. Certainly if there are spontaneous lobar intracerebral hemorrhages, this would point to a diagnosis of cerebral amyloid angiopathy. In their absence, one should perform gradient recall MRI to look for evidence of old microhemorrhages: although these are not always present in cerebral amyloid angiopathy, they are never present on the basis of Binswanger's disease, and hence they represent a significant pertinent positive finding.

Treatment

At present, there is no specific treatment; the general treatment of dementia is outlined in Section 5.1. Given that aspirin, warfarin (Rosand *et al.* 2000), and tissue plasminogen activator (Pendlebury *et al.* 1991) may all increase the risk of hemorrhage, these should be avoided. In cases in which MR scanning reveals large areas of vasogenic edema, consideration may be given to treatment with steroids (Kinnecom *et al.* 2007).

10.7 CADASIL

CADASIL is a rare autosomal dominantly inherited arteriopathy characterized by migraine, stroke, and dementia. The name CADASIL is an acronym for *c*erebral *a*utosomal *d*ominant *a*rteriopathy with *s*ubcortical *i*nfarcts and *l*eukoencephalopathy.

Clinical features

In general, the overall clinical picture of CADASIL (Bergmann *et al.* 1996; Dichgans *et al.* 1998; Jung *et al.* 1995; Kim *et al.* 2006; Malandrini *et al.* 1996; Markus *et al.* 2002; Sourander and Walinder 1977) is characterized by the onset of recurrent migraine headaches, typically with aura, in the third or fourth decade, followed by recurrent strokes or transient ischemic attacks (TIAs) in the fourth or fifth decade, and a dementia in the sixth and seventh decade; a pseudobulbar palsy may occur and, in a small minority, seizures may appear. The strokes are typically of the lacunar type, reflecting infarcts that occur primarily in the basal ganglia. The dementia, although generally reflecting the effects of multiple lacunar infarctions (Liem *et al.* 2007), at times may also be due to a progressive leukoencephalopathy, and in rare instances CADASIL may present with a dementia secondary to the leukoencephalopathy in the absence of stroke (Filley *et al.* 1999; Mellies *et al.* 1998).

Two unusual manifestations of CADASIL must also be kept in mind, namely intracerebral hemorrhage and a reversible delirium. Intracerebral hemorrhage, primarily of the thalamus or basal ganglia, may occur but is uncommon (Choi *et al.* 2006). Delirium has also been reported but appears rare. Patients present with a subacute delirium, often accompanied by seizures and fever, which may progress to coma; recovery is spontaneous and occurs after 1–2 weeks (Schon *et al.* 2003).

Magnetic resonance scanning will reveal any prior lacunar infarctions. Furthermore, most patients will also have a diffuse leukoencephalopathy and, indeed, this may be present early on, even before the first stroke. The leukoencephalopathy is evident on either T2-weighted or FLAIR imaging: patchy, confluent areas of increased signal intensity are seen in the centrum semiovale and the periventricular white matter, and also, classically, in the external capsule and, most notably, in the white matter of the anterior temporal lobe (O'Sullivan *et al.* 2001). Recent work using gradient echo imaging has also identified evidence for old microhemorrhages in the thalamus and basal ganglia (Choi *et al.* 2006; Lesnik Oberstein *et al.* 2001).

Diagnosis may be made by genetic testing. Skin biopsy may also be performed, but false negatives are common (Malandrini *et al.* 2007).

Course

The overall course is as described above; death occurs in the seventh through ninth decades, often from pneumonia (Opherk *et al.* 2004).

Etiology

As noted, CADASIL is an autosomal dominant disorder: mutations are found in the *Notch3* gene on chromosome 19 (Joutel *et al.* 1997; Tournier-Lasserve *et al.* 1993). Pathologically, there is concentric fibrous thickening of small penetrating arteries (Sourander and Walinder 1977), leading to both the subcortical infarcts and the widespread leukoencephalopathy (Baudrimont *et al.* 1993). Although peripheral nerves (Schroder *et al.* 1995) and skin (Ruchoux *et al.* 1994) may also be involved, symptoms referable to them are generally absent.

Differential diagnosis

Lacunar strokes occurring in CADASIL must be distinguished from lacunar infarctions occurring on the basis of lipohyalinosis or atherosclerosis. Similarly, the dementia occurring in CADASIL must be distinguished from the dementia occurring in lacunar dementia and in Binswanger's disease. In all these instances, a positive family history is most helpful as it points to CADASIL; however, in some cases such a history may be unavailable. Other features suggesting CADASIL are migraine with aura and, most importantly, the early appearance of leukoencephalopathy in the anterior portion of the temporal lobe, which, although common in CADASIL, is most unlikely in other disorders.

Cerebral amyloid angiopathy may cause some diagnostic difficulty, as it can present with a dementia in the setting of a diffuse leukoencephalopathy with old microhemorrhages. Here, MRI evidence of lacunar infarctions or anterior temporal leukoencephalopathy point to CADASIL, and the appearance of *lobar* intracerebral hemorrhages at any time generally indicates cerebral amyloid angiopathy.

MELAS (mitochondrial encephalomyopathy, lactic acidosis, and stroke-like episodes) may present in a fashion similar to CADASIL, but is distinguished by deafness.

Treatment

At present, there is no specific treatment for CADASIL. The general treatment of dementia is discussed in Section 5.1; genetic counselling should be offered.

10.8 GRANULOMATOUS ANGIITIS OF THE CENTRAL NERVOUS SYSTEM

Granulomatous angiitis of the central nervous system is a rare disorder characterized pathologically by a granulomatous angiitis confined to the central nervous system, and clinically by headache and delirium. An often used synonym is primary angiitis of the central nervous system; however, at times this term has also been used to refer to other vasculitic processes and hence the reader should examine any literature carefully, to ensure that, indeed, granulomatous angiitis is the disorder in question.

Clinical features

Although the disease may present at any age, from childhood to senescence, most patients are in their 30s or 40s. The onset itself is generally subacute, spanning a few weeks. Clinically (Abu-Shakara *et al.* 1994; Calabrese and Mallek 1988; Case Records 1989; Hughes and Brownell 1966; Kolodny *et al.* 1968; Koo and Massey 1988; Lie 1992; Moore 1989; Vollmer *et al.* 1993), patients typically have severe, generalized headache, and in this setting they develop a delirium that may be accompanied by focal deficits or, uncommonly, seizures. Although focal deficits, such as hemiparesis, may have a stroke-like onset, in most cases they appear gradually. In some cases, the spinal cord may be involved.

The ESR is generally either normal or only mildly elevated (Lie 1992; Moore 1989). Magnetic resonance scanning may initially be normal; however, over time areas of increased signal intensity on FLAIR or T2-weighted imaging appear in the cerebrum or cerebellum (Alhalabi and Moore 1994; Ehsan *et al.* 1995). Angiography may be normal or may disclose typical beading (Alrawi *et al.* 1999). Lumbar puncture should be performed in all suspected cases: there is typically a lymphocytic pleocytosis, an elevated protein, and a normal glucose (Vollmer *et al.* 1993). Brain biopsy, sampling both the leptomeninges and the cerebrum, is the 'gold standard' (Alrawi *et al.* 1999); however, even this may be falsely negative, missing affected tissue (Alhalabi and Moore 1994; Lie 1992).

Course

Untreated, progressive deterioration occurs in almost all cases and perhaps half of all patients will die within months, with the remainder surviving for up to two or more years.

Etiology

A granulomatous angiitis affects both small leptomeningeal vessels and small- or medium-sized parenchymal vessels (Cravioto and Feigin 1959). The cerebrum is most commonly affected, although the cerebellum, brainstem, and even the cord may also be involved. Although the cause is unknown, an autoimmune process, confined to the central nervous system, is suspected.

Differential diagnosis

Other vasculidities, such as polyarteritis nodosa or zoster arteritis, must be considered, along with subacute meningitides, as may be seen with fungal infections or syphilis.

Treatment

The general treatment of delirium is discussed in Section 5.3. Most patients are treated with a combination of prednisone and cyclophosphamide.

10.9 POLYARTERITIS NODOSA

Polyarteritis nodosa, also known as periarteritis nodosa, is a rare systemic vasculitis characterized pathologically by a segmental necrotizing panarteritis. Most patients present with constitutional symptoms and involvement of the kidneys, gastrointestinal tract or muscles; in a minority there may be a peripheral neuropathy, and in a smaller minority, central nervous system involvement, with stroke, delirium, or dementia.

Clinical features

The onset is generally subacute or gradual in middle years with constitutional symptoms and evidence of involvement of the kidneys, gastrointestinal tract or muscles; renal disease may lead to hypertension or renal failure. Importantly, the respiratory tract is not involved.

Nervous system involvement generally occurs only after other evidence of the disease is well-established (Sigal 1987). Peripheral nervous system involvement, which is most common, typically involves a mononeuritis multiplex (Lovelace 1964). In a minority of cases, central nervous system involvement may occur, most commonly presenting with lacunar strokes (Reichart *et al.* 2000); larger territorial infarctions or intracerebral hemorrhages are rare. In a very small minority delirium (Ford and Siekert 1965) or dementia (MacKay *et al.* 1950) may occur, and seizures have also been noted.

Both the peripheral white blood cell count and the ESR are elevated. Anti-neutrophil cytoplasmic antibodies (ANCA) (especially perinuclear ANCA [pANCA]) are found in the majority of cases and the Venereal Disease Research Laboratories (VDRL) test may be falsely positive. Magnetic resonance scanning will reveal infarctions. Definitive diagnosis is made by biopsy of an affected muscle or peripheral nerve.

Course

Although spontaneous remissions do occur they are rare, and most cases are characterized by relentless progression, with only about 10 percent of patients surviving past 5 years.

Etiology

There is a systemic, segmental panarteritis affecting medium and small arteries, with, at times, extension into arterioles. With intimal proliferation, thrombosis and occlusion of arteries may occur, and with involvement of the muscular layer, microaneurysms may form. These microaneurysms may occasionally rupture; however, they typically undergo fibrosis, thus creating nodules along the course of the artery, thereby providing the characteristic that gives the disease its name.

Involvement of the peripheral vasa nervorum leads to the mononeuritis multiplex. Within the central nervous system, involvement of small perforating arteries leads to lacunar infarctions; in those uncommon cases involving larger arteries, territorial infarctions may occur and, with rupture of an aneurysm, an intracerebral hemorrhage may be seen.

Although the mechanism underlying the arteritis is not known with certainty, deposition of immune complexes probably plays a role, and in this regard there is an association with hepatitis B antigenemia.

Differential diagnosis

In addition to suggesting polyarteritis nodosa, the occurrence of nervous system involvement in the context of a systemic illness also raises the possibility of systemic lupus erythematosus, indicated by a positive ANA, and Wegener's granulomatosis, which, unlike polyarteritis nodosa, also involves the respiratory tract.

Treatment

Treatment with corticosteroids and cyclophosphamide is recommended; consideration may also be given to antiplatelet agents (Reichart *et al.* 2000).

10.10 WEGENER'S GRANULOMATOSIS

Wegener's granulomatosis is an uncommon disease characterized pathologically by a systemic necrotizing granulomatous vasculitis, most commonly affecting the respiratory tract and kidneys. The nervous system is involved in a minority of cases: peripheral neuropathy is the most common manifestation; within the central nervous system there may be a vasculitis, intracerebral granulomas, and, rarely, a pachymeningitis.

Clinical features

Over 90 percent of patients have symptoms referable to granulomas within the respiratory tract. Upper respiratory tract involvement is most common, with sinusitis, epistaxis, or rhinorrhea; involvement of the nasal septum may lead to its collapse, and extension of granulomatous disease to the orbit may cause proptosis. Pulmonary involvement may be asymptomatic or lead to cough or hemoptysis. Some three-quarters of patients will have renal involvement, which may manifest initially with proteinuria and microscopic hematuria.

Nervous system involvement generally occurs in the context of respiratory or renal symptomatology (Hoffman *et al.* 1992). Clinical evidence of a mononeuritis multiplex or polyneuropathy is seen in about one-third of patients (de Groot *et al.* 2001). With central nervous system involvement (Nishino *et al.* 1993a,b; Weinberger *et al.* 1993) there may be delirium, dementia, stroke, seizures, and, with meningeal involvement, headache and cranial neuropathies; diabetes insipidus has also been reported (Rosete *et al.* 1991).

Magnetic resonance scanning will reveal intracerebral granulomatous lesions, infarcts, and meningitis. The cerebrospinal fluid may be normal or may show a lymphocytic pleocytosis and an elevated total protein.

The ESR is elevated, and over 90 percent of patients will have elevated levels of ANCA of either the pANCA or cANCA (circulating) type. Definitive diagnosis is made by biopsy of the lung or kidney.

Course

The disease is progressive and, once renal involvement occurs, death may follow within months.

Etiology

Within the central nervous system, several different pathologies may be found (Drachman 1963, Nishino *et al.* 1993a; Seror *et al.* 2006; Weinberger *et al.* 1993). Small, or rarely large, vessels may undergo a vasculitis and, with occlusion, infarction occurs. Granulomas may be found, and these may appear by extension from an extracranial source (e.g., a sinus or the orbit) or they may occur independently. Granulomatous involvement of the meninges, primarily the pachymeninges, may also occur, and cranial nerves may be entrapped and compressed; cranial neuropathies may also occur due to compression of the cranial nerves in their extracranial portions by extracranial granulomas. In some cases granulomas may appear in the hypothalamus.

Although the etiology of Wegener's granulomatosis is not known, an autoimmune response, perhaps to an inhaled substance, is suspected.

Differential diagnosis

Central or peripheral nervous system involvement in the setting of respiratory tract or renal disease should raise the possibility of Wegener's granulomatosis. Sarcoidosis may be considered, but this disease has features not seen in Wegener's granulomatosis, such as erythema nodosum, lupus pernio, hypercalcemia, etc. Polyarteritis nodosa may also be considered, although in polyarteritis nodosa one does not find the respiratory tract involvement typical of Wegener's granulomatosis.

Treatment

In most cases, treatment with a combination of prednisone and cyclophosphamide is required. The symptomatic treatment of delirium and dementia is discussed in Sections 5.3 and 5.1 respectively.

10.11 BEHÇET'S DISEASE

Behçet's disease, first described in 1937 by the Turkish dermatologist Hulusi Behçet, is characterized pathologically by a systemic, primarily venular, vasculitis, and clinically by oral aphthous ulcers, genital ulcers, uveitis, and, in anywhere from one-tenth to one-third of patients, by evidence of central nervous system involvement. Although not uncommon in Japan and the Eastern Mediterranean region, Behçet's disease is rare in Europe and the United States.

Clinical features

Behçet's disease typically presents in the twenties or thirties, and almost all patients will have oral aphthous ulcers and some form of uveitis; genital ulcers are somewhat less common. Another distinctive sign, not seen in all, is pathergy: here, within 1–2 days of minor skin trauma, for example phlebotomy, a large pustule forms at the site of the trauma. Other symptoms include furuncles, erythema nodosum, migratory thrombophlebitis, and a non-deforming polyarthritis. Within the context of these symptoms evidence of central nervous system involvement may appear.

When the central nervous system is involved, a wide variety of symptoms may appear (Akman-Demir et al. 1993, 1999; Al-Araji et al. 2003; Altinors et al. 1987; Chajek and Fainaru 1975; Farah et al. 1998; Iragui and Miravi 1986; Joseph and Scolding 2007; Kidd et al. 1999; Motomura et al. 1980; Serdaroglu et al. 1989; Wadia and Williams 1957; Wolf et al. 1965). These include delirium, dementia, pseudobulbar palsy with emotional incontinence (Pallis and Fudge 1956; Motomura et al. 1980; Rubinstein and Urich 1963; Wechsler et al. 1990), hemiplegia, ataxia, cranial nerve palsies, abnormal movements (e.g., chorea), a personality change of the frontal lobe type, and, rarely, scizures (Aykutlu et al. 2002). As noted below, in addition to vasculitis, both meningitis and dural sinus thrombosis may occur, and in such cases one may see headache; in cases of dural sinus thrombosis, one may also see signs of increased intracranial pressure, with nausea, vomiting, and papilledema.

T2-weighted or FLAIR MR scanning may reveal areas of increased signal intensity in the brainstem, cerebellum or, less commonly, cerebrum; these areas may demonstrate enhancement with gadolinium. Magnetic resonance venography may be required to demonstrate dural sinus thrombosis. The CSF may be abnormal, with an elevated total protein and/or a pleocytosis, which is generally lymphocytic (Akman-Demir et al. 1999; Farah et al. 1998). The ESR and peripheral white blood cell count may be elevated.

Course

Most cases of Behçet's disease demonstrate an episodic course. The first attack, as noted, tends to occur in the 20s or 30s, and most attacks last in the order of weeks or a month or more, after which there is a spontaneous remission. These remissions, however, are generally not complete, and most patients are left with residual symptoms. Recurrent attacks are the rule, and after each attack the overall burden of residual symptoms increases. In some cases, this typical episodic course may evolve into one of steady, waxing and waning progression; rarely Behçet's disease may pursue a chronic, non-episodic course from the outset, as was seen in a case of progressive dementia with apthous and genital ulcers (Borson 1982).

Etiology

A perivenular vasculitis occurs and, although this may be seen in any part of the central nervous system, there is a predilection for the pons, mesencephalon and diencephalon, the cerebellum, and, to a lesser degree, the frontal lobes. Meningeal inflammation may also occur, which may be accompanied by dural sinus thrombosis.

Although the etiology is not known, an autoimmune process is suspected; the vast majority of cases are sporadic.

Differential diagnosis

The relapsing and remitting course of Behçet's syndrome immediately suggests multiple sclerosis; however, in multiple sclerosis one does not find the characteristic apthous and genital ulcers, uveitis or pathergy.

Treatment

During attacks patients should be treated with prednisone and an immunosuppressant. The general management of delirium and dementia are discussed in Sections 5.3 and 5.1 respectively.

10.12 HYPERTENSIVE ENCEPHALOPATHY

Hypertensive encephalopathy, a relatively common disorder, is characterized by the occurrence of delirium and headache in the setting of severe diastolic hypertension.

Before proceeding, some words are in order regarding the syndrome known as reversible posterior leukoencephalopathy. Some authors use this as an 'umbrella' term, subsuming not only hypertensive encephalopathy but also cases that are clinically similar but which do not occur on the basis of hypertension. To this author, such a nosologic practice seems to represent inappropriate 'lumping' and, in this text, these disorders are treated separately.

Clinical features

In the setting of sustained diastolic pressure elevations, often 130 mmHg or higher, delirium and headache evolve over a matter of 1–3 days; most patients also experience nausea and vomiting, and a majority will experience bilateral visual blurring, which may progress to cortical blindness; seizures may also occur and, in a minority, focal signs such as aphasia or hemiplegia may occur (Chester et al. 1978; Healton et al. 1982; Oppenheimer and Fishberg 1928). Untreated, patients may become comatose. Funduscopic examination may reveal papilledema or retinal hemorrhages. Acute cardiac and renal failure may accompany the cerebral symptomatology.

Computed tomography scanning may reveal bilaterally symmetric areas of hypodensity in the occipitoparietal white matter. Magnetic resonance scanning is far more sensitive and, on T2-weighted or FLAIR imaging, increased signal intensity will be seen in the same areas (Hauser *et al.* 1988); gradient echo imaging may reveal evidence of petechial hemorrhages (Weingarten *et al.* 1994). Diffusion-weighted imaging is generally normal unless infarction has occurred. Rarely, these MRI findings may be found in the brainstem and cerebellum (Cruz-Flores *et al.* 2004; Kanazawa *et al.* 2005).

Course

Untreated hypertensive encephalopathy may be fatal. In cases in which blood pressure is corrected, symptoms gradually resolve over a matter of days and white matter abnormalities seen on CT or MR scanning typically clear within a week or so. In those cases in which focal findings were noted, these may persist, and MR scanning will show persistent abnormalities consistent with infarction. With a sufficient number of strategically placed infarctions, patients may be left with a multi-infarct dementia.

Etiology

As blood pressure rises above a critical level, autoregulation of small- and medium-sized cerebral arteries fails and there is extravasation of proteinaceous fluid into the surrounding white matter; some vessels may also rupture, causing petechial hemorrhages, and others may undergo fibrinoid necrosis and occlusion, causing infarction (Chester *et al.* 1978).

Differential diagnosis

Not all deliria occurring in the setting of grossly elevated diastolic pressures occur due to hypertensive encephalopathy. Indeed, in patients with chronic and gradually increasing blood pressure, such very high pressures, being very gradually reached, may be well tolerated without any immediate sequelae. As noted earlier, renal failure is not uncommon, and uremic encephalopathy must also be considered. Intracerebral hemorrhage may also be considered in the differential, but is generally of more acute onset and is easily recognized on neuroimaging. Reversible posterior leukoencephalopathy should be considered in cases that are clinically identical to hypertensive encephalopathy in all respects except for the fact that hypertension is either lacking or only mild.

Treatment

Hypertensive encephalopathy is a medical emergency and the pressure must be lowered within an hour. Normotensive levels, however, are not the goal because, with a loss of autoregulatory capacity, a systemic pressure within normal limits may be followed by cerebral hypoperfusion and watershed infarctions. Consequently, during acute treatment the diastolic pressure should be lowered to between 110 and 120 mmHg; once this has been accomplished, further treatment may be aimed at bringing the pressure down further in a more leisurely manner over the next few days. Acute treatment may be accomplished with intravenous sodium nitroprusside, labetalol or diazoxide. In cases in which intravenous access is not immediately available or when the clinical situation is not as urgent, intramuscular hydralazine may be utilized. Seizures may be treated with intravenous lorazepam and fosphenytoin, as described in Section 7.3. The general treatment of delirium is discussed in Section 5.3.

10.13 REVERSIBLE POSTERIOR LEUKOENCEPHALOPATHY SYNDROME

The reversible posterior leukoencephalopathy syndrome is a recently described disorder marked by delirium, cortical blindness, and seizures, occurring secondary to treatment with various chemotherapeutic agents. As noted in the preceding section, this disorder is clinically identical to hypertensive encephalopathy and differs only in mechanism.

Clinical features

The syndrome (Hinchey *et al.* 1996) presents acutely, over hours, and manifests with delirium or lethargy, accompanied typically by headache, nausea or vomiting, and grand mal seizures, which may have a focal onset. Cortical blindness is common and other symptoms may also occur, such as hemianopia, hemiparesis, abulia, or asterixis.

T2-weighted or FLAIR MR scanning (Lamy *et al.* 2004) reveals areas of increased signal intensity bilaterally in the white matter of the occipital and parietal lobes, with similar findings, in many cases, noted in the posterior aspects of the temporal lobes.

Course

With prompt and adequate treatment, clinical findings resolve within days to weeks.

Pathology and etiology

Vasogenic edema is seen within the white matter, as indicated by both brain biopsy (Lavigne *et al.* 2004) and MRI findings. In cases with an unfavorable outcome, infarction of the white matter occurs.

This syndrome has been noted secondary to treatment with a variety of chemotherapeutic and immunomodulatory agents, including tacrolimus, cyclosporine, vincristine, methotrexate, bevacizumab, cyclophosphamide, L-asparaginase, cisplatin, cytarabine, interferon-alpha, and immunoglobulins. Although the mechanism of toxicity is not clear, it probably involves damage to the vascular endothelium.

Differential diagnosis

The differential with hypertensive encephalopathy rests on the presence or absence of severe hypertension: although patients with the reversible posterior leukoencephalopathy syndrome may have an elevated pressure, for example a diastolic pressure of up to 105 mmHg, pressures simply do not rise to the levels seen in hypertensive encephalopathy.

Bilateral occipital infarction, as seen in the 'top of the basilar' syndrome, is distinguished by the involvement of the occipital cortex, which is in contrast to the sparing of the gray matter seen in reversible posterior leuko-encephalopathy syndrome.

Treatment

Potentially offending medications should be discontinued. Seizure may be treated with lorazepam and fosphenytoin, as described in Section 7.3. The general treatment of delirium is discussed in Section 5.3.

10.14 MELAS

MELAS (an acronym derived from *m*itochondrial *e*ncephalomyopathy, *l*actic *a*cidosis, and *s*troke-like episodes) is a rare inherited disorder characterized by varying combinations of encephalopathy, stroke-like episodes, migrainous headaches, seizures, and deafness; as with all mitochondrial disorders, it displays a maternal pattern of inheritance. Although almost all cases present before the age of 40 years, with most occurring before the age of 20 years, later onsets have been reported.

Clinical features

As noted, the clinical presentation is quite varied. Some may present with stroke-like episodes, with hemiparesis, hemianopia, cortical blindness or aphasia (Iizuka *et al.* 2003). Delirium may accompany these episodes and may persist, only to resolve into a dementia, which, in turn, may be gradually progressive (Sharfstein *et al.* 1999). In some cases, psychosis has been noted (Apostolova *et al.* 2005). Seizures may occur, and may be simple partial (Canafoglia *et al.* 2001), complex partial (including complex partial status epilepticus [Leff *et al.* 1998]) or grand mal in type. Migrainous headaches may precede, accompany, or follow any of these symptomatologies.

Hearing loss is common, and there may be an associated clinically apparent myopathy. Diabetes mellitus and either hypo- or hyperthyroidism may occur.

Diffusion-weighted MR scanning during stroke-like episodes will reveal areas of increased signal intensity; over time, these same areas will demonstrate increased signal intensity on FLAIR imaging. Importantly, these areas generally do not fall within the area of distribution of any major vessels and are most commonly seen in the occipital and parietal lobes.

The electroencephalogram (EEG) may reveal periodic lateralized epileptiform discharges (PLEDs) in patients with seizures.

Lactic acidosis is found in both the serum and CSF, and the CSF total protein is also elevated.

Muscle biopsy reveals ragged red fibers, and genetic testing for mutations in mitochondrial DNA may reveal characteristic mutations.

Course

Although the overall course is characterized by progression, the rate of progression, and the sequence with which various symptomatologies occur, is quite varied.

Etiology

Mitochondrial dysfunction occurs secondary to mutations in the gene for mitochondrial tRNA, with proliferation of abnormal mitochondria in vascular endothelial and smooth muscle cells. Infarcts, which, as noted earlier, do not conform to vascular territories, are found to affect both gray and white matter, primarily in the parietal and occipital lobes.

Differential diagnosis

MELAS should be suspected in any young person with recurrent stroke, especially when accompanied by migrainous headache or hearing loss. CADASIL is high on the differential and is suggested by the MRI finding of white matter changes in the anterior portion of the temporal lobes.

Treatment

Symptomatic treatment of delirium and dementia is described in Sections 5.3 and 5.1 respectively. Seizures may be treated with anti-epileptic drugs; however, valproic acid should be avoided as it may aggravate seizures (Lin *et al.* 2007). L-arginine, given during stroke-like episodes, may be followed by improvement (Koga *et al.* 2005).

10.15 THROMBOTIC THROMBOCYTOPENIC PURPURA

Thrombotic thrombocytopenic purpura, or TTP, is an uncommon, devastating disorder, typically occurring in young or middle-aged adults. It is marked by the subacute onset of delirium and thrombocytopenia (Druschky *et al.* 1998).

Clinical features

The delirium is marked by a pronounced fluctuation in the severity of symptoms throughout the day. Other symptomatology includes focal signs, such as hemiparesis or aphasia, which are typically transient, and seizures, with, in a small minority, complex partial status epilepticus (Blum and Drislane 1996).

The platelet count is generally reduced below $30\,000/mm^3$, and there is an accompanying microangiopathic hemolytic anemia with schistocytes or Burr cells. Renal failure with proteinuria and azotemia is common, as are fever and purpura.

Course

The disorder may persist for days to months; untreated, it is typically fatal.

Etiology

Procoagulants are released from vessel endothelial cells with the subsequent appearance of widespread platelet microthrombi in arterioles, capillaries, and venules. Presumably, the ongoing aggregation and disaggregation of platelet thrombi account for the classic waxing and waning nature of the symptomatology of this disorder. In some cases, small cortical infarctions may occur (Gruber *et al.* 2000).

Differential diagnosis

Disseminated intravascular coagulation is distinguished by a decreased fibrinogen level, an increase in fibrin split products, and a prolonged partial thromboplastin time.

Treatment

Plasma exchange is generally effective. With timely treatment most patients recover, with only a minority being left with persistent deficits. Anti-epileptic drugs may be required pending the effect of plasma exchange.

10.16 FAT EMBOLISM SYNDROME

This syndrome represents an uncommon complication of fractures or surgery to the long bones, or trauma to fatty tissues, in which showers of fat globules pass to and through the lungs, leaving the patient in respiratory distress and with a delirium.

Clinical features

Anywhere from 1 to 3 days after relevant trauma or surgery, patients develop dyspnea and confusion; there may also be seizures and strokes and in severe cases coma may develop (Dines *et al.* 1975; Jacobson *et al.* 1986). In some cases a petechial rash may appear on the trunk.

Diffusion-weighted MR scanning reveals multiple punctate areas of increased signal intensity, primarily scattered throughout the white matter with variable involvement of the cortex or subcortical structures (Marshall *et al.* 2004).

Chest radiographs will reveal bilateral 'fluffy' infiltrates and in a minority of cases fat globules may be observed on urinalysis.

Course

The mortality rate is as high as 10 percent; those who survive experience a variable degree of recovery over the following days.

Etiology

With fractures or surgery of the long bones, neutral fat is released into the venous circulation and travels to the lungs and then to the brain. A similar scenario may occur with trauma to fatty tissues. Within the brain, multiple microinfarctions occur (von Hochstetter and Friede 1977; Kamenar and Burger 1980).

Differential diagnosis

In cases secondary to trauma, head trauma may also have occurred; in post-operative cases, other causes of post-operative delirium, as discussed in Section 5.3, must be considered. When pulmonary involvement is severe, respiratory failure may occur and global cerebral hypoxia must also be considered.

Treatment

In addition to any necessary respiratory support, seizures may be treated with anti-epileptic drugs and symptomatic treatment of delirium may be provided, as outlined in Section 5.3.

10.17 MULTIPLE CHOLESTEROL EMBOLI SYNDROME

In patients with severe atheromatous disease of the ascending aorta or cerebral vessels, multiple crystals of cholesterol may break off from plaques, either spontaneously or with instrumentation, and embolize to the brain causing multiple, generally small, infarctions. Such microemboli also, of course, travel to other structures, most notably the kidneys.

Clinical features

The mode of onset appears related to whether the syndrome occurs with instrumentation or spontaneously. Cases occurring secondary to instrumentation (e.g., with coronary artery bypass grafting, cardiac catheterization, or carotid angiography [Hagiwara et al. 2004]) tend to present acutely with a full syndrome a day or so after the instrumentation. By contrast, spontaneously occurring cases may present subacutely, with the syndrome evolving over weeks or months.

Acute cases occurring after instrumentation present with delirium (Ezzeddine et al. 2000), which may or may not be accompanied by focal signs, such as hemiplegia or hemianopia. Evidence of multiple emboli to other organs (Colt et al. 1988) includes renal failure, livedo reticularis of the lower extremities, 'blue toes', petechial hemorrhages of the skin, a peripheral mononeuritis multiplex, and abdominal pain. Leukocytosis, eosinophilia, and an elevated ESR may all be present.

Subacute cases occurring spontaneously may present with TIAs or multiple cerebral infarctions; progressive renal failure is also typically present (Andreaux et al. 2007; Beal et al. 1981).

Course

In cases of acute onset, fatalities, often secondary to multiorgan failure, are common. Patients with subacute cases typically develop severe renal failure.

Differential diagnosis

Acute cases must be differentiated from other causes of post-operative delirium, as discussed in Section 5.3. Subacute cases must be distinguished from the lacunar state: here the accompanying renal failure provides a clue.

Etiology

Showers of microemboli composed of cholesterol crystals eventually lodge in small arterioles where they provoke an inflammatory response.

Treatment

The best treatment is prevention of atherosclerosis. Furthermore, extra caution should be exercised regarding instrumentation affecting the ascending aorta or cerebral vasculature in any patient with severe atherosclerosis. There is a case report suggesting that steroids given acutely may be beneficial (Andreaux et al. 2007).

10.18 TRANSIENT GLOBAL AMNESIA

Transient global amnesia, first described in the English language literature by Fisher and Adams in 1958 (Fisher and Adams 1958), is an uncommon disorder characterized by infrequent amnestic episodes. Although the etiology of this disorder is not known, it is included in this section on vascular disorders because of the strong suspicion that, as noted below, it may result from either transient ischemia or venous congestion of medial temporal structures.

Clinical features

The overall clinical features have been described in a number of papers (Bolwig 1968; Fisher and Adams 1958, 1964; Gordon and Marin 1979; Heathfield et al. 1973; Hodges and Ward 1989; Kushner and Hauser 1985; Miller et al. 1987a; Quinette et al. 2006; Regard and Landis 1984; Shuttleworth and Morris 1966).

The first episode of transient global amnesia generally occurs in the sixth or seventh decade. Episodes themselves are generally of abrupt onset, and may be associated with various precipitating events, such as strong emotion, sexual intercourse, pain, physical exertion, Valsalva maneuvers, and even immersion in cold water (Fisher 1982; Kushner and Hauser 1985; Quinette et al. 2006). Whether or not a precipitating event is present, patients suddenly experience an amnesia that has both retrograde and anterograde components. The retrograde component covers at least the previous few hours and in many cases may stretch much further into the past: typically, this retrograde amnesia displays a temporal gradient, such that whereas the amnesia may be quite dense for events of the very recent past, it become 'patchy' for events further back (Kritchevsky and Squire 1989). The anterograde component is fairly dense, and patients are unable to keep track of any ongoing events during the episode. Most patients, although not confused, are more or less alarmed at their state, and many will anxiously and repeatedly ask where they are and how they got to be where they are. Formal mental status testing reveals that patients are coherent, alert, and, as noted, not confused. Although digit span is intact, patients are unable to recall any of three words after 5 minutes; furthermore, they will be unable to recall events of the recent past leading up to the onset of the episode. In essence, cognitive ability, other than memory, remains normal, and indeed some patients may engage in quite complex activity, such as playing an organ piece, during the episode itself (Byer and Crowley 1980). The neurologic examination is generally normal. The episode itself generally lasts anywhere from 4 to 18 hours, averaging about 6 hours, and terminates gradually.

After the episode has cleared, patients are once again able to keep track of ongoing events, and their ability to recall words after 5 minutes is fully restored. When they try and recall what happened, however, they often find an 'island' of amnesia that covers not only the duration of the event itself but also any events that occurred anywhere from a few minutes to an hour or so just before the onset of the episode. Although clinically patients are thus fully restored, detailed testing may reveal some subtle decrements in memory (Guillery-Girard *et al.* 2006; Steinmetz and Vroom 1972).

Course

Long-term follow-up of approximately 5–6 years shows that only about one-fifth to one-quarter of patients have a recurrence (Gandolfo *et al.* 1992; Hinge *et al.* 1986; Miller *et al.* 1987a).

Etiology

It appears that the amnesia seen in transient global amnesia represents the effects of a similarly transient dysfunction of medial temporal lobe structures. Single photon emission computed tomography (SPECT) studies have revealed hypoperfusion of the medial aspects of both temporal lobes (Lampl *et al.* 2004), more so the left than the right, and diffusion-weighted imaging has revealed punctate areas of increased signal intensity in the hippocampus (Bartsch *et al.* 2006; Sedlaczek *et al.* 2004; Strupp *et al.* 1998); notably both of these abnormal findings clear with time. Structural MRI studies are generally normal (Bartsch *et al.* 2006); however, one high-resolution MRI study found an increased number of microcavities in the CA-1 subfield of the hippocampus, suggesting that there may be some subtle permanent damage (Nakada *et al.* 2005). Several mechanisms have been proposed to account for these changes, including epileptic activity, transient ischemia, migraine, and, recently, venous reflux. Epileptic activity appears unlikely: EEGs obtained during episodes of transient global amnesia do not display ictal activity (Miller *et al.* 1987b), and the attacks themselves, rather than ending abruptly, as is typical of a seizure, tend to clear gradually. Transient ischemia has long been an attractive hypothesis, but patients with transient global amnesia generally have few risk factors for stroke (Hodges and Warlow 1990; Lauria *et al.* 1998; Melo *et al.* 1992) and rarely end up having stroke during follow-up (Zorzon *et al.* 1995). Migraine may play a role: there is a definite association between transient global amnesia and migraine (Crowell *et al.* 1984; Hodges and Warlow 1990; Melo *et al.* 1992; Schmidtke and Ehmsen 1998; Zorzon *et al.* 1995), and an

episode of 'spreading depression of Leão' confined to medial temporal structures could, conceivably, cause amnesia. Migraine, however, would not explain the SPECT and diffusion-weighted imaging abnormalities described earlier.

The final proposed mechanism, namely venous reflux, is quite interesting. To understand the theory of venous reflux one must recall some anatomy. Normally the medial temporal structures are drained by the deep veins of Rosenthal. These veins, in turn, drain to the great vein of Galen, which drains to the straight sinus. The straight sinus, in turn, courses posteriorly to join the superior sagittal sinus at the sinus confluens. The sinus confluens gives rise to the left and right transverse sinuses, which in turn drain to the sigmoid sinuses and eventually into the internal jugular veins. Of note, and of particular importance to the venous reflux theory, in the majority of individuals, the straight sinus drains not into both transverse sinuses but only into the left transverse sinus. Given this unique drainage pattern, it is theoretically possible that venous reflux confined to the left internal jugular vein could cause venous stasis in the medial aspects of both the left *and* the right temporal lobes. Recent studies have demonstrated such reflux through incompetent valves (Maalikjy Akkawi *et al.* 2003) in the left internal jugular vein in patients with transient global amnesia, adding weight to this theory (Chung *et al.* 2006; Sander *et al.* 2000). The reflux itself could be related to a Valsalva-type maneuver, consistent with some of the precipitating events mentioned earlier, or, as indicated in one study, to intrathoracic compression of the left brachiocephalic vein (Chung *et al.* 2006).

Differential diagnosis

Transient global amnesia, as discussed in Section 5.4, is best conceived of as one of the episodic anterograde amnesias and, as such, must be distinguished from TIAs, pure epileptic amnesia, concussion, and substance-induced blackouts.

Transient ischemic attacks affecting the temporal lobes may produce a syndrome quite similar to transient global amnesia. However, when ischemia occurs in the area of distribution of the posterior cerebral arteries, in addition to amnesia one typically also sees evidence of ischemia of the occipital lobes, such as hemianopia or cortical blindness, findings not seen in transient global amnesia.

Pure epileptic amnesia is suggested by a sudden offset of the episode, in contrast to the gradual offset of transient global amnesia, and by the fact that patients in the midst of an epileptic amnestic episode generally do not engage in the anxious questioning typical of transient global amnesia. Other distinguishing features include the occurrence of other seizure types, such as complex partial or grand mal seizures, and a pattern of frequent recurrence.

Concussion is immediately suggested by a history of head injury, which, of course, must often be gained from others. Furthermore, during concussion, patients may display a degree of confusion.

Blackouts, as seen during alcohol intoxication or intoxication with benzodiazepines, are suggested by other evidence of intoxication, such as dysarthria or ataxia, and by a lack of recognition on the part of the 'blacked-out' patient that anything is amiss and a corresponding absence of any anxious questioning.

Treatment

Apart from supervision during the episode itself, and reassurance afterwards of its overall benign nature, no treatment is generally required. However, in cases in which there are obvious precipitating factors, patients should be accordingly instructed to avoid them.

REFERENCES

Abu-Shakara M, Khraishi M, Grossman H et al. Primary angiitis of the CNS diagnosed by angiography. QJ Med 1994; 87:351–8.

Alhalabi M, Moore PM. Serial angiography in isolated angiopathy of the central nervous system. Neurology 1994; 44:1221–6.

Akiguchi I, Tomimoto H, Suenega T et al. Alterations in glia and axons in the brains of Binswanger's disease patients. Stroke 1997; 28:1423–9.

Akman-Demir G, Baykan-Kurt B, Serdaroglu P et al. Seven year follow-up of neurologic involvement in Behçet syndrome. Arch Neurol 1993; 53:691–4.

Akman-Demir G, Serdaroglu P, Tasci B et al. Clinical patterns of neurological involvement in Behçet's disease: evaluation of 200 patients. Brain 1999; 122:2171–81.

Akyol A, Akyildiz UO, Tataroglu C. Vascular parkinsonism: a case of lacunar infarction localized to mesencephalic substantia nigra. Parkinsonism Relat Disord 2006; 12:459–61.

Al-Araji A, Sharquie K, Al-Rawi Z. Prevalence and patterns of neurological involvement in Behçet's disease: a prospective study from Iraq. J Neurol Neurosurg Psychiatry 2003; 74:608–13.

Alrawi A, Trobe JD, Blaivas M et al. Brain biopsy in primary angiitis of the central nervous system. Neurology 1999; 53:858–60.

Altinors N, Senveli E, Arda N et al. Intracerebral hemorrhage and hematoma in Behçet's disease: case report. Neurosurgery 1987; 21:582.

Andreaux R, Marro B, El Khoury N et al. Reversible encephalopathy associated with cholesterol embolism syndrome: magnetic resonance imaging and pathological findings. J Neurol Neurosurg Psychiatry 2007; 78:180–2.

Apostolova LG, White M, Moore SA et al. Deep white matter pathologic features in watershed regions: a novel pattern of central nervous system involvement in MELAS. Arch Neurol 2005; 62:1154–6.

Auchus AP, Chen CP, Sadagar SN et al. Single stroke dementia: insights from 12 cases in Singapore. J Neuro Sci 2002; 203–4:85–9.

Auchus AP, Brasher HR, Salloway S et al. Galantamine treatment of vascular dementia. Neurology 2007; 69:448–58.

Aykutlu E, Baykan B, Serdaroglu P et al. Epileptic seizures in Behçet disease. Epilepsia 2002; 43:832–5.

Bartsch T, Alfke K, Stingele R et al. Selective affection of hippocampal CA-1 neurons in patients with transient global amnesia. Brain 2006; 129:2874–84.

Baudrimont M, Dubas F, Joutel A et al. Autosomal dominant leukoencephalopathy and subcortical ischemic stroke. A clinicopathological study. Stroke 1993; 24:122–5.

Beal MF, Williams RS, Richardson EP et al. Cholesterol embolism as a cause of transient ischemic attacks and cerebral infarction. Neurology 1981; 31:860–5.

Bergmann M, Ebke M, Yuan Y. Cerebral autosomal dominant arteriopathy with subcortical infarcts and leukoencephalopathy (CADASIL): a morphological study of a German family. Acta Neuropathol 1996; 92:341–50.

Binswanger O. Die abgrenzung des allgemeinen progressiven. Paralysie Klin Wochenschr 1894; 31:1103–5, 1137–9, 1180–6.

Black S, Roman GC, Geldmacher DS et al. Efficacy and tolerability of donepezil in vascular dementia; positive results of a 24-week, multicenter, international, randomized, placebo-controlled trial. Stroke 2003; 34:2323–30.

Blass JP, Hoyer S, Nitsch R. A translation of Otto Binswanger's article 'The delineation of the generalized progressive paralyses'. Arch Neurol 1991; 48:961–72.

Blum AS, Drislane FW. Nonconvulsive status epilepticus in thrombotic thrombocytopenic purpura. Neurology 1996; 47:1079–81.

Bogucki A, Janczewska E, Koszewska I et al. Evaluation of dementia in subcortical arteriosclerotic encephalopathy (Binswanger's disease). Eur Arch Psychiatry Clin Neurosci 1991; 241:91–7.

Bolwig TG. Transient global amnesia. Acta Neurol Scand 1968; 44:101–6.

Borson S. Behçet's disease as a psychiatric disorder: a case report. Am J Psychiatry 1982; 139:1348–9.

Bruetsch WL, Williams CL. Arteriosclerotic muscular rigidity with special reference to gait disturbances. Am J Psychiatry 1954; 111:332–6.

Byer JA, Crowley WJ. Musical performance during transient global amnesia. Neurology 1980; 30:80–2.

Calabrese LH, Mallek JA. Primary angiitis of the central nervous system: report of 8 new cases, review of the literature, and proposal for diagnostic criteria. Medicine 1988; 67:20–39.

Canafoglia L, Franceschetti S, Antozzi C et al. Epileptic phenotypes associated with mitochondrial disorders. Neurology 2001; 56:1340–6.

Caplan LR, Schoene WC. Clinical features of subcortical arteriosclerotic encephalopathy (Binswanger disease). Neurology 1978; 28:1206–15.

Caselli RJ. Giant cell (temporal) arteritis: a treatable cause of multi-infarct dementia. Neurology 1990; 40:753–5.

Caselli RJ, Hunder GG, Whisnant JP. Neurologic disease in biopsy-proven giant cell (temporal) arteritis. Neurology 1988; 38:352–9.

Case Records of the Massachusetts General Hospital. Case 8–1989. N Engl J Med 1989; 320:514–24.

Chajek T, Fainaru M. Behçet's disease: report of 41 cases and a review of the literature. Medicine 1975; 54:179–86.

Chester EM, Agamanolis DP, Banker BQ et al. Hypertensive encephalopathy: a clinicopathologic study of 20 cases. Neurology 1978; 28:928–39.

Choi JC, Kang S-Y, Kang J-H et al. Intracerebral hemorrhages in CADASIL. Neurology 2006; 67:2042–4.

Chung C-P, Hsu H-Y, Chang F-C et al. Detection of intracranial venous reflux in patients of transient global amnesia. Neurology 2006; 66:1873–7.

Colt HG, Begg RJ, Saporito JJ et al. Cholesterol emboli after cardiac catheterization. Eight cases and a review of the literature. Medicine 1988; 67:389–400.

Cosgrove CR, Leblanc R, Meagher-Villemure K et al. Cerebral amyloid angiopathy. Neurology 1985; 38:625–31.

Cravioto H, Feigin I. Noninfectious granulomatous angiitis involving the central nervous system. Neurology 1959; 9:599–609.

Critchley M. Arteriosclerotic parkinsonism. Brain 1929; 52:23–83.

Crowell GF, Stump DA, Biller J et al. The transient global amnesia–migraine connection. Arch Neurol 1984; 41:75–19.

Cruz-Flores S, de Assis Aquino Gondim F, Leira EC. Brainstem involvement in hypertensive encephalopathy: clinical and radiological findings. Neurology 2004; 62:1417–19.

Cummings JL, Miller B, Hill MA et al. Neuropsychiatric aspects of multi-infarct dementia and dementia of the Alzheimer type. Arch Neurol 1987; 44:389–93.

Dichgans M, Mayer M, Uttner I et al. The phenotypic spectrum of CADASIL: clinical findings in 102 cases. Ann Neurol 1998; 44:731–9.

Dines DE, Burgher LW, Okazaki H. The clinical and pathologic correlation of fat embolism. Mayo Clin Proc 1975; 50:407–11.

Drachman DA. Neurological complications of Wegener's granulomatosis. Arch Neurol 1963; 8:145–55.

Druschky A, Erguth F, Strauss R et al. Central nervous system involvement in thrombotic thrombocytopenic purpura. Eur Neurol 1998; 40:220–4.

Ehsan T, Hasan S, Powers JM et al. Serial magnetic resonance imaging in isolated angiitis of the central nervous system. Neurology 1995; 45:1462–5.

Erkinjunti T, Haltia M, Palo J et al. Accuracy of the clinical diagnosis of vascular dementia: a prospective clinical and post-mortem study. J Neurol Neurosurg Psychiatry 1988; 51:1037–44.

Ezzeddine MA, Primavera JM, Rosand J et al. Clinical characteristics of pathologically proved cholesterol emboli to the brain. Neurology 2000; 54:1681–3.

Farah S, Al-Shubaili A, Montasar A et al. Behçet's syndrome: a report of 41 patients with emphasis on neurological manifestations. J Neurol Neurosurg Psychiatry 1998; 64:382–4.

Filley CM, Thompson LL, Sze CI et al. White matter dementia in CADASIL. J Neurol Sci 1999; 163:163–7.

Fisher CM. Transient global amnesia: precipitating activities and other observations. Arch Neurol 1982; 39:605–8.

Fisher CM, Adams RD. Transient global amnesia. Trans Am Neurol Assoc 1958; 83:143–6.

Fisher CM, Adams RD. Transient global amnesia. Acta Neurol Scand 1964; 40(suppl. 9):1–83.

Ford RG, Siekert RG. Central nervous system manifestations of periarteritis nodosa. Neurology 1965; 15:114–22.

Gandolfo C, Caponnetto C, Conti M et al. Prognosis of transient global amnesia: a long-term follow-up study. Eur Neurol 1992; 32:52–7.

Gilles C, Brucher JM, Khoubesserian P et al. Cerebral amyloid angiopathy as a cause of multiple intracerebral hemorrhages. Neurology 1984; 34:730–5.

Gillespie J, Jackson A. MRI and CT of the brain. London: Arnold, 2000.

Gordon B, Marin OSM. Transient global amnesia: an extensive case report. J Neurol Neurosurg Psychiatry 1979; 42:572–5.

Gray F, Dubas F, Roullet E et al. Leukoencephalopathy in diffuse hemorrhagic amyloid angiopathy. Ann Neurol 1985; 18:54–9.

Greenberg SM, Vonsattel JPG, Stakes JW et al. The clinical spectrum of cerebral amyloid angiopathy: presentations without lobar hemorrhage. Neurology 1993; 43:2073–9.

Greenberg SM, O'Donnell HC, Schaefer PW et al. MRI detection of new hemorrhages: potential marker of progression in cerebral amyloid angiopathy. Neurology 1999; 53:1135–8.

de Groot K, Schmidt DK, Arlt AC et al. Standardized neurologic evaluation of 128 patients with Wegener granulomatosis. Arch Neurol 2001; 58:1215–21.

Gruber O, Wittig L, Wiggins CJ et al. Thrombotic thrombocytopenic purpura: MRI demonstration of persistent small cerebral infarcts after clinical recovery. Neuroradiology 2000; 42:616–18.

Gudmundsson G, Halgrimsson I, Jonasson TA et al. Hereditary cerebral haemorrhage with amyloidosis. Brain 1972; 95:387–404.

Guillery-Girard B, Quinette P, Desgranges B et al. Long-term memory following transient global amnesia: an investigation of episodic and semantic memory. Acta Neurol Scand 2006; 114:329–33.

Haan J, Lanser JBK, Zigderveld I et al. Dementia in hereditary cerebral hemorrhage with amyloidosis – Dutch type. Arch Neurol 1990a; 47:965–7.

Haan J, Algra PR, Roos RAC. Hereditary cerebral hemorrhage with amyloidosis – Dutch type. Clinical and computed tomographic analysis of 24 cases. Arch Neurol 1990b; 47:649–53.

Hagiwara N, Toyoda K, Nakayama M et al. Renal cholesterol emboli in patients with carotid stenosis: a severe and underdiagnosed complication following cerebrovascular procedures. J Neurol Sci 2004; 222:109–12.

Hauser RA, Lacey M, Knight R. Hypertensive encephalopathy: magnetic resonance imaging demonstration of reversible cortical and white matter lesions. Arch Neurol 1988; 45:1078–83.

Healton EB, Brust JC, Feinfeld DA et al. Hypertensive encephalopathy and the neurologic manifestations of malignant hypertension. Neurology 1982; 32:127–31.

Heathfield K, Croft P, Swash M. The syndrome of transient global amnesia. Brain 1973; 96:729–36.

Hinchey J, Chaves C, Appignani B et al. A reversible posterior leukoencephalopathy syndrome. N Engl J Med 1996; 334:494–500.

Hinge HH, Jensen TS, Kjaer M et al. The prognosis of transient global amnesia. Results of a multicenter study. Arch Neurol 1986; 43:673–6.

Hodges JR, Ward CD. Observations during transient global amnesia: a behavioral and neuropsychological study of five cases. *Brain* 1989; **112**:595–620.

Hodges JR, Warlow CP. The aetiology of transient global amnesia. A case-control study of 114 patients with prospective follow-up. *Brain* 1990; **113**:639–57.

von Hochstetter AR, Friede RL. Residual lesions of cerebral fat embolism. *J Neurol* 1977; **216**:227–33.

Hoffman GS, Kerr GS, Leavitt RY. Wegener's granulomatosis: an analysis of 158 patients. *Ann Intern Med* 1992; **116**:488–98.

Hughes JT, Brownell B. Granulomatous giant-celled angiitis of the central nervous system. *Neurology* 1966; **16**:293–8.

Hunter R, Smith J, Thompson T *et al.* Hemiparkinsonism with infarction of the ipsilateral substantia nigra. *Neuropathol Appl Neurobiol* 1978; **4**:297–301.

Iizuka R, Sakai F, Kan S *et al.* Slowly progressive spread of the stroke-like lesions in MELAS. *Neurology* 2003; **61**:1238–44.

Iragui VJ, Miravi E. Behçet syndrome presenting as cerebrovascular disease. *J Neurol Neurosurg Psychiatry* 1986; **49**:838–9.

Ishii N, Nishihara Y, Imamura T. Why do frontal lobe symptoms predominate in vascular dementia with lacunes? *Neurology* 1986; **36**:340–5.

Jacobson DM, Terrence CF, Reinmuth OM. The neurologic manifestations of fat embolism. *Neurology* 1986; **36**:847–51.

Jayakumar PN, Taly AB, Shanmugam V *et al.* Multi-infarct dementia: a computed tomographic study. *Acta Neurol Scand* 1989; **73**:292–5.

Joseph FG, Scolding NJ. Neuro-Behçet's disease in Caucasians: a study of 22 patients. *Eur J Neurol* 2007; **14**:174–80.

Joutel A, Vahedi K, Corpechot C *et al.* Strong clustering and stereotyped nature of *Notch3* mutations in CADASIL patients. *Lancet* 1997; **350**:1511–15.

Jung HH, Bassetti C, Tournier-Lasserve E *et al.* Cerebral autosomal dominant arteriopathy with subcortical infarcts and leukoencephalopathy: a clinicopathological and genetic study of a Swiss family. *J Neurol Neurosurg Psychiatry* 1995; **59**:138–43.

Kamenar E, Burger PC. Cerebral fat embolism: a neuropathologic study of a microembolic state. *Stroke* 1980; **11**:477–84.

Kanazawa M, Sanpei K, Kasuga K. Recurrent hypertensive brainstem encephalopathy. *J Neurol Neurosurg Psychiatry* 2005; **76**:888–90.

Kansu T, Corbett JJ, Savino P *et al.* Giant cell arteritis with normal sedimentation rate. *Arch Neurol* 1977; **34**:624–5.

Katz DI, Alexander MP, Mandell AM. Dementia following strokes in the mesencephalon and diencephalon. *Arch Neurol* 1987; **44**:1127–33.

Keschner M, Sloane P. Encephalitic, idiopathic and arteriosclerotic parkinsonism: a clinicopathologic study. *Arch Neurol Psychiatry* 1931; **25**:1011–41.

Kidd D, Stever A, Denman AM *et al.* Neurological complications in Behçet's syndrome. *Brain* 1999; **122**:2183–94.

Kim Y, Choi EJ, Choi CG *et al.* Characteristics of CADASIL in Korea. a novel cysteine-sparing Notch3 mutation. *Neurology* 2006; **66**:1511–16.

Kinnecom C, Lev MH, Wendell L *et al.* Course of cerebral amyloid angiopathy-related inflammation. *Neurology* 2007; **68**:1411–16.

Knudson KA, Rosand J, Karluk D *et al.* Clinical diagnosis of cerebral amyloid angiopathy: validation of the Boston criteria. *Neurology* 2001; **56**:537–9.

Koga Y, Akita Y, Nishioka J *et al.* L-arginine improves the symptoms of strokelike episodes in MELAS. *Neurology* 2005; **64**:710–12.

Kolodny EH, Rebeiz JJ, Caveness VS *et al.* Granulomatous angiitis of the central nervous system. *Arch Neurol* 1968; **19**:510–24.

Koo EH, Massey EW. Granulomatous angiitis of the central nervous system: protean manifestations and response to treatment. *J Neurol Neurosurg Psychiatry* 1988; **51**:1126–33.

Kritchevsky M, Squire LR. Transient global amnesia: evidence for extensive, temporally graded retrograde amnesia. *Neurology* 1989; **39**:213–18.

Kushner MJ, Hauser WA. Transient global amnesia: a case-control study. *Ann Neurol* 1985; **18**:684–95.

Ladurna G, Iliff LD, Lechner H. Clinical factors associated with ischaemic stroke. *J Neurol Neurosurg Psychiatry* 1982; **45**:97–101.

Lampl Y, Sadeh M, Loberboym M. Transient global amnesia – not always a benign process. *Acta Neurol Scand* 2004; **110**:75–9.

Lamy C, Oppenheim C, Meder JF *et al.* Neuroimaging in posterior reversible leukoencephalopathy syndrome. *J Neuroimaging* 2004; **14**:89–96.

Lauria G, Gentile M, Fassetta G *et al.* Transient global amnesia and transient ischemic attack: a community-based case-control study. *Acta Neurol Scand* 1998; **97**:381–5.

Lavigne CM, Shrier DA, Letkar M *et al.* Tacrolimus leukoencephalopathy: a neuropathologic confirmation. *Neurology* 2004; **63**:1132–3.

Lazzarino LG, Nicolai A, Toppani D. Subacute parkinsonism from a single lacunar infarct in the basal ganglia. *Acta Neurol* 1990; **12**:292–5.

Leff AP, McNabb AW, Hanna MG *et al.* Complex partial status epilepticus in late-onset MELAS. *Epilepsia* 1998; **39**:438–41.

Lesnik Oberstein SAJ, van den Boom R, van Bucher MA *et al.* Cerebral microbleeds in CADASIL. *Neurology* 2001; **57**:1066–70.

Levy E, Carman MD, Fernandez Madrid IJ *et al.* Mutation of the Alzheimer's disease amyloid gene in hereditary cerebral hemorrhage, Dutch type. *Science* 1990; **248**:1124–6.

Lie JT. Primary (granulomatous) angiitis of the central nervous system: a clinicopathologic analysis of 15 new cases and a review of the literature. *Hum Pathol* 1992; **23**:164–71.

Liem MK, van den Grond J, Haan J *et al.* Lacunar infarcts are the main correlate with cognitive dysfunction in CADASIL. *Stroke* 2007; **38**:923–8.

Lin CM, Thajeb P. Valproic acid aggravates epilepsy due to MELAS in a patient with an A3243G mutation of mitochondrial DNA. *Metabol Brain Dis* 2007; **22**:105–9.

Lin JX, Tomimoto H, Akiguchi I *et al.* Vascular cell components of the medullary arteries in Binswanger's disease brains: a morphometric and immunoelectron microscopic study. *Stroke* 2000; **31**:1838–42.

Liu CK, Miller BL, Cummings JL *et al.* A quantitative MRI study of vascular dementia. *Neurology* 1992; **42**:138–43.

Lovelace RE. Mononeuritis multiplex in polyarteritis nodosa. *Neurology* 1964; **14**:434–42.

Maalikjy Akkawi N, Agosti C, Anzola GP et al. Transient global amnesia: a clinical and sonographic study. Eur Neurol 2003; **49**:67–71.

MacKay ME, McLardy T, Harris C. A case of periarteritis nodosa of the central nervous system. J Ment Sci 1950; **96**:470–5.

Malandrini A, Carrera P, Palmeri S et al. Clinicopathological and genetic studies of two further families with cerebral autosomal dominant arteriopathy. Acta Neuropathol 1996; **92**:115–22.

Malandrini A, Gaudiano C, Gambelli S et al. Diagnostic value of ultrastructural skin biopsy in CADASIL. Neurology 2007; **68**:1430–2.

Markus HS, Martin RJ, Simpson MA et al. Diagnostic strategies in CADASIL. Neurology 2002; **59**:1134–8.

Marshall GB, Heale VR, Herx L et al. Magnetic resonance diffusion weighted imaging in cerebral fat embolism. Can J Neurol Sci 2004; **31**:417–21.

Mazlumzadeh M, Hunter GG, Easley KA et al. Treatment of giant cell arteritis using induction therapy with high-dose glucocorticoids: a double-blind, placebo-controlled, randomized prospective clinical trial. Arthritis Rheum 2006; **54**:3310–18.

Mellies JK, Baumer T, Muller JA et al. SPECT study of a German CADASIL family: a phenotype with migraine and progressive dementia only. Neurology 1998; **50**:1715–21.

Melo TP, Ferro JM, Ferro H. Transient global amnesia. A case control study. Brain 1992; **115**:261–70.

Miller JW, Petersen RC, Metter EJ et al. Transient global amnesia: clinical characteristics and prognosis. Neurology 1987a; **37**:733–7.

Miller JW, Yanagihara T, Petersen RC et al. Transient global amnesia and epilepsy. Electroencephalographic distinction. Arch Neurol 1987b; **44**:629–33.

Mok VCT, Wong A, Lam WWM et al. Cognitive impairment and functional outcome after stroke associated with small vessel disease. J Neurol Neurosurg Psychiatry 2004; **75**:560–6.

Moore PM. Diagnosis and management of isolated angiitis of the central nervous system. Neurology 1989; **39**:167–73.

Mori E, Yamdori A, Mitani Y. Left thalamic infarction and disturbance of verbal memory: a clinicoanatomical study with a new method of computed tomographic stereotaxic lesion location. Ann Neurol 1986; **20**:671–6.

Motomura S, Tabira T, Kuroiwa Y. A clinical comparative study of multiple sclerosis and neuro-Behçet's syndrome. J Neurol Neurosurg Psychiatry 1980; **43**:210–13.

Murrow RW, Schweiger GD, Kepes JJ et al. Parkinsonism due to a basal ganglia lacunar state: clinicopathologic correlation. Neurology 1990; **40**:897–900.

Nakada T, Kwee IL, Fujii Y et al. High-field, T2 reversed MRI of hippocampus in transient global amnesia. Neurology 2005; **64**:1170–4.

Nesher G, Berkun Y, Mates M et al. Low-dose aspirin and prevention of cranial ischemic complications in giant cell arteritis. Arthritis Rheum 2004; **50**:1332–7.

Nightingale S, Venables GS, Bates D. Polymyalgia rheumatica with diffuse cerebral disease responding rapidly to steroid therapy. J Neurol Neurosurg Psychiatry 1982; **45**:841–3.

Nishino H, Rubino FA, DeRemee RA et al. Neurological involvement in Wegener's granulomatosis: an analysis of 324 consecutive patients at the Mayo Clinic. Ann Neurol 1993a; **33**:4–9.

Nishino H, Rubino FA, Parisi JE. The spectrum of neurologic involvement in Wegener's granulomatosis. Neurology 1993b; **43**:1334–7.

Nobuyoshi I, Nishihara Y, Horie A. Amyloid angiopathy and lobar cerebral haemorrhage. J Neurol Neurosurg Psychiatry 1984; **47**:1203–10.

Okazaki H, Reagan TJ, Campbell RJ. Clinicopathologic studies of primary cerebral amyloid: angiopathy. Mayo Clin Proc 1979; **54**:22–31.

Opherk C, Peters N, Herzog J et al. Long-term prognosis and causes of death in CADASIL: a retrospective study of 411 patients. Brain 2004; **127**:2533–9.

Oppenheimer BS, Fishberg AM. Hypertensive encephalopathy. Arch Intern Med 1928; **41**:264–78.

Orgogozo JM, Rigaud AS, Stoffer A et al. Efficacy and safety of memantine in patients with mild to moderate vascular dementia: a randomized, placebo-controlled trial (MMM 3000). Stroke 2002; **33**:1834–9.

O'Sullivan M, Jarosz JM, Martin RJ et al. MRI hyperintensities of the temporal lobe and external capsule in patients with CADASIL. Neurology 2001; **56**:628–34.

Pallis CA, Fudge BJ. The neurological complications of Behçet's syndrome. Arch Neurol Psychiatry 1956; **75**:1–14.

Palsdottir A, Abrahamson M, Thorsteinsson L et al. Mutation in cystatin C gene causes hereditary brain haemorrhage. Lancet 1988; **2**:603–4.

Pendlebury WW, Iole ED, Tracy RP et al. Intracerebral hemorrhage related to cerebral amyloid angiopathy and t-PA treatment. Ann Neurol 1991; **29**:210–13.

Quinette P, Guillery-Girard B, Dayan J et al. What does transient global amnesia really mean? Review of the literature and thorough study of 142 cases. Brain 2006; **129**:1640–58.

Regard M, Landis T. Transient global amnesia: neuropsychological dysfunction during attack and recovery in two 'pure' cases. J Neurol Neurosurg Psychiatry 1984; **47**:668–72.

Reichart MD, Bogousslavsky J, Janzer RC. Early lacunar strokes complicated polyarteritis nodosa: thrombotic microangiopathy. Neurology 2000; **54**:883–9.

Revesz T, Hawkins CP, du Boulay EPGH et al. Pathological findings correlated with magnetic resonance imaging in subcortical arteriosclerotic encephalopathy (Binswanger's disease). J Neurol Neurosurg Psychiatry 1989; **52**:1337–44.

Rosand J, Hylek EM, O'Donnell HC et al. Warfarin-associated hemorrhage and cerebral amyloid angiopathy: a genetic and pathologic study. Neurology 2000; **55**:947–51.

Rosete A, Cabral AR, Kraus A et al. Diabetes insipidus secondary to Wegener's granulomatosis: report and review of the literature. J Rheumatol 1991; **18**:761–5.

Rubinstein LJ, Urich H. Meningo-encephalitis of Behçet's disease: Case report with pathological findings. Brain 1963; **86**:151–60.

Ruchoux M-M, Chabriat H, Bousser M-G et al. Presence of ultrastructural arterial lesions in muscle and skin vessels of patients with CADASIL. Stroke 1994; **25**:2291–2.

Sander D, Winbeck K, Etgen T et al. Disturbances of venous flow patterns in patients with transient global amnesia. Lancet 2000; 356:1982–4.

Sandson TA, Daffener KR, Carvalho PA et al. Frontal lobe dysfunction following infarction of the left-sided medial thalamus. Arch Neurol 1991; 48:1300–3.

Schmidtke K, Ehmsen L. Transient global amnesia and migraine. A case control study. Eur Neurol 1998; 40:9–14.

Schon F, Martin RJ, Prevett M et al. 'CADASIL coma': an underdiagnosed acute encephalopathy. J Neurol Neurosurg Psychiatry 2003; 74:249–52.

Schroder JM, Sellhaus B, Jorg J. Identification of the characteristic vascular changes in a sural nerve biopsy of a case with cerebral autosomal dominant arteriopathy with subcortical infarcts and leukoencephalopathy (CADASIL). Acta Neuropathol (Berl) 1995; 89:116–21.

Sedlaczek O, Hirsch JG, Grips E et al. Detection of delayed focal MR changes in the lateral hippocampus in transient global amnesia. Neurology 2004; 62:2165–70.

Serdaroglu P, Yazici H, Ozdemir C et al. Neurologic involvement in Behçet's syndrome: a prospective study. Arch Neurol 1989; 46:265–9.

Seror R, Mahr A, Ramanoelina J et al. Central nervous system involvement in Wegener granulomatosis. Medicine 2006; 85:54–65.

Sharfstein SR, Gordon MF, Libman RB et al. Adult-onset MELAS presenting as herpes encephalitis. Arch Neurol 1999; 56:241–3.

Shuttleworth EC, Morris CE. The transient global amnesia syndrome. Arch Neurol 1966; 15:515–20.

Sigal LH. The neurologic presentation of vasculitic and rheumatologic syndromes. A review. Medicine 1987; 66:157–80.

Sourander P, Walinder J. Hereditary multi-infarct dementia. Acta Neuropathol (Berl) 1977; 39:247–54.

Steinmetz EF, Vroom FQ. Transient global amnesia. Neurology 1972; 22:1193–200.

Strupp M, Bruning R, Wu RH et al. Diffusion-weighted MRI in transient global amnesia: elevated signal intensity in the left medial temporal lobe in 7 of 10 patients. Ann Neurol 1998; 43:164–70.

Swartz RH, Black SE. Anterior-medial thalamic lesions in dementia: frequent, and volume dependently associated with sudden cognitive decline. J Neurol Neurosurg Psychiatry 2006; 77:1307–12.

Tolosa ES, Santamaria J. Parkinsonism and basal ganglia infarcts. Neurology 1984; 34:1515–18.

Tomlinson BE, Blessed GE, Roth M. Observations on the brains of demented old people J Neurol Sci 1970; 11:205–42.

Tournier-Lasserve E, Joutel A, Melki J et al. Cerebral autosomal dominant arteriopathy with subcortical infarcts and leukoencephalopathy maps to chromosome 19q12. Nature Genet 1993; 3:256–9.

Vollmer TL, Guarnaccia J, Harrington W et al. Idiopathic granulomatous angiitis of the central nervous system: diagnostic challenges. Arch Neurol 1993; 50:925–30.

Wadia N, Williams E. Behçet's syndrome with neurological complications. Brain 1957; 80:59–71.

Wattendorff AR, Frangione B, Luyendijk W et al. Hereditary cerebral haemorrhage with amyloidosis, Dutch type (HCHWA-D); clinicopathological studies. J Neurol Neurosurg Psychiatry 1995; 58:699–705.

Wechsler B, Dell'Isola B, Vidhaillet M et al. MRI in 31 patient's with Behçet's disease and neurological involvement: prospective study with clinical correlation. J Neurol Neurosurg Psychiatry 1990; 53:793–8.

Weinberger LM, Cohen ML, Remler BF et al. Intracranial Wegener's granulomatosis. Neurology 1993; 43:1831–4.

Weingarten K, Barbut D, Filippi C et al. Acute hypertensive encephalopathy: findings on spin-echo and gradient-echo MR imaging. Am J Roentgenol 1994; 162:665–70.

Wilcock G, Mobius HJ, Stoffer A. A double-blind, placebo-controlled multicentre study of memantine in mild to moderate vascular dementia (MMM500). Int Clin Psychopharmacol 2002; 17:297–305.

Wilkinson D, Doody R, Helme R et al. Donepezil in vascular dementia: a randomized, placebo-controlled study. Neurology 2003; 61:479–86.

Wilkinson IMS, Russell RWR. Arteries of the head and neck in giant cell arteritis. A pathological study to show the pattern of arterial involvement. Arch Neurol 1972; 27:378–91.

Winikates J, Jankovic J. Clinical correlates of vascular parkinsonism. Arch Neurol 1999; 56:98–102.

Wolf SM, Schotland DL, Phillips LL. Involvement of nervous system in Behçet's syndrome. Arch Neurol 1965; 12:315–25.

Wolfe N, Linn R, Babikian VL et al. Frontal system impairment following multiple lacunar infarcts. Arch Neurol 1990; 47:129–32.

Yamanouchi H. Loss of white matter oligodendrocytes and astrocytes in progressive subcortical vascular encephalopathy of Binswanger type. Acta Neurol Scand 1991; 83:301–5.

Yoshimura M, Yamanouchi H, Kazuhara S et al. Dementia in cerebral amyloid angiopathy: a clinicopathological study. J Neurol 1992; 239:441–50.

Yoshitake T, Kiyohara Y, Kato I et al. Incidence and risk factors of vascular dementia and Alzheimer's disease in a defined elderly Japanese population: the Hisayama study. Neurology 1995; 45:1161–8.

Zijlmans JCM, Thijssen HOM, Vogels OJM et al. MRI in patients with suspected vascular parkinsonism. Neurology 1995; 45:2183–8.

Zijlmans JC, Daniel SE, Hughes AJ et al. Clinicopathological investigation of vascular parkinsonism, including clinical criteria for diagnosis. Mov Disord 2004a; 19:630–40.

Zijlmans JC, Katzenschlager R, Daniel SE et al. The L-dopa response in vascular parkinsonism. J Neurol Neurosurg Psychiatry 2004b; 75:545–7.

Zorzon M, Antonutti L, Masc G et al. Transient global amnesia and transient ischemic attack. Natural history, vascular risk factors, and associated conditions. Stroke 1995; 26:1536–42.

Trauma

11.1 SUBDURAL HEMATOMA

Subdural hematomas, which typically, but not always, occur secondary to head trauma, may present acutely, sub-acutely, or in a chronic fashion; acute and subacute onsets may be characterized by delirium, whereas chronic sub-dural hematomas classically present with dementia. In all three varieties, blood accumulates between the dura and arachnoid; in acute subdural hematomas, this is generally due to arterial bleeding, whereas subacute and chronic sub-dural hematomas generally result from venous bleeding.

Clinical features

Acute subdural hematoma typically occurs in the setting of a traumatic brain injury, and is often accompanied by other intracranial injuries, such as diffuse axonal injury, contusions, intracerebral hemorrhages, and subarachnoid hemorrhage. Patients may develop delirium or may present in stupor or coma.

Subacute subdural hematoma tends to present with drowsiness and delirium (Black 1984), and symptoms may fluctuate for days; when the hematoma occurs secondary to trauma, the latent interval between the trauma and the onset of symptoms may last from days to a week or so. Focal signs, such as hemiparesis, may or may not be present. With progression, uncal herniation may occur with the develop-ment of an ipsilateral third nerve palsy and hemiparesis.

Chronic subdural hematoma may be caused by trivial head injury and, indeed, anywhere from one-quarter to one-half of patients may not recall any head trauma (Cameron 1978; Fogelholm and Waltimo 1975). After a latent interval of months to years patients gradually develop a dementia, which is often accompanied by headache (Arieff and Wetzel 1964; Black 1984; Ishikawa *et al.* 2002; Ramachandran and Hegde 2007); a personality change may occur (Cameron 1978) and, rarely, chronic subdural

hematoma may present with depression (Black 1984). Focal signs, such as hemiparesis, may or may not be present, and, when present, may be quite mild. Rarely seizures may occur (Annegers *et al.* 1998).

Computed tomography (CT) or magnetic resonance (MR) scanning are diagnostic. In the case of acute and sub-acute hematomas, blood may be demonstrated for a week or two, after which, with hemolysis, a proteinaceous fluid remains. In chronic cases the fluid has the same imaging characteristics as the cerebrospinal fluid. Most cases of subdural hematoma occur over the frontal or parietal con-vexities, and the hematoma itself has a convex shape; in a minority hematomas may also be found in the inter-hemispheric fissure or layering on top of the tentorium cerebelli.

Course

Acute subdural hematomas tend to rapidly enlarge and may become immediately life-threatening. Subacute sub-dural hematomas tend to evolve over a matter of weeks and may either progress to stupor or coma or may stabilize, after which there may be a greater or lesser degree of grad-ual improvement. Chronic subdural hematomas tend to undergo a very gradual progression.

Etiology

Most cases of subdural hematoma occur secondary to trauma, either due to a blow to the head or to an acceleration–deceleration injury. This may be quite obvious and severe, for example in a motor vehicle accident; however, in the elderly the trauma need not be severe and indeed may appear trivial. Acute subdural hematomas generally occur secondary to arterial bleeding, which explains their rapid evolution and grave prognosis. Subacute and chronic sub-dural hematomas, however, typically appear secondary to

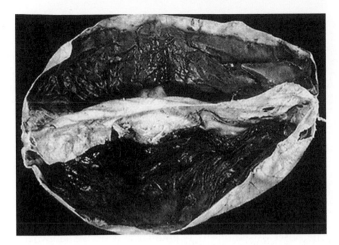

Figure 11.1 Bilateral encapsulated subdural hematomas seen over the convexities. (Reproduced from Graham and Lantos 1996.)

venous bleeding due to rupture of the delicate bridging veins that span from the surface of the cortex to the overlying dural sinuses. Regardless of the source of the bleeding, blood accumulates in the 'virtual space' between the dura and the arachnoid. As noted, hemolysis occurs and, within a week or two of the initial bleed, a relatively clear fluid remains. At this point, the further evolution may take one of two paths. In cases in which the hematoma is relatively small, the fluid may simply be resorbed, with little in the way of anatomic sequelae (Dolinskas *et al.* 1979). However, in cases of larger fluid collection, fibroblastic activity may either create a fibrotic scar that replaces the fluid or one may see the creation of a 'pseudomembrane' that encapsulates the remaining fluid, as illustrated in Figure 11.1. The appearance of a psuedomembrane sets the stage for the clinical occurrence of a chronic subdural hematoma. These encapsulated fluid collections tend to very gradually enlarge, probably as a result of bleeding from fragile capillaries found in the pseudomembrane itself (Markwalder 1981), and it is this gradual enlargement that accounts for the gradual progression of symptoms characteristic of chronic subdural hematoma.

Chronic subdural hematomas are more likely in patients who are prone to falls, such as those with alcoholism or epilepsy, and in those on warfarin or suffering from blood dyscrasias. Simple old age also increases the risk of a chronic subdural hematoma, and this may be because the normal atrophy seen with age leads to a stretching of the bridging veins, thus making them more vulnerable to rupture.

Differential diagnosis

In the case of acute and subacute subdural hematomas, the proximity of the delirium or stupor to the head trauma immediately suggests the diagnosis; however, as noted in Section 7.5 on traumatic brain injury, multiple other intracranial injuries may also be present and at times it is difficult to discern how much of the patient's clinical condition is secondary to the subdural hematoma.

With chronic subdural hematomas, given the long latency and the fact that the head trauma may have been forgotten, the diagnosis may remain obscure until, in the work-up for dementia, neuroimaging reveals the encapsulated fluid collection. Importantly, however, some judgment is required here before ascribing a dementia to a chronic subdural hematoma: whereas a thick chronic hematoma that grossly compresses the underlying cortex may reasonably be held accountable for a dementia, a thin structure that barely compresses the underlying cortex might well be incidental and in such cases it is appropriate to look for other causes of dementia.

Treatment

Symptomatic subdural hematomas generally require surgical evacuation, either by burr holes or craniotomy. Importantly, in the case of chronic subdural hematomas, after evacuation of the clot a considerable amount of time may be required for the gradual re-expansion of the chronically compressed cortex and, hence, clinical improvement may be delayed. The symptomatic treatment of dementia and delirium is discussed in Sections 5.1 and 5.3 respectively.

11.2 DIFFUSE AXONAL INJURY

With a sudden and severe acceleration–deceleration injury, axons and arterioles are subjected to substantial shearing and rotational stresses leading to widespread damage. Although this condition is referred to as 'diffuse axonal injury', given the extensive vascular injury it could also be called 'diffuse vascular injury'. These injuries are typically accompanied by other traumatic lesions, such as contusions, intracerebral hemorrhages, etc., and the reader is referred to Section 7.5 for a discussion of the overall syndrome of traumatic brain injury: this section confines itself to diffuse axonal injury.

Clinical features

Typically, patients are rendered immediately unconscious at the moment of injury. Some may never regain consciousness; those that do may develop a persistent vegetative state (Levin *et al.* 1991) or may emerge into a delirium, which, upon clearing, typically leaves patients with significant cognitive deficits, in some cases amounting to dementia (Scheid *et al.* 2006; Strich 1956). Other sequelae, as discussed in Section 7.5, may include agitation and personality change.

Computed tomography scanning may demonstrate multiple petechial hemorrhages, typically in the centrum semiovale or corpus callosum; however, in many cases the

CT scan may look unremarkable. Magnetic resonance scanning is far more sensitive in diffuse axonal injury and typically displays multiple abnormalities (Huisman *et al.* 2003) in the centrum semiovale, corpus callosum, internal capsules, dorsolateral quadrants of the brainstem, and the superior cerebellar peduncles. Although both fluid-attenuated inversion recovery (FLAIR) and diffusion-weighted imaging are helpful, gradient echo imaging, which enables identification of microhemorrhages, is the most sensitive imaging modality (Ezaki *et al.* 2006).

Course

Most improvement is seen over the first 6 months post-injury, with some further, but less substantial, progress over the following 6 months; after a year, however, little further spontaneous improvement may be expected.

Etiology

With either a sudden impact or merely a severe 'whiplash' injury the head undergoes an acceleration–deceleration injury and tremendous shearing and rotational forces are exerted intracranially, resulting in immediate damage to long axons and penetrating arterioles (Adams *et al.* 1982, 1989; Blumbergs *et al.* 1989; Ng *et al.* 1994; Strich 1956). Axons acutely display retraction balls and microglial clusters and, over time, microglial scars appear. Damage to arterioles leads to petechial hemorrhages of various sizes. Certain areas of the brain are more susceptible to such injuries, including the corpus callosum, the white matter of the centrum semiovale near the gray–white junction, the internal capsules, dorsolateral quadrants of the brainstem, and the superior cerebellar peduncles.

Differential diagnosis

As noted earlier, diffuse axonal injury occurs as part of the syndrome of traumatic brain injury and in many cases it may be very difficult to determine how great a part diffuse axonal injury plays in the overall clinical picture compared with other injuries, such as contusions, intracerebral hemorrhages, subarachnoid hemorrhage, subdural hematomas, and infarctions. In some cases, however, imaging is either normal or displays only findings consistent with diffuse axonal injury, and here one may confidently ascribe the clinical findings to this etiology.

Treatment

The overall treatment of the delirium and dementia of traumatic brain injury is discussed in Section 7.5.

11.3 DEMENTIA PUGILISTICA

Dementia pugilistica is a distinct syndrome that occurs secondary to repeated blows to the head and is characterized by dementia, ataxia, and parkinsonism. Synonyms for this disorder include 'punch drunk syndrome', 'punch drunkenness', and chronic traumatic encephalopathy.

Although dementia pugilistica is found most commonly in boxers, others may also be at risk, for example professional jockeys.

Clinical features

The onset of symptoms is gradual and occurs anywhere from 5 to 40 years after there has been an accumulation of a sufficient number of blows to the head, which, in the case of professional boxers, equates to perhaps a dozen or so knockouts. Thus, although some boxers may develop this disorder while they are still professionally active, in most cases symptoms are delayed until long after the boxer has left the ring.

Clinically (Corsellis 1989; Critchley 1957; Harvey and Davis 1974; Jordan 1987; McLatchie *et al.* 1987; Martland 1928; Mawdsley and Ferguson 1963), when the syndrome is fully developed, patients present with dementia, ataxia, some dysarthria, and parkinsonism. The presence of ataxia and dysarthria often gives the impression of alcohol intoxication, and this accounts for the synonym 'punch drunk'. The dementia itself is non-specific, except perhaps for an undue amount of irritability.

Computed tomography or MR scanning typically displays an enlarged cavum septi pellucidi, cerebral cortical atrophy, and ventricular dilation.

Etiology

Neuropathologic findings are described in the classic paper by Corsellis *et al.* (1973). As illustrated in Figure 11.2, the cavum septi pellucidi is enlarged. The cerebral cortex is atrophied and the ventricles are enlarged; cerebellar atrophy is also present. Microscopically, there are widespread neurofibrillary tangles, which are identical to those found in Alzheimer's disease (Roberts 1988; Schmidt *et al.* 2001). Senile plaques are also present; however, in contrast to the plaques seen in Alzheimer's disease, which are discrete, the plaques seen in dementia pugilistica are diffuse (Roberts *et al.* 1990). Cell loss is found in the substantia nigra and in the locus ceruleus, but Lewy bodies are absent. The mechanism whereby repeated blows to the head induce these changes is not known.

Differential diagnosis

Not all dementias occurring long after repeated head injury are due to dementia pugilistica. Some patients may have

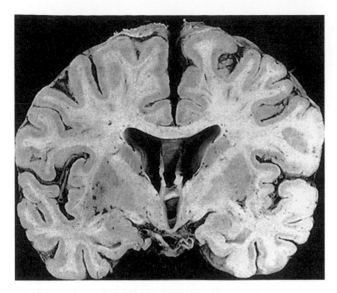

Figure 11.2   Note the wide cavum septi pellucidi in the brain of a professional boxer. (Reproduced from Graham and Lantos 1996.)

had a traumatic subarachnoid hemorrhage followed by the gradual development of a communicating hydrocephalus. Clinically, although perhaps having a 'magnetic' gait, such patients do not develop parkinsonism; furthermore, on imaging, the ventricular dilation will be out of all proportion to any cortical atrophy. Chronic subdural hematoma must also be considered but is readily diagnosed on imaging.

Treatment

The general treatment of dementia is discussed in Section 5.1. In cases in which parkinsonism is prominent, consideration may be given to a trial of levodopa.

11.4 POST-CONCUSSION SYNDROME

Concussion is characterized by a brief loss of consciousness or merely a sense of being dazed, occurring immediately after a blow to the head or, in some cases, a whiplash injury (Miller 1982); patients also experience a variable, but short, period of amnesia, with both retrograde and anterograde components. Most recover fairly promptly, however, in a minority a post-concussion syndrome will develop. Post-concussion syndrome, also known as post-concussional disorder, is characterized by headache, difficulty with concentration and memory, fatigue, dizziness, various admixtures of depression, irritability and anxiety, and other symptoms, such as photophobia.

Clinical features

As noted, concussion may be associated with a loss of consciousness and this generally lasts only a minute or so; in

other cases, patients may remain conscious but appear 'dazed' and mildly confused, with these symptoms again resolving quickly. The amnesia seen in concussion extends in a retrograde fashion for up to hours and in an anterograde fashion from minutes to, in rare cases, hours (Fisher 1966; Martland 1928). In a very small minority of cases, concussion may be associated with a grand mal seizure occurring within seconds of the impact; also known as 'concussive convulsions', these events do not recur and do not portend the development of epilepsy (McCrory *et al.* 1997). Although the grosser aspects of concussion clear immediately, there may be some subtle and mild difficulty with memory and concentration that typically resolves gradually within a week (McCrea *et al.* 2003); in those with a history of prior concussion, however, these symptoms may take longer to resolve (Guskiewicz *et al.* 2003).

In a minority of cases, concussion may be followed by the post-concussion syndrome (Lishman 1968; Mapothar 1937; Symonds 1962). In these cases, in addition to the cognitive difficulties just described, other symptoms become evident within the first day and then persist. Headache tends to be severe and may be continuous or episodic; it may be dull and continuous, or throbbing, and may be exacerbated by loud noises, coughing or sneezing. Fatigue may be constant or may become evident only when patients exert themselves. Dizziness may consist of mere light-headedness or there may be a true vertigo; when vertigo is present, patients may complain that it is exacerbated or precipitated by changes in position or by any sudden movements. Depression may occur and may be marked by severe insomnia. Irritability may be prominent, and patients may complain of great difficulty controlling their tempers. Anxiety may also be seen but appears less common. Other symptoms may occur, including photophobia, hyperacusis, and hyperhidrosis, which at times may be quite impressive. Many patients report that alcohol exacerbates their symptoms.

Course

In most cases, a gradual remission of symptoms occurs anywhere from a few weeks up to 3 years after the concussion, with the majority of patients recovering in a matter of months. When symptoms persist for more than 3 years, a chronic, indefinite, course may be anticipated.

Etiology

Although concussion probably occurs secondary to a fully reversible disruption of axonal function, the post-concussion syndrome in all likelihood occurs secondary to a mild degree of diffuse axonal injury, as indicated by MR scanning (Hofman *et al.* 2001) and in one autopsy case of a patient with the syndrome who died 7 months after the concussion of an unrelated cause (Bigler 2004).

Differential diagnosis

As discussed in Section 7.5, traumatic brain injury may be followed by a dementia, and some would argue that the difference here is merely one of degree in both the severity of the underlying diffuse axonal injury and the resulting cognitive deficits, which are, in both cases, far more profound in the dementia following traumatic brain injury.

In addition to causing the minor degree of diffuse axonal injury underlying the post-concussion syndrome, head trauma sufficient to cause a concussion may also, especially in the elderly, alcoholics, and those on warfarin, cause other injuries, such as contusions, intracerebral hemorrhages or subdural hematoma, which may all cause persistent symptoms.

Post-traumatic stress disorder may follow an assault involving a blow to the head, but here one finds evidence of a re-experiencing of the event, as in dreams or waking memories, symptoms not typical of the post-concussion syndrome.

Malingering may occur after a concussion and this is often suspected in cases in which litigation is in play. Sometimes in these cases, the diagnostic question can be resolved only on observation after resolution of the lawsuit.

Treatment

Concussion itself does not generally require specific treatment. Computed tomography scanning may be considered in the elderly, in alcoholics, those on warfarin, and in any patients with atypical symptoms, such as severe headache, focal signs or the subsequent development of delirium, lethargy or stupor. Athletes should not return to play until all symptoms, including the mild difficulty with memory and concentration, have cleared.

Treatment of the post-concussion syndrome should begin with reassurance regarding the typically benign course. Headache is treated with non-opioid analgesics. Dizziness may respond to antihistamines, but caution should be used here as these agents may exacerbate any cognitive deficits. Depression may respond to antidepressants: one single-blind study noted that treatment with sertraline was not only effective in this regard (Fann *et al.* 2000) but was also associated with cognitive improvement (Fann *et al.* 2001). Alcohol should be forbidden until recovery is complete.

11.5 RADIATION ENCEPHALOPATHY

Irradiation of the central nervous system may be followed by a radiation encephalopathy, and this may occur subsequent to either whole-brain or focal irradiation. There are three different forms of radiation encephalopathy, namely acute, early-delayed, and late-delayed: whereas the acute form is fairly common, the delayed forms are seen in only a very small minority of cases.

Clinical features

Acute radiation encephalopathy occurs within hours to days of irradiation, and probably reflects a breakdown of the blood–brain barrier. Patients may experience delirium, drowsiness, ataxia, headache, nausea and vomiting, and, in a small minority, seizures (Oliff *et al.* 1978). Symptoms undergo a gradual, spontaneous resolution.

Early-delayed radiation encephalopathy appears subacutely anywhere from 1 to 6 months post-irradiation, secondary to demyelinization. In patients who received whole-brain irradiation, there may be delirium, drowsiness, headache, and nausea. By contrast, in those subjected to focal irradiation there may be focal signs appropriate to the irradiated area. Symptoms generally resolve spontaneously within 6–8 weeks.

Late-delayed radiation encephalopathy, which probably occurs secondary to a vasculopathy, presents gradually, generally within 6–36 months post-irradiation, with most cases occurring around 14 months; in some cases, however, the latency between irradiation and the onset of symptoms may be much longer, in one case 33 years (Duffy *et al.* 1996). In patients who received whole-brain irradiation, a dementia occurs, which is often accompanied by ataxia and urinary incontinence (DeAngelis *et al.* 1989; Martins *et al.* 1977; Morris *et al.* 1994). As with the early-delayed type, focal brain irradiation may be followed by focal signs, again appropriate to the irradiated area (Kaufman *et al.* 1990; Shewmon and Masdeu 1980). Of interest, focal irradiation may be followed by a dementia when the focally irradiated area is 'strategic' for cognitive functioning, as may occur when one or both temporal lobes are damaged during irradiation of a pituitary tumor (Crompton and Layton 1961) or a nasopharyngeal carcinoma (Woo *et al.* 1988). In contrast to the other two types of radiation encephalopathy, the late-delayed type does not remit spontaneously, but rather displays a progressive course.

Magnetic resonance scanning shows an increased signal intensity on T2-weighted and FLAIR images in both the early- and late-delayed types. In cases secondary to whole-brain irradiation, this is seen diffusely in the white matter, whereas in focal cases the signal abnormalities are localized. In addition, in the late-delayed type cortical atrophy and ventricular dilation are often seen.

Before leaving this section, it is also appropriate to comment on endocrinologic changes that may occur in irradiated patients (Agha *et al.* 2005; Constine *et al.* 1993; Lam *et al.* 1991). With irradiation of the hypothalamus there may be hyperprolactinemia or tertiary forms of hypothyroidism, adrenocortical insufficiency, or growth hormone deficiency; with irradiation of the pituitary, one may in turn see the secondary forms of hypothyroidism, adrenocortical insufficiency, or growth hormone deficiency. Such changes tend to occur very gradually, with roughly the same time course as the late-delayed radiation encephalopathy; hypothyroidism is especially important to keep in mind as it may present as a dementia. Hypothalamic damage may also cause other symptomatology, as in one case of hyperphagia with severe weight gain (Christianson *et al.* 1994).

Course

This is as described above.

Etiology

As indicated above, the acute form occurs secondary to a radiation-induced breakdown of the blood–brain barrier.

The early-delayed type represents demyelinization (Lampert and Davies 1964), which probably occurs secondary to radiation damage of oligodendroglia. The half-life of myelin ranges from 5 to 8 weeks and, with loss or dysfunction of oligodendroglia, symptoms appear as myelin degrades in the absence of ongoing replacement. With a new 'crop' of oligodendroglia, replenishment of myelin gradually occurs and symptoms resolve.

Late-delayed radiation encephalopathy probably occurs on the basis of hyalinization of penetrating arterioles with fibrinoid necrosis, microthrombosis, and a myriad of microinfarctions (De Reuck and vander Eecken 1975; Pennybaker and Russell 1948).

Differential diagnosis

The history of irradiation makes the diagnosis of the acute form obvious and is highly suggestive when the delayed forms present after whole-brain irradiation with delirium (in the case of the early-delayed form) or dementia (with the late-delayed form). Difficulties may arise, however, when the delayed forms occur after focal irradiation for a central nervous system tumor, as in these cases the possibility exists that the focal findings could represent not radiation damage but rather tumor recurrence. In such cases, although MR scanning may not be helpful, positron emission tomography (PET) scanning reliably distinguishes the two possibilities, demonstrating decreased glucose utilization in radiation encephalopathy and increased utilization in cases of tumor recurrence (Glantz *et al.* 1991).

Two other differential possibilities to keep in mind are the appearance of a new tumor and large-vessel infarction. Irradiation may cause tumors (Robinson 1978) and, although this is rare, both meningiomas (Brada *et al.* 1992; Soffer *et al.* 1983) and gliomas (Zampieri *et al.* 1989) may appear. Further, in cases in which large vessels were exposed to irradiation, a vasculitis may occur, with thrombosis and large, territorial infarctions (Grattan-Smith *et al.* 1992).

Treatment

Acute radiation encephalopathy may be treated with steroids and, indeed, it is customary to give steroids prophylactically.

Early-delayed radiation encephalopathy may show some response to either dexamethasone or prednisone; the symptomatic treatment of delirium is discussed in Section 5.3.

Treatment of the late-delayed form of radiation encephalopathy is not settled: a large case series suggests improvement with either heparin or warfarin (Glantz *et al.* 1994). The symptomatic treatment of dementia is discussed in Section 5.1.

REFERENCES

Adams JH, Graham DI, Murray LS *et al.* Diffuse axonal injury due to non-missile injury in humans: an analysis of 45 cases. *Ann Neurol* 1982; **12**:557–63.

Adams JH, Doyle D, Ford I *et al.* Diffuse axonal injury in head injury: definition, diagnosis and grading. *Histopathology* 1989; **15**:49–59.

Agha A, Sherlock M, Brennan S *et al.* Hypothalamic-pituitary dysfunction after irradiation of nonpituitary brain tumors in adults. *J Clin Endocrinol Metabol* 2005; **90**:6355–60.

Annegers JF, Hauser WA, Coan SP *et al.* A population-based study of seizures after traumatic brain injury. *N Engl J Med* 1998; **338**:20–4.

Arieff AJ, Wetzel N. Subdural hematoma following epileptic convulsion. *Neurology* 1964; **14**:731–2.

Bigler Ed. Neuropsychological results and neuropathological findings at autopsy in a case of mild traumatic brain injury. *J Int Neuropsychol Soc* 2004; **10**:794–806.

Black DW. Mental changes resulting from subdural hematoma. *Br J Psychiatry* 1984; **145**:200–3.

Blumbergs PC, Jones NR, North JB. Diffuse axonal injury in head trauma. *J Neurol Neurosurg Psychiatry* 1989; **52**;838–41.

Brada M, Ford D, Ashley S *et al.* Risk of second brain tumor after conservative surgery and radiotherapy for pituitary adenoma. *BMJ* 1992; **304**:1343–6.

Cameron MM. Chronic subdural hematoma: a review of 114 cases. *J Neurol Neurosurg Psychiatry* 1978; **41**:834–9.

Christianson SA, Neppe V, Hofman H. Amnesia and vegetative abnormalities after irradiation treatment: a case study. *Acta Neurol Scand* 1994; **90**:360–6.

Constine LS, Woolf PD, Cann D *et al.* Hypothalamic-pituitary dysfunction after radiation for brain tumors. *N Engl J Med* 1993; **328**:87–94.

Corsellis JAN. Boxing and the brain. *BMJ* 1989; **298**:105–9.

Corsellis JAN, Bruton CJ, Freeman-Browne D. The aftermath of boxing. *Psychol Med* 1973; **3**:270–303.

Critchley M. Medical aspects of boxing particularly from a neurological standpoint. *BMJ* 1957; **1**:357–66.

Crompton MR, Layton DD. Delayed radionecrosis of the brain following therapeutic X-irradiation of the pituitary. *Brain* 1961; **84**:85–101.

DeAngelis LM, Delattre J-Y, Posner JB. Radiation-induced dementia in patients cured of brain metastases. *Neurology* 1989; **39**:172-7.

De Reuck J, vander Eecken H. The anatomy of late radiation encephalopathy. *Eur Neurol* 1975; **13**:481-94.

Dolinskas CS, Zimmerman RA, Bilaniuk LT *et al.* Computed tomography of post-traumatic extracerebral hematomas. *J Trauma* 1979; **19**:163-9.

Duffy P, Chari G, Cartlidge NEF *et al.* Progressive deterioration of intellect and motor function occurring several decades after cranial irradiation. *Arch Neurol* 1996; **53**:814-18.

Ezaki Y, Tsutsumi K, Morikawa M *et al.* Role of diffusion-weighted magnetic resonance imaging in diffuse axonal injury. *Acta Radiol* 2006; **47**:733-40.

Fann JR, Uomoto JM, Katon WJ. Sertraline in the treatment of major depression following mild traumatic brain injury. *J Neuropsychiatry Clin Neurosci* 2000; **12**:226-32.

Fann JR, Uomoto JM, Katon WJ. Cognitive improvement with treatment of depression following mild traumatic brain injury. *Psychosomatics* 2001; **42**:48-54.

Fisher CM. Concussion amnesia. *Neurology* 1966; **16**:826-30.

Fogelholm R, Waltimo O. Epidemiology of chronic subdural haematoma. *Acta Neurochirug* 1975; **32**:247-50.

Glantz MJ, Hoffman JM, Coleman RE *et al.* Identification of early recurrence of primary central nervous system tumors by [18F] fluorodeoxyglucose positron emission tomography. *Ann Neurol* 1991; **29**:347-55.

Glantz MJ, Burger PC, Friedman AH *et al.* Treatment of radiation-induced nervous system injury with heparin and warfarin. *Neurology* 1994; **44**:2020-7.

Graham DL, Lantos PL. *Greenfield's neuropathology*, 6th edn. London: Arnold, 1996.

Grattan-Smith PJ, Morris JG, Langlands AO. Delayed radiation necrosis of the central nervous system in patients irradiated for pituitary tumor. *J Neurol Neurosurg Psychiatry* 1992; **55**:949-55.

Guskiewicz KM, McCrea M, Marshall SW *et al.* Cumulative effects associated with recurrent concussion in collegiate football players: the NCAA Concussion Study. *JAMA* 2003; **290**:2459-55.

Harvey PKP, Davis JN. Traumatic encephalopathy in a young boxer. *Lancet* 1974; **2**:928-9.

Hofman PA, Stapert SZ, von Kroonenburgh MJ *et al.* MR imaging, single-photon emission CT, and neurocognitive performance after mild traumatic brain injury. *AJNR* 2001; **22**:441-9.

Huisman TA, Sorensen AG, Hergan K *et al.* Diffusion-weighted imaging for the evaluation of diffuse axonal injury in closed head injury. *J Comput Assist Tomogr* 2003; **27**:5-11.

Ishikawa E, Yanaka K, Sugimoto K *et al.* Reversible dementia in patients with chronic subdural hematoma. *J Neurosurg* 2002; **96**:680-3.

Jordan BD. Neurologic aspects of boxing. *Arch Neurol* 1987; **44**:453-9.

Kaufman M, Swartz BE, Mandelkern M *et al.* Diagnosis of delayed cerebral radiation necrosis following proton beam therapy. *Arch Neurol* 1990; **47**:474-6.

Lam KN, Tse VK, Wang C *et al.* Effects of cranial irradiation on hypothalamic-pituitary function – a 5-year longitudinal study in patients with nasopharyngeal cancer. *Q J Med* 1991; **78**:165-76.

Lampert PW, Davies RL. Delayed effects of radiation on the human central nervous system. *Neurology* 1964; **14**:912-17.

Levin HS, Saydjari C, Eisenberg HM *et al.* Vegetative state after closed-head injury. A traumatic coma data bank report. *Arch Neurol* 1991; **48**:580-5.

Lishman WA. Brain damage in relation to psychiatric disability after head injury. *Br J Psychiatry* 1968; **114**:373-410.

McCrea M, Guskiewicz KM, Marshall SW *et al.* Acute effects and recovery time following concussion in collegiate football players: the NCAA Concussion Study. *JAMA* 2003; **290**:2556-63.

McCrory PR, Bladin PF, Berkovic SF. Retrospective study of concussive convulsions in elite Australian rules and rugby league footballers: phenomenology, aetiology, and outcome. *BMJ* 1997; **314**:171-4.

McLatchie G, Brooks N, Galbraith S *et al.* Clinical neurologic examination and computed tomographic head scanning in active amateur boxers. *J Neurol Neurosurg Psychiatry* 1987; **50**:96-9.

Mapothar E. Mental symptoms associated with head injury: the psychiatric aspects. *BMJ* 1937; **2**:1055-61.

Markwalder T-M. Chronic subdural hematomas: a review. *J Neurosurg* 1981; **54**:637-45.

Martins AN, Johnston JS, Henry JM *et al.* Delayed radiation necrosis of the brain. *J Neurosurg* 1977; **47**:336-45.

Martland HS. Punch drunk. *JAMA* 1928; **91**:1103-7.

Mawdsley C, Ferguson FR. Neurological disease in boxers. *Lancet* 1963; **2**:795-801.

Miller CM. Whiplash amnesia. *Neurology* 1982; **32**:667-8.

Morris JG, Gratten-Smith P, Panegyres PK *et al.* Delayed cerebral radiation necrosis. *Q J Med* 1994; **87**:119-29.

Ng HK, Mahaliyana RD, Poon WS. The pathological spectrum of diffuse axonal injury in blunt head trauma: assessment with axon and myelin stains. *Clin Neurol Neurosurg* 1994; **96**:24-31.

Oliff A, Bleyer WA, Poplack DG. Acute encephalopathy after initiation of cranial irradiation for meningeal leukaemia. *Lancet* 1978; **2**:13-15.

Pennybaker J, Russell DS. Necrosis of the brain due to radiation therapy: clinical and pathological observations. *J Neurol Neurosurg Psychiatry* 1948; **11**:183-98.

Ramachandran R, Hegde T. Chronic subdural hematomas – causes of morbidity and mortality. *Surg Neurol* 2007; **67**:367-72.

Roberts GW. Immunocytochemistry of neurofibrillary tangles in dementia pugilistica and Alzheimer's disease: evidence for common genesis. *Lancet* 1988; **2**:1456-8.

Roberts GW, Allsop D, Bruton C. The occult aftermath of boxing. *J Neurol Neurosurg Psychiatry* 1990; **53**:373-8.

Robinson RG. A second brain tumor and irradiation. *J Neurol Neurosurg Psychiatry* 1978; **41**:1005-12.

Scheid R, Walther K, Guthke T *et al.* Cognitive sequelae of diffuse axonal injury. *Arch Neurol* 2006; **63**:418-24.

Schmidt ML, Zhukareva V, Newell KL *et al.* Tau isoform profile and phosphorylation state in dementia pugilistica recapitulate Alzheimer's disease. *Acta Neuropathol* 2001; **101**:518–24.

Shewmon DA, Masdeu JC. Delayed radiation necrosis of the brain contralateral to original tumor. *Arch Neurol* 1980; **37**:592–4.

Soffer D, Pittaluga S, Feiner M *et al.* Intracranial meningiomas following low-dose irradiation to the head. *J Neurosurg* 1983; **59**:1048–53.

Strich SJ. Diffuse degeneration of the cerebral white matter in severe dementia following head injury. *J Neurol Neurosurg Psychiatry* 1956; **19**:163–85.

Symonds CP. Concussion and its sequelae. *Lancet* 1962; **1**:1–5.

Woo E, Lam K, Yu YL *et al.* Temporal lobe and hypothalamo-pituitary dysfunctions after radiotherapy for nasopharyngeal carcinoma: a distinct clinical syndrome. *J Neurol Neurosurg Psychiatry* 1988; **51**:1302–7.

Zampieri P, Zorat PL, Mingrino S *et al.* Radiation-associated cerebral gliomas: a report of two cases and review of the literature. *J Neurosurg Sci* 1989; **33**:271–9.

Hypoxic disorders

12.1 POST-ANOXIC ENCEPHALOPATHY

Global cerebral ischemia or anoxia will, if sufficiently prolonged, cause coma, and those who survive may be left with a dementia, an amnesia, or a movement disorder, such as myoclonus or parkinsonism. Common causes include cardiac arrest, hemorrhagic or septic shock, carbon monoxide poisoning, strangulation, or drowning. In this text, this disorder is referred to as post-anoxic encephalopathy; other names include post-hypoxic encephalopathy, post-ischemic encephalopathy or ischemic–hypoxic encephalopathy.

Clinical features

Among those who survive the ischemic–hypoxic event and emerge from coma, some may be left in a persistent vegetative state whereas others will emerge into a delirium of variable duration. After the delirium clears, some patients may recover entirely; however, most will be left with either a dementia or an amnesia. The dementia may or may not be accompanied by delusions and hallucinations; many patients will be restless and in some cases there may be a significant degree of agitation. In some cases, rather than a dementia, patients will be left with an isolated amnestic syndrome, which has both anterograde and retrograde components (Berlyne and Strachan 1968; Bowman *et al.* 1997; Broman *et al.* 1997; Medalia *et al.* 1991).

Action (or intention) myoclonus may occur (Lance and Adams 1963; Werhahn *et al.* 1997), and may appear independently or in concert with a dementia or amnesia. Parkinsonism, dystonia or athestosis (or a combination of these) may also appear.

Magnetic resonance (MR) scanning may reveal a variety of findings, including laminar cortical necrosis, watershed infarctions, and abnormalities in the basal ganglia.

Course

Dementia and amnesia may show some improvement over the first 6 months or so, after which these features tend to remain stably chronic. Parkinsonism and dystonia, by contrast, may show a gradual progression over many years.

Etiology

After five or more minutes of global ischemia or anoxia, permanent damage occurs. In those who develop post-anoxic encephalopathy, one finds cortical atrophy, ventricular dilation, and, within the cerebral cortex, either a laminar or a multifocal pattern of cortical necrosis (Richardson *et al.* 1959; Weinberger *et al.* 1940). In cases characterized by isolated amnesia, the temporal lobes, in particular the hippocampi, are heavily involved (Cummings *et al.* 1984; Muramoto *et al.* 1979), and in cases of parkinsonism or dystonia, the basal ganglia show similar changes. In some cases of global ischemia watershed infarctions may also occur.

Differential diagnosis

As the name suggests, delayed post-anoxic encephalopathy is distinguished by the delay between the anoxic/ischemic event and the onset of the encephalopathy: in post-anoxic encephalopathy, as noted above, there is no delay and patients emerge from coma and delirium directly into the dementia or amnesia, whereas in delayed post-anoxic encephalopathy there is a latent interval, lasting from days to months, after which clinical deterioration occurs.

Treatment

The general treatment of dementia and amnesia is discussed in Sections 5.1 and 5.4 respectively. A case report suggests that agitation may respond to amitriptyline (Szlabowicz and Stewart 1990), and the author has seen dramatic results with mirtazapine in such cases. Myoclonus is traditionally treated with clonazepam, eventually in doses of 6 mg or more daily; other options include valproate (Rollinson and Gilligan 1979) or levetiracetam (Krauss et al. 2001). Parkinsonism may be treated with levodopa.

12.2 DELAYED POST-ANOXIC LEUKOENCEPHALOPATHY

After a global hypoxic or ischemic insult, patients typically develop a coma or, occasionally, merely a delirium. Upon emergence from coma some may develop a post-anoxic encephalopathy, as described in the preceding section, whereas others will recover more or less completely. In a few percent of these patients who do enjoy a more or less complete recovery, however, a delayed post-anoxic encephalopathy, characterized by delirium or a movement disorder, may appear after a lucid interval.

Clinical features

Clinically (Choi 1983, 2002; Courville 1957; Gottfried et al. 1997; Min 1986; Murata et al. 1995; Norris et al. 1982; Plum et al. 1962), the lucid interval averages about 2–3 weeks, ranging from as little as 2 days to up to 2 months. The onset of the encephalopathy itself is fairly sudden, occurring over a matter of a day or two, and patients generally present with a combination of delirium and a movement disorder. Confusion, amnesia, apathy, irritability, and incontinence are prominent, and some patients may become mute. Parkinsonism is the most common movement disorder seen, but some patients may develop dystonia and some may experience a combination of the two syndromes. Spasticity is common, with hyper-reflexia and extensor plantar responses. Delirium may occasionally be absent and patients may present only with a movement disorder, such as parkinsonism (Choi et al. 2002; Goto et al. 1997; Grinker 1926; Klawans et al. 1982; Rosenberg et al. 1989), dystonia (Valenzuela et al. 1992), or chorea (Davous et al. 1986; Schwartz et al. 1985).

T2-weighted MR scanning reveals increased signal intensity in the white matter in those with delirium (Chang et al. 1992; Gottfried et al. 1997); acutely, diffusion-weighted imaging will show increased signal intensity in the same area (Kim et al. 2003). In patients with a movement disorder, T1-weighted scanning may reveal decreased signal intensity in the striatum (Takahashi et al. 1998).

Course

In a small minority the course is fulminant, with coma and death. In most, however, the course is favorable, with patients experiencing a more or less complete recovery of cognitive abilities over 6–12 months, with only a minority being left with a residual dementia (Choi 1983; Min 1986; Plum et al. 1962; Shillito et al. 1936). The movement disorder, however, may persist, and in some cases may progressively worsen.

Etiology

At autopsy there is a massive, symmetric, diffuse demyelinization of the white matter (Plum et al. 1962), with variable involvement of the basal ganglia. Although the mechanism underlying this is not known, an autoimmune response, triggered by damage sustained during the original hypoxic/ischemic insult, is strongly suspected.

Differential diagnosis

Delayed post-anoxic encephalopathy is distinguished from post-anoxic encephalopathy by the latent interval between the hypoxic/ischemic insult and the onset of symptoms.

Treatment

Although there is no established treatment for this disorder, a case may be made, given the suspected mechanism, for acute treatment with methylprednisolone or prednisone. The general treatment of delirium is discussed in Section 5.3; in cases characterized by parkinsonism, a trial of levodopa may be considered.

12.3 CARBON MONOXIDE POISONING

Carbon monoxide poisoning may be accidental, as may occur with poorly ventilated gas, wood, or charcoal stoves, or by suicidal intent, such as when patients hook a hose to the car exhaust and then funnel it into the tightly windowed car, or simply leave the car running in an enclosed garage.

Clinical features

The onset of intoxication may be gradual or sudden, and, given that carbon monoxide is colorless and odorless, victims may be unaware of their plight. In general (Sayers and Davenport 1930), although the correlation between carboxyhemoglobin level and clinical symptomatology is only a rough one, headache and delirium appear at a carboxyhemoglobin level between 10 and 30 percent, worsening and being joined by nausea and vomiting as the level rises to 40 percent. At levels of 40–50 percent, stupor and ataxia appear, and cyanosis may be seen. When the level rises above 50 percent, coma and convulsions occur, and levels over 60 percent are often fatal. Although it is traditional to

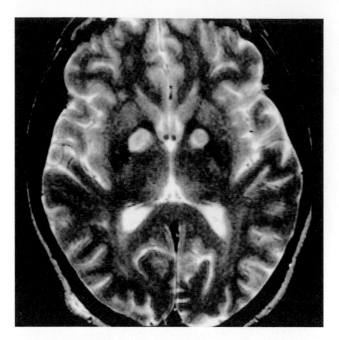

Figure 12.1　T2-weighted magnetic resonance imaging scan in a case of carbon monoxide poisoning, demonstrating increased signal intensity in the globus pallidus. (Reproduced from Graham and Lantos 2002.)

associate carbon monoxide poisoning with a cherry-red discoloration of the lips, nails and skin, this is in fact rare: if anything, most patients will display a degree of cyanosis.

In those who survive, characteristic changes may be seen in the globus pallidus on MR scanning, as illustrated in Figure 12.1.

Course

In general, if intoxication ceases before the onset of stupor, recovery is typically complete within anywhere from hours to weeks (Smith and Brandon 1970). Should coma occur, and even in some cases in which only delirium has occurred, a minority of patients may experience significant sequelae, such as a post-anoxic encephalopathy or a delayed post-anoxic encephalopathy.

Etiology

The affinity of carbon monoxide for hemoglobin is over 200 times greater than that of oxygen and, when a high fraction of hemoglobin exists as carboxyhemoglobin, tissue anoxia supervenes. Anoxia may not, however, be the only mechanism of toxicity. Carbon monoxide also binds to mitochondrial cytochrome oxidase and thus impairs cellular respiration; furthermore, carbon monoxide also binds to areas of the central nervous system rich in iron, for example the globus pallidus and the substantia nigra. In fatal cases widespread petechial hemorrhages are found throughout the cerebrum (Finck 1966).

Differential diagnosis

The circumstances in which the patient is found usually leave little doubt as to the diagnosis; in cases of attempted suicide, however, one must keep in mind that the patient may also have overdosed.

Treatment

The goal of treatment is to eliminate the carbon monoxide as rapidly as possible. The half-life of carboxyhemoglobin ranges from 4 to 6 hours; with inhalation of 100 percent oxygen, however, this is cut to about 1 hour, and with hyperbaric oxygen it falls to 30 minutes or less; consequently hyperbaric oxygen is preferred in virtually all cases (Weaver *et al.* 2002).

REFERENCES

Berlyne N, Strachan M. Neuropsychiatric sequelae of attempted hanging. *Br J Psychiatry* 1968; **114**:411–22.

Bowman M, Rose AL, Hotson G *et al.* Severe anterograde amnesia with onset in childhood as a result of anoxic encephalopathy. *Brain* 1997; **120**:417–33.

Broman M, Rose AL, Hotson G *et al.* Severe anterograde amnesia with onset in childhood as a result of anoxic encephalopathy. *Brain* 1997; **120**:417–33.

Chang KH, Han MH, Kim HS *et al.* Delayed encephalopathy after acute carbon monoxide intoxication: MR imaging features and distribution of cerebral white matter lesions. Radiology 1992; **184**:117–22.

Choi IS. Delayed neurologic sequelae in carbon monoxide intoxication. *Arch Neurol* 1983; **40**:433–5.

Choi IS. Parkinsonism following carbon monoxide poisoning. *Eur Neurol* 2002; **48**:30–3.

Courville CB. The process of demyelination in the central nervous system. IV. Demyelination as a delayed residual of carbon monoxide asphyxiation. *J Nerv Ment Dis* 1957; **125**:534–46.

Cummings JL, Tomiyasu U, Read S *et al.* Amnesia with hippocampal lesions after cardiopulmonary arrest. *Neurology* 1984; **24**:679–81.

Davous P, Rondot P, Marion MH *et al.* Severe chorea after acute carbon monoxide poisoning. *J Neurol Neurosurg Psychiatry* 1986; **49**:206–8.

Finck PA. Exposure to carbon monoxide: review of the literature and 567 autopsies. *Milit Med* 1966; **131**:1513–39.

Goto S, Kunitoku N, Suyama N *et al.* Posteroventral pallidotomy in a patient with parkinsonism caused by hypoxic encephalopathy. *Neurology* 1997; **49**:707–10.

Gottfried JA, Mayer SA, Shungu DC *et al.* Delayed posthypoxic demyelination: association with arylsulfatase A deficiency and lactic acidosis on proton MR spectroscopy. *Neurology* 1997; **49**:1400–4.

Graham DL, Lantos PL. *Greenfield's neuropathology*, 7th edn. London: Arnold, 2002.

Grinker RR. Parkinsonism following carbon monoxide poisoning. *J Nerv Ment Dis* 1926; **64**:18–28.

Kim JH, Chang KH, Song IC *et al.* Delayed encephalopathy of acute carbon monoxide intoxication: diffusivity of cerebral white matter lesions. *AJNR* 2003; **24**:1592–7.

Klawans HL, Stein RW, Tanner CM *et al.* A pure parkinsonian syndrome following acute carbon monoxide intoxication. *Arch Neurol* 1982; **39**:302–4.

Krauss GL, Bergin A, Kramer RE *et al.* Suppression of post-hypoxic and post-encephalitic myoclonus with levetiracetam. *Neurology* 2001; **56**:1144–5.

Lance JW, Adams RD. The syndrome of intention or action myoclonus as a sequel to hypoxic encephalopathy. *Brain* 1963; **86**:111–36.

Medalia AA, Merriam AE, Ehrenreich JH. The neuropsychological sequelae of attempted hanging. *J Neurol Neurosurg Psychiatry* 1991; **54**:546–8.

Min SK. A brain syndrome associated with delayed neuropsychiatric sequelae following acute carbon monoxide intoxication. *Acta Psychatr Scand* 1986; **73**:80–6.

Muramoto O, Kuru Y, Sugishita M *et al.* Pure memory loss with hippocampal lesions: a pneumoencephalographic study. *Arch Neurol* 1979; **36**:54–6.

Murata T, Itoh S, Koshino Y *et al.* Serial proton magnetic resonance spectroscopy in a patient with the interval form of carbon monoxide poisoning. *J Neurol Neurosurg Psychiatry* 1995; **58**:100–3.

Norris CR, Trench JM, Hook R. Delayed carbon monoxide encephalopathy: clinical and research implications. *J Clin Psychiatry* 1982; **43**:294–5.

Plum F, Posner JB, Hain RF. Delayed neurological deterioration after anoxia. *Arch Intern Med* 1962; **110**:56–63.

Richardson JC, Chambers RA, Heywood PM. Encephalopathies of anoxia and hypoglycemia. *Arch Neurol* 1959; **1**:178–90.

Rollinson RD, Gilligan BS. Post-anoxic myoclonus (Lance-Adams syndrome) responding to valproate. *Arch Neurol* 1979; **36**:44–5.

Rosenberg NL, Myers JA, Martin WRW. Cyanide-induced parkinsonism: clinical MRI and 6-fluorodopa PET studies. *Neurology* 1989; **39**:142–4.

Sayers PR, Davenport SJ. Review of carbon monoxide poisoning. Public Health Bulletin No. 195. Washington DC: US Government Printing Office, 1930.

Schwartz A, Hennerici M, Wegener OH. Delayed choreoathetosis following acute carbon monoxide poisoning. *Neurology* 1985; **35**:98–9.

Shillito FH, Drinker CK, Shaughnessy TJ. The problem of nervous and mental sequelae in carbon monoxide poisoning. *JAMA* 1936; **106**:669–74.

Smith JS, Brandon S. Acute carbon monoxide poisoning – 3 years experience in a defined population. *Postgrad Med J* 1970; **46**:65–70.

Szlabowicz JW, Stewart JT. Amitriptyline treatment of agitation associated with anoxic encephalopathy. *Arch Phys Med Rehabil* 1990; **71**:612–13.

Takahashi W, Ohnuki Y, Takizawa S *et al.* Neuroimaging on delayed postanoxic encephalopathy with lesions localized in the basal ganglia. *Clin Imaging* 1998; **22**:188–91.

Valenzuela R, Court J, Godoy J. Delayed cyanide induced dystonia. *J Neurol Neurosurg Psychiatry* 1992; **55**:198–9.

Weaver LK, Hopkins RD, Chan KJ *et al.* Hyperbaric oxygen for acute carbon monoxide poisoning. *N Engl J Med* 2002; **347**:1057–67.

Weinberger LM, Gibbon MH, Gibbon JH. Temporary arrest of the circulation to the central nervous system. II. Pathologic effects. *Arch Neurol Psychiatry* 1940; **43**:961–86.

Werhahan KJ, Brown P, Thompson PD *et al.* The clinical features and prognosis of chronic posthypoxic myoclonus. *Mov Disord* 1997; **12**:216–20.

13

Nutritional, toxic, and metabolic disorders

13.1 VITAMIN B12 DEFICIENCY

Vitamin B12 deficiency may lead to demyelinization in the cerebrum, with, among other disturbances, dementia, or in the cord, leading to a syndrome known as subacute combined degeneration; a macrocytic anemia is also common; however, as stressed below, neuropsychiatric symptomatology may occur in patients with normal red blood cell counts and red blood cell indices. Although vitamin B12 deficiency is most commonly due to pernicious anemia, multiple other causes must also be considered.

Clinical features

Symptoms referable to the cerebrum or spinal cord tend to appear subacutely over weeks or months.

Cerebral involvement (Healton *et al.* 1991; Lindenbaum *et al.* 1988) manifests most commonly with a dementia, which may be marked by hallucinations and delusions (Lurie 1919). Personality change may also occur, and, rarely, one may also see depression (Fraser 1960) or mania (Goggans 1984). Another rare manifestation is psychosis, referred to in the past as 'megaloblastic madness': in one case (Smith 1929), a 46-year-old woman developed delusions of persecution and jealousy, and was only correctly diagnosed when symptoms of subacute combined degeneration became evident; in another (Evans *et al.* 1983), a 47-year-old woman became withdrawn, guarded, and suspicious, heard the voice of God commanding her to board a spaceship, and prayed fervently, with all symptoms resolving upon B12 administration. There is also a case report of tremor and chorea occurring as a manifestation of B12 deficiency (Pacchetti *et al.* 2002).

Subacute combined degeneration (Healton *et al.* 1991; Russell *et al.* 1900) reflects demyelinization of the peripheral nerves, posterior columns, and lateral corticospinal tracts. Patients present with acral parasthesiae, followed by ataxia, a positive Romberg test, and eventually spasticity: the plantar responses are generally extensor, but the deep tendon reflexes may be either increased or depressed, depending on the severity of the peripheral neuropathy.

Macrocytosis, with or without anemia, is common; however, as noted above, it must be stressed that both these findings may be absent. Indeed, in one large study both the red blood cell count and the mean corpuscular volume were normal in approximately one-fifth of all patients (Lindenbaum *et al.* 1988).

Magnetic resonance imaging (MRI) scanning reveals patchy, confluent areas of increased signal intensity in the centrum semiovale in patients with cerebral symptomatology (Chatterjee *et al.* 1996; Stojsavljevic *et al.* 1997). The electroencephalogram (EEG) may show generalized slowing (Watson *et al.* 1954).

It is customary to obtain a serum B12 level; although this custom should be observed, it is also appropriate to obtain levels of both methylmalonic acid and homocysteine. In B12 deficiency, both methylmalonic acid and homocysteine levels are elevated, and this combination of findings is extremely sensitive and specific for B12 deficiency (Lindenbaum *et al.* 1988); when the serum B12 level is 'borderline', these two findings should be relied on when deciding whether intracellular B12 deficiency is present.

Before leaving this section, it is appropriate to note that clinical B12 deficiency can be precipitated by inhalation of nitrous oxide, as may occur during dental procedures or in drug abusers. In cases in which there is already a 'subclinical' B12 deficiency, nitrous oxide inhalation can acutely precipitate symptoms (Beltramello *et al.* 1998; Kinsella and Green 1995; Marie *et al.* 2000); in other cases, for example in young, well-nourished drug abusers, symptoms may not occur until nitrous oxide has been abused for a long time.

Course

Most cases of B12 deficiency are gradually progressive.

Etiology

Vitamin B12, or cobalamin, is formed only by certain plant-associated bacteria, and humans generally obtain their supply indirectly by eating liver, other organ meats, beef, pork, milk, or eggs. Once ingested, cobalamin is first bound within the stomach to gastric R binder; this complex is digested by pancreatic enzymes in the duodenum and the liberated cobalamin is then bound to intrinsic factor, a glycoprotein that is secreted by gastric parietal cells. This cobalamin–intrinsic factor complex then passes to the ileum, where it is bound to a receptor on the cell wall and taken into the cell. Inside the ileal epithelial cell, cobalamin is released from intrinsic factor and bound to a carrier protein known as transcobalamin II. The cobalamin–transcobalamin II complex is then released into the systemic circulation. A substantial amount of cobalamin is stored in the liver and, because of extensive enterohepatic recirculation, years must pass before hepatic stores are depleted.

As noted earlier, the most common cause of B12 deficiency is pernicious anemia (Healton *et al.* 1991). In this disease, anti-parietal cell antibodies lead to the destruction of gastric parietal cells, with a consequent lack of intrinsic factor and a deficient uptake of ingested B12 by the ileal cells. In addition to anti-parietal cell antibodies, the majority of patients also have anti-intrinsic factor antibodies, and it is customary to test for both of these. Other antibodies may also be present in patients with pernicious anemia, including antibodies against the thyroid and the adrenal gland, and patients may develop Hashimoto's thyroiditis with hypothyroidism, or adrenocortical insufficiency.

Other causes of B12 deficiency include strict vegetarianism, severe malnutrition (as may be seen in chronic alcoholics), total or partial gastrectomy, inherited abnormalities of the R binder or intrinsic factor, achlorhydria, pancreatic insufficiency, steatorrhea or malabsorption of any cause, tapeworms, bacterial overgrowth (as may occur after a Billroth II operation), ileal diseases (e.g., Crohn's disease), ileal resection, and chronic treatment with either omeprazole (Marcuard *et al.* 1994) or metformin (Andres *et al.* 2002). All of the preceding causes lead to intracellular B12 deficiency because of a failure of B12 absorption, and all are associated with decreased serum B12 levels. It is important to keep in mind, however, that in addition to these causes there are also some very rare diseases characterized by intracellular B12 deficiency or malutilization, and that in these disorders the serum B12 level will be normal, but the serum methylmalonic acid and homocysteine levels will be elevated. Examples include inherited abnormalities in transcobalamin II and abnormalities in the intracellular metabolism of cobalamin (Bodamar *et al.* 2001; Boxer *et al.* 2005; Powers *et al.* 2001). Finally, there may also be an association between acquired autoimmune deficiency syndrome (AIDS) and B12 deficiency (Herzlich and Schiano 1993; Shor-Posner *et al.* 1995).

When B12 deficiency has been confirmed by elevated methylmalonic acid and homocysteine levels, efforts should be made to determine the cause of this deficiency. In the past, the Schilling test was utilized to determine whether or not B12 absorption could be increased by the addition of hog-derived intrinsic factor: if this test was positive, then one inferred that the deficiency was due to destruction of parietal cells, as seen in pernicious anemia. With the availability of assays for anti-parietal cell and anti-intrinsic factor antibodies, however, this test is generally no longer required. Given that pernicious anemia is the most common cause of B12 deficiency, all patients should be tested for these antibodies. If these are absent, then the other causes noted above should be considered.

Neuropathologically, demyelinization is seen within the centrum semiovale (Ferraro *et al.* 1945; Lurie 1919), and in the posterior columns and the lateral corticospinal tracts within the spinal cord (Russell *et al.* 1900).

Differential diagnosis

Vitamin B12 deficiency may be almost perfectly mimicked by folic acid deficiency, and the differential rests on the results of testing for homocysteine and methylmalonic acid levels: in B12 deficiency both are elevated, whereas in folic acid deficiency the homocysteine level is elevated but the methylmalonic acid level is normal.

Progressive multiple sclerosis may also mimic B12 deficiency, and the differential again rests on testing for homocysteine and methylmalonic acid levels.

Treatment

Traditionally, treatment involves the administration of intramuscular cyanocobalamin at a dose of 1000 μg daily for 1 week, then weekly for 4 weeks, then monthly thereafter until maximum recovery has occurred. In those rare cases in which the underlying cause has been corrected, treatment may then cease; however, given that most of the underlying causes are not treatable, chronic treatment is typically required. After patients have been treated for 2 weeks, folic acid, at a dose of 2 mg daily, should be added; importantly, folic acid should not be administered earlier than this as it may lead to an exacerbation of symptoms. Potassium levels should be checked periodically, as hypokalemia may develop early in the course of treatment with cyanocobalamin.

Although, as noted, traditional treatment involves parenteral administration of B12, recent work has indicated that oral treatment with 1 or 2 mg daily may be just as effective (Kuzminski *et al.* 1998; Rajan *et al.* 2002). Most physicians, however, continue to use intramuscular B12, at least early on, switching to oral treatment only after patients have recovered.

With B12 treatment improvement may not occur for months, and up to 18 months may be required for full improvement. If treatment is begun early, before axonal loss has occurred, recovery may be complete; however, if symptoms have been present for months prior to treatment, irreversible damage may already have occurred and the recovery will only be partial.

13.2 FOLIC ACID DEFICIENCY

Although there has been controversy over whether folic acid deficiency can cause disease of the central nervous system, it appears that, albeit rarely, dementia and subacute combined degeneration of the cord do in fact occur on this basis.

Clinical features

The onset of symptoms appears to be gradual over weeks or months. Reynolds *et al.* (1973) demonstrated an association of folate deficiency with dementia, and Strachan and Henderson (1967) described two very convincing cases of dementia secondary to folate deficiency, one occurring in combination with a peripheral neuropathy and the other without any other symptoms. Furthermore, Pincus *et al.* (1972) reported a convincing case of a folate-induced combination of dementia and subacute combined degeneration. Folic acid deficiency, of course, is also a cause of megaloblastic anemia.

The serum homocysteine level is elevated.

Course

It appears that, in the absence of treatment, the course is progressive.

Etiology

Folic acid is a necessary factor in DNA synthesis and is found in fresh green vegetables, some fruits, yeast, kidney, and liver. Dietary deficiency, as may be seen in chronic alcoholics, is the most common cause of folic acid deficiency; intestinal malabsorption, for example in sprue, may also be a factor. Given the limited hepatic storage of folic acid, symptoms of deficiency may appear within a few months of poor oral intake or malabsorption. Certain medicines also reduce folate levels, including oral contraceptives, phenytoin, primidone, phenobarbital, carbamazepine, pyrimethamine, trimethoprim, pentamidine, sulfasalazine, and methotrexate. Marginal folic acid reserves may be rapidly depleted in conditions of increased metabolic demand, for example during pregnancy and lactation, and during the reticulocytosis seen with treatment of B12-induced anemia.

The underlying neuropathology is not known.

Differential diagnosis

As noted in the preceding chapter, it may not be possible clinically to differentiate folic acid deficiency from B12 deficiency, and the diagnosis here rests on homocysteine and methylmalonic acid levels: in folate deficiency only homocysteine levels are increased, whereas in B12 deficiency, both homocysteine and methylmalonic levels are elevated.

Treatment

Parenteral treatment is almost never required, even in cases of intestinal disease, and an oral dose of 1–2 mg daily is generally sufficient.

13.3 PELLAGRA

Niacin, also known as nicotinic acid or vitamin B3, is a water-soluble B vitamin found in liver, yeast, poultry, fish, and meat. Another source of this vitamin is tryptophan, which is converted endogenously into niacin.

Niacin deficiency causes pellagra, and this may occur clinically in one of two forms: acute pellagra, also known as 'encephalopathic' pellagra, is characterized by delirium, whereas gradually developing, chronic pellagra is characterized by dementia. In developed countries, pellagra is seen most commonly in malnourished alcoholics as the encephalopathic form; chronic pellagra, although once endemic in the American South, is now only rarely seen.

Clinical features

Encephalopathic pellagra presents fairly acutely, over days to a week, and, when fully developed, is characterized by delirium, dysarthria, cogwheel rigidity, gegenhalten, and myoclonus (Ishii and Nishihara 1981; Jolliffe *et al.* 1940; Serdaru *et al.* 1988).

Pellagra of gradual onset appears insidiously over many months, and, when fully developed, is characterized by the classic 'three Ds' of dementia, dermatitis, and diarrhea (Spivak and Jackson 1977). The dementia may present with apathy, depression, or anxiety; however, over time typical cognitive deficits, such as decreased memory and poor concentration, eventually appear. The dementia at times may also be marked by delusions or hallucinations (Pierce 1924). The dermatitis is characterized initially by erythematous lesions in sun-exposed areas. Eventually, the skin becomes hyperpigmented and roughened, and it is from the Italian for rough (*pelle*) skin (*agra*) that the disease gains its name. Diarrhea may be severe, and the fluid may be blood tinged. It must be stressed that most cases of pellagra do not, however, present with the full 'three Ds'; some patients with pellagrous dementia may have only one of the other 'Ds', and in some cases there may only be dementia, without any rash or diarrhea.

MRI scanning is unremarkable and the EEG shows generalized slowing.

Although the serum niacin level is low, a more reliable, if rarely ordered, test is a 24-hour urine test for niacin metabolites.

Course

The encephalopathic form may be rapidly progressive, and coma and death may occur in a matter of weeks. The chronic form pursues a slower course, with death in a matter of years.

Etiology

Niacin deficiency occurs most commonly as a result of dietary deficiency. As noted earlier, in current practice in developed countries this is seen primarily in malnourished alcoholics as the encephalopathic form. The chronic form of pellagra was endemic in the American South among those individuals who subsisted primarily on corn. As corn contains niacin in a bound, biologically less active form, and also lacks tryptophan, these individuals very gradually became niacin deficient. Since corn flour was 'enriched' with niacin, however, the chronic form of pellagra has almost disappeared in the United States. Other causes of niacin deficiency include bowel resection, Crohn's disease (Zaki and Millard 1995), and anorexia nervosa (Rapaport 1985).

In addition to dietary lack, pellagra has also been noted in conditions in which the normal endogenous conversion of tryptophan to niacin is, for one reason or another, impaired. Perhaps the most common example of this is in patients treated with isoniazid. The normal enzymatic conversion of tryptophan to niacin is dependent on the activated

form of pyridoxine (vitamin B6); isoniazid impairs the conversion of the inactive form of B6 to the active form and by this indirect mechanism reduces the endogenous production of niacin (Ishii and Nishihara 1985). Another example is in cases of carcinoid tumor, in which the gross overutilization of tryptophan by the tumor leaves less available for conversion to niacin.

Within the central nervous system (Hauw *et al.* 1988; Ishii and Nishihara 1981; Langworthy 1931), neurons are swollen and display chromatolysis with eccentric nuclei and a loss of Nissl substance. These chromatolytic changes may be seen in neurons of the cerebral cortex, basal ganglia, dentate nuclei, brainstem motor nuclei, and the anterior horn of the spinal cord.

Differential diagnosis

The acute encephalopathic form may be confused with other disorders seen in chronic alcoholics, such as delirium tremens or Wernicke's encephalopathy. Prominent tremor, of course, favors a diagnosis of delirium tremens. Nystagmus, a sixth cranial nerve palsy, or ataxia favors Wernicke's encephalopathy. Cogwheel rigidity favors encephalopathic pellagra. In practice, however, it may be difficult to differentiate between these disorders, and indeed they may appear concurrently (Serdaru *et al.* 1988).

The chronic form of pellagra is difficult to miss when all three of the 'Ds' are present; however, as noted earlier, many patients have only two of these, and some may have only one. Consequently, a high index of suspicion is required, and chronic pellagra should always be suspected in any chronically malnourished patient who gradually develops a dementia.

Treatment

Niacin may be given orally in doses from 250 to 500 mg daily. In the encephalopathic form, the response is rapid and often robust; in the chronic form recovery is slower and may be incomplete. Once full benefit has occurred, patients may be maintained on 50–100 mg of niacin daily. In cases due to isoniazid, administration of pyridoxine, in doses of 50 mg daily, is generally sufficient; however, in some cases symptoms may persist and in these cases isoniazid must be discontinued (Burke and Hiangabeza 1977).

13.4 WERNICKE'S ENCEPHALOPATHY

Wernicke's encephalopathy, also known as Wernicke's disease, occurs secondary to thiamine (vitamin B1) deficiency and, in its fully developed classic form, it presents with the triad of delirium, nystagmus, and ataxia. It occurs most frequently in malnourished alcoholics and is a common cause of delirium in general hospital practice.

Before proceeding further, a word on nomenclature is in order. In the literature, one often sees the term 'Wernicke–Korsakoff syndrome'; however, this practice should be avoided as Wernicke's encephalopathy and Korsakoff's syndrome are, from a clinical point of view, fundamentally different. Wernicke's encephalopathy, as just noted, is characterized by delirium. Korsakoff's syndrome, although occurring as a sequela to Wernicke's encephalopathy, is an amnestic disorder in which there is no confusion. Lumping the two together under one name serves only to confuse the diagnostic picture.

Clinical features

In general the onset is subacute, spanning several days, and nystagmus is often one of the earliest signs. Occasionally, however, one may see an acute onset over hours and this may follow a glucose load, either orally or intravenously, in a thiamine-deficient patient.

Delirium is characterized by confusion and disorientation, and is often accompanied by a degree of lethargy or drowsiness. With progression, stupor or coma may occur (Wallis et al. 1978).

Nystagmus, although generally horizontal, may at times be vertical. With progression, a bilateral and typically asymmetric sixth cranial nerve palsy may appear and patients may complain of diplopia. In extreme cases, a total ophthalmoplegia may occur.

Ataxia typically follows nystagmus and may be evident as an ataxia of gait or as a truncal ataxia, which, in turn, may be so severe that patients are unable to sit up in bed.

It must be emphasized that this classic triad of symptoms is the exception rather than the rule. Autopsy studies have revealed that the full triad is found in only 14–16 percent of cases (Cravioto et al. 1961; Harper et al. 1986). By far the most common presentation is with delirium alone, or with a combination of delirium and either nystagmus or ataxia (Harper et al. 1986).

In addition to delirium, nystagmus, and ataxia, a minority of patients will have grand mal seizures. The temperature is often decreased and there may be tachycardia and postural hypotension.

Various laboratory and imaging findings occur in Wernicke's encephalopathy but these are rarely required for the diagnosis, and, in any case, treatment of suspected Wernicke's encephalopathy should never wait upon test results.

The EEG may show generalized slowing, but in many cases it is within normal limits. Although the cerebrospinal fluid (CSF) is generally normal, an elevated total protein, rarely more than 100 mg/dL, may be found. Red blood cell transketolase activity may be decreased (Dreyfus 1962), and blood pyruvate and lactate levels may be increased.

MRI scanning may reveal increased signal intensity on T2-weighted, fluid-attenuated inversion recovery (FLAIR), and diffusion-weighted images in the mammillary bodies, medial aspects of the thalami, periaqueductal gray, and the midbrain tectum (Chu et al. 2002; Weidauer et al. 2003); with gadolinium, enhancement may be seen in some cases in the mammillary bodies (Zuccoli et al. 2007).

Course

Untreated, approximately 50 percent of patients die, in some cases suddenly (Harper 1979). Among those who survive, sequelae are common. With resolution of the delirium, confusion clears and patients may be left with a Korsakoff's syndrome (Malamud and Skillicorn 1956), which, as discussed in Section 13.5, is characterized by an amnesia with both anterograde and retrograde components. In those with a sixth nerve palsy, residual nystagmus is very common, and in those with ataxia, only a partial clearing is seen in a majority.

Etiology

Thiamine is found in many foods and 1–2 mg daily is generally sufficient to meet most daily needs. Total body stores of thiamine range from 20 to 100 mg, and the half-life of thiamine ranges from 10 to 20 days; thus, with severely reduced thiamine intake, significant deficiency may appear in 1–3 months.

Once absorbed, thiamine is converted to its active form, thiamine pyrophosphate; this molecule functions as an essential co-factor for transketolase, which plays a critical role in the hexose monophosphate shunt pathway. With significant thiamine deficiency, transketolase activity is lost, and the characteristic lesions, described below, develop.

Although most cases of Wernicke's encephalopathy are seen in malnourished alcoholics, cases have also been noted in a number of other conditions (Ogershok et al. 2002), including hunger strikes (Frantzen 1966), anorexia nervosa (Handler and Perkin 1982), prolonged parenteral nutrition (Vortmeyer et al. 1992) with inadequate thiamine supplementation, bariatric surgery (Abarbanel et al. 1987; Paulson et al. 1985; Singh and Kumar 2007) with subsequent prolonged vomiting, peritoneal dialysis or hemodialysis (Jagadha et al. 1987), hyperemesis gravidarum (Gardian et al. 1999), and prolonged vomiting occurring after liver transplantation (DiMartini 1996) or as a side-effect of digitalis (Richmond 1959). Importantly, two or more of these factors may at times be required to produce the encephalopathy. There are, for example, case reports of patients developing Wernicke's encephalopathy anywhere from 2 to 20 years post-gastrectomy, the precipitant being a modestly decreased thiamine intake, for example secondary to a loss of appetite during an upper respiratory infection (Shimomura et al. 1998).

Although, generally, at least a month must pass before a significant deficiency occurs, there are exceptions to this rule. Glucose loads, either orally or parenterally, may rapidly precipitate symptoms. Furthermore, some individuals have an inherited form of transketolase that displays a decreased affinity for thiamine pyrophosphate (Blass and Gibson 1977), and these individuals are at higher risk of developing Wernicke's encephalopathy and may do so even if their thiamine reserves are only marginally depleted.

In acute cases petechial hemorrhages are seen in gray matter adjacent to the third ventricle, aqueduct of Sylvius, and the fourth ventricle, including the dorsomedial and anterior nuclei of the thalamus, the mammillary bodies, the periaqueductal gray, the oculomotor and abducens nuclei, and the superior vermis (Cravioto *et al.* 1961; Harper 1983; Malamud and Skillicorn 1956; Victor *et al.* 1971). In those who survive, neuronal loss and gliosis are seen in the same areas.

Differential diagnosis

The diagnosis of Wernicke's encephalopathy should be entertained in any malnourished patient who develops delirium; although from a diagnostic point of view it is comforting to also see nystagmus and ataxia, it must be forcefully kept in mind that, as noted above, these are typically not present.

Among alcoholics, consideration must also be given to delirium tremens, encephalopathic pellagra, and hepatic encephalopathy. Prominent tremor suggests delirium tremens, cogwheel rigidity points to pellagra, and myoclonus suggests hepatic encephalopathy. These disorders, however, often appear simultaneously, and it is appropriate to treat all alcoholics with thiamine, as described below.

Rarely, a clinical picture identical to Wernicke's encephalopathy may occur secondary to a cytomegalovirus ventriculoencephalitis, for example in patients with AIDS (Torgovnik *et al.* 2000).

Treatment

Whenever Wernicke's encephalopathy is suspected, patients should emergently be given 100 mg thiamine intravenously or intramuscularly. Barring a severe degree of hypoglycemia, food and glucose-containing fluids should be withheld for at least several hours. Thiamine is then continued at a dose of 100 mg twice daily parenterally until substantial improvement is seen, after which patients may be continued on the same dose of oral thiamine for at least a month.

The response to treatment is at times spectacular. Nystagmus may begin to clear within hours, and delirium and ataxia improve over a matter of days; maximum improvement generally takes about a month.

On a political note, it is remarkable, given the devastation of Wernicke's encephalopathy and its major sequela Korsakoff's syndrome, that governments have not mandated the addition of thiamine to alcoholic beverages. The results could be as spectacular as those that occurred when flour was 'enriched' with niacin and the plague of endemic pellagra was eradicated.

13.5 KORSAKOFF'S SYNDROME

Korsakoff's syndrome is a chronic amnestic disorder with prominent anterograde and variable retrograde components that occurs as sequela to Wernicke's encephalopathy.

Some words are in order regarding nomenclature. As noted in Section 13.4, the term 'Wernicke–Korsakoff' syndrome is often seen; however, this should probably be abandoned as, from a clinical point of view, Wernicke's encephalopathy and Korsakoff's syndrome are fundamentally different: Wernicke's encephalopathy is marked by a delirium, whereas Korsakoff's syndrome is characterized by an amnesia that is not accompanied by confusion. There is an additional difficulty regarding nomenclature and this has to do with the definition of Korsakoff's syndrome. In some texts this term is used to refer to any chronic amnestic disorder, regardless of cause. In this text, however, the term refers only to the chronic amnestic disorder that occurs as a sequela to Wernicke's encephalopathy.

Clinical features

As noted in Section 13.4, Wernicke's encephalopathy is characterized by delirium with or without nystagmus and ataxia. In those who survive, the delirium gradually resolves and patients may then be left with an amnestic disorder.

These patients, as pointed out by Korsakoff himself (Victor and Yakovlev 1955), may not, at least to casual inspection, appear ill at all. They are typically able to carry on a conversation and may be reasonably sociable. However, formal testing reveals that, although immediate recall, as with a digit span, is intact, short-term memory, tested by asking the patient to recall three objects after 5 minutes, is severely deficient. Indeed, patients may not be able to recall a conversation they had with the physician just minutes before. A degree of disorientation to time and place inevitably accompanies this anterograde amnesia. The retrograde component of the amnesia becomes apparent on asking patients about their lives before the Wernicke's encephalopathy: answers often display a 'temporal gradient' (Albert *et al.* 1979; Seltzer and Benson 1974), such that patients, although having no recall of the events occurring for perhaps months before the Wernicke's encephalopathy, may have a hazy or partial recall of events occurring years earlier and a fairly clear memory of childhood events. In questioning patients about recent events, one often encounters the phenomenon of confabulation: here, the patient blithely makes up responses, as if to 'fill in' the amnestic gap. Thus, if a patient were asked whether he or she had ever met the physician before, the patient might respond in the affirmative and go on to talk about meeting the physician at a local tavern the week before, where they had a 'few' beers, played some pool, etc.

Course

Over the first year, approximately one-quarter of patients will show improvement, which in some cases may be substantial; in the remainder a stable chronicity is seen.

Etiology

As stressed above, Korsakoff's syndrome occurs as a sequela to Wernicke's encephalopathy (Malamud and Skillicorn 1956).

Neuropathologically, one sees atrophy and fibrosis in the mediodorsal and anterior nuclei of the thalamus (Halliday et al. 1994; Malamud and Skillicorn 1956; Victor et al. 1971).

Differential diagnosis

As discussed in detail in Section 5.4, Korsakoff's syndrome is one of the chronic anterograde amnesias that also have a retrograde component and as such must be distinguished from other disorders capable of producing such an amnesia. When the history of an immediately preceding Wernicke's encephalopathy is present, the diagnosis is fairly clear; however, in cases in which the patient's prior history is unknown, consideration must be given to other disorders, such as infarctions or tumors.

Treatment

Some form of supervision is generally required and, in severe cases, institutionalization may be necessary. Pharmacologic treatment seems of no avail: double-blind studies fail to support a role for donepezil (Sahin et al. 2002), fluvoxamine (O'Carroll et al. 1994), or clonidine (O'Carroll et al. 1993).

13.6 MANGANISM

Chronic exposure to manganese may be followed by the development of a personality change, an atypical parkinsonism, and, less commonly, a dementia or psychosis. Although most cases occur as a result of inhalation among manganese miners and those who work in steel or battery factories, cases have also been reported secondary to drinking contaminated well water or, very rarely, to prolonged intravenous total parenteral nutrition with manganese-containing solutions (Nagatomo et al. 1999).

Clinical features

The onset of symptoms is typically gradual, occurring after months or years of exposure, and patients may present with a personality change, parkinsonism, or both (Abd El Naby and Hassanein 1965).

The personality change (Abd El Naby and Hassanein 1965; Cook et al. 1974) typically consists of asthenia, fatigue, irritability, emotional lability, and a peculiar kind of 'incongruous' laughter, reminiscent of the emotional incontinence seen in pseudobulbar palsy: patients may smile without cause, or burst out in laughter, again for no apparent reason (Charles 1927). Insomnia or hypersomnia may accompany these changes (Abd El Naby and Hassanein 1965; Cook et al. 1974).

The parkinsonism (Abd El Naby and Hassanein 1965; Calne et al. 1994; Cook et al. 1974; Huang et al. 1989) is characterized by rigidity, bradykinesia, postural instability, and a tendency to 'freeze' and fall upon turning. Cogwheeling is often seen and, although tremor may also be present, it is generally not of the 'pill-rolling' type. The parkinsonism may also be accompanied by dystonia, often affecting the cervical musculature or the face. The most characteristic feature of manganese-induced parkinsonism is, however, a distinctive dystonic gait abnormality known as a 'cock-walk'. Here, patients walk on their metatarsophalangeal joints as if they were wearing high heels; at times, the elbows may be flexed, creating the overall appearance of the walk of a rooster. Such a 'cock-walk' has been reported in anywhere from a small minority (Cook et al. 1974; Huang et al. 1993) to up to one-third (Abd El Naby and Hassanein 1965) of patients.

Dementia may occur concurrent with the parkinsonism, and may be characterized by a marked degree of memory loss (Cook et al. 1974).

Psychosis, known as 'manganese madness', may occur, and is characterized by excitation, hallucinations, and delusions (Abd El Naby and Hassanein 1965).

T1-weighted MRI scanning may reveal increased signal intensity within the globus pallidus bilaterally. Manganese levels are increased in the serum, hair or a 24-hour urine sample.

Course

As one might expect, with ongoing exposure, symptoms gradually worsen. With cessation of exposure, however, rather than a gradual reduction of parkinsonian signs and symptoms, these actually continue to gradually worsen over the next 10 years or so (Huang et al. 1993, 1998), after which they persist in a stable chronicity (Huang et al. 2007). A similar progression has been noted for the 'cock-walk' (Huang et al. 1997).

Etiology

Neuronal loss and gliosis, although most prominent in the globus pallidus, are also found in the putamen, the pars reticulata of the substantia nigra, the thalamus, hypothalamus, and the cerebral cortex (Yamada et al. 1986).

Differential diagnosis

Lacking a history of manganese exposure, the differential generally involves a consideration of other causes of parkinsonism, as discussed in Section 3.8. In this regard, special attention should be given to those disorders that can cause a combination of parkinsonism and dystonia, such as late-onset pantothenate kinase-associated neurodegeneration, Wilson's disease, corticobasal ganglionic degeneration, and progressive supranuclear palsy.

Treatment

The general treatment of personality change, dementia, and psychosis are outlined in Sections 7.2, 5.1, and 7.1 respectively. If antipsychotics are required, consideration should be given to second-generation agents, such as quetiapine, in an effort to avoid exacerbating parkinsonism. Regarding the parkinsonism, although case reports suggest a usefulness for levodopa (Huang *et al.* 1993) (sometimes in high doses of up to 3 g or more daily [Mena *et al.* 1970]), placebo-controlled studies cast doubt on this (Koller *et al.* 2004; Lu *et al.* 1994). In practice, however, it is reasonable to give it a trial.

Manganese is stored in bone and has a long half-life, extending to 1 month or more. Although the role of chelating agents during the first few months is not established, case reports suggest their utility (Discalzi *et al.* 2000).

13.7 THALLIUM INTOXICATON

Although thallium can be absorbed through either the lungs or the skin, industrial exposure is rare, and most cases of thallium intoxication are by ingestion. Since thallium was banned as a rodenticide, current cases generally represent a deliberate, often homicidal, poisoning.

Clinical features

The onset of symptoms may be either acute or gradual, depending on the amount ingested.

Acute intoxication (Bank *et al.* 1972; Moore *et al.* 1993; Reed *et al.* 1963; Thompson *et al.* 1988; Wainwright *et al.* 1988) generally presents with abdominal pain, vomiting, and diarrhea. Within days or a week or so, patients develop a delirium and a painful peripheral sensorimotor polyneuropathy, which may progress to a quadriplegia. Cranial neuropathies, with facial palsy or ophthalmoplegia, may also develop, and, rarely, grand mal seizures may occur. Within 1–3 weeks patients then develop the most characteristic feature of thallium intoxication, namely a severe, generalized alopecia.

Gradual intoxication presents with dementia, a sensorimotor polyneuropathy, and alopecia; gastrointestinal symptomatology may or may not be present.

Thallium may be found in the urine and serum, and, in long-standing cases, the hair.

Course

Acute intoxications may be fatal in up to one-tenth of cases. In those who survive, there is a gradual, more or less complete recovery; in some cases there may be persistent cognitive deficits (which may be severe enough to produce a dementia [Reed *et al.* 1963; Thompson *et al.* 1988]) or a personality change (McMillan *et al.* 1997). Gradual intoxications likewise show a variable degree of recovery.

Etiology

In acute cases there is cerebral edema, often with petechial hemorrhages; in more gradual onset cases, and in those who have recovered, there is a variable degree of neuronal loss in the cortex, basal ganglia, and thalamus (Cavanagh *et al.* 1974). In the peripheral nerves axonal degeneration and demyelinization are seen (Davis *et al.* 1981).

Differential diagnosis

Acute cases may be confused with arsenic intoxication or, when symptoms are confined primarily to a polyneuropathy, with the Guillain–Barré syndrome. The eventual appearance of severe alopecia, however, indicates the correct diagnosis.

Treatment

Thallium undergoes enterohepatic recirculation and, consequently, laxatives and activated charcoal should be given. Prussian blue binds to thallium in the gut, and this is part of standard treatment. Both forced diuresis and hemodialysis hasten excretion. Chelation therapy is contraindicated as it may be followed by a deterioration in the patient's condition (Wainwright *et al.* 1988).

13.8 ARSENIC INTOXICATION

Although elemental arsenic causes relatively little central nervous system toxicity, arsenic salts are toxic; with acute intoxication one may see a delirium, whereas with chronic, low-level exposure a dementia may occur. Arsenic salts are found in certain herbicides and rodenticides, and ingestion may occur accidentally or with suicidal or homicidal intent.

Clinical features

Acute ingestion is followed rapidly by delirium (Freeman and Couch 1978), nausea, vomiting, and diarrhea, which may be bloody; convulsions may also occur. Classically there is also an odor of garlic on the breath. Arrhythmias, renal failure, and hypotension may occur. Within 1–3 weeks a painful peripheral sensorimotor polyneuropathy appears.

Chronic exposure to small amounts of arsenic salts may cause both a dementia and a polyneuropathy. Hyperkeratosis of the palms and soles may occur, and Mees' lines may appear, which are transverse white discolorations of the nails. Occasionally there may be a mild degree of alopecia.

Arsenic may be found in a 24-hour urine sample, and, within weeks of exposure, is also found in the hair and nails.

Course

Acute arsenic intoxication is often fatal. In those who survive either acute or chronic intoxication, there may be either cognitive deficits or a peripheral neuropathy, both of which may show a greater or lesser degree of resolution over long-term follow-up (Fincher et al. 1987).

Etiology

In acute cases, widespread petechial hemorrhages within the white matter are seen (Hurst 1959; Russell 1937). Within the peripheral nervous system, axonal degeneration occurs.

Differential diagnosis

Thallium intoxication is suggested by the prominent alopecia.

Treatment

Acute intoxication is treated with gastric lavage, osmotic diuresis, and intensive supportive care. Chelation therapy is appropriate for both acute and chronic cases.

13.9 BISMUTH INTOXICATION

Bismuth is found in a number of preparations and is used for the control of diarrhea and in the treatment of *Helicobacter pylori* infection. Although generally quite safe, high dosage may be followed by a delirium.

Clinical features

The onset may be gradual or acute, depending on the dosage. Gradual onsets (Supino-Viterbo et al. 1977) are marked by insomnia and mood changes, with depression, irritability, or, uncommonly, euphoria; rarely, delusions or hallucinations may occur. With high dosage, there may be an acute onset of delirium, accompanied by myoclonus, ataxia, and, in a minority, seizures (Buge et al. 1981; Burns et al. 1974; Supino-Viterbo et al. 1977).

Computed tomography (CT) scanning may reveal patchy areas of radiolucency in the cortex (Gardeur et al. 1978).

Course

Recovery is gradual, occurring over many months.

Etiology

In one autopsied case neuronal loss was noted among the Purkinje cells of the cerebellum and in the hippocampus (Liessens et al. 1978).

Differential diagnosis

When the history of bismuth ingestion is lacking, the differential includes other deliria associated with myoclonus, as discussed in Section 3.2.

Treatment

Supportive care is provided; there is no specific treatment.

13.10 TIN INTOXICATION

Exposure to tin compounds may occur in certain industries or by ingestion, and may be followed by delirium.

Clinical features

Delirium and seizures have been reported after intoxication with trimethyltin (Feldman et al. 1993; Fortemps et al. 1978) and triethyltin (Alajouanine et al. 1958); with phenyltin ingestion, delirium and ataxia occur (Wu et al. 1990).

Course

Although most patients survive trimethyltin intoxication (Besser et al. 1987; Feldman et al. 1993), the mortality rate after triethyltin intoxication is approximately 50 percent (Alajouanine et al. 1958). Among patients who do survive tin intoxication, residual symptoms are common and may be severe.

Etiology

With trimethyltin, neuronal loss has been observed in the temporal cortex, amygdala, basal ganglia, and cerebellum

(Besser *et al.* 1987; Kreyberg *et al.* 1992). In contrast, with triethyltin intoxication, the myelin becomes edematous and vacuolization may be seen in the white matter (Cossa *et al.* 1958).

Differential diagnosis

When the history of exposure is lacking the differential becomes quite wide, as discussed in Section 5.3.

Treatment

There is no known specific treatment.

13.11 LEAD ENCEPHALOPATHY

Toxic accumulations of lead may occur in a number of ways. Children may eat lead-based paint chips. Among adults, exposure may occur in certain occupations, for example in welders or those who work in battery factories or lead smelters; 'moonshine' whiskey, made with the help of old car radiators, may also be a source (Akelaitis 1941; Morris *et al.* 1964; Whitfield *et al.* 1972). Other less common sources include lead-glazed pottery (Matte *et al.* 1994), certain 'alternative' medications (Fisher and Le Couteur 2000), and retained bullets. Leaded gasoline used to be a major source, but since lead additives were banned this has essentially ceased to be a problem.

A sudden massive exposure in either children or adults may cause an acute lead encephalopathy with, among other symptoms, a delirium. Enduring, low-level exposure may produce a chronic lead encephalopathy: in children one may see cognitive decline and symptoms similar to those of attention deficit/hyperactivity disorder, whereas in adults there may be a dementia, a motor polyneuropathy, and colicky abdominal pain.

Clinical features

In children, acute lead encephalopathy may be preceded by a prodrome of irritability, abdominal pain, and lethargy that lasts for weeks. In both children (Jenkins and Mellins 1957; Mellins and Jenkins 1955) and adults (Akelaitis 1941; Morris *et al.* 1964; Whitfield *et al.* 1972), the full syndrome is marked by delirium, which may be accompanied by excitation, hallucinations and delusions, ataxia, and seizures; classically, patients complain of a metallic taste. Hemolysis and renal failure may occur.

Chronic lead encephalopathy in children (Baghurst *et al.* 1992; Bellinger *et al.* 1987; Canfield *et al.* 2003; Needleman *et al.* 1990) may present with a very gradual cognitive decline, which may range in severity from a drop of a few IQ points to a dementia. There is also an association between lead exposure in children and the development of a syndrome virtually identical to attention deficit/hyperactivity disorder. Occasionally seizures may occur.

Chronic lead encephalopathy in adults may present with either a personality change or a dementia of variable severity; patients also may complain of colicky abdominal pain and a metallic taste. In some cases, depressive symptoms may be seen (Schottenfeld and Cullen 1984). A motor peripheral neuropathy may occur, with, classically, wrist and foot drop.

Whole blood lead levels of over 80 μg/dL are associated with an acute presentation, whereas levels of 10–20 μg/dL, if chronically maintained, produce a chronic encephalopathy. The zinc protoporphyrin level is also increased. In both children and adults 'lead lines' may be seen at the border of the gingiva and teeth, and in childhood cases lead lines may also be seen in radiographs of the tibia or other long bones.

Course

Acute lead encephalopathy runs a rapid course, with mortality rates approaching 25 percent. Those who survive may be left with dementia (Jenkins and Mellins 1957), seizures, or spasticity. Chronic lead encephalopathy shows little improvement over time.

Etiology

In acute encephalopathy there is widespread cerebral edema associated with petechial hemorrhages and microinfarctions (Pentschew 1965; Smith *et al.* 1960). In chronic cases there is cortical atrophy and widespread neuronal loss.

Differential diagnosis

Colicky abdominal pain and complaints of a metallic taste in patients with delirium or dementia should always suggest lead encephalopathy. When these symptoms are absent, or go unrecognized, the differential widens, as discussed in Sections 5.1 and 5.3.

Treatment

Acute lead encephalopathy is a medical emergency. Steroids and mannitol may be required for cerebral edema, and patients should undergo chelation treatment with dimercaptosuccinic acid, calcium sodium diacetate, dimercaprol, or penicillamine. The half-life for lead in blood ranges from 25 to 35 days, whereas in the brain it is 2 years and in bone it is decades. Chelation therapy is of unproven benefit in chronic lead encephalopathy. Public health measures to remove lead paint are imperative.

13.12 MERCURY INTOXICATION

Three forms of mercury are potentially toxic to humans, namely elemental mercury, salts of mercury, and organic mercury.

Elemental mercury at room temperature is a liquid. Ingestion is generally non-toxic as it is poorly absorbed through the gastrointestinal tract. Elemental mercury, however, readily volatizes with warming or merely with shaking, and may be inhaled. Once inhaled, it readily passes across the alveoli and into the blood, where it is taken up into erythrocytes and oxidized to a mercuric salt. This mercuric salt, and any unoxidized elemental mercury, then cross the blood–brain barrier and are taken up by neurons. Exposure to elemental mercury generally occurs in gold miners and in certain other industries.

Salts of mercury may be either monovalent (mercurous) or divalent (mercuric). Salts of mercury may be absorbed through the gastrointestinal tract or transdermally and, as just noted, once absorbed they may cross the blood–brain barrier. Mercury salts were once used medicinally, as in the case of calomel, also called mercurous chloride (Davis *et al.* 1974). Currently, however, most exposure occurs in those employed in the manufacture of plastics, fungicides, and electronics. In the nineteenth century, mercuric nitrate was used in the manufacture of felt, and chronic exposure among hat makers led to the 'mad hatter syndrome', made famous in Lewis Carroll's *Alice's Adventures in Wonderland*.

Organic mercury is found as methylmercury, ethylmercury (Hay *et al.* 1963), and phenylmercury (O'Carroll *et al.* 1995), and, of these, methylmercury is the most toxic. Organic mercury, especially methylmercury, is readily taken up through the gastrointestinal tract and easily crosses the blood–brain barrier. Exposure occurs generally by accidental ingestion. Perhaps the most notorious example of this is the Minamata epidemic, named after the town in Japan where it occurred (Kurland *et al.* 1960). Industrial waste containing elemental mercury was discharged into Minamata bay where it was converted by bacteria into methylmercury; fish became contaminated and, when residents ate the fish, the stage was set for disaster. Other incidents have involved methylmercury used as a fungicide on seed grain. In one example, treated seed grain was sent to Iraq (Amin-Zaki *et al.* 1978; Rustam and Hamri 1974). Although civilians had been warned not to eat the grain but only to plant it, the contaminated grain was nevertheless made into flour and bread, leading to hundreds of deaths. In another example, hogs were fed with treated seed grain, and those that then ate the hogs became ill (Snyder 1972).

Clinical features

With acute exposure to elemental mercury via inhalation, a pneumonitis may occur. Acute exposure to either mercury salts or to organic mercury may cause vomiting, which may be quite severe in the case of mercury salts and which may also be accompanied by renal failure.

Among patients who survive the acute exposure, and in cases of chronic, low-level exposure, various sequelae may gradually ensue, including a personality change, a dementia, and various abnormal movements. The personality change, known as erethism, is classically characterized by emotional lability, shyness, and anxiety, all of which may be accompanied by insomnia. The dementia, occurring generally only with greater exposure, does not appear to have any specific distinguishing features. Of the abnormal movements seen with mercury intoxication, tremor is perhaps the most classic, and this may affect the hands, lips, and tongue. Ataxia is common and may be accompanied by an intention tremor and dysarthria. Choreoathetosis may occur, as may parkinsonian features. A sensorimotor polyneuropathy may also appear, which may be quite painful. Visual scotoma or tunnel vision may also occur.

Whole blood levels of mercury are elevated, but the correlation between blood levels and clinical symptomatology is rough at best. In chronic cases, neuroimaging may reveal atrophy of the cerebral cortex (most prominently the calcarine cortex) and the cerebellar cortex (Tokuomi *et al.* 1982).

Course

For the most part the sequelae described are chronic.

Etiology

Pathologically, there is widespread neuronal loss throughout the cerebral and cerebellar cortex, especially involving the calcarine cortex and, in the cerebellum, the granule cell layer (Davis *et al.* 1974; Hunter and Russell 1954).

Differential diagnosis

The diagnosis rests heavily on a history of exposure.

Treatment

Acute exposure to salts of mercury or to organic mercury may be treated with gastric lavage and activated charcoal. Chelation treatment is also indicated.

13.13 DIALYSIS DEMENTIA

Dialysis dementia, also known as progressive dialysis encephalopathy, might better be termed 'aluminum dementia' or 'aluminum intoxication' given that it is the accumulation of aluminum in the central nervous system that causes the dementia. This used to be a not uncommon cause of dementia and death in patients undergoing chronic hemodialysis, and in such cases the aluminum intoxication occurred secondary to aluminum in the dialysate (Davison *et al.* 1982) and perhaps also to the use of aluminum-containing phosphate binders. With the routine purification of the dialysate, this disorder has almost disappeared; occasional cases, however, still occur, for example with the use of aluminum-containing medications in patients with chronic renal failure who are not on hemodialysis (Andreoli *et al.* 1984; Shirabe *et al.* 2002).

Clinical features

The onset of the dementia is gradual, occurring on average after 37–40 months of dialysis (Garrett *et al.* 1988; Lederman and Henry 1978). Typically (Burks *et al.* 1976; Chokroverty *et al.* 1976; Garrett *et al.* 1988; Lederman and Henry 1978; O'Hare *et al.* 1983), patients present with a peculiar, stuttering type of aphasia, followed by myoclonus, seizures, and dementia. In a minority (Garrett *et al.* 1988), psychotic symptoms may occur, with delusions, hallucinations, and bizarre behavior (Chokroverty *et al.* 1976; Scheiber and Ziesat 1976); in one case mania occurred (Jack *et al.* 1983).

The EEG reveals periodic spikes or spike-and-wave complexes on a background of slowing; there may also be bursts of frontally dominant slow activity (Hughes and Schreeder 1980).

Course

Untreated, the disease is progressive, with death on average within 6 months.

Etiology

The brain aluminum content is elevated (Alfrey *et al.* 1976) and there is widespread neuronal loss in the cerebral cortex, with, in some cases, laminar spongiform change (Shirabe *et al.* 2002; Winkelman and Ricanti 1986).

Differential diagnosis

Other disorders that are not uncommon in dialysis patients and which are capable of causing dementia include intracerebral hemorrhage, infarctions, and subdural hematoma. Patients on dialysis may also develop thiamine deficiency, with a resulting Wernicke's encephalopathy (Hung *et al.* 2001).

Treatment

Dialysate purity must be maintained and patients should not be given any aluminum-containing medications.

Diazepam may reduce the severity of many of the symptoms of dialysis dementia (Nadel and Wilson 1976) but does not alter the course of the disease. Chelation with deferoxamine may be considered; however, in some patients this may lead to a mobilization of aluminum from bone with a consequent worsening of the cerebral symptomatology (Sherrard *et al.* 1988).

13.14 DIALYSIS DISEQUILIBRIUM SYNDROME

The dialysis disequilibrium syndrome (Mawdsley 1972; Peterson and Swanson 1964; Raskin and Fishman 1976; Tyler 1965) is a transient disorder seen in approximately 5 percent of patients undergoing hemodialysis, especially early on or during rapid dialyses.

Clinical features

The syndrome usually appears several hours after the start of a dialysis run, but may sometimes be delayed for up to a day. The most common symptom is headache, which is generalized and may be severe. Other symptoms, seen in a minority of cases, include nausea, muscle cramping, delirium, and grand mal seizures; rarely one may find papilledema or exophthalmos. The EEG shows generalized slowing.

Course

Typically the syndrome resolves spontaneously within a matter of hours or, at the very most, a few days.

Etiology

Normally in hemodialysis an osmotic gradient occurs between the blood and CSF (Yoshida *et al.* 1987) and cerebral edema occurs (Walters *et al.* 2001). In all likelihood the syndrome occurs secondary to a pronounced degree of these changes.

Differential diagnosis

Consideration should be given to subdural hematoma or intracerebral hemorrhage.

Treatment

Symptomatic treatment of delirium is discussed in Section 5.3; if necessary seizures may be treated with lorazepam, as described in Section 7.3. Future episodes may be prevented by slowing the dialysis run.

13.15 HYPOGLYCEMIA

Hypoglycemia may cause autonomic symptoms, such as tremor, and may also cause 'neuroglycopenic' symptoms, such as delirium or seizures; when severe enough, coma may ensue and patients may be left with dementia.

Clinical features

As the blood glucose level falls below 2.5 mmol/L (45 mg/dL), autonomic symptoms appear fairly promptly. These include anxiety, palpitations, tremulousness, and diaphoresis; patients may also complain of hunger and nausea, headache, and generalized weakness.

Neuroglycopenic symptoms (Hart and Frier 1998; Malouf and Brust 1985) are associated with blood glucose levels of 1.67 mmol/L (30 mg/dL) or lower, but, unlike the autonomic symptoms, these tend to appear only after this degree of hypoglycemia has been sustained for approximately 30 minutes. Initially, patients may experience light-headedness or depersonalization. A delirium is common and this may be associated with unusual behavior: in one case (Bosboom et al. 1996), the patient 'was restless, opening and closing his eyes, and thrashing about with his arms and legs, occasionally hitting onlookers and spitting in their faces'; in another case (Zivin 1970), the patient, a soldier, 'walked into the mess hall . . . [dressed] in his underwear'. Seizures may occur, and these may be either partial seizures or grand mal in type. A very small minority of patients will also have focal findings, such as hemiplegia (Malouf and Brust 1985) or aphasia (Shintani et al. 1993; Wallis et al. 1985). With sustained hypoglycemia, coma may ensue (Ben-Ami et al. 1999).

Of note, although in most cases neuroglycopenic symptoms are preceded by autonomic symptoms, exceptions to this rule occur, and some patients may present with neuroglycopenic symptoms alone (Case Records 1988; Malouf and Brust 1985; Moersch and Kernohan 1938). This may occur in diabetics who have developed a diabetic autonomic neuropathy or in patients under treatment with beta-blockers, which mask autonomic symptoms. Such a scenario may also occur in cases in which the blood glucose level drops very slowly, for example as may occur with fasting.

In cases of coma, diffusion-weighted MRI scanning may reveal areas of increased signal intensity in the cerebral cortex, white matter, and basal ganglia (Jung et al. 2005). EEGs obtained during neuroglycopenic delirium will display generalized slowing.

Course

Whereas autonomic symptoms respond promptly to treatment with glucose, delirium may take up to an hour to subside. Patients who have developed coma may not recover consciousness and those that do may be left with a dementia. In cases characterized by a residual dementia, a greater or lesser degree of recovery may occur over the following year or two.

Etiology

Symptomatic hypoglycemia may occur in the fasting state, for example early in the morning before breakfast or in those who skip meals, or post-prandially, several hours after a meal. Fasting hypoglycemia is seen most commonly in diabetics on insulin or oral antidiabetic agents; it may also occur in patients with insulinomas (Dizon et al. 1999) or in those who undertake a prolonged fast, for example during hunger strikes or in patients with anorexia nervosa (Rich et al. 1990). Liver disease, by impairing gluconeogenesis, may also set the stage for fasting hypoglycemia. Gluconeogenesis is also inhibited by alcohol and, after a bout of binge drinking when little food is consumed, hypoglycemia is common. Post-prandial hypoglycemia may be seen in early type II diabetes; after vagotomy, gastrectomy, pyloroplasty, or gastrojejunostomy; and in a rare (Palardy et al. 1989) and somewhat controversial condition known as 'functional' or 'essential' post-prandial hypoglycemia.

Hypoglycemia may also be intentionally produced by malingerers who inject themselves with insulin or take high doses of oral antidiabetic agents (Price et al. 1986). Whenever this is suspected, as well as checking the glucose level one should also determine the insulin and C-peptide levels and obtain a toxicology screen for oral agents. C-peptide is normally excreted in conjunction with insulin and, under physiologic conditions, when the insulin is elevated so too is the C-peptide level. In cases of exogenous insulin administration, however, whereas the insulin level is elevated, the C-peptide level will be normal or low (Scarlett et al. 1977). In cases in which the elevated insulin level is produced by an oral agent, both the insulin and C-peptide level will be increased, but the toxicology will be positive.

Autonomic symptoms reflect an immediate physiologic sympathetic response to hypoglycemia. Neuroglycopenic symptoms, by contrast, reflect a complex series of events triggered by intraneuronal hypoglycemia. The half-hour or so delay in the onset of neuroglycopenic symptoms reflects the time required for the depletion of intraneuronal glucose stored as glycogen. In cases in which coma occurs, neuronal death occurs, and, if sufficient, this constitutes the cause of any persistent coma or residual dementia. In such cases pathologic studies have revealed (Auer et al. 1989; Kalimo and Olsson 1980; Lawrence et al. 1942; MacKeith and Meyer 1939) neuronal loss and gliosis in the cerebral cortex, the hippocampus (especially the dentate gyrus), and the basal ganglia; in severe cases laminar cortical necrosis was found.

Differential diagnosis

In cases in which the symptomatology is restricted to autonomic symptoms, the diagnosis is immediately suggested by associated hunger and the prompt relief gained by eating or drinking glucose-rich fluids. Consideration may also be given to the possibility of an anxiety attack, hyperventilation, or a simple partial seizure, as discussed in Section 6.5.

In cases characterized by autonomic symptoms followed by delirium, consideration may be given to other deliria associated with tremor, such as delirium tremens, thyroid storm, amphetamine intoxication, and either the serotonin syndrome or the neuroleptic malignant syndrome. In some cases, however, as noted above, autonomic symptoms may be lacking, and here the differential becomes quite wide, as discussed in Section 5.3; special attention should be given to complex partial seizures.

In doubtful cases, consideration may be given to demonstrating 'Whipple's triad' by performing a glucose tolerance test. Whipple's triad consists of:

1. the presence of typical symptoms;
2. the concurrent presence of significant hypoglycemia;
3. the relief of symptoms with glucose administration.

The duration of the glucose tolerance test may range from 5 hours in cases with a post-prandial pattern to up to 12 hours in those with a fasting pattern.

Treatment

If the patient is able to take fluids, a glass of orange juice or soda mixed with two or three tablespoonfuls of sugar is often adequate. Patients unable to take fluids should be given 50 mL of a 50 percent solution of glucose intravenously. In cases in which intravenous access is lacking, one may stimulate gluconeogenesis by giving glucagon in a dose of 1 mg intramuscularly, keeping in mind, of course, that glucagon is ineffective in patients with significant liver damage. Regardless of which therapy is given, patients should be closely monitored to see if repeat doses are required. An exception to this approach occurs in alcoholics, in whom a glucose load may precipitate a Wernicke's encephalopathy. In such a situation one should given 100 mg of thiamine intravenously and refrain from administering glucose for several hours or as long as clinically possible; clearly, much clinical judgment is required in this situation.

13.16 HYPERVISCOSITY SYNDROME

Significantly increased viscosity will cause microcirculatory sludging within the central nervous system leading to, among other symptoms, a dementia. This is a very rare syndrome and is generally seen in patients with a paraproteinemia such as Waldenstrom's macroglobulinemia (Mehta and Singhal 2003).

Clinical features

Patients may present with a dementia (Mueller *et al.* 1983) and lethargy. Other symptoms include headache, blurry vision, dizziness, ataxia, and dysarthria. Stroke may occur (Pavy *et al.* 1980), and seizures have been reported.

Serum viscosity is measured in centipoises, and in most symptomatic cases the viscosity is elevated above 4 centipoises.

Course

As might be expected, the course parallels changes in serum viscosity. With progression, coma and death may occur.

Etiology

The presence of excess or variously deformed proteins, usually immunoglobulins, increases serum viscosity with, as noted, literal sludging of blood flow within capillaries. In some cases, it appears that this sludging is also accompanied by microthrombus formation.

As noted, the most common cause of hyperviscosity is Waldenstrom's macroglobulinemia; cases may also be seen in multiple myeloma (Camacho *et al.* 1985), cryoglobulinemia, and, rarely, in rheumatoid arthritis (Bach *et al.* 1989).

Differential diagnosis

Given the non-specific nature of the syndrome, the index of suspicion must be high.

Treatment

Daily plasmapheresis should be performed until symptoms clear.

13.17 CENTRAL PONTINE MYELINOLYSIS

Central pontine myelinolysis, originally described by Adams and Foley in 1953, is classically characterized clinically by the development of a combination of flaccid quadriplegia and delirium, and pathologically by demyelinization in the central portion of the pons, all occurring within 2–3 days of overly rapid correction of chronic hyponatremia. Exceptions to this classic picture, as described further below, do occur, with prominent demyelinization in extrapontine sites associated with movement disorders or delirium in the absence of quadriplegia. The existence of these exceptions has led some authors to propose alternative names for this syndrome, such as 'central pontine and extrapontine myelinolysis' or, more generally, 'osmotic demyelination syndrome'.

Clinical features

In classic cases, a flaccid symmetric quadriparesis develops within 2–3 days of rapid correction of chronic hyponatremia, accompanied by a delirium or lethargy (Karp and Laureno 1993), which in turn may be marked by both visual and auditory hallucinations (Sterns *et al.* 1986). Symptoms gradually worsen over about a week and, in severe cases, patients may be left in a 'locked in' state and totally paralyzed except for vertical eye movements. Over time the flaccidity resolves, to be replaced by spasticity with hyperreflexia. Within the first day, diffusion-weighted MRI scanning may reveal increased signal intensity within the central portion of the pons, and over the following days the same area will reveal increased signal intensity on FLAIR and T2-weighted imaging and decreased signal intensity on T1-weighted imaging (Ruzek *et al.* 2004). Importantly, CT scanning is very insensitive here and may be normal despite florid symptomatology.

Exceptions to this classic picture occur when demyelinization occurs in extrapontine locations. Thus, one may see delirium alone (without quadriplegia) (Hadfield and Kubal 1996; Karp and Laureno 1993) or a movement disorder such as dystonia (Maraganore *et al.* 1992; Yoshida *et al.* 2000) or parkinsonism (Dickoff *et al.* 1988; Seiser *et al.* 1998; Sullivan *et al.* 2000; Tomita *et al.* 1997); importantly, in cases characterized by a movement disorder, these symptoms may be delayed for weeks or months.

Course

In classic cases, death may occur within a matter of days. In those who survive, recovery may begin within a week or two of the syndrome reaching its peak intensity, with maximum recovery taking up to a year; enduring deficits may include a variable degree of quadriparesis or dementia (Menger and Jorg 1999). In cases characterized by a movement disorder, symptoms may either resolve over many months or be chronic, or, in the case of dystonia, may actually gradually worsen.

Etiology

As noted earlier, the classic precipitant for central pontine myelinolysis is the overly rapid correction of a chronic hyponatremia (Brunner *et al.* 1990; Karp and Laureno 1993; Messert *et al.* 1979; Norenberg *et al.* 1982; Sterns *et al.* 1986). In cases of chronic hyponatremia, intracellular osmolarity gradually falls to maintain an osmotic balance with the hypo-osmolar extracellular fluid. If the hyponatremia is corrected gradually, there is time for the intracellular osmolarity to 'catch up', so that an excessive osmotic gradient does not appear between the intracellular and extracellular fluids. However, when the hyponatremia is rapidly corrected, an osmotic gradient does occur, with a substantial fluid shift from the intracellular to extracellular compartments. Oligodendrocytes appear particularly affected by this osmotic shift, and these cells, in particular those located within the pons, become damaged or die, leading

to demyelinization. Although such a scenario is most likely in chronic alcoholics given intravenous fluids (Lampl and Yazdi 2002), other groups at risk include the recipients of liver transplants (Estol *et al.* 1989), those suffering from severe malnutrition, and patients hyponatremic because of protracted vomiting (Dickoff *et al.* 1988) or diarrhea (Price and Mesulam 1987).

Although this mechanism appears operative for the vast majority of cases, other mechanisms may also be found. For example, central pontine myelinolysis has been noted in severe burn patients who were not hyponatremic but who had developed a severe hyperosmolar state (McKee *et al.* 1988), leading, presumably, to the same kind of osmotic shift.

Pathologically, in classic cases one finds symmetric demyelinization within the basis pontis (Adams *et al.* 1959). This is most prominent within the central portion of the pons and spreads outward but does not involve the periphery of the pons where a rim of intact white matter survives. This demyelinization may at times extend to the pontine tegmentum and occasionally also into the mesencephalon, but the medulla is generally spared. In severe cases, cavitation may occur. Extrapontine myelinolysis, as noted, may also occur, and has been noted in the centrum semiovale, internal capsule, striatum, thalamus, subthalamic nucleus, and the lateral geniculate body (Wright *et al.* 1979). In pathologic material, the most common pattern is myelinolysis confined to the pons, followed by myelinolysis involving both the pons and extrapontine sites; the least common pattern consists of myelinolysis solely in extrapontine sites (Gocht and Colmant 1987).

Differential diagnosis

Classic cases must be distinguished from stroke secondary to infarction in the area of distribution of the basilar artery. Stroke is suggested by a more rapid onset and by an asymmetry of signs; furthermore, MRI scanning will reveal a lesion that, in contrast to central pontine myelinolysis, involves the periphery of the pons. In cases characterized by delirium alone, the clue, of course, would be the history of rapid correction of hyponatremia 2 or 3 days earlier.

Treatment

As there is no specific treatment for acute central pontine myelinolysis, prevention is essential. It must be borne in mind that, when chronic, hyponatremia is often relatively well-tolerated and indeed some patients may be asymptomatic. Consequently, even in cases in which the serum sodium is as low as 115 mEq/L, simple fluid restriction to perhaps 800–1200 mL/24 hours is adequate. In cases, however, in which significant symptoms of hyponatremia are present or anticipated and treatment with normal or hypertonic saline is required, it is essential to temper one's therapeutic enthusiasm and to limit the rise in sodium to no more than approximately 0.4 mEq/L/hour (Norenberg *et al.* 1982; Sterns *et al.* 1986) and to aim only for a level of 120 mEq/L: once that level is reached, further correction may be made at a much more leisurely pace. Patients left with a dementia may be treated as described in Section 5.1; parkinsonism may respond to levodopa (Sullivan *et al.* 2000).

13.18 UREMIC ENCEPHALOPATHY

In severe renal failure, patients may develop a delirium due to a condition known as uremic encephalopathy.

Clinical features

The mode of onset, as might be expected, reflects the rapidity with which the kidneys fail, and hence the onset of uremic encephalopathy may range from acute to gradual. Patients may initially experience some lassitude or a mild degree of somnolence; however, eventually a delirium appears that is often marked by visual hallucinations. Asterixis (Raskin and Fishman 1976; Tyler 1968) and multifocal myoclonus are common, and in some cases one may see diffuse multifocal muscle twitching; dysarthria may also occur. In a minority seizures, typically grand mal in type, may appear. In one rare case, uremia presented with mania alone, without any other symptoms (El-Mallakh *et al.* 1987).

A sensorimotor polyneuropathy may occur (Ropper 1993; Thomas *et al.* 1971) and, as with the encephalopathy, this may be acute or gradual in onset; the motor component may be quite severe and patients may become quadriparetic. In a little under 50 percent of patients with a polyneuropathy there may be prominent dysesthesiae and restlessness, similar to that seen in the restless legs syndrome.

The severity of the encephalopathy correlates not only with the level of the blood urea nitrogen (BUN) but also with the rapidity with which the BUN rises. For example, although in cases of acute renal failure levels of 35.7 mmol/L (100 mg/dL) are typically associated with delirium, in renal failure of very gradual onset, levels of 71.4 mmol/L (200 mg/dL) may be tolerated with few if any symptoms.

The EEG typically shows generalized slowing; triphasic waves may also be seen.

Course

Typically the symptoms of the delirium show marked fluctuations throughout the day. The overall course parallels that of the renal failure, and in some progressive cases coma may ensue.

Etiology

Although the level of the BUN serves as a rough guide to the presence and severity of the encephalopathy, urea itself is not the cause of the central nervous system dysfunction and in all likelihood the delirium results from an 'auto-intoxication' by as yet unidentified substances. In chronic cases that come to autopsy, an excess of protoplasmic astrocytes has been found.

Differential diagnosis

Not all deliria occurring in the context of an elevated BUN represent uremic encephalopathy. Certain disorders, such as polyarteritis nodosa and systemic lupus erythematosus, may not only cause renal failure but also directly affect the central nervous system. Another example is malignant hypertension, which may cause a concurrent hypertensive encephalopathy and renal failure.

Renal failure is also associated with subdural hematoma (Fraser and Arieff 1988), hypocalcemia, and hypomagnesemia, each of which may also cause delirium. Finally, attention must be paid to toxicity from drugs excreted primarily via the kidneys.

Treatment

If the underlying cause of the renal failure is untreatable and spontaneous improvement is not expected, then uremic encephalopathy constitutes an indication for dialysis. With dialysis, the delirium typically resolves in a matter of days.

13.19 HEPATIC ENCEPHALOPATHY

With significant disease or dysfunction of hepatocytes, or with significant shunting of blood past the liver and directly into the systemic circulation, toxins normally removed by the liver reach the brain and a hepatic encephalopathy may occur.

Clinical features

The mode of onset of hepatic encephalopathy mirrors the rapidity with which hepatic failure occurs, and thus may range from acute, as in fulminant hepatic failure in some cases of viral hepatitis, to gradual, as in slowly progressive alcoholic cirrhosis.

Acute-onset hepatic encephalopathy typically presents with a delirium; in gradual-onset cases, although a delirium eventually occurs, this development is often preceded by a more or less lengthy prodrome characterized by impaired judgment, difficulty with abstracting, and mood changes, which often tend toward euphoria. The delirium (Adams and Foley 1953; Fraser and Arieff 1985; Read *et al.* 1961; Summerskill *et al.* 1956) is characterized by confusion, drowsiness, sleep reversal, asterixis, and myoclonus; a small minority may have seizures, which may be partial or grand mal, and a minority may also have focal signs, such as hemiparesis (Cadranel *et al.* 2001). Rarely, catatonic symptoms, such as waxy flexibility, may occur (Jaffe 1967). *Fetor hepaticus*, a sickly-sweet musty odor to the breath, is seen in about half of the cases. With progression of the hepatic failure, stupor and coma may occur, accompanied by rigidity and bilateral Babinski signs.

The EEG shows generalized slowing, which is often accompanied by triphasic waves; interictal epileptiform discharges may be seen in a small minority (Ficker *et al.* 1997).

Although the blood ammonia level is elevated in the vast majority of cases, there is only a rough correlation between the degree of elevation and the severity of the encephalopathy (Ong *et al.* 2003); indeed, although rare, in some cases the ammonia level may be normal (Sherlock 1993).

Course

In the absence of treatment, the course of the encephalopathy mirrors the severity of the underlying hepatic failure. With treatment, provided that coma has not supervened, the recovery is generally quite good; in cases that have progressed to coma, however, the mortality rate is high.

With repeated episodes patients may develop acquired hepatocerebral degeneration, as described in Section 13.20.

Etiology

As indicated earlier, hepatic encephalopathy occurs when the brain is exposed to toxins found in the portal vessels, toxins that are normally removed by the liver. Although ammonia itself is the most likely culprit here, other candidates have also been considered, including mercaptans, various aromatic amino acids, and short-chain fatty acids. In chronic cases, there may be an increased number of Alzheimer type II astrocytes (Adams and Foley 1953). In acute cases characterized by coma, cerebral edema occurs, with, in some instances, transtentorial herniation (Donovan *et al.* 1998).

The most common causes of hepatic failure are viral hepatitis and alcoholic cirrhosis. In many cases, the onset of the delirium may be traced to an event that increased the nitrogenous load in the gut beyond the diminished detoxifying capacity of the liver. Examples include high protein meals, blood (as may occur with bleeding esophageal varices or peptic ulcer disease), and constipation. Other precipitants include infection, anesthesia, hypokalemia, uremia, and exposure to alcohol or sedative–hypnotics, especially benzodiazepines.

Differential diagnosis

In alcoholics, consideration must be given to delirium tremens, Wernicke's encephalopathy, hypoglycemia, encephalopathic pellagra, and subdural hematoma. The differential for delirium accompanied by asterixis is discussed in Section 3.12, and for delirium with myoclonus in Section 3.2.

Rarely, valproic acid may cause an encephalopathy associated with an elevated ammonia level (Baver *et al.* 2005); however, the relation of this encephalopathy to hepatic encephalopathy is not entirely clear. In any case, treatment of valproic acid encephalopathy consists of discontinuing the drug and administering carnitine (Bohan *et al.* 2001).

Treatment

In addition to treating any precipitating events, efforts are made to reduce the nitrogenous load in the gut. This may be accomplished using three methods, individually or in combination: a low-protein diet, lactulose, and treatment with rifaximin. Reducing dietary protein to 20–60 g/day is helpful, but many patients find this unpalatable. In acute situations, lactulose may be started at a dose of 20–45 mL hourly until the patient starts to have bowel movements, after which the dose may be decreased to a maintenance dose of 30–45 mL q.i.d.; in less urgent situations, one may simply start with a maintenance dose, with dosage adjustments as required to ensure three to four soft bowel movements daily. Rifaximin is a non-absorbable intestinal antibiotic that targets nitrogenous bacteria, and this may be given in a dose of 400 mg t.i.d.

The general symptomatic treatment of delirium is discussed in Section 5.3. With regard to symptomatic pharmacologic treatment, benzodiazepines are contraindicated; if antipsychotics are required the dose should be low, as all of these agents are metabolized in the liver.

Patients in coma may require treatment with mannitol and monitoring of intracranial pressure.

13.20 ACQUIRED HEPATOCEREBRAL DEGENERATION

Acquired hepatocerebral degeneration is a rare disorder that occurs secondary to repeated or prolonged bouts of hepatic encephalopathy and is characterized by variable mixtures of cognitive deficits and abnormal movements.

Clinical features

Clinical features have been described in a number of reports (Finlayson and Superville 1981; Graham *et al.* 1970; Raskin *et al.* 1984; Victor *et al.* 1965). The onset is typically gradual and is often punctuated by repeated episodes of hepatic encephalopathy. Cognitive deficits may occur, which may be quite mild or, in some cases, amount to a dementia. The movement disorder is often complex, with variable admixtures of chorea, facial grimacing, postural tremor, parkinsonism, and ataxia. Chorea, when present, often affects the head and neck, and the resulting movements may be tic-like in character.

T1-weighted MRI scanning (Burkhard *et al.* 2003; Krieger *et al.* 1995) typically reveals increased signal intensity in the globus pallidus; similar changes may be seen in the striatum and in the substantia nigra.

Course

In general, the overall course is marked by slow progression.

Etiology

At autopsy (Finlayson and Superville 1981; Victor *et al.* 1965), spongiform change or laminar cortical necrosis may be found in the cerebral and cerebellar cortices; spongiform change is also noted in the basal ganglia and this may be accompanied by microcavitation. Alzheimer type II astrocytes are present in the cortex and basal ganglia.

The occurrence of these changes in the context of repeated episodes of hepatic encephalopathy strongly suggests that they are toxic in nature and, of the various candidate toxins, manganese stands out. Elevated manganese levels are found in the basal ganglia and cerebral cortex (Klos *et al.* 2006; Krieger *et al.* 1995) and also in the CSF and blood (Burkhard *et al.* 2003); furthermore, one study found a correlation between the elevation in blood manganese and the increase in signal intensity on T1-weighted scanning in the globus pallidus (Krieger *et al.* 1995).

Differential diagnosis

Hepatic encephalopathy is distinguished by the presence of delirium and asterixis, alcoholic dementia by the absence of abnormal movements, and Wilson's disease by copper studies.

Treatment

Remarkably, symptoms may remit after liver transplantation (Powell *et al.* 1990; Servin-Abad *et al.* 2006; Stracciari *et al.* 2001). In cases in which transplantation is not possible, consideration may be given to treatment with branched-chain amino acids, which in case reports led to a reduction in abnormal movements and a partial resolution of MRI abnormalities (Ueki *et al.* 2002); furthermore, in cases in which parkinsonism is prominent, case series suggest an effectiveness for levodopa (Burkhard *et al.* 2003).

13.21 HEPATIC PORPHYRIA

Of the hepatic porphyrias, four can cause delirium. Three of these are inherited in an autosomal dominant pattern, namely acute intermittent porphyria, variegate porphyria, and hereditary coproporphyria, whereas the fourth, delta-aminolevulinic acid (ALA) dehydratase deficiency, is an autosomal recessive disorder. Acute intermittent porphyria is found worldwide and may have a prevalence as high as 5–10 cases per 100 000 population. Variegate porphyria, although rare in the United States, may be found in Sweden and among white people in South Africa. Hereditary coproporphyria is quite rare, and ALA dehydratase deficiency is so extraordinarily rare that it is not considered further in this text.

From a clinical viewpoint the three autosomal dominantly inherited hepatic porphyrias are essentially the same, with the exception that both variegate porphyria and hereditary coproporphyria may cause a photosensitive rash, a symptom not seen in acute intermittent porphyria.

Of interest, it appears that the periodic 'madness' of King George III represented attacks of hepatic porphyria (Cox *et al.* 2005; Macalpine and Hunter 1966; Macalpine *et al.* 1968).

Clinical features

The hepatic porphyrias are episodic disorders and the first episode usually appears in late adolescence or early adult years. The attacks themselves tend to present fairly acutely and are often precipitated by one of the factors discussed below, such as infection, menstruation, or pregnancy.

The overall symptomatology of the episodes has been reported in a number of papers (Becker and Kramer 1975; Goldberg 1959; Rowland 1961; Stein and Tschudy 1970). Classically, episodes are characterized by abdominal pain with vomiting, constipation, or diarrhea, accompanied, in about half of the cases, by a delirium. The delirium is often marked by affective lability, delusions of persecution, and visual hallucinations, which may be quite compelling (Cross 1956; Paredes and Jones 1959); in some cases, stupor or coma may supervene. Uncommonly, rather than a delirium there may be a psychosis with auditory hallucinations, delusions of persecution, and bizarre behavior, all occurring in a 'clear sensorium' without confusion or cognitive deficits (Hirsch and Dunsworth 1955; Mandoki and Sumner 1994). Other symptoms, seen in a minority, include a primarily motor polyneuropathy (which may progress to a quadriparesis), a cranial neuropathy (most commonly with ophthalmoplegia or facial palsy), partial or grand mal seizures, hypertension, tachycardia, and fever. A small minority of patients may also have significant hyponatremia, which in turn may be due either to a syndrome of inappropriate antidiuretic hormone (ADH) secretion or to intestinal or renal sodium loss.

As noted earlier, patients with variegate porphyria and hereditary coproporphyria may have a rash: this is a photosensitive rash that may or may not coincide with the episodes just described.

T2-weighted MR scanning may reveal scattered areas of increased signal intensity within the subcortical white matter (Bylesjo *et al.* 2004; King and Bragdon 1991).

During episodes, a 24-hour urine test will reveal elevated levels of both porphobilinogen and ALA in all three of these porphyrias, and the diagnosis rests on this finding. In addition to these findings, both variegate porphyria and hereditary coproporphyria will also display an elevated urinary coproporphyrin. Distinguishing between variegate porphyria and hereditary coproporphyria requires a 24-hour stool collection for protoporphyrin and coproporphyrin. In variegate porphyria, protoporphyrin levels are higher than those of coproporphyrin, whereas in hereditary coproporphyria the converse holds true. Importantly, in between episodes all of these measurements may be normal.

Course

The duration of episodes usually ranges from days to weeks, although sometimes they can be much longer. Although most patients recover completely, death may occur as a result of respiratory failure due to the motor neuropathy, or an arrhythmia. Repeat episodes are common and typically occur in response to a specific precipitating factor.

Etiology

All of these hepatic porphyrias occur secondary to mutations in genes that code for various enzymes involved in the heme biosynthetic pathway: acute intermittent porphyria occurs secondary to mutations in the gene for porphobilinogen deaminase on chromosome 11; variegate porphyria to mutations in the gene for protoporphyrinogen oxidase on chromosome 1; and hereditary coproporphyria to mutations in the gene for coproporphyrinogen oxidase on chromosome 3. When the heme biosynthetic pathway becomes stressed in the presence of these mutated proteins, 'upstream' proteins, such as porphobilinogen and ALA, accumulate and an episode occurs. Although the mechanism by which central nervous system dysfunction occurs is not clear, one theory suggests that ALA acts as an agonist at GABAergic sites. Although most autopsy studies of the brain (reviewed by Suarez et al. [1997]) have been negative, some have found diffuse neuronal loss and diffuse perivascular demyelination within the central nervous system. Within the peripheral nervous system, axonal damage (Cavanagh and Mellick 1965; Sweeney et al. 1970) with associated chromatolysis of the spinal motor neurons (Hierons 1957) has been noted.

As noted earlier, most episodes are precipitated by various factors including infection, menstruation, pregnancy, fasting (or merely a low-carbohydrate diet), surgery, and a host of drugs including barbiturates, phenytoin, valproic acid, carbamazepine, nortriptyline, sulfonamides, griseofulvin, meprobamate, glutethimide, methyprylon, ethchlorvynol, ergot derivatives, synthetic estrogens and progestins, danazol, alpha-methyldopa, chlorpropamide,

and alcohol. Importantly, the following drugs appear to be safe: phenothiazines (e.g. chlorpromazine or trifluoperazine), opioid analgesics, chloral hydrate, gabapentin, levetiracetam, diazepam, diphenhydramine, aspirin, and acetaminophen.

Differential diagnosis

Both thallium and arsenic intoxication may produce a similar clinical picture.

Treatment

Acute episodes may respond to a high carbohydrate diet or, if patients cannot take food or fluid (as is often the case), to intravenous glucose in a dose of 400 g/day. In cases resistant to this, consideration should be given to intravenous hemin (formerly known as hematin), which suppresses the heme biosynthetic pathway and provides relief generally within 3 days. Pending resolution of the episode, symptomatic treatment, in addition to general supportive care, may include chlorpromazine or propranolol. Chlorpromazine, in doses of 25–50 mg intramuscularly or intravenously every 4–6 hours, may not only control symptoms of the delirium but also reduce abdominal pain (Calvy et al. 1957). Propranolol, in doses ranging from 20 to 200 mg total daily, will control both blood pressure and tachycardia (Menawat et al. 1979). If seizures occur and require treatment, consideration may be given to either gabapentin (Hahn et al. 1997; Tatum and Zachariah 1995) or levetiracetam (Paul and Meencke 2004); in emergent situations, diazepam may be given intravenously.

Prevention is critical and this may generally be accomplished by maintaining a high carbohydrate diet and, when possible, avoiding precipitating factors. In cases of menstrually induced attacks, consideration may be given to leuteinizing hormone-releasing hormone to suppress menstruation. In instances in which episodes recur despite these measures, consideration may be given to prophylactic use of hemin.

13.22 FAHR'S SYNDROME

Fahr's syndrome is characterized by a movement disorder, generally parkinsonism, or a neuropsychiatric syndrome, most commonly dementia, or both, occurring secondary to brain calcification, which, although most common in the basal ganglia, may also be found in the dentate nuclei, thalamus, and at the gray–white junction of the cerebral and cerebellar cortices. This calcification may be either secondary to some other disorder, such as hypoparathyroidism, or may occur on a primary basis as either an idiopathic or inherited disorder, in which case one speaks of Fahr's disease. Synonyms for Fahr's disease include idiopathic striopallidodentate calcinosis and idiopathic calcification of the basal ganglia (ICBG).

Although, as noted below, asymptomatic basal ganglia calcification is a not uncommon incidental finding, especially in the elderly, Fahr's syndrome, by contrast, is rare.

Clinical features

The presentation is generally gradual and may be characterized by either a movement disorder or a neuropsychiatric syndrome. Regardless of the presentation, over long-term follow-up most patients will display a combination of these symptoms.

Of the movement disorders seen in Fahr's syndrome, the most common is parkinsonism (Klawans et al. 1976; Margolin et al. 1980; Tambyah et al. 1993); choreathetosis or dystonia (Larsen et al. 1985; Saiki et al. 2007) may also occur and in a small minority there may be ataxia or dysarthria.

Neuropsychiatric syndromes most commonly include dementia (Kobari et al. 1997; Slyter 1979; Wszolek et al. 2006). Personality change, which may be of the frontal lobe type (Lam et al. 2007; Weisman et al. 2007), may also occur. A psychosis, similar to that seen in schizophrenia (Chabot et al. 2001; Francis and Freeman 1984), has also been reported, especially in the elderly (Ostling et al. 2003). Other presentations include depression or mania (Trautner et al. 1988) and obsessions and compulsions (Lopez-Villegas et al. 1996). Seizures have also been noted, and in cases occurring secondary to hypoparathyroidism these may occur on the basis of hypocalcemia.

Computed tomography scanning is superior to both MRI and skull radiography and in all cases displays bilateral calcification in the basal ganglia; in most cases, as illustrated in Figure 13.1, one also sees bilateral calcification in other structures, such as the dentate nuclei, the thalamus, and the gray–white junction of the cerebral and cerebellar cortices.

Course

Fahr's syndrome is generally gradually progressive.

Etiology

The majority of cases occur on a primary basis. These may be either idiopathic (Trautner et al. 1988) or inherited (Boller et al. 1977; Kobari et al. 1997); of the inherited cases, although most occur on an autosomal dominant basis (Manyam et al. 2001), a recessive pattern has also been noted (Smits et al. 1983). At present, the genetic basis of the autosomal dominant cases is not known; although linkage has been demonstrated to the IBGC1 locus on chromosome 14 in some cases (Geschwind et al. 1999), such linkage was not found in others (Oliveira et al. 2004).

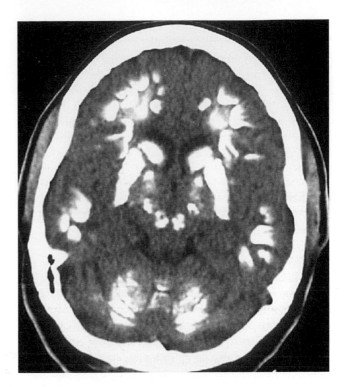

Figure 13.1   Computed tomography (CT) scan showing extensive calcium deposition in a case of Fahr's syndrome. (Reproduced from Gillespie and Jackson 2000.)

Secondary cases may occur on the basis of hypoparathyroidism (either surgical [Berger and Ross 1981; Klawans et al. 1976, Tambyah et al. 1993] or idiopathic [Kazis 1985; Slyter 1979]), pseudohypoparathyroidism (Mathews 1957), pseudo-pseudohypoparathyroidism (Nyland and Skre 1977), or, rarely, hyperparathyroidism (Margolin et al. 1980). Fahr's syndrome may also occur in concert with bone cysts of the hands and feet in the very rare autosomal recessive Nasu–Hakola disease (Kluneman et al. 2005; Kondo et al. 2002).

Differential diagnosis

In practice, the question of this diagnosis arises when, in the evaluation of patients with one of the clinical syndromes described above, neuroimaging reveals calcification. Care must be taken at this point, however, given that a degree of calcification of the basal ganglia, primarily in the globus pallidus, is not uncommon in asymptomatic individuals, being found in approximately 0.5 percent of the general population (Harrington et al. 1981; Koller et al. 1979) and up to 19 percent of 85 year olds (Ostling et al. 2003). In general, the diagnosis should therefore be reserved either for cases in which there is massive calcification involving not only the basal ganglia but also the other structures noted above (Manyam et al. 2001) or for cases in which no other cause may be found for the patients' symptomatology despite an exhaustive evaluation.

Treatment

If present hypoparathyroidism should be treated as this may prompt a partial remission of symptoms (Berger and Ross 1981; Slyter 1979). Parkinsonism may respond to levodopa. The general treatment of dementia is described in Section 5.1. In cases characterized by depression, mania, or obsessions or compulsions, treatment may be attempted as described in Sections 6.1, 6.3, and 4.17 respectively.

REFERENCES

Abarbanel JM, Berginer VM, Osimani A *et al*. Neurologic complications after gastric restriction surgery for morbid obesity. *Neurology* 1987; **37**:196–200.

Abd El Naby S, Hassanein M. Neuropsychiatric manifestations of chronic manganese poisoning. *J Neurol Neurosurg Psychiatry* 1965; **28**:282–8.

Adams RD, Foley JM. The neurological disorder associated with liver disease. *Assoc Res Nerv Ment Dis Proc* 1953; **32**:198–237.

Adams RD, Victor M, Mancall EL. Central pontine myelinolysis: a hitherto undescribed disease occurring in alcoholic and malnourished patients. *Arch Neurol Psychiatry* 1959; **81**:154–72.

Akelaitis AJ. Lead encephalopathy in children and adults. *J Nerv Ment Dis* 1941; **93**:313–32.

Alajouanine T, DeRobert L, Thieffry S. Etude clinique d'ensemble de 210 cas d'intoxication par les sels organiques d'etain. *Rev Neurol* 1958; **98**:85–96.

Albert MS, Butters N, Levin J. Temporal gradients in the retrograde amnesia of patients with alcoholic Korsakoff's disease. *Arch Neurol* 1979; **36**:211–16.

Alfrey AC, LeGendre GR, Kaehny WD. The dialysis encephalopathy syndrome. Possible aluminium intoxication. *N Engl J Med* 1976; **294**:184–8.

Amin-Zaki L, Majeed MA, Traxon TW *et al*. Methyl mercury poisoning in Iraqi children: clinical observations of two years. *BMJ* 1978; **1**:613–16.

Andreoli SP, Bergstein JM, Sherrard DJ. Aluminum intoxication from aluminum-containing phosphate binders in children with azotemia not undergoing dialysis. *N Engl J Med* 1984; **310**:1079–84.

Andres E, Noel e, Goichot B. Metformin-associated vitamin B12 deficiency. *Arch Int Med* 2002; **162**:2251–2.

Auer RN, Hugh J, Cosgrove E *et al*. Neuropathologic findings in three cases of profound hypoglycemia. *Clin Neuropathol* 1989; **8**:63–8.

Bach LA, Buchanan RR, Scarlett JD *et al*. Hyperviscosity syndrome secondary to rheumatoid arthritis. *Aust NZ J Med* 1989; **19**:710–12.

Baghurst PA, McMichael AJ, Wigg NR *et al*. Environmental exposure to lead and children's intelligence at the age of seven years – the Port Pirie Cohort Study. *N Engl J Med* 1992; **327**:1279–84.

Bank WJ, Pleasure DE, Suzuki K *et al*. Thallium poisoning. *Arch Neurol* 1972; **26**:456–64.

Baver MS. Fatal hepatic failure and valproate. *Am J Psychiatry* 2005; **162**:192.

Becker DM, Kramer S. The neurological manifestations of porphyria: a review. *Medicine* 1975; **56**:411–23.

Bellinger D, Leviton A, Waternaux C *et al*. Longitudinal analysis of prenatal and postnatal lead exposure and early cognitive development. *N Engl J Med* 1987; **316**:1037–43.

Beltramello A, Puppini G, Cerini R *et al*. Subacute combined degeneration of the spinal cord after nitrous oxide anaesthesia: role of magnetic resonance imaging. *J Neurol Neurosurg Psychiatry* 1998; **64**:563–4.

Ben-Ami H, Nagachandran P, Mendelson A *et al*. Drug-induced hypoglycemic coma in 102 diabetic patients. *Arch Intern Med* 1999; **159**:281–4.

Berger JR, Ross DB. Reversible Parkinson syndrome complicating postoperative hypoparathyroidism. *Neurology* 1981; **31**:881–2.

Besser R, Kramer G, Thumler R *et al*. Acute trimethyltin limbic–cerebellar syndrome. *Neurology* 1987; **37**:945–50.

Blass JP, Gibson GE. Abnormality of a thiamine-requiring enzyme in patients with the Wernicke–Korsakoff syndrome. *N Engl J Med* 1977; **297**:1367.

Bodamar OAF, Rosenblatt DS, Appel SH *et al*. Adult-onset combined methylmalonic aciduria and homocystinuria. *Neurology* 2001; **56**:1113.

Bohan TP, Helton E, McDonald I *et al*. Effect of l-carnitine treatment for valproate-induced hepatotoxicity. *Neurology* 2001; **56**:1405–9.

Boller F, Boller M, Gilbert J. Familial idiopathic cerebral calcifications. *J Neurol Neurosurg Psychiatry* 1977; **40**:280–5.

Bosboom WMJ, Frijns CJM, Gijn J. Yelling attacks and wasted hands. *Lancet* 1996; **348**:238.

Boxer AL, Kramer JH, Johnston N *et al*. Executive dysfunction in hyperhomocystinemia responds to homocysteine-lowering treatment. *Neurology* 2005; **64**:1431–4.

Brunner JE, Redmond JM, Haggar AM *et al*. Central pontine myelinolysis and pontine lesions after rapid correction of hyponatremia: a prospective magnetic resonance imaging study. *Ann Neurol* 1990; **27**:61–6.

Buge A, Supino-Viterbo V, Rancurel G *et al*. Epileptic phenomena in bismuth toxic encephalopathy. *J Neurol Neurosurg Psychiatry* 1981; **44**:62–7.

Burke GJ, Hiangabeza T. Isoniazid-induced pellagra in a patient on vitamin B supplement. *S Afr Med J* 1977; **51**:719.

Burkhard PR, Delavelle J, Du Pasquier R *et al*. Chronic parkinsonism associated with cirrhosis: a distinct subset of acquired hepatocerebral degeneration. *Arch Neurol* 2003; **60**:521–8.

Burks JS, Alfrey AC, Huddlestone J *et al*. A fatal encephalopathy in chronic hemodialysis patients. *Lancet* 1976; **1**:764–8.

Burns R, Thomas DQ, Barron VJ. Reversible encephalopathy possibly associated with bismuth subgallate ingestion. *BMJ* 1974; **1**:220–3.

Bylesjo I, Brekke OL, Prytz J *et al*. Brain magnetic resonance imaging white-matter lesions an cerebrospinal fluid findings in patients with acute intermittent porphyria. *Eur Neurol* 2004; **51**:1–5.

Cadranel JF, Lebiz E, Di Martino V *et al*. Focal neurologic signs in hepatic encephalopathy in cirrhotic patients: an underestimated entity? *Am J Gastroenterol* 2001; **96**:515–18.

Calne DB, Chu NS, Huang CC *et al*. Manganese and idiopathic parkinsonism: similarities and differences. *Neurology* 1994; **44**:1583–6.

Calvy GL, Leeper RD, Monaco RN *et al*. Intermittent acute porphyria treated with chlorpromazine. *N Engl J Med* 1957; **256**:309–11.

Camacho J, Arnalich F, Anciones B *et al*. The spectrum of neurological abnormalities in myeloma. *J Med* 1985; **16**:597–611.

Canfield RL, Henderson CP, Cory-Slechta DA *et al*. Intellectual impairment in children with blood lead concentrations below 10 microgr per deciliter. *N Engl J Med* 2003; **348**:1517–26.

Case Records of the Massachusetts General Hospital. *N Engl J Med* 1988; **318**:1523–8.

Cavanagh JB, Mellick RS. On the nature of the peripheral nerve lesions with acute intermittent porphyria. *J Neurol Neurosurg Psychiatry* 1965; **28**:320–72.

Cavanagh JB, Fuller NH, Johnson HRM *et al*. The effects of thallium salts, with particular reference to the nervous system changes. *Q J Med* 1974; **43**:293–319.

Chabot B, Roulland C, Dollfus S. Schizophrenia and familial idiopathic basal ganglia calcification: a case report. *Psychol Med* 2001; **31**:741–7.

Charles JR. Manganese toxaemia, with special reference to the effects of liver feeding. *Brain* 1927; **50**:30–43.

Chatterjee A, Yapundich R, Palmer CA *et al*. Leukoencephalopathy associated with cobalamin deficiency. *Neurology* 1996; **46**:832–4.

Chokroverty S, Bruetman ME, Berger V *et al*. Progressive dialytic encephalopathy. *J Neurol Neurosurg Psychiatry* 1976; **39**:411–19.

Chu K, Kang DW, Kim HJ *et al*. Diffusion-weighted imaging abnormalities in Wernicke encephalopathy: reversible cytotoxic edema? *Arch Neurol* 2002; **59**:123–7.

Cook DG, Fahn S, Brairt KA. Chronic manganese intoxication. *Arch Neurol* 1974; **30**:59–64.

Cossa P, Duplay J, Fischgold A *et al*. Encephalopathies toxiques au Stalinon. Aspects anatomo-cliniques et electroencephalographiques. *Rev Neurol* 1958; **98**:97–108.

Cox TN, Jack N, Lofthouse S *et al*. King George III and porphyria: an elemental hypothesis and investigation. *Lancet* 2005; **366**:332–5.

Cravioto H, Korein J, Silberman J. Wernicke's encephalopathy: a clinical and pathological study of 28 autopsied cases. *Arch Neurol* 1961; **4**:510–19.

Cross TN. Porphyria – a deceptive syndrome. *Am J Psychiatry* 1956; **112**:1010–14.

Davis LE, Wands JR, Weiss SA *et al*. Central nervous system intoxication from mercurous chloride laxative. *Arch Neurol* 1974; **30**:428–31.

Davis LE, Standefer JC, Kornfeld M *et al*. Acute thallium poisoning: toxicological and morphological studies of the nervous system. *Ann Neurol* 1981; **10**:38–44.

Davison AM, Walker GS, Oh H *et al*. Water supply aluminum concentration dialysis dementia, and effect of reverse-osmosis water treatment. *Lancet* 1982; **2**:785–7.

Dickoff DJ, Raps M, Yahr MD. Striatal syndrome following hyponatremia and its rapid correction: a manifestation of extrapontine myelinolysis confirmed by magnetic resonance imaging. *Arch Neurol* 1988; **45**:112–14.

DiMartini A. Wernicke–Korsakoff syndrome in a liver transplant recipient. *Psychosomatics* 1996; **37**:564–7.

Discalzi G, Pira E, Herrero Hernandez E *et al*. Occupational Mn parkinsonism: magnetic resonance imaging and clinical patterns following CaNa2-EDTA chelation. *Neurotoxicology* 2000; **21**:863–6.

Dizon AM, Kowaly S, Hoogwerf BJ. Neuroglycopenic and other symptoms in patients with insulinomas. *Am J Med* 1999; **106**:307–10.

Donovan JP, Schaefer DF, Shaw BW *et al*. Cerebral oedema and increased intracranial pressure in chronic liver disease. *Lancet* 1998; **351**:719–21.

Dreyfus PM. The clinical applications of blood transketolase determinations. *N Engl J Med* 1962; **267**:596–8.

El-Mallakh RS, Shrader SA, Widger E. Single case study: mania as a manifestation of end-stage renal disease. *J Nerv Ment Dis* 1987; **175**:243–5.

Estol CJ, Faris AA, Martinez J *et al*. Central pontine myelinolysis after liver transplantation. *Neurology* 1989; **39**:493–8.

Evans DL, Edelsohn GA, Golden RN. Organic psychosis without anemia or spinal cord symptoms in patients with B12 deficiency. *Am J Psychiatry* 1983; **140**:218–21.

Feldman RG, White RF, Eriator II. Trimethyltin encephalopathy. *Arch Neurol* 1993; **50**:1320–4.

Ferraro A, Arieti S, English WH. Cerebral changes in the course of pernicious anemia and their relationship to psychic changes. *J Neuropathol Exp Neurol* 1945; **4**:217–39.

Ficker DM, Westmoreland BF, Sharbrough FW. Epileptiform abnormalities in hepatic encephalopathy. *J Clin Neurophysiol* 1997; **14**:230–4.

Fincher RM, Koerker RM. Long-term survival in acute arsenic encephalopathy. Follow-up using newer measures of electrophysiologic parameters. *Am J Med* 1987; **82**:549–52.

Finlayson MH, Superville B. Distribution of cerebral lesions in acquired hepatocerebral degeneration. *Brain* 1981; **104**:79–85.

Fisher AA, Le Couteur DG. Lead poisoning from complementary and alternative medicine in multiple sclerosis. *J Neurol Neurosur Psychiatry* 2000; **69**:687–9.

Fortemps E, Amand G, Bomboir A *et al*. Trimethyltin poisoning. Report of two cases. *Int Arch Occup Environ Health* 1978; **41**:1–6.

Francis A, Freeman H. Psychiatric abnormality and brain calcification over four generations. *J Nerv Ment Dis* 1984; **172**:166–70.

Frantzen E. Wernicke's encephalopathy: 3 cases occurring in connection with severe malnutrition. *Acta Neurol Scand* 1966; **42**:426–41.

Fraser CL, Arieff AI. Hepatic encephalopathy. *N Engl J Med* 1985; **313**:865–73.

Fraser CL, Arieff AI. Nervous system complications in uremia. *Ann Intern Med* 1988; **109**:143–9.

Fraser TN. Cerebral manifestations of addisonian pernicious anemia. *Lancet* 1960; **2**:458–9.

Freeman JW, Couch JR. Prolonged encephalopathy with arsenic poisoning. *Neurology* 1978; **28**:853–5.

Gardeur D, Buge A, Rancurel G *et al.* Bismuth encephalopathy and cerebral computed tomography. *J Comput Assist Tomogr* 1978; **2**:436–8.

Gardian G, Voros E, Jardanhazy T *et al.* Wernicke's encephalopathy induced by hyperemesis gravidarum. *Acta Neurol Scand* 1999; **95**:196–8.

Garrett PJ, Mulcahey D, Carmody M *et al.* Aluminum encephalopathy: clinical and immunologic features. *Q J Med* 1988; **69**:775–83.

Geschwind DH, Loginov M, Stern JM. Identification of a locus on chromosome 14q for idiopathic basal ganglia calcification (Fahr disease). *Am J Hun Genet* 1999; **65**:764–72.

Gillespie J, Jackson A. *MRI and CT of the brain.* London: Arnold, 2000.

Gocht A, Colmant HJ. Central pontine and extrapontine myelinolysis: a report of 58 cases. *Clin Neuropathol* 1987; **6**:262–70.

Goggans FC. A case of mania secondary to vitamin B12 deficiency. *Am J Psychiatry* 1984; **141**:300–1.

Goldberg A. Acute intermittent porphyria. *Q J Med* 1959; **28**:183–209.

Graham DI, Adams JH, Caird FI *et al.* Acquired hepatocerebral degeneration: report of an atypical case. *J Neurol Neurosurg Psychiatry* 1970; **23**:656–62.

Hadfield MG, Kubal WS. Extrapontine myelinolysis of the basal ganglia without central pontine myelinolysis. *Clin Neuropathol* 1996; **15**:96–100.

Hahn M, Gildemeister OS, Krauss GL *et al.* Effects of new anticonvulsant medications on porphyrin synthesis in cultured liver cells: potential implications for patients with acute porphyria. *Neurology* 1997; **49**:97–106.

Halliday G, Cullen K, Harding A. Neuropathological correlates of memory dysfunction in the Wernicke–Korsakoff syndrome. *Alcohol Alcoholism Suppl* 1994; **2**:247–53.

Handler CE, Perkin GD. Anorexia nervosa and Wernicke's encephalopathy: an underdiagnosed association. *Lancet* 1982; **2**:771–2.

Harper C. Wernicke's encephalopathy: a more common disease than realized: a neuropathological study of 51 cases. *J Neurol Neurosurg Psychiatry* 1979; **42**:226–31.

Harper C. The incidence of Wernicke's encephalopathy in Australia – a neuropathological study of 131 cases. *J Neurol Neurosurg Psychiatry* 1983; **46**:593–8.

Harper CG, Giles M, Finlay-Jones R. Clinical signs in the Wernicke–Korsakoff complex: a retrospective analysis of 131 cases diagnosed at necropsy. *J Neurol Neurosurg Psychiatry* 1986; **49**:341–5.

Harrington MG, MacPherson P, McIntosh WB *et al.* The significance of the incidental finding of basal ganglia calcification on computed tomography. *J Neurol Neurosurg Psychiatry* 1981; **44**:1168–70.

Hart SP, Frier BM. Causes, management and morbidity of acute hypoglycaemia in adults requiring hospital admission. *Q J Med* 1998; **91**:505–10.

Hauw J-J, De Baecque C, Hausser-Hauw C *et al.* Chromatolysis in alcoholic encephalopathies. *Brain* 1988; **111**:843–57.

Hay WJ, Rickards AG, McMenemey WH *et al.* Organic mercurial encephalopathy. *J Neurol Neurosurg Psychiatry* 1963; **26**:199–202.

Healton EH, Savage DG, Brust JCM *et al.* Neurologic aspects of cobalamin deficiency. *Medicine* 1991; **70**:228–45.

Herzlich BC, Schiano TD. Reversal of apparent AIDS dementia complex following treatment with vitamin B12. *J Intern Med* 1993; **233**:495–7.

Hierons R. Changes in the nervous system in acute porphyria. *Brain* 1957; **80**:176–92.

Hirsch S, Dunsworth FA. An interesting case of porphyria. *Am J Psychiatry* 1955; **111**:703.

Huang C-C, Chu N-S, Lu C-S *et al.* Chronic manganese intoxication. *Arch Neurol* 1989; **46**:1104–6.

Huang C-C, Lu C-S, Chu N-S *et al.* Progression after chronic manganese exposure. *Neurology* 1993; **43**:1479–83.

Huang C-C, Chus N-S, Lu C-S *et al.* Cock gait in manganese intoxication. *Mov Disord* 1997; **12**:807–8.

Huang C-C, Chu N-S, Lu C-S *et al.* Long-term progression in chronic manganism: ten years of follow-up. *Neurology* 1998; **50**:698–700.

Huang C-C, Chu N-S, Lu C-S *et al.* The natural history of neurological manganism over 18 years. *Parkinsonism Relat Disord* 2007; **13**:143–5.

Hughes JR, Schreeder MT. EEG in dialysis encephalopathy. *Neurology* 1980; **30**:1148–54.

Hung SC, Hung SH, Tarug DC *et al.* Thiamine deficiency and unexplained neuropathology in hemodialysis and peritoneal dialysis patients. *Am J Kidney Dis* 2001; **38**:941–7.

Hunter D, Russell DS. Focal cerebral and cerebellar atrophy in a human subject due to organic mercury compounds. *J Neurol Neurosurg Psychiatry* 1954; **17**:235–41.

Hurst EW. The lesions produced in the central nervous system by certain organic arsenical compounds. *J Pathol Bacteriol* 1959; **77**:523–34.

Ishii N, Nishihara Y. Pellagra among chronic alcoholics: clinical and pathological study of 20 necropsy cases. *J Neurol Neurosurg Psychiatry* 1981; **44**:209–15.

Ishii N, Nishihara Y. Pellagra encephalopathy among tuberculous patients: its relation to isoniazid therapy. *J Neurol Neurosurg Psychiatry* 1985; **48**:628–34.

Jack RA, Rivers-Bulkeley NT, Rabin PL. Single case study: secondary mania as a presentation of progressive dialysis encephalopathy. *J Nerv Ment Dis* 1983; **171**:193–5.

Jaffe N. Catatonia and hepatic dysfunction. *Dis Nerv Syst* 1967; **28**:606–8.

Jagadha V, Deck JHN, Halliday WL *et al.* Wernicke's encephalopathy in patients on peritoneal dialysis or hemodialysis. *Ann Neurol* 1987; **21**:78–84.

Jenkins CD, Mellins RB. Lead poisoning in children. *Arch Neurol Psychiatry* 1957; **77**:70–8.

Jolliffe N, Bowman K, Rosenblum L *et al.* Nicotinic acid deficiency encephalopathy. *J Am Med Assoc* 1940; **114**:307–9.

Jung SL, Kim BS, Lee KS *et al.* Magnetic resonance imaging and diffusion-weighted imaging changes after hypoglycemic coma. *J Neuroimaging* 2005; **15**:193–6.

Kalimo H, Olsson Y. Effect of severe hypoglycemia on the human brain. *Acta Neurol Scand* 1980; **62**:345–56.

Karp BI, Laureno R. Pontine and extrapontine myelinolysis: a neurologic disorder following rapid correction of hyponatremia. *Medicine* 1993; **72**:359–73.

Kazis AD. Contribution of CT scan to the diagnosis of Fahr's syndrome. *Acta Neurol Scand* 1985; **71**:206–11.

King PH, Bragdon AC. MRI reveals multiple reversible cerebral lesions in an attack of acute intermittent porphyria. *Neurology* 1991; **41**:1300–2.

Kinsella LJ, Green R. 'Anesthesia paresthetica' nitrous oxide-induced cobalamin deficiency. *Neurology* 1995; **45**:1608–10.

Klawans HL, Lipton M, Simon L. Calcification of the basal ganglia as a cause of levodopa-resistant parkinsonism. *Neurology* 1976; **26**:221–5.

Klunemann HH, Ridha BH, Magy L et al. The genetic causes of basal ganglia calcification, dementia, and bone cysts. *DAP12* and *TREM2. Neurology* 2005; **64**:1502–7.

Klos KJ, Ahlskog JE, Kumar N et al. Brain metal concentrations in chronic liver failure patients with pallidal T1 MRI hyperintensity. *Neurology* 2006; **67**:1984–9.

Kobari M, Nogawa S, Sugimoto Y et al. Familial idiopathic brain calcification with autosomal dominant inheritance. *Neurology* 1997; **48**:645–9.

Koller WC, Cochran JW, Klawans HL. Calcification of the basal ganglia: computerized tomography and clinical correlation. *Neurology* 1979; **29**:328–33.

Koller WC, Lyons KE, Truly W. Effect of levodopa treatment for parkinsonism in welders. *Neurology* 2004; **62**:730–3.

Kondo T, Takahashi K, Kohara N et al. Heterogeneity of presenile dementia with bone cysts (Nasu–Hakola disease). *Neurology* 2002; **59**:1105–7.

Kreyberg S, Torvik A, Bjorneboe A et al. Trimethyltin poisoning: report of a case with postmortem examination. *Clin Neuopathol* 1992; **11**:256–9.

Krieger D, Krieger S, Jansen O et al. Manganese and chronic hepatic encephalopathy. *Lancet* 1995; **346**:270–4.

Kurland LT, Faro SN, Siedler H. Minamata disease. *World Neurol* 1960; **1**:370–95.

Kuzminski AM, Del Giacco EJ, Allen RH et al. Effective treatment of cobalamin deficiency with oral cobalamin. *Blood* 1998; **92**:1191–8.

Lam JS, Fong SY, Yiu GC et al. Fahr's disease: a differential diagnosis of frontal lobe syndrome. *Hong Kong Med J* 2007; **13**:75–7.

Lampl C, Yazdi K. Central pontine myelinolysis. *Eur Neurol* 2002; **47**:3–10.

Langworthy OR. Lesions of the central nervous system characteristic of pellagra. *Brain* 1931; **54**:291–302.

Larsen TA, Dunn HG, Jae JE et al. Dystonia and calcification of the basal ganglia. *Neurology* 1985; **35**:533–7.

Lawrence RD, Meyer R, Nevin S. The pathological changes in fatal hypoglycemia. *Q J Med* 1942; **11**:181–201.

Lederman RJ, Henry CE. Progressive dialysis encephalopathy. *Ann Neurol* 1978; **4**:199–204.

Liessens JL, Monstrui J, Vanden Eeckhout E et al. Bismuth encephalopathy. A clinical case and anatomicopathological report of one case. *Acta Neurol* 1978; **78**:301–9.

Lindenbaum J, Healton EB, Savage DG et al. Neuropsychiatric disorders caused by cobalamin deficiency in the absence of anemia or macrocytosis. *N Engl J Med* 1988; **318**:1720–8.

Lopez-Villegas D, Kulisevsky J, Deus J et al. Neuropsychological alterations in patients with computed tomography-detected basal ganglia calcification. *Arch Neurol* 1996; **53**:251–6.

Lu C-S, Huang C-C, Chu N-S et al. Levodopa failure in chronic manganism. *Neurology* 1994; **44**:1600–2.

Lurie LA. Pernicious anemia with mental symptoms: observations on the variable extent and probable duration of central nervous system lesions in four autopsied cases. *Arch Neurol Psychiatry* 1919; **2**:67–109.

Macalpine I, Hunter R. The 'insanity' of King George III: a classic case of porphyria. *BMJ* 1966; **1**:65–71.

Macalpine I, Hunter R, Rimington C. Porphyria in the royal houses of Stuart, Hanover and Prussia: a follow-up study of George III's illness. *BMJ* 1968; **1**:7–8.

MacKeith SA, Meyer A. A death during insulin treatment of schizophrenia; with pathological report. *J Ment Sci* 1939; **85**:96–105.

Malamud N, Skillicorn SA. Relationship between the Wernicke and the Korsakoff syndrome. *Arch Neurol Psychiatry* 1956; **76**:585–96.

Malouf R, Brust JCM. Hypoglycemia: causes, neurological manifestations, and outcome. *Ann Neurol* 1985; **17**:421–30.

Mandoki MW, Sumner GS. Psychiatric manifestations of hereditary coproporphyria in a child. *J Nerv Ment Dis* 1994; **182**:117–18.

Manyam BV, Walters AS, Narla KR. Bilateral striopallidodentate calcinosis: clinical characteristics of patients seen in a registry. *Mov Disord* 2001; **16**:258–64.

Maraganore DM, Folger WN, Swanson JW et al. Movement disorders as sequelae of central pontine myelinolysis: report of three cases. *Mov Disord* 1992; **7**:142–8.

Marcuard SP, Albernaz L, Khazanie PG. Omeprazole therapy causes malabsorption of cyanocobalamin (vitamin B12). *Ann Intern Med* 1994; **120**:211–15.

Margolin D, Hammerstad J, Orwoll E et al. Intracranial calcification in hyperparathyroidism associated with gait apraxia and parkinsonism. *Neurology* 1980; **30**:1005–7.

Marie R-M, Le Biez E, Busson P et al. Nitrous oxide anesthesia-associated myelopathy. *Arch Neurol* 2000; **57**:380–2.

Mathews WB. Familial calcification of the basal ganglia with response to parathormone. *J Neurol Neurosurg Psychiatry* 1957; **20**:172–7.

Matte TD, Proops D, Palazuelos E et al. Acute high-dose lead exposure from beverage contaminated by traditional Mexican pottery. *Lancet* 1994; **344**:1064.

Mawdsley C. Neurological complications of haemodialysis. *Proc R Soc Med* 1972; **65**:871–3.

McKee AC, Winkleman MD, Banker BQ. Central pontine myelinolysis in severely burned patients: relationship to serum hyperosmolality. *Neurology* 1988; **38**:1211–17.

McMillan TM, Jacobson RR, Gross M. Neuropsychology of thallium poisoning. *J Neurol Neurosurg Psychiatry* 1997; **63**:247–50.

Mehta J, Singhal S. Hyperviscosity syndrome in plasma cell dyscrasias. *Semin Thromb Hemost* 2003; **29**:467–471.

Mellins RB, Jenkins CD. Epidemiologic and psychological study of lead poisoning in children. *J Am Med Assoc* 1955; **158**:15–20.

Mena I, court J, Fuenzalida S *et al*. Modification of chronic manganese poisoning. Treatment with L-dopa or 5-OH tryptophan. *N Engl J Med* 1970; **282**:5–10.

Menawat AS, Panwar RB, Kochar DK *et al*. Propranolol in acute intermittent porphyria. *Postgrad Med J* 1979; **55**:546–7.

Menger H, Jorg J. Outcome of central pontine and extrapontine myelinolysis (n= 44). *J Neurol* 1999; **246**:700–5.

Messert B, Orrison WM, Quaglieri CE. Central pontine myelinolysis. *Neurology* 1979; **29**:147–60.

Moersch FP, Kernohan JW. Hypoglycemia: neurologic and neuropathologic studies. *Arch Neurol Psychiatry* 1938; **39**:242–57.

Moore D, House I, Dixon A. Thallium poisoning. Diagnosis may be elusive but alopecia is the clue. *BMJ* 1993; **306**:1527–9.

Morris CE, Heyman A, Pozersky T. Lead encephalopathy caused by ingestion of illicitly distilled whiskey. *Neurology* 1964; **14**:493–9.

Mueller J, Hotson JR, Langston JW. Hyperviscosity-induced dementia. *Neurology* 1983; **33**:101–3.

Nadel AM, Wilson WP. Dialysis encephalopathy: a possible seizure disorder. *Neurology* 1976; **26**:1130–2.

Nagatomo S, Umehara F, Hanada K *et al*. Manganese intoxication during total parenteral nutrition: report of two cases and review of the literature. *J Neurol Sci* 1999; **162**:102–5.

Needleman HL, Shell A, Ballinger D *et al*. The long-term effects of exposure to low doses of lead in childhood: an 11-year follow up report. *N Engl J Med* 1990; **322**:83–8.

Norenberg MD, Leslie KO, Robertson AS. Association between rise in serum sodium and central pontine myelinolysis. *Ann Neurol* 1982; **11**:128–35.

Nyland H, Skre H. Cerebral calcinosis with late onset encephalopathy. *Acta Neurol Scand* 1977; **56**:309–25.

O'Carroll RE, Moffoot A, Ebmeir KP *et al*. Korsakoff's syndrome, cognition and clonidine. *Psychol Med* 1993; **23**:341–7.

O'Carroll RE, Moffoot APR, Ebmeier KP *et al*. Effects of fluvoxamine on cognitive functioning in the alcoholic Korsakoff syndrome. *Psychopharmacology* 1994; **116**:85–8.

O'Carroll RE, Masterton G, Dougall N *et al*. The neuropsychiatric sequelae of mercury poisoning: the Mad Hatter's disease revisited. *Br J Psychiatry* 1995; **167**:95–8.

Ogershok PR, Rahman A, Nestor S *et al*. Wernicke encephalopathy in nonalcoholic patients. *Am J Med Sci* 2002; **323**:107–11.

O'Hare JA, Callaghan NM, Murnaghan DJ. Dialysis encephalopathy. Clinical, electroencephalographic, and interventional aspects. *Medicine* 1983; **62**:129–41.

Oliveira JR, Spiteri E, Sobrio MJ *et al*. Genetic heterogeneity in familial idiopathic basal ganglia calcification (Fahr disease). *Neurology* 2004; **63**:2165–7.

Ong JP, Aggarwal A, Krieger D *et al*. Correlation between ammonia levels and the severity of hepatic encephalopathy. *Am J Med* 2003; **114**:188–93.

Ostling S, Andreasson LA, Skoog I. Basal ganglia calcification and psychotic symptoms in the very old. *Int J Geriatr Psychiatry* 2003; **18**:983–7.

Pacchetti C, Cristina S, Nappi G. Reversible chorea and focal dystonia in vitamin B12 deficiency. *N Engl J Med* 2002; **347**:295.

Palardy J, Havrankova J, Lepage R *et al*. Blood glucose measurements during symptomatic episodes in patients with suspected postprandial hypoglycemia. *N Engl J Med* 1989; **321**:1421–5.

Paredes A, Jones H. Psychopathology of acute intermittent porphyria: case report. *J Nerv Ment Dis* 1959; **129**:291–301.

Paul F, Meencke H-J. Levetiracetam in focal epilepsy and hepatic porphyria: a case report. *Epilepsia* 2004; **45**:559–60.

Paulson GW, Martin EW, Mojzisik C *et al*. Neurologic complications of gastric partitioning. *Arch Neurol* 1985; **42**:675–7.

Pavy MD, Murphy PL, Virella G. Paraprotein-induced hyperviscosity. A reversible cause of stroke. *Postgrad Med* 1980; **68**:109–12.

Pentschew A. Morphology and morphogenesis of lead encephalopathy. *Acta Neuropathol* 1965; **5**:133–60.

Peterson H, Swanson AG. Acute encephalopathy occurring during hemodialysis. *Arch Int Med* 1964; **113**:877–80.

Pierce LB. Pellagra: report of a case. *Am J Psychiatry* 1924; **81**:237–43.

Pincus JH, Reynolds EH, Glaser GH. Subacute combined system degeneration with folate deficiency. *J Am Med Assoc* 1972; **221**:496–7.

Powell EE, Pender MP, Chalk JB *et al*. Improvement in chronic hepatocerebral degeneration following liver transplantation. *Gastroenterology* 1990; **98**:1079–82.

Powers JM, Rosenblatt DS, Schmidt RE *et al*. Neurological and neuropathologic heterogeneity in two brothers with cobalamin C deficiency. *Ann Neurol* 2001; **49**:396–400.

Price BH, Mesulam M-M. Behavioral manifestation of central pontine myelinolysis. *Arch Neurol* 1987; **44**:671–3.

Price WA, Zimmer B, Conway R *et al*. Insulin-induced factitious hypoglycemic coma. *Gen Hosp Psychiatry* 1986; **8**:291–3.

Rajan S, Wallache JI, Brodkin KI *et al*. Response of elevated methylmalonic acid to three dose levels of oral cobalamin in older adults. *J Am Geriatr Soc* 2002; **50**:1789–95.

Rapaport MJ. Pellagra in a patient with anorexia nervosa. *Arch Dermatol* 1985; **121**:255–7.

Raskin NH, Fishman RA. Neurologic disorders in renal failure. *N Engl J Med* 1976; **294**:143–8, 204–10.

Raskin NH, Bredesen D, Ehrenfeld WK *et al*. Periodic confusion caused by congenital extrahepatic portocaval shunt. *Neurology* 1984; **34**:666–9.

Read AE, Laidlaw J, Sherlock S. Neuropsychiatric complications of portocaval anastamosis. *Lancet* 1961; **1**:961–4.

Reed D, Crawley J, Faro SN *et al*. Thallotoxicosis. *J Am Med Assoc* 1963; **183**:516–22.

Reynolds EH, Rothfeld P, Pincus JH. Neurological disease associated with folate deficiency. *BMJ* 1973; **2**:398–400.

Rich LM, Caine MR, Findling JW *et al*. Hypoglycemic coma in anorexia nervosa. Case report and review of the literature. *Arch Int Med* 1990; **150**:894–5.

Richmond J. Wernicke's encephalopathy associated with digitalis poisoning. *Lancet* 1959; **1**:344–5.

Ropper AH. Accelerated neuropathy of renal failure. *Arch Neurol* 1993; **50**:536–9.

Rowland LP. Acute intermittent porphyria: search for an enzymatic defect with implications for neurology and psychiatry. *Dis Nerv Syst* 1961; **22**(suppl.):1–12.

Russell DS. Changes in the central nervous system following arsphenamine medication. *J Pathol* 1937; **45**:357–66.

Russell JSR, Batten FE, Collier J. Subacute combined degeneration of the spinal cord. *Brain* 1900; **23**:39–110.

Rustam H, Hamri T. Methyl mercury poisoning in Iraq. *Brain* 1974; **97**:499–510.

Ruzek KA, Campeau NG, Miller GM. Early diagnosis of central pontine myelinolysis with diffusion-weighted imaging. *AJNR* 2004; **25**:210–13.

Sahin HA, Gurvit IH, Bilgic B et al. Therapeutic effects of an acetylcholinesterase inhibitor (donepezil) on memory in Wernicke-Korsakoff's disease. *Clin Neuropharmacol* 2002; **25**:16–20.

Saiki M, Saiki S, Saiki K et al. Neurological deficits are associated with increased brain calcinosis, hypoperfusion and hypometabolism in idiopathic basal ganglia calcification. *Mov Disord* 2007; **22**:1027–30.

Scarlett JA, Mako ME, Rubenstein AH et al. Factitious hypoglycemia: diagnosis by measurement of serum C-peptide immunoreactivity and insulin-binding antibodies. *N Engl J Med* 1977; **297**:1029–32.

Scheiber SC, Ziesat H. Brief communication: clinical and psychological test findings in cerebral dyspraxia associated with hemodialysis. *J Nerv Ment Dis* 1976; **162**:212–14.

Schottenfeld RS, Cullen MR. Organic affective illness associated with lead intoxication. *Am J Psychiatry* 1984; **141**:1425–6.

Seiser A, Schwarz S, Aichinger-Steiner MM et al. Parkinsonism and dystonia in central pontine and extrapontine myelinolysis. *J Neurol Neurosurg Psychiatry* 1998; **65**:119–21.

Seltzer B, Benson DF. The temporal pattern of retrograde amnesia in Korsakoff's disease. *Neurology* 1974; **24**:527–30.

Serdaru M, Hausser-Hauw C, Laplane D et al. The clinical spectrum of alcoholic pellagra encephalopathy. A retrospective analysis of 22 cases studied pathologically. *Brain* 1988; **111**:829–42.

Servin-Abad L, Tzakis A, Schiff ER et al. Acquired hepatocerebral degeneration in a patient with HCV cirrhosis: complete resolution with subsequent recurrence after liver transplantation. *Liver Transpl* 2006; **12**:1161–5.

Sherlock S. Fulminant hepatic failure. *Adv Intern Med* 1993; **38**:245–67.

Sherrard DJ, Walker JV, Boykin JL. Precipitation of dialysis dementia by deferoxamine treatment of aluminum-related bone disease. *Am J Kidney Dis* 1988; **12**:12–30.

Shimomura T, Mori E, Hirono N et al. Development of Wernicke–Korsakoff syndrome after long intervals following gastrectomy. *Arch Neurol* 1998; **55**:1242–5.

Shintani S, Tsuruoka S, Shiigai T. Hypoglycemic hemiplegia: a repeat SPECT study. *J Neurol Neurosurg Psychiatry* 1993; **56**:700–1.

Shirabe T, Irie K, Uchida M. Autopsy cases of aluminum encephalopathy. *Neuropathology* 2002; **22**:206–10.

Shor-Posner G, Morgan R, Wilkie F et al. Plasma cobalamin levels affect information processing speed in a longitudinal study of HIV-1 disease. *Arch Neurol* 1995; **52**:195–8.

Singh S, Kumar A. Wernicke encephalopathy after obesity surgery. A systematic review. *Neurology* 2007; **68**:807–11.

Slyter H. Idiopathic hypoparathyroidism presenting as dementia. *Neurology* 1979; **29**:393–4.

Smith JF, McLaurin RL, Nichols JP et al. Studies in cerebral oedema and cerebral swelling. 1. The changes in lead encephalopathy in children compared with those in alkyl tin poisoning in animals. *Brain* 1960; **83**:411–24.

Smith LH. Mental and neurologic changes in pernicious anemia. *Arch Neurol Psychiatry* 1929; **22**:551–7.

Smits MG, Gabreels FJ, Thijssen HO et al. Progressive idiopathic strio-pallido-dentate calcinosis (Fahr's disease) with autosomal recessive inheritance. Report of three siblings. *Eur Neurol* 1983; **22**:58–64.

Snyder RD. The involuntary movements of chronic mercury poisoning. *Arch Neurol* 1972; **26**:379–81.

Spivak JL, Jackson DL. Pellagra: an analysis of 18 patients and a review of the literature. *Johns Hopkins Med J* 1977; **140**:295–309.

Stein JA, Tschudy DP. Acute intermittent porphyria. A clinical and biochemical study of 46 patients. *Medicine* 1970; **49**:1–16.

Sterns RH, Riggs JE, Schochet SS. Osmotic demyelination syndrome following correction of hyponatremia. *N Engl J Med* 1986; **314**:1535–42.

Stojsavljevic N, Levic Z, Drulovic J et al. A 44-month clinical-brain MRI follow-up in a patient with B12 deficiency. *Neurology* 1997; **49**:878–81.

Stracciari A, Guarino M, Pazzaglia P et al. Acquired hepatocerebral degeneration: full recovery after liver transplantation. *J Neurol Neurosurg Psychiatry* 2001; **70**:136–70.

Strachan RW, Henderson JG. Dementia and folate deficiency. *Q J Med* 1967; **36**:189–204.

Suarez JI, Cohen ML, Larkin J et al. Acute intermittent porphyria: clinicopathologic correlation. Report of a case and review of the literature. *Neurology* 1997; **48**:1678–83.

Sullivan AA, Chervin RD, Albin RL. Parkinsonism after correction of hyponatremia with radiological central pontine myelinolysis and changes in the basal ganglia. *J Clin Neurosci* 2000; **7**:256–9.

Summerskill WHJ, Davidson EA, Sherlock S et al. The neuropsychiatric syndrome associated with hepatic cirrhosis and extensive portal collateral circulation. *Q J Med* 1956; **25**:245–66.

Supino-Viterbo V, Sicard C, Risvegliato M et al. Toxic encephalopathy due to ingestion of bismuth salts: clinical and EEG studies of 45 patients. *J Neurol Neurosurg Psychiatry* 1977; **40**:748–52.

Sweeney VP, Pathak MA, Asbury AK et al. Acute intermittent porphyria. Increased ALA-synthetase activity during an acute attack. *Brain* 1970; **93**:369–80.

Tambyah PA, Ong BKC, Lee KO. Reversible parkinsonism and asymptomatic hypocalcemia with basal ganglia calcification from hypoparathyroidism 26 years after thyroid surgery. *Am J Med* 1993; **94**:444–5.

Tatum WO, Zachariah SB. Gabapentin treatment of seizures in acute intermittent porphyria. *Neurology* 1995; **45**:1216–17.

Thomas PK, Hollinrake K, Lascelles RG *et al.* The polyneuropathy of chronic renal failure. *Brain* 1971; **94**:761–80.

Thompson C, Dent J, Saxby P. Effect of thallium poisoning on intellectual function. *Br J Psychiatry* 1988; **153**:396–9.

Tokuomi H, Uchino M, Imamura S *et al.* Minamata disease (organic mercury poisoning): neuroradiologic and electrophysiologic studies. *Neurology* 1982; **32**:1369–75.

Torgovnik J, Arsura EL, Lala D. Cytomegalovirus ventriculoencephalitis presenting as Wernicke's encephaloathy-like syndrome. *Neurology* 2000; **55**:1910–13.

Tomita I, Satoh H, Satoh A *et al.* Extrapontine myelinolysis presenting with parkinsonism as a sequel of rapid correction of hyponatremia. *J Neurol Neurosurg Psychiatry* 1997; **62**:422–3.

Trautner RJ, Cummings JL, Read SL *et al.* Idiopathic basal ganglia calcification and organic mood disorders. *Am J Psychiatry* 1988; **145**:350–3.

Tyler RH. Neurological complications of dialysis, transplantation and other forms of treatment in chronic uremia. *Neurology* 1965; **15**:1081–8.

Tyler RH. Neurologic disorders in renal failure. *Am J Med* 1968; **44**:734–48.

Ueki Y, Isozaki E, Miyazaki Y *et al.* Clinical and neuroradiological improvement in chronic acquired hepatocerebral degeneration after branched-chain amino acid therapy. *Acta Neurol Scand* 2002; **106**:113–16.

Victor M, Yakovlev PI. Korsakoff's psychic disorder in conjunction with peripheral neuritis: a translation of Korsakoff's original article with brief comments on the author and his contribution to clinical medicine. *Neurology* 1955; **5**:394–406.

Victor M, Adams RD, Cole M. The acquired 'non-Wilsonian' type of chronic hepatocerebral degeneration. *Medicine* 1965; **44**:345–96.

Victor M, Adams RD, Collins GH. *The Wernicke–Korsakoff syndrome*. Oxford: Blackwell, 1971.

Vortmeyer AO, Hagel C, Laas R. Haemorrhagic thiamine deficient encephalopathy following prolonged parenteral nutrition. *J Neurol Neurosurg Psychiatry* 1992; **55**:826–9.

Wainwright AP, Kox WJ, House IM *et al.* Clinical features and therapy of acute thallium poisoning. *Q J Med* 1988; **69**:939–44.

Wallis WE, Willoughby E, Baker P. Coma in the Wernicke–Korsakoff syndrome. *Lancet* 1978; **2**:400–1.

Wallis WE, Donaldson I, Scott RS *et al.* Hypoglycemia masquerading as cerebrovascular disease (hypoglycemic hemiplegia). *Ann Neurol* 1985; **18**:510–12.

Walters RJ, Fox NC, Crum WR *et al.* Hemodialysis and cerebral oedema. *Nephron* 2001; **87**:143–7.

Watson JN, Kiloh LG, Osselton JW *et al.* The electroencephalogram in pernicious anemia and subacute combined degeneration of the spinal cord. *Electroencephalogr Clin Neurophysiol* 1954; **6**:45–64.

Weidauer S, Nichtweiss M, Lanfermann H *et al.* Wernicke encephalopathy: MR findings and clinical presentation. *Eur Radiol* 2003; **13**:1001–9.

Weisman DC, Yaari R, Hansn LA *et al.* Density of the brain, decline of the mind. An atypical case of Fahr disease. *Arch Neurol* 2007; **64**:756–7.

Whitfield CL, Ch'ien LT, Whitehead JD. Lead encephalopathy in adults. *Am J Med* 1972; **52**:289–98.

Winkelman MD, Ricanti ES. Dialysis encephalopathy: neuropathologic aspects. *Hum Pathol* 1986; **17**:82–33.

Wright DG, Laureno R, Victor M. Pontine and extrapontine myelinolysis. *Brain* 1979; **102**:361–85.

Wszolek ZK, Baba Y, Mackenzie IR *et al.* Autosomal dominant dystonia-plus with cerebral calcifications. *Neurology* 2006; **67**:620–5.

Wu R-M, Chang Y-C, Chiu H-C. Acute triphenyltin intoxication: a case report. *J Neurol Neurosurg Psychiatry* 1990; **53**:356–7.

Yamada M, Ohno S, Okayasu I *et al.* Chronic manganese poisoning: a neuropathological study with determination of managanese distribution in the brain. *Acta Neuropathol* 1986; **70**:273–8.

Yoshida S, Tajika T, Yamasaki N *et al.* Dialysis disequilibrium syndrome in neurosurgical patients. *Neurosurgery* 1987; **20**:716–21.

Yoshida Y, Akanuma J, Tochikubo S *et al.* Slowly progressive dystonia following central pontine and extrapontine myelinolysis. *Intern Med* 2000; **39**:956–60.

Zaki I, Millard L. Pellagra complicated Crohn's disease. *Postgrad Med J* 1995; **71**:496–7.

Zivin I. The neurological and psychiatric aspects of hypoglycemia. *Dis Nerv Syst* 1970; **31**:604–7.

Zuccoli G, Gallucci M, Capellades J *et al.* Wernicke encephalopathy: MR findings at clinical presentation in twenty-six alcoholic and non-alcoholic patients. *AJNR* 2007; **28**:1328–31.

14

Infectious and related disorders

14.1 ACQUIRED IMMUNODEFICIENCY SYNDROME (AIDS)

AIDS may affect the nervous system in a variety of ways. Cerebral involvement may manifest with an early mononucleosis-like syndrome, and, later, with dementia or seizures; there may also be a myelopathy with paraparesis and a peripheral sensorimotor polyneuropathy. Fatigue and depression are also common, and, rarely, mania may be seen.

Clinical features

Although nervous system involvement, such as AIDS dementia, may rarely be the presenting symptom of AIDS (Navia and Price 1987), in most cases patients already have other evidence of the illness, such as generalized lymphadenopathy, constitutional symptoms, thrush, diarrhea, shingles, cytopenia (including thrombocytopenia) Kaposi's sarcoma, and *Pneumocystis* pneumonia.

Early on in the infection, often concurrent with seroconversion, patients may develop a mononucleosis-like syndrome, which may be accompanied by an aseptic meningitis. Cranial nerve palsies, particularly affecting the fifth, seventh, and eighth nerves, may accompany the meningitis, and there may rarely also be an encephalitis with delirium (McArthur 1987; Malouf *et al.* 1990).

AIDS dementia typically appears about 10 years after the initial infection, generally only when the CD4+ count has fallen below 200 cells/mm^3 Clinically speaking (Navia *et al.* 1986a; Price *et al.* 1988), the dementia is of subacute or gradual onset and is characterized by apathy, poor concentration, and forgetfulness; in some cases there may be agitation, delusions, and visual hallucinations. Accompanying the dementia one often sees dysarthria, ataxia, and long-tract signs, such as hyper-reflexia and Babinski signs; in one case, the dementia was accompanied by chorea (Pardo *et al.* 1998). With progression, there may be muteness, confusion, seizures, and myoclonus (Maher *et al.* 1997).

Seizures occur in a small minority of patients (Pascual-Sedano *et al.* 1999; Wong *et al.* 1990), and these may be due to human immunodeficiency virus (HIV) infection itself or to opportunistic infections (e.g., toxoplasmosis) or metabolic abnormalities (e.g., hypomagnesemia or hypocalcemia). Although grand mal seizures are most common, both simple partial and complex partial seizures may also occur.

The spinal cord may be affected by a vacuolar myelopathy (Navia *et al.* 1986b; Sharer *et al.* 1986), with paraparesis and sensory ataxia; within the peripheral nervous system there may be a sensorimotor polyneuropathy (de la Monte *et al.* 1988; Morgello *et al.* 2004), which may be quite painful.

Fatigue is common in AIDS and may be debilitating. Depression is likewise common; however, it is unclear whether this syndrome occurs as a direct effect of central nervous system involvement or rather reflects other factors. Mania, although rare in AIDS, may, by contrast, occur directly as a result of the infection (Kieburtz *et al.* 1991).

Serologic testing generally becomes positive within 2–12 weeks of the initial infection and is inevitably positive by 6 months; thus, in patients with AIDS dementia, the

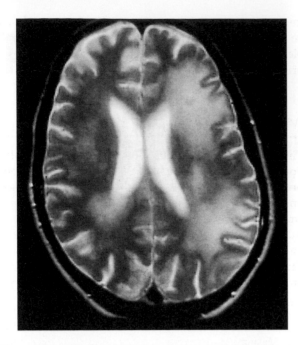

Figure 14.1 This T2-weighted magnetic resonance imaging scan shows both patchy and confluent areas of increased signal intensity in the centrum semiovale of a patient with AIDS dementia. (Reproduced from Gillespie and Jackson 2000.)

enzyme-linked immunosorbent assay (ELISA) test will be positive, as will the confirmatory Western blot test.

Magnetic resonance imaging (MRI) in AIDS dementia generally reveals a degree of cortical atrophy and ventricular dilation, and there may also be multiple areas, some confluent, of increased signal intensity in the centrum semiovale on T2-weighted scans (Dooneief *et al.* 1992; Navia *et al.* 1986a), as illustrated in Figure 14.1.

The cerebrospinal fluid (CSF) in AIDS dementia generally displays a mild mononuclear pleocytosis, a mildly elevated total protein level, an increased IgG index, and oligoclonal bands.

Course

In the natural course of events, AIDS dementia is relentlessly progressive, and death usually occurs within 3–6 months (Bouwman *et al.* 1998).

Etiology

AIDS is caused by infection with HIV. This RNA virus is found in blood, semen, vaginal fluid, breast milk, and colostrum, and may be spread via all these fluids. In the United States, spread occurs most commonly with homosexual contact, in particular anal intercourse; however, as the virus spreads among females, it is likely that the most common mode of transmission in the United States will eventually become heterosexual contact, as is the case in Africa. With improved screening of blood products,

transfusion-related transmission is now becoming quite rare, but blood-borne transmission remains a significant problem among intravenous drug users who fail to sterilize their needles. Although the virus is also found in saliva, urine, and tears, there is as yet no convincing evidence that it can be spread by these.

HIV gains attachment to cells such as lymphocytes, monocytes, and macrophages by virtue of the CD4 molecule found on the cell membrane (Pantaleo *et al.* 1993). Once inside the cell, the enzyme reverse transcriptase catalyzes the reverse transcription of genomic viral RNA into DNA, which eventually becomes inserted into the chromosomes of the host cell. With cell activation, this inserted DNA is copied, which is eventually followed by the production of mature HIV virus particles.

Subsequent to infection there is an intense viremia followed by a vigorous cellular and humoral immune response, such that, in most cases, the viremia is substantially contained within about 3 months. The virus, however, is not eradicated but rather continues to reproduce within lymphoid tissue. Tragically, the cell most likely to be infected is the CD4+ T-lymphocyte, with the result that, over many years, there is a gradual loss of these 'helper' lymphocytes and the body's defenses are subverted to the point at which a significant viremia again occurs. In addition, with the loss of these CD4+ helper lymphocytes, opportunistic infections begin to appear.

It is not entirely clear how HIV gains entry into the central nervous system. One theory holds that free viruses pass directly through a disrupted blood–brain barrier; another, known as the 'Trojan horse' theory, suggests that infected peripheral monocytes carry the virus with them as they cross the blood–brain barrier. Although at autopsy approximately 90 percent of patients have evidence of HIV within the central nervous system, the frequency of AIDS dementia is not as high, ranging from 15 percent (McArthur *et al.* 1993) to 65 percent (Navia *et al.* 1986a). Once inside the central nervous system HIV is found primarily in monocytes, macrophages, and microglia: although astrocytes and neurons may also be infected, this is far less prominent. In cases of AIDS dementia, the primary pathologic changes include diffuse myelin pallor (in some cases with vacuolization), scattered microglial nodules, and multinucleated giant cells (Glass *et al.* 1993; Gray *et al.* 1988; Navia *et al.* 1986b); there may also be a relatively minor degree of neuronal loss within the cerebral cortex (Wiley *et al.* 1991). Of note, in patients with AIDS dementia, definite microscopic pathology may be lacking, and it is hypothesized that the dementia in these cases, and perhaps also in those with definite pathology, results from the toxic effects of cytokines released by inflammatory cells (Glass *et al.* 1993).

Differential diagnosis

Opportunistic central nervous system infections are very common and may cause dementia, delirium, focal signs, or seizures. These include toxoplasmosis, cytomegalovirus (CMV) encephalitis, progressive multifocal leukoencephalopathy, mycoses (e.g., candidiasis), tuberculosis, varicella-zoster encephalitis or vasculopathy, herpes simplex encephalitis, and neurosyphilis. With regard to the possibility of neurosyphilis, it must be kept in mind that, in patients with AIDS, treatment of primary syphilis with benzathine penicillin may not prevent the development of neurosyphilis. Primary central nervous system lymphoma (Hochberg and Miller 1988) and, rarely, Kaposi's sarcoma may also appear as space-occupying lesions.

For unclear reasons, vitamin B12 deficiency is not uncommon in patients with AIDS (Herzlich and Schiano 1993), and as it may produce a dementia or a spinal cord syndrome similar to that of vacuolar myelopathy it should always be checked for (Beach *et al.* 1992).

Concurrent drug addiction (e.g., to cocaine) and alcoholism are also common, and these must be attended to. With regard to alcoholism, special attention must be paid to such alcohol-related disorders as Wernicke's encephalopathy and alcoholic dementia.

Treatment

The advent of highly active antiretroviral treatment (HAART) has revolutionized the treatment of AIDS, and may lead to stabilization or improvement of its central nervous system manifestations. Given the complex and rapidly evolving nature of antiretroviral treatment, referral to a specialist is always essential.

The general treatment of dementia is discussed in Section 5.1 In addition to the measures noted there, there is some evidence that selegiline may improve cognitive performance (Dana Consortium 1998); a dose no higher than 10 mg should be used to avoid the risk of a hypertensive crisis. If antipsychotics are required, either for the dementia or for delirium, low doses are used as patients with AIDS seem particularly likely to develop extrapyramidal side-effects (Hriso *et al.* 1991); in this regard, second-generation agents, such as quetiapine or risperidone, are preferable to the first-generation agents such as haloperidol. Anti-epileptic drugs may be used for seizures; although phenytoin is often used, side-effects may dictate one of the other agents discussed in Section 7.3. Painful peripheral neuropathy may respond to gabapentin (Hahn *et al.* 2004), lamotrigine (Simpson *et al.* 2003), or smoked cannabis (Abrams *et al.* 2007), but amitriptyline does not appear to be effective (Kieburtz *et al.* 1998). Fatigue may respond to treatment with methylphenidate (Breitbart *et al.* 2001); however, this should not be given to patients who might abuse it. Depression may be treated with antidepressants such as fluoxetine (Rabkin *et al.* 1999).

All patients should be reminded to practice 'safe sex', with an emphasis on latex condoms and the use of nonoxynol-9 spermicide. Patients should also be reminded that AIDS may be spread via fellatio and cunnilingus. All intravenous drug users, if unable to stop, should be instructed to sterilize their needles with household bleach. Blood and organ donation are prohibited, as is breastfeeding.

14.2 CYTOMEGALOVIRUS ENCEPHALITIS

The great majority of adults show evidence of prior infection with cytomegalovirus (CMV), and in immunocompromised patients, for example those with AIDS or those undergoing transplantation, the virus may reactivate and, among other syndromes, produce a delirium. Autopsy studies have demonstrated evidence of CMV infection of the central nervous system in approximately one-third of patients with AIDS, making it one of the most common opportunistic infections seen in this condition (Vintners *et al.* 1989).

Clinical features

The delirium typically presents subacutely and is of variable severity (Berman and Kim 1994; Holland *et al.* 1994); in some cases, however, the onset may be fulminant and the delirium quite severe, and in such cases there are often signs of brainstem involvement, such as nystagmus, ophthalmoplegia, and ataxia (Kalayjian *et al.* 1993; Torgovnik *et al.* 2000). Some patients may also have cord involvement or a peripheral neuropathy.

In most cases, immunocompromised patients with CMV encephalitis will also have evidence of systemic infection, such as retinitis, esophagitis, gastritis, colitis, hepatitis, and, importantly, adrenalitis, which may cause adrenocortical insufficiency.

In most cases the CD4+ count is below 100 cells/mm^3.

T2-weighted or fluid-attenuated inversion recovery (FLAIR) MR scanning may reveal patchy, confluent areas of increased signal intensity both in the centrum semiovale and in a periventricular distribution.

The CSF may be normal or may display a mild lymphocytic pleocytosis and a mildly elevated total protein. Polymerase chain reaction (PCR) assay for CMV will generally be positive.

Before leaving this section on clinical features, it is appropriate to note that CMV infection of the central nervous system may rarely occur in immunocompetent adults. In such cases there may be either a meningitis (Causey 1976) or an encephalitis (Studahl *et al.* 1994), occurring in the context of a mononucleosis-like syndrome.

Course

In severe cases of fulminant onset, death may occur within weeks or months.

Etiology

In most cases there are widespread microglial nodules and inclusion-positive cytomegalic cells (Morgello *et al.* 1987); in those cases characterized by a fulminant delirium there is marked periventricular inflammation, with, in some cases, necrotic changes (Berman and Kim 1994; Kalayjian *et al.* 1993).

Differential diagnosis

Both AIDS dementia and other opportunistic infections must be considered; fulminant cases with brainstem signs may mimic Wernicke's encephalopathy.

Treatment

The general treatment of dementia and delirium are discussed in Sections 5.1 and 5.3 respectively. Ganciclovir and foscarnet are typically prescribed; however, in some cases CMV encephalitis has occurred despite ongoing treatment with these agents (Berman and Kim 1994).

14.3 PROGRESSIVE MULTIFOCAL LEUKOENCEPHALOPATHY

Progressive multifocal leukoencephalopathy occurs secondary to an opportunistic infection of the central nervous system by the JC virus (Padgett *et al.* 1971). Multifocal areas of demyelinization occur, producing various focal signs and, in some, a dementia. In almost all cases patients have depressed cell-mediated immunity, most commonly due to AIDS, in which 2–5 percent of patients are afflicted.

Clinical features

The onset is typically subacute, generally over approximately 2 weeks. In most cases, patients present with a slowly progressive focal sign, such as hemianopia, aphasia, apraxia, hemisensory loss, or hemiplegia (Astrom *et al.* 1958; Krupp *et al.* 1985; Richardson 1961); rarer focal findings such as Balint's syndrome (Ayuso-Peralta *et al.* 1994) have also been reported. Over time, these initially unilateral deficits become bilateral, and many patients then go on to develop a personality change, a dementia or, rarely, a delirium. Seizures may occur in up to 20 percent of patients and may be simple partial, complex partial, or grand mal (Lima *et al.* 2006; Moulignier *et al.* 1995). Rarely, progressive multifocal leukoencephalopathy may present with a dementia (Sellal *et al.* 1996; Zunt *et al.* 1997), delirium (Davies *et al.* 1973), or personality change (Astrom *et al.* 1958). Cerebellar signs may occur but are not common (Parr *et al.* 1979). Other rare signs include quadriparesis

secondary to brainstem involvement (Kastrup *et al.* 2002), and dystonia (Factor *et al.* 2003), chorea (Piccolo *et al.* 1999), or parkinsonism (Bhatia *et al.* 1996).

The electroencephalogram (EEG) may show diffuse or focal slowing.

Magnetic resonance scanning (Guilleux *et al.* 1986; Kuker *et al.* 2006) will reveal one or more focal lesions, generally in the subcortical white matter. On T1-weighted imaging these display decreased signal intensity, and on FLAIR or T2-weighted imaging, increased signal intensity is seen. Diffusion-weighted imaging may demonstrate mild increased signal intensity in some cases and, again, in some cases there may be enhancement with gadolinium (Huang *et al.* 2007).

The CSF, although characteristically normal, may occasionally reveal a mild lymphocytic pleocytosis. The PCR assay for JC virus is generally, but not always, positive (Hensen *et al.* 1991; Koralnik *et al.* 1999). Serum testing for antibodies to JC virus is not helpful, given, as noted below, that most adults will be positive. In doubtful cases brain biospy may be required.

Course

In the natural course of events the disease is generally relentlessly progressive, with death occurring after about 4 months on average. Rarely the course may stretch out for years, and even more rarely there may be spontaneous remissions (Price *et al.* 1983).

Etiology

Approximately 80 percent of the adult population of the United States has latent infection with the JC virus. In a very small minority of patients with depressed cell-mediated immunity, this virus reactivates and spreads to the brain. Although by far the most common cause of immunoincompetence in these patients is AIDS, progressive multifocal leukoencephalopathy has also been noted in patients with Hodgkin's disease, other lymphomas, leukemia, other cancers, tuberculosis, sarcoidosis, systemic lupus erythematosus (Krupp *et al.* 1985), and in patients undergoing therapeutic immunosuppression after transplantation (Sponzilli *et al.* 1975). Progressive multifocal leukoencephalopathy may also, albeit rarely, occur in patients treated with natalizumab (Yousry *et al.* 2006). Finally, it also appears that, very rarely, progressive multifocal leukoencephalopathy may occur in otherwise healthy individuals (Fermaglich *et al.* 1970; Guillaume *et al.* 2000).

Within the central nervous system, oligodendrocytes and, to a lesser degree, astrocytes are infected by the JC virus. With destruction of oligodendrocytes, demyelinization with only relative axonal sparing occurs, and foci of demyelinization begin to appear. Within and surrounding these foci there is a variable, and typically quite slight, degree of inflammation. At least initially, these foci are generally few in number and confined to one hemisphere; most commonly they are seen in the subcortical white matter and the centrum semiovale; however, rarely they may be prominent in the cerebellar white matter or the brainstem. Over time, the foci increase in size and number, and bilateral involvement occurs.

Differential diagnosis

In patients with AIDS, consideration must be given to AIDS dementia and to other opportunistic infections, such as CMV or toxoplasmosis, and to primary central nervous system lymphoma.

Treatment

No specific treatment is available. In patients with AIDS it is clear that treatment with HAART slows the progression of the disease. The general treatment of dementia is discussed in Section 5.1.

14.4 ARBOVIRUS MENINGOENCEPHALITIS

Viruses transmitted by arthropods are known as arboviruses, a term derived from the fact that they are all *arthropod borne*. In North America, there are seven arboviruses known to cause meningoencephalitis, including six mosquito-borne viruses (eastern equine, western equine, Venezualan, St. Louis, La Crosse, and the newest member, West Nile) and one tick-borne virus (Powassan virus). Most cases occur in the late summer and early fall, when mosquitoes are most active. Mention should also be made of Japanese encephalitis, which, although not endemic in North America, is a very common cause of meningoencephalitis in the Far East (Lewis *et al.* 1947; Solomon *et al.* 2000, 2002) and may be contracted by travellers there.

Clinical features

The onset is typically acute, over a matter of days or, exceptionally, merely hours. Patients present with delirium, fever, and, typically, meningeal signs such as headache, stiff neck, and photophobia. Seizures, focal signs, and abnormal movements may or may not occur, and some patients may develop a syndrome of inappropriate antidiuretic hormone (ADH) secretion. Patients may progress to stupor or coma. Although distinguishing among the various pathogens on clinical grounds is difficult, some features may be helpful: St. Louis encephalitis may be marked by a coarse tremor (Wasay *et al.* 2000); West Nile encephalitis by a rash, flaccid paralysis, and cranial nerve palsies (Davis *et al.* 2006); and Japanese virus by parkinsonism (Pradhan *et al.* 1999) or dystonia (Kalita and Misra 2000).

The peripheral white blood cell count is typically elevated.

Magnetic resonance scanning may be normal early on; however, eventually both T2-weighted and FLAIR imaging will reveal areas of increased signal intensity, which may be seen in the thalami, basal ganglia, and the cortex.

The CSF may be under increased pressure. The white blood cell count is typically increased. Early on, polymorphonuclear cells may predominate; however, over time the pleocytosis becomes lymphocytic. The total protein is increased but the glucose is normal. Both PCR assay and assays for specific IgM antibodies are available for all of the arboviruses.

The EEG typically shows generalized slowing, at times with focal predominances; in some cases interictal epileptiform discharges may be present.

Course

The mortality rate varies from as little as 1 percent for La Crosse virus to close to 50 percent for eastern equine encephalitis. For those who survive, the encephalitis tends to run its course within a matter of a few weeks, sometimes longer. A minority of patients will be left with sequelae, such as dementia, personality change, or a persistence of any focal signs or abnormal movements seen during the acute illness (Herzon *et al.* 1957; Przelomski *et al.* 1988; Smardel *et al.* 1958); in this regard, post-encephalitic parkinsonism has been noted after western equine encephalitis (Mulder *et al.* 1951; Schultz *et al.* 1977) and dementia after Japanese encephalitis (Solomon *et al.* 2002), which, in some cases, may have prominent psychotic symptoms (Richter and Shimojyo 1961).

Etiology

After the mosquito or tick bite, hematogenous spread carries the virus to the brain. Although the severity of the pathologic changes varies widely depending on the responsible virus, in general one finds widespread perivascular inflammation and areas of focal cerebritis in the leptomeninges, cortical gray matter, cerebral white matter, subcortical gray structures, and, in some cases, brainstem. At times, thrombus formation may occur in the vessels involved, with infarction (Leech and Harris 1977; Reyes *et al.* 1981).

Differential diagnosis

As discussed in Section 7.6, arboviral meningoencephalitis represents just one cause of acute encephalitis, and the reader is directed to that section for a discussion of the differential possibilities.

Treatment

There is no specific treatment. In many cases, aggressive supportive care is required and osmotic agents may be indicated to lower intracranial pressure. Some authors recommend prophylactic use of anti-epileptic drugs such as phenytoin or fosphenytoin. The routine treatment of delirium is discussed in Section 5.3.

A vaccine is available for Japanese encephalitis, and travellers may wish to consider this.

14.5 HERPES SIMPLEX ENCEPHALITIS

Although herpes simplex infection accounts for only about one-tenth of all cases of acute encephalitis, it is by far the most common cause of sporadic encephalitis and, given its treatability, it should be strongly considered in the differential of any adult suspected of having acute encephalitis.

Clinical features

Herpes simplex encephalitis can occur at any age but most patients are middle-aged or older (Koskiniemi *et al.* 1996).

The onset itself generally spans several days; however, the range is wide, from explosive onsets over several hours to gradual ones lasting weeks or more. In some cases the onset may be preceded be a prodrome, lasting several days, of malaise, headache, irritability, and mild fever.

Typically (Kennedy 1988; Marton *et al.* 1996; McGrath *et al.* 1997; Whitley *et al.* 1986; Williams and Lerner 1978), patients present with fever, headache, and delirium. In this setting a majority of patients will also develop focal signs, such as hemiparesis or aphasia, and approximately two-thirds will have seizures, which may be either complex partial or grand mal in type. Although meningeal signs, such as a stiff neck or photophobia, are common, they are generally not at all severe. Notably, bizarre behavior is common and, although this usually occurs in the context of the delirium, there are rare reports of the encephalitis presenting with either mania (Fisher 1996) or a psychosis (Wilson 1976). Untreated, coma develops in about one-third of patients.

Computed tomographic (CT) scanning may show radiolucent areas in the medial aspects of one or both temporal lobes, but it may be normal for up to a week. Magnetic resonance scanning is much more sensitive, showing increased signal intensity on FLAIR or T2-weighted scans in the medial temporal lobe (Figure 14.2), although this too may be normal for the first few days. Diffusion-weighted imaging may show increased signal intensity in the same areas, and this abnormality may be evident earlier than that seen on T2-weighted or FLAIR imaging. Gadolinium enhancement may also occur.

The EEG (Upton and Gumpert 1970) is usually normal for the first few days but will eventually show delta slowing in one temporal area, which may be accompanied by

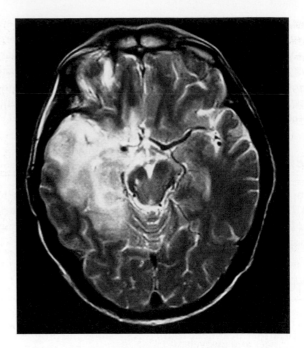

Figure 14.2   This T2-weighted magnetic resonance imaging scan shows increased signal intensity in the left temporal lobe (especially its medial aspect) of a patient with herpes simplex encephalitis. (Reproduced from Gillespie and Jackson 2000.)

periodic complexes; with progression of the disease, bilateral involvement may be seen.

Polymerase chain reaction assay of the CSF (Aurelius *et al.* 1991) is almost 100 percent sensitive for herpes simplex DNA and is the diagnostic procedure of choice. The CSF itself may be normal during the first few days but will in most cases show an elevated total protein with a lymphocytic and polymorphonuclear pleocytosis; red cells may also be present, reflecting the hemorrhagic nature of the inflammatory process. Although the glucose level is typically normal, it may rarely be reduced.

If lumbar puncture is not possible, brain biopsy may be necessary to make a definitive diagnosis; however, as noted below, treatment rarely waits upon such a procedure.

Course

Untreated, over 50 percent of patients will die in days or a few weeks. In those who survive, the clinical picture usually stabilizes in a matter of weeks; exceptionally the acute illness may be prolonged for months (Sage *et al.* 1985) or even longer (Yamada *et al.* 2003).

Although most patients have only one episode, recurrences may appear in a small minority.

Among those who do survive, the vast majority will be left with significant sequelae, most commonly a chronic amnestic syndrome (Hokkanen *et al.* 1996; Kapur *et al.* 1994; Young *et al.* 1992), dementia (Hokkanen *et al.* 1996; McGrath *et al.* 1997), or a personality change (Caparros-Lefebvre *et al.* 1996). Other sequelae include focal signs (e.g., aphasia or hemiplegia) (McGrath *et al.* 1997) or epilepsy (McGrath *et al.* 1997); rarely there may be a Kluver–Bucy syndrome (Greenwood *et al.* 1983; Lilly *et al.* 1983; Marlowe *et al.* 1975). There is also a case report in which complex motor and vocal tics occurred as a sequela (Northam and Singer 1991).

Etiology

There are two types of herpes simplex virus: type 1 and type 2. Type 1 virus usually causes orolabial infections and type 2 virus generally causes genital infections. Although the vast majority of cases of herpes simplex encephalitis are caused by type 1 virus, type 2 virus may be at fault in a small minority (Koskiniemi *et al.* 1996). The majority of the adult population has at some time been infected with herpes simplex type 1, and the virus may remain in a latent state in various sites, including the trigeminal ganglion (Baringer and Swoveland 1973).

Although it is known that the virus can undergo retrograde axonal transport, it is not clear precisely how the virus gains entry into the central nervous system. One theory suggests that, after the reactivation of a latent infection in the trigeminal ganglion, the virus undergoes transport through the ophthalmic division of the trigeminal nerve to the olfactory mucosa, where it gains access to the olfactory filia and undergoes retrograde transport through the olfactory nerve and then to the temporal lobes; another holds that, after reactivation in the trigeminal ganglion, the virus spreads along sensory fibers to the meninges of the middle and anterior fossae where it then gains entry.

Pathologically (Adams and Miller 1973; Esiri 1982) there is intense inflammation (which may progress to hemorrhagic necrosis) affecting initially the medial portions of the temporal lobe, with, in most cases, eventual spread to other areas, including the lateral aspects of the temporal lobe, the insula, inferior portions of the frontal lobes, and the cingulate cortex. Although involvement is typically unilateral early on, with time both temporal lobes become involved. There may be substantial edema, and both uncal and subfalcine herniation may occur. In those who survive, scarring, cavitation, and cystic change is seen in the involved areas.

Differential diagnosis

A delirium accompanied by headache and fever immediately suggests the diagnosis of an acute encephalitis, and, as discussed in Section 7.6, consideration must be given not only to herpes simplex encephalitis but also to various other encephalitides, for example arboviral infections. Magnetic resonance scanning is helpful here as medial temporal lobe involvement strongly suggests herpes simplex encephalitis; however, as noted above, MR findings may be normal early

on. Polymerase chain reaction assay of the CSF for herpes simplex DNA is critical and should be promptly performed. In instances in which a reliable differential between herpes simplex encephalitis and other encephalitides cannot be made, either because MRI findings are equivocal or lumbar puncture cannot be performed, most clinicians will make a presumptive diagnosis of herpes simplex encephalitis and treat the patient accordingly. Given that herpes simplex encephalitis is treatable whereas the other viral encephalitides are not, and given the generally benign side-effect profile of acyclovir, such a course is justifiable.

In those rare cases in which the presentation is with mania or a psychosis, the differential is wide, as discussed in Sections 6.3 and 7.1 respectively; however, the eventual development of fever, headache, and delirium will settle the issue.

Treatment

In addition to aggressive supportive care, patients should be treated with acyclovir using a dose of 10 mg/kg intravenously every 8 hours for a course of 2–3 weeks. It also appears that concurrent treatment with dexamethasone or methylprednisolone will enhance recovery (Kamei *et al.* 2005). Seizures may be treated with a standard anti-epileptic drug, such as phenytoin or fosphenytoin, and it is prudent to continue treatment with an anti-epileptic until the patient has been seizure free for at least a year. The general treatment of delirium is further discussed in Section 5.3.

14.6 ENCEPHALITIS LETHARGICA

Encephalitis lethargica, also known as von Economo's disease or European sleeping sickness, was first described by Baron Constantin von Economo at a meeting of the Vienna Psychiatric Society in April 1917 (Dickman 2001; Wilkins and Brody 1968). This disease swept the world in an epidemic that lasted from 1917 to 1928 and, although there have been no further epidemics, sporadic cases still occur (Dale *et al.* 2004; Howard and Lees 1987), making a familiarity with this disease of more than academic interest.

Clinical features

Acute encephalitis lethargica (Hohman 1921; Kirby and Davis 1921) is characterized by headache, fever, sleep reversal (nocturnal wakefulness and diurnal somnolence), delirium, various oculomotor pareses, and, classically, oculogyric crises; some patients also displayed euphoria or psychosis (Kirby and Davis 1921; Meninger 1926; Sands 1928), or stuporous catatonia (Bond 1920; Shill and Stacy 2000).

The CSF may be normal or may reveal a lymphocytic pleocytosis and an elevated total protein; oligoclonal bands may also be present (Dale *et al.* 2004; Howard and Lees 1987).

Course

The mortality rate for acute encephalitis was about 25 percent; among those who survived, the encephalitis gradually cleared over about a month. Of great importance, neuropsychiatric sequelae, most notably post-encephalitic parkinsonism, occurred in the majority of cases.

Post-encephalitic parkinsonism occurred in over 50 percent of survivors after a latent interval of from 1 to over 20 years (Duvoisin and Yahr 1965). Patients gradually developed a syndrome similar to that seen in idiopathic Parkinson's disease (Rail *et al.* 1981). In addition, other motor abnormalities, including dystonia, blepharospasm (Alpers and Patten 1927), and, most importantly, oculogyric crises (Taylor and McDonald 1928), were often present. Interestingly, these transient oculogyric crises could also be accompanied by classic obsessions or compulsions (Jelliffee 1929); in some cases, palilalia (Van Bogaert 1934) or agitation and excitation (McCowan *et al.* 1928) were noted to accompany the oculogyric crises. Oculogyric crises, although most commonly seen in conjunction with post-encephalitic parkinsonism, at times occurred independently (McCowan *et al.* 1928).

Other sequelae, seen in a minority, included dementia, narcoleptic and cataplectic attacks (Adie 1926; Fournier and Helguera 1934), and, in children, restlessness and inattentiveness (Hohman 1922).

Etiology

Autopsies of those dying in the acute stage revealed inflammation with a perivascular accumulation of lymphocytes and plasma cells in the midbrain, basal ganglia, and cortex (Buzzard and Greenfield 1919; Howard and Lees 1987). In those with sequelae, autopsy studies (Geddes *et al.* 1993; Ishii and Nakamura 1981; Rail *et al.* 1981) have revealed neuronal loss, gliosis, and, in the remaining neurons, neurofibrillary tangles similar to those seen in Alzheimer's disease, in the substantia nigra, locus ceruleus, hippocampus, basal ganglia, thalamus, and cerebral cortex. Macroscopically, there was cortical atrophy and depigmentation of the substantia nigra and locus ceruleus.

Given that the pandemic of encephalitis lethargica coincided with the Spanish influenza epidemic, it was long suspected that encephalitis lethargica was secondary to influenza. Recent work on archived specimens, however, failed to find any evidence of influenza RNA (McCall *et al.* 2001), and consideration is now being given to the possibility that encephalitis lethargica, rather than resulting directly from a viral infection, may represent an autoimmune disease with antibodies directed at the midbrain, basal ganglia, and other structures, with the autoimmune

assault having been triggered by a preceding viral or bacterial pharyngitis (Dale *et al.* 2004).

Differential diagnosis

Encephalitis lethargica must be distinguished from other acute encephalitides, as discussed in Section 7.6. One clue here is the presence of sleep reversal and, especially, oculogyric crises, which are very rare in other cases of acute viral encephalitis.

With regard to sequelae, the diagnosis is fairly straightforward when they are present immediately after resolution of the acute syndrome. Difficulty, however, may arise when, as in the case of post-encephalitic parkinsonism, there is a prolonged latent interval between the encephalitis and the onset of the parkinsonism. In such cases, the presence of oculogyric crises is again an important clue.

Treatment

In addition to routine supportive care, consideration may be given to corticosteroids.

14.7 INFECTIOUS MONONUCLEOSIS

In up to a little over 5 percent of cases of infectious mononucleosis (Gautier-Smith 1965), the central or peripheral nervous system may be involved, producing, variously, delirium, seizures, meningismus, ataxia, a cord syndrome, or a cranial or peripheral neuropathy.

Clinical features

Although mononucleosis may occur in adults (Fujimoto *et al.* 2003), it is most commonly seen in children or adolescents. Typically there is a prodrome, lasting for 1–2 weeks, of fatigue, malaise, and headache, after which one sees the classic development of sore throat, fever, and cervical adenopathy; splenomegaly and hepatomegaly may also occur.

Although nervous system involvement generally occurs in the context of this typical clinical picture, at times it may be the presenting feature of the disease. Meningism with stiff neck is the most common manifestation, followed by delirium (Bergin 1960; Schlesinger and Crelinsten 1977; Schnell *et al.* 1966; Tselis *et al.* 1997). Seizures may occur (Doja *et al.* 2006; Freedman *et al.* 1953; Silverstein *et al.* 1972) and status epilepticus has been reported (Russell *et al.* 1985). Other features include acute cerebellar ataxia (Gautier-Smith 1965; Leavell *et al.* 1986), a transverse myelitis, a cranial neuropathy (with either a unilateral or bilateral Bell's palsy), and a primarily motor peripheral polyneuropathy that may resemble the Guillan–Barré syndrome.

In most cases there is a lymphocytosis with atypical lymphocytes, and the 'monospot' test will be positive in over 90 percent of cases. When the diagnosis remains in doubt, one may also test for IgM anti-viral capsid antigen (anti-VCA) and anti-early antigen (anti-EA). In cases of central nervous system involvement, PCR assay of the CSF for Epstein–Barr virus DNA may be positive (Tselis *et al.* 1997). The anti-nuclear antibody (ANA) test and Venereal Disease Research Laboratories (VDRL) test may transiently be falsely positive.

In delirious patients the EEG may show generalized slowing (Doja *et al.* 2006), with, rarely, periodic complexes (Greenberg *et al.* 1982).

Course

Symptoms typically resolve after about a month. Although most patients recover completely, a minority will be left with persistent fatigue (Petersen *et al.* 2006) or sleepiness (Guilleminault and Mondini 1986).

Etiology

Infectious mononucleosis is caused by the Epstein–Barr virus (Epstein and Achong 1977) and is transmitted primarily via oral secretions passed during intimate contact such as kissing. The virus gains access to the bloodstream and infects lymphocytes, spreading later to various other organs, including the brain. Scarce autopsy reports have revealed a widespread lymphocytic or monocytic inflammation of the cerebrum (Roulet Perez *et al.* 1993; Sworn and Urich 1970).

Differential diagnosis

A similar syndrome may occur during seroconversion in HIV infection.

Treatment

At present, treatment is supportive; there is no good evidence for the effectiveness of antiviral medications or corticosteroids.

14.8 MUMPS

Although over 50 percent of patients with mumps will have a CSF pleocytosis (Russell and Donald 1958), only a minority will have clinical evidence of central nervous system involvement, with 15 percent developing a meningitis and less than 1 percent with evidence of an encephalitis. Currently, thanks to widespread vaccination, mumps is quite rare in developed countries; although overall mumps is equally common in males and females, males are far more likely to develop symptomatology reflecting infection of the central nervous system.

Clinical features

Mumps typically occurs in children or adolescents, generally during the winter or spring, and presents with a prodrome of fever, myalgia, and malaise, followed within 1–7 days by the typical parotitis; males may also develop a unilateral or bilateral orchitis.

Meningitis manifests with headache, drowsiness, and a stiff neck, and typically follows the parotitis after a latency of from 2 to 20 days; occasionally the meningitis will precede the parotitis (Levitt *et al.* 1970) and rarely parotitis may be absent.

Encephalitis presents with an increasing fever and either delirium or stupor; seizures, ataxia, and various focal signs may also occur (Azimi *et al.* 1969; Bistrian *et al.* 1972; Finklestein 1938; Koskiniemi *et al.* 1983; Levitt *et al.* 1970).

Serum anti-mumps IgM antibody is present acutely, and acute and convalescent serum IgG antibody displays a fourfold or greater rise. The CSF usually shows a lymphocytic pleocytosis and an elevated protein, and the mumps-specific IgG index is generally increased; mumps virus RNA may also be detected via PCR assay.

Course

Overall, mumps usually runs its course in 3–4 weeks, and meningitis or encephalitis typically resolve after a week or two. Rarely, it appears that the encephalitis may remain chronic (Vaheri *et al.* 1982).

Although most recover from meningitis or encephalitis without sequelae, some post-encephalitic patients may be left with chronic cognitive deficits, ataxia, seizures or deafness; rarely hydrocephalus, secondary to aqueductal stenosis (Thompson 1979), may occur.

Etiology

The mumps virus is spread via the respiratory route and is trophic for salivary glands, gonads, and the nervous system. Within the meninges and cerebrum there may be a widespread perivascular lymphocytic and mononuclear inflammation.

Differential diagnosis

Mumps encephalitis must be distinguished from other acute viral encephalitides, as discussed in Section 7.6; the occurrence of parotitis or orchitis constitute obvious clues. Importantly, either a history of mumps or mumps vaccination effectively rules out the diagnosis, given that both of these generally confer lifelong immunity.

Treatment

There is no specific treatment for mumps; the general treatment of delirium is discussed in Section 5.3.

14.9 VARICELLA–ZOSTER

Infection with the varicella-zoster virus may cause two different illnesses (Strauss *et al.* 1984). Acute infection causes chickenpox, also known as varicella. After resolution of chickenpox, the virus undergoes latency in the sensory ganglia of the cord and also in the gasserian ganglion of the trigeminal nerve and the geniculate ganglion of the facial nerve (Mahalingam *et al.* 1990). In the aged or immunocompromised, the virus may reactivate to cause shingles (also known as herpes zoster) or one of the other forms of zoster noted below.

Clinical features

Chickenpox is a disease of childhood or adolescence that is spread via respiratory droplets. The pharynx is the initial seat of the infection; subsequently, a viremia occurs, resulting in a characteristic rash. Rarely, the central nervous system may be affected during the viremia, producing either an encephalitis (with various symptoms, including delirium [Applebaum *et al.* 1953] or ataxia [Johnson and Milbourn 1970]) or a meningitis.

Reactivation of the latent varicella-zoster virus may occur during the immune 'senescence' that occurs with aging (Miller 1980), during certain illnesses, such as AIDS (Gilden *et al.* 1988), Hodgkin's disease (McCormick *et al.* 1969) or other cancers, or during treatment with corticosteroids or various immunosuppressants, and the form of the resulting zoster is determined by the site of the reactivation.

With reactivation of virus latent within the sensory ganglia of the cord, anterograde spread of the virus down the sensory nerve results in a classic dermatomal rash. Typically there is a prodrome of malaise, lasting several days, followed by the occurrence of dermatomal pain; over the next 3 or 4 days, a typical vesicular rash follows. In almost all cases the rash is unilateral and typically occurs in one of the thoracic dermatomes. Resolution occurs gradually after a matter of weeks. In a very small minority of cases, the virus may spread retrogradely to the cord with the delayed and gradual appearance of myelitic symptoms (Devinsky *et al.* 1991; Hogan and Krigman 1973); involvement of the ventral horn may lead to a segmental sensory loss whereas involvement of the anterior horn may lead to segmental weakness and amyotrophy. Occasionally the white matter of the cord may be involved and in such cases

there may be a transverse myelitis or, rarely, a Brown–Sequard syndrome.

When virus latent within the gasserian ganglion of the trigeminal nerve undergoes reactivation, anterograde spread leads to a zosteriform rash within the area of distribution of one of the divisions of the trigeminal nerve, almost always the first or ophthalmic division. The resulting herpes zoster ophthalmicus may disastrously also involve the eye. Patients who have suffered a herpes zoster ophthalmicus are also at risk for a rare complication, namely a zoster vasculopathy (Doyle *et al.* 1982; Linnemann and Alvira 1980). In these cases, the virus spreads anterogradely along sensory fibers to the meninges, resulting in infection of either the middle or anterior cerebral arteries: after a latency of from weeks to months, thrombus formation in these arteries may lead to ischemic infarction of subserved areas, with the development of focal syndromes, such as hemiparesis contralateral to the side where the zoster rash occurred (Hilt *et al.* 1983).

In cases in which the geniculate ganglion is the site of reactivation, the Ramsey Hunt syndrome (also known as zoster oticus) may occur, with a rash in the external auditory canal or the pinna, and a peripheral seventh cranial nerve palsy (Sweeney and Gliden 2001).

Rarely, and generally only in debilitated patients, there may be a hematogenous dissemination of the reactivated virus with the development of a severe, generalized vesicular rash, and in such cases hematogenous spread of the virus may also occur to the brain, causing an encephalitis (Applebaum *et al.* 1962; Jemsek *et al.* 1983; Krumholz and Luhan 1945). Typically in such cases, within days to weeks (or exceptionally months [Weaver *et al.* 1999]) of the onset of the generalized rash, a delirium develops that may be accompanied by seizures, focal signs, ataxia, or meningismus. In such cases the EEG shows generalized slowing, and FLAIR or T2-weighted MR scanning will reveal multifocal areas of increased signal intensity within both the white matter and the cortex. The CSF is typically, but not always, abnormal, with a lymphocytic pleocytosis and an elevated total protein; anti-varicella-zoster IgG antibodies are commonly found and, although somewhat less sensitive, PCR assay may reveal varicella-zoster DNA (Nagel *et al.* 2007). Although the encephalitis usually resolves in a matter of weeks, chronic courses may be seen, especially in severely immunocompromised patients, such as those with AIDS.

Before leaving this section on clinical features, note must also be made of a variant of zoster known as zoster sine herpete (Gilden *et al.* 1994). In such cases the rash does not appear, and hence one may have dermatomal pain, spinal cord symptoms, vasculopathy or encephalitis without this all-important diagnostic clue (Mayo and Booss 1989).

Course

The course of zoster is dependent on the immunological competence of the patient. In immunocompetent patients, symptoms generally resolve within a matter of weeks; in the immunocompromised, however, protracted, and at times fatal, courses may be seen.

One complication of a zoster rash, whether dermatomal or cranial, is post-herpetic neuralgia, in which the pain persists beyond resolution of the rash. This neuralgic pain may be lancinating or burning in quality and may cause considerable disability; although in some cases a gradual remission may occur after many months, in others the pain proves to be chronic.

Etiology

As indicated above, zoster may be complicated by a myelitis, a cerebral vasculopathy or an encephalitis. The myelitis results from retrograde spread from the sensory ganglia. In all likelihood, the cerebral vasculopathy occurs secondary to seeding of such large pial vessels as the middle or anterior cerebral arteries by virus that spreads from the gasserian ganglion up along sensory nerves destined for the meninges; in such cases, there is often segmental narrowing of the involved vessels (MacKenzie et al. 1981) and virus has been found within the vessel walls (Linnemann and Alvira 1980; Melanson et al. 1996); in some cases thrombotic occlusion has been noted with little or no associated inflammation (Eidelberg et al. 1986). As noted earlier, the encephalitis occurs secondary to hematogenous seeding of the cerebrum, generally occurring only during a disseminated rash. In such cases one may find multifocal areas of cerebritis (Weaver et al. 1999), primarily affecting the white matter, with, at times, multiple areas of microinfarction occurring secondary to small vessel vasculitis (Kleinschmidt-DeMasters et al. 1996).

Differential diagnosis

The occurrence of a myelopathy, stroke or encephalitic symptoms (e.g., delirium, seizures, etc.) in the setting of a recent rash should immediately suggest a varicella-zoster infection. As noted earlier, some of these manifestations may occur in the absence of a rash, and in such cases one would have to closely question the patient and family regarding any complaints of pain, either in a dermatomal pattern or in the ophthalmic division of the fifth cranial nerve.

Treatment

Treatment with an antiviral agent, such as acyclovir, valacyclovir, famciclovir, or brivudin, should be immediately instituted for all forms of zoster, and, in the case of large-vessel vasculopathy, antiplatelet agents should also be started.

With regard to post-herpetic neuralgia, a number of agents have been shown to be effective in double-blind studies, including nortriptyline, amitriptyline, gabapentin, and pregabalin. Importantly, with regard to nortriptyline

and amitriptyline, patients get relief regardless of whether they are depressed or not. Nortriptyline and amitriptyline are equally effective, but nortriptyline is better tolerated (Watson et al. 1998); nortriptyline may be given in doses ranging from 10 to 75 mg, and amitriptyline in doses ranging from 10 to 100 mg. Gabapentin is roughly equivalent in effectiveness to nortriptyline but better tolerated (Chandra et al. 2006); it may be given in doses ranging from 1200 to 3600 mg. Pregabalin is the most recently introduced agent and it is unclear how effective it is compared with the others; it may be given in doses ranging from 150 to 600 mg (Dworkin et al. 2003). Regardless of which agent is used, a week or more may be required before some relief is seen.

14.10 RABIES

Rabies typically occurs after being bitten by a rabid animal, for example a dog, cat, wolf, fox, skunk, raccoon, or vampire bat; cases have also been reported secondary to respiratory transmission in spelunkers within bat-infested caves and in a veterinarian who was working with the homogenized brain of a rabid animal (Conomy et al. 1977); recently rabies was also reported secondary to solid organ transplantation from a donor with an unsuspected case (Srinivasan et al. 2005). Although very rare in developed countries, rabies remains a significant problem in India and parts of Asia.

Clinical features

After being bitten by an infected animal there is a latent, asymptomatic period, generally of 1–3 months, with a range of weeks to a year or more; the duration of the latency appears related not only to the severity of the bite but also to the distance from the bitten area to the brain, with bites on the feet having the longest latency and facial bites the shortest.

With resolution of the latent interval, there is usually a prodrome, lasting days, characterized by headache and malaise; pain or parasthesiae may also develop at the site of the original bite. Subsequently, the illness may evolve in one of two forms, namely 'furious' rabies or 'dumb' (also known as 'paralytic') rabies.

Furious rabies (Adle-Biassette et al. 1996; Blatt et al. 1938; Dupont and Earle 1965) is seen in perhaps 80 percent of cases and is characterized by restlessness, agitation, excitability, excessive startability, and convulsions; delirium is typical and patients may engage in bizarre behavior, including biting. The combination of excessive salivation and dysphagia caused by pharyngeal spasm may literally cause the patient to 'foam at the mouth'. Pharyngeal spasm may also be provoked by swallowing water or even by the sight of water, giving rise to the classic symptom of hydrophobia.

Dumb rabies (Chopra et al. 1980) is characterized by a flaccid paralysis that typically begins in one limb and rapidly becomes generalized and symmetric.

The CSF shows a lymphocytic pleocytosis, elevated protein level, and anti-rabies antibodies. Rabies virus RNA may also be detected by PCR assay. T2-weighted magnetic resonance scanning may reveal multiple foci of increased signal intensity in both the gray and white matter of the cerebrum and cerebellum (Laothamatas *et al.* 2003).

Course

Although survival has been reported (Porras *et al.* 1976; Willoughby *et al.* 2005), this is exceptional and the overwhelming majority of patients die within days to a couple of weeks.

Etiology

In the typical case of rabies secondary to a bite by a rabid animal, the virus slowly travels up a peripheral nerve to finally gain access to the central nervous system. Within the brain and spinal cord there is a widespread inflammatory response, with a predilection for the limbic system and the cerebellum. Within neurons, one finds cytoplasmic eosinophilic inclusions, known as Negri bodies (Chopra *et al.* 1980; Dupont and Earle 1965).

Differential diagnosis

Lacking the history of exposure, the differential in the case of furious rabies includes other causes of acute encephalitis, as discussed in Section 7.6; the presence of excessive salivation and dysphagia, and certainly hydrophobia, however, would suggest the correct diagnosis. In cases of dumb rabies, consideration must be given to Guillan–Barré syndrome.

Treatment

There is no specific treatment for either furious or dumb rabies; intensive supportive care, as described in a recent case (Willoughby *et al.* 2005), may rarely enable a patient to survive.

Given this lack of treatment, the focus must be on prevention. In cases of animal bites, the wound should be thoroughly cleansed and consideration should be given to the injection of rabies immune globulin followed by vaccination with human diploid cell anti-rabies vaccine. Those caring for patients with rabies must avoid any contact with saliva.

14.11 ACUTE DISSEMINATED ENCEPHALOMYELITIS

Acute disseminated encephalomyelitis (ADEM) is a monophasic illness that occurs as a result of an autoimmune assault on the cerebrum, primarily the white matter, triggered by a preceding infectious illness or vaccination. It is characterized clinically by multifocal lesions within the cerebrum. This disease was formerly called post-infectious encephalomyelitis (PIE) or, if it occurred after a vaccination, post-vaccinial encephalomyelitis, and these names, although no longer current, have much to recommend them, as they not only refer to the clinical picture, namely an encephalomyelitis, but also to the etiology, namely a reaction to a preceding infection or vaccination. By contrast, the term acute disseminated encephalomyelitis encompasses only the clinical picture and, as such, it may, in the minds of some authors, perhaps inappropriately broaden the concept to include encephalomyelitides that occur on the basis of other causes.

Responsible infections include measles, mumps, rubella, pertussis, chickenpox, infectious mononucleosis, influenza, arboviruses, herpes simplex virus, HIV, hepatitis, non-specific viral infections, scarlet fever, mycoplasma, *Borrelia*, and typhoid (Fisher *et al.* 1983; Hart and Earle 1975; Moscovich *et al.* 1995; Paskavitz *et al.* 1995). Vaccinations associated with ADEM include those for measles, mumps, rubella, chickenpox, influenza, rabies, hepatitis, typhoid, and tetanus. Both smallpox and smallpox vaccination (Dolgopol *et al.* 1955) were once very common causes, but with this disease now apparently eradicated they are no longer of immediate concern.

Clinical features

Although ADEM is most common in children and adolescents, it also occurs in adults and the elderly.

In general, between the preceding infection or vaccination and the onset of ADEM there is a latent interval lasting about a week or two, with a range of from 2 to 30 days. Clinically (Hollinger *et al.* 2002; Marchioni *et al.* 2005; Miller *et al.* 1956; Tenembaum *et al.* 2002), the onset is generally acute, with the full picture evolving over a day or so. The symptomatology may be quite varied, depending on which part of the central nervous system bears the brunt of the autoimmune assault. Thus, with cerebral involvement there may be headache, delirium, seizures, and various focal signs, such as hemiparesis; meningismus may be present, but is usually mild, and there may be fever, but again this too is generally mild; rarely, mania may occur (Moscovich *et al.* 1995; Paskavitz *et al.* 1995). Cerebellar involvement may cause an ataxia, and with spinal involvement there may be a transverse myelitis with paraplegia. The cranial nerves (most commonly the optic nerve) may be affected, and patients may develop visual obscurations or blindness. Rarely the basal ganglia are involved with chorea or dystonia.

MRI scanning may be normal for the first day or two although, eventually, T2-weighted imaging will reveal multiple areas of increased signal intensity (Kesserling *et al.* 1990); these are typically found in the cerebral white matter

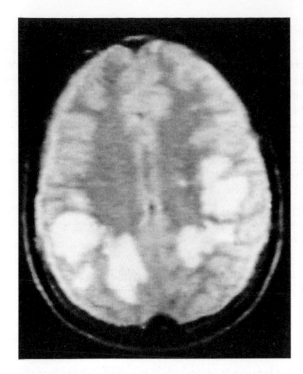

Figure 14.3 Multiple bilateral areas of increased signal intensity on a T2-weighted magnetic resonance imaging scan of a patient with acute disseminated encephalomyelitis. (Reproduced from Marsden and Fowler 1998.)

(as illustrated in Figure 14.3) but may also appear in the gray matter of the cerebral cortex, the basal ganglia, and the thalamus; other potentially affected areas include the cerebellar white matter, the brainstem, and the cord. A minority of these lesions will also demonstrate gadolinium enhancement. Of note, T2-weighted signal abnormalities may persist far beyond clinical resolution of ADEM, often for many months (O'Riordan *et al.* 1999).

The EEG typically displays generalized slowing with or without more focal areas of accentuated slowing.

The CSF is generally, but not always, abnormal. Findings include a lymphocytic pleocytosis, an elevated total protein, an elevated myelin basic protein, and oligoclonal bands. In severe cases there may be both polymorphonuclear and red blood cells.

Course

The outcome is fatal in roughly 20 percent of cases; those who survive tend to recover gradually over a week or two. Although most appear to recover completely, sequelae, reflecting the initial clinical picture, may occur, including dementia, epilepsy, and various focal signs.

As noted earlier, ADEM is a 'monophasic' illness that, in the natural course of events, does not recur unless the patient is again exposed to one of the precipitating infections or vaccinations.

Etiology

As noted earlier, ADEM occurs secondary to an autoimmune attack on the cerebrum. Pathologically (Greenfield 1929; Hart and Earle 1975), there are multiple foci of perivenous mononuclear inflammation with associated demyelinization and relative axonal sparing: although these are most common in the white matter of the cerebrum, cerebellum, and cord, the gray matter, as noted earlier, may also be involved. In severe cases, known as acute hemorrhagic leukoencephalitis (Hart and Earle 1975; Russell 1955), widespread petechial hemorrhages are also seen.

Differential diagnosis

Differential consideration must be given to acute viral encephalitides and to a first episode of multiple sclerosis (MS).

Most of the viral illnesses capable of causing ADEM can also directly cause an encephalitis in their own right, and the differential in such cases rests primarily on the existence of a clear latent interval. In cases presumably triggered by measles, consideration must also be given to subacute measles encephalitis, as discussed in Section 14.13.

Multiple sclerosis often enters into the differential; however, in most cases a clinical distinction between ADEM and MS is possible on several counts. First, although MS may present with multiple acute areas of demyelinization, more commonly one finds only one or a few, in marked contrast to the common picture in ADEM, which is characterized by multiple lesions (Schwarz *et al.* 2001). Second, consideration should be given to whether or not the patient may have had prior lesions that perhaps were clinically 'silent', as may often occur in MS. Here, MR imaging is quite helpful, as T1-weighted scanning may disclose old 'burnt-out' lesions known as 'black holes'; although these may occur in MS they are classically absent in ADEM, which, as noted earlier, is typically a monophasic illness. Finally, in cases in which there is still doubt, the diagnosis may rest on long-term follow-up: MS is typically a relapsing illness and thus one expects to see future clinical episodes or MRI evidence of new lesions, whereas in ADEM no new lesions, either clinical or 'silent', occur, unless of course the patient is again exposed to a precipitating illness or vaccination.

Treatment

Methylprednisolone should be immediately started using a dose for adults of 250 mg intravenously every 6 hours; this is continued for approximately 2 weeks after which the patient may be switched to prednisone, which may then be tapered over a month or so. Although the response to steroids is often prompt (and at times dramatic), some patients fail to respond and in such cases consideration may be given to intravenous immune globulins, plasmapheresis or immuno-suppression with, for example, cyclophosphamide.

14.12 SUBACUTE SCLEROSING PANENCEPHALITIS

Subacute sclerosing panencephalitis (SSPE), also known as Dawson's disease, results from a reactivation of a defective measles virus and is typically characterized by dementia, myoclonus, and ataxia. This is a very rare disorder, occurring in 5–10 out of 1 000 000 with a history of measles and in approximately 1 out of 1 000 000 who receive the measles vaccine; it is three to four times more common in males than females.

Clinical features

The vast majority of cases occur in children; in these cases the average latency between the preceding infection or vaccination is about 8 years, and the average age of onset is about 13 years. In adults, the latency ranges from 8 to 33 years and the average age of onset is in the early 20s.

The onset itself is generally gradual, even insidious, and typically the disease evolves through three stages (Dawson 1934; Ozturk et al. 2002; Prashanth et al. 2006). In the first stage, the patient may become restless, distractable, and forgetful, and irritability and moodiness may be noted. In some cases, particularly in those with adult onset, this first stage may be characterized by a psychosis (Cape et al. 1973; Salib 1988) that may faithfully mimic schizophrenia, with delusions (including Schneiderian first-rank symptoms [Duncalf et al. 1989]) and stuporous catatonia (Koehler and Jakumeit 1976). In the second stage a dementia evolves, which is accompanied by myoclonus, ataxia, and seizures, which may be partial or grand mal in type; abnormal involuntary movements, such as chorea, athetosis, or dystonia, are occasionally seen at this point. In the third and final stage there is stupor and generalized rigidity, and eventually coma. It must be borne in mind that there are many exceptions to this typical picture (Risk and Haddad 1979). In some cases the onset may be relatively fulminant, with severe symptomatology seen in a matter of months, and, furthermore, there may be considerable overlap among the various stages.

Magnetic resonance scanning may reveal cortical atrophy and, on T2-weighted imaging, multiple areas of increased signal intensity in the gray and white matter of the cerebrum, with a predilection for the periventricular area (Anlar et al. 1996).

The EEG in the second and third stages will display a classic burst-suppression pattern in the majority of cases (Wulf 1982).

The CSF is generally acellular with a mildly elevated total protein. The IgG level is increased, sometimes greatly so, oligoclonal bands may be found, and, most importantly, anti-measles antibodies are present.

Course

Although the course is variable, most patients pass through the three stages and die within 1–3 years; in fulminant cases, however, a fatal outcome may occur within several months. Occasionally the course is prolonged, up to a decade or more, and there may at times be periods of relative stability (Risk et al. 1978), lasting many years (Cobb et al. 1984; Donner et al. 1972; Landau and Luse 1958); however, these inevitably give way to further progression.

Etiology

SSPE occurs secondary to a reactivation of a 'dormant' measles virus that has the peculiarity of lacking a normal M protein; rather than undergoing 'budding', these defective viruses spread by means of cell fusion within the central nervous system. Pathologically there is widespread perivascular inflammation accompanied by patchy demyelinization and neuronal loss (Ohya et al. 1974). Within surviving neurons inclusions are found within nuclei, which, by electron microscopy, appear similar to measles nucleocapsids.

Differential diagnosis

Subacute measles encephalitis, like subacute sclerosing panencephalitis, also occurs as a sequela to measles; however, in subacute measles encephalitis the latent interval between the preceding measles and the onset of the illness is much shorter than in subacute sclerosing panencephalitis, being measured in months and not years. In adult-onset cases, consideration may be given to other dementias associated with myoclonus, such as Creutzfeldt–Jakob disease or possibly AIDS dementia.

Treatment

Various treatments have been advocated. However, in the only randomized study to date it appears that oral inosiplex was equivalent to a combination of oral inosiplex and intraventricular interferon-alpha (Gascon et al. 2003); the benefit, however, was not great. The general treatment of dementia is discussed in Section 5.1; in cases with marked myoclonus, consideration may be given to either clonazepam or carbamazepine.

14.13 SUBACUTE MEASLES ENCEPHALITIS

Subacute measles encephalitis, also known as measles inclusion body encephalitis, is a rare disorder occurring generally, but not always, in immunocompromised patients who have recently recovered from the measles. Although, given the epidemiology of measles, most cases occur in children, adult-onset cases have been reported (Croxson et al. 2002).

Clinical features

Clinically (Agamanolis *et al.* 1979; Aicardi *et al.* 1977), after an asymptomatic latent interval ranging from 1 to 6 months after a measles infection, there is a subacute onset of delirium over days or a week or so, accompanied, variously, by myoclonus, focal signs, and seizures, which may be either grand mal or partial; in some cases simple partial motor status epilepticus has been noted.

Although the CSF is generally normal, in some cases there may be a mild lymphocytic pleocytosis or a mildly elevated total protein; anti-measles antibodies may or may not be present.

Course

The disease is relentlessly progressive to coma and death within weeks to months.

Etiology

This disease probably occurs secondary to reactivation of a defective measles virus within neurons and oligodendrocytes; pathologically, there is very little or no inflammation, and measles-containing inclusion bodies may be found within both the nuclei and cytoplasm of both types of cells (Aicardi *et al.* 1977; Gazzola *et al.* 1999).

Although most patients have been children with leukemia, cases have occurred in adults with Hodgkin's disease (Wolinsky *et al.* 1977), adults undergoing therapeutic immunosuppression (Gazzola *et al.* 1999), patients with AIDS (Budka *et al.* 1996), and, rarely, apparently immunocompetent adult patients (Chadwick *et al.* 1982; Croxson *et al.* 2002).

Differential diagnosis

Subacute measles encephalitis must be distinguished from other measles-related disorders. Acute measles may be complicated by an encephalitis; however, in these cases symptoms occur in the context of a measles rash. Acute disseminated encephalomyelitis, like subacute measles encephalitis, also has a latent interval but it is shorter, in the order of weeks; furthermore, there is no myoclonus in acute disseminated encephalomyelitis. Subacute sclerosing panencephalitis also has a latent interval but this is much longer, in the order of years.

Treatment

The general treatment of delirium is discussed in Section 5.3; anecdotally, ribavirin was beneficial.

14.14 PROGRESSIVE RUBELLA PANENCEPHALITIS

Progressive rubella panencephalitis is a vanishingly rare disorder occurring as a result of a reactivation of rubella infection, generally in a patient with the congenital rubella syndrome.

Clinical features

The congenital rubella syndrome is characterized by mental retardation, microcephaly, deafness, and cataracts, and most cases of progressive rubella panencephalitis occur in this setting in patients aged from 4 to 19 years (Townsend *et al.* 1975a; Weil *et al.* 1975). Rarely, progressive rubella panencephalitis has occurred as a sequela to an uncomplicated case of German measles in an otherwise healthy individual (Lebon and Lyon 1974; Wolinsky *et al.* 1976), again after a long latent interval.

Clinically (Townsend *et al.* 1975a, 1976) there is a gradual onset of dementia, which is typically accompanied by ataxia; seizures are uncommon and myoclonus is generally absent.

The EEG shows generalized slowing and, in some cases, a burst-suppression pattern may eventually appear. Neuroimaging reveals cortical atrophy and ventricular dilation. The CSF is generally abnormal, with a lymphocytic pleocytosis, an elevated total protein, oligoclonal bands, and anti-rubella antibodies.

Course

This is a relentlessly progressive disease; spasticity and quadriparesis eventually appear and death occurs after 8–10 years.

Etiology

Pathologically (Townsend *et al.* 1975a, 1976, 1982; Weil *et al.* 1975; Wolinsky *et al.* 1976), there is a widespread perivascular inflammatory response, with prominent demyelinization and gliosis; although rubella virus may be found in neurons, there are no inclusion bodies. Furthermore, immunoglobulin deposits are found on cerebral vessels.

Differential diagnosis

When the syndrome occurs in the setting of the congenital rubella syndrome, there is little doubt as to the diagnosis. When, however, it occurs in an otherwise healthy child or adolescent, consideration may be given to subacute sclerosing panencephalitis, which is distinguished by prominent myoclonus.

Treatment

The general treatment of dementia is discussed in Section 5.1; there is no specific treatment for this disease.

14.15 NEUROSYPHILIS

Infection by the spirochete *Treponema pallidum* may cause primary, secondary, or tertiary syphilis. Primary syphilis typically presents with a painless chancre that remits spontaneously. Secondary syphilis may appear weeks to months after resolution of the chancre and is characterized by a widespread rash, which may or may not be accompanied by an acute syphilitic meningitis. Following resolution of the rash there is a long latency interval, lasting years, after which about 10 percent of patients go on to develop tertiary syphilis. Tertiary syphilis may manifest in a variety of organs, including the central nervous system, in which case one speaks of neurosyphilis.

Neurosyphilis may occur in any one of several forms (Merritt *et al.* 1946), including meningovascular syphilis, gummas, general paresis, and tabes dorsalis, each discussed below. Meningovascular neurosyphilis is characterized by a chronic, indolent basilar meningitis; both arteries and cranial nerves that cross the meninges may be affected and there may be infarctions and cranial nerve palsies. Gummas are granulomatous tumors that are typically found in association with meningovascular syphilis and which may range in size from minute to quite large, in which case they may present as any other mass lesion. General paresis is characterized pathologically by a direct invasion of the brain by the spirochete and clinically by a dementia. Tabes dorsalis is characterized by inflammation of the posterior spinal roots and softening of the posterior columns with ataxia and, in some, severe pain.

Although tertiary syphilis was common in the pre-antibiotic era, after World War II, with the widespread use of penicillin, the incidence fell dramatically to the point where it appeared to have almost vanished in developed countries. Over the past couple of decades, however, it has been enjoying something of a resurgence, particularly among those with AIDS.

Clinical features

As noted, some patients with secondary syphilis may develop *acute syphilitic meningitis*. Whether or not this condition should be subsumed under the rubric of neurosyphilis is not clear, although given that it does, of course, involve the nervous system it appears reasonable to do so; however, many authors reserve the term 'neurosyphilis' for nervous system manifestations occurring after a long latent interval as part of tertiary syphilis. Of these traditional forms of neurosyphilis, *meningovascular neurosyphilis* is currently the most common (Conde-Sendin *et al.* 2004)

and has an onset after a latency of about 6 or 7 years, with a range of 1 to 12 years. *Gummas* are currently quite rare and present with the same latency as meningovascular syphilis. *General paresis* has a longer latency, ranging from 15 to 20 years, and *tabes dorsalis* has potentially the longest latency, ranging from 10 to 30 years. Each of these will be discussed below, and consideration will also be given to *laboratory findings*, to the effect of concurrent *AIDS and neurosyphilis*, and to *congenital neurosyphilis*. It must be borne in mind that, although the various forms of tertiary neurosyphilis may occur in isolation, more commonly patients will have elements of two or more forms.

ACUTE SYPHILITIC MENINGITIS

In close relation to the rash of secondary syphilis, a minority of patients may develop a meningitis with typical symptoms such as malaise, headache, stiff neck, and, in some, a delirium. Although these symptoms generally undergo a gradual spontaneous remission, a small minority of patients may develop obstructive hydrocephalus.

MENINGOVASCULAR SYPHILIS

The symptomatology of meningovascular syphilis depends on which arteries and which cranial nerves are affected. When large arteries, such as the middle or posterior cerebral arteries, are involved, one sees a thrombotic stroke with the gradual evolution of appropriate focal deficits, such as hemiparesis or hemianopia (Holmes *et al.* 1984). In cases in which small arteries are involved, there may be small lacunar infarctions with appropriate lacunar syndromes, as discussed in Section 7.4; with an accrual of a significant number of these a lacunar dementia, as discussed in Section 10.2, may occur. Of the various cranial nerves, the most commonly involved are the third and sixth, with diplopia; the seventh, with unilateral or bilateral facial palsy; and the first, with unilateral or bilateral blindness. Rarely, obstructive hydrocephalus may appear. Most cases of meningovascular syphilis will also be characterized by the Argyll Robertson pupil, in which, although pupillary constriction to direct illumination is lost, constriction upon accommodation testing is preserved.

GUMMAS

Gummas tend to occur at the base of the brain or over the convexities; occasionally they may be deep-seated. They tend to present similarly to any gradually enlarging mass lesion and, if large enough, may cause dementia (Bianchi and Frera 1957).

GENERAL PARESIS

General paresis, also known as general paresis of the insane (GPI), dementia paralytica, or paretic neurosyphilis, is not necessarily associated with meningovascular syphilis and, indeed, it may be the only manifestation of tertiary neurosyphilis. General paresis typically manifests with a dementia of gradual onset and slow progression (Gomez and Aviles 1984; Storm-Mathisen 1969). Although the dementia may be non-specific in nature, certain cases may be marked by a personality change of the frontal lobe type; by mood changes, tending either toward mania or toward depression; or by delusions and hallucinations. Rarely, general paresis may present with a psychosis (Rothschild 1940; Schube 1934). Regardless of the typology of the dementia, other signs and symptoms gradually accrue. Seizures, either partial or grand mal, are common. Dysarthria and anomia may occur, and handwriting becomes very poor. Coarse tremor is common and may be present not only in the hands but also in the lips and tongue. Very typically the facial musculature loses its tone, giving the patient a vacant, dull facial expression. The Argyll Robertson pupil, described earlier, is present in most cases. With further progression the gait becomes unsteady and a true 'general paresis' occurs, with profound widespread weakness of almost all of the voluntary musculature. The plantar responses become extensor and, unless tabes dorsalis is present, there is a generalized hyper-reflexia.

TABES DORSALIS

Tabes dorsalis is characterized by ataxia, diminished vibratory sense, a positive Romberg test, urinary incontinence, and erectile dysfunction. There may also be 'tabetic pains' in the lower extremities that tend to be lightning-like and lancinating. 'Visceral crises' may also occur with abdominal pain similar to that seen in the 'acute abdomen'.

LABORATORY FINDINGS

Magnetic resonance scanning may reveal a basal pachymeningitis in meningovascular syphilis, along with evidence for any concurrent infarctions. In general paresis both cortical atrophy and ventricular dilation are seen, and if gummas are present they will immediately be apparent as space-occupying lesions.

Examination of the CSF is critical and must be interpreted in light of the results of testing for VDRL and fluorescent treponemal antibody (FTA). The pressure of the CSF is generally normal. There is usually a mild lymphocytic pleocytosis and the total protein is generally elevated as is the IgG index; oligoclonal bands may also be seen. The serum VDRL is positive in only about 70 percent of cases of neurosyphilis (Simon 1985), and the CSF VDRL is less sensitive: one study found a sensitivity of only 27 percent (Davis and Schmitt 1989). The serum FTA is positive in almost 100 percent of cases, whereas the CSF FTA, like the CSF VDRL, is less sensitive, being positive in about 75 percent of patients. False-positive serum VDRLs may occur in collagen vascular diseases, such as lupus, and also in heroin addicts; generally these false-positive VDRLs are low titer (e.g., less than 1:8). False-positive serum FTAs may occur under the same circumstances but are much less common.

In practice, demented patients are often screened with a serum VDRL and, if this is positive, with a serum FTA for confirmation. Given, however, the relative insensitivity of the serum VDRL, it is more appropriate to skip the VDRL and proceed directly to a serum FTA. If the serum FTA is negative, then neurosyphilis is effectively ruled out. In cases in which the serum FTA is positive and there is clinical evidence of neurosyphilis, then CSF should be obtained. If the CSF VDRL is positive, then the diagnosis of neurosyphilis is almost certain. If the CSF VDRL is negative but there is other CSF evidence of infection (e.g., lymphocytic pleocytosis or an elevated total protein), then it may be prudent to obtain a CSF FTA, as this is more sensitive than the CSF VDRL. Obtaining a CSF FTA, however, is controversial, as even minute contamination of the CSF by blood may create a false-positive FTA (Davis and Sperry 1979); caution is therefore required when interpreting this result. In the rare cases in which both the CSF VDRL and the CSF FTA are negative (Ch'ien et al. 1970) but the clinical picture is highly suggestive of neurosyphilis and there is evidence of infection in the CSF, then some clinicians will treat the patient as if neurosyphilis is present; if there is clinical improvement on follow-up, and if other CSF abnormalities resolve (e.g., the cell count falls), then it is reasonable to assume that a correct 'diagnosis by treatment response' has been made.

Given the frequency with which neurosyphilis is seen in AIDS, it is prudent to check all patients with neurosyphilis for HIV infection.

AIDS AND NEUROSYPHILIS

Some 15 percent of patients with AIDS are seropositive for syphilis and about 1 percent have neurosyphilis. Immunoincompetence in AIDS has probably altered the clinical picture of neurosyphilis in these patients: the latencies may be shorter and the evolution of the various forms may be more rapid (Johns et al. 1987).

CONGENITAL NEUROSYPHILIS

Infected mothers may pass the spirochete to the fetus, and congenitally infected children may or may not have the classic 'Hutchinson's triad' of cataracts, sensorineuronal deafness, and 'Hutchinson's teeth', in which the central incisors are notched, widely spaced, and often tapering. Neurosyphilis may present in these children after the normal latency periods and, in such cases, a dementia secondary to general paresis may present in teenage years.

Course

All forms of neurosyphilis are gradually progressive; untreated, both meningovascular neurosyphilis and general paresis are fatal within 3–5 years.

Etiology

The spirochete *T. pallidum* first gains access to the central nervous system during the course of secondary syphilis. Indeed, CSF studies indicate infection in up to one-third of patients at this stage (Lukehart *et al.* 1988). In most cases, however, host defenses are adequate to eradicate *T. pallidum* before tissue damage occurs. However, in about one-tenth of cases, host defenses fail and the stage is set for the appearance of one or more forms of neurosyphilis after the latent intervals noted earlier.

In meningovascular neurosyphilis, a granulomatous basilar meningitis is present. Cranial nerves traversing these meninges may become inflamed and undergo degenerative changes. Traversing arteries develop an endarteritis that may be followed by thrombotic occlusion and infarction of subserved tissues. Obstruction of the outflow foramina of the fourth ventricle may lead to hydrocephalus.

Gummas are granulomatous tumors that probably represent 'localized' forms of meningovascular neurosyphilis.

In general paresis, cortical atrophy is prominent, more so in the frontal and temporal areas than elsewhere. The ventricles are dilated and generally display a granular ependymitis. Spirochetes are found throughout the cortex, and neurons are lost with a disruption of the normal cortical architecture. Microglia and astrocytes are present in abundance, and there may be some perivascular cuffing by lymphocytes of small penetrating vessels.

In tabes dorsalis, inflammation is present in the ventral spinal roots, and the posterior columns display atrophy and softening.

Differential diagnosis

Importantly, a history of treatment of primary or secondary syphilis with benzathine penicillin does not rule out a diagnosis of neurosyphilis, given that benzathine penicillin is not capable of consistently inducing treponemocidal levels of penicillin within the CSF (Holmes *et al.* 1984).

Meningovascular syphilis may be mimicked by other disorders capable of causing an indolent basilar meningitis, such as sarcoidosis, tuberculosis, and mycotic infections. Gummas may be difficult to distinguish on clinical grounds from other granulomatous mass lesions. General paresis may mimic other dementias of gradual or subacute onset, as discussed in Section 5.1; in this regard, particular attention must be paid to the possibility of concurrent AIDS dementia.

One clinical finding may be very helpful in the differential diagnosis, namely the Argyll Robertson pupil, which is very rare in other disorders.

Treatment

A 2-week course of intravenous penicillin G is the treatment of choice, and in patients allergic to penicillin consideration should be given to desensitization. In a minority of patients, institution of antibiotic treatment will immediately be followed by what is known as the Jarisch–Herxheimer reaction, with malaise and fever and, in some, a transient exacerbation of the clinical symptomatology (Hahn *et al.* 1959), which in one extraordinary case characterized by a large gumma was fatal (Zifko *et al.* 1994); this Jarisch–Herxheimer reaction probably represents an inflammatory reaction to dying spirochetes, and may be treated by a short course of steroids. Because a course of penicillin G is not universally effective (especially in patients with AIDS [Gordon *et al.* 1994]), it is necessary to follow patients with serial examinations of the CSF every 3–6 months until there has been a satisfactory response. In general, the first evidence of improvement is a fall in the cell count, the total protein level falling later. The VDRL titer is the last to fall, a fourfold fall being seen as significant. As treatment failure is most common in patients with AIDS, serial CSF examinations are particularly important in this group.

Treatment with penicillin halts the progression of the symptoms of neurosyphilis, and in the case of general paresis there may be a partial remission. Gummas may or may not respond. In treatment-resistant cases the addition of steroids may be beneficial (Fleet *et al.* 1986); however, in some cases surgical resection is required.

With regard to the dementia that may occur with a lacunar state in meningovascular syphilis or with general paresis, symptomatic treatment is discussed in Section 5.1. Tabetic pains may respond to carbamazepine (Gimenez-Roldan and Martin 1981).

14.16 LYME DISEASE

Lyme disease is caused by the spirochete *Borrelia burgdorferi* and is transmitted to humans via the bite of an ixodid tick (Burgdorfer *et al.* 1982). The disease itself may be loosely divided into three stages. Stage I is characterized by a rash, known as erythema chronicum migrans. Stage II is characterized by cardiac conduction defects, polyarthralgia, and, in a minority, nervous system involvement with, variously, meningitis, cranial neuritis, and radiculitis; a small percentage may also develop an encephalitis. Stage III may present with an oligoarthritis, a mild dementia, or both. When Lyme disease is characterized by nervous system involvement, the term 'neuroborreliosis' is often used.

Although *Borrelia* is endemic in certain parts of North America, particularly the Northeast and the Midwest, Lyme disease itself is uncommon.

Clinical features

In considering the various stages of Lyme disease it must be borne in mind that there may be some overlap between them and that not all patients will experience all three stages: stage I is seen in about 75 percent and stage II nervous system involvement occurs in about 15 percent; the percentage of patients who develop stage III disease is not clear, but is probably low. Each of these stages is discussed in turn, followed by a consideration of laboratory testing.

STAGE I

Erythema chronicum migrans appears anywhere from 3 days to a month after the tick bite. The rash is characterized by a gradually enlarging, ring-like erythematous lesion, which as it enlarges leaves a pale, indurated central portion, thus creating an overall 'bull's-eye' effect. Smaller, 'satellite' lesions may also occur. In general, the rash resolves spontaneously in a matter of weeks.

STAGE II

Stage II typically follows stage I within weeks to months. Cardiac involvement most frequently manifests with an atrioventricular block; evidence of pericarditis or even myocarditis may also be found. As noted earlier, polyarthralgia may also occur. Nervous system involvement classically manifests with the triad of meningitis, cranial neuritis, and radiculoneuritis (Hansen and Lebech 1992; Pachner and Steere 1985). The meningitis presents with headache, neck stiffness, and malaise. Although cranial neuritis may affect virtually any of the cranial nerves, by far the most common manifestation is a unilateral or bilateral peripheral facial palsy. When radiculitis occurs it is often accompanied by significant pain. The occurrence of encephalitis is heralded by somnolence and delirium, and, in a small minority, seizures or chorea. In addition to this classic triad, one may also find evidence of a mononeuritis multiplex, a primarily sensory polyneuropathy, or, rarely, a myelitis. In general, symptoms gradually remit over 3–18 months.

STAGE III

Stage III Lyme disease may appear anywhere from months to up to a decade after stage I, and may be characterized by a large-joint oligoarthritis or, in a minority, by a dementia. The dementia tends to be quite mild and manifests with poor short-term memory, poor concentration, mild somnolence, fatigue, and either depression or irritability (Halperin et al. 1989; Logigian et al. 1990; Shadick et al. 1994); a peripheral polyneuropathy may also be present and in a minority there may also be focal signs such as ataxia, aphasia, or hemiplegia; seizures have also been noted. In one very rare case, stage III Lyme disease presented with a psychosis characterized by delusions of persecution, auditory hallucinations, and stuporous catatonia (Pfister et al. 1993). Although some patients may show gradual progression, it appears that in most cases the course is characterized by a stable chronicity.

LABORATORY TESTING

Serum should be tested for both IgG and IgM anti-*Borrelia* antibodies: IgG antibodies are found in almost all patients with neurologic involvement, and IgM antibodies may be found in those with stage I and stage II disease.

The CSF may display a lymphocytic pleocytosis, an elevated protein, and oligoclonal bands; anti-*Borrelia* antibodies may or may not be present. PCR assay is generally less sensitive than testing for antibodies. Although the CSF is typically clearly abnormal in stage II disease, findings may be equivocal in stage III.

Magnetic resonance scanning in stage III may reveal multifocal areas of demyelinization in the subcortical and periventricular white matter, or multifocal areas of cerebritis.

Course

This is as noted above.

Etiology

Erythema chronicum migrans represents a local reaction to the infection; hematogenous spread then occurs to the heart, joints, and nervous system. Various findings have been reported in the nervous system, including a lymphocytic vasculitis in stage II (Meurers et al. 1990), and, in addition to a small-vessel vasculitis, multifocal areas of either demyelinization or cerebritis in stage III (Kobayashi et al. 1997; Oksi et al. 1996).

Differential diagnosis

In classic cases with a well-documented progression from stage I to stage II and beyond, the diagnosis is fairly straightforward. Unfortunately, however, as noted earlier, up to one-quarter of patients do not have erythema chronicum migrans, and those who do may not recall having it. Consequently, diagnosis may rest on a high index of suspicion. In this regard, however, prudence must be exercised in evaluating the results of serum testing for anti-*Borrelia* antibodies. Although the absence of IgG antibodies argues strongly against the diagnosis, their presence cannot be seen as strongly confirmatory: in some parts of North America, 5 percent or more of inhabitants will be seropositive, with absolutely no evidence of active disease.

Treatment

For stage II, intravenous ceftriaxone is recommended; in a small minority, a Jarisch–Herxheimer-like reaction may develop soon after the initiation of treatment, with malaise, fever, and, in some, an exacerbation of the presenting symptomatology. Treatment of stage III is a matter of debate. Although some patients with marked dementia and clearly positive CSF findings definitely respond to ceftriaxone (Steinbach et al. 2005), it appears that patients with only mild cognitive complaints do no better with ceftriaxone than with placebo (Klempner *et al.* 2001; Krupp *et al.* 2003). In my opinion, when the diagnosis of stage III disease is clinically suspected, antibiotic treatment should probably be offered only to patients with positive CSF or MRI findings.

14.17 TUBERCULOSIS

Mycobacterium tuberculosis is an acid-fast intracellular bacillus that in most cases is spread by droplets from patients with pulmonary tuberculosis. In many patients a focus of infection may be held in check by adequate host defenses for many years or even decades until some loss of immunocompetence, for example in AIDS or after treatment with steroids or immunosuppressants, is followed by reactivation. Hematogenous spread may carry the bacillus to various organs, including the brain, where it may cause a meningitis or present with one or more tuberculomas.

In North America the incidence of tuberculosis has increased dramatically over the past decades, in large part because of its occurrence in patients with AIDS; indeed in some cases tubercular meningitis has constituted the presentation of AIDS (Barnes *et al.* 1979).

Clinical features

The meningitis seen in tuberculosis is generally basilar in location and typically presents subacutely, over a matter of weeks. When fully developed (Davis *et al.* 1993; Kennedy and Fallon 1979; Sanchez-Portocarrero *et al.* 1996; Traub *et al.* 1984; Williams and Smith 1954), patients have delirium or stupor, headache, stiff neck, and fever. Cranial nerves may be entrapped and palsies of cranial nerves III, IV, VI, and VII are common (McKendrick and Grose 1957). Arteries traversing the inflamed meninges may undergo an arteritis with thrombus formation and infarction of subserved tissue: the basal ganglia are most vulnerable in this regard and there may be focal signs or abnormal movements, such as tremor, chorea, or dystonia (Alacon *et al.* 2000). Involvement of the hypothalamus or pituitary may lead to either the syndrome of inappropriate ADH secretion or diabetes insipidus. Obstruction of the outflow foramina of the fourth ventricle is common and produces obstructive hydrocephalus, with a dramatic worsening of the clinical picture.

Tuberculomas may be single or, more commonly, multiple, may occur either in the cerebellum or cerebrum, and present as would any mass lesion, with focal signs or seizures (Damergis *et al.* 1978).

The spinal cord may also be involved. Spinal meningitis may lead to entrapment of nerve roots, and arteritis of spinal arteries may lead to infarction of the cord.

In cases of meningitis, MR scanning typically reveals enhancement of the basilar meninges. In addition, the CSF is often under increased pressure. There is a pleocytosis that may be either lymphocytic from the start or characterized initially by polymorphonuclear cells, which eventually give way to lymphocytes. The total protein is increased and the glucose is decreased. All specimens should be stained for acid-fast rods, but the search may be fruitless. Culture results, although positive in perhaps one-half of cases, may take weeks, and treatment decisions should never wait upon them. PCR assay is generally positive (Lin *et al.* 1995) and results are available promptly.

The PPD skin test may be falsely negative, and this is particularly likely in those with AIDS (Sanchez-Portocarrero *et al.* 1996).

Course

Untreated, tubercular meningitis is generally fatal within weeks to months, and those who survive may be left with dementia, cranial nerve palsies, or focal signs (Kalita *et al.* 2007). Tuberculomas generally show some progression but may eventually stabilize, in some cases undergoing calcification.

Etiology

With hematogenous spread, bacilli may infect the meninges with the formation of minute tuberculomas; these may subsequently rupture with spread of the bacilli throughout the subarachnoid space, prompting the development of a thick, almost gelatinous exudate that, as noted earlier, is typically basilar in location (Rich and McCordock 1933). Cranial nerves and arteries traversing the exudate may become inflamed with cranial nerve palsies or infarctions. In some cases the parenchyma directly subjacent to the inflamed meninges may also become infiltrated.

Hematogenous spread may also carry bacilli to the brain parenchyma, with the subsequent development of tuberculomas, which, like tuberculomas anywhere, may undergo caseation necrosis. As noted earlier, these tuberculomas tend to be multiple and exhibit a broad range in size, from minute to so large that they destroy an entire lobe.

Differential diagnosis

Tubercular meningitis may be confused with basilar meningitides seen with fungal infections, tertiary neurosyphilis, sarcoidosis, and meningeal carcinomatosis. Tuberculomas may be mimicked by gliomas or other mass lesions.

Treatment

Tuberculous meningitis requires urgent treatment and a multiple-drug regimen is typically utilized, often consisting of isoniazid, rifampin, pyrazinamide, and ethambutol. Given the recent emergence of drug-resistant strains (Frieden *et al.*

1993), sensitivity testing should be undertaken. If isoniazid is used, consideration should be given to supplementation with vitamin B6 to prevent the development of pellagra (Ishii and Nishihara 1985), as discussed in Section 13.3.

Tuberculomas may be treated with the same drug regimen. In some cases, excision is required.

14.18 WHIPPLE'S DISEASE

Whipple's disease, first described by George Hoyt Whipple in 1907 (Whipple 1907), is a rare disorder found mostly in white males, which occurs secondary to infection with a bacillus known as *Tropheryma whippelii*. Although Whipple's disease most commonly causes arthralgia and abdominal complaints, the nervous system may be involved with, as described below, a wide variety of signs and symptoms.

Clinical features

Whipple's disease typically presents in middle years. Migratory large-joint polyarthralgia is common and patients also typically have abdominal pain, diarrhea, weight loss, and mild fever. In a minority of cases the central nervous system is involved and, although such involvement generally occurs within the context of long-standing arthralgia or abdominal symptomatology, there are definite cases in which Whipple's disease has presented with central nervous system involvement alone (Adams *et al.* 1987; Lampert *et al.* 1962; Pruss *et al.* 2007; Romanul *et al.* 1977).

When the central nervous system is involved (Gerard *et al.* 2002; Louis *et al.* 1996; Manzel *et al.* 2000; Matthews *et al.* 2005), patients typically present with a gradually progressive dementia, delirium or personality change. In most cases other symptoms are also present, including upper motor neuron signs, ataxia, nystagmus, myoclonus, seizures, supranuclear ophthalmoplegia, and various manifestations of hypothalamic dysfunction including sleep disturbance (with either hypersomnolence or, less commonly, insomnia), hyperphagia, decreased libido or diabetes insipidus. A small minority of patients may also display a very distinctive abnormal movement known as oculomasticatory myorhythmia, in which pendular eye movements occur in concert with rhythmic jaw movements (Schwartz *et al.* 1986).

T2-weighted MRI may reveal multifocal areas of increased signal intensity within the cerebral cortex, the basal ganglia, thalamus, midbrain, and cerebellar cortex; in some cases these lesions may show enhancement with gadolinium.

The CSF may show either a lymphocytic pleocytosis or an elevated total protein, or both, with a normal glucose. In rare instances some of the white cells may be periodic acid–Schiff (PAS) positive. PCR assay is typically, but not always, positive for *T. whippelii* DNA.

The diagnosis may also be established by small bowel biopsy, which may reveal not only PAS-positive macrophages but also a positive PCR assay; in this regard, however, it must be kept in mind that, albeit rarely, central nervous system Whipple's disease can occur with a negative small bowel biopsy (Pollock *et al.* 1981).

Course

Central nervous system involvement is a grave sign in Whipple's disease; in most cases there is a steady progression, with death occurring within 6–12 months.

Etiology

Whipple's disease, as noted, occurs secondary to infection by *T. whippelii* (Raoult *et al.* 2000; Relman *et al.* 1992). Within the central nervous system (Powers and Rawe 1979; Smith *et al.* 1965), focal areas of inflammation and necrosis, along with glial scars, are found in the cerebral cortex, basal ganglia, hypothalamus, brainstem (especially the periaqueductal gray), and cerebellar cortex. PAS-positive macrophages are found in these areas, and electron microscopy may reveal the bacillus within the macrophage.

Differential diagnosis

The appearance of dementia, delirium, or personality change in the context of long-standing polyarthralgia or abdominal complaints is highly suggestive; in these cases, consideration might also be given to Lyme disease or to cerebrotendinous xanthomatosis. The differential for dementia or delirium occurring with myoclonus is discussed in Sections 5.1 and 5.3 respectively. Oculomasticatory myorhythmia, although present in only a minority of cases, is a particularly valuable sign as it is virtually pathognomonic for this disease.

Vitamin B12 deficiency may occur in cases characterized by severe diarrhea, making an independent contribution to central nervous system symptomatology.

Treatment

The general treatment of dementia, delirium, and personality change is discussed in Sections 5.1, 5.3, and 7.2 respectively. Although there are no controlled trials of antibiotic treatment, most clinicians will begin with a 2-week course of ceftriaxone, followed by treatment with trimethoprim–sulfamethoxazole. The CSF should be monitored and treatment continued until the patient is clinically stable and the CSF has normalized; in many cases this may take up to 2 years. If antibiotics are discontinued the patient should be closely monitored as relapses may occur; in some cases indefinite treatment is required.

14.19 ROCKY MOUNTAIN SPOTTED FEVER

Rocky Mountain spotted fever is a rare disorder secondary to infection by a tick-borne obligate intracellular parasite, *Rickettsia rickettsii*, which manifests classically with fever, rash, and delirium. Rocky Mountain spotted fever is generally found in the Rocky Mountain area and the Appalachians, and is most common in the spring or early summer.

Clinical features

After the tick bite, which is recalled by only about three-quarters of patients, there is a latent interval of from days to a couple of weeks, after which there is a fairly abrupt onset of fever, headache, malaise, and myalgia. After a few days, a characteristic maculopapular rash appears: this is initially present at the ankles and wrists but then spreads to involve the extremities and, in over 50 percent of cases, the soles and palms. In this setting, most patients become delirious or lethargic, and this may be accompanied by seizures and various focal signs; coma may supervene (Bell and Lascari 1970; Horney and Walker 1988; Kirk *et al.* 1990). Pulmonary and hepatic involvement may also occur.

The CSF typically shows a mild lymphocytic pleocytosis and an elevated total protein; the glucose is generally normal.

Serologic testing may reveal anti-rickettsial IgM or, with serial testing, a fourfold or greater rise in IgG antibodies. Prompter diagnosis may be obtained via a punch biopsy of affected skin.

Course

Untreated, the mortality rate is as high as 20 percent. Among those who survive, recovery occurs gradually in a matter of weeks; various sequelae may be found, including dementia or any focal signs present during the acute illness.

Etiology

Rickettsia rickettsii undergoes hematogenous spread to the brain. Within the cortex and the subcortical gray matter there are multiple petechial hemorrhages and areas of perivascular inflammation; small arteries may become occluded, resulting in multiple mini-infarcts (Green *et al.* 1978; Miller and Price 1972).

Differential diagnosis

Typhus may be virtually indistinguishable from Rocky Mountain spotted fever; however, this disease is virtually extinct in North America.

Treatment

In adults, treatment is with tetracycline or doxycycline.

14.20 MALARIA

Malaria occurs secondary to infection with any one of four species of the protozoon *Plasmodium*, including *P. malariae*, *P. vivax*, *P. ovale*, and *P. falciparum*. Of these four species, only one, *P. falciparum*, invades the central nervous system, thereby causing cerebral malaria.

Malaria is endemic in Haiti, much of Asia and Oceania, and in tropical and subtropical areas of Africa and South America; although it has been eradicated from most of North America and Europe, cases may still be seen in those returning from travel in endemic areas who did not take adequate prophylactic medication.

Clinical features

Anywhere from 1 to 4 weeks after infection via the bite of an *Anopheles* mosquito, patients fall ill with fever, headache, malaise, and myalgia. A small minority of those patients whose malaria has occurred secondary to *P. falciparum* may then develop cerebral malaria (Blocker *et al.* 1968; Idro *et al.* 2005), with delirium, stupor or coma, and seizures. Focal signs, such as hemiparesis, may occur, but are uncommon.

The CSF may be normal or may show a mild pleocytosis and a mildly elevated total protein.

Diagnosis is made by examination of peripheral blood smears.

Course

Cerebral malaria is fatal in perhaps one-third of all cases; among those who survive, sequelae may occur in 10–20 percent of children, including dementia, hemiparesis, aphasia, ataxia, and blindness (Brewster *et al.* 1990). Sequelae are less common in adults, but may include dementia (Roze *et al.* 2001) and epilepsy (Ngoungou *et al.* 2006).

Recently, a 'post-malaria neurological syndrome' has been described (Schnorf *et al.* 1998; Zambito Marsala *et al.* 2006). Here, after recovering from malaria there is an asymptomatic latent interval of several weeks, after which patients fall ill with various symptoms, including delirium, myoclonus, tremor, aphasia, ataxia, and seizures. The syndrome responds promptly to treatment with corticosteroids, and it is suspected that it represents an example of acute disseminated encephalomyelitis.

Etiology

Erythrocytes infected with *P. falciparum* develop 'knobs' on their cell membranes, which promote the adhesion of the erythrocyte to the vascular endothelium; within the brain, capillaries and post-capillary venules are packed with infected red cells (Oo *et al.* 1987). Petechial and ring hemorrhages are found scattered throughout the parenchyma and in chronic cases there may be widespread gliotic areas, known as Durck's granulomas (Oo *et al.* 1987; Toro and Roman 1978). Cerebral edema is common, and in some cases there may be herniation.

Differential diagnosis

The differential diagnosis of acute encephalitis is discussed in Section 7.6. In North America and Europe, the diagnosis should be suspected in travellers who have returned from an endemic area; in this regard it must be kept in mind that mosquitoes can gain access to airplanes during stopovers, and hence it is not necessary for travellers to actually disembark in endemic areas to become infected.

Treatment

Although chloroquine was once considered adequate treatment, drug-resistant strains of malaria are emerging, and various combination treatments are now recommended. Steroids are not recommended (Warrell *et al.* 1982) and, although anti-epileptic drugs may be required, they should not be given prophylactically.

14.21 TOXOPLASMOSIS

Infection by *Toxoplasma gondii* is common in birds and mammals; cats serve as the definitive hosts and oocysts found in cat feces may remain viable for up to a year. Primary infection in humans occurs secondary to eating contaminated food or undercooked lamb, pork or beef from infected animals, and is very common: serologic studies indicate that about one-third of adults in North America and Europe have been infected. In the vast majority of cases, host defenses are capable of rapidly controlling the infection and, during primary infection, patients are either asymptomatic or suffer a self-limited mononucleosis-like syndrome. Toxoplasma, however, may not be eradicated but remain latent in cysts, often in muscle.

Infection of the central nervous system is very rare in immunocompetent adults. In immunocompromised patients, however, central nervous system toxoplasmosis does occur, either during a primary infection or, more commonly, with reactivation of a latent infection. In the pre-AIDS era this was noted in patients with cancer or those undergoing therapeutic immunosuppression, but was rare (Townsend *et al.* 1975b); with the advent of AIDS, however, central nervous system toxoplasmosis has become common and indeed is the most common opportunistic infection in AIDS patients, where it typically appears only when the CD4+ count falls below 200/mm^3.

Clinical features

Although fulminant onsets have been noted, in most cases central nervous system toxoplasmosis presents subacutely, over a matter of weeks. The presentation is variable (Navia *et al.* 1986c; Porter and Sande 1992), depending on the number and location of toxoplasma abscesses, and may include headache, fever, delirium, dementia, seizures (Pascual-Sedano *et al.* 1999), and various focal signs, including hemianopia, hemiparesis, aphasia, or, uncommonly, abnormal movements such as dystonia (Factor *et al.* 2003) or chorea (Piccolo *et al.* 1999).

Magnetic resonance scanning reveals toxoplasma abscesses as areas of increased signal intensity on T2-weighted or FLAIR imaging, which typically show ring enhancement with gadolinium. Typically, multiple lesions are present in the cortex, white matter, and subcortical structures, but the number varies from a solitary lesion to such a high number as to constitute a miliary presentation. The CSF may be normal or may display a mild lymphocytic pleocytosis and a mildly elevated total protein. Polymerase chain reaction assay for toxoplasma DNA is generally positive, and occasionally the organism may be detected in the CSF by staining with Wright's or Giesma's stain.

Serologic testing may or may not be helpful. Finding a positive IgG, of course, proves little, given the high prevalence of past infection among adults; in addition, although a negative serum IgG anti-toxoplasma antibody would argue against the diagnosis, in immunocompromised patients toxoplasmosis may not be accompanied by either the appearance of IgM antibodies or a fourfold rise in the IgG titer. In one large study (Porter and Sande 1992) about one-fifth of patients with AIDS and central nervous system toxoplasmosis were negative for IgG.

Course

Untreated, central nervous system toxoplasmosis is generally fatal in a matter of months.

Etiology

Although toxoplasma abscesses may occur anywhere in the brain, favored sites include the junction of the cerebral cortex and subcortical white matter, and the basal ganglia (Navia *et al.* 1986c). These abscesses, as noted earlier, vary widely both in number and size; in some cases they may become quite large. Rarely, an abscess may obstruct CSF outflow, causing obstructive hydrocephalus, and, also rarely, the pituitary may be involved with subsequent endocrinologic disturbances.

Differential diagnosis

Although toxoplasmosis is the most common opportunistic central nervous system infection in AIDS, it must nevertheless be distinguished from other opportunistic infections, such as tuberculosis, fungal infections, and progressive multifocal leukoencephalopathy. A solitary toxoplasma must also be distinguished from primary central nervous system lymphoma. In practice, the differential here is often based on a 'diagnosis by treatment response' strategy: when lesions fail to regress with adequate anti-toxoplasma therapy then one or more of the other possibilities is strenuously investigated.

Treatment

A 2-week course of combination treatment with pyrimethamine and sulfadiazine is generally sufficient to prompt a regression of the lesions; chronic treatment, however, is typically required to prevent relapses.

14.22 FUNGAL INFECTIONS

Fungal, or mycotic, infection of the central nervous system (Mori *et al.* 1992; Walsh *et al.* 1985a) generally occurs only in immunocompromised patients, such as those with AIDS, and includes candidiasis, histoplasmosis, cryptococcosis, coccidioidomycosis, aspergillosis, and, much less commonly, mucormycosis, nocardiosis, or blastomycosis. In general, the primary site of infection is the respiratory tract, most often the lung, and this may represent either an initial infection or a reactivation of a latent one. In either case, the brain is typically reached via hematogenous spread; aspergillosis at times, however, may spread directly from a sinus infection.

Clinical features

Typically, the onset is subacute, over days or weeks, and patients may or may not be febrile. As noted below, the pathology seen in these fungal infections may include either a basilar meningitis or multiple abscesses or granulomas, or both. In candidiasis, granulomas and abscesses predominate (Parker *et al.* 1981; Roessman and Friede 1967), whereas in histoplasmosis (Cooper and Goldstein 1963), cryptococcosis (Chuck and Sande 1989; Edwards *et al.* 1970) and coccidiomycosis (Caudill *et al.* 1970), the clinical picture is often dominated by a basilar meningitis. In aspergillosis (Walsh *et al.* 1985b), abscesses and granulomas are dominant, but here one may also see mycotic aneurysms.

Abscesses and granulomas may either present as mass lesions, with focal signs determined by their location, or, if there are a large number of lesions, a delirium may occur.

Basilar meningitis typically presents with headache and delirium. With entrapment of cranial nerves and arteries that traverse the inflamed meninges, there may be cranial nerve palsies or infarctions; when infarctions do occur they preferentially involve the penetrating arteries and produce

lacunar syndromes, discussed in Section 7.4. With obstruction of the outflow foramina of the fourth ventricle, an obstructive hydrocephalus may occur, with a dramatic worsening of the overall clinical picture.

Magnetic resonance scanning reveals both abscesses and granulomas and evidence of a basilar meningitis.

The CSF may be normal when pathology is confined to abscesses or granulomas. When basilar meningitis is present, the fluid may be under increased pressure and there is a pleocytosis, which may be lymphocytic, polymorphonuclear, or mixed; the total protein is increased, sometimes greatly so, and the glucose is decreased. India ink staining may reveal cryptococci. Assays for cryptococcal or coccidioidomycoccal antigen may be positive, and pan-fungal PCR assay appears to hold great promise.

Course

In the natural course of events, symptoms progress gradually, typically over months, with a fatal outcome in roughly one-half of all cases.

Etiology

Abscesses or granulomas may be single or multiple and may occur in any part of the cerebrum. Basilar meningitis is characterized by a thick exudate at the base of the brain, which, as noted earlier, may entrap arteries or cranial nerves.

Differential diagnosis

Fungal abscesses and granulomas must be distinguished from other opportunistic infections, such as toxoplasmosis or tuberculosis. A fungal basilar meningitis may be mimicked by tuberculosis, tertiary neurosyphilis, and sarcoidosis.

Treatment

Treatment involves amphotericin B, either singly or in combination with other anti-fungals.

REFERENCES

Abrams DI, Jay CA, Shade SB *et al.* Cannabis in painful HIV-associated sensory neuropathy: a randomized placebo-controlled trial. *Neurology* 2007; **68**:515–21.

Adams JH, Miller D. Herpes simplex encephalitis: a clinical and pathological analysis of twenty-two cases. *Postgrad Med J* 1973; **49**:393–7.

Adams M, Rhyner PA, Day J *et al.* Whipple's disease confined to the central nervous system. *Ann Neurol* 1987; **21**:104–8.

Adie WJ. Idiopathic narcolepsy: a disease *sui generis* with remarks on the mechanism of sleep. *Brain* 1926; **49**:257–306.

Adle-Biassette H, Bourhy H, Gisselbrecht M *et al.* Rabies encephalitis in a patient with AIDS: a clinicopathological study. *Acta Neuropathol* 1996; **92**:415–20.

Agamanolis DP, Tan JS, Parker DL. Immunosuppressive measles encephalitis in a patient with a renal transplant. *Arch Neurol* 1979; **36**:686–90.

Aicardi J, Goutieres F, Arsenio-Nunes HL *et al.* Acute measles encephalitis in children with immunosuppression. *Pediatrics* 1977; **55**:232–5.

Alacon F, Duenas G, Cevallos N *et al.* Movement disorders in 30 patients with tuberculous meningitis. *Mov Disord* 2000; **15**:561–9.

Alpers BJ, Patten CA. Paroxysmal spasm of the eyelids as a postencephalitic manifestation. *Arch Neurol Psychiatry* 1927; **18**:427–32.

Anlar B, Saatci I, Kose G *et al.* MRI findings in subacute sclerosing panencephalitis. *Neurology* 1996; **47**:1278–83.

Applebaum E, Rachelson MH, Dolgopol VB. Varicella encephalitis. *Am J Med* 1953; **15**:233–6.

Applebaum E, Krebs SI, Sunshine A. Herpes zoster encephalitis. *Am J Med* 1962; **32**:25–31.

Astrom KE, Mancall EL, Richardson EP. Progressive multifocal leuko-encephalopathy: a hitherto unrecognized complication of chronic lymphatic leukaemia and Hodgkin's disease. *Brain* 1958; **81**:93–111.

Aurelius E, Johansson G, Skoldenberg B *et al.* Rapid diagnosis of herpes simplex encephalitis by nested polymerase chain reaction assay of cerebrospinal fluid. *Lancet* 1991; **337**:189–92.

Ayuso-Peralta L, Jimenez-Jimenez FJ, Tejeiro J *et al.* Progressive multifocal leukoencephalopathy in HIV infection presenting as Balint's syndrome. *Neurology* 1994; **44**:1339–40.

Azimi PH, Cramblett HG, Haynes RE. Mumps meningoencephalitis in children. *JAMA* 1969; **207**:509–12.

Baringer JR, Swoveland P. Recovery of herpes simplex virus from human trigeminal ganglions. *N Engl J Med* 1973; **228**:648–50.

Barnes PF, Bloch AB, Davidson PT *et al.* Tuberculosis in patients with human immunodeficiency virus. *N Engl J Med* 1979; **301**:126–30.

Beach RS, Morgan R, Wilkie F *et al.* Plasma vitamin B12 level as a potential cofactor in studies of human immunodeficiency virus type 1-related cognitive changes. *Arch Neurol* 1992; **49**:501–6.

Bell WE, Lascari AD. Rocky Mountain spotted fever. Neurologic manifestations in the acute phase. *Neurology* 1970; **20**:841–7.

Bergin JD. Fatal encephalopathy in glandular fever. *J Neurol Neurosurg Psychiatry* 1960; **23**:69–73.

Berman SM, Kim RC. The development of cytomegalovirus encephalitis in AIDS patients receiving ganciclovir. *Am J Med* 1994; **96**:415–19.

Bhatia KP, Morris JH, Frackowiak RS. Primary progressive multifocal leukoencephalopathy presenting as an extrapyramidal syndrome. *J Neurol* 1996; **243**:91–5.

Bianchi M, Frera C. A case of brain gumma. *J Neurol Neurosurg Psychiatry* 1957; **20**:133–5.

Bistrian B, Phillips CA, Kaye IS. Fatal mumps meningoencephalitis. *JAMA* 1972; **222**:478–9.

Blatt ML, Hoffman SJ, Schneider M. Rabies: report of twelve cases, with a discussion of prophylaxis. *JAMA* 1938; **111**:688–91.

Blocker WW, Kasil AJ, Daroff RB. The psychiatric manifestations of cerebral malaria. *Am J Psychiatry* 1968; **125**:192–6.

Bond ED. Epidemic encephalitis and katatonic symptoms. *Am J Insanity* 1920; **76**:261–4.

Bouwman FH, Skolasky RL, Hes D *et al.* Variable progression of HIV-associated dementia. *Neurology* 1998; **50**:1814–20.

Breitbart W, Rosenfeld B, Kaim M *et al.* A randomized, double-blind, placebo-controlled trial of psychostimulants for the treatment of fatigue in ambulatory patients with human immunodeficiency virus disease. *Arch Int Med* 2001; **161**:411–20.

Brewster DR, Kwiatkowski D, White NJ. Neurological sequelae of cerebral malaria in children. *Lancet* 1990; **336**:1039–43.

Budka H, Urbanits S, Liberski PP *et al.* Subacute measles virus encephalitis: a new and fatal opportunistic infection in a patient with AIDS. *Neurology* 1996; **46**:586–7.

Burgdorfer W, Barbour AF, Hayes SF *et al.* Lyme disease – a tick-borne spirochetosis. *Science* 1982; **216**:1317–19.

Buzzard EF, Greenfield JG. Lethargic encephalitis: its sequelae and morbid anatomy. *Brain* 1919; **42**:305–38.

Caparros-Lefebvre D, Girard-Buttaz I, Rebout S *et al.* Cognitive and psychiatric impairment in herpes simplex virus encephalitis suggest involvement of the amygdalo-frontal pathways. *J Neurol* 1996; **243**:248–56.

Cape CA, Martinez AI, Robertson JJ *et al.* Adult onset of subacute sclerosing panencephalitis. *Arch Neurol* 1973; **28**:124–7.

Caudill RG, Smith CE, Reinharz JA. Coccidioidal meningitis. A diagnostic challenge. *Am J Med* 1970; **49**:360–5.

Causey JQ. Spontaneous cytomegalovirus mononucleosis-like syndrome and aseptic meningitis. *South Med J* 1976; **69**:1384–7.

Chadwick DW, Martin S, Buxton PH *et al.* Measles virus and subacute neurological disease: an unusual presentation of measles inclusion body encephalitis. *J Neurol Neurosurg Psychiatry* 1982; **45**:680–4.

Chandra K, Shafiq N, Pandhi P *et al.* Gabapentin versus nortriptyline in post-herpetic neuralgia patients: a randomized, double-blind clinical trial – the GONIP Trial. *Int J Clin Pharmacol Ther* 2006; **44**:358–63.

Ch'ien L, Hathaway BM, Israel CW. Seronegative dementia paralytica: report of a case. *J Neurol Neurosurg Psychiatry* 1970; **33**:376–80.

Chopra JS, Banerjee AK, Murthy JMK *et al.* Paralytic rabies: a clinicopathological study. *Brain* 1980; **103**:789–802.

Chuck SL, Sande MA. Infections with *Cryptococcus neoformans* in the acquired immunodeficiency syndrome. *N Engl J Med* 1989; **321**:580–4.

Cobb WA, Marshall J, Scaravilli F. Long survival in subacute sclerosing panencephalitis. *J Neurol Neurosurg Psychiatry* 1984; **47**:176–83.

Conde-Sendin MA, Amela-Paris R, Aladro-Benito Y *et al.* Current clinical spectrum of neurosyphilis in immunocompetent patients. *Eur Neurol* 2004; **52**:29–35.

Conomy JP, Leibovitz A, McCombs W et al. Airborne rabies encephalitis: demonstration of rabies virus in the human central nervous system. Neurology 1977; 27:67–9.

Cooper RA, Goldstein E. Histoplasmosis of the central nervous system. Report of two cases and review of the literature. Am J Med 1963; 35:45–57.

Croxson MC, Anderson NE, Vaughn AA et al. Subacute measles encephalitis in an immunocompetent adult. J Clin Neurosci 2002; 9:600–4.

Dale RC, Church AJ, Surtees RA et al. Encephalitis lethargica syndrome: 20 new cases and evidence of basal ganglia autoimmunity. Brain 2004; 127:21–33.

Damergis JA, Leftwich EI, Curtin JA et al. Tuberculoma of the brain. JAMA 1978; 239:413–15.

Dana Consortium on the Therapy of HIV Dementia and Related Cognitive Disorders. A randomized, double-blind, placebo-controlled trial of deprynel and thioctic acid in human immunodeficiency virus-associated cognitive impairment. Neurology 1998; 50:645–51.

Davies JA, Hughes JT, Oppenheimer DR. Richardson's disease (progressive multifocal leukoencephalopathy). Q J Med 1973; 42:481–93.

Davis LE, Schmitt JW. Clinical significance of cerebrospinal fluid tests for neurosyphilis. Ann Neurol 1989; 25:50–5.

Davis LE, Sperry S. The CSF-FTA test and the significance of blood contamination. Ann Neurol 1979; 6:68–9.

Davis LE, Rastogi KR, Lambert LC et al. Tuberculous meningitis in the southwest United States: a community-based study. Neurology 1993; 43:1775–8.

Davis LE, DeBiasi R, Goade DE et al. West Nile virus neuroinvasive disease. Ann Neurol 2006; 60:286–300.

Dawson JR. Cellular inclusions in cerebral lesions of epidemic encephalitis. Arch Neurol Psychiatry 1934; 31:685–700.

Devinsky O, Cho E-S, Petito CK et al. Herpes zoster myelitis. Brain 1991; 114:1991–9.

Dickman MS. von Economo encephalitis. Arch Neurol 2001; 58:1696–8.

Doja A, Bitnun A, Ford Jones EL et al. Pediatric Epstein–Barr virus-associated encephalitis: 10-year review. J Child Neurol 2006; 21:384–91.

Dolgopol VB, Greenberg M, Aronoff R. Encephalitis following smallpox vaccination. Arch Neurol Psychiatry 1955; 73:216–23.

Donner M, Waltimo O, Poros J et al. Subacute sclerosing panencephalitis as a cause of chronic dementia and relapsing brain disorder. J Neurol Neurosurg Psychiatry 1972; 35:180–5.

Dooneief G, Bello J, Todak G et al. A prospective controlled study of magnetic resonance imaging of the brain in gay men and parenteral drug users with human immunodeficiency virus infection. Arch Neurol 1992; 49:38–43.

Doyle P, Gibson GM, Dolman CL. Proved herpes zoster arteritis with cerebral infarct. J Neuropathol Exp Neurol 1982; 41:351.

Duncalf CM, Kent JNG, Harbord M et al. Subacute sclerosing panencephalitis presenting as schizophreniform psychosis. Br J Psychiatry 1989; 155:557–9.

Dupont JR, Earle KM. Human rabies encephalitis: a study of forty-nine fatal cases with a review of the literature. Neurology 1965; 15:1023–34.

Duvoisin RC, Yahr MD. Encephalitis and parkinsonism. Arch Neurol 1965; 12:227–39.

Dworkin RH, Corbin AE, Young JP et al. Pregabalin for the treatment of postherpetic neuralgia: a randomized, placebo-controlled trial. Neurology 2003; 60:1274–83.

Edwards VE, Sutherland JM, Tyrer JH. Cryptococcosis of the central nervous system. J Neurol Neurosurg Psychiatry 1970; 33:415–25.

Eidelberg D, Sotrel A, Hooupian DS et al. Thrombotic cerebral vasculopathy associated with herpes zoster. Ann Neurol 1986; 19:7–14.

Epstein MA, Achong BG. Pathogenesis of infectious mononucleosis. Lancet 1977; 2:1270–3.

Esiri MM. Herpes simplex encephalitis. An immunohistological study of the distribution of viral antigen within the brain. J Neurol Sci 1982; 54:209–26.

Factor SA, Troche-Panetto M, Weaver SA. Dystonia in AIDS: report of four cases. Mov Disord 2003; 18:1492–8.

Fermaglich J, Hardman JM, Earle KM. Spontaneous progressive multifocal leukoencephalopathy. Neurology 1970; 20:479–85.

Finklestein H. Meningoencephalitis in mumps. JAMA 1938; 111:17–19.

Fisher CM. Hypomanic symptoms caused by herpes simplex encephalitis. Neurology 1996; 47:1374–8.

Fisher RS, Clark AW, Wolinsky JS et al. Post-infectious leukoencephalitis complicating Mycoplasma pneumoniae infection. Arch Neurol 1983; 40:109–13.

Fleet WS, Watson RT, Ballinger WE. Resolution of gumma with steroid therapy. Neurology 1986; 36:1104–7.

Fournier JCM, Helguera RAL. Postencephalitic narcolepsy and cataplexy: muscles and motor nerves inexcitability during the attack of cataplexy. J Nerv Ment Dis 1934; 80:159–62.

Freedman MJ, Odland LT, Cleve EA. Infectious mononucleosis with diffuse involvement of nervous system: report of a case. Arch Neurol Psychiatry 1953; 69:49–54.

Frieden TR, Sterling T, Pables-Mendes A et al. The emergence of drug-resistant tuberculosis in New York City. N Engl J Med 1993; 328:521–6.

Fujimoto H, Asaoka K, Imaizumi T et al. Epstein-Barr infections of the central nervous system. Intern Med 2003; 42:33–40.

Gascon GG, International Consortium on Subacute Sclerosing Panencephalitis. Randomized treatment study of inosiplex versus combined inosiplex and intraventricular inteferon-alfa in subacute sclerosing panencephalitis (SSPE): international multicenter study. J Child Neurol 2003; 18:819–27.

Gautier-Smith PC. Neurological complications of glandular fever. Brain 1965; 88:323–34.

Gazzola P, Cocito L, Capello E et al. Subacute measles encephalitis in a young man immunocompromised for ankylosing spondylitis. Neurology 1999; 52:1074–7.

Geddes JF, Hughes AJ, Lees AJ et al. Pathological overlap in cases of parkinsonism associated with neurofibrillary tangles. A study of recent cases of postencephalitic parkinsonism and comparison with progressive supranuclear palsy and

Guamanian parkinsonism–dementia complex. *Brain* 1993; **116**:281–302.

Gerard A, Sarrot-Reynauld F, Liozon E *et al.* Neurologic presentation of Whipple disease: report of 12 cases and review of the literature. *Medicine* 2002; **81**:443–57.

Gilden DH, Murray RS, Wellish M *et al.* Chronic progressive varicella-zoster virus encephalitis in an AIDS patient. *Neurology* 1988; **38**:1150–3.

Gilden DH, Wright RR, Schneck SA *et al.* Zoster sine herpete, a clinical variant. *Ann Neurol* 1994; **35**:530–3.

Gillespie J, Jackson A. *MRI and CT of the brain.* London: Arnold, 2000.

Gimenez-Roldan S, Martin M. Tabetic lightning pains: high-dosage intravenous penicillin versus carbamazepine therapy. *Eur Neurol* 1981; **20**:424–8.

Glass JD, Wesselingh SL, Selnes OA *et al.* Clinical-neuropathologic correlation in HIV-associated dementia. *Neurology* 1993; **43**:2230–7.

Gomez EA, Aviles M. Neurosyphilis in community mental health clinics: a case series. *J Clin Psychiatry* 1984; **45**:127–9.

Gordon SM, Eaton ME, George R *et al.* The response of symptomatic neurosyphilis to high-dose intravenous penicillin G in patients with human immunodeficiency virus infection. *N Engl J Med* 1994; **331**:1469–73.

Gray F, Gherardi R, Scaravilli F. The neuropathology of the acquired immune deficiency syndrome (AIDS): a review. *Brain* 1988; **11**:245–66.

Green WR, Walker DH, Cain BG. Fatal viscerotropic Rocky Mountain spotted fever. Report of a case diagnosed by immunofluorescence. *Am J Med* 1978; **64**:523–8.

Greenberg DA, Weinkle DI, Aminoff MJ. Periodic EEG complexes in infectious mononucleosis encephalitis. *J Neurol Neurosurg Psychiatry* 1982; **45**:648–51.

Greenfield JG. The pathology of measles encephalomyelitis. *Brain* 1929; **52**:171–95.

Greenwood R, Bhalla A, Gordon A *et al.* Behavior disturbances during recovery from herpes simplex encephalitis. *J Neurol Neurosurg Psychiatry* 1983; **46**:809–17.

Guillaume B. Sindic CJ, Weber T. Progressive multifocal leukoencephalopathy: simultaneous detection of JCV DNA and anti-JCV antibodies in cerebrospinal fluid. *Eur J Neurol* 2000; **7**:101–6.

Guilleminault C, Mondini S. Mononucleosis and chronic daytime sleepiness. A long-term follow-up study. *Arch Int Med* 1986; **146**:1333–5.

Guilleux MH, Steneir RE, Young IR. MR imaging in progressive multifocal leukoencephalopathy. *AJNR* 1986; **7**:1033–5.

Hahn K, Arendt G, Braun JS *et al.* A placebo-controlled trial of gabapentin for painful HIV-associated sensory neuropathies. *J Neurol* 2004; **251**:1260–6.

Hahn RD, Webster B, Weickhardt G *et al.* Penicillin treatment of general paresis (dementia paralytica). *Arch Neurol Psychiatry* 1959; **81**:557–90.

Halperin JJ, Luft BJ, Anand AK *et al.* Lyme neuroborreliosis: central nervous system manifestations. *Neurology* 1989; **39**:753–9.

Hansen K, Lebech AM. The clinical and epidemiological profile of Lyme neuroborreliosis in Denmark 1985–1990. A prospective study of 187 patients with *Borrelia burgdorferi* specific intrathecal antibody production. *Brain* 1992; **115**:399–423.

Hart MN, Earle KM. Haemorrhagic and perivenous encephalitis: a clinical–pathological review of 38 cases. *J Neurol Neurosurg Psychiatry* 1975; **38**:585–91.

Hensen J, Rosenblum M, Armstrong D *et al.* Amplification of JC virus DNA from brain and cerebrospinal fluid of patients with progressive multifocal leukoencephalopathy. *Neurology* 1991; **41**:1967–71.

Herzlich BC, Schiano TD. Reversal of apparent AIDS dementia complex following treatment with vitamin B12. *J Intern Med* 1993; **233**:495–7.

Herzon H, Shelton JT, Bruyn HG. Sequelae of western equine and other arthropod-borne encephalitides. *Neurology* 1957; **7**:535–48.

Hilt DC, Bucholz D, Krumholz A *et al.* Herpes zoster ophthalmicus and delayed contralateral hemiparesis caused by cerebral angiitis: diagnosis and management approaches. *Ann Neurol* 1983; **14**:543–53.

Hochberg FH, Miller DC. Primary central nervous system lymphoma. *J Neurosurg* 1988; **68**:835–53.

Hogan EL, Krigman MR. Herpes zoster myelitis: evidence for viral invasion of spinal cord. *Arch Neurol* 1973; **29**:309–13.

Hohman LB. Epidemic encephalitis (lethargic encephalitis): its psychotic manifestations with a report of twenty-three cases. *Arch Neurol Psychiatry* 1921; **6**:295–333.

Hohman LB. Post-encephalitic behavior disorders in children. *Bull Johns Hopkins Hosp* 1922; **33**:372–5.

Hokkanen L, Salonen O, Launes J. Amnesia in acute herpetic and nonherpetic encephalitis. *Arch Neurol* 1996; **53**:972–8.

Holland NR, Power C, Mathews VP *et al.* Cytomegalovirus encephalitis in acquired immunodeficiency syndrome (AIDS). *Neurology* 1994; **44**:507–14.

Hollinger P, Sturzenegger M, Mathis J *et al.* Acute disseminated encephalomyelitis in adults: a reappraisal of clinical, CSF, EEG and MRI findings. *J Neurol* 2002; **249**:320–9.

Holmes MD, Brant-Zawadzki MM, Simon RP. Clinical features of meningovascular syphilis. *Neurology* 1984; **34**:553–6.

Horney LF, Walker DH. Meningoencephalitis as a major manifestation of Rocky Mountain spotted fever. *South Med J* 1988; **81**:915–18.

Howard RS, Lees AJ. Encephalitis lethargica: a report of four recent cases. *Brain* 1987; **110**:19–33.

Hriso E, Kuhn T, Masdeu JC *et al.* Extrapyramidal symptoms due to dopamine-blocking agents in patients with AIDS encephalopathy. *Am J Psychiatry* 1991; **148**:1558–61.

Huang D, Cossoy M, Li M *et al.* Inflammatory progressive multifocal leukoencephalopathy in human immunodeficiency virus-negative patients. *Ann Neurol* 2007; **62**:34–9.

Idro R, Jenkins NE, Newton CR. Pathogenesis, clinical features, and neurological outcome of cerebral malaria. *Lancet Neurol* 2005; **4**:827–40.

Ishii N, Nishihara Y. Pellagra encephalopathy among tuberculosis patients: its relation to isoniazid therapy. *J Neurol Neurosurg Psychiatry* 1985; **48**:628–34.

Ishii T, Nakamura Y. Distribution and ultrastructure of Alzheimer's neurofibrillary tangles in postencephalitic parkinsonism of Economo type. *Acta Neuropathol* 1981; **55**:59–62.

Jelliffee SE. Oculogyric crises as compulsion phenomena in postencephalitis: their occurrence, phenomenology and meaning. *J Nerv Ment Dis* 1929; **69**:59–68, 165–84, 278–97, 415–26, 531–51, 666–9.

Jemsek J, Greenberg SB, Tabor L *et al.* Herpes zoster-associated encephalitis: clinicopathologic report of twelve cases and review of the literature. *Medicine* 1983; **62**:81–97.

Johns DR, Tierney M, Felsenstein D. Alteration in the natural history of neurosyphilis by concurrent infection with the human immunodeficiency virus. *N Engl J Med* 1987; **316**:1569–72.

Johnson RT, Milbourn PE. Central nervous system manifestations of chickenpox. *Can Med Assoc J* 1970; **102**:831–6.

Kalayjian RC, Cohen ML, Bonomo RA *et al.* Cytomegalovirus ventriculoencephalitis in AIDS. A syndrome with distinct clinical and pathologic features. *Medicine* 1993; **72**:67–77.

Kalita J, Misra UK. Markedly severe dystonia in Japanese encephalitis. *Mov Disord* 2000; **15**:1168–72.

Kalita J, Misra UK, Ranjan P. Predictors of long-term neurological sequelae of tuberculous meningitis: a multivariate analysis. *Eur J Neurol* 2007; **14**:33–7.

Kamei S, Sekizawa T, Shiota H *et al.* Evaluation of combination therapy using aciclovir and corticosteroid in adult patients with herpes simplex virus encephalitis. *J Neurol Neurosurg Psychiatry* 2005; **76**:1544–9.

Kapur N, Barker S, Burrows EH *et al.* Herpes simplex encephalitis: long term magnetic resonance imaging and neuropsychological profile. *J Neurol Neurosurg Psychiatry* 1994; **57**:1334–42.

Kastrup O, Maschke M, Diener HC *et al.* Progressive multifocal leukoencephalopathy limited to the brainstem. *Neuroradiology* 2002; **44**:227–9.

Kennedy DH, Fallon RJ. Tuberculous meningitis. *J Am Med Assoc* 1979; **241**:264–8.

Kennedy PGE. A retrospective study of forty-six cases of herpes simplex encephalitis seen in Glasgow between 1962 and 1985. *Q J Med* 1988; **68**:533–40.

Kesserling J, Miller DH, Robb SA *et al.* Acute disseminated encephalomyelitis. MRI findings and the distinction from multiple sclerosis. *Brain* 1990; **113**:291–302.

Kieburtz K, Zettelmaier AE, Ketonen L *et al.* Manic syndrome in AIDS. *Am J Psychiatry* 1991; **148**:1068–70.

Kieburtz K, Simpson D, Yiannoutsos C *et al.* A randomized trial of amitriptyline and mexiletine for painful neuropathy in HIV infection. AIDS Clinical Trial Group 242 Protocol Team. *Neurology* 1998; **51**:1682–8.

Kirby GH, Davis TK. Psychiatric aspects of epidemic encephalitis. *Arch Neurol Psychiatry* 1921; **5**:491–551.

Kirk JL, Fine DP, Sexton DJ *et al.* Rocky Mountain spotted fever. A clinical review based on 48 confirmed cases, 1943–1986. *Medicine* 1990; **69**:35–45.

Kleinschmidt-DeMasters BK, Amlie-Lefond C, Gilden DH. The patterns of varicella zoster encephalitis. *Hum Pathol* 1996; **27**:927–38.

Klempner MS, Hu LT, Evans J *et al.* Two controlled trials of antibiotic treatment in patients with persistent symptoms and a history of Lyme disease. *N Engl J Med* 2001; **345**:85–92.

Kobayashi K, Mizukoshi C, Aoki T *et al.* Borrelia-burgdorferi-seropositive encephalomyelopathy: Lyme neuroborreliosis? An autopsied report. *Dement Geriatr Cogn Disord* 1997; **8**:384–90.

Koehler K, Jakumeit U. Subacute sclerosing panencephalitis presenting as Leonhard's speech-prompt catatonia. *Br J Psychiatry* 1976; **129**:29–31.

Koralnik IJ, Boden O, Mai VX *et al.* JC virus DNA load in patients with and without progressive multifocal leukoencephalopathy. *Neurology* 1999; **52**:253–60.

Koskiniemi M, Donner M, Pettay O. Clinical appearance and outcome in mumps encephalitis in children. *Acta Paediatr Scand* 1983; **72**:603–9.

Koskiniemi M, Piiparinen H, Mannonen L *et al.* Herpes encephalitis is a disease of middle aged and elderly people: polymerase chain reaction for detection of herpes simplex virus in the CSF of 516 patients with encephalitis. *J Neurol Neurosurg Psychiatry* 1996; **60**:174–8.

Krumholz S, Luhan JA. Encephalitis associated with herpes zoster. *Arch Neurol Psychiatry* 1945; **53**:59–67.

Krupp LB, Lipton RB, Swerdlow ML *et al.* Progressive multifocal leukoencephalopathy: clinical and demographic features. *Ann Neurol* 1985; **17**:344–9.

Krupp LB, Hyman LG, Grimson R *et al.* Study and treatment of post Lyme disease (STOP-LD). A randomized double masked clinical trial. *Neurology* 2003; **60**:1923–30.

Kuker W, Mader I, Nagele T *et al.* Progressive multifocal leukoencephalopathy; value of diffusion-weighted and contrast-enhanced magnetic resonance imaging for diagnosis and treatment control. *Eur J Neurol* 2006; **13**:819–26.

Lampert P, Tom MI, Cumings JN. Encephalopathy in Whipple's disease: a histochemical study. *Neurology* 1962; **12**:65–71.

Landau WM, Luse SA. Relapsing inclusion encephalitis (Dawson type) of eight years' duration. *Neurology* 1958; **8**:669–76.

Laothamatas J, Hemachudha T, Mitrabhakdi E *et al.* MR imaging in human rabies. *AJNR* 2003; **24**:1102–9.

Leavell R, Ray CG, Ferry PC *et al.* Unusual acute neurologic presentations with Epstein–Barr virus infection. *Arch Neurol* 1986; **43**:186–8.

Lebon P, Lyon G. Non-congenital rubella encephalitis. *Lancet* 1974; **2**:468.

Leech RW, Harris JC. The neuropathology of Western equine and St Louis encephalitis: a review of the 1975 North Dakota epidemic. *J Neuropathol Exp Neurol* 1977; **36**:611.

Levitt LP, Rich TA, Kinde SW *et al.* Central nervous system mumps: a review of 64 cases. *Neurology* 1970; **20**:829–34.

Lewis L, Taylor HG, Sorem MB. Japanese B encephalitis: clinical observations in an outbreak on Okinawa Shima. *Arch Neurol Psychiatry* 1947; **57**:430–63.

Lilly R, Cummings JL, Benson DF *et al.* The human Kluver–Bucy syndrome. *Neurology* 1983; **33**:1141–5.

Lima MA, Drislane FW, Koralink IJ. Seizures and their outcome in progressive multifocal leukoencephalopathy. *Neurology* 2006; **66**:262–4.

Lin JJ, Harn HJ, Hsue YD *et al.* Rapid diagnosis of tuberculous meningitis by polymerase chain reaction assay of cerebrospinal fluid. *J Neurol* 1995; **242**:147–52.

Linnemann CC, Alvira MM. Pathogenesis of varicella-zoster angiitis in the CNS. *Arch Neurol* 1980; **37**:239–40.

Logigian EL, Kaplan RF, Steere AC. Chronic neurologic manifestations of Lyme disease. *N Engl J Med* 1990; **323**:1438–44.

Louis ED, Lynch T, Kaufman P *et al.* Diagnostic guidelines in central nervous system Whipple's disease. *Ann Neurol* 1996; **40**:561–8.

Lukehart SA, Hook EW, Baker-Zander SA *et al.* Invasion of the central nervous system by *Treponema pallidum*: implications for diagnosis and treatment. *Ann Int Med* 1988; **109**:855–62.

Mahalingam R, Wellis M, Wolf W *et al.* Latent varicella-zoster viral DNA in human trigeminal and thoracic ganglia. *N Engl J Med* 1990; **323**:627–9.

Maher J, Choudri S, Halliday W *et al.* AIDS dementia complex with generalized myoclonus. *Mov Disord* 1997; **12**:593–7.

Malouf R, Jacquette G, Dobkin J *et al.* Neurologic disease in human immunodeficiency virus-infected drug abusers. *Arch Neurol* 1990; **47**:1002.

Manzel K, Tranel D, Cooper G. Cognitive and behavioral abnormalities in a case of central nervous system Whipple disease. *Arch Neurol* 2000; **57**:399–403.

Marchioni E, Ravaglia S, Piccolo G *et al.* Postinfectious inflammatory disorders. Subgroups based on prospective follow-up. *Neurology* 2005; **65**:1057–65.

Marlowe WB, Mancall EL, Thomas TJ. Complete Kluver–Bucy syndrome in man. *Cortex* 1975; **11**:53–9.

Marsden CD, Fowler TJ. *Clinical neurology*, 2nd edn. London: Arnold, 1998.

Marton R, Gotlieb-Steimatsky T, Klein C *et al.* Acute herpes simplex encephalitis: clinical assessment and prognostic data. *Acta Neurol Scand* 1996; **93**:149–55.

Matthews BR, Jones LK, Saad DA *et al.* Cerebellar ataxia and central nervous system Whipple disease. *Arch Neurol* 2005; **62**:618–20.

Mayo DR, Booss J. Varicella zoster-associated neurologic disease without skin lesions. *Arch Neurol* 1989; **46**:313–15.

McArthur JC. Neurologic manifestations of AIDS. *Medicine* 1987; **66**:407–11.

McArthur JC, Hoover DR, Bacellar H *et al.* Dementia in AIDS patients: incidence and risk factors. *Neurology* 1993; **43**:2245–52.

McCall S, Henry JM, Reid AH *et al.* Influenza RNA not detected in archival brain tissues from acute encephalitis lethargica cases or in postencephalitic Parkinson cases. *J Neuropathol Exp Neurol* 2001; **60**:696–704.

McCormick WF, Rodnitzky RL, Schochet SS *et al.* Varicella-zoster encephalomyelitis. *Arch Neurol* 1969; **21**:559–70.

McCowan PK, Cook LC, Cantab BA. Oculogyric crises in chronic epidemic encephalitis. *Brain* 1928; **51**:285–309.

McGrath N, Anderson NE, Croxson MC *et al.* Herpes simplex encephalitis treated with acyclovir: diagnosis and long term outcome. *J Neurol Neurosurg Psychiatry* 1997; **63**:321–6.

McKendrick GDW, Grose RJ. Tuberculous meningitis. *J Neurol Neurosurg Psychiatry* 1957; **20**:198–201.

MacKenzie RA, Forbes GS, Karnes WE. Angiographic findings in herpes zoster arteritis. *Ann Neurol* 1981; **10**:458–64.

Melanson M, Chalk C, Georgevich L *et al.* Varicella-zoster virus DNA in CSF and arteries in delayed contralateral hemiplegia: evidence for viral invasion of cerebral arteries. *Neurology* 1996; **47**:569–70.

Meninger KA. Influenza and schizophrenia. *Am J Psychiatry* 1926; **82**:469–529.

Merritt HH, Adams RD, Solomon HC. *Neurosyphilis*. New York: Oxford University Press, 1946.

Meurers B, Kohlepp WRG, Rohrbach E *et al.* Histopathological findings in the central and peripheral nervous system in neuroborreliosis. A report of three cases. *J Neurol* 1990; **327**:113–16.

Miller AE. Selective decline in cellular immune response to varicella-zoster in the elderly. *Neurology* 1980; **30**:582–7.

Miller HG, Stanton JB, Gibbons JL. Para-infectious encephalomyelitis and related syndromes. *Q J Med* 1956; **25**:427–505.

Miller JQ, Price TR. The nervous system in Rocky Mountain spotted fever. *Neurology* 1972; **22**:561–70.

de la Monte SM, de la Gabuzda DH, Ho DD *et al.* Peripheral neuropathy in the acquired immunodeficiency syndrome. *Ann Neurol* 1988; **23**:485–92.

Morgello S, Cho ES, Nielsen S *et al.* Cytomegalovirus encephalitis in patients with acquired immunodeficiency syndrome: an autopsy study of 30 cases and a review of the literature. *Hum Pathol* 1987; **18**:289–97.

Morgello S, Estanislao L, Simpson D *et al.* HIV-associated distal sensory polyneuropathy in the era of highly active antiretroviral therapy: the Manhattan HIV Brain Bank. *Arch Neurol* 2004; **61**:546–51.

Mori T, Ebe T. Analysis of cases of central nervous system fungal infections reported in Japan between January 1979 and June 1989. *Intern Med* 1992; **31**:174–9.

Moscovich DG, Singh MB, Eva FJ *et al.* Acute disseminated encephalomyelitis presenting as an acute psychotic state. *J Nerv Ment Dis* 1995; **183**:116–17.

Moulignier A, Mikol J, Pialoux G *et al.* AIDS-associated progressive multifocal leukoencephalopathy revealed by new-onset seizure. *Am J Med* 1995; **99**:64–8.

Mulder DW, Parrott M, Thaler M. Sequelae of Western equine encephalitis. *Neurology* 1951; **1**:318–27.

Nagel MA, Forghani B, Mahalingam R *et al.* The value of detecting anti-VZV IgG antibody in CSF to diagnose VZV vasculopathy. *Neurology* 2007; **68**:1069–73.

Navia BA, Price RW. The acquired immunodeficiency syndrome dementia complex as the presenting or sole manifestation of human immunodeficiency virus infection. *Ann Neurol* 1987; **44**:656–9.

Navia BA, Jordan BD, Price RW. The AIDS dementia complex. I. Clinical features. *Ann Neurol* 1986a; **19**:517–24.

Navia BA, Jordan BD, Price RW. The AIDS dementia complex. II. Neuropathology. *Ann Neurol* 1986b; **19**:525–35.

Navia BA, Petito CK, Gold JWM *et al.* Cerebral toxoplasmosis complicating the acquired immune deficiency syndrome: clinical and neuropathological findings in 27 patients. *Ann Neurol* 1986c; **19**:224–38.

Ngoungou EB, Koko J, Druet-Cabanac M et al. Cerebral malaria and sequelar epilepsy: first matched case-control study in Gabon. Epilepsia 2006; 47:2147–53.

Northam RS, Singer HS. Postencephalitic acquired Tourette-like syndrome in a child. Neurology 1991; 41:592–3.

Ohya T, Martinez AJ, Jabbour JT et al. Subacute sclerosing panencephalitis. Neurology 1974; 24:211–18.

Oksi J, Kalimo H, Marttila RJ et al. Inflammatory brain changes in Lyme borreliosis. A report on three patients and review of the literature. Brain 1996; 119:2143–54.

Oo MM, Aikawa M, Than T et al. Human cerebral malaria: pathological study. J Neuropathol Exp Neurol 1987; 46:223–31.

O'Riordan JI, Gomez-Anson B, Moseley IF et al. Long term MRI follow-up of patients with post infectious encephalomyelitis: evidence for a monophasic disease. J Neurol Sci 1999; 167:132–6.

Ozturk A, Gurses C, Baykan B et al. Subacute sclerosing panencephalitis: clinical and magnetic resonance imaging evaluation of 36 patients. J Child Neurol 2002; 17:25–9.

Pachner AR, Steere AC. The triad of neurologic manifestations of Lyme disease: meningitis, cranial neuritis and radiculoneuritis. Neurology 1985; 35:47–53.

Padgett BL, Walker DL, Zurheim GM et al. Cultivation of papova-like virus from human brain with progressive multifocal leukoencephalopathy. Lancet 1971; 1:1257–60.

Pantaleo G, Graziosi C, Fauci AS. The immunopathogenesis of human immunodeficiency virus infection. N Engl J Med 1993; 328:327–35.

Pardo J, Marcos A, Bhathal H et al. Chorea as a form of presentation of human immunodeficiency virus-associated dementia complex. Neurology 1998; 50:568–9.

Parker JC, McCloskey JJ, Lee RS. Human cerebral candidosis. A post mortem evaluation of 19 patients. Hum Pathol 1981; 12:23–8.

Parr J, Horoupian DS, Winkelman AC. Cerebellar form of progressive multifocal leukoencephalopathy (PML). Can J Neurol Sci 1979; 6:123–8.

Pascual-Sedano B, Iranzo A, Marti-Fabregas J et al. Prospective study of new-onset seizures in patients with human immunodeficiency virus infection. Arch Neurol 1999; 56:609–12.

Paskavitz JF, Anderson CA, Filley CM et al. Acute arcuate fiber demyelination encephalopathy following Epstein–Barr virus infection. Ann Neurol 1995; 38:127–31.

Petersen I, Thomas JM, Hamilton WT et al. Risk and predictors of fatigue after infectious mononucleosis in a large primary-care cohort. Q J Med 2006; 99:49–55.

Pfister H-W, Preac-Mursic V, Wilske B et al. Catatonic syndrome in acute severe encephalitis due to Borrelia burgdorferi infection. Neurology 1993; 43:433–5.

Piccolo I, Causarano R, Sterzi R et al. Chorea in patients with AIDS. Acta Neurol Scand 1999; 100:332–6.

Pollock S, Lewis PD, Kendall B. Whipple's disease confined to the central nervous system. J Neurol Neurosurg Psychiatry 1981; 44:1104–9.

Porras C, Barboza JJ, Fuenzalida E et al. Recovery from rabies in man. Ann Intern Med 1976; 85:44–8.

Porter SB, Sande MA. Toxoplasmosis of the central nervous system in the acquired immunodeficiency syndrome. N Engl J Med 1992; 327:1643–8.

Powers JM, Rawe SE. A neuropathological study of Whipple's disease. Acta Neuropathol 1979; 48:223–6.

Pradhan S, Pandey N, Shashank S et al. Parkinsonism due to predominant involvement of substantia nigra in Japanese encephalitis. Neurology 1999; 53:1781–6.

Prashanth LK, Taly AB, Ravi V et al. Adult subacute sclerosing panencephalitis: clinical profile of 39 patients from a tertiary care center. J Neurol Neurosurg Psychiatry 2006; 77:630–3.

Price RW, Nielsen S, Horten B et al. Progressive multifocal leukoencephalopathy: a burnt-out case. Ann Neurol 1983; 13:485–9.

Price RW, Berew B, Sidtis J et al. The brain in AIDS: central nervous system HIV-1 infection and AIDS dementia complex. Science 1988; 239:586–91.

Pruss H, Katchanov J, Zschederlein R et al. A patient with cerebral Whipple disease with gastric involvement but not gastrointestinal symptoms: a consequence of local protective immunity? J Neurol Neurosurg Psychiatry 2007; 78:896–8.

Przelomski MM, O'Rourke E, Grady GF et al. Eastern equine encephalitis in Massachusetts. Neurology 1988; 38:736–9.

Rabkin JG, Wagner GJ, Rabkin R. Fluoxetine treatment for depression in patients with HIV and AIDS: a randomized, placebo-controlled trial. Am J Psychiatry 1999; 156:101–7.

Rail D, Scholtz C, Swash M. Post-encephalitic parkinsonism: current experience. J Neurol Neurosurg Psychiatry 1981; 44:670–6.

Raoult D, Birg ML, La Scola B et al. Cultivation of the bacillus of Whipple's disease. N Engl J Med 2000; 342:620–5.

Relman DA, Schmidt TM, MacDermott RP et al. Identification of the uncultured bacillus of Whipple's disease. N Engl J Med 1992; 327:293–301.

Reyes MG, Gardner JJ, Poland JD et al. St Louis encephalitis: quantitative, histologic and immunofluorescent studies. Arch Neurol 1981; 38:329–34.

Rich AR, McCordock HA. The pathogenesis of tuberculous meningitis. Bull Johns Hopkins Hosp 1933; 52:5–37.

Richardson EP. Progressive multifocal leukoencephalopathy. N Engl J Med 1961; 265:815–23.

Richter RW, Shimojyo S. Neurologic sequelae of Japanese B encephalitis. Neurology 1961; 11:553–9.

Risk WS, Haddad FS. The variable natural history of subacute sclerosing panencephalitis: a study of 118 cases from the middle east. Arch Neurol 1979; 36:610–14.

Risk WS, Haddad FS, Chemali R. Substantial spontaneous long-term improvement in subacute sclerosing panencephalitis: six cases from the middle east and overview of the literature. Arch Neurol 1978; 35:495–502.

Roessman U, Friede RL. Candidal infection of the brain. Arch Pathol 1967; 48:495–8.

Romanul FCA, Radvany J, Rosales RK. Whipple's disease confined to the brain: a case confirmed clinically and pathologically. J Neurol Neurosurg Psychiatry 1977; 40:901–9.

Rothschild D. Dementia paralytica accompanied by manic-depressive and schizophrenic psychoses. Am J Psychiatry 1940; 96:1043–60.

Roulet Perez E, Mader P, Cotting J et al. Acute fatal parainfectious cerebellar swelling in two children. A rare or an overlooked situation? Neuropediatrics 1993; 24:346–51.

Roze E, Thiebault MM, Mazevet D et al. Neurologic sequelae after severe falciparum malaria in adult travelers. Eur Neurol 2001; 46:192–7.

Russel J, Fisher M, Zivin JA et al. Status epilepticus and Epstein-Barr virus encephalopathy. Diagnosis by modern serologic techniques. Arch Neurol 1985; 42:789–92.

Russell DS. The nosological unity of acute haemorrhagic leucoencephalitis and acute disseminated encephalomyelitis. Brain 1955; 78:369–76.

Russell RR, Donald JC. The neurological complications of mumps. BMJ 1958; 2:27–30.

Sage JI, Weinstein MP, Miller DC. Chronic encephalitis possibly due to herpes simplex virus: two cases. Neurology 1985; 35:1470–2.

Salib EA. Subacute sclerosing panencephalitis (SSPE) presenting at the age of 21 as a schizophrenia-like state with bizarre dysmorphophobic features. Br J Psychiatry 1988; 152:709–10.

Sanchez-Portocarrero J, Perez-Cecilia F, Jimenez-Escrig A et al. Tuberculous meningitis: clinical characteristics and comparison with cryptococcal meningitis in patients with human immunodeficiency virus infection. Arch Neurol 1996; 53:671–6.

Sands IJ. The acute psychiatric type of epidemic encephalitis. Am J Psychiatry 1928; 84:975–87.

Schlesinger RD, Crelinsten GL. Infectious mononucleosis dominated by neurologic symptoms and signs. Can Med Assoc J 1977; 117:652–3.

Schnell RG, Dyck PJ, Bowie EJW et al. Infectious mononucleosis: neurologic and EEG findings. Medicine 1966; 45:51–63.

Schnorf H, Diserens K, Schnyder H et al. Corticosteroid-responsive postmalaria encephalopathy characterized by motor aphasia, myoclonus, and postural tremor. Arch Neurol 1998; 55:417–20.

Schube PG. Emotional states of general paresis. Am J Psychiatry 1934; 91:625–38.

Schultz DR, Barthal JS, Garrett C. Western equine encephalitis with rapid onset parkinsonism. Neurology 1977; 27:1095–6.

Schwartz MA, Selhorst JB, Ochs AI et al. Oculomasticatory myorhythmia: a unique movement disorder occurring in Whipple's disease. Ann Neurol 1986; 20:677–83.

Schwarz S, Mohr A, Knauth M et al. Acute disseminated encephalomyelitis. A follow-up study of 40 adult patients. Neurology 2001; 56:1313–18.

Sellal F, Mohr M, Collard M. Dementia in a 58-year-old woman. Lancet 1996; 347:236.

Shadick NA, Phillis CB, Logigian EL et al. The long-term clinical outcomes of Lyme disease. Ann Intern Med 1994; 121:560–7.

Sharer LR, Epstein LG, Cho ES et al. HTLV-III and vacuolar myelopathy in AIDS. N Engl J Med 1986; 315:62–3.

Shill HA, Stacy MA. Malignant catatonia secondary to sporadic encephalitis lethargica. J Neurol Neurosurg Psychiatry 2000; 69:402–3.

Silverstein A, Steinberg G, Nathanson M. Nervous system involvement in infectious mononucleosis. Arch Neurol 1972; 26:353–8.

Simon RP. Neurosyphilis. Arch Neurol 1985; 42:606–13.

Simpson DM, McArthur JC, Olney R et al. Lamotrigine for HIV-associated painful sensory neuropathies: a placebo-controlled trial. Neurology 2003; 60:1508–14.

Smardel JE, Bailey P, Baker AB. Sequelae of the arthropod-borne encephalitides. Neurology 1958; 8:873–96.

Smith WT, Frency JM, Guttsmann M et al. Cerebral complications of Whipple's disease. Brain 1965; 88:137–50.

Solomon T, Dung NM, Kneen R et al. Japanese encephalitis. J Neurol Neurosurg Psychiatry 2000; 68:405–15.

Solomon T, Dung NM, Kneen R et al. Seizures and raised intracranial pressure in Vietnamese patients with Japanese encephalitis. Brain 2002; 125:1084–93.

Sponzilli EE, Smith JK, Malamud N et al. Progressive multifocal leukoencephalopathy: a complication of immunosuppressive treatment. Neurology 1975; 25:664–8.

Srinivasan A, Burton EC, Kuehnert MJ et al. Transmission of rabies virus from an organ donor to four transplant recipients. N Engl J Med 2005; 352:1103–11.

Steinbach JP, Melms A, Skalej M et al. Delayed resolution of white matter changes following therapy of B burgdorferi encephalitis. Neurology 2005; 64:758–9.

Storm-Mathisen A. General paresis: a follow-up study of 203 patients. Acta Psychiatr Scand 1969; 45:118–32.

Strauss SE, Reinhold W, Smith HA et al. Endonuclease analysis of viral DNA from varicella and subsequent zoster infections in the same patients. N Engl J Med 1984; 311:1362–4.

Studahl M, Rickstein A, Sandberg T et al. Cytomegalovirus infection of the CNS in non-compromised patients. Acta Neurol Scand 1994; 89:451–7.

Sweeney CJ, Gilden DG. Ramsey Hunt syndrome. J Neurol Neurosurg Psychiatry 2001; 71:149–54.

Sworn MJ, Urich H. Acute encephalitis in infectious mononucleosis. J Pathol 1970; 100:201–5.

Taylor EW, McDonald CA. Forced conjugate upward movement of the eyes following epidemic encephalitis. Arch Neurol Psychiatry 1928; 19:95–103.

Tenembaum S, Chamoles N, Fejerman N. Acute disseminated encephalomyelitis. A long-term follow-up of 84 pediatric patients. Neurology 2002; 59:1224–31.

Thompson JA. Mumps: a cause of acquired aqueductal stenosis. J Pediatr 1979; 94:923–4.

Torgovnik J, Arsura EL, Lala D. Cytomegalovirus ventriculoencephalitis presenting as a Wernicke's encephalopathy-like syndrome. Neurology 2000; 55:1910–13.

Toro G, Roman G. Cerebral malaria. A disseminated vasculomyelopathy. Arch Neurol 1978; 35:271–5.

Townsend JJ, Baringer JR, Wolinsky JS et al. Progressive rubella panencephalitis: late onset after congenital rubella. N Engl J Med 1975a; 292:990–3.

Townsend JJ, Wolinsky JS, Baringer JR et al. Acquired toxoplasmosis: a neglected cause of treatable central nervous system disease. Arch Neurol 1975b; 32:335–43.

Townsend JJ, Wolinsky JS, Baringer JR. The neuropathology of progressive rubella panencephalitis of late onset. Brain 1976; 99:81–90.

Townsend JJ, Stroop WG, Baringer JR et al. Neuropathology of progressive rubella panencephalitis after childhood rubella. Neurology 1982; **32**:185–90.

Traub M, Colchester ACF, Kingsley DPE et al. Tuberculosis of the central nervous system. Q J Med 1984; **53**:81–100.

Tselis A, Duman R, Storch GA et al. Epstein–Barr virus encephalomyelitis diagnosed by polymerase chain reaction: detection of the genome in the CSF. Neurology 1997; **48**:1351–5.

Upton A, Gumpert J. Electroencephalography in diagnosis of herpes-simplex encephalitis. Lancet 1970; **1**:650–2.

Vaheri A, Julkunen I, Koskiniemi M. Chronic encephalomyelitis with specific increase in intrathecal mumps antibodies. Lancet 1982; **2**:685–8.

Van Bogaert L. Ocular paroxysms and palilalia. J Nerv Ment Dis 1934; **80**:48–61.

Vintners HV, Kwok MK, Ho HW et al. Cytomegalovirus in the nervous system of patients with the acquired immunodeficiency syndrome. Brain 1989; **112**:245–68.

Walsh TJ, Hier DB, Caplan LR. Fungal infections of the central nervous system: comparative analysis of risk factors and clinical signs in 57 patients. Neurology 1985a; **35**:1654–7.

Walsh TJ, Hier DB, Caplan LR. Aspergillosis of the central nervous system: clinicopathological analysis of 17 patients. Ann Neurol 1985b; **18**:574–82.

Warrell DA, Loorareesuwan S, Warrell MJ et al. Dexamethasone proves deleterious in cerebral malaria. A double-blind trial in 100 comatose patients. N Engl J Med 1982; **306**:313–19.

Wasay M, Diaz-Arrastia R, Suss RA et al. St Louis encephalitis. A review of 11 cases in a 1995 Dallas, Tex, epidemic. Arch Neurol 2000; **57**:114–18.

Watson CP, Vernich L, Chipman M et al. Nortriptyline versus amitriptyline in postherpetic neuralgia: a randomized trial. Neurology 1998; **51**:1166–71.

Weaver S, Rosenblum MK, DeAngelis LM. Herpes varicella zoster encephalitis in immunocompromised patients. Neurology 1999; **52**:193–5.

Weil ML, Itibashi HH, Cremer NE et al. Chronic progressive panencephalitis due to rubella virus simulating subacute sclerosing panencephalitis. N Engl J Med 1975; **292**:994–8.

Whipple GH. A hitherto undescribed disease characterized anatomically by deposits of fat and fatty acids in the intestinal and mesenteric lymphatic tissues. Johns Hopkins Hosp Bull 1907; **18**:382–91.

Whitley RJ, Alford CA, Hirsch MS et al. Vadarabine versus acyclovir therapy in herpes simplex encephalitis. N Engl J Med 1986; **314**:144–9.

Wiley CA, Masliah E, Morey M et al. Neocortical damage during HIV infection. Ann Neurol 1991; **29**:651–7.

Wilkins RH, Brody IA. Encephalitis lethargica. Arch Neurol 1968; **18**:324–8.

Williams BB, Lerner AM. Some previously unrecognized features of herpes simplex encephalitis. Neurology 1978; **28**:1193–6.

Williams M, Smith HV. Mental disturbances in tuberculous meningitis. J Neurol Neurosurg Psychiatry 1954; **17**:173–82.

Willoughby RE, Tieves KS, Hoffman GM et al. Survival after treatment of rabies with induction of coma. N Engl J Med 2005; **352**:2508–14.

Wilson LG. Viral encephalopathy mimicking functional psychosis. Am J Psychiatry 1976; **133**:165–70.

Wolinsky JS, Berg BO, Maitland CJ. Progressive rubella panencephalitis. Arch Neurol 1976; **33**:722–3.

Wolinsky JS, Swoveland P, Johnson KP et al. Subacute measles encephalitis complicating Hodgkin's disease in an adult. Ann Neurol 1977; **1**:452–4.

Wong MC, Suite ND, Labar DR. Seizures in human immunodeficiency virus infection. Arch Neurol 1990; **47**:640–2.

Wulf CH. Subacute sclerosing panencephalitis: serial electroencephalographic studies. J Neurol Neurosurg Psychiatry 1982; **45**:418–21.

Yamada S, Kaneyama T, Nagaya S et al. Relapsing herpes simplex encephalitis: pathological confirmation of viral reactivation. J Neurol Neurosurg Psychiatry 2003; **74**:262–4.

Young CA, Humphrey DM, Ghadiali EJ et al. Short-term memory impairment in an alert patient as a presentation of herpes simplex encephalitis. Neurology 1992; **42**:260–1.

Yousry TA, Major EO, Ryschkewitsch C et al. Evaluation of patients treated with natalizumab for progressive multifocal leukoencephalopathy. N Engl J Med 2006; **354**:924–33.

Zambito Marsala S, Ferracci F, Cecotti L et al. Post-malaria neurological syndrome: clinical and laboratory findings in one patient. Neurol Sci 2006; **27**:442–4.

Zifko U, Linder K, Wimberger D et al. Jarisch–Herxheimer reaction in a patient with neurosyphilis. J Neurol Neurosurg Psychiatry 1994; **57**:865–7.

Zunt JR, Tu RK, Anderson DM et al. Progressive multifocal leukoencephalopathy presenting as human immunodeficiency virus type 1 (HIV)-associated dementia. Neurology 1997; **49**:263–5.

15

Prion diseases

15.1 CREUTZFELDT–JAKOB DISEASE

Creutzfeldt–Jakob disease, also known as transmissible spongiform encephalopathy, is characterized by a fairly rapidly progressive dementia accompanied, in most cases, by myoclonus. In the past, this disease was also termed a 'slow virus' infection; however, it is now known that it is caused not by a virus but by a unique agent known as a prion. This is a rare disorder, occurring at a yearly rate of 1–2 cases per 1 000 000, and is equally common in males and females. About 85 percent of cases occur on a sporadic basis, 10 percent are inherited on an autosomal dominant basis, and the remainder represent iatrogenic infections, as has occurred with dura mater grafts for example.

Clinical features

On average, sporadic cases appear in the early sixties, but the range is wide, from late teenage years to the tenth decade. Inherited cases tend to appear a bit earlier, mostly in the early fifties. Iatrogenic cases appear anywhere from 1 to 30 years after the infectious event. Although most cases appear subacutely, over weeks to months, fulminant onsets spanning only a few days have been reported.

The overall symptomatology of Creutzfeldt–Jakob disease has been described in several studies (Brown et al. 1986, 1994; Collins et al. 2006; Cooper et al. 2006; Glatzel et al. 2005; Roos et al. 1973). The presentation may be with dementia, personality change, psychosis (Dervaux et al. 2004; Zeng et al. 2001), cerebellar ataxia, or visual symptomatology, such as hemianopia or cortical blindness; rare presentations include aphasia (Mandell et al. 1989), the alien hand sign (MacGowan et al. 1997), or mania (Lendvai et al. 1999). With progression almost all patients become profoundly demented, and the dementia is accompanied by myoclonus (which may be stimulus responsive) in almost 90 percent of cases. Parkinsonism of the rigid,

akinetic variety may occur, as may upper motor neuron signs, and, in a small minority, evidence of lower motor neuron dysfunction, such as fasciculations, may be seen. Seizures occur in a small minority.

Magnetic resonance imaging (MRI) generally discloses cortical atrophy, the progression of which may be monitored with serial scans. T2-weighted and fluid-attenuated inversion recovery (FLAIR) imaging, and, with greater sensitivity, diffusion-weighted imaging, may display increased signal intensity in the striatum and in the cerebral and cerebellar cortices; within the cortex the increased signal intensity follows the cortical ribbon, displaying a 'gyriform' pattern (Shiga et al. 2004; Tschampa et al. 2005).

The electroencephalogram (EEG) may show generalized slowing (Burger et al. 1972) and in some cases frontal intermittent rhythmic delta activity (FIRDA) has been noted (Wieser et al. 2004). The most characteristic EEG findings, however, are periodic spike-and-slow-wave complexes (Collins et al. 2006; Levy et al. 1986; May 1986; Steinhoff et al. 2004), which are eventually seen in anywhere from one-half to three-quarters of all cases. Importantly, the EEG may become abnormal only as the disease progresses, and consequently, when the initial EEG fails to reveal this finding, it may be appropriate to perform serial EEGs.

The cerebrospinal fluid (CSF) is acellular with a normal glucose; in a very small minority the total protein level may show a mild elevation. Most importantly, the 14-3-3 protein is found in anywhere from 50 to 95 percent of cases (Collins et al. 2006; Geschwind et al. 2003; Hsich et al. 1996; Lemstra et al. 2000; Rosenmann et al. 1997; Van Everbroeck et al. 2005; Zerr et al. 1998a).

Although, at present, a definitive ante-mortem diagnosis may be made only by brain biopsy, this is rarely performed.

Course

This disease progresses rapidly, with death occurring within about 6 months on average. The overall range, however, is wide, with some dying in as little as a month and others surviving for up to 3 years (Masters and Richardson 1978; Pocchiara *et al.* 2004; Will and Mathews 1984). The rapid progression is one of the hallmarks of Creutzfeldt–Jakob disease, and often one may seen a decline from week to week.

Etiology

Microscopically there is widespread spongiform change within the gray matter of the cerebral cortex, basal ganglia, thalamus, and cerebellar cortex (Masters and Richardson 1978), which in turn is accounted for by grossly swollen dendrites and axons (Beck *et al.* 1982; Chou *et al.* 1980). In a small minority, perhaps 5–10 percent of cases, plaques resembling the amyloid plaques seen in Alzheimer's disease may be found. In contrast to the plaques of Alzheimer's disease, however, these plaques are not composed of beta-amyloid but appear to be, at least in part, composed of prions (Kitamoto *et al.* 1986). There is also neuronal loss and astrogliosis, but very little, if any, inflammation. It must be emphasized that prions are found not only in the central nervous system but also in peripheral nerves (Favereaux *et al.* 2004), olfactory neuroepithelium (Tabaton *et al.* 2004; Zanusso *et al.* 2003), spleen, and muscle (Glatzel *et al.* 2003).

The prion protein is a normally occurring cellular protein that is coded for by the *PRNP* gene on chromosome 20. It is a constituent of the neuronal cell membrane and undergoes recycling from the exterior surface of the cell membrane into the cytoplasm, where it is digested by lysozymes. The agent responsible for Creutzfeldt–Jakob disease is a pathologic form of the prion protein The normal prion protein exists in an alpha-helical conformation, whereas the pathologic prion protein exists for the most part in a beta-sheet conformation (Pan *et al.* 1993). This beta-sheet conformation allows for aggregation of these pathologic prion proteins once they recycle into the cytoplasm and, as they aggregate and coalesce, a particle known as a prion is formed. Eventually, with an accumulation of prions, spongiform change occurs.

As an aside, in the literature the normal form of the prion protein is often referred to as PrPc, with the 'c' derived from the fact that these are normal 'cellular' components. The pathologic form, however, is often referred to as PrPsc, with the 'sc' derived from 'scrapie', which is the name given to a disease similar to Creutzfeldt–Jakob disease that is found in sheep.

As noted earlier, Creutzfeldt–Jakob disease may occur sporadically, as an autosomal dominantly inherited disease, or iatrogenically, and each of these is now discussed in turn.

The etiology of the sporadic cases is not clear. Some believe that they represent spontaneous, age-related transformations of normal cellular prion proteins into pathogenic prion proteins, whereas others suspect that they may represent infections with a long incubation period (Galvez

et al. 1980). The finding of prions within the olfactory neuroepithelium is intriguing in this regard, as their presence could be accounted for either by spread from the brain down the olfactory tracts and filia, in which case they might merely be seen as epiphenomenal, or by contact with airborne prions from an infected person, in which case they could represent the bridgehead of an infection. Recent work has further subdivided sporadic cases according to the type of pathologic prion protein present and to a polymorphism at codon 129 of *PRNP* (Parchi *et al.* 1999a). The pathologic prion protein actually exists in two isoforms, type 1 and type 2, and in each patient it appears that only one type is present. At codon 129 of *PRNP* there is a normal isomorphism with either a methionine or a valine allele, thus there are potentially three genotypes, namely MM, MV, and VV. Combining both the type of pathologic prion protein and the genotype gives six potential variants of sporadic Creutzfeldt–Jakob disease, namely MM1, MM2, MV1, MV2, VV1, and VV2. At present, it is not clear how useful this classification scheme is for clinical work.

Inherited cases occur secondary to any one of a large number of mutations in the *PRNP* gene (Goldfarb *et al.* 1990; Hsiao *et al.* 1991a; Owen *et al.* 1989). Importantly, in many cases mutations may occur spontaneously, and here, of course, the family history will be negative (Ladogana *et al.* 2005).

Iatrogenic cases have occurred upon inadvertent exposure to tissue from patients with Creutzfeldt–Jakob disease via the following procedures: corneal transplants (Duffy *et al.* 1974; Heckmann *et al.* 1997); dura mater grafts (Brown *et al.* 2000; Hannah *et al.* 2001; Heath *et al.* 2006; Miyashita *et al.* 1991); the use of contaminated electrodes during neurosurgical procedures (Bernouilli *et al.* 1977); injections of human growth hormone (Billette de Villemeur *et al.* 1991, 1996; Brown *et al.* 2000); and the injection of human pituitary gonadotrophins (Cochius *et al.* 1992; Healy and Evans 1993); it is of especial interest that a case also occurred secondary to the use of lyophilized dura mater in the treatment of a nasopharyngeal angiofibroma, a procedure in which the dura mater remained extracranial (Antoine *et al.* 1997). The persistence of prions cannot be overemphasized: in one case (Gibbs *et al.* 1994), electrodes that had been used during neurosurgery on a patient with Creutzfeldt–Jakob disease 2 years earlier were cleaned three times and repeatedly sterilized in ethanol and formaldehyde vapor yet were still able to transmit the disease to a chimpanzee. Presumably, in these iatrogenic cases, the pathogenic prion protein acts as a template that alters the conformation of the patient's normal prion protein into the pathologic beta-sheet protein.

Differential diagnosis

The diagnosis of Creutzfeldt–Jakob disease is often suspected in cases of a fairly rapidly progressive dementia when accompanied by myoclonus. As discussed in Section 5.1, however, the combination of dementia and myoclonus is not specific for Creutzfeldt–Jakob disease, and other possibilities must be considered, including Hashimoto's encephalopathy, AIDS dementia, Whipple's disease, subacute sclerosing panencephalitis, and two other prion diseases, namely new-variant Creutzfeldt–Jakob disease and fatal familial insomnia. New-variant Creutzfeldt–Jakob disease is only rarely associated with periodic complexes on the EEG (Binelli et al. 2006), and also displays a distinctive 'pulvinar' sign on MRI, with increased signal intensity seen in the pulvinar of the thalamus. Fatal familial insomnia is marked, as the name dramatically suggests, by severe insomnia (which is only rarely prominent in Creutzfeldt–Jakob disease [Landolt et al. 2006; Taratuto et al. 2002]) and lacks periodic complexes. Other disorders may also enter the differential, such as diffuse Lewy body disease or Alzheimer's disease, but these rarely show the rapid progression characteristic of Creutzfeldt–Jakob disease.

Periodic spike-and-slow-wave complexes, although highly suggestive of Creutzfeldt–Jakob disease, may also, as noted in Section 1.2, be seen in other disorders, including not only post-anoxic encephalopathy and subacute sclerosing panencephalitis but also herpes simplex viral encephalitis.

The presence of 14-3-3 protein reflects acute damage, and it may be seen not only in Creutzfeldt–Jakob disease but also in new-variant Creutzfeldt–Jakob disease; it is rarely seen in fatal familial insomnia, Hashimoto's encephalopathy, limbic encephalitis, viral encephalitis, acute stroke (as may occur in the course of a multi-infarct dementia), and multiple sclerosis (Hsich et al. 1996; Lemstra et al. 2000; Martinez et al. 2001; Saiz et al. 1999; Sanchez-Juan et al. 2006; Van Everbroeck et al. 2005).

Treatment

The general treatment of dementia is discussed in Section 5.1. To date, the only medication shown to have any specific usefulness in a double-blind study is flupirtine, which may slow the progression of the disease (Otto et al. 2004); quinacrine is not useful (Haik et al. 2004). Early uncontrolled reports suggested a usefulness for amanatadine (Braham 1971; Sanders 1979; Sanders and Dunn 1973; Terzano et al. 1983), but these have not been validated. In familial cases, genetic counselling should be offered.

The question inevitably arises as to what sorts of precautions should be in place to guard against transmission of the disease. Although isolation does not appear to be necessary, routine universal precautions are appropriate. It is critical to avoid contamination via CSF, blood, or biopsy specimens, and it must be borne in mind that routine sterilization procedures, including autoclaving and alcohol immersion, are not effective. In cases of accidental contact, consideration may be given to washing with a 1:10 solution of 5 percent common hypochlorite bleach, which is effective. Pins used for sensory testing in any patient should never be used twice.

15.2 NEW-VARIANT CREUTZFELDT–JAKOB DISEASE

New-variant Creutzfeldt–Jakob disease is a very rare infectious prion disease acquired by eating meat derived from cows that had bovine spongiform encephalopathy, or 'mad cow disease'. Although most cases have occurred in the UK, at least one has been reported in the United States (Belay et al. 2005).

Clinical features

The incubation period between the ingestion of contaminated meat and the development of the disease is probably less than 20 years. The onset of the disease is subacute, and although most patients have been in their late 20s, the range of age of onset is wide, from early adolescence to the eighth decade.

Most patients present with behavioral changes such as depression or, less commonly, personality change, withdrawal, agitation, insomnia, apathy, emotional lability, or psychosis, which in turn may comprise visual and auditory hallucinations and Schneiderian first-rank symptoms (Will et al. 2000; Zeidler 1997a,b); the remainder present with ataxia, dysesthesiae or memory loss, or a combination of these and behavioral changes. With progression a dementia eventually appears that is often accompanied by myoclonus (Allroggen et al. 2000; Collinge and Rossor 1996; Will et al. 1996; Zeidler et al. 1997a).

FLAIR MR scanning displays a distinctive 'pulvinar' sign in approximately three-quarters of all patients, characterized by increased signal intensity in the pulvinar of the thalamus (Zeidler et al. 2000). In addition to this pulvinar sign, increased signal intensity may also occur in the basal ganglia and the cerebral and cerebellar cortices (Collie et al. 2003).

The EEG may demonstrate generalized slowing (Zeidler et al. 1997a). With rare exceptions (Binelli et al. 2006), periodic spike-and-slow-wave complexes are absent (Zeidler et al. 1997a).

The CSF is acellular with a normal total protein; the 14-3-3 protein is found in about 50 percent of cases (Green et al. 2001; Sanchez-Juan et al. 2006; Will et al. 2000).

Tonsilar biopsy appears to be both sensitive and specific (Hill et al. 1999).

Course

The disease is relentlessly progressive, with most patients dying within a little over a year, with a range of 18 months to 3 years (Will et al. 2000).

Etiology

As noted earlier, new-variant Creutzfeldt–Jakob disease occurs secondary to eating beef from cows that had bovine spongiform encephalopathy (Bruce *et al.* 1997); in turn, cows contract the disease by eating meal made from the offal of sheep that had a transmissible spongiform encephalopathy known as scrapie. Host factors appear to play a role in susceptibility among humans in that, with rare exceptions (Ironside *et al.* 2006), all patients have been homozygous for methionine at codon 129 of *PRNP*, the gene for normal prion proteins found on chromosome 20 (Collinge *et al.* 1996; Will *et al.* 2000).

Within the thalamus, basal ganglia, and also the cerebral and cerebellar cortices there are widespread prion plaques surrounded by spongiform change (Will *et al.* 1996). In this disease prions are not restricted to the brain but are also found in tonsils, lymph nodes, and the spleen (Hill *et al.* 1999). It also appears that prions are present in the blood, and, alarmingly, there have been cases of new-variant Creutzfeldt–Jakob disease occurring secondary to blood transfusion (Wroe *et al.* 2006).

Differential diagnosis

The differential diagnosis is as described for Creutzfeldt–Jakob disease in Section 15.1. As noted here, the pulvinar sign is quite important, but it must be borne in mind that it is not specific for new-variant Creutzfeldt–Jakob disease and has been reported in cases of limbic encephalitis (Mihara *et al.* 2005) and, albeit rarely, in sporadic Creutzfeldt–Jakob disease (Petzold *et al.* 2004).

Treatment

There is no specific treatment for this disease; general treatment recommendations are as discussed for Creutzfeldt–Jakob disease in Section 15.1. Strenuous efforts are in place to prevent bovine spongiform encephalopathy; however, given the difficulty in monitoring the food chain, continual vigilance is necessary.

15.3 GERSTMANN–STRÄUSSLER–SCHEINKER DISEASE

Gerstmann–Sträussler–Scheinker disease is a very rare, autosomal dominantly inherited prion disease characterized classically by ataxia and, eventually, dementia.

Clinical features

The onset is subacute or gradual, and usually in the sixth decade, with a wide range from the third to the eighth decades. Classically (Barbanti *et al.* 1996; Farlow *et al.* 1989), patients present with a progressive ataxia with the eventual development of a dementia; in some cases parkinsonism or long-tract signs may also occur.

The EEG may show generalized slowing but there are no periodic complexes; the CSF is normal and the 14-3-3 protein is absent.

Course

For a prion disease the course is relatively slow, with death, on average, after 5–6 years.

Etiology

Gerstmann–Sträussler–Scheinker disease may occur secondary to any one of several mutations in the *PRNP* gene. Mutations have been noted at codons 102 (Arata *et al.* 2006; Brown *et al.* 1991; Goldhammer *et al.* 1993; Hsiao *et al.* 1989; Kretzchmar *et al.* 1992; Young *et al.* 1995), 105 (Kitamoto *et al.* 1993; Yamada *et al.* 1993), 117 (Hsiao *et al.* 1991b; Nochlin *et al.* 1989), 198 (Farlow *et al.* 1989; Ghetti *et al.* 1989), and 217 (Hsiao *et al.* 1992).

Pathologically, regardless of which mutation is at fault, all cases of Gerstmann–Sträussler–Scheinker disease share a common feature, namely the presence of multicentric amyloid plaques that stain positively for prion proteins (Kitamoto *et al.* 1986; Roberts *et al.* 1986). In some cases, unicentric spiky plaques, similar to those seen in kuru, may also occur, and in others neurofibrillary tangles may be seen. Spongiform change is either minimal or absent. Although the distribution of these microscopic changes varies, the cerebellar cortex, basal ganglia, and cerebral cortex are generally involved.

Differential diagnosis

The differential diagnosis of dementia occurring in the context of ataxia is discussed in Section 5.1.

Treatment

There is no specific treatment; genetic counselling should be offered, and the general treatment of dementia is discussed in Section 5.1.

15.4 FATAL FAMILIAL INSOMNIA

Fatal familial insomnia is a rare prion disease, characterized, as the name suggests, by severe insomnia, which is typically accompanied by a dementia and prominent autonomic disturbances.

Clinical features

Onset is typically subacute or gradual and occurs in middle years, with a wide range from late adolescence to the seventh decade. In general (Almer *et al.* 1999; Gallassi *et al.* 1996; Manetto *et al.* 1992; Medori *et al.* 1992a,b; Nagayama *et al.* 1996; Reder *et al.* 1995; Silburn *et al.* 1996; Tabernero *et al.* 2000), patients develop intractable insomnia, followed in many cases by 'oneiroid' states in which they appear confused, experience visual hallucinations, and behave as if they were acting out dreams; in one case (Almer *et al.* 1999) 'the patient performed movements of sawing with a virtual saw and stopped bewildered when told there was no saw'. Rarely, the presentation may be with a psychosis coupled with insomnia (Dimitri *et al.* 2006). Paroxysms of autonomic disturbance often occur, with hyperhidrosis, tachycardia, hypertension, and irregular respiration. Over time dementia appears, accompanied, variously, by ataxia, myoclonus, and spasticity. Importantly, although insomnia is the initial hallmark of this disease, in some cases it may appear late in the course and, rarely, it may be absent (Zerr *et al.* 1998b).

The EEG shows slowing but there are no periodic complexes. The CSF is generally normal although in a small minority the 14-3-3 protein may be found (Sanchez-Juan *et al.* 2006).

Course

The disease is relentlessly progressive, with the development of stupor and coma; on average, death occurs after 12–18 months.

Etiology

Pathologically (Almer *et al.* 1999; Lugaresi *et al.* 1986; Manetto *et al.* 1992), there is extensive neuronal loss and astrocytosis in the anterior and mediodorsal nuclei of the thalamus and in the inferior olives; in some cases, mild cell loss and spongiform change may also be seen in the cerebral and cerebellar cortices and in the dorsal raphe and superior central nuclei (Almer *et al.* 1999).

Most cases of fatal familial insomnia occur on an autosomal dominant basis, with mutations found at codon 178 of the *PRNP* gene (Medori *et al.* 1992a,b). Interestingly, this mutation causes fatal familial insomnia only if there is a methionine polymorphism at codon 129 of the same allele; if the polymorphism at codon 129 is valine, then one sees familial Creutzfeldt–Jakob disease rather than fatal familial insomnia (Goldfarb *et al.* 1992). It also appears that the same clinical and neuropathologic picture may occur on a sporadic basis (Parchi *et al.* 1999b).

Differential diagnosis

The diagnosis is typically suspected in cases marked by intractable insomnia. Severe depression in the elderly may be marked by dementia and by insomnia, but in such cases the autonomic disturbances are absent and one also sees a depressed mood.

Treatment

There is no known specific treatment; general measures may be undertaken, as described for Creutzfeldt–Jakob disease in Section 15.1, and sequential trials of various hypnotics should be attempted.

15.5 KURU

Kuru is a unique human prion disease, spread by cannibalism and present only in the Fore people of New Guinea (Gajdusek 1977). With the elimination of cannibalism in the 1950s new infections stopped, but, given the long incubation period, the disease itself is still present.

Clinical features

After a long incubation period, spanning from 4 to 50 years or more (Collinge *et al.* 2006), patients gradually develop ataxia and tremor, followed, in a minority, by dementia.

Course

The disease is slowly progressive.

Etiology

The disease was spread by ritual cannibalism, which included ingestion of brain. Pathologically (Gajdusek and Zigas 1959; Kakulas *et al.* 1967) there is atrophy of the cerebellar vermis and flocculonodular lobe, and microscopically there is widespread spongiform change, neuronal loss, and astrocytosis, together with 'kuru plaques'. These are distinguished from the amyloid plaques found in Alzheimer's disease, for example, by the presence of 'spikes' that radiate out around the circumference of the plaque.

Differential diagnosis

The diagnosis is only relevant in those Fore tribespeople who engaged in cannibalism.

Treatment

There is no known treatment.

REFERENCES

Allroggen H, Dennis G, Abbott RJ et al. New-variant Creutzfeldt–Jakob disease: three case reports from Leicestershire. *J Neurol Neurosurg Psychiatry* 2000; **68**:375–8.

Almer G, Hainfellner JA, Brucke T et al. Fatal familial insomnia: a new Austrian family. *Brain* 1999; **122**:5–16.

Antoine JC, Michel D, Bertholon P et al. Creutzfeldt–Jakob disease after extracranial dura mater embolization for a nasopharyngeal angiofibroma. *Neurology* 1997; **48**:1451–3.

Arata H, Takashima H, Hirano R et al. Early clinical signs and imaging findings in Gerstmann–Straussler–Scheinker syndrome (Pro102Leu). *Neurology* 2006; **66**:1672–8.

Barbanti P, Fabbrini G, Salvatore M et al. Polymorphism at codon 129 or codon 219 of PRNP and clinical heterogeneity in a previously unreported family with Gerstmann–Straussler–Scheinker disease (Prp-P102L mutation). *Neurology* 1996; **47**:734–41.

Beck E, Danile PM, Davey AJ et al. The pathogenesis of transmissible spongiform encephalopathy – an ultrastructural study. *Brain* 1982; **105**:755–86.

Belay ED, Sejvar JJ, Shieh WJ et al. Variant Creutzfeldt–Jakob disease death, United States. *Emerg Infect Dis* 2005; **11**:1351–4.

Bernouilli C, Siegfried J, Baumgartner G et al. Danger of accidental person to person transmission of Creutzfeldt–Jakob disease by surgery. *Lancet* 1977; **1**:478–9.

Billette de Villemeur T, Beuavais P, Gourmelon M et al. Creutzfeldt–Jakob disease in children treated with growth hormone. *Lancet* 1991; **337**:864–5.

Billette de Villemeur T, Beslys J-P, Pradel A et al. Creutzfeldt–Jakob disease from contaminated growth hormone extracts in France. *Neurology* 1996; **47**:690–5.

Binelli S, Agazzi P, Giaccone G et al. Periodic electroencephalogram complexes in a patient with variant Creutzfeldt–Jakob disease. *Ann Neurol* 2006; **59**:423–7.

Braham J. Jakob–Creutzfeldt disease: treatment by amantadine. *BMJ* 1971; **4**:212–13.

Brown P, Cathala F, Castaigne P et al. Creutzfeldt–Jakob disease: clinical analysis of a consecutive series of 230 neuropathologically verified cases. *Ann Neurol* 1986; **20**:597–602.

Brown P, Goldfarb LG, Brown WT et al. Clinical and molecular genetic study of a large German kindred with Gerstmann–Straussler–Scheinker syndrome. *Neurology* 1991; **41**:375–9.

Brown P, Gibbs CJ, Rodgers-Johnson P et al. Human spongiform encephalopathy: the National Institutes of Health series of 300 cases of experimentally transmitted disease. *Ann Neurol* 1994; **35**:513–29.

Brown P, Preece M, Brandel JP et al. Iatrogenic Creutzfeldt-Jacob disease at the millennium. *Neurology* 2000; **55**:1075–81.

Bruce ME, Will RG, Ironside JW et al. Transmissions to mice indicate that 'new variant' CJD is caused by the BSE agent. *Nature* 1997; **389**:498–501.

Burger LJ, Rowan J, Goldensohn E. Creutzfeldt-Jacob disease. *Arch Neurol* 1972; **26**:428–33.

Chou SM, Payne WN, Gibbs CG et al. Transmission and scanning electron microscopy of spongiform change in Creutzfeldt–Jakob disease. *Brain* 1980; **103**:885–904.

Cochius JI, Hyman N, Esiri MM. Creutzfeldt–Jakob disease in a recipient of human pituitary-derived gonadotrophin: a second case. *J Neurol Neurosurg Psychiatry* 1992; **55**:1094–5.

Collie DA, Summers DM, Sellar RJ et al. Diagnosing variant Creutzfeldt–Jakob disease with the pulvinar sign: MR imaging findings in 86 neuropathologically confirmed cases. *AJNR* 2003; **24**:1560–9.

Collinge J, Rossor M. A new-variant of prion disease. *Lancet* 1996; **347**:916–17.

Collinge J, Sidle KCL, Meads J et al. Molecular analysis of prion strain variation and the aetiology of 'new-variant' CJD. *Nature* 1996; **383**:685–90.

Collinge J, Whitfield J, McIntosh E et al. Kuru in the 21st century – an acquired human prion disease with very long incubation periods. *Lancet* 2006; **367**:2068–74.

Collins SJ, Sanchez-Juan P, Masters CL et al. Determinants of diagnostic investigation sensitivities across the clinical spectrum of sporadic Creutzfeldt–Jakob disease. *Brain* 2006; **129**:2278–87.

Cooper SA, Murray KL, Will RG et al. Sporadic Creutzfeldt–Jakob disease with cerebellar ataxia at onset in the UK. *J Neurol Neurosurg Psychiatry* 2006; **77**:1273–5.

Dervaux A, Laine H, Czermak M et al. Creutzfeldt–Jakob disease presenting as psychosis. *Am J Psychiatry* 2004; **161**:1307–8.

Dimitri D, Jehel L, Durr A et al. Fatal familial insomnia presenting as psychosis in an 18-year-old man. *Neurology* 2006; **67**:363–4.

Duffy P, Wolf J, Collins G et al. Possible person to person transmission of Creutzfeldt–Jakob disease. *N Engl J Med* 1974; **290**:692–3.

Farlow MR, Yee RD, Dlouhy SR et al. Gerstmann–Straussler–Scheinker disease. I. Extending the clinical spectrum. *Neurology* 1989; **39**:1446–52.

Favereaux A, Quadrio I, Vital C et al. Pathologic prion protein spreading in the peripheral nervous system of a patient with sporadic Creutzfeldt–Jakob disease. *Arch Neurol* 2004; **61**:747–50.

Gajdusek DC. Unconventional viruses and the origin and disappearance of Kuru. *Science* 1977; **197**:943–60.

Gajdusek DC, Zigas V. Clinical, pathological and epidemiological study of the central nervous system among natives of the eastern highlands of New Guinea. *Am J Med* 1959; **26**:442–69.

Gallassi R, Morreale A, Montagna P et al. Fatal familial insomnia: behavioral and cognitive features. *Neurology* 1996; **46**:935–9.

Galvez S, Masters C, Gajdusek C. Descriptive epidemiology of Creutzfeldt–Jakob disease in Chile. *Arch Neurol* 1980; **37**:11–14.

Geschwind MD, Martindale J, Miller D et al. Challenging clinical utility of the 14-3-3 protein for the diagnosis of sporadic Creutzfeldt–Jakob disease. *Arch Neurol* 2003; **60**:813–16.

Ghetti B, Tagliavini F, Masters CL et al. Gerstmann–Straussler–Scheinker disease. II. Neurofibrillary tangles and plaques with PrP-amyloid coexist in an affected family. *Neurology* 1989; **39**:1453–61.

Gibbs CJ, Asher DM, Kobrine A *et al*. Transmission of Creutzfeldt–Jakob disease to a chimpanzee by electrodes contaminated during neurosurgery. *J Neurol Neurosurg Psychiatry* 1994; **57**:757–8.

Glatzel M, Abela E, Maissen M *et al*. Extraneural pathologic prion protein in sporadic Creutzfeldt–Jakob disease. *N Engl J Med* 2003; **349**:1812–20.

Glatzel M, Stoeck K, Seeger H *et al*. Human prion disease. Molecular and clinical aspects. *Arch Neurol* 2005; **62**:545–52.

Goldfarb LG, Mitrova E, Brown P *et al*. Mutation in codon 200 of scrapie amyloid protein gene in two clusters of Creutzfeldt–Jakob disease in Slovakia. *Lancet* 1990; **336**:514–15.

Goldfarb LG, Petersen RB, Tabaton M *et al*. Fatal familial insomnia and familial Creutzfeldt–Jakob disease: disease phenotype determined by a DNA polymorphism. *Science* 1992; **258**:806–8.

Goldhammer Y, Gabison R, Meiner Z *et al*. An Israeli family with Gerstmann–Straussler–Scheinker disease manifesting the codon 102 mutation in the prion protein gene. *Neurology* 1993; **43**:2718–19.

Green AJE, Thompson EJ, Stewart GE *et al*. Use of 14-3-3 protein and other brain-specific proteins in CSF in the diagnosis of variant Creutzfeldt–Jakob disease. *J Neurol Neurosurg Psychiatry* 2001; **70**:744–8.

Haik S, Brandel JP, Salomon D *et al*. Compassionate use of quinacrine in Creutzfeldt–Jakob disease fails to show significant effects. *Neurology* 2004; **63**:2413–15.

Hannah EL, Belay ED, Gambetti P *et al*. Creutzfeldt–Jakob disease after receipt of a previously unimplicated brand of dura mater graft. *Neurology* 2001; **56**:1080–3.

Healy D, Evans J. Creutzfeldt–Jakob disease after pituitary gonadotrophins. *BMJ* 1993; **307**:517–18.

Heath CA, Barver RA, Esmonde TFG *et al*. Dura mater associated Cretuzfeldt–Jakob disease: experience from surveillance in the UK. *J Neurol Neurourg Psychiatry* 2006; **77**:880–1.

Heckmann JG, Lang CJG, Petruch F *et al*. Transmission of Creutzfeldt–Jakob disease via a corneal transplant. *J Neurol Neurosurg Psychiatry* 1997; **63**:388–90.

Hill AF, Butterworth RJ, Joiner S *et al*. Investigation of variant Creutzfeldt–Jakob disease and other human prion diseases with tonsil biopsy specimens. *Lancet* 1999; **353**:183–9.

Hsiao K, Doh-ura K, Kitamoto T *et al*. A prion protein amino acid substitution in ataxic Gerstmann–Straussler–Scheinker syndrome. *Ann Neurol* 1989; **26**:137.

Hsiao K, Meiner Z, Kahana E *et al*. Mutation of the prion protein gene in Libyan Jews with Creutzfeldt–Jakob disease. *N Engl J Med* 1991a; **324**:1091–7.

Hsiao K, Cass C, Schellenberg GD *et al*. A prion protein variant in a family with the telencephalic form of Gerstmann–Straussler–Scheinker syndrome. *Neurology* 1991b; **41**:681–4.

Hsiao K, Dlouhy S, Farlow MR *et al*. Mutant prion proteins in Gerstmann–Straussler–Scheinker disease with neurofibrillary tangles. *Nat Genet* 1992; **1**:68–71.

Hsich G, Kenney K, Gibbs CJ *et al*. The 14-3-3 brain protein in cerebrospinal fluid as a marker for transmissible spongiform encephalopathies. *N Engl J Med* 1996; **335**:924–30.

Ironside JW, Bishop MT, Connolly K *et al*. Variant Creutzfeldt–Jakob disease: prion protein genotype analysis of positive appendix tissue samples from a retrospective prevalence study. *BMJ* 2006; **332**:1186–8.

Kakulas BA, Lecours AR, Gajdusek DC. Further observations on the pathology of Kuru (a study of two cerebra in serial section). *J Neuropathol Exp Neurol* 1967; **26**:85–97.

Kitamoto T, Tateishi J, Tashima I *et al*. Amyloid plaques in Creutzfeldt–Jakob disease stain with prion protein antibodies. *Ann Neurol* 1986; **20**:204–8.

Kitamoto T, Amano N, Terao Y *et al*. A new inherited prion disease (PrP-P105L mutation) showing spastic paraparesis. *Ann Neurol* 1993; **34**:808–13.

Kretzchmar HA, Kufer P, Reithmuller G *et al*. Prion protein mutation at codon 102 in an Italian family with Gerstmann–Straussler–Scheinker syndrome. *Neurology* 1992; **42**:809–10.

Ladogana A, Puopolo D, Poleggi A *et al*. High incidence of genetic human transmissible spongiform encephalopathies in Italy. *Neurology* 2005; **64**:1592–7.

Landolt H-P, Gratzel M, Blatter T *et al*. Sleep-wake disturbances in sporadic Creutzfeldt–Jakob disease. *Neurology* 2006; **66**:1418–24.

Lemstra AW, van Meegen MT, Vreyling JP *et al*. 14-3-3 testing in diagnosing Creutzfeldt–Jakob disease. A prospective study in 112 patients. *Neurology* 2000; **55**:514–16.

Lendvai I, Saravay SM, Steinberg MD. Creutzfeldt–Jakob disease presenting as secondary mania. *Psychosomatics* 1999; **40**:524–5.

Levy SR, Chiappa KH, Burke CJ *et al*. Early evolution and incidence of electroencephalographic abnormalities in Cretuzfeldt–Jakob disease. *J Clin Neurophysiol* 1986; **3**:1–21.

Lugaresi E, Medori R, Montagna P *et al*. Fatal familial insomnia and dysautonomia with selective degeneration of thalamic nuclei. *N Engl J Med* 1986; **315**:997–1003.

MacGowan DJL, Delanty N, Petito F *et al*. Isolated myoclonic alien hand as the sole presentation of pathologically established Creutzfeldt–Jakob disease: a report of two patients. *J Neurol Neurosurg Psychiatry* 1997; **63**:404–7.

Mandell AM, Alexander MP, Carpenter S. Creutzfeldt–Jakob disease presenting as isolated aphasia. *Neurology* 1989; **39**:55–8.

Manetto V, Medori R, Cortelli P *et al*. Fatal familial insomnia: clinical and pathological study of five new cases. *Neurology* 1992; **42**:312–19.

Martinez-Yelamos A, Saiz A, Sanchez-Valle R *et al*. 14-3-3 protein in the CSF as prognostic marker in early multiple sclerosis. *Neurology* 2001; **57**:722–4.

Masters CL, Richardson EP. Subacute spongiform encephalopathy (Creutzfeldt–Jakob disease) – the nature and progression of spongiform change. *Brain* 1978; **101**:333–44.

May WW. Creutzfeldt–Jakob disease. *Acta Neurol Scand* 1986; **44**:1–32.

Medori R, Tritschler HJ, LeBlanc A *et al*. Fatal familial insomnia with a mutation at codon 178 of the prion protein gene. *N Engl J Med* 1992a; **326**:444–9.

Medori R, Montagna P, Tritschler HJ *et al*. Fatal familial insomnia: a second kindred with mutation of prion protein gene at codon 178. *Neurology* 1992b; **42**:669–70.

Mihara M, Sgase S, Konaka K et al. The 'pulvinar sign' in a case of paraneoplastic limbic encephalitis associated with non-Hodgkin's lymphoma. J Neurol Neurosurg Psychiatry 2005; 76:882–4.

Miyashita K, Inuzuka T, Kondo H et al. Creutzfeldt–Jakob disease in a patient with a cadaveric dural graft. Neurology 1991; 41:940–1.

Nagayama M, Shinohara Y, Furukawa H et al. Fatal familial insomnia with a mutation at codon 178 of the prion protein gene: first report from Japan. Neurology 1996; 47:1313–16.

Nochlin D, Sumi SM, Bird TD et al. Familial dementia with PrP-positive amyloid plaques: a variant of the Gerstmann–Straussler syndrome. Neurology 1989; 39:910–18.

Otto M, Cepek L, Ratzka R et al. Efficacy of flupirtine on cognitive function in patients with CJD: A double blind study. Neurology 2004; 62:714–18.

Owen F, Poulter M, Lofthouse R et al. Insertion in prion protein gene in familial Creutzfeldt–Jakob disease. Lancet 1989; 1:51–2.

Pan K-M, Baldwin M, Nguyen J et al. Conversion of alpha-helices into beta-sheets features in the formation of the scrapie prion proteins. Proc Natl Acad Sci USA 1993; 90:962–6.

Parchi P, Gise A, Capelleri S et al. Classification of sporadic Creutzfeldt–Jakob disease based on molecular and phenotypic analysis of 300 subjects. Ann Neurol 1999a; 46:224–33.

Parchi P, Capellari S, Chin S et al. A subtype of sporadic prion disease mimicking fatal familial insomnia. Neurology 1999b; 52:1757–63.

Petzold GC, Westner I, Bohner G et al. False-positive pulvinar sign on MRI in sporadic Creutzfeldt–Jakob disease. Neurology 2004; 62:1235–6.

Pocchiara M, Pupolo M, Croes EA et al. Predictors of survival in sporadic Creutzfeldt-Jakob disease and other transmissible spongiform encephalopathies. Brain 2004; 127:2348–59.

Reder AT, Mednick AS, Brown P et al. Clinical and genetic studies of fatal familial insomnia. Neurology 1995; 45:1068–75.

Roberts GW, Lofthouse R, Brown R et al. Prion-protein immunoreactivity in human transmissible dementias. N Engl J Med 1986; 315:1231–3.

Roos R, Cajdusek DC, Gibbs CJ. The clinical characteristics of transmissible Creutzfeldt–Jakob disease. Brain 1973; 96:1–20.

Rosenmann H, Meiner Z, Kahana E et al. Detection of 14-3-3 protein in the CSF of genetic Creutzfeldt–Jakob disease. Neurology 1997; 49:593–5.

Saiz A, Graus F, Dalmau J et al. Detection of 14-3-3 brain protein in the cerebrospinal fluid of patients with paraneoplastic neurological disorders. Ann Neurol 1999; 46:774–7.

Sanchez-Juan P, Green A, Ladogana A et al. CSF tests in the differential diagnosis of Cretuzfeldt–Jakob disease. Neurology 2006; 67:637–43.

Sanders WL. Creutzfeldt–Jakob disease treated with amantadine. J Neurol Neurosurg Psychiatry 1979; 42:960–1.

Sanders WL, Dunn TL. Creutzfeldt–Jakob disease treated with amantadine. J Neurol Neurosurg Psychiatry 1973; 36:581–4.

Shiga Y, Miyazawa K, Sato S et al. Diffusion-weighted MRI abnormalities as an early diagnostic marker for Creutzfeldt–Jakob disease. Neurology 2004; 63:443–9.

Silburn P, Cervenakova L, Varghese P et al. Fatal familial insomnia: a seventh family. Neurology 1996; 47:1326–8.

Steinhoff BJ, Zerr I, Glatting M et al. Diagnostic value of periodic complexes in Creutzfeldt–Jakob disease. Ann Neurol 2004; 56:702–8.

Tabaton M, Monaco S, Cordone MP et al. Prion deposition in olfactory biopsy of sporadic Creutzfeldt–Jakob disease. Ann Neurol 2004; 55:294–6.

Tabernero C, Polo JM, Sevillano MD et al. Fatal familial insomnia: clinical, neuropathological, and genetic description of a Spanish family. J Neurol Neurosurg Psychiatry 2000; 68:774–7.

Taratuto AL, Piccardo P, Reich EG et al. Insomnia associated with thalamic involvement in E220K Creutzfeldt–Jakob disease. Neurology 2002; 58:362–7.

Terzano MG, Montanari E, Calzetti S et al. The effect of amantadine on arousal and EEG patterns in Creutzfeldt–Jakob disease. Arch Neurol 1983; 40:555–9.

Tschampa H, Kallenberg K, Urbach H et al. MRI in the diagnosis of sporadic Creutzfeldt–Jakob disease: a study on inter-observer agreement. Brain 2005; 128:2026–33.

Van Everbroeck BRJ, Boons J, Cras P. 14-3-3 gamma-isoform detection distinguishes sporadic Creutzfeldt–Jakob disease from other dementias. J Neurol Neurosurg Psychiatry 2005; 76:100–2.

Wieser HG, Schwarz U, Blatter T et al. Serial EEG findings in sporadic and iatrogenic Creutzfeldt–Jakob disease. Clin Neurophysiol 2004; 115:2467–78.

Will RG, Mathews WB. A retrospective study of Creutzfeldt–Jakob disease in England and Wales 1970–1979 I. Clinical features. J Neurol Neurosurg Psychiatry 1984; 47:134–40.

Will RG, Ironside JW, Zeidler M et al. A new-variant of Creutzfeldt–Jakob disease in the UK. Lancet 1996; 347:921–5.

Will RG, Zeidler M, Stewart GE et al. Diagnosis of new variant Creutzfeldt–Jakob disease. Ann Neurol 2000; 47:575–82.

Wroe SJ, Pal S, Siddique D et al. Clinical presentation and pre-mortem diagnosis of variant Creutzfeldt–Jakob disease associated with blood transfusion; a case report. Lancet 2006; 368:2061–7.

Yamada M, Itoh Y, Fujigasaki H et al. A missense mutation at codon 105 with codon 129 polymorphism of the prion protein gene in a new-variant of Gerstmann–Straussler–Scheinker disease. Neurology 1993; 43:2723–4.

Young K, Jones CK, Piccardo P et al. Gerstmann–Straussler–Scheinker disease with mutation at codon 102 and methionine at codon 129 of PRNP in previously unreported patients. Neurology 1995; 45:1127–34.

Zanusso G, Ferrari S, Cardone F et al. Detection of pathologic prion protein in the olfactory epithelium in sporadic Creutzfeldt-Jacob disease N Engl J Med 2003; 348:711–19.

Zeidler M, Stewart GE, Barraclough CR et al. New-variant Creutzfeldt–Jakob disease: neurological features and diagnostic tests. Lancet 1997a; 350:903–7.

Zeidler M, Johnstone EC, Bamber RWK et al. New-variant Creutzfeldt–Jakob disease: psychiatric features. Lancet 1997b; 350:908–10.

Zeidler M, Sellar RJ, Collie DA. The pulvinar sign on magnetic resonance imaging in variant Creutzfeldt–Jakob disease. *Lancet* 2000; **355**:1412–18.

Zeng S, Kim CH, Rahman H. Psychotic symptoms presented in familial Creutzfeldt–Jakob disease, subtype E220K. *J Clin Psychiatry* 2001; **62**:734–5.

Zerr I, Bodemer M, Gefeller O *et al.* Detection of 14-3-3 protein in the cerebrospinal fluid supports the diagnosis of Creutzfeldt–Jakob disease. *Neurology* 1998a; **43**:32–40.

Zerr I, Giese A, Windl O *et al.* Phenotypic variability in fatal familial insomnia (D178N-129M) genotype. *Neurology* 1998b; **51**:1398–405.

Endocrinologic disorders

16.1 CUSHING'S SYNDROME

Cushing's syndrome typically manifests with various neuropsychiatric features (e.g., depression), classically in a patient with a 'Cushingoid' habitus consisting of 'moon' facies, truncal obesity, and violaceous abdominal striae (Orth 1995). This syndrome occurs secondary to the effects of sustained hypercortisolemia, which in turn may be due to either administration of exogenous steroids (e.g., prednisone) or endogenous overproduction of steroids.

Normally, cortisol levels are maintained within normal limits by the hypothalamic–pituitary–adrenal axis. The hypothalamus secretes corticotrophin-releasing hormone (CRH), which in turn stimulates the pituitary to produce adrenocorticotrophic hormone (ACTH); ACTH then stimulates the adrenal cortex to produce cortisol, which in turn exerts a negative feedback effect on the hypothalamus and pituitary. A sustained, excessive production of endogenous cortisol by the adrenal gland may result from the following causes: an enhanced release of CRH from the hypothalamus or from CRH-secreting ectopic tumors; an ACTH-secreting pituitary adenoma; ectopic ACTH production (e.g., by an oat cell carcinoma of the lung); and, finally, adrenal tumors.

The term 'Cushing's syndrome' refers to cases of symptomatic hypercortisolemia of any cause; the term 'Cushing's disease', however, is restricted to cases caused by pituitary adenomas.

Clinical features

The mode of onset of Cushing's syndrome is dependent on the underlying cause. Cases due to exogenous steroid use are of the most rapid onset, and may appear within days. Cushing's disease secondary to a pituitary adenoma may present very gradually, over years, and cases of Cushing's syndrome secondary to ectopic ACTH production may present over months.

The neuropsychiatric features of Cushing's syndrome include depression, mania or hypomania, anxiety, psychosis, dementia, or delirium. Depression is the most prominent neuropsychiatric feature of Cushing's syndrome (Spillane 1951); it has been noted in between one-half (Haskett 1985; Jeffcoate et al. 1979; Kelly 1996) and three-quarters (Cohen 1980; Starkman et al. 1981) of patients with Cushing's syndrome and indeed may be the presenting feature (Kelly 1996). Anxiety commonly accompanies the depression creating the picture of an 'agitated depression'. The depression at times may be severe, with psychotic features (Cohen 1980), which may be either mood-congruent (Anderson and McHugh 1971; Maclay and Stokes 1939) or mood-incongruent (Trethowan and Cobb 1952), with Schneiderian first-rank symptoms of thought broadcasting and thought insertion. Both suicide attempts and completed suicides may occur (Jeffcoate et al. 1979).

Mania is less common than depression in Cushing's syndrome of endogenous origin (Haskett 1985; Jeffcoate et al. 1979; Kelly 1996), but the converse holds true in exogenous cases, in which mania is common (Wolkowitz et al. 1990).

Anxiety of pathologic degree has been noted in about one-tenth of patients (Kelly 1996), but is most often seen in the context of depression.

Psychosis, although rare, can occur secondary to Cushing's syndrome. One patient presented with delusions of persecution, auditory and visual hallucinations, and bizarre behavior, all of which cleared with adrenalectomy (Hickman et al. 1961); another experienced agitation, auditory hallucinations, and religious and grandiose delusions, which again cleared with adrenalectomy (Hertz et al. 1955).

Delirium may occur (Kawashima et al. 2004) but is rare, being noted in only about 1 percent of cases (Kelly 1996). Dementia is likewise rare and is often characterized by prominent memory loss (Varney et al. 1984).

These neuropsychiatric features classically occur in the setting of a Cushingoid habitus, with, as noted earlier, 'moon' facies, truncal obesity, and violaceous abdominal striae. Other features include acne, hirsutism, proximal myopathy, easy bruisability, hypertension, diabetes mellitus, amenorrhea, and, rarely, pseudotumor cerebri. All of these features, however, take time to develop and thus may not be present in cases of Cushing's syndrome secondary to exogenous steroid use, which, as noted earlier, may develop over days. Furthermore, in cases of Cushing's syndrome secondary to ectopic ACTH secretion by an oat cell carcinoma, one may see emaciation rather than obesity.

When Cushing's syndrome occurs secondary to exogenous steroid administration the diagnosis is fairly obvious, as symptoms appear within days of using high dosage steroids, for example ⩾60 mg/day of prednisone. However, when endogenous steroid overproduction is suspected, laboratory testing is essential to confirm the diagnosis. Confirmation of suspected endogenous hypercortisolemia is sought via a 24-hour urine test for free cortisol. Serum cortisol levels show pulsatile fluctuations during the day, and hence should not be relied on. If the 24-hour urine free cortisol level is normal, the diagnosis is effectively ruled out.

In cases in which the 24-hour urinary free cortisol level is elevated, further testing is required to determine the cause. The first step is to obtain an ACTH level. In hypercortisolemia secondary to an adrenal tumor, the ACTH is low, whereas in all other cases it is elevated. If the ACTH is elevated, the next step is to determine whether the ACTH is derived from an ectopic source, for example lung carcinoma, or from a pituitary tumor, and this is accomplished with the 'high dose' dexamethasone suppression test (Tyrell et al. 1986). In this test, patients are given 2 mg of dexamethasone orally every 6 hours over 2 days, and during the second day a 24-hour urine sample is collected for measurement of free cortisol. In cases of ectopic ACTH production, the tumor secreting the ACTH is not sensitive to the feedback of dexamethasone and hence continues to secrete ACTH, resulting in an increased free cortisol level in the 24-hour urine sample: in such cases one speaks of 'non-suppression' of cortisol by dexamethasone. By contrast, pituitary adenomas do remain sensitive to dexamethasone and in these cases ACTH output falls with a resulting fall in the 24-hour urine free cortisol level: in such cases one speaks of 'suppression' of cortisol by dexamethasone. An alternative, or supplementary, test is the CRH stimulation test. Here, one gives 1 µg/kg of ovine CRH intravenously and determines both ACTH and cortisol levels 15 minutes before the infusion and 15, 30, 60, 90, and 120 minutes afterward. Ectopic ACTH-secreting tumors are not sensitive to CRH, and cortisol and ACTH levels do not rise significantly. Pituitary adenomas, however, are sensitive, and in such cases cortisol and ACTH levels do rise.

In some cases the dexamethasone test may be equivocal, and differentiating between an ectopic ACTH-secreting tumor and a pituitary tumor may depend on sampling venous blood flow from the pituitary. As might be expected, in cases of pituitary tumors, the ACTH level in venous blood from either the superior petrosal sinus or the internal jugular vein will be higher than that in venous blood drawn at phlebotomy; conversely, when the source of ACTH is an ectopic tumor, this 'gradient' between superior petrosal or internal jugular blood and systemic venous blood will not be present. Sampling the superior petrosal sinus is difficult and not without risk, but is more sensitive than sampling the internal jugular vein; hence, one should begin with sampling the internal jugular vein, reserving petrosal sampling for cases in which this is negative (Doppman et al. 1998).

In cases in which a pituitary tumor is suspected, high-resolution magnetic resonance imaging (MRI) with gadolinium enhancement is in order, and, if positive, may obviate the need for superior petrosal or internal jugular sampling. Unfortunately, however, most ACTH-secreting pituitary tumors are microadenomas and about 50 percent will escape detection by MRI (Kaskarelis et al. 2006).

Course

The course is determined by the underlying cause. Once cortisol levels are returned to normal, either by stopping exogenous steroids or by virtue of treatment of endogenous causes, neuropsychiatric features gradually resolve; although such resolution may occur within weeks to days in cases secondary to relatively short-term treatment with high-dose exogenous steroids, months may be required in endogenous cases (Kelly et al. 1983).

Etiology

The mechanism by which hypercortisolemia causes the neuropsychiatric features noted above is not known.

As noted earlier, there are various causes for endogenous hypercortisolemia, including adrenal tumors, ectopic ACTH-secreting tumors, and pituitary tumors (Erem et al. 2003). Adrenal tumors, which may be either adenomas or carcinomas, account for about 15 percent of cases. Ectopic ACTH-secreting tumors likewise account for about 15 percent of cases; although small-cell lung cancer is the most common of these, other tumors may also be at fault, including cancer of the thymus, pancreas, or thyroid, and pheochromocytoma. Pituitary adenomas are by far the most common cause of endogenous hypercortisolemia, accounting for about 70 percent of all cases. There are also very rare reports of CRH-secreting tumors, which may be located in either the hypothalamus or ectopically, as for example in thyroid cancer.

Differential diagnosis

The appearance of neuropsychiatric symptomatology in a patient receiving relatively high doses of exogenous corticosteroids immediately implicates the drug. Diagnostic uncertainty may arise, however, in cases in which the condition that prompted the treatment with corticosteroids may itself affect the central nervous system, as is the case with multiple sclerosis or systemic lupus erythematosus. In such cases, a careful history, with due attention to the existence of neuropsychiatric symptoms before steroid treatment, may resolve the issue. In other cases it may be necessary to change the corticosteroid dose significantly: if the dose is increased and symptoms worsen (or, conversely, if the dose is decreased and symptoms lessen), the steroid is implicated.

As noted earlier, mood disturbances are the most common neuropsychiatric feature, and the diagnosis of Cushing's syndrome may be missed in depressed or manic patients unless one keeps in mind the typical Cushingoid habitus.

Treatment

In exogenous cases, the dose of the steroid should, if possible, be reduced. In endogenous cases, the tumor should be resected if possible. In cases of pituitary tumors, the transphenoidal approach is utilized; however, if this is not possible, radiation treatment may be considered. When the tumor cannot be treated, one may consider adrenalectomy or, alternatively, a 'chemical' adrenalectomy may be performed by administering daily doses of drugs such as ketoconazole or metyrapone, which inhibit enzymes responsible for steroidogenesis in the adrenal glands. After adrenalectomy, whether surgical or 'chemical', daily maintenance doses of steroids will be required. Furthermore, one must be alert to the development of Nelson's syndrome, in which ACTH tumors of the pituitary may develop with the appearance of hyperpigmentation in cases in which inhibitory feedback is lacking.

Symptomatic treatment of neuropsychiatric features may be required in cases in which etiologic treatment is unsuccessful or not possible or, in cases when it is, when symptoms are severe and resolution is slow. Depression may be treated with antidepressants, mania with mood stabilizers, and psychosis with antipsychotics, as discussed in Sections 6.1, 6.3, and 7.1 respectively.

16.2 ADRENOCORTICAL INSUFFICIENCY

Adrenocortical insufficiency may be primary, due to actual destruction of the adrenal gland, or secondary, due to pituitary failure or to abrupt discontinuation of long-term treatment with corticosteroids. Adrenocortical insufficiency, whether primary or secondary, may be further subdivided into acute and chronic forms.

Before proceeding, a word is in order regarding the term 'Addison's disease'. Some authors use this term to refer to all cases of adrenocortical insufficiency, regardless of cause, whereas others restrict it to primary cases, specifically those due to autoimmune destruction of the adrenal gland. Given this unfortunate definitional ambiguity, the term is not used further in this text.

Clinical features

Acute adrenocortical insufficiency presents with nausea, vomiting, and abdominal pain, with a rapidly falling blood pressure, postural dizziness, and eventually hypovolemic shock: delirium develops, followed by stupor and coma.

Chronic adrenocortical insufficiency presents gradually with fatigue, listlessness, poor concentration, anorexia, nausea, diarrhea or constipation, and abdominal pain. Depression may occur (Engel and Margolin 1941; Varadaraj and Cooper 1986) and, rarely, there may be delirium (Engel and Margolin 1941; Fang and Jaspan 1989) or psychosis (Anglin et al. 2006; Cleghorn 1951; McFarland 1963). Blood pressure is low and postural dizziness is common. In primary cases, with a lack of cortisol feedback on the pituitary, excessive stimulation of melanocytes by ACTH may lead to hyperpigmentation, especially prominent in sun-exposed areas and on the buccal and gingival mucosa. Chronic adrenocortical insufficiency may also be complicated by an acute episode, for example as may occur when chronic patients are subjected to a significant physiologic stress such as surgery.

Laboratory testing begins with a serum cortisol level, which is reduced. An ACTH level is also obtained: in primary cases ACTH levels are increased because of a lack of feedback inhibition on the pituitary, whereas in secondary cases the ACTH level is low. In cases in which ACTH levels are equivocal, further testing may be conducted with cosyntropin, a synthetic ACTH analogue, to determine whether such cases are primary or secondary. Cosyntropin is given intravenously in a dose of 0.25 mg, and cortisol levels are obtained 15 minute pre-injection and 30 and 60 minutes post-injection. In primary cases there is little or no rise in ACTH, whereas in secondary cases, presuming that the adrenal glands have not atrophied due to chronic non-stimulation, there should be a robust rise in ACTH.

Further laboratory abnormalities may be seen in primary cases in which destruction of the adrenal glands causes decreased mineralocorticoid levels, with resulting hyponatremia and hyperkalemia.

Course

Acute adrenocortical insufficiency is a life-threatening emergency. The course of chronic adrenocortical insufficiency is determined by the underlying cause: in the case of primary chronic adrenocortical insufficiency due to autoimmune destruction of the adrenals, there is a gradual progression of symptoms, with death occurring in perhaps 2 years.

Etiology

Primary adrenocortical insufficiency is most commonly due to autoimmune destruction of the adrenal glands.

In this disorder, other endocrine glands may also be targeted by the autoimmune process, and patients may develop Hashimoto's thyroiditis (with either hyperthyroidism or hypothyroidism), pernicious anemia with vitamin B12 deficiency, hypoparathyroidism with hypocalcemia, or diabetes mellitus. Other causes of primary adrenocortical insufficiency include adrenoleukodystrophy, tuberculosis, cytomegalovirus infection (as may occur in AIDS), sarcoidosis, amyloidosis, metastatic disease, and hemorrhagic infarction (as may occur during septicemia or with overvigorous anticoagulation). With the exception of hemorrhagic infarction, all of these forms of primary adrenocortical insufficiency cause a chronic presentation.

Secondary adrenocortical insufficiency, as noted earlier, most commonly occurs secondary to abrupt discontinuation of long-term treatment with corticosteroids. Any patient taking supraphysiologic doses of a corticosteroid (e.g., 10 mg or more daily of prednisone) for more than 1 month will have some suppression of ACTH output from the pituitary coupled with some atrophy of the adrenal cortex. Other causes of secondary adrenocortical insufficiency include infarction, and tumors or granulomas of either the pituitary or, rarely, the hypothalamus. These secondary cases may present either acutely (as for example with abrupt discontinuation of steroid treatment) or chronically (as may be seen with slowly growing pituitary tumors).

Differential diagnosis

Delirium occurring in acute adrenocortical insufficiency is suggested by concurrent nausea, vomiting, and postural dizziness. In cases occurring in the course of sepsis, the delirium may be erroneously attributed to the systemic effects of the infection.

Depression, delirium, or psychosis occurring during chronic adrenocortical insufficiency are each suggested by the overall fatigue and listlessness of the patient and by the associated gastrointestinal symptomatology and postural dizziness.

Treatment

Chronic adrenocortical insufficiency is generally treated with hydrocortisone in a dose of 20–30 mg/day, with two-thirds of the dose given in the morning and one-third in the afternoon, with dose increases during periods of physiologic stress. In primary cases this should be supplemented with fludrocortisone in a dose of 0.05–0.1 mg/day.

Acute adrenocortical insufficiency often requires treatment in an intensive care unit; normal saline with 5 percent glucose is given, along with a bolus of 100 mg of hydrocortisone intravenously, followed by repeat doses of 10 mg hourly.

16.3 HYPERTHYROIDISM

Sustained elevation of thyroxine (T_4) typically causes a syndrome characterized by anxiety and autonomic hyperactivity; most cases are due to Graves' disease or toxic multinodular goiter. Although in routine clinical work most clinicians refer to all of these cases as 'hyperthyroidism', this practice, technically, is not correct. Strictly speaking, hyperthyroidism refers to conditions in which the thyroid gland is producing excess amounts of thyroid hormone, and the term 'thyrotoxicosis' refers to the clinical syndrome itself. Although this may seem to be splitting hairs, it does call attention to the fact that, although most cases are due to diseases that cause excess thyroid hormone production, for example Graves' disease, there are diseases, such as Hashimoto's thyroiditis, in which the elevated serum T_4 concentrations occur not because of increased production of hormone but rather because of a 'leakage' of hormone from the inflamed gland. Clinicians' habits, however, are hard to break, and in this text the term 'hyperthyroidism' is used to refer to the syndrome.

Clinical features

The age of onset varies according to the underlying etiology: Graves' disease typically appears in the twenties or thirties and toxic multinodular goiter generally has an onset in old age. Although in most cases symptoms appear gradually, over weeks or months, subacute onsets may be seen, especially in relation to various physiologic stressors.

The discussion of clinical features will begin with a description of the typical picture of hyperthyroidism, followed by a discussion of an important variant known as apathetic hyperthyroidism. Subsequently, neuropsychiatric features seen only in a minority of cases of hyperthyroidism are discussed, including depression, mania, psychosis, dementia, and delirium. Finally, 'thyroid storm' is considered.

Typically, patients are apprehensive and anxious and, although fatigued and tired, they often experience restlessness and an inability to sit still. Anxiety often stands out (Greer et al. 1973; MacCrimmon et al. 1979) and in some cases may represent the presenting complaint (Dietch 1981). Patients typically complain of diaphoresis, heat intolerance, and an increased frequency of bowel movements, and, despite an often increased appetite with increased caloric intake, there may be substantial weight loss. On examination, one finds tachycardia, widened palpebral fissures and proptosis, a fine postural tremor, and generalized hyperreflexia; there may also be a proximal myopathy. Women may complain of menstrual irregularity and men may experience erectile dysfunction. Rarely, there may be chorea (Fidler et al. 1971; Fishbeck and Layzer 1979; Van Uitert and Russakoff 1979), grand mal seizures (Jabbari and Huott 1980), or a motor peripheral neuropathy (Pandit et al. 1998).

Apathetic hyperthyroidism (Brenner 1978; Lahey 1931; Thomas et al. 1970) represents a peculiar variant of hyperthyroidism that is generally only seen in the elderly and which is characterized by apathy and, in some, lethargy. Remarkably, of the 'autonomic' signs and symptoms seen in typical cases, only tachycardia is common in this apathetic variant: diaphoresis, tremor, and hyper-reflexia are generally absent. Many patients will also develop atrial fibrillation and congestive failure.

Of the neuropsychiatric features seen in hyperthyroidism, depression is the most common and is seen in a substantial minority of patients (Kathol and Delahunt 1986; Trzepacz et al. 1988), especially in those with apathetic hyperthyroidism (Thomas et al. 1970), in whom the only clue to the correct diagnosis, as just noted, may be tachycardia or congestive heart failure (Arnold et al. 1974; Brenner 1978). Depression in hyperthyroidism may be accompanied by mood-congruent delusions (Taylor 1975) or considerable agitation (Van Uitert and Russakoff 1979).

Mania is less common than depression in hyperthyroidism (Trzepacz et al. 1988), and in some cases may be of the 'mixed' variety (Ingham and Nielsen 1931).

Psychosis, although only rarely due to hyperthyroidism, may occur (Lazarus and Jaffe 1986; Steinberg 1994): one patient developed a delusion of jealousy and, convinced that his wife was having an affair, had her followed; when his hyperthyroidism was treated, his psychosis resolved (Hodgson et al. 1992).

Dementia may occur in typical hyperthyroidism (Bulens 1981; Fukui et al. 2001) but is rare; by contrast, a significant minority of patients with the apathetic variant will develop cognitive deficits that may be severe enough to constitute a dementia (Martin and Deam 1996). Delirium may also occur, but appears to be very rare.

Thyroid storm is a dreaded complication of hyperthyroidism and typically appears in a patient with untreated hyperthyroidism who is subjected to some significant physiologic stress, such as surgery or an infection. In this setting there is a rapid escalation of all of the typical signs and symptoms followed by hyperthermia, delirium, stupor, and coma. In some cases seizures may occur and, rarely, thyroid storm has presented with a psychosis (Bursten 1961; Greer and Parsons 1968). Thyroid storm may also occur in the setting of apathetic hyperthyroidism, and in such cases may present with coma in the absence of any autonomic features (Ghobrial and Ruby 2002).

In almost all cases of hyperthyroidism the free T_4 level will be elevated and the thyroid-stimulating hormone (TSH) level will be reduced. Exceptions occur in cases of 'T_3 (triiodothyronine) thyrotoxicosis', in which the free T_4 level is normal; in cases in which the clinical suspicion of hyperthyroidism is high and the free T_4 is normal, the free T_3 level should be determined. Other exceptions include the very rare cases of a hypothalamic tumor secreting thyrotropin-releasing hormone (TRH) or a pituitary adenoma secreting TSH: in both of these cases both the free T_4 and the TSH levels are elevated.

Course

The course is dictated by the underlying cause. Thyroid storm, regardless of the underlying cause, may pursue a fulminant course, with death in hours or days.

Etiology

The vast majority of cases are due to Graves' disease. Other causes include toxic multinodular goiter, toxic solitary adenoma, and the thyroiditides, including lymphocytic thyroiditis, subacute (De Quervain's) thyroiditis, and Hashimoto's thyroiditis. The thyroiditides are characterized by a 'leakage' of T_4 from the inflamed thyroid and, typically, cause a hyperthyroidism that is time limited and that may, depending on the amount of inflammatory damage and scarring, be followed by hypothyroidism. Rare causes include hypothalamic tumors, pituitary adenomas (Carlson et al. 1983; Wynne et al. 1992), inherited pituitary resistance to T_4, production of ectopic TSH by various tumors (hydatidiform mole, choriocarcinoma of the uterus, and choriocarcinoma of the testis), and production of T_4 by various tumors (struma ovarii or metastatic follicular carcinoma of the thyroid). Finally, hyperthyroidism may occur as a side-effect of amiodarone, and may also be intentional, as in 'thyrotoxicosis factitia'.

Differential diagnosis

As noted earlier, anxiety is a prominent feature of hyperthyroidism and, of the various other causes of persistent anxiety discussed in Section 6.5, the one that often comes to mind is generalized anxiety disorder. One clue to the differential here may be found on shaking the patient's hand: in both hyperthyroidism and generalized anxiety disorder the hand is moist with sweat, but in hyperthyroidism the skin is warm whereas in generalized anxiety disorder it is cool, yielding a 'cold and clammy' impression.

The differential diagnosis for depression is discussed in Section 6.1. One feature of depression secondary to hyperthyroidism that sets it apart from depression due to other causes is the presence of weight loss in the face of increased eating; by contrast, weight loss occurring in depression due to other causes is generally associated with anorexia.

Mania, psychosis, dementia, or delirium occurring secondary to hyperthyroidism, as discussed in Sections 6.3, 7.1, 5.1, and 5.3, respectively, is suggested by concurrent proptosis and autonomic signs, such as tremor and tachycardia.

Treatment

If necessary, autonomic features may be controlled with propranolol, in doses of 20–40 mg orally every 4–6 hours. In cases characterized by increased production of T_4, as occurs in Graves' disease, toxic multinodular goitre, and solitary adenomas, anti-thyroid drugs such as propylthiouracil or methimazole are generally indicated; in some cases radioactive iodine treatment or surgery may also be required. Once T_4 levels are normalized, most of the symptoms of hyperthyroidism gradually resolve. Symptomatic treatment of depression and other neuropsychiatric features may or may not be required pending this resolution; if so, this may be accomplished as discussed in the respective sections.

Thyroid storm constitutes a medical emergency and requires treatment in an intensive care unit. In addition to propranolol and anti-thyroid drugs, sodium or potassium iodide, hydrocortisone, and cooling blankets are often required.

16.4 HYPOTHYROIDISM

Hypothyroidism is the clinical syndrome that occurs secondary to a persistently low level of circulating thyroxine, or T_4. A synonym for this is myxedema, a name that calls attention to the mucinous edema that gives rise to the typical facial appearance seen in hypothyroidism, described below. Hypothyroidism is a common condition, found in a little under 1 percent of the general population; it is 10–20 times more common in females than males.

Thyroxine levels are maintained within normal limits by virtue of the hypothalamic–pituitary–thyroid axis. The hypothalamus produces TRH, which in turn stimulates the anterior pituitary to produce TSH; TSH then stimulates the thyroid gland to produce T_4, which in turn exerts a negative feedback effect on both the pituitary and the hypothalamus. The various causes of hypothyroidism may be grouped according to which element of the hypothalamic–pituitary–thyroid axis is affected. Tertiary hypothyroidism occurs as a result of hypothalamic disease (e.g., tumors) and is characterized by a low TSH and a low T_4. Secondary hypothyroidism occurs with pituitary disease (e.g., tumors or infarction) and likewise displays both a low TSH and low T_4. Primary hypothyroidism, which is by far the most common type, occurs with disease of the thyroid itself (e.g., Hashimoto's thyroiditis or post-thyroidectomy) and, here, the TSH is elevated whereas the T_4 is low.

Clinical features

The age of onset of hypothyroidism is determined by the underlying cause. Cases occurring secondary to Hashimoto's thyroiditis typically appear in the late thirties or early forties, and cases occurring after thyroidectomy may first appear within weeks post-operatively. The onset and evolution of symptoms is typically gradual.

The clinical picture includes not only typical features, such as psychomotor retardation, but also, in a significant minority, neuropsychiatric features including depression, psychosis, and dementia.

Typically, patients develop psychomotor retardation, with slowed speech and movements; in some cases lethargy and somnolence may occur. When asked a question, up to a minute may pass before the patient responds, and the response itself, when it does come, is slow. Simple activities, such as unfastening a button, may likewise take an inordinate amount of time to complete. Patients may appear apathetic and lacking in initiative, and often there may be difficulty with concentration and a certain 'fogginess' of thought and memory (Nickel and Frame 1958). The overall appearance of hypothyroid patients is often distinctive: skin becomes thickened, puffy, and even boggy, and this is particularly obvious on the face, in the supraclavicular fossae, and on the dorsal surfaces of the hands and feet. The hair becomes thin and brittle and there may be considerable hair loss; interestingly there may also be a loss of hair on the lateral thirds of the eyebrows. Other symptoms include a voice change towards hoarseness, cold intolerance, constipation, weight gain, decreased libido, erectile dysfunction, and menorrhagia. Vibratory sense may be lost and the deep tendon reflexes are often reduced; the ankle jerk is often 'hung up', with a delayed relaxation phase. Cranial nerves may be involved, with partial deafness and, rarely, a peripheral facial palsy; cerebellar ataxia ('myxedema staggers') (Jellinek and Kelly 1960) occurs in up to 20 percent of cases. Very rarely, seizures may occur (Bryce and Poyner 1992). Myxedematous infiltration may cause a carpal or tarsal tunnel syndrome; macroglossia may also occur and, if severe, may be followed by obstructive sleep apnea. Bradycardia and hypotension are common, and there may be a degree of hypothermia; pericardial and pleural effusions may also occur. In a small minority of cases, a syndrome of inappropriate antidiuretic hormone (ADH) secretion may occur, with hyponatremia.

In severe cases of hypothyroidism a condition known as 'myxedema coma' may develop. Typically this occurs in patients with long-standing hypothyroidism who are subjected to a physiologic stress, such as surgery or a significant infection, or who are given phenothiazines (Mitchell et al. 1959) or any medications with prominent sedative effects. Stupor or coma develops, accompanied by hypothermia (which may be severe), significant bradycardia, respiratory depression, and, in a significant minority, grand mal seizures.

Of the neuropsychiatric features seen in hypothyroidism, depression is most common; this may be severe and may be accompanied by hallucinations and delusions (Whybrow et al. 1969).

Psychosis occurring secondary to hypothyroidism has traditionally been referred to as 'myxedema madness' (Asher 1949) and is often characterized by delusions of persecution and reference, as well as auditory hallucinations (Crowley 1940; de Fine Olivarius and Roder 1970; Karnosh and Stout 1935; Logothetis 1963; Reed and Bland 1977). One case of myxedema madness (Ziegler 1930) deserves to be quoted at length, as it illustrates the sometimes exquisite nature of the dependence of the psychosis on the level of circulating thyroid hormone. The patient had undergone radiation treatment for hyperthyroidism 3 years earlier and had subsequently done well with an appropriate dosage of supplemental thyroid hormone. At the age of 48 years, however, she became non-compliant and soon thereafter:

> she began to feel that her husband was paying attention to another woman and that he was trying to do away with her by means of gas or the electric chair. During a game at a party in her own home during the holidays in 1928, she refused to sit in a chair designated for her, thinking it might be a plot to kill her. She also felt that her husband was trying to poison her and refused to take desiccated thyroid gland at home on account of such a belief. On several occasions subsequently, when desiccated thyroid was administered in sufficient quantity, at the repeated and urgent request of her physician, the delusions entirely disappeared and she felt so much better that she concluded that it was foolish to be taking medicine and discontinued taking it. On such occasions, the psychosis would slowly return in the same form as before.

Dementia (Akelaitis 1936; de Fine Olivarius and Roder 1970; Uyematsu 1920) may present with failing memory, followed by deficits in calculation and orientation; in some cases, the dementia may be accompanied by delusions of persecution and auditory hallucinations.

The electroencephalogram (EEG) typically shows generalized slowing.

Thyroxine levels are available as both 'total' T_4, including both bound and free fractions, and 'free' T_4, and in all instances a free T_4 level should be obtained. This free T_4, as noted earlier, is reduced in all cases. The TSH level, however, may be elevated or decreased, depending on the cause of the hypothyroidism. In primary hypothyroidism, the TSH is increased; in both secondary and tertiary cases, however, it is reduced. Distinguishing secondary from tertiary cases generally requires a TRH stimulation test. In this test, TRH is given intravenously and TSH levels are determined just before and 20 minutes after the infusion. In cases of secondary hypothyroidism, given a lack of pituitary cells capable of producing TSH, the response to exogenous TRH is blunted. By contrast, in tertiary hypothyroidism, in which a chronic lack of endogenous TRH allows for an up-regulation of TRH receptors on pituitary cells, there is an enhanced response of TSH to TRH.

Before leaving this section some words are in order regarding the condition known as 'subclinical' primary hypothyroidism. Here, although the free T_4 level is within normal limits, the TSH level is mildly elevated. Such a combination of laboratory values indicates that, although the free T_4 may be within broadly defined limits of normal, it is nevertheless below the individual patient's 'normal' as indicated by the rise in TSH. Although patients may not have symptoms directly related to these findings, they are significant for

two reasons. First, such findings may indicate that the patient is in the very early stages of what will become clinically evident hypothyroidism and, given this, close monitoring is required. Second, such subclinically reduced free T_4 levels, although not causing symptoms *per se*, will nevertheless blunt the response to antidepressants or mood-stabilizing agents in patients with major depression or bipolar disorder.

Course

The course of hypothyroidism is determined by the underlying cause.

Etiology

As noted earlier, the various causes of hypothyroidism are divided into primary, secondary, and tertiary types.

Primary hypothyroidism is by far the most common type, accounting for over 90 percent of cases. The most common cause of primary hypothyroidism is Hashimoto's thyroiditis, indicated by the presence of anti-thyroid antibodies: anti-thyroid peroxidase antibody (also known as anti-microsomal antibody) is most common, but anti-thyroglobulin antibodies may also be present. Other causes include thyroidectomy, radioactive iodine treatment, neck irradiation, iodine deficiency, and various medications, including amiodarone, rifampin (Takasu *et al.* 2005), ethionamide (McDonnell *et al.* 2005), and, most especially, lithium (Lindstedt *et al.* 1977), in which case the occurrence of hypothyroidism is most likely in patients who have anti-thyroid antibodies (Calabrese *et al.* 1985).

Secondary hypothyroidism may occur with tumors or infarction of the pituitary.

Tertiary hypothyroidism may occur with tumors or infarction of the hypothalamus; other causes include granulomatous disease and carbamazepine.

Differential diagnosis

The differential diagnoses of the syndromes of depression, psychosis, and dementia are discussed in Sections 6.1, 7.1 and 5.1 respectively. In all these cases, the chief clues to the diagnosis are the typical symptoms seen in hypothyroidism, especially the psychomotor retardation, lethargy, and the distinctive 'myxedematous' appearance.

In cases of primary hypothyroidism secondary to Hashimoto's thyroiditis, it must be kept in mind that the underlying autoimmune process may cause additional disorders including primary adrenocortical insufficiency and pernicious anemia with vitamin B12 deficiency. Given that both of these disorders may cause psychosis, and that B12 deficiency, in addition, may cause depression and dementia, it is appropriate in all cases of Hashimoto's thyroiditis to check cortisol and B12 levels. Checking the cortisol level is also important because the treatment of hypothyroidism with T_4 in a patient with adrenocortical insufficiency may precipitate a life-threatening Addisonian crisis.

Cases of secondary or tertiary hypothyroidism may also be associated with other endocrinopathies, such as hyperprolactinemia or secondary adrenocortical insufficiency.

Finally, one must clearly distinguish between Hashimoto's thyroiditis and Hashimoto's encephalopathy. Both of these disorders are associated with anti-thyroid antibodies. In Hashimoto's thyroiditis, however, the thyroid alone is targeted, whereas in Hashimoto's encephalopathy, as discussed in Section 17.9, the thyroid is usually spared and the autoimmune onslaught is directed against the cerebrum.

Treatment

Treatment with once-daily T_4 is generally curative. In cases of hypothyroidism of relatively recent onset in young patients who are otherwise healthy and lack heart disease, one may begin with 50–75 μg daily, increasing in 25–50 μg increments every 2 or 3 weeks. In cases of long-standing hypothyroidism, however, or in elderly patients or those in poor health or with significant heart disease, the starting dose should be lower, in the range of 12.5–25 μg, and the increases should be in increments of 12.5–25 μg every 4–6 weeks. Serial T_4 determinations are made, and the dose should be increased until the free T_4 is within the normal range. In cases of primary hypothyroidism, TSH levels should also be obtained, with the goal of bringing TSH down to within normal limits; in this regard it must be kept in mind that the TSH level falls very slowly and that 4–8 weeks may be required at any given dose of T_4 for the TSH level to plateau out. For most adult females, anywhere from 75 to 100 μg of T_4 is generally an adequate maintenance dose; in males the range is from 100 to 150 μg. In the elderly, however, the maintenance dose is generally 75 μg or less. In females given conjugated estrogens an increase in thyroid-binding globulins may decrease the free T_4, necessitating a dose increase (Arafah 2001).

It has been suggested that a combination of T_4 and T_3 produced better symptomatic relief than T_4 alone (Bunevicius et al. 1999); however, subsequent work has failed to confirm this (Gorzinsky-Glasberg et al. 2006).

Myxedema coma constitutes a medical emergency and patients should be admitted to an intensive care unit. Treatment involves giving intravenous T_4 in a dose of 300 μg, followed by daily intravenous doses of 50–100 μg. Intravenous hydrocortisone is also given, along with vigorous supportive care.

REFERENCES

Akelaitis AJE. Psychiatric aspects of myxedema. *J Nerv Ment Dis* 1936; **83**:22–36.

Anderson AE, McHugh PR. Oat cell carcinoma with hypercortisolemia presenting to a psychiatric hospital as a suicide attempt. *J Nerv Ment Dis* 1971; **152**:427–31.

Anglin RE, Rosebush PI, Mazurek MF. The neuropsychiatric profile of Addison's disease: revisiting a forgotten phenomenon. *J Neuropsychiatry Clin Neurosci* 2006; **18**:450–9.

Arafah BM. Increased need for thyroxine in women with hypothyroidism during estrogen therapy. *N Engl J Med* 2001; **344**:1743–9.

Arnold BM, Casal G, Higgins HP. Apathetic thyrotoxicosis. *Can Med Assoc J* 1974; **111**:957–8.

Asher R. Myxoedematous madness. *BMJ* 1949; **2**:555–62.

Brenner I. Apathetic hyperthyroidism. *J Clin Psychiatry* 1978; **39**:479–80.

Bryce GM, Poyner F. Myxoedema presenting with seizures. *Postgrad Med J* 1992; **68**:35–6.

Bulens C. Neurologic complications of hyperthyroidism: remission of spastic paralysis, dementia, and optic neuropathy. *Arch Neurol* 1981; **38**:669–70.

Bunevicius R, Kazanavicius G, Zalinkevicius R et al. Effects of thyroxine as compared with thyroxine plus triiodothyronine in patients with hypothyroidism. *N Engl J Med* 1999; **340**:424–9.

Bursten B. Psychosis associated with thyrotoxicosis. *Arch Gen Psychiatry* 1961; **4**:267–73.

Calabrese JR, Gulledge AD, Hahn K et al. Autoimmune thyroiditis in manic-depressive patients treated with lithium. *Am J Psychiatry* 1985; **142**:1318–21.

Carlson HE, Linfoot JA, Burnstein GD et al. Hyperthyroidism and acromegaly due to a TSH- and GH-secreting tumor: lack of hormonal response to bromocriptine. *Am J Med* 1983; **74**:915–23.

Cleghorn RA. Adrenal cortical insufficiency: psychological and neurological observations. *Can Med Assoc J* 1951; **65**:449–54.

Cohen SI. Cushing's syndrome: a psychiatric study of 29 patients. *Br J Psychiatry* 1980; **136**:120–4.

Crowley RM. Psychoses with myxedema. *Am J Psychiatry* 1940; **96**:1105–16.

Dietch JT. Diagnosis of organic anxiety disorders. *Psychosomatics* 1981; **22**:661–9.

Doppman JL, Oldfield EH, Nieman LK. Bilateral sampling of the internal jugular vein to distinguish between mechanisms of adrenocorticotropic hormone-dependent Cushing syndrome. *Ann Intern Med* 1998; **128**:33–6.

Engel GL, Margolin SG. Neuropsychiatric disturbances in Addison's disease and the role of impaired carbohydrate metabolism in the production of abnormal cerebral function. *Arch Neurol Psychiatry* 1941; **45**:881–4.

Erem C, Algun E, Osbey N et al. Clinical laboratory findings and results of therapy in 55 patients with Cushing's syndrome. *J Endocrinol Invest* 2003; **26**:65–72.

Fang VBS, Jaspan JB. Delirium and neuromuscular symptoms in an elderly man with isolated corticotroph deficiency syndrome completely reversed with glucocorticoid replacement. *J Clin Endocrinol Metab* 1989; **69**:1073–7.

Fidler SM, O'Rourke RA, Buschbaum HW. Choreoathetosis as a manifestation of thyrotoxicosis. *Neurology* 1971; **21**:55–7.

de Fine Olivarius B, Roder E. Reversible psychosis and dementia in myxedema. *Acta Psychiatr Scand* 1970; **46**:1–13.

Fishbeck KH, Layzer RB. Paroxysmal choreoathetosis associated with thyrotoxicosis. *Ann Neurol* 1979; **6**:453–4.

Fukui T, Hasegawa Y, Takenaka H. Hyperthyroid dementia: clinicoradiological findings and response to treatment. *J Neurol Sci* 2001; **184**:81–8.

Ghobrial MW, Ruby EB. Coma and thyroid storm in apathetic thyrotoxicosis. *South Med J* 2002; **95**:552–4.

Greer S, Parsons V. Schizophrenia-like psychosis in thyroid crisis. *Br J Psychiatry* 1968; **114**:1357–62.

Greer S, Ramsay I, Bagley C. Neurotoxic and thyrotoxic anxiety: clinical, psychological and physiological measurements. *Br J Psychiatry* 1973; **122**:549–54.

Gorzinsky-Glasberg S, Fraser A, Nahsoni E et al. Thyroxine-triiodothyronine combination therapy versus thyroxine monotherapy for clinical hypothyroidism: meta-analysis of randomized controlled trials. *J Clin Endocrinol Metab* 2006; **91**:2592–9.

Haskett RF. Diagnostic categorization of psychiatric disturbance in Cushing's syndrome. *Am J Psychiatry* 1985; **142**:911–16.

Hertz PE, Nadas E, Wojtkowiki H. Case report: Cushing's syndrome and its management. *Am J Psychiatry* 1955; **112**:144–5.

Hickman JW, Atkinson RP, Flint LD et al. Transient schizophrenic reaction as a major symptom of Cushing's syndrome. *N Engl J Med* 1961; **264**:797–800.

Hodgson RE, Murray D, Woods MR. Othello's syndrome and hyperthyroidism. *J Nerv Ment Dis* 1992; **180**:663–4.

Ingham SD, Nielsen JM. Thyroid psychosis: difficulties in diagnosis. *J Nerv Ment Dis* 1931; **74**:271–7.

Jabbari B, Huott AD. Seizures in thyrotoxicosis. *Epilepsia* 1980; **21**:91–6.

Jeffcoate WJ, Silverstone JT, Edwards CRW et al. Psychiatric manifestations of Cushing's syndrome: response to lowering of plasma cortisol. *Q J Med* 1979; **191**:465–72.

Jellinek EH, Kelly RE. Cerebellar syndrome in myxoedema. *Lancet* 1960; **2**:225–7.

Karnosh LJ, Stout RE. Psychoses of myxedema. *Am J Psychiatry* 1935; **91**:1263–74.

Kaskarelis IS, Tsatalou EG, Benakis SV et al. Bilateral inferior petrosal sinuses sampling in the routine investigation of Cushing's syndrome: a comparison with MRI. *AJR* 2006; **187**:562–70.

Kathol RG, Delahunt JW. The relationship of anxiety and depression to symptoms of hyperthyroidism using operational criteria. *Gen Hosp Psychiatry* 1986; **8**:23–8.

Kawashima T, Oda M, Kund T et al. Metyrapone for delirium due to Cushing's syndrome induced by occult ectopic adrenocorticotropic hormone secretion. *J Clin Psychiatry* 2004; **65**:1019–20.

Kelly WF. Psychiatric aspects of Cushing's syndrome. *Q J Med* 1996; **89**:543–51.

Kelly WF, Checkley SA, Bender DA et al. Cushing's syndrome and depression – a prospective study of 26 patients. *Br J Psychiatry* 1983; **142**:16–19.

Lahey FH. Non-activated (apathetic) type of hyperthyroidism. *N Engl J Med* 1931; **204**:747–8.

Lazarus A, Jaffe R. Resolution of thyroid-induced schizophreniform disorder following subtotal thyroidectomy: case report. *Gen Hosp Psychiatry* 1986; **8**:29–31.

Lindstedt G, Nilsson L, Walinder J et al. On the prevalence, diagnosis and management of lithium-induced hypothyroidism in psychiatric patients. *Br J Psychiatry* 1977; **130**:452–8.

Logothetis J. Psychotic behavior as the initial indicator of adult myxedema. *J Nerv Ment Dis* 1963; **136**:561–8.

MacCrimmon DJ, Wallace JE, Goldberg WM et al. Emotional disturbances and cognitive deficits in hyperthyroidism. *Psychosom Med* 1979; **41**:331–40.

Maclay WS, Stokes AB. Mental disorder in Cushing's syndrome. *J Neurol Neurosurg Psychiatry* 1939; **1**:110–18.

Martin FI, Deam DR. Hyperthyroidism in elderly hospitalized patients. Clinical features and treatment outcomes. *Med J Aust* 1996; **164**:200–3.

McDonnell ME, Braverman JE, Bernardo J. Hypothyroidism due to ethionamide. *N Engl J Med* 2005; **352**:2757–9.

McFarland HR. Addison's disease and related psychoses. *Compr Psychiatry* 1963; **4**:90–5.

Mitchell JRA, Surridge DHC, Willison RG. Hypothermia after chlorpromazine in myxoedematous psychosis. *BMJ* 1959; **2**:932–3.

Nickel SN, Frame B. Neurologic manifestations of myxedema. *Neurology* 1958; **8**:511–17.

Orth DN. Cushing's syndrome. *N Engl J Med* 1995; **332**:791–803.

Pandit L, Shankar SK, Gayathri N et al. Acute thyrotoxic neuropathy – Basedow's paraplegia revisited. *J Neurol Sci* 1998; **155**:211–4.

Reed K, Bland RC. Masked 'myxedema madness'. *Acta Psychiatr Scand* 1977; **56**:421–6.

Spillane JD. Nervous and mental disorders in Cushing's syndrome. *Brain* 1951; **74**:72–94.

Starkman MN, Schteingart DE, Schork MA. Depressed mood and other psychiatric manifestations of Cushing's syndrome: relationship to hormone levels. *Psychosom Med* 1981; **43**:3–18.

Steinberg PI. A case of paranoid disorder associated with hyperthyroidism. *Can J Psychiatry* 1994; **39**:153–6.

Takasu N, Takara M, Komiya I. Rifampin-induced hypothyroidism in patients with Hashimoto's thyroiditis. *N Engl J Med* 2005; **352**:518–19.

Taylor JW. Depression in thyrotoxicosis. *Am J Psychiatry* 1975; **132**:552–3.

Thomas FB, Mazzaferri EL, Skillman TG. Apathetic thyrotoxicosis: a distinctive clinical and laboratory entity. *Ann Intern Med* 1970; **72**:679–85.

Trethowan WH, Cobb S. Neuropsychiatric aspects of Cushing's syndrome. *Arch Neurol Psychiatry* 1952; **67**:283–309.

Trzepacz P, McCue M, Klein I et al. A psychiatric and neuropsychological study of patients with untreated Graves' disease. *Gen Hosp Psychiatry* 1988; **10**:49–55.

Tyrell JB, Findling JW, Aron EDC et al. An overnight high-dose dexamethazone suppression test for rapid differential diagnosis of Cushing's syndrome. *Ann Intern Med* 1986; **104**:180–6.

Uyematsu S. A case of myxedematous psychosis. *Arch Neurol Psychiatry* 1920; **3**:252–76.

Van Uitert RL, Russakoff LM. Hyperthyroid chorea mimicking psychiatric disease. *Am J Psychiatry* 1979; **136**:1208–10.

Varadaraj R, Cooper AJ. Addison's disease presenting with psychiatric features. *Am J Psychiatry* 1986; **143**:553–4.

Varney NR, Alexander B, MacIndoe JH. Reversible steroid dementia in patients without steroid psychosis. *Am J Psychiatry* 1984; **141**:369–72.

Whybrow PC, Prange AJ, Treadway CR. Mental changes affecting thyroid gland dysfunction: a reappraisal using objective psychological measurement. *Arch Gen Psychiatry* 1969; **20**:48–63.

Wolkowitz OM, Rubinow D, Doran AR *et al.* Prednisone effects on neurochemistry and behavior. *Arch Gen Psychiatry* 1990; **47**:963–8.

Wynne AG, Gharib H, Scheithauer BW *et al.* Hyperthyroidism due to inappropriate secretion of thyrotropin in 10 patients. *Am J Med* 1992; **92**:15–24.

Ziegler LH. Psychosis associated with myxedema. 1930; **11**:20–7.

Immune-related disorders

17.1 MULTIPLE SCLEROSIS

Multiple sclerosis (MS) is characterized pathologically by the more or less sequential occurrence of lesions known as plaques in various parts of the white matter of the central nervous system, and clinically by the appearance of signs and symptoms appropriate to the location of the plaques. This is a fairly common disorder, occurring in about 0.1 percent of the general population, and is roughly two to three times more common in females than males.

Clinical features

Although the range of age of onset is wide, from childhood to the seventh decade, the vast majority of patients first fall ill in their twenties or thirties. As discussed further below (see Course, below), in most cases, at least initially, MS pursues an episodic course, and the episodes typically have a subacute onset, over days or a week or so. Exceptions to this rule, however, do occur, with some onsets spanning less than a day and others being quite leisurely, occurring over weeks or months. The duration of individual episodes varies widely, from weeks to months, after which there is a gradual defervescence of symptomatology of variable degree. The severity of symptoms varies widely, and in some cases may be so mild that patients fail to recognize them as such.

The most common symptoms are motor or sensory in type. Spastic weakness may occur in one limb, or there may be a hemiparesis or paraparesis. Sensory symptoms, similar in distribution, may include numbness and tingling, and, in a minority, dysesthesiae or actual pain. Visual symptomatology is also common and may include optic neuritis with unilateral blurring of vision or blindness; not uncommonly one may see the combination of optic neuritis and paraplegia

secondary to a transverse myelitis, in which case one speaks of Devic's disease or neuromyelitis optica. Cerebellar and brainstem involvement is also common and may produce ataxia, intention tremor, dysarthria or scanning speech, nystagmus, diplopia, and vertigo. Internuclear ophthalmoplegia may also occur, and this should be carefully sought for as it is of great diagnostic significance: although internuclear ophthalmoplegia may occur with other mesencephalic lesions, such as tumors, infarctions or Wernicke's encephalopathy, these are all quite rare in young adults and, hence, this finding in a young person is almost specific for MS (Keane 2005). Bladder dysfunction is quite common with various symptoms including urgency and frequency, incontinence or urinary retention. Bowel dysfunction is also common and most frequently presents with constipation. Sexual dysfunction is very common, with decreased libido, erectile dysfunction or decreased vaginal lubrication. Uncommon symptoms and signs include aphasia (Achiron et al. 1992; Devere et al. 2000; Lacour et al. 2004; Olmos-Lau et al. 1977) and seizures, which may be either partial or grand mal in type (Nicoletti et al. 2003), and various paroxysmal phenomena, such as hemifacial spasm, Lhermitte's sign, trigeminal neuralgia, and lancinating pains in the extremities. Fatigue may also occur in MS and may be quite severe.

Dementia of variable severity, ranging from mild, almost subclinical impairment to debilitating, is eventually seen in the majority of patients (Franklin et al. 1989; Surridge 1969). In rare cases, dementia may constitute the sole, or predominant, presenting feature of MS (Bergin 1957; Hotopf et al. 1994; Koenig 1968; Young et al. 1976). In one case, for example, the only symptom in addition to the dementia was optic neuritis (Jennekens-Schinkel and Sanders 1986), and in two others it was unsteady gait (Mendez and Frey 1992). In one very rare case a gradually progressive dementia constituted the *only* clinical evidence of MS (Fontaine *et al.* 1994). Although the correlation of dementia and plaque location and number has not been definitively worked out, it appears that cognitive deficits correlate both with the total burden of plaques within the cerebral white matter (Comi *et al.* 1999; Franklin *et al.* 1988; Ron *et al.* 1991) and with atrophy of the corpus callosum (Huber *et al.* 1987), which in turn may merely reflect overall disease activity in the hemispheric white matter (Barnard and Triggs 1974).

Depression is eventually seen in perhaps one-quarter of patients (Surridge 1969). Depression may occur on a reactive basis in any debilitating disease, and MS is no exception. Certain facts, however, suggest strongly that depression in MS may also be a direct result of plaque formation. Patients with MS are more likely to experience depression than are normal control subjects (Fassbender *et al.* 1998) or those with comparably disabling neurologic diseases that generally spare the cerebrum, such as amyotrophic lateral sclerosis (Schiffer and Babigian 1984; Whitlock and Siskind 1980). Furthermore, in contrast to what one might expect if the depression were reactive, there is little or no correlation between the occurrence of depression and the extent of the patient's disability (Moller *et al.* 1994), and, regardless of the degree of overall disability, patients are more likely to experience depression when the plaques are in the cerebrum than when they are in the cerebellum or spinal cord (Rabins *et al.* 1986; Schiffer *et al.* 1983). Furthermore, a correlation has been noted between depression and the presence of plaques in the inferior left frontal white matter (Feinstein *et al.* 2004), the left arcuate fasciculus (Pujol *et al.* 1997), and the white matter of the right temporal lobe (Berg *et al.* 2000).

Euphoria may also occur in MS, and this is typically of the 'bland' or non-infectious type; it has been noted in anywhere from one-quarter (Surridge 1969) to the vast majority of patients (Cottrell and Wilson 1926), and is correlated with cerebral rather than spinal plaque formation (Rabins *et al.* 1986). The contrast between this euphoria and the patient's actual condition can be quite dramatic: one of S.A.K. Wilson's (1955) patients, 'bedridden and unable to stand, remarked, "you will not believe me when I say I feel thundering well."' This bland euphoria is typically not accompanied by hyperactivity or pressure of speech and is often seen in concert with some degree of intellectual impairment (Surridge 1969). Although they are unusual, definite manic episodes may also occur in addition to this bland euphoria (Joffe *et al.* 1987; Schiffer *et al.* 1986); indeed, out of all of the reasons for admission to psychiatric hospital for patients with MS, mania is the most common (Pine *et al.* 1995).

Emotional incontinence, with uncontrollable laughter or crying in the absence of a corresponding affect, is seen in about one-tenth of patients (Feinstein *et al.* 1997; Surridge 1969), generally only in far-advanced cases.

Psychosis may rarely dominate the clinical picture (Mathews 1979; Parker 1956), and in one very rare case MS presented with a psychosis characterized by social

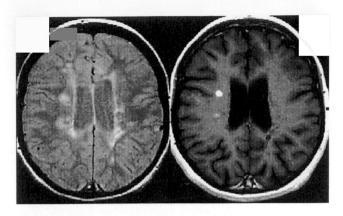

Figure 17.1 In the T2-weighted magnetic resonance imaging scan on the left, there are multiple areas of increased signal intensity corresponding to both chronic and active plaques; in the T1-weighted scan with gadolinium enhancement on the right, however, only the active lesions enhance. (Reproduced from Graham and Lantos 1996.)

withdrawal, 'mystic' visual hallucinations, and various delusions (Fontaine *et al.* 1994).

Magnetic resonance (MR) scanning has assumed a dominant role in the evaluation of patients with suspected MS. Almost all plaques demonstrate increased signal intensity on T2-weighted or fluid-attenuated inversion recovery (FLAIR) imaging, and active plaques show enhancement with gadolinium, as demonstrated in Figure 17.1. In some cases, as noted below (see Etiology), severe plaques may undergo cystic change, and on T1-weighted imaging such plaques will appear as 'black holes' with greatly reduced signal intensity. Plaques are typically found in the centrum semiovale and in a periventricular distribution, where they tend to favor the occipital horns.

The cerebrospinal fluid (CSF) is abnormal in almost all cases. A mild lymphocytic pleocytosis, in the range of 6–30 cells/mm³, is seen in about one-third of cases, and the total protein is mildly elevated (rarely over 100 mg/dL) in about one-half of cases. The IgG index is elevated in over two-thirds of cases, and oligoclonal bands are present in over 90 percent. The myelin basic protein is elevated in over three-quarters of cases. Of note, the 14-3-3 protein may be found in a little over one-tenth of all cases (Martinez-Yelamos *et al.* 2001).

Evoked potentials, including somatosensory, brainstem, and visual-evoked potentials, were once widely used to demonstrate lesions within the respective white matter pathways; however, with the advent of MR scanning, these are generally no longer required.

Course

As noted earlier, most cases of MS are characterized by episodes of illness, and this course is referred to as relapsing and remitting. The interval between episodes is extremely variable, ranging from months to two decades. Subsequent episodes may consist of exacerbations of symptoms seen in previous episodes, or completely new symptoms, depending on whether old plaques become reactivated or new plaques form. With the resolution of any episode, remission of symptoms is rarely complete and most patients are left with residuals; over time and with recurrent episodes, this burden of residual symptoms gradually increases. Predicting the overall pattern in patients with a relapsing and remitting course is very difficult, and in some cases, even after long observation, it may still not be possible to make accurate predictions.

In addition to this relapsing and remitting pattern, the overall course of MS may also be characterized by a chronic progression of symptoms, and this 'progressive' course may be further subdivided into a 'secondary' or 'primary' type. A secondary progressive course emerges within the context of an initially relapsing and remitting course, and this pattern eventually appears in the majority of relapsing and remitting cases. A primary progressive course, that is an illness characterized by relentless and uninterrupted progression from the start, is much less common, being seen in perhaps one-tenth of all cases.

As noted earlier, the severity of symptoms seen in MS varies quite widely and, in some cases, active plaques, which can be seen on MRI, may escape clinical detection (Thompson et al. 1992; Willoughby et al. 1989). With the routine use of MRI, more and more cases of 'benign MS' are being discovered. On the other hand, some patients may experience devastatingly severe episodes. Such cases of MS are often referred to as 'Marburg' variants and are characterized by large and multiple plaques, and severe symptomatology, with, in some cases, death in a matter of weeks or months.

Although pregnancy itself does not seem to predispose to new episodes, the first 3 months post-partum do seem to be associated with an increased risk.

Symptoms of MS may undergo transient exacerbation with stress, infection, or temperature elevation, as may occur with a hot bath, fever, or exercise. These exacerbations do not reflect inflammatory plaque activity but rather impaired conduction through partially damaged axons, and thus they should not be interpreted as relapses. Interestingly, in the past this kind of transient exacerbation was used as a diagnostic test for MS: in such a 'hot bath' test, the patient was immersed in hot water and observed for the emergence of signs or symptoms.

Etiology

As indicated earlier, the pathologic hallmark of MS is the plaque. Classically, active plaques consist of an area of perivenular mononuclear inflammation with loss of oligodendrocytes and demyelinization, with relative axonal sparing (Greenfield and King 1936). Recently, however, it has become apparent that this classic view may not apply in all cases, and that in a minority the active plaque may be characterized by apoptosis of oligodendrocytes with relatively little inflammation (Barnett and Prineas 2004). In time, the active plaque resolves into a chronic plaque, which is composed of a relatively well-circumscribed area of demyelinization and gliosis, with, in severe cases, a degree of cavitation. The size of plaques varies widely, from as little as a few millimeters up to several centimeters in diameter. As noted earlier, most plaques are found in the centrum semiovale and in a periventricular location (Brownell and Hughes 1962); plaques, of course, are also found in the cerebellar white matter, the brainstem, and the cord. Although the vast majority of plaques are found in the white matter, small gray matter plaques are seen at times.

Although the cause of MS remains unknown, several lines of evidence suggest that it represents an autoimmune disorder in genetically susceptible individuals triggered by a relatively common childhood viral infection.

The incidence of MS rises from that seen in the general population to that seen in first-degree relatives and finally to monozygotic twins. As noted earlier, the incidence of MS in the general population is about 0.1 percent; this rises to about 2–4 percent in first-degree relatives up to 25–40 percent in monozygotic twins (Ebers et al. 1986; Mumford et al. 1994). Although this could conceivably be explained on the basis of a shared environment, adoption studies support a genetic cause (Ebers et al. 1995). Furthermore, there is significant linkage between MS and certain human leukocyte antigen (HLA) haplotypes.

The evidence for an infectious agent acting on this fertile genetic background rests on several facts. First, although found at all latitudes, MS is more common in temperate zones. Furthermore, if individuals remain in a high-risk temperate zone past the age of 15 years and then migrate to a tropical area, they 'carry' their increased risk with them (Dean 1967), indicating that the increased risk relates to some environmental exposure that is more common in temperate zones. Second, although not without controversy, it appears that there have been 'epidemics' of MS in the Faroe Islands and in Iceland, and that these epidemics may have been related to the presence of British troops stationed there during World War II. Although the nature of the presumed infection is not clear, certain evidence points toward such common viral infections as mononucleosis (DeLorenze et al. 2006). It must be clearly noted, however, that the deleterious effect of any such infection is not direct: there is no evidence for an actual viral infection in MS plaques. Rather, it is suspected that a childhood infection sensitizes the immune system in genetically susceptible individuals and that some event in adult life, perhaps a reactivation of a latent viral infection, triggers off an immune response that incorrectly targets oligodendrocytes and myelin.

Differential diagnosis

In large part, the differential diagnosis of MS depends on where in the course of the disease the patient happens to be. In cases in which the patient is encountered during the first episode of illness, the prime consideration is given to acute disseminated encephalomyelitis (ADEM). As discussed in Section 14.11, ADEM is a monophasic illness and the first step is to determine, by MR scanning, whether or not there are white matter lesions consistent with old plaques that may have been asymptomatic. If these are found, then the diagnosis of ADEM is effectively ruled out. In cases in which they are absent, the acute findings on MRI may be helpful. In ADEM one typically finds multiple, large white matter lesions and, although such a picture may be seen in some cases of MS, it is far more common to find a few relatively small lesions. If the differential still remains in doubt, then one may have to settle for long-term clinical observation. If there are no further episodes, then ADEM remains high on the differential; by contrast, the appearance of a new episode argues strongly for a diagnosis of MS.

In cases characterized by progressive white matter disease from the onset, MS of the primary progressive type must be distinguished from vitamin B12 deficiency and adrenoleukodystrophy, a differential readily accomplished by testing for vitamin B12 and plasma long-chain fatty acid levels.

In cases in which there is an established pattern of relapses and remissions, consideration may be given to Behçet's syndrome, systemic lupus erythematosus, and polyarteritis nodosa. In each of these three disorders, however, one also finds systemic signs that are lacking in MS: in Behçet's disease there are oral and genital ulcers; and in lupus and polyarteritis nodosa, in addition to constitutional signs one finds evidence of other organ involvement, such as the joints, kidneys, or gastrointestinal tract. In older patients consideration may also be given to lacunar infarctions; however, here the clinical episodes are generally of acute onset, over perhaps minutes or hours at the most, and the lesions are typically found in the internal capsule and basal ganglia; this is in contrast to MS in which the episodes are of more gradual onset and the lesions are more commonly found higher up in the white matter, surrounding the lateral ventricles and extending into the centrum semiovale.

Treatment

Treatment of MS may be divided into that directed at the *acute episode*, *preventive treatments* designed to forestall future episodes or to limit secondary progression, and *symptomatic treatments*. Each of these aspects of treatment is now considered in turn, followed by some *summary* recommendations.

ACUTE EPISODES

Acute episodes may be treated with intravenous methylprednisolone, followed by oral prednisone. Although there is no unanimity regarding dosage, a reasonable regimen consists of 250 mg of methylprednisolone every 6 hours for

3–7 days, followed by prednisone in a dose of approximately 1 mg/kg/day for 4 days, with this dose gradually tapered over the following 2–3 weeks, with due consideration being given to the clinical response. Mania may complicate such a course of prednisone, and this may require treatment with antipsychotics or a mood stabilizer such as lithium or valproate, as discussed in Section 6.3. In cases in which patients have received prior courses of steroids that were complicated by mania, it may be appropriate to consider prophylactic treatment with one of these mood stabilizers.

PREVENTIVE TREATMENTS

Preventive treatments may be considered in patients with a relapsing and remitting course and also in those whose course is marked by secondary progression.

In relapsing and remitting MS, preventive treatment may be accomplished with several agents, including interferons, glatiramer, and natalizumab.

Interferons are immunomodulatory agents, and three are effective: interferon beta-1b (Betaseron, given subcutaneously every other day) (European Study Group 1998) and two preparations of interferon beta-1a (Rebif, given subcutaneously three times weekly [PRISMS Study Group 1998], and Avonex, given intramuscularly once weekly [Rudick et al. 1997]). Each of these three interferons reduces relapse rates by about one-third. Choosing among them is not straightforward. All three may induce the formation of neutralizing antibodies after anywhere from 6 to18 months, which may blunt their response; this occurs in about one-third of patients on Betaseron, one-fifth of patients on Rebif, and less than one-tenth of patients on Avonex. On this count, Avonex appears attractive; however, recent work has demonstrated that both Betaseron (Durelli et al. 2002) and Rebif (Panitch et al. 2002) are more effective than Avonex.

Glatiramer (Copaxone, given subcutaneously daily) (Comi et al. 2001; Johnson et al. 1998) is a mixture of polypeptides that mimics myelin basic protein, thereby presumably blunting the autoimmune assault on myelin. Like the interferons, it reduces relapse rates by about one-third and may also induce neutralizing antibodies.

Natalizumab (Tysabri, given intravenously once monthly) is a humanized monoclonal antibody directed at human alpha-4 integrin. This molecule exists on the surface of lymphocytes and serves to bind them to vascular cell adhesion molecules (VCAM) on vascular endothelial cells, thus allowing their transport across the vessel wall. When integrin is blocked, this 'trafficking' into the interstitial fluid is inhibited and the inflammatory response is blunted. Natalizumab appears to reduce relapse rates by roughly two-thirds (Miller et al. 2003); neutralizing antibodies occur in about one-tenth of cases. Enthusiasm for natalizumab has been tempered, however, by the appearance of progressive multifocal leukoencephalopathy in treated patients; although this is a very rare complication, it is potentially fatal.

Overall, in choosing a preventive treatment for relapsing and remitting MS it is probably reasonable to begin with an interferon, such as Betaseron. Should this offer little benefit, consideration may be given to glatiramer. In clearly treatment-resistant cases, natalizumab is a reasonable option. Other, less well-established options for treatment-resistant cases include intravenous immunoglobulins or immunosuppressants such as azathioprine.

In secondary progressive MS one may use an interferon, either interferon beta-1b (Betaseron) (European Study Group 1998) or intramuscular interferon beta-1a (Avonex) (Cohen *et al.* 2002). If the patient is already on one of these agents while the course undergoes transformation from relapsing and remitting to secondary progression, then consideration may be given to an immunosuppressant, such as mitoxantrone (Hartung *et al.* 2002) or low-dose methotrexate (Goodkin *et al.* 1995).

SYMPTOMATIC TREATMENT

Spasticity has traditionally been treated with baclofen, diazepam, or tizanidine; gabapentin represents a recent addition to this armamentarium (Cutter *et al.* 2000). Painful dysesthesiae, trigeminal neuralgia, or lancinating pains may respond to either carbamazepine or gabapentin. Intention tremor may be reduced by either clonazepam or, in some cases, propranolol. Bladder dysfunction is often a focus of treatment: urinary retention may respond to bethanechol, and spastic bladder with urinary urgency and frequency may be relieved by oxybutynin or tolterodine; in some cases a Foley catheter or more invasive measures may be required. Bowel dysfunction usually consists of constipation, which may be managed with a bowel program. Erectile dysfunction may be managed with a phosphodiesterase inhibitor, such as sildenafil, and decreased vaginal lubrication may be helped by lubricating agents. Seizures may be managed with standard anti-epileptic drugs. Fatigue may respond to amantadine in a dose of 100 mg b.i.d. (Krupp *et al.* 1995; Rosenberg and Appenzeller 1988); recent enthusiasm for modafinil should be tempered by a negative double-blind study (Stankoff *et al.* 2005).

Dementia is treated as discussed in Section 5.1. Recent work suggests that donepezil may improve cognitive functioning in MS (Krupp *et al.* 2004).

Depression should be treated with an antidepressant. Remarkably, there has been only one double-blind study in this regard, which found desipramine to be superior to placebo (Schiffer and Wineman 1990); unfortunately, as might have been predicted, this was poorly tolerated. In practice, most patients are given a selective serotonin reuptake inhibitor (SSRI) such as escitalopram but, if this is not effective, other agents such as duloxetine might be considered.

Euphoria of the 'bland' type rarely requires any treatment. Should mania occur, however, treatment is conducted as described in Section 6.3.

As discussed in Section 4.7, emotional incontinence may respond to amitriptyline or to a combination of dextromethorphan and quinidine. Whether it would respond to some of the other agents used in emotional incontinence resulting from other disorders (e.g., citalopram in vascular cases) is not clear.

Psychosis is treated as outlined in Section 7.1.

SUMMARY

The overall treatment of patients with MS is difficult and at times quite complex, and it is often best carried out by a specialized team. Except in cases of very benign MS, most patients will receive preventive treatment; whenever an episode does occur, consideration should be given to prompt acute treatment with steroids to lessen the chance of any permanent damage and residual symptoms. Given the number of medications involved for symptomatic treatment, the potential for drug–drug interactions and cumulative side-effects is large, and constant vigilance is required.

17.2 SYSTEMIC LUPUS ERYTHEMATOSUS

Systemic lupus erythematosus (SLE or, colloquially, lupus) is a systemic autoimmune disease that involves multiple organs, including the brain. Cerebral lupus (or as it is also referred to, neuropsychiatric systemic lupus erythematosus) occurs in the vast majority of cases, and may occur secondary to either a direct autoimmune assault on neurons (in which case one may speak of 'lupus cerebritis') or multiple infarctions, which may be either cardioembolic or secondary to a vasculopathy.

SLE occurs in 0.015–0.05 percent of the general population. It is far more common among females than males, and among black populations than white populations, and in black females the prevalence rises to 0.4 percent.

Clinical features

Although lupus may appear at almost any age, including in the elderly, the majority of patients fall ill between puberty and 40 years of age.

As noted, lupus is a systemic disease and in most cases cerebral lupus occurs in the setting of other symptoms, including constitutional symptoms (fatigue, fever, weight loss) and those referable to other organ systems, such as the musculoskeletal system, skin, heart, lungs, or kidneys (Johnson and Richardson 1968). Musculoskeletal symptomatology is very common and includes myalgia, arthralgia, and a non-deforming polyarthritis. Cutaneous manifestations include photosensitivity, rashes (especially a malar rash), and alopecia. Cardiac symptomatology incorporates pericarditis and Libman–Sacks endocarditis. Pulmonary involvement may manifest with pleurisy, which may or may not be accompanied by pleural effusion. Renal involvement may manifest initially with proteinuria and cellular casts; over time renal failure may occur. Various cytopenias, including anemia, leukopenia, or thrombocytopenia, may also occur.

Cerebral lupus (Brey *et al.* 2002; Feinglass *et al.* 1976; Johnson and Richardson 1968) may manifest with depression, mania, psychosis, delirium or dementia, seizures, chorea, or focal signs, such as hemiparesis. Although these findings may occur independently, patients often have a mixture (Devinsky *et al.* 1988).

Depression, in some cases accompanied by hallucinations or delusions, has been found commonly by some (Ganz *et al.* 1972; Miguel *et al.* 1994), but not all (Guze 1967; Hugo *et al.* 1996), authors. Mania, although reported (Johnson and Richardson 1968), appears rare. Psychosis is relatively uncommon (Guze 1967; Lim *et al.* 1988; Miguel *et al.* 1994) and, although typically characterized by delusions and hallucinations, may rarely present with stuporous catatonia (Lanham *et al.* 1985; Mac and Pardo 1983). Rarely, psychosis may constitute the presenting feature of lupus (Agius *et al.* 1997).

Delirium may occur (Devinsky *et al.* 1988; Hugo *et al.* 1996; Miguel *et al.* 1994) and is often accompanied by hallucinations, either visual or auditory (Lief and Silverman 1960; O'Connor and Musher 1966). Dementia may also be seen (Kirk *et al.* 1991; Johnson and Richardson 1968; MacNeil *et al.* 1976; Robin *et al.* 1995) but is relatively uncommon (Devinsky *et al.* 1988).

Seizures are relatively common (Devinsky *et al.* 1988) and may be partial (complex partial or simple partial) or grand mal in type (Mikdashi *et al.* 2005). Chorea may occur and indeed may constitute the presentation of SLE (Donaldson and Espiner 1971; Fermaglich *et al.* 1973). Focal deficits (Devinsky *et al.* 1988) are common and may include hemiparesis, aphasia, or hemianopia. Thrombotic thrombocytopenic purpura has been noted but this is usually a terminal event (Devinsky *et al.* 1988).

In addition to cerebral involvement, the peripheral nervous system may also be involved, with either a peripheral polyneuropathy (McCombe *et al.* 1987) or a mononeuritis multiplex (Hughes *et al.* 1982).

The anti-nuclear antibody (ANA) test is positive in approximately 95 percent of cases (Venables 1993), and the serum Venereal Disease Research Laboratories (VDRL) test may be falsely positive. As the ANA lacks specificity, however, a positive result here must be followed up by a more specific test, such as anti-native DNA (also known as anti-double stranded DNA) or anti-Sm. During active disease, the erythrocyte sedimentation rate (ESR) is often elevated and one or more complement levels (C3, C4, CH50) are generally decreased. Consideration may also be given to testing for the presence of serum anti-ribosomal P antibodies and for the anti-phospholipid syndrome, including lupus anticoagulant and anti-cardiolipin antibodies of both the IgG and IgM types. Anti-ribosomal P antibodies may be associated with the occurrence of psychosis (Agius *et al.* 1997; Bonfa *et al.* 1987; Isshi and Hirohata 1998; Nojima *et al.* 1992; Schneebaum *et al.* 1991), and anti-phospholipid antibodies may be associated with infarction.

Magnetic resonance scanning may be normal or may show evidence of infarction. When infarctions are present, they tend to occur in one of two patterns. Either there are multiple small infarcts in either the cerebral cortex or the subcortical white matter, or one may find relatively large territorial infarctions in the areas of distribution of large pial vessels.

The electroencephalogram (EEG) may be normal or show slowing, which may be generalized or focal (Sibley *et al.* 1992). In patients with seizures, interictal epileptiform discharges may or may not be present.

The CSF (Johnson and Richardson 1968; McLean *et al.* 1995; West *et al.* 1995) may be normal or there may be a mild lymphocytic pleocytosis or a mildly elevated total protein. Other abnormalities, primarily in patients with lupus cerebritis (West *et al.* 1995), include an elevated IgG index, oligoclonal bands, and the presence of anti-neuronal antibodies.

In cases in which infarction is suspected, a work-up, as described in Section 7.4, is required: appropriate tests may include an echocardiogram, computed tomographic angiography, or magnetic resonance angiography, and, as noted earlier, testing for anti-phospholipid antibodies.

Course

Overall, the course is characterized by a gradual waxing and waning of symptoms; full remissions are unusual and generally not permanent. Although SLE is in general compatible with long-term survival, the appearance of cerebral (Rubin *et al.* 1985) or renal disease is an ominous sign.

Etiology

Lupus is characterized by the presence of a large number of autoantibodies directed at various tissues in multiple organ systems. Although the cause is not known, it is strongly suspected that the autoimmune response occurs secondary to some environmental trigger in genetically susceptible individuals.

It must be stated at the outset that the mechanism or mechanisms underlying many of the syndromes seen in cerebral lupus are not clearly understood. With this caveat in mind, however, it appears that two global mechanisms may be operative (West *et al.* 1995): a direct autoimmune attack on neurons, and multiple infarctions, occurring on a variety of different bases.

It is clear from autopsy studies that in some cases of cerebral lupus there is no evidence of infarction (O'Connor and Musher 1966; Tsokos *et al.* 1986) and, in such cases, it is suspected that a cerebritis occurs secondary to anti-neuronal antibodies (Bluestein *et al.* 1981; Isshi and Hirohata 1998; Kelly and Denburg 1987); the finding of immune complexes in the choroid plexus (Atkins *et al.* 1972) lends support to this idea.

Infarctions appear commonly in lupus and may occur on any one of several bases. Cardioembolic emboli may arise from Libman–Sacks endocarditis, valvulitis, or mural thrombi (Devinsky *et al.* 1988; Mitsias and Levine 1994; Tsokos *et al.* 1986). If these emboli are large, then large vessels, such as the middle cerebral or anterior cerebral artery, may be occluded, with resulting large territorial infarctions; if small there may be widespread microinfarctions throughout the cortex and subcortical white matter. Thrombotic infarctions of large- or medium-sized vessels may also occur, on the basis of either a fibrinoid vasculopathy (Ellis and Verity 1979; Hanley *et al.* 1992; Johnson and Richardson 1968; Malamud and Saver 1954) or the anti-phospholipid syndrome. True vasculitis may occur (Weiner and Allen 1991) but this appears to be rare (Devinsky *et al.* 1988). Cerebral venous thrombosis may also occur but this too seems rare.

It appears that most cases of depression, mania, psychosis, and delirium occur on the basis of cerebritis; however, these syndromes may also occur with appropriately placed infarctions (e.g., depression with frontal lobe; mania with frontal or temporal lobe, thalamus or caudate; psychosis with temporal lobe or thalamus; and delirium with temporal lobe or thalamus). Dementia may occur on the basis of cerebritis but appears more commonly due to multiple infarctions. Seizures may likewise occur with cerebritis or with infarction. Chorea may occur with cerebritis or infarction (e.g., of the basal ganglia or thalamus) and is also associated with the presence of anti-phospholipid antibodies. Focal signs generally occur on the basis of appropriately placed infarctions.

Differential diagnosis

Polyarteritis nodosa, sarcoidosis, and, in older patients, cranial arteritis may all mimic lupus to a certain degree, and it is good practice to check for ANA in any case in which the neuropsychiatric symptoms described above occur in the setting of constitutional symptoms or multi-organ disease.

In evaluating neuropsychiatric syndromes in patients with established lupus, care must be taken to be sure that the syndrome is, in fact, due to lupus rather than some other cause. In this regard, special care must be taken in the evaluation of patients with depression. As discussed in Section 6.1, although it is normal for patients to be depressed in the face of adverse events, such as the occurrence of lupus, the severity of such 'normal' depressions is proportionate to the severity of the adverse event; furthermore, such 'normal' depressions are typically not accompanied by hallucinations or delusions. Consequently, the appearance of a non-psychotic depression in the context, say, of imminent renal failure might be considered normal. On the other hand, the occurrence of a severe depression in a patient whose lupus manifested only with a rash probably does not represent a normal depression, and the occurrence of a depression with hallucinations and delusions, even in patients with severe extracerebral lupus, would never represent a normal reaction. Although important in the case of depression, this concern with teasing out 'normal' reactions to stressful events does not apply to patients with mania, psychosis, or delirium, as none of these syndromes ever occurs as a 'normal' reaction.

Patients with lupus may develop renal failure with uremia, which may be accompanied by hypertension, and uremic encephalopathy or hypertensive encephalopathy may occur (Wong *et al.* 1991). Uremia may cause mania, delirium or seizures, and hypertensive encephalopathy is characterized by delirium and seizures. Steroid treatment may also cause neuropsychiatric side-effects, including depression, mania, and psychosis. Finally, treatment with either steroids or immunosuppressants opens the way to opportunistic central nervous system infections (Futrell *et al.* 1992; Wong *et al.* 1991), which may also be associated with delirium, seizures, or focal signs.

On a final differential diagnostic note, care must be taken to distinguish naturally occurring lupus from drug-induced lupus. This syndrome is most commonly seen secondary to use of procainamide, hydralazine, or, less frequently, alpha-methyl dopa; it has also been rarely noted secondary to use of other medications, including chlorpromazine, carbamazepine, phenytoin, and primidone. Importantly, unlike naturally occurring lupus, drug-induced lupus rarely causes cerebral symptoms. When there is doubt as to whether any given case of lupus is drug-induced or not, antibody levels may be helpful. Although all patients with drug-induced lupus have a positive ANA, very few will have the more specific antibodies to native DNA or Sm. Obtaining an anti-histone antibody level may also be helpful: whereas patients with drug-induced lupus typically have this, it is unusual in patients with naturally occurring lupus.

Treatment

Treatment of the various features of cerebral lupus is dictated by the presumed underlying etiology, as discussed above. In this regard, a reasonable strategy is to obtain an MR scan to determine whether or not infarction has occurred, and, if so, to then decide whether the identified infarction or infarctions could reasonably be expected to explain the patient's symptomatology. If this is the case, treatment is directed at the cause of the underlying infarction, as discussed in Section 7.4. In cases of infarction occurring in the context of the anti-phospholipid syndrome, preventive treatment with warfarin is probably in order.

In the remaining cases, which are presumably due to a cerebritis, consideration may be given to treatment with steroids or cyclophosphamide, either individually or in combination. Initial treatment with steroids generally involves a 3- to 7-day course of methylprednisolone, 250 mg intravenously four times daily, followed by prednisone in a dose of 1 mg/kg/day, with the dose of prednisone gradually tapered over a few weeks depending on the clinical response. With regard to cyclophosphamide, some clinicians will utilize this as single-agent therapy from the start, whereas others will add it to the course of steroids, generally several days into treatment with methylprednisolone. Repeat courses of steroids or monthly infusions of cyclophosphamide are generally required to maintain remission. Remarkably, at the time of this writing there has been only one double-blind study comparing steroids alone with the combination of steroids and cyclophosphamide (Barile-Fabris et al. 2005). This study found that the addition of cyclophosphamide to an initial course of steroids, followed by monthly cyclophosphamide, was greatly superior to initial treatment with steroids alone, followed by repeat courses of methylprednisolone. However, this study primarily included patients with seizures and excluded patients with depression, mania, psychosis, delirium, or dementia, and hence it is not clear whether the results would apply to these syndromes.

Symptomatic treatment of depression, mania, psychosis, delirium, dementia, and seizures may or may not be required, and is discussed in Sections 6.1, 6.3, 7.1, 5.3, 5.1, and 7.3 respectively.

17.3 SJÖGREN'S SYNDROME

Sjögren's syndrome is an autoimmune disease characterized by keratoconjunctivitis sicca and xerostomia (dry eyes and dry mouth: the 'sicca syndrome'), and, in a small minority, by disease of the nervous system. Once thought to be rare, it is now known to occur in up to 2 percent of those over 60 years. It is far more common in woman than men, by a ratio of 9:1.

Clinical features

The onset is very gradual and typically occurs in middle or later adult years. Although the sicca syndrome is present in all cases it may be relatively mild, and direct questioning is often required to elicit these symptoms. Extraglandular involvement occurs in about one-third of patients, a polyarthralgia or polyarthritis is seen in about two-thirds, and Raynaud's phenomenon is seen in about one-third.

The proportion of patients who develop central nervous system involvement is not known with certainty, but it probably represents a very small minority (Anaya et al. 2002). Multiple areas of the nervous system may be involved (Delalande et al. 2004) and there may be stroke (Bragoni et al. 1994), a gradually progressive dementia (Caselli et al. 1991, 1993; Kawashima et al. 1993), subacute aseptic meningitis, seizures, optic neuritis, myelopathy, and, in a very small minority, parkinsonism (Walker et al. 1999). Peripheral nervous system involvement may also occur and is far more common than central nervous system involvement (Goransson et al. 2006); a cranial neuropathy may also occur, affecting the V, VII or VIII cranial nerves.

T2-weighted or FLAIR MR scanning often reveals multiple small areas of increased signal intensity in the white matter (Coates et al. 1999) and, in cases of dementia, increased signal intensity in the white matter may be confluent and widespread. In patients with meningitis, contrast enhancement is seen in the meninges, as expected.

The CSF may be normal or may display oligoclonal bands or an increased IgG index (Vrethem et al. 1990).

Serologic abnormalities are found in almost all patients. Over 90 percent will have a positive ANA and some 75 percent will have a positive rheumatoid factor. Anti-SS-A (formerly known as anti-Ro) is found in 60–75 percent, and anti-SS-B (formerly known as anti-La) in about 40 percent. In doubtful cases, a lip biopsy will reveal lymphocytic infiltrates.

Course

Overall, the course is characterized by gradual progression.

Etiology

Although autoimmune factors are clearly at play in Sjögren's syndrome, the precise nature of the responsible antibodies, and their genesis, is not known. Lymphocytic infiltration is seen in exocrine glands and, in those with central nervous system disease, similar infiltrates may be found in a perivascular location, both in the parenchyma and the meninges (Caselli et al. 1991, 1993; de la Monte et al. 1983).

Differential diagnosis

The sicca syndrome may be seen in other connective tissue diseases, such as systemic lupus erythematosus, systemic sclerosis, rheumatoid arthritis, and polymyositis. In patients with involvement of the nervous system the most important consideration is lupus, and here the differential rests on testing for anti-native DNA, which is present in lupus but absent in Sjögren's syndrome.

Multiple sclerosis enters into the differential, especially in patients with optic neuritis and/or myelopathy. Here the differential rests on finding the typical serologic abnormalities mentioned above; in doubtful cases, a lip biopsy may be required.

The sicca syndrome, of course, may also be caused by multiple different medications.

Treatment

Central nervous system involvement generally requires treatment with steroids or immunosuppressants, such as cyclophosphamide.

17.4 SNEDDON'S SYNDROME

First described by Sneddon in 1965 (Sneddon 1965), this syndrome is characterized by livedo reticularis and cerebrovascular disease. This is a rare disorder, more common in woman than men, with an onset in early to middle adult years.

Clinical features

Livedo reticularis is generally present for years before other symptoms appear. Typically, it is seen not only on the lower extremities but also the trunk.

Transient ischemic attack (TIA) and stroke are common, and, with multiple strokes, a typical multi-infarct dementia may occur. Patients may also present with a gradually progressive cognitive decline and in these cases one typically finds significant white matter disease (Adair et al. 2001; Boesch et al. 2003; Stockhammer et al. 1993; Tourbah et al. 1997).

Magnetic resonance scanning will reveal both areas of infarction and white matter disease. Echocardiography may reveal valvular disease. Anti-phospholipid antibodies, either lupus anticoagulant or anti-cardiolipin antibodies, are present in a minority of cases and are often transient. The ANA may be positive; however, anti-native DNA and extractable nuclear antigen (ENA) antibodies are absent (Kalashnikova et al. 1990). Skin biopsy generally reveals typical vascular lesions (Stockhammer et al. 1993).

Course

The course may be marked by recurrent stroke or, in cases with leukoencephalopathy, by a gradually progressive decline.

Etiology

Within the central nervous system there is a widespread, non-inflammatory vasculopathy affecting primarily small- to medium-sized arteries, with subendothelial proliferation and eventual fibrosis (Geschwind et al. 1995; Hilton and Footitt 2003; Rebollo et al. 1983). Although territorial infarctions may occur, smaller subcortical infarctions are far more common; furthermore, in many cases there is also widespread white matter disease involving the periventricular area and the centrum semiovale. Although most of these lesions probably reflect in situ thrombosis and occlusion of involved vessels, valvular disease has also been noted and embolization may play a role in some cases (Sitzer et al. 1995). A similar vasculopathy underlies the livedo reticularis.

The mechanism underlying the vasculopathy is not clear. As noted above, anti-phospholipid antibodies may be present but their pathogenic role is uncertain. Although most cases are sporadic, familial cases have been noted (Pettee et al. 1994).

Differential diagnosis

The diagnosis should always be suspected in any adult with livedo reticularis and cerebrovascular disease. The primary anti-phospholipid syndrome is distinguished by the constant presence of anti-phospholipid antibodies and by the absence of white matter changes. Systemic lupus erythematosus is suggested by finding anti-native DNA or ENA antibodies. Binswanger's disease is distinguished by the later age of onset and the absence of livedo reticularis. It must also be borne in mind that livedo reticularis may occur as a side-effect to certain drugs, most notably amantadine.

Treatment

Long-term anticoagulation may be considered.

17.5 PRIMARY ANTI-PHOSPHOLIPID SYNDROME

This is a rare syndrome, found much more commonly in women than men, which has an onset in early or middle adult years. It is characterized by recurrent arterial or venous thromboses, and constitutes an important cause of stroke in younger adults (Asherson et al. 1989; Levine et al. 1990).

Clinical features

Stroke, secondary to either ischemic infarction or, much less commonly, venous infarction, is common (Chancellor et al. 1991), and with a multiplicity of these a multi-infarct dementia may occur (Coull et al. 1987; Kurita et al. 1994). Transient ischemic attacks may also occur, and amaurosis fugax is often seen. With occlusion of the retinal artery, blindness may occur. Chorea has also been noted (Cervera et al. 1997).

Deep venous thromboses are common, and pulmonary embolism may occur. Another characteristic feature is recurrent miscarriage.

Anti-phospholipid antibodies, either the lupus anticoagulant or anti-cardiolipin antibodies, or both, are present in every case. Anti-cardiolipin antibodies include IgG, IgM, and IgA, and the IgG antibody is most strongly associated with thrombosis. Other abnormalities include a prolonged activated partial thromboplastin time, thrombocytopenia, and a false-positive VDRL. The ANA may be positive, but anti-native DNA and anti-Sm antibodies are absent.

Course

Recurrent thrombotic events are the rule.

Etiology

In this syndrome, circulating anti-phospholipid antibodies attach to vessel walls, either arterial or venous, and induce thrombus formation and fibrosis (Hughson *et al.* 1993). With arteries, the cerebral vasculature is preferentially attacked, resulting in ischemic infarction. Veins subject to attack include not only the cerebral veins but also peripheral veins, resulting in deep venous thromboses. In about one-third of patients, Libman–Sacks endocarditis may occur, affecting the mitral and aortic valves, with subsequent embolization.

Differential diagnosis

The diagnosis should always be suspected in any young person with stroke (Brey *et al.* 1990), especially in those with a history of deep venous thrombosis or recurrent miscarriage. Anti-phospholipid antibodies may also be seen in systemic lupus erythematosus, Sjögren's syndrome, Sneddon's syndrome, and various malignancies, and with treatment with certain drugs, including procainamide, quinidine, hydralazine, phenytoin, valproic acid, and phenothiazines. Of these causes of the 'secondary' anti-phospholipid antibody syndrome, lupus is the most important, and the differential here is made by finding either anti-native DNA or anti-Sm antibodies.

Treatment

Long-term anticoagulation is required.

17.6 SUSAC'S SYNDROME

Susac's syndrome, first described by Susac in 1979 (Susac *et al.* 1979), is a rare disorder, typically seen in young adult females. The syndrome is also referred to as retinocochleocerebral vasculopathy, a term that, although cumbersome, nicely summarizes the structures involved.

Clinical features

Classically one sees the subacute onset of a delirium, often accompanied by headache, in the setting of sensorineuronal hearing loss and visual disturbances (Aubart-Cohen *et al.* 2007; Papo *et al.* 1998, Petty *et al.* 1998).

Magnetic resonance scanning (Susac *et al.* 2003) typically reveals multiple areas of increased signal intensity on FLAIR and T2-weighted images, scattered throughout the white and gray matter with a predilection for the corpus callosum. In some cases these lesions may demonstrate contrast enhancement.

Course

In the natural course of events there is a more or less complete remission of symptoms after 2–4 years; recurrences, although not common, may occur.

Etiology

In the setting of a widespread cerebral microangiopathy there are multiple microinfarcts affecting the white matter (especially the corpus callosum) and the gray matter (Heiskala *et al.* 1988; Monteiro *et al.* 1985). Retinal and cochlear infarctions also occur.

Although the etiology of the angiopathy is not known, an autoimmune mechanism is suspected.

Differential diagnosis

Both multiple sclerosis and systemic lupus erythematosus may be considered; however, the hearing loss and visual disturbances suggest the correct diagnosis.

Treatment

Steroids or immunosuppressants, such as cyclophosphamide, are beneficial.

17.7 LIMBIC ENCEPHALITIS

Limbic encephalitis, first described in 1960 (Brierly *et al.* 1960), is an autoimmune disorder, characterized pathologically by the presence of anti-neuronal antibodies and inflammatory changes in the medial aspects of the temporal lobes, and clinically, in most but not all cases, by delirium and seizures. In the vast majority of cases, limbic encephalitis occurs on a paraneoplastic basis, most often in patients with small-cell lung cancer, and serum samples will be positive for typical anti-neuronal antibodies, such as anti-Hu. Recent work has demonstrated, however, that in a very small minority, limbic encephalitis exists as a non-paraneoplastic disorder associated with the presence of anti-voltage-gated potassium channel antibodies.

Limbic encephalitis is a rare disorder, occurring in less than 0.1 percent of all patients with cancer.

Clinical features

The onset of symptoms is typically subacute, spanning days or weeks (Alamowitch *et al.* 1997). Importantly, limbic encephalitis is often the presenting symptom of cancer (Alamowitch *et al.* 1997; Dalmau *et al.* 1992), and in some cases the tumor itself may remain undetected for years after the onset of the encephalitis (Ahern *et al.* 1994).

The most common presentation is with delirium marked by prominent anterograde and retrograde amnesia, often accompanied by seizures and personality change or hallucinations (Alamowitch *et al.* 1997; Antoine *et al.* 1995; Bakheit *et al.* 1990; Gultekin *et al.* 2000; Lawn *et al.* 2003). Other, less common presentations include depression (Brierly *et al.* 1960; Corsellis *et al.* 1968; Glaser and Pincus 1969), isolated amnesia (Bak *et al.* 2001; Nokura *et al.* 1997; Sutton *et al.* 2000), seizures (Corsellis *et al.* 1968), somnolence (Byrne *et al.* 1997), and catatonia (with 'confusion, stereotypy, echolalia, stiffness, verbigeration, formal thought disorder, and negativism' [Tandon *et al.* 1988]). Rare symptoms include abnormal movements, such as chorea (Croteau *et al.* 2001; Vernino *et al.* 2002), narcoleptic attacks with cataplexy (Rosenfeld *et al.* 2001), rapid eye movement (REM) sleep behavior disorder (Iranzo *et al.* 2006), and, especially in association with ovarian cancer, hypoventilation with respiratory failure (Dalmau *et al.* 2007; Vitaliani *et al.* 2005).

In cases that occur on a paraneoplastic basis, one may also see other paraneoplastic syndromes (Alamowitch *et al.* 1997), including the following: cerebellar degeneration with ataxia; brainstem encephalitis with nystagmus, ataxia, oculomotor palsies, and vertigo; opsoclonus–myoclonus; sensory neuropathy; Lambert–Eaton myasthenic syndrome; and the stiff-person syndrome.

Early in the course, MR scanning is often normal; over time, however, most cases will have increased signal intensity in the medial aspects of the temporal lobes on T2-weighted or FLAIR imaging; these abnormalities, although initially unilateral, typically become bilateral (Alamowitch *et al.* 1997; Bakheit *et al.* 1990; Gultekin *et al.* 2000; Lawn *et al.* 2003; Tsukamoto *et al.* 1993).

The EEG is abnormal in almost all cases and typically shows temporal slowing, which, similarly to the MRI findings, may initially be unilateral, only to later become bilateral. Interictal epileptiform discharges may or may not be present.

The CSF may be normal or may display any one of a number of findings, including a mild lymphocytic pleocytosis, a mildly elevated total protein, or oligoclonal bands (Alamowitch *et al.* 1997; Gultekin *et al.* 2000).

Although in the vast majority of cases of limbic encephalitis abnormalities will be found on MRI, EEG, or CSF assay, exceptions do occur, especially early on, and in cases in which the clinical findings are strongly suggestive of the diagnosis but these tests are negative, positron emission tomography (PET) scanning should be considered; even in cases in which all other tests are negative, PET may reveal focal hypermetabolism in one or both temporal lobes.

A wide variety of anti-neuronal antibodies have been identified (Bataller *et al.* 2007; Pittock *et al.* 2005), including anti-Hu (also known as ANNA-1), anti-Ri (also known as ANNA-2), ANNA-3, anti-Ma1, anti-Ma2 (also known as anti-Ta), anti-amphiphysin, anti-CRMP-5, and anti-voltage-gated potassium channel (also known as anti-VGKC). In paraneoplastic cases, various tumors have been found, including cancer of the lung (most commonly of the

small-cell type) (Alamowitch *et al.* 1997), breast, testicle (Ahern *et al.* 1994; Burton *et al.* 1988; Voltz *et al.* 1999), colon (Tsukamoto *et al.* 1993), pancreas, ovary (Nokura *et al.* 1997), thymus (Antoine *et al.* 1995; Ingenito *et al.* 1990), prostate, and bladder; cases have also been associated with lymphoma. Although there is an association between certain anti-neuronal antibodies and certain types of cancer (e.g., anti-Hu with lung cancer [Anderson *et al.* 1988; Alamowitch *et al.* 1997]; anti-Ma2 with testicular cancer [Gultekin *et al.* 2000; Pruss *et al.* 2007; Voltz *et al.* 1999]) there is a wide overlap (Pittock *et al.* 2004, 2005); for example, anti-Hu, in addition to being found in association with lung cancer, may also be found with cancer of the breast, prostate, colon, and ovary (Graus *et al.* 2001). Given this overlap, it is appropriate to test for the entire range of known anti-neuronal antibodies. It must also be kept in mind that new anti-neuronal antibodies are routinely discovered and, consequently, negative tests for known anti-neuronal antibodies do not rule out the diagnosis (Ances *et al.* 2005).

Once the diagnosis of limbic encephalitis has been made, it is essential to find the tumor. In this regard, if routine investigations are unrevealing, many clinicians will undertake computed tomography (CT) scans of the chest, abdomen, and pelvis, and, in young males, ultrasound of the testes. If the tumor escapes detection by these methods, consideration may be given to whole-body PET scanning.

Course

Although the overall course is one of progression, there may at times be 'plateaus'; however, these almost always give way to further decline (Alamowitch *et al.* 1997). True spontaneous remissions, although reported (Byrne *et al.* 1997), are rare, and most patients die within months to a year or more, either of complications of the limbic encephalitis or from the underlying cancer.

Etiology

Pathologically (Henson *et al.* 1965) there is a lymphocytic perivascular inflammation, with neuronal loss and gliosis within the limbic system, primarily involving medial temporal structures, such as the hippocampus and the amygdala. As noted earlier, in the vast majority of cases this inflammation occurs on a paraneoplastic basis, with antibodies raised against the cancer cross-reacting with normal neuronal tissue. However, there are cases of limbic encephalitis occurring in the context of anti-VGKC antibodies in which no cancer is found, and the mechanism underlying the genesis of this autoimmune response remains unknown (Vincent *et al.* 2004).

Differential diagnosis

Although limbic encephalitis immediately comes to mind in patients with known cancer who develop delirium with seizures, other disorders that are not uncommon in cancer must also be considered, including metastatic disease, Cushing's syndrome, and opportunistic infections, such as cytomegaloviral encephalitis or progressive multifocal leukoencephalopathy.

As noted earlier, in most cases limbic encephalitis precedes other evidence of cancer and hence in most cases the differential is wider, as discussed in Section 5.1. Special consideration may be given to herpes simplex viral encephalitis, hypertensive encephalopathy, the posterior reversible leukoencephalopathy syndrome, Hashimoto's encephalopathy, and Creutzfeldt–Jakob disease.

Treatment

Although treatment of the underlying cancer in paraneoplastic cases should be undertaken, it appears that, even with successful treatment, limbic encephalitis undergoes remission in only a minority of cases (Burton *et al.* 1988). Consequently, other modalities must be considered; although there are no controlled studies, various treatments, alone or in combination, are utilized, including steroids, immunosuppressants (e.g., cyclophosphamide), intravenous immunoglobulins, and plasmapheresis (Bataller *et al.* 2007). The symptomatic treatment of delirium is discussed in Section 5.3, and of seizures in Section 7.3.

17.8 SARCOIDOSIS

Sarcoidosis is an uncommon disease characterized pathologically by the presence of sarcoid granulomas in multiple organ systems, including, in a minority, the nervous system, in which case one may speak of neurosarcoidosis. In addition to a granulomatous basilar meningitis, granulomas may also be found scattered throughout the cerebrum, with a special predilection for the hypothalamus and pituitary.

Sarcoidosis is somewhat more common in females than males; in the United States it is far more common in black people than white people, and in Europe those from northern countries are more commonly affected.

Clinical features

Although onset in adolescence or the middle or later years may occur, most patients fall ill in their twenties or thirties. The onset itself is often gradual, and many cases are discovered serendipitously when a chest radiograph reveals pulmonary findings characteristic of the disease.

Although sarcoidosis may be protean in its manifestations, certain presentations deserve note. Perhaps 90 percent of patients will have pulmonary involvement, which may manifest clinically with symptoms such as cough or dyspnea, or may be asymptomatic and discovered only incidentally by chest radiograph, which may reveal

bilateral hilar lymphadenopathy or a diffuse reticulonodular appearance. Other symptoms include erythema nodosum, lupus pernio, lymphadenopathy, arthropathy, and parotid gland enlargement. Hepatic involvement occurs in almost three-quarters of patients although hepatic failure is rare. Hypercalcemia occurs in a majority of cases, and some patients may develop nephrocalcinosis and eventual renal failure.

Involvement of the nervous system occurs in anywhere from 5 to 25 percent of patients, and in a very small minority of cases it may represent the only manifestation of sarcoidosis. The overall symptomatology of neurosarcoidosis has been described in a number of reports (Chapelon *et al.* 1990; Delaney 1977; Manz 1983; Oksanen 1986; Sharma and Sharma 1991; Stern *et al.* 1985). With a basilar meningitis, cranial neuropathies may occur, and with obstruction of the outflow foramina of the fourth ventricle, hydrocephalus may occur; involvement of arteries may be followed by stroke. Cerebral involvement may be characterized by multiple granulomas or by relatively few large lesions, or even by a solitary lesion; in these cases there may be dementia, delirium, seizures, or focal signs. Hypothalamic or pituitary granulomas may present with endocrinologic syndromes. The cord may also be compressed and the peripheral nervous system is often involved.

Cranial neuropathies occur in approximately one-half of all cases and, although various of the cranial nerves may be involved (Symonds 1958), one most commonly sees a peripheral facial palsy, which may be unilateral or bilateral (Scott 1993; Sharma and Sharma 1991). The eighth cranial nerve may also be involved with deafness, as may the optic nerve or chiasm with blindness or hemianopia.

Hydrocephalus occurs in about 5 percent of cases and may present with dementia and a gait disturbance.

Stroke is rare in sarcoidosis and appears to generally present with a lacunar syndrome (Brown *et al.* 1989; Michotte *et al.* 1991), reflecting granulomatous involvement of the penetrating arteries.

Dementia does occur in sarcoidosis (Camp and Frierson 1962; Cordingly *et al.* 1981; Miller *et al.* 1988; Sanson *et al.* 1996) and may be accompanied by a frontal lobe syndrome (Hook 1954) or by delusions and hallucinations (Thompson and Checkley 1981). Although the prevalence of this syndrome is uncertain, one study found cognitive deficits of variable degree in close to 50 percent of all patients with neurosarcoidosis (Scott *et al.* 2007). Delirium has also been noted (Douglas and Maloney 1973; Silverstein and Siltzbach 1965; Wiederholt and Siekers 1965) but appears to be rare.

Seizures occur in about 15 percent of cases and may be grand mal or partial in type (Krumholz *et al.* 1991). Focal signs may occur, and reflect the location of any cerebral granulomas.

Endocrinologic changes have been noted in up to one-third of patients, and may consist of diabetes insipidus, hyperprolactinemia, hypothyroidism, hypogonadism, and adrenocortical insufficiency (Scott *et al.* 1987). Hypothalamic involvement may also manifest with disturbances of appetite or with somnolence; rarely symptomatic narcolepsy may occur (Rubinstein *et al.* 1988).

Spinal cord compression by granulomas may lead to various symptomatologies, including paraplegia.

The peripheral nervous system is involved in up to 50 percent of patients, and may manifest with a mononeuropathy, a mononeuritis multiplex, or a primarily sensory polyneuropathy.

Magnetic resonance scanning with T2-weighted or FLAIR imaging typically reveals any basilar meningitis or macroscopic parenchymal granulomas; with gadolinium, enhancement is seen in most of these.

The CSF is abnormal in only about 50 percent of cases. Various abnormalities may occur (Kinnman and Link 1984; McLean *et al.* 1995), including a mild lymphocytic pleocytosis, a mildly elevated total protein, and, in a minority, oligoclonal bands or an elevated IgG index; in a very small minority the glucose level is mildly reduced. The level of CSF angiotensin-converting enzyme is elevated in a little over 50 percent of cases (Oksanen 1986). The serum angiotensin-converting enzyme level is likewise elevated in over 50 percent of cases.

Definitive diagnosis requires biopsy evidence of typical sarcoid granulomas, and in most cases lung biopsy is performed.

Course

The course is variable. Spontaneous remission of neurosarcoidosis occurs after many months in about one-half of cases, although relapses may occur; in the remaining cases the disease pursues a chronic, often fluctuating course (Pentland *et al.* 1985).

Etiology

The cardinal lesion in sarcoidosis is a non-caseating granuloma, and the pathology of neurosarcoidosis has been described in a number of studies (Delaney 1977; Herring and Urich 1969; Jefferson 1957). As noted above, one typically sees a granulomatous basilar meningitis, with entrapment and inflammation of cranial nerves, penetrating arteries, and, in a small minority, obstruction of the outflow foramina of the fourth ventricle. Granulomatous infiltration of the hypothalamus is very common, and further infiltration down the pituitary stalk may lead to granuloma formation in the posterior or anterior lobe of the pituitary gland. Of note, it appears that most of the endocrinologic disturbances seen in neurosarcoidosis result primarily from hypothalamic disease, with pituitary function being secondarily disturbed by the lack of releasing or inhibiting factors normally secreted by the hypothalamus (Winnacker *et al.* 1968). Parenchymal granulomas may be found not only in the white matter of the cerebrum but also in the cortex and, as noted earlier, they may range

widely in size and number, from miliary lesions to large masses mimicking gliomas (Powers and Miller 1981).

Although the mechanism underlying the appearance of these granulomas is not known, it is strongly suspected that sarcoidosis represents an autoimmune disorder that is triggered in genetically susceptible individuals by an exogenous, inhaled substance.

Differential diagnosis

Neurosyphilis, tuberculosis, and fungal infections may all closely mimic sarcoidosis. Multiple sclerosis is often mentioned on the differential; however, this possibility would only arise in cases of neurosarcoidosis in which lesions were essentially restricted to the cerebral white matter.

Treatment

Active neurosarcoidosis may be treated with prednisone in a dose of approximately 1 mg/kg/day for 4–6 weeks, after which the dose may be gradually tapered over the following months, depending on the clinical evolution. Importantly, steroids, although often effective, do not alter the natural course of the disease, and repeat courses may be required. In treatment-resistant cases, some clinicians will give a course of intravenous methylprednisolone, whereas others will turn to hydroxycholoquine (Sharma 1998) or to an immunosuppressant, such as cyclophosphamide, azathioprine or methotrexate (Scott *et al.* 2007). Unfortunately, there are no blind studies of the treatment of neurosarcoidosis to guide these choices. Hydrocephalus may require shunting.

17.9 HASHIMOTO'S ENCEPHALOPATHY

Hashimoto's encephalopathy, first described by Lord Brain in 1966 (Brain *et al.* 1966), is an uncommon cause of delirium which occurs secondary to an autoimmune process that targets the brain.

Before proceeding further some words are in order regarding the confusion that may exist between Hashimoto's encephalopathy and Hashimoto's thyroiditis, which are two very different diseases. The name 'Hashimoto' is generally associated not with an encephalopathy but with thyroiditis. Hashimoto's thyroiditis, first described by Hakaru Hashimoto in 1912 (Hashimoto 1912), is the most common cause of thyroiditis and is characterized by the presence of anti-thyroid antibodies and by a lymphocytic infiltration of the thyroid gland; affected patients may be euthyroid, transiently hyperthyroid, or, more commonly, hypothyroid. Dr. Hashimoto did not note delirium in any of these patients with thyroiditis. In 1966, however, Lord Brain described a patient with thyroiditis and anti-thyroid antibodies who also had delirium and stroke-like episodes, and it was this association of Hashimoto's thyroiditis with delirium that prompted the new term, 'Hashimoto's encephalopathy'. Importantly, however, as noted below, although anti-thyroid antibodies are present in all cases of Hashimoto's encephalopathy, there is no association between the encephalopathy and thyroid disease, and it appears that the anti-thyroid antibodies are merely 'innocent bystanders' that serve as markers of a more widespread autoimmune disorder; in addition to autoantibodies directed at the thyroid, other autoantibodies directed at the brain are also present.

A recently coined synonym for Hashimoto's encephalopathy is 'steroid-responsive encephalopathy associated with autoimmune thyroiditis' or 'SREAT'. Whether this new terminology is helpful or will gain currency remains to be seen.

Clinical features

The clinical features have been most clearly described in two case series from the Mayo Clinic (Castillo et al. 2006; Sawka et al. 2002). Although most patients are in their forties, the age of onset varies widely, from childhood to the eighth decade; the onset itself is typically subacute, over days or perhaps weeks.

The overwhelming majority of patients have a delirium, which in most cases is accompanied by any or all of tremor, myoclonus, ataxia, or seizures; seizures may be grand mal, complex partial or, rarely, simple partial, and grand mal status epilepticus may occur in a small minority. Stroke-like episodes are common and are typically characterized by aphasia (Bohnen et al. 1997; Ghika-Schmid et al. 1996; Henchey et al. 1995; Shaw et al. 1991; Thrush and Boddie 1974); hemiplegia or hemisensory loss may also occur. These stroke-like episodes are of brief duration, lasting in the order of hours or a day or more, and typically undergo a full remission. Very rarely Hashimoto's encephalopathy may present with a psychosis (Bostantjopoulou et al. 1996) or with a dementia (Galluzzi et al. 2002).

Magnetic resonance scanning is normal in the majority of cases; in the remainder, T2-weighted or FLAIR imaging may disclose diffusely increased signal intensity in the cerebral white matter (Bohnen et al. 1997) and, in a small minority, subcortical infarctions may be noted. (Henchey et al. 1995). Computed tomography scanning is almost always normal.

The EEG shows generalized slowing in the vast majority of cases, and this may be accompanied by other changes in a small minority, including triphasic waves and interictal epileptiform discharges (Schauble et al. 2003).

The CSF typically, but not always, displays various abnormalities. An elevated total protein is most common; in a small minority there may be a mild lymphocytic pleocytosis. Rarely, there may be oligoclonal bands or the 14-3-3 protein (Hernandez Echebarria et al. 2000).

A small minority may have a mildly elevated ANA or ESR. Thyroid indices are generally normal; if abnormal one typically sees only a mildly reduced thyroxine (T4) and a mildly elevated thyroid-stimulating hormone (TSH) (Henchey et al. 1995; Shaw et al. 1991).

Elevations of anti-thyroid antibodies, either anti-thyroid peroxidase or anti-thyroglobulin, are present in all cases. Although in the vast majority of cases both of these are elevated, exceptions do occur and patients may have elevation of only one; consequently, both should be routinely tested for. Typically the levels of these antibodies are elevated tenfold or greater; importantly, however, there is no correlation between the degree of elevation and the severity of the clinical syndrome

Course

Although the course of Hashimoto's encephalopathy has not been clearly delineated, it appears to be an episodic disease. The episodes themselves tend to persist for anywhere from weeks up to 6 months, after which there is generally a remission. Repeat episodes can occur; however, it is not clear whether this is the case for all, or even most, patients, nor is it clear how long the intervals are between episodes.

Etiology

Neuropathologically there is widespread perivascular lymphocytic inflammation, microglial activation, and gliosis (Castillo et al. 2006; Chong et al. 2003; Doherty et al. 2002; Duffey et al. 2003; Nolte et al. 2000).

Although the mechanism underlying this inflammatory change has not been positively identified, an autoimmune process is strongly suggested both by the association with anti-thyroid antibodies and by the good response to steroids. In all likelihood, however, the anti-thyroid antibodies are not pathogenic but merely represent part of a wider autoimmune response, with other antibodies directed at the brain; in this regard serum anti-neuronal antibodies have been demonstrated (Oide et al. 2004) and one study identified a particular autoantibody directed at alpha-enolase (Ochi et al. 2002).

Differential diagnosis

Various other causes of delirium, as discussed in Section 5.3, must be considered, including toxic deliria (serotonin syndrome, neuroleptic malignant syndrome, delirium tremens), metabolic deliria (Wernicke's encephalopathy, uremic encephalopathy, hepatic encephalopathy), other autoimmune disorders (systemic lupus erythematosus, limbic encephalitis), intracranial disorders (hypertensive encephalopathy, posterior reversible leukoencephalopathy syndrome), viral encephalitis, complex partial status epilepticus, and Creutzfeldt–Jakob disease (which may closely mimic Hashimoto's encephalopathy [Doherty et al. 2002]).

In cases in which there is an associated Hashimoto's thyroiditis, consideration may be given to delirium secondary to either hyperthyroidism or hypothyroidism, but these are very rare; Hashimoto's thyroiditis may also be associated with adrenocortical insufficiency, which, again very rarely, may cause delirium.

In pursuing this differential, it must also be kept in mind that anti-thyroid antibodies may be found in about 3 percent of children and adolescents (Kabelitz et al. 2003) and 8 percent of those over 60 years (Roti et al. 1992); consequently the entire clinical picture must be taken into account.

Treatment

Although there are no blind treatment studies, most patients are given 1000 mg/day of intravenous methylprednisolone for 5–7 days, followed by 60–100 mg/day of oral prednisone in a tapering dose over the following weeks (Castillo et al. 2006). In most cases the response is prompt, within days, and most patients do well with tapering. In some cases, however, prolonged treatment with steroids is required, and it appears also that some patients are resistant to steroids and require treatment with immunosuppressants (azathioprine, methotrexate, or cyclophosphamide), plasma exchange, or intravenous immunoglobulins. Although intuitively it makes sense to monitor levels of anti-thyroid antibodies to gauge treatment response, in practice this is not useful, as in some cases levels may actually rise despite a good clinical response.

The general treatment of delirium is discussed in Section 5.3; seizures may be treated as described in Section 7.3.

17.10 SYDENHAM'S CHOREA

Sydenham's chorea, also known as Saint Vitus' dance, rheumatic chorea, or chorea minor, is one of the major manifestations of rheumatic fever (Anonymous 1992; Bland and Jones 1951, 1952), occurring in about one-quarter of all cases (Cardoso et al. 1997). In addition to chorea, these patients also display other neuropsychiatric features, most notably obsessions and compulsions.

Because of the widespread treatment of streptococcal pharyngitis with penicillin, Sydenham's chorea is currently uncommon; it occurs more frequently in females than males with a ratio of approximately 7:3.

Clinical features

The diagnosis of rheumatic fever is made according to the 'Jones criteria' (Anonymous 1992), which demand the presence of: (i) laboratory evidence of recent pharyngeal infection with group A beta-hemolytic streptococci; and (ii) either two 'major' criteria or one 'major' criterion plus two 'minor' criteria. Major criteria include carditis, migratory polyarthritis, Sydenham's chorea, subcutaneous nodules, and erythema marginatum. Minor criteria include fever, arthralgia, a prolonged PR interval on electrocardiography, and either an elevated ESR or an elevated C-reactive protein level. Acceptable laboratory evidence of recent pharyngeal infection includes a positive throat culture or an elevated anti-DNAase B, anti-streptolysin O, or anti-hyaluronidase titer; of these three titers, anti-DNAase B tends to remain elevated for the longest period of time, in some cases up to 6 months after the pharyngitis.

Although most of the clinical manifestations of rheumatic fever appear about 10 days after the pharyngitis (Taranta 1959), Sydenham's chorea is an exception in that the latency between the pharyngitis and the onset of the chorea is, on average, in the order of 2 or 3 months (Taranta 1959; Taranta and Stollerman 1956). Consequently, it is not unusual to see a case of 'pure' chorea (Feinstein and Spagnuola 1962; Taranta and Stollerman 1956) in which the other manifestations of rheumatic fever have already undergone a full remission, leaving the chorea as the sole manifestation of the disease.

Sydenham's chorea generally presents subacutely, over several weeks (McCullogh 1938; Nausieda et al. 1980), in children aged from 8 to 15 years (Cardoso et al. 1997; Kilic et al. 2007; Thayer 1906); later onsets, however, are certainly possible, as late, indeed, as the ninth decade (Goyal and Williams 1967). The onset itself is typically characterized by symptoms reminiscent of attention deficit/hyperactivity disorder, such as restlessness, fidgetiness, irritability, and emotional lability; choreiform movements, if present, are mild and evanescent (Diefendorf 1912; Gerstley et al. 1935). When the chorea does settle in, it is usually generalized but most prominent in the limbs and face; alternatively, one may occasionally see hemichorea (Abt and Levinson 1916; Nausieda et al. 1980); rarely, rather than chorea there may be a profound weakness, known as 'chorea mollis'.

Neuropsychiatric features are very common during Sydenham's chorea and include obsessions and compulsions, tics, delirium, mania or, less commonly, depression and psychosis. In addition to these features, seizures (Ch'ien et al. 1978; Nausieda et al. 1980), either complex partial or grand mal, may be seen in a small minority, along with various signs, such as a positive Babinski reflex (Ganji et al. 1988).

Obsessions and compulsions occur most notably in Sydenham's chorea (Swedo et al. 1989): one prospective study reported them in 70 percent of patients (Asbahr et al. 1998), another in 82 percent (Swedo et al. 1993). The course of these obsessions and compulsions is of interest. Although they tend to peak in severity along with the worsening of the chorea and to remit before the chorea does, in fact they generally make their appearance before the chorea sets in (Swedo et al. 1993); importantly, it appears that in cases of rheumatic fever it is only those patients who develop Sydenham's chorea who develop obsessions and compulsions; those without chorea remain free of them (Asbahr et al. 1998).

Tics, similar to those seen in Tourette's syndrome, may also occur during Sydenham's chorea (Creak and Guttmann 1935).

Delirium is seen in fewer than 10 percent of patients (Nausieda *et al.* 1980) but may be profound (Diefendorf 1912).

Mania is a rare manifestation of Sydenham's chorea (Abt and Levinson 1916; MacKenzie 1887) and may present as either pure mania or mixed mania (Bradley 1904; Ebaugh 1926; Gay 1889; Lewis and Minski 1935; Powell 1889; Reaser 1940; Shaskan 1938) or, rarely, be coupled with a depression (Abt and Levinson 1916; Haskell 1914). Depression is even rarer than mania in Sydenham's chorea (Abt and Levinson 1916).

Psychosis, with hallucinations and delusions, may occur in a small minority (Hammes 1922) and may symptomatically resemble the psychosis seen in schizophrenia (Leys 1946; Putzel 1879).

On average, an episode of Sydenham's chorea gradually remits after 5–9 months, the range being a week up to 2 years or more (Aron *et al.* 1965; Kilic *et al.* 2007; Lessof 1958; Swedo *et al.* 1993); very rarely Sydenhams' chorea may be chronic, even lifelong (Gibb *et al.* 1985). Although there may be some very mild residual chorea, especially evident when the patient is under stress (Lessof 1958; Swedo *et al.* 1993), in most cases recovery is essentially complete. The mortality rate is less than 1 percent (Abt and Levinson 1916; Bussiere and Rhea 1926; Lessof and Bywaters 1956).

T2-weighted or FLAIR MR scanning may show increased signal intensity in the caudate and in the cerebral white matter (Castillo *et al.* 1999; Emery and Vicco 1997; Moreau *et al.* 2005; Robertson and Smith 2002).

The EEG is abnormal in the majority of cases, demonstrating either posterior slowing or, in a minority, sharp waves or interictal epileptiform discharges (Ch'ien *et al.* 1978).

Course

The overall course of Sydenham's chorea parallels that of the underlying rheumatic fever, and if there are recurrences of rheumatic fever the patient is at risk for another episode of Sydenham's chorea. Indeed, it appears that with repeated bouts of rheumatic fever the likelihood that future episodes of rheumatic fever will be characterized by Sydenham's chorea increases (Aron *et al.* 1965; Bland and Jones 1951; Jones and Bland 1935). Although most recurrences of Sydenham's chorea occur after about 2 years (Nausieda *et al.* 1980; Schwartzman *et al.* 1948), in some cases a very long interval may separate individual episodes, in one case up to 52 years (Gibb and Lees 1989).

Although most cases of recurrent episodes of Sydenham's chorea are associated with laboratory evidence of a recent streptococcal pharyngitis, there are exceptions and some cases may appear in the absence of such indicators (Berrios *et al.* 1985; Korn-Lubetzki *et al.* 2004); whether this implies that other factors may be involved in recurrences or that the preceding infection was of such low intensity as to leave no laboratory trace is not clear.

In addition to relapses of chorea consequent upon recurrent group A beta-hemolytic pharyngitis, patients who have recovered from Sydenham's chorea are also at risk for other sequelae. Females with a history of Sydenham's chorea may develop chorea gravidarum during pregnancy (Beresford and Graham 1950; Wilson and Preece 1932a) and are also at increased risk for developing chorea during treatment with oral contraceptives (Nausieda *et al.* 1983). There is also suggestive evidence that some cases of obsessive–compulsive disorder (Swedo 1994; Swedo *et al.* 1994), Tourette's syndrome (Kerbeshian *et al.* 1990; Swedo *et al.* 1994), and even schizophrenia (Casanova *et al.* 1995; Wilcox and Nasrallah 1986, 1988) occur as sequelae.

Etiology

Autopsy studies of patients dying during acute Sydenham's chorea have revealed two kinds of damage: vasculitic and encephalitic. Vasculitic changes affecting small vessels (Buchanen 1941; Buchanen *et al.* 1942; Poynton and Holmes 1906; Van Bogaert and Bertrand 1932; Winkelman and Eckel 1932) have been noted in the cerebral cortex and basal ganglia; encephalitic changes (Bradley 1904; Buchanen *et al.* 1942; Colony and Malamud 1956; Coombs 1912; Gordon and Norman 1934; Greenfield and Wolfsohn 1922; Ziegler 1927), with inflammation and neuronal loss, have been found throughout the cerebral cortex and the basal ganglia, without any corresponding vasculitis. Autopsies of patients who died from unrelated causes long after recovering from the chorea have revealed evidence of old endarteritis (Benda 1949) and patchy gliosis and neuronal loss (Lange *et al.* 1976).

It appears that these vasculitic and encephalitic changes occur secondary to an autoimmune assault on the central nervous system, which is triggered by the preceding group A beta-hemolytic streptococcal pharyngitis. Serum antineuronal antibodies have been detected (Kiessling *et al.* 1993; Swedo *et al.* 1991), specifically targeting the following structures: pial arteries and parenchymal capillaries (Kingston and Glynn 1971); white matter astrocytes (Kingston and Glynn 1976); neurons, in particular those of the basal ganglia (Church *et al.* 2002; Husby *et al.* 1976) and certain brainstem nuclei (Husby *et al.* 1976); and the ependyma (Kingston and Glynn 1976).

Differential diagnosis

As discussed in Section 3.4, there are few other disorders capable of causing self-limited episodes of chorea in childhood or adolescence. Consideration should be given to toxicity of various medications, such as phenytoin, and to Wilson's disease, systemic lupus erythematosus, and hyperthyroidism.

Treatment

Patients should be given penicillin VK in a dose of 500 mg twice daily for 10 days, regardless of whether there is any clinical evidence of an active pharyngitis, as it is critical to eradicate all of the offending streptococci. Erythromycin may be substituted in patients allergic to penicillin. Various treatments have been proposed, including steroids (e.g., prednisone), valproic acid, carbamazepine, haloperidol, and plasma exchange or intravenous immunoglobulins. Of these, only prednisone has been subjected to a double-blind trial.

Treatment with steroids makes sense in that it targets the underlying mechanism of the disease and could conceivably, if effective, prevent the occurrence of some of the sequelae noted above, such as obsessive–compulsive disorder. In the double-blind study that demonstrated the effectiveness of prednisone, patients were given 2 mg/kg/day for 4 weeks, after which the dose was gradually tapered (Paz et al. 2006).

In contrast to steroids, valproic acid, carbamazepine, and haloperidol all represent purely symptomatic treatments. One open study found valproic acid to be superior to carbamazepine, which in turn was superior to haloperidol (Pena et al. 2002); another open study, however, found valproic acid and carbamazepine to be equally effective (Genel et al. 2002). Valproic acid and carbamazepine are given in customary doses; haloperidol has been given in doses ranging from 1 to 4 mg/day (Axley 1981; Shenker et al. 1973).

A reasonable strategy would be to initiate treatment with prednisone and observe the patient. In cases in which there is a response but it is slow and the chorea is of such severity as to threaten the patient, consideration may then be given to adding a symptomatic treatment, beginning with valproic acid. In cases in which there is no response to prednisone, symptomatic treatment may also, of course, be considered, but some authors would recommend further etiologic treatment, with consideration given to a course of intravenous methylprednisolone (Cardoso et al. 2003) or to treatment with plasmapheresis or intravenous immunoglobulins (Garvey et al. 2005).

Patients should also be treated with injections of penicillin G benzathine, using a dose of 1.2 million units every 3–4 weeks, to prevent recurrences of streptococcal pharyngitis. For children or adolescents, such treatment should probably continue for 5 years or until the age of 21 years, whichever comes later. For adults, the decision must be individualized, with special attention given to those at risk of contracting further streptococcal pharyngitides, such as teachers or pediatricians.

17.11 CHOREA GRAVIDARUM

As a result of the endocrinologic changes occurring during pregnancy, women with certain disorders may develop chorea. Chorea gravidarum is a rare disorder, occurring in anywhere from 0.001 percent (Wilson and Preece 1932a) to 0.003 percent (Beresford and Graham 1950) of pregnancies. In the past, the most common of the pre-existing disorders was Sydenham's chorea; with the greatly decreased incidence of this disorder, however, other conditions, such as the anti-phospholipid syndrome and systemic lupus erythematosus, have become more important.

Clinical features

The onset of the chorea is usually during the first half of pregnancy, and symptoms resolve either toward the end of the third trimester or during the puerperium. In cases occurring in women with a history of Sydenham's chorea, anywhere from 7 percent (Wilson and Preece 1932b) to 26 percent (Thiele 1935) may also experience hallucinations or delusions; furthermore, mania or delirium may also occur (Wilson and Preece 1932b).

Course

With subsequent pregnancies, recurrences may occur, and this appears to be common in those with a history of Sydenham's chorea (Wilson and Preece 1932a).

Etiology

Sydenham's chorea greatly increases the chances of chorea gravidarum, which may occur in anywhere from 4 percent (Beresford and Graham 1950) to an astounding 26 percent (Wilson and Preece 1932a) of patients with a history of this condition. Chorea gravidarum has also been noted in association with the anti-phospholipid syndrome (Cervera et al. 1997; Omdal and Roalso 1992) and systemic lupus erythematosus (Wolf and McBeath 1985). There has been one autopsy case, which revealed neuronal loss and gliosis within the caudate nucleus (Ichikawa et al. 1980).

Differential diagnosis

Of the multiple causes of chorea discussed in Section 3.4, several may occur coincidentally with pregnancy. For example, women with schizophrenia being treated with antipsychotics may stop taking the antipsychotics upon learning of a pregnancy, only to then go on to develop tardive dyskinesia; another example might be the coincidental onset of a neurodegenerative disease, such as Huntington's disease.

Treatment

Although termination of pregnancy is followed by a resolution of the symptoms, chorea gravidarum, given its essentially benign nature, is generally not considered an indication for abortion. If symptomatic treatment is required, consideration may be given to an antipsychotic, such as haloperidol (Patterson 1979) or risperidone; however, in most cases it is prudent to simply let the disease run its course.

REFERENCES

Abt IA, Levinson A. A study of two-hundred twenty-six cases of chorea. *JAMA* 1916; **67**:1342–7.

Achiron A, Ziv I, Djaldetti R *et al.* Aphasia in multiple sclerosis: clinical and radiologic correlation. *Neurology* 1992; **42**:2195–7.

Adair JC, Digre KB, Swanda RM *et al.* Sneddon's syndrome: a cause of cognitive decline in young adults. *Neuropsychiatry Neuropsychol Behav Neurol* 2001; **14**:197–204.

Agius MA, Chan JW, Chung S *et al.* Role of antiribosomal P protein antibodies in the diagnosis of lupus isolated to the central nervous system. *Arch Neurol* 1997; **54**:862–4.

Ahern GL, O'Connor M, Dalmau J *et al.* Paraneoplastic temporal lobe epilepsy with testicular neoplasm and atypical amnesia. *Neurology* 1994; **44**:1270–4.

Alamowitch S, Graus F, Uchuya M *et al.* Limbic encephalitis and small cell lung cancer: clinical and immunological features. *Brain* 1997; **120**:923–8.

Anaya JM, Villa LA, Restrepo L *et al.* Central nervous system compromise in primary Sjögren's syndrome. *J Clin Rheumatol* 2002; **8**:189–96.

Ances BM, Vitaliani R, Taylor RA *et al.* Treatment-responsive limbic encephalitis identified by neuronal antibodies: MRI and PET correlates. *Brain* 2005; **128**:1764–77.

Anderson NE, Rosenblum MK, Graus F *et al.* Autoantibodies in paraneoplastic syndromes associated with small-cell lung cancer. *Neurology* 1988; **38**:1391–8.

Anonymous. Guidelines for the diagnosis of rheumatic fever: Jones criteria, 1992 update. *JAMA* 1992; **268**:2069–73.

Antoine JC, Honnorat J, Anterion CT *et al.* Limbic encephalitis and immunological perturbations in two patients with thymoma. *J Neurol Neurosurg Psychiatry* 1995; **58**:706–10.

Aron AM, Freeman JM, Carter S. The natural history of Sydenham's chorea. *Am J Med* 1965; **38**:83–95.

Asbahr FR, Negrao AB, Gentil V *et al.* Obsessive-compulsive and related symptoms in children and adolescents with and without chorea: a prospective 6-month study. *Am J Psychiatry* 1998; **155**:1122–4.

Asherson RA, Khamashta MA, Ordis-Ros J *et al.* The 'primary' antiphospholipid syndrome: major clinical and serological features. *Medicine* 1989; **68**:366–74.

Atkins CJ, Kondon JJ, Quismorio FP *et al.* The choroid plexus in systemic lupus erythematosus. *Ann Intern Med* 1972; **76**:65–72.

Aubart-Cohen F, Klein I, Alexandra JF *et al.* Long-term outcome in Susac syndrome. *Medicine* 2007; **96**:93–102.

Axley J. Rheumatic chorea controlled with haloperidol. *J Pediatr* 1981; **72**:1216–17.

Bak TH, Antoun N, Balan KK *et al.* Memory lost, memory regained: neuropsychological findings and neuroimaging in two cases of paraneoplastic limbic encephalitis with radically different outcomes. *J Neurol Neurosurg Psychiatry* 2001; **71**:40–7.

Bakheit AMO, Kennedy PGE, Behan PO. Paraneoplastic limbic encephalitis: clinico-pathological correlation. *J Neurol Neurosurg Psychiatry* 1990; **53**:1084–8.

Barile-Fabris L, Ariza-Andraca R, Olguin-Ortega L *et al.* Controlled clinical trial of cyclophosphamide versus IV methylprednisolone in severe neurological manifestations in systemic lupus erythematosus. *Ann Rheum Dis* 2005; **64**:620–5.

Barnard RO, Triggs M. Corpus callosum in multiple sclerosis. *J Neurol Neurosurg Psychiatry* 1974; **37**:1259–64.

Barnett MH, Prineas JW. Relapsing and remitting multiple sclerosis: pathology of the newly forming lesions. *Ann Neurol* 2004; **55**:458–60.

Bataller L, Kleopa KA, Wu GF *et al.* Autonomic limbic encephalitis in 39 patients: immunophenotypes and outcomes. *J Neurol Neurosurg Psychiatry* 2007; **78**:381–5.

Benda CA. Chronic rheumatic encephalitis, torsion dystonia, and Hallervorden–Spatz disease. *Arch Neurol Psychiatry* 1949; **61**:137–63.

Beresford OD, Graham AM. Chorea gravidarum. *J Obs Gynaecol Br Emp* 1950; **57**:616–25.

Berg D, Supprian T, Thomas J *et al.* Lesion patterns with multiple sclerosis and depression. *Mult Scler* 2000; **6**:156–62.

Bergin JD. Rapidly progressive dementia in disseminated sclerosis. *J Neurol Neurosurg Psychiatry* 1957; **20**:285–92.

Berrios X, Quesney F, Morales A *et al.* Are all recurrences of 'pure' Sydenham chorea true recurrence of acute rheumatic fever? *J Pediatr* 1985; **107**:867–72.

Bland EF, Jones TD. Rheumatic fever and rheumatic heart disease: a twenty-year report on 1000 patients followed since childhood. *Circulation* 1951; **4**:836–43.

Bland EF, Jones TD. The natural history of rheumatic fever: a 20 year perspective. *Ann Intern Med* 1952; **37**:1006–26.

Bluestein HG, Williams GW, Stebeg AD. Cerebrospinal fluid antibodies to neuronal cells: association with neuropsychiatric manifestations of systemic lupus erythematosus. *Am J Med* 1981; **70**:240–6.

Boesch SM, Plorer AL, Auer AJ *et al.* The natural course of Sneddon's syndrome: clinical and magnetic resonance imaging findings in a prospective six year observation study. *J Neurol Neurosurg Psychiatry* 2003; **74**:542–4.

Bohnen NILJ, Parnell KJ, Harper CM. Reversible MRI findings in a patient with Hashimoto's encephalopathy. *Neurology* 1997; **49**:246–7.

Bonfa E, Golembek SJ, Kaufman LD *et al.* Association between lupus psychosis and anti-ribosomal P antibodies. *N Engl J Med* 1987; **317**:265–71.

Bostantjopoulou S, Zafiriou D, Katsarou Z *et al.* Hashimoto's encephalopathy: clinical and laboratory findings. *Funct Neurol* 1996; **11**:247–51.

Bradley IA. A case of chorea insaniens with autopsy. *Am J Insanity* 1904; **60**:777–85.

Bragoni M, Di Piero V, Priori R et al. Sjögren's syndrome presenting as ischemic stroke. Stroke 1994; 25:2276–9.

Brain L, Jellinek EH, Ball K. Hashimoto's disease and encephalopathy. Lancet 1966; 2:512–14.

Brey RL, Hart RG, Sherman DG et al. Antiphospholipid antibodies and cerebral ischemia in young people. Neurology 1990; 40:190–6.

Brey RL, Holliday SL, Saklad AR et al. Neuropsychiatric syndromes in lupus. Prevalence using standardized definitions. Neurology 2002; 58:1214–20.

Brierly JB, Corsellis JAN, Hierons R et al. Subacute encephalitis of later adult life. Brain 1960; 83:357–68.

Brown MM, Thompson AJ, Wedzicha JA et al. Sarcoidosis presenting with stroke. Stroke 1989; 20:400–5.

Brownell B, Hughes JT. The distribution of plaques in the cerebrum in multiple sclerosis. J Neurol Neurosurg Psychiatry 1962; 25:315–20.

Buchanen DN. Pathologic change in chorea. Am J Dis Child 1941; 62:443–4.

Buchanen DN, Walker AK, Case TJ. The pathogenesis of chorea. J Pediatr 1942; 20:555–75.

Burton GE, Bullard DE, Walther PJ et al. Paraneoplastic limbic encephalopathy with testicular carcinoma. A reversible neurologic syndrome. Cancer 1988; 62:2248–51.

Bussiere HC, Rhea LJ. Acute rheumatic fever and chorea in children. Can Med Assoc J 1926; 16:35–40.

Byrne T, Mason WP, Posner JB et al. Spontaneous neurologic improvement in anti-Hu associated encephalomyelitis. J Neurol Neurosurg Psychiatry 1997; 62:276–8.

Camp WA, Frierson JG. Sarcoidosis of the central nervous system. Arch Neurol 1962; 7:432–41.

Cardoso F, Eduardo C, Silva AP et al. Chorea in 50 consecutive patients with rheumatic fever. Mov Disord 1997; 12:701–3.

Cardoso F, Maia D, Cunningham MC et al. Treatment of Sydenham chorea with corticosteroids. Mov Disord 2003; 18:1374–7.

Casanova MF, Crapanzano KA, Mannheim G et al. Sydenham's chorea and schizophrenia: a case report. Schizophr Res 1995; 16:73–6.

Caselli RJ, Scheithauer BW, Bowles CA et al. The treatable dementia of Sjögren's syndrome. Ann Neurol 1991; 30:98–101.

Caselli RJ, Scheithauer BW, O'Duffy JD et al. Chronic inflammatory meningoencephalitis should not be mistaken for Alzheimer's disease. Mayo Clin Proc 1993; 68:846–53.

Castillo M, Kwock L, Arbelaez A. Sydenham's chorea: MRI and proton spectroscopy. Neuroradiology 1999; 41:943–5.

Castillo P, Woodruff B, Caselli R et al. Steroid-responsive encephalopathy associated with autoimmune thyroiditis. Arch Neurol 2006; 63:197–202.

Cervera R, Asherson RA, Font J et al. Chorea in the antiphospholipid syndrome. Clinical, radiologic, and immunologic characteristics of 50 patients from our clinics and the recent literature. Medicine 1997; 76:203–12.

Chancellor AM, Cull RE, Kilpatrick DC et al. Neurological disease associated with anticardiolipin antibodies in patients without systemic lupus erythematosus: clinical and immunological features. J Neurol 1991; 238:401–7.

Chapelon C, Ziza JM, Piette JC et al. Neurosarcoidosis: signs, course and treatment in 36 confirmed cases. Medicine 1990; 69:261–76.

Ch'ien LT, Economides AH, Lemmi H. Sydenham's chorea and seizures: clinical and electroencephalographic studies. Arch Neurol 1978; 35:382–5.

Chong JY, Rowland LP, Utiger RD. Hashimotos's encephalopathy: syndrome or myth? Arch Neurol 2003; 60:164–71.

Church AJ, Cardoso F, Dale RC et al. Anti-basal ganglia antibodies in acute and persistent Sydenham's chorea. Neurology 2002; 59:227–31.

Coates T, Slavotinek JP, Rischmueller M et al. Cerebral white matter lesions in primary Sjögren's syndrome: a controlled study. J Rheumatol 1999; 26:1301–5.

Cohen JA, Cutter GR, Fischer JS et al. Benefit of interferon beta-1a on MSFC progression in secondary progressive MS. Neurology 2002; 59:679–87.

Colony HS, Malamud N. Sydenham's chorea: a clinicopathologic study. Neurology 1956; 6:672–6.

Comi G, Rovaris M, Falautano M et al. A multiparametric study of frontal lobe dementia in multiple sclerosis. J Neurol Sci 1999; 171:135–44.

Comi G, Filippi M, Wolinsky JS et al. European/Canadian multicenter, double-blind, randomized, placebo-controlled study of the effects of glatiramer acetate on magnetic resonance imaging-measured disease activity and burden in patients with relapsing multiple sclerosis. Ann Neurol 2001; 49:290–7.

Coombs C. Cerebral rheumatism. Practitioner 1912; 88:99–106.

Cordingly G, Navarro C, Brust JCM et al. Sarcoidosis presenting as senile dementia. Neurology 1981; 31:1148–51.

Corsellis JAN, Goldberg GJ, Norton AR. 'Limbic encephalitis' and its association with carcinoma. Brain 1968; 91:481–96.

Cottrell SS, Wilson SAK. The affective symptomatology of disseminated sclerosis: a study of 100 cases. J Neurol Psychopathology 1926; 7:1–30.

Coull BM, Bourdette DM, Goodnight SH et al. Multiple cerebral infarctions and dementia associated with anticardiolipin antibodies. Stroke 1987; 18:1107–12.

Creak M, Guttmann E. Chorea, tics, compulsive utterances. J Ment Sci 1935; 81:834–9.

Croteau d, Owainati A, Dalmau J et al. Response to cancer therapy in a patient with paraneoplastic choreiform disorder. Neurology 2001; 57:719–22.

Cutter NC, Scott DD, Johnson JC et al. Gabapentin effect on spasticity in multiple sclerosis: a placebo-controlled, randomized trial. Arch Phys Med Rehabil 2000; 81:164–9.

Dalmau J, Graus F, Rosenblum MK et al. Anti-Hu-associated paraneoplastic encephalomyelitis/sensory neuropathy. A clinical study of 71 patients. Medicine 1992; 71:59–72.

Dalmau J, Tuzun E, Wu H-Y et al. Paraneoplastic anti-N-methyl-D-aspartate receptor encephalitis associated with ovarian teratoma. Ann Neurol 2007; 61:25–36.

Dean G. Annual incidence, prevalence and mortality in white South African-born and in white immigrants to South Africa. BMJ 1967; 2:724–30.

Delalande S, de Seze J, Fauchais AL et al. Neurologic manifestations in primary Sjögren syndrome: a study of 82 patients. Medicine 2004; 83:280–91.

Delaney P. Neurologic manifestations in sarcoidosis. Ann Intern Med 1977; 87:336–45.

DeLorenze GN, Munger KL, Lennette EI et al. Epstein-Barr virus and multiple sclerosis. Evidence of association from a prospective study with long-term follow-up. Arch Neurol 2006; 63:839–44.

Devere TD, Trotter JL, Cross AH. Acute aphasia in multiple sclerosis. Arch Neurol 2000; 57:1207–9.

Devinsky O, Petito CK, Alonso DR. Clinical and neuropathological findings in systemic lupus erythematosus: the role of vasculitis, heart emboli, and thrombotic thrombocytopenic purpura. Ann Neurol 1988; 23:380–4.

Diefendorf AR. Mental symptoms of acute chorea. J Nerv Ment Dis 1912; 39:161–72.

Doherty CP, Schlossmacher M, Torres N et al. Hashimoto's encephalopathy mimicking Creutzfeldt–Jakob disease: brain biopsy findings. J Neurol Neurosurg Psychiatry 2002; 73:601–2.

Donaldson IM, Espiner EA. Disseminated lupus erythematosus presenting as chorea gravidarum. Arch Neurol 1971; 25:240–4.

Douglas AC, Maloney AFJ. Sarcoidosis of the central nervous system. J Neurol Neurosurg Psychiatry 1973; 36:1024–33.

Duffey P, Yee S, Rein IN et al. Hashimoto's encephalopathy: postmortem findings after fatal status epilepticus. Neurology 2003; 61:1124–6.

Durelli L, Verdun E, Barbero P et al. Every-other-day interferon beta-1b versus once-weekly interferon beta-1a for multiple sclerosis: results of a 2-year prospective randomized multicentre study (INCOMIN). Lancet 2002; 359:1453–60.

Ebaugh FG. Neuropsychiatric aspects of chorea in children. JAMA 1926; 87:1083–8.

Ebers GC, Bulman DE, Sodovnik AD et al. Population-based studies of multiple sclerosis in twins. N Engl J Med 1986; 315:1638–42.

Ebers GC, Sadovnik AD, Risch NJ. A genetic basis for familial aggregation in multiple sclerosis. Canadian Collaborative Study Group. Nature 1995; 377:150–1.

Ellis SG, Verity MA. Central nervous system involvement in systemic lupus erythematosus: a review of neuropathologic findings in 57 cases. Semin Arthritis Rheum 1979; 8:212–21.

Emery ES, Vieco PT. Sydenham chorea: magnetic resonance imaging reveals permanent basal ganglia injury. Neurology 1997; 48:531–3.

European Study Group on Interferon Beta-1b in Secondary Progressive MS. Placebo-controlled multicentre randomized trial of interferon beta-1b in treatment of secondary progressive multiple sclerosis. Lancet 1998; 352:1491–7.

Fassbender K, Schmidt R, Mofsner R et al. Mood disorders and dysfunction of the hypothalamic-pituitary-adrenal axis in multiple sclerosis. Arch Neurol 1998; 55:66–72.

Feinglass EJ, Arnett FC, Dorsch CA. Neuropsychiatric manifestations of systemic lupus erythematosus: diagnosis,

clinical spectrum, and relationship to other features of the disease. Medicine 1976; 55:323–39.

Feinstein AR, Spagnuola M. The clinical pattern of acute rheumatic fever. Medicine 1962; 41:279–305.

Feinstein A, Feinstein K, Gray T et al. Prevalence and neurobehavioral correlates of pathological laughing and crying in multiple sclerosis. Arch Neurol 1997; 54:1116–21.

Feinstein A, Roy P, Lobaugh N et al. Structural brain abnormalities in multiple sclerosis patients with major depression. Neurology 2004; 62:586–90.

Fermaglich J, Streib E, Auth T. Chorea associated with systemic lupus erythematosus. Arch Neurol 1973; 28:276–7.

Fontaine B, Seilhean D, Tourbah A et al. Dementia in two histologically confirmed cases of multiple sclerosis: one case with isolated dementia and one case associated with psychiatric symptoms. J Neurol Neurosurg Psychiatry 1994; 57:353–9.

Franklin GM, Heaton RK, Nelson LM et al. Correlations of neuropsychological and MRI findings in chronic-progressive multiple sclerosis. Neurology 1988; 38:1826–9.

Franklin GM, Nelson LM, Filley CM et al. Cognitive loss in multiple sclerosis: case reports and review of the literature. Arch Neurol 1989; 46:162–7.

Futrell N, Schultz LR, Millikan C. Central nervous system disease in patients with systemic lupus erythematosus. Neurology 1992; 42:1649–57.

Galluzzi S, Geroldi C, Zanetti O et al. Hashimoto's encephalopathy in the elderly: relationship to cognitive impairment. J Geriatr Psychiatry Neurol 2002; 15:175–9.

Ganji S, Duncan MC, Frazier E. Sydenham's chorea: clinical, CT scan, and evoked potential studies. Clin Electroencephalogr 1988; 19:114–22.

Ganz VH, Gurland BJ, Deming WE et al. The study of the psychiatric symptoms of systemic lupus erythematosus: a biometric study. Psychosom Med 1972; 34:207–20.

Garvey MA, Snider LA, Leitman SF et al. Treatment of Sydenham's chorea with intravenous immunoglobulin, plasma exchange or prednisone. J Child Neurol 2005; 20:424–9.

Gay W. Chorea insaniens. Brain 1889; 12:150–6.

Genel F, Arslanoglu S, Uran N et al. Sydenham's chorea: clinical findings and comparison of the efficacies of sodium valproate and carbamazepine regimens. Brain Dev 2002; 24:73–6.

Gerstley JR, Wile SA, Falstein E et al. Chorea: is it a manifestation of rheumatic fever? J Pediatr 1935; 6:42–50.

Geschwind DH, FitzPatrick M, Mischel PS et al. Sneddon's syndrome is a thrombotic vasculopathy: neuropathologic and neuroradiologic evidence. Neurology 1995; 43:557–60.

Ghika-Schmid F, Ghika J, Regli F et al. Hashimoto's myoclonic encephalopathy: an underdiagnosed treatable condition? Mov Disord 1996; 11:555–62.

Gibb WRG, Lees AJ. Tendency to late recurrence following rheumatic chorea. Neurology 1989; 39:999.

Gibb WR, Lees AJ, Scadding JW. Persistent rheumatic chorea. Neurology 1985; 35:101–2.

Glaser G, Pincus JH. Limbic encephalitis. J Nerv Ment Dis 1969; 149:59–67.

Goodkin DE, Rudick RA, VanderBrug Medendorp S *et al.* Low-dose (7.5 mg) oral methotrexate reduces the rate of progression in chronic progressive multiple sclerosis. *Ann Neurol* 1995; **37**:30–40.

Goransson LG, Herigstad A, Tjensvoll AB *et al.* Peripheral neuropathy in primary Sjögren syndrome: a population-based study. *Arch Neurol* 2006; **63**:1612–15.

Gordon RG, Norman RM. A case of acute toxic chorea. *J Neurol Psychopathology* 1934; **15**:313–19.

Goyal BK, Williams BJ. Sydenham's chorea in an octogenarian. *Gerontologica Clinica* 1967; **9**:176–81.

Graham DI, Lantos PL. *Greenfield's neuropathology*, 6th edn. London: Arnold, 1996.

Graus F, Keime-Guibert F, Rene R *et al.* Anti-Hu-associated paraneoplastic encephalomyelitis: analysis of 200 patients. *Brain* 2001; **124**:1138–48.

Greenfield JG, King LS. Observations on the histopathology of the cerebral lesions in disseminated sclerosis. *Brain* 1936; **59**:445–58.

Greenfield JG, Wolfsohn JM. The pathology of Sydenham's chorea. *Lancet* 1922; **2**:603–6.

Gultekin SH, Rosenfeld MR, Voltz R *et al.* Paraneoplastic limbic encephalitis: neurological symptoms, immunological findings and tumour association in 50 patients. *Brain* 2000; **123**:1481–94.

Guze SB. The occurrence of psychiatric illness in systemic lupus erythematosus. *Am J Psychiatry* 1967; **123**:1562–70.

Hammes EM. Psychoses associated with Sydenham's chorea. *JAMA* 1922; **79**:804–7.

Hanley JG, Walsh NMG, Sangalang V. Brain pathology in systemic lupus erythematosus. *J Rheumatol* 1992; **19**:732–41.

Hartung HP, Gonsetta R, Konig N *et al.* Mitoxantrone in progressive multiple sclerosis: a placebo-controlled, double-blind, randomised, multicentre trial. *Lancet* 2002; **360**:2018–25.

Hashimoto H. Zur kenntnis der lymphomatosan veranderung der schilddruse (struma ymphomatosa). *Arch Klin Chir* 1912; **97**:219–48.

Haskell RH. Mental disturbance associated with acute articular rheumatism. *Am J Insanity* 1914; **71**:361–81.

Heiskala H, Somer H, Kovanen J *et al.* Microangiopathy with encephalopathy, hearing loss and arteriolar occlusions: two new cases. *J Neurol Sci* 1988; **8**:239–50.

Henchey R, Cibula J, Helveston W *et al.* Electroencephalographic findings in Hashimoto's encephalopathy. *Neurology* 1995; **45**:977–81.

Henson RA, Hofman HL, Ulrich H. Encephalomyelitis with carcinoma. *Brain* 1965; **88**:449–64.

Hernandez Echebarria LE, Saiz A, Graus F *et al.* Detection of 14-3-3 protein in the CSF of a patient with Hashimoto's encephalopathy. *Neurology* 2000; **54**:1539–40.

Herring AB, Urich H. Sarcoidosis of the central nervous system. *J Neurol Sci* 1969; **9**:405–22.

Hilton DA, Footitt D. Neuropathological findings in Sneddon's syndrome. *Neurology* 2003; **60**:1181–2.

Hook O. Sarcoidosis with involvement of the nervous system. *Arch Neurol Psychiatry* 1954; **71**:554–75.

Hotopf MH, Pollock S, Lishman WA. An unusual presentation of multiple sclerosis. *Psychol Med* 1994; **24**:525–8.

Huber SJ, Paulson GW, Shuttleworth EC *et al.* Magnetic resonance imaging correlates of dementia in multiple sclerosis. *Arch Neurol* 1987; **44**:732–6.

Hughes RAC, Cameron JS, Hall SM *et al.* Multiple mononeuropathy as the initial presentation of SLE. *J Neurol* 1982; **228**:239–47.

Hughson MD, McCarty GA, Sholer CM *et al.* Thrombotic cerebral angiopathy in patients with the antiphospholipid syndrome. *Mod Pathol* 1993; **6**:644–53.

Hugo FJ, Halland AM, Spangenberg JJ *et al.* DSM-III-R classification of psychiatric symptoms in systemic lupus erythematosus. *Psychosomatics* 1996; **37**:262–9.

Husby G, van de Rijn I, Zabriskie JB *et al.* Antibodies reacting with cytoplasm of subthalamic and caudate neurons in chorea and acute rheumatic fever. *J Exp Med* 1976; **144**:1094–110.

Ichikawa K, Kim RC, Givelbar H *et al.* Chorea gravidarum. Report of a fatal case with neuropathological observations. *Arch Neurol* 1980; **37**:429–32.

Ingenito GG, Berger JR, David NJ *et al.* Limbic encephalitis associated with benign thymoma. *Neurology* 1990; **40**:382.

Iranzo A, Graus F, Clover L *et al.* Rapid eye movement sleep disorder and potassium channel antibody-associated limbic encephalitis. *Ann Neurol* 2006; **59**:178–82.

Isshi K, Hirohata S. Differential roles of the anti-ribosomal P antibody and antineuronal antibody in the pathogenesis of central nervous system involvement in systemic lupus erythematosus. *Arthritis Rheum* 1998; **41**:1819–27.

Jefferson M. Sarcoidosis of the central nervous system. *Brain* 1957; **80**:540–56.

Jennekens-Schinkel A, Sanders EACM. Decline of cognition in multiple sclerosis: dissociable artifacts. *J Neurol Neurosurg Psychiatry* 1986; **49**:1354–60.

Joffe RT, Lippert GP, Gray TA *et al.* Mood disorder and multiple sclerosis. *Arch Neurol* 1987; **44**:376–8.

Johnson KP, Brooks BR, Cohen JA *et al.* Extended use of glatiramer acetate (Copaxone) is well tolerated and maintains its clinical effect on multiple sclerosis relapse and degree of disability. *Neurology* 1998; **50**:701–8.

Johnson RT, Richardson EP. The neurological manifestations of systemic lupus erythematosus: a clinical–pathological study of 24 cases and review of the literature. *Medicine* 1968; **47**:337–69.

Jones TD, Bland EF. Clinical significance of chorea as a manifestation of rheumatic fever: a study in prognosis. *JAMA* 1935; **105**:571–7.

Kabelitz M, Liesenkotter KP, Stach B *et al.* The prevalence of anti-thyroid antibodies and autoimmune thyroiditis in children and adolescents in an iodine replete area. *Eur J Endocrinol* 2003; **148**:301–7.

Kalashnikova LA, Noasonov EL, Kushekbaeva AE *et al.* Anticardiolipin antibodies in Sneddon's syndrome. *Neurology* 1990; **40**:464–7.

Kawashima N, Shindo R, Kohno M. Primary Sjögren's syndrome with subcortical dementia. *Intern Med* 1993; **32**:561–4.

Keane JR. Internuclear ophthalmoplegia. Unusual causes in 114 of 410 patients. *Arch Neurol* 2005; **62**:714–17.

Kelly MC, Denburg JA. Cerebrospinal fluid immunoglobulins and neuronal antibodies in neuropsychiatric systemic lupus erythematosus and related conditions. *J Rheumatol* 1987; **14**:740–4.

Kerbeshian J, Burd L, Pettit R. A possible post-streptococcal movement disorder with chorea and tics. *Dev Med Child Neurol* 1990; **32**:642–4.

Kiessling LS, Marotte AC, Culpepper L. Antineuronal antibodies in movement disorders. *Pediatrics* 1993; **92**:39–43.

Kilic A, Unuvar E, Tatli B *et al.* Neurologic and cardiac findings in children with Sydenham chorea. *Pediatr Neurol* 2007; **36**:159–64.

Kingston G, Glynn LE. A cross-reaction between *Str. pyogenes* and human fibroblasts, endothelial cells and astrocytes. *Immunology* 1971; **21**:1003–16.

Kingston G, Glynn LE. Anti-streptococcal antibodies reacting with brain tissue I. Immunofluorescent studies. *Br J Exp Pathology* 1976; **57**:114–28.

Kinnman J, Link H. Intrathecal production of oligoclonal IgM and IgG in CNS sarcoidosis. *Acta Neurol Scand* 1984; **69**:97–106.

Kirk A, Kertesz A, Polk MJ. Dementia with leukoencephalopathy in systemic lupus erythematosus. *Can J Neurol Sci* 1991; **18**:344–8.

Koenig H. Dementia associated with the benign form of multiple sclerosis. *Trans Am Neurol Assoc* 1968; **93**:227–31.

Korn-Lubetzki I, Brand A, Steiner I. Recurrence of Sydenham chorea: implications for pathogenesis. *Arch Neurol* 2004; **61**:1261–4.

Krumholz A, Stern BJ, Stern EG. Clinical implications of seizures in neurosarcoidosis. *Arch Neurol* 1991; **48**:842–4.

Krupp LB, Coyle PK, Doescher C *et al.* Fatigue therapy in multiple sclerosis: results of a double-blind, randomized, parallel trial of amantadine, pemoline, and placebo. *Neurology* 1995; **45**:1956–61.

Krupp LB, Christodoulou C, Melville P *et al.* Donepezil improved memory in multiple sclerosis in a randomized clinical trial. *Neurology* 2004; **63**:1579–85.

Kurita A, Hasunuma T, Mochio S *et al.* A young case with multi-infarct dementia associated with lupus anticoagulant. *Intern Med* 1994; **33**:373–5.

Lacour A, de Seze J, Revenco E *et al.* Acute aphasia in multiple sclerosis. *Neurology* 2004; **62**:974–7.

Lange H, Thorner G, Hopf A *et al.* Morphometric studies of the neuropathological changes in choreatic disease. *J Neurol Sci* 1976; **28**:401–25.

Lanham JG, Brown MM, Hughes GRV. Cerebral systemic lupus erythematosus presenting with catatonia. *Postgrad Med J* 1985; **61**:329–30.

Lawn ND, Westmoreland BF, Kiely MJ *et al.* Clinical, magnetic resonance imaging, and electroencephalographic findings in paraneoplastic limbic encephalitis. *Mayo Clinic Proc* 2003; **78**; 1363–8.

Lessof MH. Sydenham's chorea. *Guys Hospital Reports* 1958; **107**:185–206.

Lessoff MH, Bywaters EGL. The duration of chorea. *BMJ* 1956; **1**:1520–3.

Levine SR, Deegan MJ, Futrell N *et al.* Cerebrovascular and neurologic disease associated with antiphospholipid antibodies: 48 cases. *Neurology* 1990; **40**:1181–9.

Lewis A, Minskl L. Chorea and psychosis. *Lancet* 1935; **1**:536–8.

Leys D. Rheumatic encephalopathy. *Edinburgh Med J* 1946; **53**:444–9.

Lief VF, Silverman T. Psychosis associated with lupus erythematosus disseminatus. *Arch Gen Psychiatry* 1960; **3**:608–11.

Lim L, Ron MA, Ormerod IEC *et al.* Psychiatric and neurological manifestations in systemic lupus erythematosus. *Q J Med* 1988; **66**:27–38.

Mac DS, Pardo MP. Systemic lupus erythematosus and catatonia: a case report. *J Clin Psychiatry* 1983; **44**:155–6.

MacKenzie S. Report on inquiry: II. Chorea. *BMJ* 1887; **1**:425–36.

MacNeil A, Grennan DM, Ward D *et al.* Psychiatric problems in systemic lupus erythematosus. *Br J Psychiatry* 1976; **128**:442–5.

Malamud N, Saver G. Neuropathologic findings in disseminated lupus erythematosus. *Arch Neurol Psychiatry* 1954; **71**:723–31.

Manz HJ. Pathobiology of neurosarcoidosis and clinicopathologic correlation. *Can J Neurol Sci* 1983; **10**:50–5.

Martinez-Yelamos A, Saiz A, Sanchez-Valle R *et al.* 14-3-3 protein in the CSF as prognostic marker in early multiple sclerosis. *Neurology* 2001; **57**:722–4.

Mathews WB. Multiple sclerosis presenting with acute remitting psychiatric symptoms. *J Neurol Neurosurg Psychiatry* 1979; **42**:859–63.

McCombe PA, McLeod JG, Pollard JG *et al.* Peripheral sensorimotor and autonomic neuropathy associated with systemic lupus erythematosus. *Brain* 1987; **110**:533–50.

McCullogh H. Encephalitis rheumatica: chorea minor of Sydenham. *J Pediatr* 1938; **13**:741–7.

McLean BN, Miller D, Thompson D. Oligoclonal banding of IgG in CSF; blood–brain barrier function, and MRI findings in patients with sarcoidosis, systemic lupus erythematosus, and Behçet's disease involving the nervous system. *J Neurol Neurosurg Psychiatry* 1995; **58**:548–54.

Mendez MF, Frey WH. Multiple sclerosis dementia. *Neurology* 1992; **42**:696.

Michotte A, Dequenne P, Jacobovitz D *et al.* Focal neurological deficit with sudden onset as the first manifestation of sarcoidosis: a case report with MRI follow-up. *Eur Neurol* 1991; **31**:376–9.

Miguel EC, Rodriguez Pereira RM, de Braganca Pereira CA *et al.* Psychiatric manifestations of systemic lupus erythematosus: clinical features, symptoms, and signs of central nervous system activity in 43 patients. *Medicine* 1994; **73**:224–32.

Mikdashi J, Krumholz A, Handwerger B. Factors at diagnosis predict subsequent occurrence of seizures in systemic lupus erythematosus. *Neurology* 2005; **64**:2102–7.

Miller DH, Kendall BE, Barter S *et al.* Magnetic resonance imaging in central nervous system sarcoidosis. *Neurology* 1988; **38**:378–83.

Miller DH, Khan OA, Sheremata WA *et al.* A controlled trial of natalizumab for relapsing multiple sclerosis. *N Engl J Med* 2003; **348**:15–23.

Mitsias P, Levine SR. Large cerebral vessel occlusive disease in systemic lupus erythematosus. *Neurology* 1994; **44**:385–93.

Moller A, Wiedemann G, Rohde U *et al.* Correlates of cognitive impairment and depressive mood disorder in multiple sclerosis. *Acta Psychiatr Scand* 1994; **89**:117–21.

de la Monte SM, Hutchins GM, Gupta PK. Polymorphous meningitis with atypical mononuclear cells in Sjögren's syndrome. *Ann Neurol* 1983; **14**:455–61.

Monteiro ML, Swanson RA, Coppeto JR *et al.* A microangiopathic syndrome of encephalopathy, hearing loss, and retinal arteriolar occlusions. *Neurology* 1985; **35**:1113–21.

Moreau C, Devos D, Delmaire C *et al.* Progressive MRI abnormalities in late recurrence of Sydenhams chorea. *J Neurol* 2005; **252**:1341–4.

Mumford CJ, Wood NW, Kellar-Wood HF *et al.* The British Isles Survey of multiple sclerosis in twins. *Neurology* 1994; **44**:11–15.

Nausieda PA, Grossman BJ, Koller WC *et al.* Sydenham chorea: an update. *Neurology* 1980; **30**:331–4.

Nausieda PA, Bielauskas LA, Bacon LD *et al.* Chronic dopaminergic sensitivity after Sydenham's chorea. *Neurology* 1983; **33**:750–4.

Nicoletti A, Sofia V, Biondi R *et al.* Epilepsy and multiple sclerosis in Sicily: a population-based study. *Epilepsia* 2003; **44**:1445–8.

Nojima Y, Sinota S, Yamada A *et al.* Correlation of antibodies to ribosomal P protein with psychosis in patients with systemic lupus erythematosus. *Ann Rheum Dis* 1992; **51**:1053–5.

Nokura K, Yamamoto H, Okawara Y *et al.* Reversible limbic encephalitis caused by ovarian teratoma. *Acta Neurol Scand* 1997; **95**:367–73.

Nolte KW, Undehaun A, Sieker H *et al.* Hashimoto's encephalopathy: a brainstem vasculitis? *Neurology* 2000; **54**:769–70.

O'Connor JF, Musher DM. Central nervous system involvement in systemic lupus erythematosus. *Arch Neurol* 1966; **14**:157–64.

Ochi H, Horiuchi I, Araki N *et al.* Proteonomic analysis of human brain identifies alpha-enolase as a novel autoantigen in Hashimoto's encephalopathy. *FEBS Lett* 2002; **528**:197–202.

Oide T, Tokuda T, Yazaki M *et al.* Anti-neuronal antibody in Hashimoto's encephalopathy: neuropathological, immunochemical, and biochemical analysis of two patients. *J Neurol Sci* 2004; **217**:7–12.

Oksanen V. Neurosarcoidosis: clinical presentations and course in 50 patients. *Acta Neurol Scand* 1986; **73**:283–90.

Olmos-Lau N, Ginsberg MD, Geller JB. Aphasia in multiple sclerosis. *Neurology* 1977; **27**:623–6.

Omdal R, Roalso S. Chorea gravidarum and chorea associated with oral contraceptives – diseases due to antiphospholipid antibodies? *Acta Neurol Scand* 1992; **86**:219–20.

Panitch H, Goodin DS, Francis G *et al.* Randomized, comparative study of interferon beta-1a treatment regimens in MS: the EVIDENCE trial. *Neurology* 2002; **59**:1496–506.

Papo T, Biousse V, Lehoang P *et al.* Susac syndrome. *Medicine* 1998; **77**:3–11.

Parker N. Disseminated sclerosis presenting as schizophrenia. *Med J Aust* 1956; **1**:405–7.

Patterson JF. Treatment of chorea gravidarum with haloperidol. *South Med J* 1979; **72**:1220–1.

Paz JA, Silva CA, marques-Dias MJ. Randomized double-blind study with prednisone in Sydenham's chorea. *Pediatr Neurol* 2006; **34**:264–9.

Pena J, Mora E, Cardozo J *et al.* Comparison of the efficacy of carbamazepine haloperidol and valproic acid in the treatment of children with Sydenham's chorea: clinical follow-up of 18 patients. *Arq Neuropsiquitr* 2002; **60**:374–7.

Pentland B, Mitchell JD, Cull RE *et al.* Central nervous system sarcoidosis. *Q J Med* 1985; **56**:457–65.

Pettee AD, Wasserman BA, Adams NL *et al.* Familial Sneddon's syndrome: clinical, hematologic, and radiographic findings in two brothers. *Neurology* 1994; **44**:399–405.

Petty GW, Engel AG, Younge BR *et al.* Retinocochleocerebral vasculopathy. *Medicine* 1998; **77**:12–40.

Pine DS, Douglas CJ, Charles E *et al.* Patients with multiple sclerosis presenting to psychiatric hospitals. *J Clin Psychiatry* 1995; **56**:297–306.

Pittock SJ, Kryzer TJ, Lennon VA. Paraneoplastic antibodies coexist and predict cancer, not neurological syndrome. *Ann Neurol* 2004; **56**:715–19.

Pittock SJ, Lucchinetti CF, Parisi JE *et al.* Amphiphysin autoimmunity: paraneoplastic accompaniments. *Ann Neurol* 2005; **58**:96–107.

Powell E. Two fatal cases of acute chorea with insanity. *Brain* 1889; **12**:157–60.

Powers WJ, Miller EM. Sarcoidosis mimicking glioma: case report and review of intracranial sarcoid mass lesions. *Neurology* 1981; **31**:907–10.

Poynton FJ, Holmes GM. A contribution to the study of chorea. *Lancet* 1906; **2**:982.

PRISMS (Prevention of Relapses and Disability by Interferon Beta-1a Subcutaneously in Multiple Sclerosis) Study Group. Randomized, double-blind, placebo-controlled study of interferon beta-1a in relapsing/remitting multiple sclerosis. *Lancet* 1998; **352**:1498–504.

Pruss H, Voltz R, Flath B *et al.* Anti-ta-associated paraneopastic encephalitis with occult testicular intratrabecular germ cell neoplasia. *J Neurol Neurosurg Psychiatry* 2007; **78**: 651–2.

Pujol J, Bello J, Deus J *et al.* Lesions in the left arcuate fasciculus region and depressive symptomatology in multiple sclerosis. *Neurology* 1997; **49**:1105–10.

Putzel L. Cerebral complications of chorea. *Medical Record* 1879; 220–2.

Rabins PV, Brooks BR, O'Donnell P *et al.* Structural brain correlates of emotional disorder in multiple sclerosis. *Brain* 1986; **109**:585–97.

Reaser EF. Chorea of infectious origin. *South Med J* 1940; **33**:1324–8.

Rebollo M, Val JF, Garijo F *et al.* Livedo reticularis and cerebrovascular lesions (Sneddon's syndrome). Clinical, radiological and pathological features in eight cases. *Brain* 1983; **106**:965–79.

Robertson WC, Smith CD. Sydenham's chorea in the age of MRI: a case report and review. *Pediatr Neurol* 2002; **27**:6–7.

Robin C, Gonnaud P-M, Durieu I *et al*. Demence lupique progressive: deux cas avec anticorps antiphospholipides ou non. *Rev Neurol* 1995; **151**:699–707.

Ron MA, Callanan MM, Warrington EK. Cognitive abnormalities in multiple sclerosis: a psychometric and MRI study. *Psychol Med* 1991; **21**:59–68.

Rosenberg GA, Appenzeller O. Amantadine, fatigue and multiple sclerosis. *Arch Neurol* 1988; **45**:1104–6.

Rosenfeld MR, Eichen JG, Wade DF *et al*. Molecular and clinical diversity in paraneoplastic immunity to Ma proteins. *Ann Neurol* 2001; **50**:339–48.

Roti E, Gardini F, Minelli R *et al*. Prevalence of anti-thyroid peroxidase antibodies in serum in the elderly: comparison with other tests for anti-thyroid antibodies. *Clin Chem* 1992; **38**:88–92.

Rubin LA, Urowitz MB, Gladman DD. Mortality in systemic lupus erythematosus: the bimodal pattern revisited. *Q J Med* 1985; **55**:87–98.

Rubinstein I, Gray TA, Moldofsky H *et al*. Neurosarcoidosis associated with hypersomnolence treated with corticosteroids and brain irradiation. *Chest* 1988; **94**:205–6.

Rudick RA, Goodkin DE, Jacobs LD *et al*. Impact of interferon beta-1a on neurologic disability in relapsing multiple sclerosis. *Neurology* 1997; **49**:358–63.

Sanson M, Duyckaerts C, Thibault J-L *et al*. Sarcoidosis presenting as late-onset dementia. *J Neurol* 1996; **243**:484–7.

Sawka AM, Fatourechi V, Boeve BF *et al*. Rarity of encephalopathy associated with autoimmune thyroiditis: a case series from Mayo Clinic from 1950 to 1996. *Thyroid* 2002; **12**:227–8.

Schauble B, Castillo PR, Boeve BF *et al*. EEG findings in steroid-responsive encephalopathy associated with autoimmune thyroiditis. *Clin Neurophysiol* 2003; **114**:32–7.

Schiffer RB, Babigian H. Behavioral disorders in multiple sclerosis, temporal lobe epilepsy and amyotrophic lateral sclerosis. An epidemiologic study. *Arch Neurol* 1984; **41**:1067–9.

Schiffer RB, Wineman NM. Antidepressant pharmacotherapy of depression associated with multiple sclerosis. *Am J Psychiatry* 1990; **147**:1493–7.

Schiffer RB, Caine ED, Bamford KA *et al*. Depressive episodes in patients with multiple sclerosis. *Am J Psychiatry* 1983; **140**:1498–500.

Schiffer RB, Wineman M, Weitkamp LR. Association between bipolar affective disorder and multiple sclerosis. *Am J Psychiatry* 1986; **143**:94–5.

Schneebaum AB, Singleton JD, West SG *et al*. Association of psychiatric manifestations with antibodies to ribosomal P proteins in systemic lupus erythematosus. *Am J Med* 1991; **90**:54–62.

Schwartzman J, McDonald DH, Derillo L. Sydenham's chorea: report of 140 cases and review of the recent literature. *Arch Pediatr* 1948; **65**:6–24.

Scott IA, Stocks AE, Saines N. Hypothalamic/pituitary sarcoidosis. *Aust NZ J Med* 1987; **17**:243–5.

Scott TF. Neurosarcoidosis: progress and clinical aspects. *Neurology* 1993; **43**:8–12.

Scott TF, Yandora K, Valeri A *et al*. Aggressive therapy for neurosarcoidosis. *Arch Neurol* 2007; **64**:691–6.

Sharma OP. Effectiveness of chloroquine and hydroxychloroquine in treated selected patients with sarcoidosis with neurological involvement. *Arch Neurol* 1998; **55**:1248–54.

Sharma OP, Sharma AM. Sarcoidosis of the nervous system: a clinical approach. *Arch Int Med* 1991; **151**:1317–21.

Shaskan D. Mental changes in chorea minor. *Am J Psychiatry* 1938; **95**:193–202.

Shaw PJ, Walls TJ, Newman PK *et al*. Hashimoto's encephalopathy: a steroid-responsive disorder associated with high anti-thyroid antibody titers – report of 5 cases. *Neurology* 1991; **41**:228–33.

Shenker DM, Grossman HJ, Klawans HL. Treatment of Sydenham's chorea with haloperidol. *Dev Med Child Neurol* 1973; **15**:19–24.

Sibley JT, Olszynski WP, DeCoteau WE *et al*. The incidence and prognosis of central nervous system disease in systemic lupus erythematosus. *J Rheumatol* 1992; **19**:47–52.

Silverstein A, Siltzbach LE. Neurologic sarcoidosis: a study of 18 cases. *Arch Neurol* 1965; **12**:1–11.

Sitzer M, Sohngen D, Siebler M *et al*. Cerebral microembolism in patients with Sneddon's syndrome. *Arch Neurol* 1995; **52**:271–5.

Sneddon JB. Cerebrovascular lesions and livedo reticularis. *Br J Dermatol* 1965; **77**:180–5.

Stankoff B, Waubant E, Confavreux C *et al*. Modafinil for fatigue in MS. A randomized placebo-controlled double-blind study. *Neurology* 2005; **64**:1139–43.

Stern BJ, Krumholz A, Johns C *et al*. Sarcoidosis and its neurological manifestations. *Arch Neurol* 1985; **42**:909–17.

Stockhammer G, Felber SR, Zelger B *et al*. Sneddon's syndrome: diagnosis by skin biopsy and MRI in 17 patients. *Stroke* 1993; **24**:685–90.

Surridge D. An investigation into some psychiatric aspects of multiple sclerosis. *Br J Psychiatry* 1969; **115**:749–64.

Susac JO, Hardman JM, Selhorst JB. Microangiopathy of the brain and retina. *Neurology* 1979; **29**:313–16.

Susac JO, Murtagh FR, Egan RA *et al*. MRI findings in Susac's syndrome. *Neurology* 2003; **61**:1783–7.

Sutton I, Winer J, Rowlands D *et al*. Limbic encephalitis and antibodies to Ma2: a paraneoplastic presentation of breast cancer. *J Neurol Neurosurg Psychiatry* 2000; **69**:266–8.

Swedo SE. Sydenham's chorea: a model for childhood autoimmune neuropsychiatric disorders. *JAMA* 1994; **272**:1788–91.

Swedo SE, Rapoport JL, Cheslow DL *et al*. High prevalence of obsessive–compulsive symptoms in patients with Sydenham's chorea. *Am J Psychiatry* 1989; **146**:246–9.

Swedo SE, Kilpatrick K, Schapiro M *et al*. Antineuronal antibodies (AnA) in Sydenham's chorea (SC) and obsessive-compulsive disorder (OCD). *Pediatr Res* 1991; **29**:364A

Swedo SE, Leonard HL, Schapiro MB *et al*. Sydenham's chorea: physical and psychological symptoms of St Vitus dance. *Pediatrics* 1993; **91**:706–13.

Swedo SE, Leonard HL, Kiessling LS. Speculations on antineuronal antibody-mediated neuropsychiatric disorders of childhood. *Pediatrics* 1994; **93**:323–6.

Symonds C. Recurrent multiple cranial nerve palsies. *J Neurol Neurosurg Psychiatry* 1958; **21**:95–100.

Tandon R, Walden M, Falcon S. Catatonia as a manifestation of paraneoplastic encephalopathy. *J Clin Psychiatry* 1988; **49**:121–2.

Taranta A. Relation of isolated recurrences of Sydenham's chorea to preceding streptococcal infection. *N Engl J Med* 1959; **260**:1204–10.

Taranta A, Stollerman GH. Relationship of Sydenham's chorea to infection with Group A streptococcus. *Am J Med* 1956; **20**:170–5.

Thayer WS. An analysis of 808 cases of chorea with special reference to cardiovascular manifestations. *J Am Med Assoc* 1906; **47**:1352–4.

Thiele R. Clinical observations on chorea of pregnancy. *Arch Neurol Psychiatry* 1935; **39**:1077.

Thompson AJ, Miller D, Youl B *et al.* Serial gadolinium-enhanced MRI in relapsing/remitting multiple sclerosis of varying disease duration. *Neurology* 1992; **42**:60–3.

Thompson C, Checkley S. Short term memory deficit in a patient with cerebral sarcoidosis. *Br J Psychiatry* 1981; **139**:160–1.

Thrush DC, Boddie HG. Episodic encephalopathy associated with thyroid disorders. *J Neurol Neurosurg Psychiatry* 1974; **37**:697–700.

Tourbah A, Piette JC, Iba-Zizen MT *et al.* The natural course of cerebral lesions in Sneddon syndrome. *Arch Neurol* 1997; **54**:53–60.

Tsokos GC, Tsokos M, LeRiche NGH *et al.* A clinical and pathological study of cerebrovascular disease in patients with systemic lupus erythematosus. *Semin Arthritis Rheum* 1986; **16**:70–8.

Tsukamoto T, Mochizuki R, Mochizuki H *et al.* Paraneoplastic cerebellar degeneration and limbic encephalitis in a patient with adenocarcinoma of the colon. *J Neurol Neurosurg Psychiatry* 1993; **56**:713–16.

Van Bogaert L, Bertrand I. Hemorrhagic affection of cortico-neostriatal site revealed clinically by acute and fatal chorea. *J Neurol Psychopathology* 1932; **13**:1–13.

Venables PJW. Diagnosis and treatment of systemic lupus erythematosus. *BMJ* 1993; **307**:663–6.

Vernino S, Tuite P, Adler CH *et al.* Paraneoplastic chorea associated with CRMP-5 neuronal antibody and lung carcinoma. *Ann Neurol* 2002; **51**:625–30.

Vincent A, Buckley C, Schott JM *et al.* Potassium channel antibody-associated encephalopathy: a potentially immunotherapy-responsive form of limbic encephalitis. *Brain* 2004; **127**:701–12.

Vitaliani R, Mason W, Ances B *et al.* Paraneoplastic encephalitis, psychiatric symptoms, and hypoventilation in ovarian teratoma. *Ann Neurol* 2005; **58**:594–604.

Voltz R, Gultekin H, Rosenfeld MR *et al.* A serologic marker of paraneoplastic limbic and brain-stem encephalitis in patients with testicular cancer. *N Engl J Med* 1999; **340**:1788–95.

Vrethem E, Ernerudh J, Lindstrom F *et al.* Immunoglobulins within the central nervous system in primary Sjögren's syndrome. *J Neurol Sci* 1990; **100**:186–92.

Walker RH, Spiera H, Brin MF *et al.* Parkinsonism associated with Sjögren's syndrome: three cases with a review of the literature. *Mov Disord* 1999; **14**:262–8.

Weiner DK, Allen NB. Large vessel vasculitis of the central nervous system in systemic lupus erythematosus: report and review of the literature. *J Rheumatol* 1991; **18**:748–51.

West SG, Emlen W, Wener MH *et al.* Neuropsychiatric lupus erythematosus: a 10-year prospective study on the value of diagnostic tests. *Am J Med* 1995; **99**:153–63.

Whitlock FA, Siskind MM. Depression as a major symptom of multiple sclerosis. *J Neurol Neurosurg Psychiatry* 1980; **43**:861–5.

Wiederholt WC, Siekert RG. Neurological manifestations of sarcoidosis. *Neurology* 1965; **15**:1147–54.

Wilcox JA, Nasrallah HA. Sydenham's chorea and psychosis. *Neuropsychobiology* 1986; **15**:13–14.

Wilcox JA, Nasrallah HA. Sydenham's chorea and psychopathology. *Neuropsychobiology* 1988; **19**:6–8.

Willoughby EW, Growchowski E, Li DKB *et al.* Serial magnetic resonance scanning in multiple sclerosis. A second retrospective study in relapsing patients. *Ann Neurol* 1989; **25**:43–9.

Wilson P, Preece M. Chorea gravidarum. *Arch Intern Med* 1932a; **49**:471–533.

Wilson P, Preece M. Chorea gravidarum. *Arch Intern Med* 1932b; **49**:671–97.

Wilson SAK. *Neurology*, 2nd edn. London: Butterworth & Co, 1954.

Winnacker JL, Becker KL, Katz S. Endocrine aspects of sarcoidosis. *N Engl J Med* 1968; **278**:483–92.

Winkelman NW, Eckel JL. The brain in acute rheumatic fever. *Arch Neurol Psychiatry* 1932; **28**:844–70.

Wolf RE, McBeath JG. Chorea gravidarum in systemic lupus erythematosus. *J Rheumatol* 1985; **12**:992–3.

Wong KL, Woo EKW, Yu YL *et al.* Neurologic manifestations of systemic lupus erythematosus. *Q J Med* 1991; **81**:857–70.

Young AC, Saunders J, Ponsford JR. Mental change as an early feature of multiple sclerosis. *J Neurol Neurosurg Psychiatry* 1976; **39**:1008–13.

Ziegler LH. The neuropathological findings in a case of acute Sydenham's chorea. *J Nerv Ment Dis* 1927; **65**:273–81.

SLEEP DISORDERS

18.1 SOMNAMBULISM

Isolated episodes of sleepwalking are common in children, occurring in about 15 percent (Kales *et al.* 1987). Recurrent, frequent episodes, however, are not normal, and in these instances one speaks of somnambulism or, as it is also called, 'sleepwalking disorder'. Somnambulism is not common, being found in 2–3 percent of children and far fewer adolescents or adults.

Clinical features

Somnambulism generally has an onset in children, sometime between the ages of 3 and 6 years; onsets in adolescence are uncommon, and in adult years are rare.

Sleepwalking arises from non-rapid eye movement (NREM) sleep, generally in the first third of the night (Kales and Kales 1974; Kavey *et al.* 1990). Typically (Kales *et al.* 1966), the patient sits up in bed; the eyes may be closed or open and, if open, the patient may look about the room with a blank stare. Some patients merely engage in simple, stereotyped behavior, such as fumbling with pyjamas or sheets, but most will get out of bed and begin to walk. Although some patients may bump into furniture or walls, many are able to navigate in such a way as to avoid obstacles. Some patients may simply wander, whereas others may attempt to climb out of windows or go down stairs. Rarely, patients may engage in complex activities such as eating, writing, or even driving a car. Patients may be mute or mumble incoherently; some may respond to requests with a few simple words.

Attempts to redirect patients or lead them back to bed may or may not be met with success; some patients actively resist any attempts to interfere with them. If a patient is awakened, there is no dream recall. Most episodes end spontaneously within 15–30 minutes; some patients may make it back to bed, whereas others will lie down on a couch, or even the floor, and resume sleep. Upon awakening the next day, patients are either amnestic for the episode or, at most, have only a patchy recall of the events that transpired.

Childhood-onset cases are generally not associated with other neuropsychiatric disturbances; by contrast, some (Kales *et al.* 1980a; Sours *et al.* 1963), but not all (Parkes 1986), authors have found an association between adult-onset cases and various forms of abnormal personality trait.

Polysomnography reveals the onset of sleepwalking in stage IV or, at times, stage III sleep. If polysomnography is required, it is useful to precede it with 38 hours of sleep deprivation, which greatly increases the chances of catching an episode (Joncas *et al.* 2002). Importantly, there are no ictal discharges and no interictal epileptiform discharges.

Course

If the onset is in early childhood, a remission is likely by early adolescence (Kales *et al.* 1980a); later-onset cases, however, may persist into adult years. After a remission there may rarely be a recurrence of sleepwalking.

Overall, the frequency of sleepwalking in somnambulism is increased during febrile illnesses, with sleep disruption (as may be seen with shift work [Driver and Shapiro 1993]), and, as noted above, with sleep deprivation.

Etiology

Somnambulism probably occurs on a hereditary basis; it is clearly familial (Kales *et al.* 1980b) and the concordance rate is higher for monozygotic than for dizygotic twins (Bakwin 1970; Hublin *et al.* 1997).

Differential diagnosis

At first glance, rapid eye movement (REM) sleep behavior disorder may appear quite similar to somnambulism; however, the differential is easily made by awakening the patient and asking if he or she were dreaming during the episode. In REM sleep behavior disorder there is always a dream present and the patient's behavior during the episode is 'explained' by the dream content; by contrast, in somnambulism there is no associated dreaming.

Night terrors are distinguished from sleepwalking both by the extreme terror evident in the sleeping patient and by the lack of any actual walking about.

Sleep drunkenness may resemble sleepwalking; however, the episodes of sleep drunkenness are seen in the morning as the patient struggles to awaken, in contrast to sleepwalking in which episodes occur in the early part of the night and are not associated with awakening.

Nocturnal complex seizures may be difficult to distinguish from episodes of sleepwalking (Pedley and Guilleminault 1977). A history of complex partial or other types of seizures during waking hours is helpful, but in limiting cases polysomnography may be required.

Various medications may cause sleepwalking, including paroxetine (Kawashima and Yamada 2003), bupropion (Khazaal *et al.* 2003), olanzapine (Kolivakis *et al.* 2001), zolpidem (Harazin and Berigan 1999), and the combinations of antipsychotics with lithium (Charney *et al.* 1979) and zolpidem with valproic acid (Sattar *et al.* 2003). Sleepwalking may also occur during hyperthyroidism (Ajlouni *et al.* 2005).

Treatment

Patients and parents should be reassured regarding the essentially benign nature of somnambulism, and common sense precautions, such as locking windows or doors and removing potentially dangerous objects, should be taken to reduce the risk of any injury. Should these measures fail, consideration may be given to 'anticipatory awakenings' (Tobin 1993). Here, one monitors the patient to determine when episodes are most likely to occur and then awakens the patient just beforehand; in many cases this may provide lasting relief after only a few nights. In limiting cases, medications may be utilized. The only blind study carried out found diazepam, in

a dose of 10 mg nightly, to be effective in adults (Reid *et al.* 1984). Anecdotally, clonazepam (Kavey *et al.* 1990) and imipramine (Cooper 1987) were also effective.

18.2 REM SLEEP BEHAVIOR DISORDER

REM sleep behavior disorder is a remarkable condition in which patients, while asleep and dreaming, literally 'act out' their role in the dream, with the bedroom serving as the 'stage'. Although in the general population this is a rare disorder, it is found in a significant minority of patients with parkinsonian conditions and in these cases it is often the presenting feature of the disease, preceding the parkinsonism by years. It is far more common in males than females.

Clinical features

The onset is generally in middle or later years, and episodes occur with variable frequency, from multiple episodes nightly to isolated episodes occurring every few months (Olson *et al.* 2000).

Schenck and colleagues have comprehensively described this condition (Schenck and Mahowald 1990; Schenck *et al.* 1986, 1987, 1989). Episodes typically arise out of REM sleep, in the middle or last third of the night. Violent or potentially dangerous behavior is not at all uncommon, and patients may suffer bruises, lacerations, or even fractures; in one case (Dyken *et al.* 1995) a subdural hematoma was sustained. Patients are generally difficult to awaken and, if they do come to full consciousness, they may relate a vivid dream that, in retrospect, clearly provides the context for their behavior.

Some examples will help to convey a sense of the remarkable phenomenology of this disorder. In one case (Schenck *et al.* 1986) a 67-year-old man described his dream and what he found when he woke up:

> I was a halfback playing football, and after the quarterback received the ball from the center he lateraled it sideways to me and I'm supposed to go around end and cut back over tackle and – this is very vivid – as I cut back over tackle there is this big 280-pound tackle waiting, so I, according to football rules, was to give him my shoulder and bounce him out of the way, supposedly, and when I came to I was standing in front of our dresser and I had knocked lamps, mirrors, and everything off the dresser, hit my head against the wall and my knee against the dresser.

Damage to property is not the only danger here: during one incident (Schenck *et al.* 1989), the patient 'was awakened one night by his wife's yelling as he was choking her. He was dreaming of breaking the neck of a deer he had just knocked down'; during another (Culebras and Moore 1989), a 70-year-old man 'dreamed that an alligator was trying to get into his car, and in order to prevent it, he held the animal's snout with great force . . .' After finally being awakened by his wife calling him, he found himself 'strongly grabbing her arm'.

Importantly, although the dream content, and resulting behavior, are often aggressive, the waking behavior of these patients is not characterized by any increased aggressiveness (Fantini et al. 2005).

There may be an association between REM sleep behavior disorder and other sleep disorders, including narcolepsy (Schenck and Mahowald 1992) and periodic leg movements (Fantini et al. 2002).

Polysomnography is diagnostic and reveals REM sleep during the episode, without, obviously, the expected atonia.

Course

In the natural course of events, REM sleep behavior disorder appears to be chronic.

Etiology

REM sleep behavior disorder most commonly occurs either on an idiopathic basis or secondary to certain parkinsonian conditions; other rare causes are noted below.

Idiopathic REM sleep behavior is diagnosed when the disorder occurs in an isolated fashion. This diagnosis, however, must be tentative, given that a large percentage of these patients will eventually develop a parkinsonian condition. For example, diffuse Lewy body disease may follow 6–8 years later, and Parkinson's disease some 3–5 years later (Schenck et al. 1996a; Tan et al. 1996). Indeed, in one autopsied case, REM sleep behavior disorder was the only manifestation of diffuse Lewy body disease (Uchiyama et al. 1995).

Parkinsonian conditions capable of causing REM sleep behavior disorder include diffuse Lewy body disease (Boeve et al. 2003a), Parkinson's disease (Olson et al. 2000), and the striatonigral variant of multiple system atrophy (Boeve et al. 2003a; Plazzi et al. 1997).

Rare causes of REM sleep behavior disorder include Alzheimer's disease (Schenck et al. 1996b), spinocerebellar ataxia type 3 (Iranzo et al. 2003), limbic encephalitis with anti-voltage-gated potassium channel antibodies (Iranzo et al. 2006), and certain focal lesions. Focal lesions capable of causing REM sleep behavior disorder have all been found in the pontine tegmentum, and include paramedian infarction (Kimura et al. 2000), plaques of multiple sclerosis (Plazzi and Montagna 2002; Tippmann-Peikert et al. 2006), and peritumoral edema (Zambelis et al. 2002).

Although the precise structures involved in the genesis of REM sleep behavior disorder are not known, attention has been focused on certain brainstem nuclei. In cases occurring secondary to diffuse Lewy body disease, neuronal loss and Lewy bodies have been noted in both the locus ceruleus and the substantia nigra (Turner et al. 2000). This, of course, is not unexpected; however, in cases in which REM sleep behavior disorder was the only manifestation of Lewy body disease, this too was where the pathology was found (Uchiyama et al. 1995). Other investigators, however, have cast doubt on this localization, finding only minimal changes in these nuclei in a patient with diffuse Lewy body disease who also had REM sleep behavior disorder (Boeve et al. 2007).

Differential diagnosis

Somnambulism is readily differentiated from REM sleep behavior disorder by simply waking the patient during the episode and asking about dreaming: somnambulists will have no recall of any dreaming, whereas those with REM sleep behavior disorder will recall the dream vividly. If there is any doubt, polysomnography will reveal episodes arising from NREM sleep in somnambulism and from REM sleep in REM sleep behavior disorder.

Complex partial seizures arising from sleep may likewise be distinguished from REM sleep behavior disorder by asking about dreaming, which is absent in the patient having a seizure. Furthermore, one typically also finds a history of other types of seizures, such as grand mal seizures, or of seizures during the day. In doubtful cases, polysomnography may reveal ictal activity during the episode. Importantly, not too much weight should be placed on finding interictal epileptiform discharges, as these are not uncommon incidental findings in elderly patients with REM sleep behavior disorder (Manni et al. 2006).

Obstructive sleep apnea may at times enter into the differential. In some cases of obstructive sleep apnea, patients, during arousals from an apneic episode, may appear confused and engage in complex activity (Iranzo and Santamaria 2005). Polysomnography may be required here and reveals that these episodes do not arise from REM sleep.

Treatment

Although there are no blind studies of the treatment of REM sleep behavior disorder, clonazepam (Schenck and Mahowald 1990), in doses ranging from 0.5 to 2 mg nightly, has become the accepted first-line treatment. Melatonin, in doses ranging from 3 to 12 mg, constitutes an acceptable alternative (Boeve et al. 2003b), and in my opinion should in fact be tried first as it does not carry with it any risk of falls. In cases in which both of these agents are either ineffective or not well tolerated, consideration may be given to pramipexole (found to be effective in one report [Schmidt et al. 2006] but only minimally so in another [Fantini et al. 2003]) or donepezil (Ringman and Simmons 2000). Certain medications should probably be avoided as they may aggravate the condition, including selegiline (Louden et al. 1995) and mirtazapine (Onofrj et al.

2003). Pending effective treatment, the bedroom should be made as safe as possible.

18.3 NIGHTMARE DISORDER

Occasional nightmares, occurring at a frequency of no more than once every few weeks, are not abnormal. When nightmares occur frequently, however, on at least a weekly basis, one may speak of 'nightmare disorder'.

Clinical features

The nightmares of nightmare disorder typically first appear in childhood or adolescence, often after an emotionally troubling event.

During a nightmare (Kales *et al.* 1980c), patients typically lie quite still; rarely is there much movement at all, and one never sees any thrashing about or complex behavior. During the nightmare, patients may be chased, attacked, tortured, or preyed upon by any number of unspeakable apparitions. Typically, as the fear crescendos, patients awaken with a cry of fright and are shaky, mildly diaphoretic, and tachycardic. Within moments, full alertness and orientation are achieved, and patients are then able to provide a vivid and emotional recount of the frightening dream. Although some are able to go directly back to sleep, most, fearful of another nightmare, have some difficulty in this regard and may lie awake for a half-hour or more.

Nightmares arise from REM sleep, typically in the middle and last thirds of the night.

Course

As noted above, the nightmares in nightmare disorder occur at least on a weekly basis and in some cases may occur multiple times a night. Fever, fatigue, emotional stress, and watching frightening shows before bed may all aggravate this condition. Although in most cases the disorder eventually remits, in a minority it may be lifelong.

Etiology

Apart from a suggestion that frequent nightmares may be inherited (Hublin *et al.* 1999), little is known about the etiology of nightmare disorder.

Differential diagnosis

Night terrors may be distinguished from nightmares in that night terrors are associated with overt signs of fright while the patient is asleep (e.g., crying out), arise from NREM sleep in the first third of the night, and are not associated with any clear dream recall; by contrast, nightmares are not associated with any movement, arise from REM sleep in the last two-thirds of the night, and are clearly and readily recalled.

Nocturnal panic attacks are easily distinguished from nightmares in that the panic attacks are not associated with frightening dreams; although patients with nocturnal panic attacks awaken into panic, they do not awaken out of a frightening dream.

Nightmares are very common in post-traumatic stress disorder and may also be seen during a depressive episode of a major depressive disorder or bipolar disorder, in the course of schizophrenia, or during delirium of any cause.

Various medications may cause nightmares, including tricyclic antidepressants, selective serotonin reuptake inhibitors (SSRIs), antipsychotics, levodopa, and beta-blockers. Nightmares may also occur during the 'REM rebound' seen during withdrawal from sedative–hypnotics or alcohol.

Very rarely, nightmares may constitute the only symptomatology of a seizure (Boller *et al.* 1975). Clues to this would be a history of other seizure types and a lack of any other reasonable explanation. Polysomnography may not be helpful here, as ictal electroencephalograms (EEGs) during simple partial seizures are typically normal. In doubtful cases one may consider attempting a 'diagnosis by treatment response' to an anti-epileptic drug.

Treatment

Avoidance of fatigue, frightening stories or shows, and, whenever possible, emotional stress, along with prompt treatment of any febrile illness, are all in order.

Behavioral treatments, such as densensitization or dream rehearsal, appear to be effective (Kellner *et al.* 1992; Neidhardt *et al.* 1992). When such treatment is not feasible or is ineffective, one may consider suppressing REM sleep with a benzodiazepine, such as diazepam, or using cyproheptadine in a dose of 16–24 mg h.s. (Harsch 1986). Consideration may also be given to prazosin, which is effective in the treatment of nightmares seen in post-traumatic stress disorder.

18.4 NIGHT TERRORS

Night terrors, also known as sleep terrors, sleep terror disorder, or pavor nocturnus, occurs in 1–4 percent of children and is somewhat more common in boys than girls.

Clinical features

The onset is generally in childhood, between the ages of 4 and 12 years; rarely the onset may be delayed until early adult years.

Attacks (Fisher *et al.* 1973a; Kales and Kales 1974) arise from stage III or IV NREM sleep in the first third of the night, typically before the first episode of REM sleep. Patients typically scream or cry out in terror, sit bolt upright, and appear dazed; the heart rate is increased, sometimes greatly so, and respiration is rapid and panting. The sheets may be grasped and patients may cry out for help. Attempts to awaken the child are generally unsuccessful, and the episode generally runs its course in a matter of minutes. Afterwards, patients may simply fall back into sleep or they may awaken; those who do awaken, although recalling the sense of terror, find either no memory of a dream or merely fragments of one. Remarkably, in contrast to their parents, who are generally quite shaken at witnessing the episode, the children themselves are generally able to fall back to sleep without any difficulty.

Otherwise typical attacks may rarely occur during daytime naps, thus constituting a 'pavor diurnus'.

Course

The frequency of attacks varies widely, from daily or weekly attacks to widely-spaced attacks occurring at monthly or longer intervals; in most cases attacks eventually cease, generally after about 4 years or so; uncommonly they may persist into adolescence or even adult years (DiMario and Emery 1987). Anxiety, stress, fatigue, and irregular sleep habits may all increase the frequency of attacks.

Etiology

Apart from the fact that sleep terrors are familial (Kales et al. 1980b), little is known of their etiology.

Differential diagnosis

Nightmares are quite different from night terrors. Nightmare sufferers typically have a vivid recall of the nightmare and are reluctant to go back to sleep for fear of having another one; in contrast, patients with night terrors have little or no recall of any dream and, if awakened, can fall back asleep with little anxiety. Furthermore, nightmares arise from REM sleep in the middle or last third of the night, whereas night terrors arise from NREM sleep in the first third of the night.

Nocturnal panic attacks are often included on the differential, but these are also quite different from night terrors. In nocturnal panic attacks, patients awaken from sleep into the panic attack and are awake and alert during the attack, with a full recall of it afterward. By contrast, patients with night terrors stay asleep during the attack and have little, if any, recall of it if they can be awakened. Most patients with nocturnal panic attacks will also have typical attacks during waking hours (Mellman and Uhde 1989a), and this history, of course, is very helpful; exceptions do occur, however, and some patients with panic disorder may have only nocturnal attacks (Mellman and Uhde 1990). Polysomnography is not very helpful in this differential, given that nocturnal panic attacks arise from NREM sleep (Mellman and Uhde 1989b), just as night terrors do.

Nocturnal complex partial seizures may closely resemble night terrors. In one case (Tinuper et al. 1990), a teenager had nocturnal seizures characterized by 'episodes of sudden arousal, screaming, grimacing, and violent, repetitive movements of the trunk and all four limbs' lasting for 5–10 minutes. The occurrence of seizures during waking hours, or a family history of epilepsy, is an important clue. In doubtful cases, polysomnography will be required.

Finally, there is a case report of adult-onset night terrors occurring secondary to a thalamic tumor (Di Gennaro et al. 2004).

Treatment

Parents should be reassured regarding the benign nature of night terrors, and, in most cases, as the episodes do not appear to bother patients much, this is all that is required. Should suppression of the episodes be necessary, open studies and case reports suggest effectiveness for diazepam (2.5–106 mg) (Fisher et al. 1973b), imipramine (25–506 mg) (Burstein et al. 1983; Cooper 1987), paroxetine (Wilson et al. 1997), and trazodone (Balon 1994).

18.5 NOCTURNAL HEAD BANGING

Nocturnal head banging, also known as jactatio nocturna capitis, is characterized by repetitive head banging or bumping during the transition into sleep. This is a common disorder in infants, seen in about 15 percent.

Clinical features

Head banging usually begins around the age of 9 months and typically occurs during stage I or II of sleep; the head movements are rhythmic, occurring several times a minute, with the head repeatedly making contact with the bed, bedrails, or headboard (Kravitz et al. 1960). The contact itself is generally not very forceful, and injuries are rare.

Course

The vast majority of cases resolve by the age of 4 years; persistence into adolescence (Hashizume et al. 2002) or adult years (Chisolm and Morehouse 1996; Whyte et al. 1991) is very rare.

Etiology

The etiology is not known.

Differential diagnosis

Nocturnal head banging must be distinguished from head banging seen during wakefulness, as may occur in mental retardation, autism, and schizophrenia. There is also a case report of acquired nocturnal head banging occurring after traumatic brain injury (Drake 1986).

Treatment

In most cases treatment is not required. Anecdotally, behavior therapy and nightly clonazepam (0.5–26 mg) or imipramine (10–25 mg) are effective.

18.6 ENURESIS

In the normal course of events, 90 percent or more of children become dry during the night by the age of 5 or 6 years. Persistent, recurring bedwetting past this age is considered abnormal and is termed enuresis (Forsythe and Redmond 1974) or, more precisely, nocturnal enuresis. Enuresis is nearly twice as common in males as females.

The vast majority of cases of enuresis occur on an idiopathic or primary basis; secondary causes of enuresis, such as diabetes mellitus, are relatively uncommon.

Clinical features

The achievement of nocturnal continence of urine is a normal developmental event, and, in most cases of primary enuresis, this developmental milestone is simply never attained at the expected age. In a minority of cases of primary enuresis, however, continence is attained and maintained, sometimes for long periods up to a year, after which it is lost. Secondary enuresis may have an onset at any time, from middle childhood to adult years, depending on the underlying cause.

In primary enuresis bedwetting typically occurs in the first half of the night. Children may or may not awaken during the bedwetting; if they do, it is always after urination has begun. Although wetting tends to be more common in NREM sleep and is generally not associated with dreaming, (Pierce et al. 1961), it may occur during REM sleep (Mikkelsen et al. 1980; Neveus et al. 1999).

In primary enuresis there are no associated symptoms. In secondary enuresis, however, one may find polyuria, dribbling, or dysuria, depending on the underlying cause.

Course

In the natural course of events, primary enuresis typically undergoes a spontaneous remission: by the age of 12 years, only 3 percent of children are still bedwetting, and by adult years the figure drops to 1 percent (Forsythe and Redmond 1974; Forsythe and Butler 1989). The course of secondary enuresis is determined by the underlying cause.

Etiology

In about two-thirds of cases primary enuresis is inherited on an autosomal dominant basis (von Gontard et al. 2001). Although it is not exactly clear what is inherited, several mechanisms have been proposed, including delays in the normal neuromuscular maturation that allows for continence, a smaller than normal bladder capacity, or either a reduced secretion of vasopressin or a decreased sensitivity of renal tubule cells to vasopressin. There is no evidence for any association with personality variables or particular methods of toilet training.

Secondary enuresis may be seen in diabetes mellitus, diabetes insipidus, urinary tract infections, cystic medullary disease, sickle cell disease, bladder or urethral obstructions, spastic bladder (as in cerebral palsy), compression of the bladder by pelvic masses or impacted stool, treatment with sedating drugs, clozapine or SSRIs, obstructive sleep apnea, and nocturnal seizures.

Differential diagnosis

In mental retardation of moderate or greater degree, a developmental age of 4 or more years may simply never be attained and, hence, in the normal course of events nocturnal continence does not occur.

Some authors include awake wetting in children over the age of 5 or 6 years under the rubric of enuresis; however, this may not be appropriate as in these cases the wetting is usually intentional or secondary to a resistance on the child's part to make the trip to the bathroom, as may be seen in young children who are reluctant to leave their friends in the playground and simply cannot 'hold it'.

Treatment

Primary enuresis may respond to a number of different treatments. Behavioral treatments should probably be tried first. Caffeinated beverages are eliminated and, except for ice chips for thirst or small sips of water for toothbrushing, fluids are withheld for the 3 hours leading up to bedtime, and the bladder is emptied just before going to bed. If the child remains dry through the night, a reward, perhaps a 'gold star' or a small present, is given the next morning. If bedwetting does occur the child should strip the bed but parents should take care of cleaning the sheets and bed and there should be no punishment. Many children respond favorably to this program in about a month. If it is unsuccessful, it should be supplemented with an 'enuresis alarm' (Forsythe and Butler 1989). Use of these alarms, which are inexpensive devices triggered by minute amounts of urine, is generally followed by gradual improvement over weeks or months. Once dryness has been maintained for a month, the program and, if utilized, the alarm, may be discontinued; should a relapse occur, a repeat course may be given.

If behavioral measures fail, medications may be considered; of the various medications shown to be effective in double-blind trials, imipramine and desmopressin are both considered first-line treatments. Overall, imipramine takes longer to work and tends to cause more side-effects; desmopressin, although easier to use, is not without liabilities, however, in that it carries a small risk of hyponatremia, with delirium or seizures (Dehoorne et al. 2006; Odeh and Oliven 2001). Imipramine may be started at a dose of approximately 1 mg/kg and increased in 0.5 mg/kg increments every 2 weeks until control is established, limiting side-effects occur, or a maximum dose of about 2.5 mg/kg is reached (Fritz et al. 1994). Desmopressin is given orally at bedtime in a dose of 0.2–0.6 mg (Schulman et al. 2001). Once continence has been achieved with either imipramine or desmopressin, treatment should be continued until continence has been maintained for anywhere from 1 to 3 months, after which the medication may be tapered over the following 3 months; relapses may be treated with reinstitution of the previously effective regimen.

Treatment of secondary enuresis is directed at the underlying cause.

18.7 NARCOLEPSY

Narcolepsy is characterized by narcoleptic attacks and, in most case, cataplexy; sleep paralysis and either hypnagogic or hypnopompic hallucinations may also occur in a minority. In addition to this classic tetrad, a minority of patients will also experience episodes of 'automatic behavior'.

Narcolepsy occurs in 0.025–0.05 percent of the general population and is equally common in males and females.

Clinical features

The basic clinical features of narcolepsy have been described in a number of reports (Adie 1926; Kales et al. 1982; Parkes et al. 1975; Wilson 1928). Of the classic tetrad of symptoms, narcoleptic attacks occur in all patients, cataplexy in about three-quarters, sleep paralysis in one-third, and hypnagogic or hypnopompic hallucinations in about one-third; only about 1 in 10 patients experience the full tetrad. In over 90 percent of cases, the first manifestation of the illness is a narcoleptic attack and, although this may appear anywhere from childhood to the middle years, most patients fall ill in their late teens or early adult years.

Narcoleptic attacks are ushered in by an overwhelming and irresistible desire to sleep; although such attacks are most likely to occur in situations conducive to drowsiness, such as long-distance driving or sitting through a boring lecture or meeting, they can occur at any time, even during otherwise lively and engaging conversations at the dinner table. Undisturbed, patients may sleep for minutes or even up to half an hour, after which they awaken, feeling more or less refreshed. Importantly, waking patients from a narcoleptic attack is not at all difficult and may be accomplished by a light touch or simply by calling the patient's name. Distinctively, the narcoleptic attack itself consists of REM sleep (Dement et al. 1964, 1966; Hishikawa and Kaneko 1965; Hishikawa et al. 1968), and most patients will be able to recall dreams upon awakening. Narcoleptic attacks are most frequent in the afternoon or evening and may recur anywhere from once to dozens of times per day. Nocturnal sleep is often broken and some patients may complain of insomnia; indeed, for most patients, the total 24-hour sleep time is actually not increased.

Cataplectic attacks tend to begin several years after the narcoleptic attacks make their appearance and may be either generalized or focal. Typically, the cataplectic attack is precipitated by some strong emotion, such as laughter, fear, anger, or a sudden surprise. In the generalized form, all voluntary muscle power, except for that of the diaphragm and, at times, the extraocular muscles, is diminished or lost, and the head droops forward, the jaw sags, the knees buckle, and patients may sink and collapse to the floor. In the focal type, the sudden muscle weakness is confined to one part, for example the neck musculature, with consequent head droop, the forearm and hand musculature, with items being dropped, or the extraocular muscles, with diplopia. Most attacks last for about a minute. During the attack, patients, even if fully paralyzed, remain conscious and alert, and are able, upon recovery, to give a full description of the event. In some cases, cataplectic attacks may be prolonged, lasting 5 minutes or more, and during such lengthy attacks, patients may experience vivid visual hallucinations. Very prolonged attacks, lasting 20 minutes or more, are referred to as 'status cataplecticus', and these may be precipitated by the sudden discontinuation of certain medications, such as fluoxetine (Poryazova et al. 2005). The frequency with which cataplexy occurs varies widely, from a mere handful of attacks through the patient's lifetime to multiple attacks daily.

Sleep paralysis may occur upon either falling asleep or awakening. Although fully conscious, patients find themselves unable to move. Most attacks last only a minute or so, and some may be accompanied by visual hallucinations. Importantly, although patients appear to the observer to be sound asleep, they may nevertheless be easily awakened by simply calling their names or lightly touching them.

Hypnagogic hallucinations appear upon falling asleep, being generally visual and quite vivid and complex, as if the patient were dreaming while still awake. Hypnopompic hallucinations are quite similar and appear upon awakening.

In addition to the classic tetrad just described, perhaps one-third or so of patients will also experience episodes of 'automatic behavior'. During these episodes, patients appear to be half-asleep and, although they may continue to engage in complex behavior, such as driving a car, there is generally a decrement in the quality of behavior: if writing, patients may write a gibberish scrawl, and, if speaking, they may engage in incoherent muttering. Importantly, upon coming to full alertness, these patients generally have no recall of what they did during the event; thus, a patient who drove automatically may, upon 'coming to', have no idea of how many exits were passed.

Furthermore, a small minority of patients with narcolepsy will also have other sleep disorders, including periodic limb movements of sleep, sleep apnea, and REM sleep behavior disorder.

The clinical diagnosis of narcolepsy may be confirmed with the multiple sleep latency test (MSLT). In narcolepsy, REM sleep occurs soon after sleep onset (Rechtschaffen et al. 1963), and the MSLT is designed to capture this. The results, however, must be interpreted in light of the overall clinical picture, as false negatives may occur. False positives may also be found in various conditions, including psychomotorically retarded, hypersomnic depressions, sleep apnea, and alcohol or sedative/hypnotic withdrawal.

Some clinicians will also test patients to see if they are positive for the HLA-DQB1*0602 haplotype. This haplotype is found in about 20 percent of the general population but in almost all patients with narcolepsy; consequently, whereas a negative test for this haplotype argues against the diagnosis, a positive test is of little diagnostic value.

Course

Although in a small minority there may be temporary remissions and, rarely, permanent remissions, for the vast majority of patients narcolepsy is a chronic, lifelong disease.

Etiology

The various clinical features of narcolepsy each seem to represent an 'intrusion' of REM sleep into waking life. The narcoleptic attack itself appears to be nothing but an episode of REM sleep, and the other features appear to represent a fragment of REM sleep, namely atonia, with or without associated dream imagery. Consequently, research has focused on those structures involved in sleep, namely the hypothalamus and various brainstem nuclei. Neuropathologic studies have demonstrated a loss of hyocretin-containing neurons in the lateral hypothalamus (Blouin et al. 2005; Crocker et al. 2005), and cerebrospinal fluid (CSF) studies have shown low hypocretin levels in almost all patients (Ebrahim et al. 2003; Mignot et al. 2002). The mechanism underlying these changes, however, is not clear. Although the prevalence of narcolepsy is increased among family members of patients with narcolepsy, it still remains low, at approximately 5 percent (Guilleminault et al. 1989), and although there has been one atypical case associated with a mutation in the gene for hypocretin (Peyron et al. 2000), there is no evidence for

Mendelian inheritance in the remaining vast majority of cases. Recent work has focused on the possibility that these hypocretin-containing neurons may be lost on an autoimmune basis, and it is felt that such an autoimmune attack may be triggered by some, as yet unknown, environmental trigger in genetically susceptible patients; to date, however, autoantibodies have not been detected. With this theory in mind, some patients have been openly treated with intravenous immunoglobulins, and in such cases a reduction in the frequency of cataplexy was reported (Dauvilliers 2006).

Differential diagnosis

The combination of narcolepsy and cataplexy is virtually pathognomonic for narcolepsy. As noted earlier, however, in most patients the illness begins with narcolepsy alone and, consequently, early in the course of the disease, when only narcoleptic attacks are present, other causes of 'excessive daytime sleepiness' must be considered, including, especially, sleep apnea, the Pickwickian syndrome, periodic leg movements of sleep, restless legs syndrome, the Kleine–Levin syndrome, psychomotorically retarded depressions, and alcohol or sedative–hypnotic withdrawal. All of these other disorders have distinctive features, as described in the respective sections, and the sleepiness seen in them rarely occurs as discrete attacks.

True sleep attacks may be seen as a side-effect of direct dopamine agonists, such as bromocriptine, pergolide, pramipexole, and ropinirole (Ferreira et al. 2000; Frucht et al. 1999; Hauser et al. 2000), and secondary to various hypothalamic lesions, including tumors (Aldrich and Naylor 1989), sarcoid granulomas (Aldrich and Naylor 1989), and infarction (Scammell et al. 2001). The combination of sleep attacks and cataplexy has been reported secondary to hypothalamic irradiation (Dempsey et al. 2003), lesions in the upper brainstem or floor of the third ventricle (Clavelou et al. 1995), and brainstem gliomas (Stahl et al. 1980), as a symptom of limbic encephalitis (Rosenfeld et al. 2001), and as a sequela to traumatic brain injury (Lankford et al. 1994) and encephalitis lethargica (Adie 1926; Fournier and Helguera 1934).

Treatment

Activities such as driving or operating hazardous machinery should be prohibited until narcoleptic and cataplectic attacks have been brought under control.

Narcoleptic attacks may be partially eliminated by brief scheduled naps (Roehrs et al. 1986; Rogers et al. 2001), judiciously spread out during the day. In most cases, however, pharmacologic treatment is required, and this generally involves the use of modafinil or methylphenidate. Modafinil is currently preferred and may be started at a dose of 200 mg once daily in the morning; in some cases, a total of 400 mg may be required (Broughton et al. 1997; US

Modafinil in Narcolepsy Multicenter Study Group 1998, 2000), generally divided into a morning and early afternoon dose (Schwartz *et al.* 2005a). Methylphenidate (Mitler *et al.* 1986a) may be used as a second-line agent and is given in a total daily dose of 20–60 mg, equally divided into a morning and early afternoon schedule. Tolerance to methylphenidate may occur, and in these cases the drug should be gradually tapered over a few days followed by a 'drug holiday' for another day or two, after which it may be gradually restarted, with a resumption of effect. Importantly, neither modafinil nor methylphenidate are effective against cataplexy. Alternatives to modafinil or methylphenidate include selegiline (in a dose of 20–40 mg) (Hublin *et al.* 1994; Mayer *et al.* 1995) and sodium oxybate (Black and Houghton 2006).

Cataplectic attacks may be prevented by selegiline (Hublin *et al.* 1994) and by sodium oxybate (Black and Houghton 2006). Open studies or case reports also suggest usefulness for clomipramine (Schacter and Parkes 1980), fluvoxamine (Schacter and Parkes 1980), fluoxetine (Frey and Darbonne 1994), citalopram (Thirumalai and Shubin 2000), escitalopram (Sonka *et al.* 2006), and venlafaxine (Guilleminault *et al.* 2000).

Overall, the vast majority of patients are treated with either modafinil or methylphenidate. When cataplexy requires treatment it would appear logical to add either selegiline or sodium oxybate, given that they have 'double-blind support'; however, in practice, these are not often used. Selegiline, in the doses required, is no longer a selective monoamine oxidase B (MAO-B) inhibitor, and hence the low tyramine diet is required, making this problematic. Sodium oxybate has high abuse potential and must be taken in the middle of the night, and is rarely used. In practice, when cataplexy does require treatment, most patients seem to do quite well on one of the antidepressants, such as escitalopram or venlafaxine.

18.8 SLEEP APNEA

Sleep apnea, sometimes also referred to as 'breathing-related sleep disorder', may manifest in one of three different types, namely obstructive, central, and mixed. The common denominator in all of these types is the appearance of frequent apneic episodes during sleep, and complaints of either daytime sleepiness or, less commonly, insomnia. Cognitive deficits (including delirium and dementia) and depression are also common.

During episodes of obstructive sleep apnea the oropharyngeal airway closes and, despite ongoing vigorous inspiratory efforts of the diaphragmatic and intercostal musculature, air flow at the mouth and nares ceases. By contrast, in central sleep apnea, cessation of air flow occurs not because of any obstruction but because of a lack of inspiratory effort due to inappropriate relaxation of the diaphragmatic and intercostal musculature. In the mixed type of sleep apnea, there is, as the name suggests, a combination

of the preceding two types: initially one sees a lack of inspiratory effort, as in the central type; this is soon followed by inspiratory effort of the diaphragmatic and intercostal musculature, which, due to oropharyngeal obstruction, is not followed by inspiration.

Of these three types, obstructive sleep apnea is the most common, followed by the mixed type; pure central types are relatively rare.

Sleep apnea is a common disorder, found in anywhere from 2 to 4 percent of the adult population over 40 years; it is at least twice as common in males as in females.

Clinical features

Although sleep apnea can occur at any age, it generally appears in middle years.

Apneic episodes last anywhere from 10 seconds up to 2 minutes, and may occur anywhere from 30 to several hundred times a night. In addition to episodes of complete apnea, patients will often also have hypopneic episodes, in which, although some inspiration occurs, it is at least 50 percent less than that seen with a normal breath. The severity of sleep apnea is often quantified by the 'apnea index' or the 'apnea–hypopnea index', which is equal to either the total number of apneic episodes per night or the total number of apneic plus hypopneic episodes per night divided by the number of hours spent in sleep. At a minimum, one wishes to see an apnea index of greater than 5 or an apnea–hypopnea index greater than 10.

In obstructive sleep apnea episodes (Strollo and Rogers 1996; Whyte *et al.* 1989), the patient, often an obese, middle-aged man, presents with a chief complaint of daytime sleepiness, which may or may not be accompanied by complaints of broken sleep. Almost universal is a history of frequent loud snoring, which may have prompted equally loud complaints from the patient's bed partner. Upon observing these patients while they sleep, for example while making rounds early in the morning, one may see a characteristic episode: oral and nasal airflow ceases despite increasingly vigorous diaphragmatic and intercostal muscular activity, until finally the obstruction resolves with a loud, gasping snort, at which point the patient may or may not awaken; should awakening occur it lasts only seconds, after which sleep once again occurs.

In central sleep apnea, patients tend to complain of insomnia and restless sleep, and there may or may not be any daytime drowsiness. As snoring is typically absent, there may be no complaints from the patient's bed partner, who may be unaware of the problem. The typical episode of central sleep apnea is far less dramatic than an obstructive one, as patients with central sleep apnea simply stop breathing: the chest and diaphragm are relaxed and there is no airflow. Eventually, inspiratory effort occurs with easy inspiration, and, at this point, the patient often has a transient awakening.

Mixed apneic episodes pursue a biphasic course. After an initial period of central apnea an inspiratory effort begins but is met by oropharyngeal obstruction, causing a period of obstructive apnea. Clinically, these patients resemble more the obstructive than the central type, and one often hears complaints of snoring and daytime sleepiness.

In addition to complaints of daytime sleepiness or insomnia, patients with sleep apnea typically also experience a dry mouth and a dull headache in the morning. There may also be sleep drunkenness, in which patients experience a brief period of confusion as they struggle to awaken in the morning. Enuresis may occur (Kramer *et al.* 1998) and erectile dysfunction is common (Goncalves *et al.* 2005).

Cognitive deficits are common. There may be difficulty with concentration and patients may complain of feeling 'fuzzy' or 'wooden-headed' during the day; there may also be minor deficits in short-term memory and difficulty in making decisions. Mechanical ability is impaired, and traffic accidents are more frequent in patients with obstructive sleep apnea than in the general public (George *et al.* 1987). In an uncertain percentage of patients, delirium may occur (Dyken *et al.* 2004; Lee 1998; Munoz *et al.* 1998; Sandberg *et al.* 2001; Whitney and Gannon 1996); in my experience this has not been at all uncommon. Rarely, rather than delirium there may be a dementia (Scheltens *et al.* 1991; Steiner *et al.* 1999).

Depressive symptoms are also common (Millman *et al.* 1989; Schwartz *et al.* 2005b), with indecisiveness, low self-esteem, helplessness, tearfulness, and, in some cases, suicidal ideation.

During episodes of sleep apnea, hypercapnia and hypoxia occur, and cyanosis may be seen. With frequent episodes of hypercapnia, pulmonary hypertension may occur, leading to cor pulmonale. Systemic hypertension is common. Arrhythmias may occur during episodes, including sinus bradycardia, sinus tachycardia, sinus arrest, atrial flutter, premature ventricular contractions, and ventricular tachycardia.

Sleep apnea may also aggravate epilepsy (Malow *et al.* 2000) and increase the risk of stroke and death (Yaggi *et al.* 2005).

Polysomnography should be considered in all cases of suspected sleep apnea, not only to document its presence and the type of sleep apneic episodes but also to determine the presence of arrhythmias. Often, overnight oximetry is performed as a screening test; however, this does not appear to be as sensitive as polysomnography.

Course

Sleep apnea is chronic.

Etiology

Obstructive episodes may occur secondary to various conditions, either singly or in combination, including the following: hypertrophy of the adenoids or tonsils; micrognathia (in which the tongue falls back to occlude the airway); lingual hypertrophy (as may be seen in hypothyroidism, acromegaly, or Down's syndrome); and, most commonly, obesity. Occasionally, no obvious cause is found for the obstruction, and in such cases it is suspected that there is a failure of the brainstem mechanisms responsible for maintaining the patency of the airway during sleep.

Central episodes are seen in association with obesity and congestive heart failure and may also occur in multiple system atrophy and with medullary lesions, for example infarctions, tumors, multiple sclerosis, or syringobulbia.

Differential diagnosis

The Pickwickian syndrome may resemble obstructive sleep apnea in that most Pickwickian patients are middle-aged or older obese men with a history of excessive daytime sleepiness. Waking blood gases, however, tell the tale, as they reveal hypercarbia in the Pickwickian syndrome but are normal in patients with obstructive sleep apnea while they are awake. It must be borne in mind, however, that these two syndromes often co-exist.

Narcolepsy is distinguished by the fact that in this condition daytime sleepiness comes in discrete attacks, in contrast to the chronic, waxing and waning sleepiness seen in obstructive sleep apnea.

Treatment

In obstructive sleep apnea, correction of the underlying cause, such as obesity (Smith *et al.* 1985), may be followed by significant relief. In very mild cases, some relief may also be gained by having patients sleep on their sides, a position that favors airway patency (Cartwright *et al.* 1985, 1991). Mild cases may also be treated with either protriptyline, 10–20 mg at bedtime (Brownell *et al.* 1982), or paroxetine, 20 mg at bedtime (Kraiczi *et al.* 1999). In most cases, however, a continuous positive airway pressure (CPAP) or bi-level positive airway pressure (BIPAP) device is required, and the relief gained with these devices may be pronounced: not only daytime sleepiness but also cognitive difficulties (including delirium or dementia), depression, erectile dysfunction, and enuresis are all improved or cleared. In those who cannot tolerate one of these devices, or in those in whom they are ineffective, the use of orthodontic devices or surgery may be contemplated. Orthodontic devices serve to keep the jaw advanced, thus preventing the tongue from occluding the airway. Surgical options include uvulopalatopharyngoplasty or uvuloplasty, and, in severe and limiting cases, tracheostomy. Another option in cases in which the devices are not tolerated or not fully effective is modafinil, which, in doses of 200–400 mg daily, may partially relieve daytime sleepiness (Kingshott *et al.* 2001).

In central sleep apnea, acetazolamide, in a dose of 250 mg four times daily, may provide some relief (White *et al.* 1982);

however, its effectiveness often wanes. In severe cases, diaphragmatic pacing may be required.

The treatment of mixed episodes is similar to that of the obstructive type.

Regardless of the type of sleep apnea present, care must be taken to avoid alcohol (Scrima *et al.* 1982) or any medication that might depress respiratory drive, including sedative–hypnotics (Mendelson *et al.* 1981), anxiolytics, sedating antidepressants, opioids, etc. Of note, sildenafil, which may be prescribed for the erectile dysfunction seen in obstructive sleep apnea, may also worsen the apnea (Roizenblatt *et al.* 2006) and consequently care must be taken in its use.

18.9 PICKWICKIAN SYNDROME (OBESITY–HYPOVENTILATION SYNDROME)

The constellation of extreme obesity, a ruddy complexion, and somnolence has long been recognized and was exemplified by the fat boy in Charles Dickens's *The Pickwick Papers*. Following the lead given by Dickens, Burwell *et al.* (1956) coined the term 'Pickwickian syndrome'; a more recent name is 'obesity–hypoventilation syndrome' and, although this is gaining currency, it lacks the color and flair of the eponym. As noted below, the extreme obesity in this syndrome leads to waking hypoventilation.

Clinical features

Patients are extremely obese and often have a ruddy complexion; they are typically somnolent and lethargic and have difficulty paying attention or concentrating on things (Burwell *et al.* 1956; Drachman and Gumnit 1962; Nowbar *et al.* 2004; Sieker *et al.* 1955; Ward and Kelsey 1962). Arterial blood gases drawn while patients are awake reveal significant hypercapnia and hypoxemia; erythrocytosis may occur as may pulmonary hypertension and cor pulmonale. Although, as might be expected, most patients also have obstructive sleep apnea, this is not inevitable, and some patients with the Pickwickian syndrome may have normal sleep (Kessler *et al.* 2001).

Course

In general, this parallels the course of the underlying obesity. These extremely obese patients are prone to venous stasis and deep venous thrombosis, and any acute worsening of their clinical status should always prompt a search for pulmonary emboli.

Etiology

The burden of excess adipose tissue encircling the chest and also pushing up the diaphragm from the obese abdomen

below leads to chronic alveolar hypoventilation. The resulting hypercapnia causes the somnolence.

Differential diagnosis

As noted, most patients with the Pickwickian syndrome also have obstructive sleep apnea, and the somnolence that they experience is often attributed entirely to the sleep apnea. The differential between the combination of the Pickwickian syndrome plus sleep apnea and sleep apnea alone rests on measurement of daytime arterial blood gases: in the combination, one finds waking hypercapnia and hypoxemia, whereas in sleep apnea alone, waking blood gases are normal.

Treatment

Weight loss is critical and effective (Chiang *et al.* 1980). Alcohol, sedative–hypnotics, and any other medications that may reduce respiratory drive, such as antihistamines or opioids, should be avoided. Concurrent obstructive sleep apnea is treated as described in the preceding section. Supplemental oxygen is sometimes recommended but this must be administered with caution as it may precipitate respiratory failure. In some cases oral medroxyprogesterone may improve daytime ventilatory status (Sutton *et al.* 1975). The usefulness, if any, of modafinil or stimulants such as methylphenidate is unclear.

18.10 KLEINE–LEVIN SYNDROME

The Kleine–Levin syndrome, first described by Kleine (1925) and Levin (1936), is a rare disorder characterized by episodes of hypersomnolence and associated symptoms (most notably hyperphagia), which occurs primarily in adolescence and most commonly in males.

Clinical features

The clinical features of the Kleine–Levin syndrome have been described in a number of case series (Critchley 1962; Critchley and Hoffman 1942; Dauvilliers *et al.* 2002; Gadoth *et al.* 2001) and a recent comprehensive review (Arnulf *et al.* 2005). As noted, this is an episodic disorder, and the first episode, although able to occur at almost any age, from early childhood to the ninth decade, appears in late adolescence in the vast majority. Although in the majority of cases the first episode is preceded by an infection, often viral, subsequent episodes generally occur without any precipitating factors. The episodes themselves generally last in the order of two weeks; however, the range is wide, from days up to 3 months.

Episodes may be ushered in by a brief prodrome, lasting perhaps days, of malaise, headache, and lethargy. During the episode proper, all patients experience hypersomnia, often sleeping 18 or more hours per day. During waking hours, about three-quarters of patients will also experience hyperphagia. Mood changes are seen in over half of all patients and typically consist of depression. Cognitive changes, such as confusion, are also seen in the majority. Hypersexuality occurs in a little less than half of patients and may manifest with exhibitionism, unwelcome sexual advances, and frequent, and at times public, masturbation. Delusions and hallucinations may appear in a small minority, as may unusual behaviors such as persistent humming and singing.

As noted, hypersomnia and hyperphagia constitute the primary symptomatology seen during an episode. Levin (1936) noted that 'the patient sleeps excessively day and night, in extreme instances waking only to eat and go to the toilet. He can always be roused. When roused he is usually irritable and wants to be left alone so that he can go back to sleep. He is abnormally hungry and eats excessively'. The hyperphagia seen during the episode is often indiscriminate, and patients may eat whatever is at hand (Critchley 1962), beg for food from other patients (Garland et al. 1965), or indulge in unusual food preferences (Will et al. 1988).

Mood changes tend toward depression, often tinged with irritability. Critchley (1962) noted that 'in the majority . . . the patient when awake is intensely irritable and resentful . . . a few patients are actually hostile in their behavior . . . in his attitude toward others he may be uninhibited, insolent, and quarrelsome'.

Cognitive changes most frequently manifest with confusion; however, there may also be short-term memory loss and incoherence.

Hypersexuality may be very problematic: one patient masturbated in public (Fernandez et al. 1990) and another continued his 'vigorous attempts at masturbation' during the interview, refusing laboratory testing unless 'the house physician was prepared to "come into bed and give me a feel over"'(Garland et al. 1965).

Delusions, which are typically of persecution, and hallucinations, which may be either auditory or visual, are seen in a small minority and tend to be fragmentary.

Unusual behaviors may also be seen. Some authors have commented that patients would 'sing inappropriately' (Chiles and Wilkus 1976); in one case the patient 'frequently burst into song' but sang the same song over and over again (Garland et al. 1965). In other cases patients may pace, wring their hands, tear out their hair, or engage in body rocking.

As noted earlier, most episodes last in the order of 2 weeks. Upon recovery, most patients are more or less amnestic for the events that occurred during the episode (Critchley 1962; Levin 1936), and some may experience a residual mood disturbance (Critchley 1962), tending towards either depression (Gallinek 1954) or elation (Gilbert 1964), which passes within a week or so.

Magnetic resonance scanning is normal, as is assay of the CSF. In the majority of cases the EEG displays diffuse slowing during an episode, with at times an accentuation of this in the temporal or frontotemporal areas. There are no ictal or interictal epileptiform discharges, and in between episodes the EEG normalizes. Polysomnography may reveal reduced REM latency, frequent awakenings, and decreased delta sleep (Pike and Stores 1994; Reynolds et al. 1980), and the MSLT may reveal sleep-onset REM (Reynolds et al. 1984).

Course

Although the long-term course has not been clearly delineated, it appears that in about two-thirds of patients there are recurrent episodes, with the intervals between episodes ranging from weeks to years but averaging about 6 months; in many of the cases in which there are recurrences, the subsequent episodes become less severe and more widely spaced out and, after perhaps 4 or more years, episodes finally cease to occur.

In the intervals between episodes, although it appears that the vast majority of patients return to normal, there is some suggestive evidence that there may be some residual quarrelsomeness and slightly reduced academic ability (Sagar et al. 1990).

Etiology

I could find three autopsy reports: one (Carpenter et al. 1982) noted widespread microgliosis in the thalamus, with little neuronal loss; another (Fenzi et al. 1993) found microgliosis not only in the thalamus but also in the midbrain; and the third (Koerber et al. 1984) reported only mild depigmentation of the substantia nigra and locus ceruleus, without evidence of Lewy bodies. The role of the thalamus in this disorder is further highlighted by a single photon emission computed tomography (SPECT) study (Huang et al. 2005) that found hypoperfusion of the thalami in seven out of seven patients tested, with resolution of this abnormality upon recovery.

Although the mechanism underlying these changes is not clear, the frequency with which the first episode follows an infectious illness has suggested an autoimmune basis (Dauvilliers et al. 2002), with the infection triggering an immune attack on diencephalic or mesencephalic structures.

Differential diagnosis

The overall clinical picture of one or more episodes of hypersomnolence and hyperphagia is fairly distinctive. Consideration might be given to a diagnosis of depression as depressive episodes in major depressive disorder or, especially, bipolar disorder may be characterized by depressed mood, increased need for sleep, and increased appetite, thus mimicking the episodes seen in the Kleine–Levin syndrome. Certain features of the Kleine–Levin syndrome, however, remain distinctive, including the indiscriminate nature of the hyperphagia and, especially, the hypersexuality.

Treatment

There are no controlled treatment studies. Anecdotally, lithium may reduce the severity or frequency of episodes (Dauvilliers *et al.* 2002; Goldberg 1983; Muratori *et al.* 2002; Ogura *et al.* 1976; Poppe *et al.* 2003), and success has also been reported with carbamazepine (Dauvilliers *et al.* 2002). Modafinil (Dauvilliers *et al.* 2002) and amphetamines (Gallinek 1962) have also been used to reduce the somnolence seen during an episode.

18.11 RESTLESS LEGS SYNDROME

The restless legs syndrome, also known as Ekbom's syndrome, is a common disorder, with a lifetime prevalence of about 5 percent. As the name implies it is characterized by the experience of restlessness in the legs, an experience so disagreeable and uncomfortable that it keeps patients from falling asleep. This disorder occurs in two forms: a primary form, which in all likelihood is inherited, and a secondary form, which occurs on the basis of numerous other disorders such as iron deficiency anemia or various sensory polyneuropathies.

Clinical features

In both primary and secondary forms the onset is generally gradual. Primary forms typically first appear in early adult years, whereas the age of onset of secondary forms is determined by the underlying condition; for the most part, however, the onset of the secondary form tends to be in middle or later years.

Clinically (Ekbom 1960; Montplaisir *et al.* 1997; Ondo and Jankovic 1996), patients report that when they lie down, or even merely sit down, they feel a restlessness deep within the legs, especially in the calves; some may also experience formication, with a sense of crawling under the skin, or an aching discomfort. Often the experience is so uncomfortable that patients feel impelled to get up and walk about, which brings some relief. Over time, the restlessness may begin to involve the upper extremities.

At night, falling asleep may be almost impossible, and patients may either try and lay still and bear the discomfort or spend hours out of bed, pacing about. Typically, symptoms lessen by early morning hours and patients may then be able to get some sleep.

The majority of patients will also experience periodic movements of sleep (Montplaisir *et al.* 1997; Ondo and Jankovic 1996), described in Section 18.12.

Course

Primary restless legs syndrome is generally chronic, and symptoms may either wax and wane in intensity over time or progressively worsen. The course of the secondary form is determined by the underlying cause. Certain medications, such as the SSRIs paroxetine (Sanz-Fuentenebro *et al.* 1996) and citalopram (Perroud *et al.* 2007), may exacerbate symptoms.

Etiology

The primary, or idiopathic, form of restless legs syndrome is familial and displays genetic heterogeneity, with both autosomal dominant and recessive patterns being recognized (Levchenko *et al.* 2006; Trenkwalder *et al.* 1996; Winkelmann *et al.* 2000, 2002). Although the underlying mechanism has not been clearly delineated, it appears that this primary form occurs secondary to a disturbance in iron transport in the substantia nigra. Both magnetic resonance imaging (MRI) (Allen *et al.* 2001) and transcranial sonographic (Schmidauer *et al.* 2005) studies have demonstrated a lack of iron in the substantia nigra, and CSF studies have disclosed decreased ferritin and increased transferrin levels (Earley *et al.* 2000). Although neuropathologic studies have not demonstrated any cell loss or gliosis in the substantia nigra, or any tau or synuclein pathology in neuromelanin cells (Pittock *et al.* 2004), there does appear to be a deficiency of transferrin receptors on these cells (Connor *et al.* 2003, 2004), which is consistent with a functional derangement of iron transport into them. Importantly, this putative disturbance in iron transport in the central nervous system is not mirrored by any systemic disturbances in iron transport or metabolism, and there is no association between the primary form of restless legs syndrome and iron deficiency anemia.

Secondary restless legs syndrome, by contrast, is associated with iron deficiency anemia (Rangarajan and D'Souza 2007). Other causes include sensory polyneuropathies (Gemignani *et al.* 2006; Polydefkis *et al.* 2000), uremia (Winkelmann *et al.* 1996, 2000), chronic hemodialysis (Kawauchi *et al.* 2006), Parkinson's disease (Krishnan *et al.* 2003), multiple sclerosis (Manconi *et al.* 2007), spinal cord lesions (Hartmann *et al.* 1999), spinal anesthesia with either bupivacaine or mepivacaine (Hogl *et al.* 2002), mirtazapine (Agargun *et al.* 2002), and pregnancy (Manconi *et al.* 2004). Most of these causes are either obvious or readily determined, with the exception of sensory polyneuropathy. In some cases secondary to polyneuropathy, the restless legs syndrome may be the only clinical evidence, and hence it is appropriate to consider nerve conduction velocity studies in doubtful cases (Ondo and Jankovic 1996). In the case of pregnancy, symptoms typically resolve shortly after delivery.

Differential diagnosis

The chief differential possibility is akathisia. In akathisia, as described in Section 3.10, patients experience a restlessness when seated or lying down and may feel impelled to get up; hence, they present a picture similar to that of the restless legs syndrome. Two features, however, enable a differentiation to be made (Walters *et al.* 1991). First, when patients with the restless legs syndrome get up they tend to pace about, whereas those with akathisia often 'march in place'. Second, patients with the restless legs syndrome often get some relief by massaging their calves, a manuever that is useless in akathisia.

Treatment

In secondary cases the underlying cause should, if possible, be treated, as this may bring relief. In secondary cases in which treatment of the underlying cause is either not possible or ineffective, and in primary cases, various medications may be considered, including the following: levodopa, direct-acting dopaminergic agents, gabapentin, clonazepam, oxycodone, and clonidine. Each is discussed in turn, followed by some overall recommendations.

Levodopa, in combination with carbidopa (Benes *et al.* 1999; Brodeur *et al.* 1988), may be started at a dose of 100 mg levodopa and 25 mg carbidopa, which may be doubled if needed after 3–7 days. Of the direct-acting dopaminergic agents that are effective in the restless legs syndrome, pramipexole (Montplaisir *et al.* 1999; Winkelmann *et al.* 2006) and ropinirole (Trenkwalder *et al.* 2004) are currently used. Starting doses are 0.125 mg of pramipexole or 0.5 mg of ropinirole, and the dose may be increased in similar increments every 3–7 days up to a maximum of 0.75 mg of pramipexole or 4 mg of ropinirole. All of these dopaminergic agents may be either given as a single dose 1–3 hours before bedtime or divided into two doses, given in the early evening and then at bedtime. Importantly, treatment with all of these dopaminergic agents may be associated with the phenomenon of 'augmentation', in which, over long periods of time, the symptoms of restless legs syndrome worsen. Although this is most commonly seen as a side-effect of levodopa (Allen and Earley 1996), it may also occur with direct-acting agents (Ondo *et al.* 2004). Another drawback associated with direct-acting agents is the possible emergence of pathological gambling, as has been noted with pramipexole (Tippmann-Peikert *et al.* 2007).

Gabapentin (Garcia-Borreguero *et al.* 2002) may be started at a low dose of 300–400 mg and increased every few days in similar increments up to a maximum of 3600 mg; the dose should be divided into an early evening dose, equal to one-third of the total, and a bedtime dose of the remainder; most patients respond to a total daily dose of 1800 mg.

Clonazepam (Saletu *et al.* 2001) may be started at a dose of 0.5 mg per hour before bedtime, with similar increments every 3–7 days up to a maximum of 2 mg.

Oxycodone (Walters *et al.* 1993) is effective in a dose of about 15 mg at bedtime, and clonidine in a dose of 0.025–0.05 mg (Wagner *et al.* 1996).

Although most texts recommend trying a dopaminergic agent first, the possibility of 'augmentation', which is unique to this group, may give one pause. In my experience gabapentin has proved quite satisfactory as a first-line agent. If a dopaminergic agent is used, either pramipexole or ropinirole should be used first, as they are probably more effective than levodopa and are less likely to cause augmentation. Clonazepam is another reasonable choice. Enthusiasm for oxycodone is tempered by its abuse potential, and clonidine carries a significant side-effect burden.

18.12 PERIODIC LIMB MOVEMENTS IN SLEEP

Periodic limb movements in sleep is characterized by multiple jerkings of one or both legs during sleep. This disorder has traditionally been referred to as nocturnal myoclonus; however, this is a misnomer because, as pointed out below, the abnormal movements seen in this disorder are not truly myoclonic in character but, when fully developed, resemble more a 'triple flexion' response.

Patients may or may not be awakened by the abnormal movements; if they are awakened and also complain of either insomnia or daytime sleepiness, then it is customary to speak not of 'periodic limb movements in sleep' but rather 'periodic limb movement disorder'; this in turn may occur on either an idiopathic basis or secondary to various other disorders. Periodic limb movement disorder is common, seen in at least 4 percent of the general population.

Clinical features

The onset of the disorder may occur at any time from early adult years to old age.

The jerking movement itself may occur in one or both of the lower extremities. Upon observation, one sees dorsiflexion at the ankle accompanied in most cases by dorsiflexion of the great toe; in many cases these movements are accompanied by flexion at the knee and hip, thus mimicking a classic triple flexion response (Coleman *et al.* 1980; Smith 1985; de Weerd *et al.* 2004). The jerkings evolve over anywhere from 0.5 to 4 seconds, and repeat every 20–120 seconds during episodes that last from minutes to hours. Episodes occur during NREM sleep and may recur throughout the night. The jerkings may or may not be accompanied by an awakening and, if they are, patients may complain of either insomnia or daytime sleepiness. Despite these complaints, patients themselves may be unaware of the jerkings, and an accurate history of these nocturnal events may depend on their description by a bed partner, who may complain of being repeatedly 'kicked' during the night.

A minority of patients will also have the restless legs syndrome.

Course

Idiopathic periodic limb movement disorder appears to be chronic; the course of the secondary form is determined by the underlying cause. Tricyclic antidepressants may exacerbate this disorder (Ware *et al.* 1984).

Etiology

The idiopathic form appears to be inherited and, as indicated by single photon emission computed tomography (SPECT) studies, is associated with a deficiency of postsynaptic dopamine receptors in the striatum (Staedt *et al.* 1995). Although the mechanism underlying the abnormal movements is not known, their strong resemblance to a Babinski response suggests that they result from a lack of normal supraspinal inhibition (Smith 1985).

Secondary forms have been associated with congestive heart failure (Hanley and Zuberi-Khokhar 1996), chronic hemodialysis (Rijsman *et al.* 2004), alcohol withdrawal (Gann *et al.* 2002), and spinal cord lesions (Lee *et al.* 1996). Rare cases have also been reported secondary to lacunar infarctions in the corona radiata (Kang *et al.* 2004) and in the pons (Kim *et al.* 2003).

Differential diagnosis

Isolated jerkings, occurring at a frequency of up to five per hour, may be an incidental finding on polysomnography (Mendelson 1996) and are not associated with any symptoms.

Hypnic jerks (Oswald 1959), also known as 'sleep starts', are a normal accompaniment of the transition into sleep. They differ from the jerkings seen in periodic limb movements in that they are very brief, typically involve all four extremities, and occur only as the individual is falling asleep.

Myoclonus, discussed in Section 3.2, is distinguished from the jerkings of periodic limb movements by its 'shock-like' rapid onset, in contrast to the relatively leisurely evolution of the jerking movement.

Treatment

Various medications are effective, including levodopa/carbidopa (Becker *et al.* 1993; Brodeur *et al.* 1988; Kaplan *et al.* 1993), pramipexole (Montplaisir *et al.* 1999), gabapentin (Garcia-Borreguero *et al.* 2002), clonazepam (Mitler *et al.* 1986b; Ohanna *et al.* 1985; Peled and Lavie 1987; Saletu *et al.* 2001), and oxycodone (Walters *et al.* 1993). The choice among these and their method of use are similar to that noted for restless legs syndrome in Section 18.11; of note, 'augmentation', as may be seen with dopaminergic agents in the restless legs syndrome, has not been reported in periodic limb movement disorder. Interestingly, in an open

study bupropion was also effective (Nofzinger *et al.* 2000), as was selegiline (Grewal *et al.* 2002).

18.13 PAINFUL LEGS AND MOVING TOES

As the name implies, this syndrome is characterized by pain in the legs (which may be quite severe) and involuntary movements of the toes, all resulting in insomnia. This is a rare but potentially devastating condition.

Clinical features

The syndrome (Dressler *et al.* 1994; Spillane *et al.* 1971) generally has an onset in the sixth or seventh decades. In most cases pain appears first and, although symptoms may begin unilaterally, bilateral involvement eventually ensues. As noted by Spillane *et al.* (1971), the pain varies 'in intensity from discomfort to a pain of great severity . . . an ache, an intense pressure, a tightness, a feeling that the toes were pulling or being pulled, a throbbing, bursting, crushing . . . [or] a deep burning' and the movements consist of a 'sinuous clawing and re-straightening, fanning and circular movements of the toes'. The effect of the toe movements can be remarkable: one of Spillane *et al.*'s patients 'was surprised to see that the toes were actually moving "as though they were playing a piano on their own"'. The symptoms are not relieved by walking about and insomnia can be severe (Montagna *et al.* 1983). When sleep does come, the abnormal movements cease.

Course

In most case this syndrome appears to be chronic.

Etiology

The syndrome has been noted secondary to lesions of the cord, posterior lumbar roots, and peripheral nerves, and with trauma to the back or feet (Dressler *et al.* 1994; Ikeda *et al.* 2004; Montagna *et al.* 1983; Nathan 1978; Pla *et al.* 1996; Schott 1981). Interestingly, lesions or trauma need not be bilateral; unilateral lesions may be followed initially by an ipsilateral onset, but eventually the contralateral extremity becomes involved.

Differential diagnosis

The restless legs syndrome is distinguished by an absence of pain and abnormal movements, and by the characteristic relief obtained by walking about. Reflex sympathetic dystrophy is distinguished by the lack of abnormal movements.

Treatment

There are no controlled treatment studies. Case reports indicate relief with gabapentin and clonazepam, and with epidural block, lumbar sympathectomy, and utilization of transcutaneous electrical nerve stimulation (TENS).

18.14 CIRCADIAN RHYTHM SLEEP DISORDER

The onset and duration of sleep, as is the case with most biological rhythms, is under the control of the suprachiasmatic nucleus of the hypothalamus, which functions as the body's 'internal clock'. Under its influence, most people begin to feel sleepy in the evening, go to sleep between the hours of 2000 and 2400, sleep for 7 or 8 hours, and then awaken, generally feeling refreshed. Social demands for work and other functions are built around this biologically determined schedule.

Whenever there is a mismatch between social demands for sleep and wakefulness and this biologically determined rhythm, one speaks of a circadian rhythm sleep disorder. Such mismatches may occur in one of two ways: either the timing of social demands changes or the internal 'clock' changes. Examples of the first type of change include the sleep disturbance that comes with transmeridian jet travel ('jet lag') or with shift work. Examples of the second type of change include the delayed sleep phase syndrome, the advanced sleep phase syndrome, the non-24-hour sleep syndrome, and the irregular sleep–wake syndrome.

As a whole, circadian rhythm sleep disorders are very common. 'Jet lag' occurs routinely in air travelers and some seven million Americans are exposed to the deleterious effects of shift work. The delayed sleep phase syndrome occurs in roughly 7 percent of adolescents; the non-24-hour sleep syndrome and the irregular sleep–wake syndrome, by contrast, are uncommon.

Clinical features

Jet lag occurs with air travel that crosses five or more meridians. With eastward flight, the traveler's internal clock is phase-delayed relative to the local schedule, and travelers tend to feel awake long past the local 'bedtime', with resulting insomnia. With westward travel, which is generally better tolerated, the traveler's internal clock is phase-advanced relative to the local time, and travelers find themselves sleepy quite early in the evening.

Shift work sleep disorder occurs when individuals, normally accustomed to working during the day and sleeping at night, are shifted to night-time work. Although a minority of individuals adjust to this change fairly rapidly, most do not, and, under the influence of their internal clock, they feel sleepy during the night while at work and have trouble sleeping during their daytime off-hours.

The delayed sleep phase syndrome (Weitzman *et al.* 1981, Wyatt 2004) is characterized by an inability to fall asleep at socially approved times. Patients often stay awake until the early morning hours and are then unable to awaken early enough in the morning to get to school or work on time. Importantly, if such 'night owls' are allowed to 'sleep in' they get a normal amount of sleep and awaken refreshed. In most cases, this syndrome has an onset in adolescence.

The advanced sleep phase syndrome, which is generally restricted to the elderly, is characterized by an urge to go to sleep very early in the evening. Such individuals then awaken some 7 or so hours later, in the very early morning. These 'morning larks' awaken refreshed and get a start on the day long before their companions.

In the non-24-hour sleep syndrome there is a failure of entrainment of the internal clock to the normally occurring 24-hour schedule. Given that the internal clock, when allowed to 'run free', has a cycle length some 15–30 minutes longer than 24 hours, such patients experience progressively worsening insomnia, followed by hypersomnia, until their free-running internal clock finally completes enough cycles to bring it into alignment with the normal environmental 24-hour cycle.

In the irregular sleep–wake syndrome the urge to sleep seems to come at random, with no clear-cut relationship to any cycle, whether environmental or internal.

Etiology

Jet lag and the shift work type of sleep disorder occur secondary to the environmental changes, which create a mismatch between the newly enforced sleep–wake schedule and the ongoing workings of the internal clock.

The delayed sleep phase syndrome may have a genetic basis. Associations have been found with polymorphisms of the 'circadian clock gene' *hPER3* (Pereira *et al.* 2005), polymorphisms of the gene encoding an enzyme that is responsible for phosphorylation of clock proteins (Takano *et al.* 2004), and polymorphisms of the gene coding for the rate-limiting enzyme responsible for melatonin synthesis (Hohjoh *et al.* 2003). Uncommonly, this syndrome may occur after closed head injury (Ayalon *et al.* 2007; Quinto *et al.* 2000).

The advanced sleep phase syndrome occurs most commonly on a sporadic basis in the elderly, and, in these cases, is presumed to be secondary to age-related changes in the suprachiasmatic nucleus or related structures. Rarely, the syndrome may occur on a familial basis, with autosomal dominant inheritance (Reid *et al.* 2001); in some such cases, mutations have been found in *hPER2* (Xu *et al.* 2005).

The non-24-hour sleep syndrome generally occurs in patients who are blind secondary to lesions affecting the optic chiasm, optic nerves, or eyes. Anatomically, entrainment of the suprachiasmatic nucleus to the environmental light–dark schedule is dependent on fibers of the retino-hypothalamic tract, which arise in the retina and then traverse the optic nerves to the optic chiasm from where they ascend into the hypothalamus. With bilateral lesions of these tracts, the internal clock 'runs free'. Less commonly, this syndrome may occur in sighted patients, and such cases have been noted after head trauma (Boivin *et al.* 2003) and in otherwise normal individuals with disorders of melatonin metabolism (McArthur *et al.* 1996, Nakamura *et al.* 1997).

The irregular sleep–wake syndrome is generally seen only in patients with diffuse brain disease, whether congenital or acquired (e.g., after traumatic brain injury [Ayalon *et al.* 2007]), and in such cases it is presumed that the suprachiasmatic nucleus has been damaged or destroyed.

Differential diagnosis

The diagnosis of the jet lag and shift work types of sleep disorder is usually self-evident. In the other types, routine history taking alone generally suffices; however, in some cases it may be necessary to have the patient or a caretaker keep a 'sleep log' for a couple of weeks; polysomnography is rarely required.

In evaluating patients with suspected delayed sleep phase syndrome, non-24 hour sleep syndrome or irregular sleep–wake syndrome, consideration should be given to the effects of alcohol or stimulants, and to the presence of various psychiatric disorders that can disturb sleep, especially depression, anxiety, mania, and schizophrenia.

Treatment

Both bedtime melatonin and appropriately timed exposure to bright light are useful in most of these disorders. If melatonin is used, the immediate-release type should be prescribed, in doses ranging from 3 to 6 mg.

Jet lag is approached by rigidly adhering to the local bed time; an additional strategy is to adjust one's internal clock before departure by adhering progressively closer, over 2 or 3 days, to the anticipated bedtime at one's destination. Upon arrival, melatonin use for 5 days may also help. Zolpidem, in a dose of 5–10 mg, also appears to be effective; however, melatonin and zolpidem should not be used in combination as this may result in confusion (Suhner *et al.* 2001).

Shift work sleep disorder is treated by use of bright light during night-time work (5000 Lux or more) and use of sunglasses or goggles during daytime hours (Crowley *et al.* 2003; Czeisler *et al.* 1990). Melatonin does not appear to be robustly effective (Cavallo *et al.* 2005), however, it is worth a try. Many individuals also utilize hypnotics, such as zolpidem; although there are no data to support this use, it is probably preferable to drinking oneself to sleep. Use of modafinil during the day is marginally helpful (Czeisler *et al.* 2005).

Delayed sleep phase syndrome may be treated with a combination of modalities including administration of melatonin sometime between the hours of 1900 and 2100 (Kayumov *et al.* 2001), dim lights in the evening, rigid adherence to a normal wake-up time, and exposure to bright light for 2 or 3 hours after arising (Watanabe *et al.* 1999). Another method of resetting the internal clock involves what is known as 'chronotherapy' (Czeisler *et al.* 1981). Here, patients advance their sleep time progressively by 3 hours every day until, after 5 or 6 days (depending on when their original sleep time was), their new sleep time coincides with environmental demands, which are then rigidly adhered to. Although effective, this procedure is difficult to implement.

Advanced sleep phase syndrome rarely requires treatment, as it rarely causes significant problems. Evening bright light treatment may be considered, but there are no controlled studies regarding such use.

In case reports, the non-24-hour sleep syndrome has been successfully treated with melatonin (Hayakawa *et al.* 1998, Palm *et al.* 1991). In sighted patients, and in those whose blindness is due to retrochiasmal lesions, morning bright-light treatment may be considered.

Anecdotally, the irregular sleep–wake syndrome has been improved with melatonin (Pillar *et al.* 1998).

18.15 PRIMARY INSOMNIA

Primary insomnia remains a diagnosis of exclusion and should be withheld until other causes of insomnia, discussed below, are ruled out. Primary insomnia occurs in one of two forms. The most common form, psychophysiologic insomnia, occurs in anywhere from 1 to 10 percent of the general population and in up to 25 percent of the elderly. The other form, referred to as idiopathic insomnia, is quite rare.

Clinical features

Psychophysiologic insomnia (Hauri and Fisher 1986) typically has an onset in middle or later years, and, generally, but not always, follows upon some stressful life event. Idiopathic insomnia, by contrast, appears much earlier, either in childhood or infancy.

Patients typically have trouble falling asleep, experience multiple awakenings, and have an overall reduced total sleep time. Most patients are fretful about their insomnia and, while lying in bed, may find themselves worrying constantly over their inability to achieve sleep.

Course

Psychophysiologic insomnia remits in about 50 percent of patients within a year; in the remainder it tends to persist, with its severity waxing and waning over time.

Idiopathic insomnia tends to be chronic.

Pathology and etiology

Psychophysiologic insomnia, as noted earlier, generally occurs after some stressful life event. When stressed, most individuals will experience some insomnia, but, in the overwhelming majority, this is transient. In those destined to develop psychophysiologic insomnia, however, a certain anxiety appears over whether or not sleep will come. This anxiety then makes sleep less likely to occur and a vicious cycle may be established in which a failure to sleep engenders more anticipatory anxiety, which in turn makes the insomnia worse. Once this pattern is firmly established, the bed, rather than being seen as a place for relaxation and restoration, becomes an anxiety-provoking stimulus in itself. Interestingly, in such cases patients may sleep better on the couch or in a hotel. Whether or not other etiologic factors exist in psychophysiologic insomnia is not clear; a recent report, however, did note reduced nocturnal melatonin levels in patients compared with control subjects (Riemann *et al.* 2002a).

Idiopathic insomnia is presumed to be secondary to dysfunction of hypothalamic or brainstem structures involved in sleep.

Differential diagnosis

Other sleep disorders, discussed in other sections in this chapter, must be considered, including sleep apnea, restless legs syndrome, periodic leg movements of sleep, and the syndrome of painful legs and moving toes.

Depression is perhaps one of the most common causes of insomnia, and one should always inquire about the presence of other vegetative symptoms. Generalized anxiety disorder, post-traumatic stress disorder, and schizophrenia must also be considered.

Caffeine and other stimulants taken too late in the day cause insomnia, and insomnia is universal and often very severe and long-lasting in alcohol withdrawal.

Painful conditions, such as heartburn or arthritis, routinely disturb sleep.

Finally, one must consider whether the patient suffers from 'sleep state misperception' or is merely an otherwise normal 'short sleeper'. Sleep state misperception is said to exist in cases in which, despite often bitter complaints of insomnia, polysomnography reveals normal sleep. Before making this diagnosis, however, it must be borne in mind that some patients with psychophysiologic insomnia sleep better when they are away from home. When this is suspected, it may be appropriate to perform polysomnography at the patient's home before making the diagnosis. 'Short sleepers' are individuals who, despite getting little sleep, awake refreshed and have no complaints.

Treatment

Good sleep hygiene is essential. Naps should not be taken, and patients should get some exercise every day. Caffeine and other stimulants should be reserved for morning use only. Evenings should be reserved for relaxing activities, the bedroom should be darkened and quiet, and the bed should be reserved for sleep or sexual activity. If sleep does not come, patients should do something else, perhaps reading, until drowsiness occurs. Whether insomnia occurs or not, the wake-up time should be strictly adhered to.

Should insomnia persist despite good sleep hygiene, consideration may be given to cognitive behavioral therapy, which is not only effective acutely (Edinger *et al.* 2001) but also confers enduring benefits (Backhaus *et al.* 2001). Should cognitive behavioral therapy be ineffective or impractical, pharmacologic treatment may be considered.

Zolpidem, 10 mg h.s., is effective (Perlis *et al.* 2004) and is perhaps the most widely prescribed hypnotic for primary insomnia; it generally has no residual effects the next day (Staner *et al.* 2005) or any rebound insomnia upon discontinuation after chronic use; there have, however, been rare reports of somnambulism with zolpidem (Morgenthaler and Silber 2002, Yang *et al.* 2005). Eszopiclone is an alternative choice (Zammit *et al.* 2004).

Melatonin was effective in one double-blind study (Zhdanova *et al.* 2001) but not another (Almeida Montes *et al.* 2003), in doses ranging from 0.1 to 6 mg given in the evening. Ramelteon, a selective melatonin receptor agonist, also appears to be effective (Erman *et al.* 2006).

Doxepin, in doses of 25 to 50 mg h.s., is effective, but in a small minority may be followed by severe rebound insomnia upon discontinuation after chronic use (Hajak *et al.* 2001). Trimipramine, another tricyclic antidepressant, is also effective in doses of 100–200 mg h.s. (Hohagen *et al.* 1994, Riemann *et al.* 2002b), and does not appear to suppress REM sleep or cause rebound insomnia. Trazodone is very widely used in doses ranging from 25–100 mg h.s.; however, there is little evidence for its effectiveness (Mendelson 2005).

Benzodiazepines (e.g., lorazepam, diazepam) and antihistamines (e.g., hydroxyzine, diphenhydramine) are often prescribed, but there are no double-blind studies supporting their use in primary insomnia.

Choosing among these various agents requires considerable clinical judgment. Given the excellent tolerability of melatonin, starting with this agent, using a dose of 3–6 mg in the evening, is a reasonable choice. At present, there are no comparative studies of melatonin and ramelteon; the latter agent, however, represents another reasonable first choice. Should melatoninergic agents fail, consideration may be given to zolpidem or eszopiclone; doxepin and trimipramine, although effective, tend to cause considerable side-effects. Trazodone should also be considered if melatoninergic agents fail.

The foregoing discussion of pharmacologic treatment concerns the psychophysiologic form of primary insomnia; in cases of idiopathic insomnia in children, melatonin, 5 mg in the evening, appears to be effective (Smits *et al.* 2001).

18.16 PRIMARY HYPERSOMNIA

Primary or essential hypersomnia is a rare disorder characterized by chronic persistent hypersomnolence (Bassetti and Aldrich 1997, Billiard *et al.* 1998).

Clinical features

The onset is gradual, typically occurring in late adolescence. Nocturnal sleep is prolonged to anywhere from 8 to 14 hours, and, upon awakening in the morning, patients are typically groggy and have trouble 'getting going'; a minority may also experience sleep drunkenness. Patients report persistent drowsiness during the day and often take long naps, which, as with their nocturnal sleep, leave them unrefreshed. Importantly, these naps do not occur as irresistible attacks but rather are preceded by a gradually increasing drowsiness, which can often be resisted.

The MSLT, although characterized by a reduced sleep latency, does not reveal sleep-onset REM.

Course

For most, primary hypersomnia is a chronic condition; spontaneous improvement is seen in only about 10 percent.

Etiology

Primary hypersomnia may occur sporadically or on a familial basis. Recent work has demonstrated reduced levels of hypocretin in the CSF (Ebrahim *et al.* 2003), suggesting hypothalamic dysfunction.

Differential diagnosis

Although some authorities subsume not only chronic but also intermittent forms of hypersomnia under the rubric of 'primary hypersomnia', in this text the diagnosis of primary hypersomnia is reserved for chronic cases only. Consequently, the first task in differential diagnosis is to determine whether the hypersomnolence is chronic or occurs in episodes. Episodic hypersomnolence may occur in the Kleine–Levin syndrome, in association with menstruation (Sachs *et al.* 1982), with intermittent use of sedating medications, and, most importantly, in certain depressive illnesses. Depressive episodes of bipolar disorder are often characterized by severe hypersomnia, and in taking the history one must be alert to other vegetative symptoms and to any history of mania.

Once it is established that the patient indeed has chronic hypersomnia, other disorders must be distinguished. Sleep disorders characterized by excessive daytime sleepiness include sleep apnea, the Pickwickian syndrome, restless legs syndrome, periodic limb movement disorder, painful legs and moving toes, and the advanced sleep phase type of circadian rhythm sleep disorder. Narcolepsy is also often considered; however, the naps seen in narcolepsy, unlike those of primary hypersomnia, come in irresistible attacks and, when they are over, leave the patient feeling refreshed; furthermore, the MSLT in narcolepsy typically demonstrates sleep-onset REM.

Excessive daytime sleepiness may also be seen in myotonic muscular dystrophy, hypothyroidism, as a sequela to infectious mononucleosis, and with lesions of the hypothalamus (Eisensehr *et al.* 2003), thalamus (Bassetti *et al.* 1996), or pons (Ganji *et al.* 1996). Chronic use of sedating medications, such as benzodiazepines, tricyclic antidepressants, certain anti-epileptic drugs, antihistamines, and opioids must also be considered on the differential.

Finally, there are individuals known as 'long sleepers' who require more than 8 hours of sleep a night. In contrast to patients with primary hypersomnia, however, these individuals awaken refreshed and are not subject to unrefreshing naps during the day.

Treatment

There are no controlled studies; case series (Bassetti and Aldrich 1997) suggest that some patients improve with stimulants, and consideration may be given to either methylphenidate or modafinil.

REFERENCES

Adie WJ. Idiopathic narcolepsy: a disease *sui generis*; with remarks on the mechanism of sleep. *Brain* 1926; **49**:257–306.

Agargun MY, Kara H, Ozbek H *et al.* Restless legs syndrome induced by mirtazapine. *J Clin Psychiatry* 2002; **63**:1179.

Ajlouni KM, Ahmad AT, El-Zaheri MM *et al.* Sleepwalking associated with hyperthyroidism. *Endocr Pract* 2005; **11**:5–10.

Aldrich MS, Naylor MW. Narcolepsy associated with lesions of the diencephalon. *Neurology* 1989; **39**:1505–8.

Allen RP, Earley CJ. Augmentation of the restless legs syndrome with carbidopa/levodopa. *Sleep* 1996; **19**:205–13.

Allen R, Barker PB, Wehrl F *et al.* MRI measurements of brain iron in patients with restless legs syndrome. *Neurology* 2001; **56**:263–5.

Almeida Montes LG, Ontiveros Uribe MP, Cortes Sotres J *et al.* Treatment of primary insomnia with melatonin: a double-blind, placebo-controlled, crossover study. *J Psychiatry Neurosci* 2003; **28**:191–6.

Arnulf I, Zeitzer JM, File J *et al.* Kleine–Levin syndrome: a systematic review of 186 cases in the literature. *Brain* 2005; **128**:2763–76.

Ayalon L, Borodkin K, Dishon L *et al.* Circadian rhythm sleep disorders following mild traumatic brain injury. *Neurology* 2007; **68**:1136–40.

Backhaus J, Hohagen F, Voderholzer U *et al.* Long-term effectiveness of a short-term cognitive-behavioral group treatment for primary insomnia. *Eur Arch Psychiatry Clin Neurosci* 2001; **251**:35–41.

Bakwin HI. Sleepwalking in twins. *Lancet* 1970; **2**:446–7.

Balon R. Sleep terror disorder and insomnia treated with trazodone: a case report. *Ann Clin Psychiatry* 1994; **6**:161–3.

Bassetti C, Aldrich MS. Idiopathic hypersomnia. A series of 42 patients. *Brain* 1997; **120**:1423–35.

Bassetti C, Mathis J, Gugger M *et al*. Hypersomnia following paramedian thalamic stroke: a report of 12 patients. *Ann Neurol* 1996; **39**:471–80.

Becker PM, Jamieson AO, Brown WD. Dopaminergic agents in restless legs syndrome and periodic limb movements of sleep: response and complications of extended treatment in 49 cases. *Sleep* 1993; **16**:713–16.

Benes H, Kurella B, Kummer J *et al*. Rapid onset of action of levodopa in restless legs syndrome: a double-blind, randomized, multicenter, crossover trial. *Sleep* 1999; **22**:1073–81.

Billiard M, Merle C, Carlander B *et al*. Idiopathic hypersomnia. *Psychiatry Clin Neurosci* 1998; **52**:125–9.

Black J, Houghton WC. Sodium oxybate improves excessive daytime sleepiness in narcolepsy. *Sleep* 2006; **29**:939–46.

Blouin AM, Thannickal TC, Worley PF *et al*. NARP immunostaining of human hypocretin (orexin) neurons. Loss in narcolepsy. *Neurology* 2005; **65**:1189–92.

Boeve BF, Silber MH, Parisi JE *et al*. Synucleinopathy pathology and REM sleep behavior disorder plus dementia or parkinsonism. *Neurology* 2003a; **61**:40–5.

Boeve BF, Silber MH, Ferman TJ. Melatonin for treatment of REM sleep behavior disorder in neurologic disorders: results in 14 patients. *Sleep Med* 2003b; **4**:281–4.

Boeve BF, Dickson DW, Olson EJ *et al*. Insights into REM sleep behavior disorder pathophysiology in brainstem-predominant Lewy body disease. *Sleep Med* 2007; **8**:60–4.

Boivin DB, James FO, Santo JB *et al*. Non-24-hour sleep-wake syndrome following a car accident. *Neurology* 2003; **60**:1841–3.

Boller F, Wright DG, Cavalieri R *et al*. Paroxysmal 'nightmares'. Sequel of a stroke responsive to diphenylhydantoin. *Neurology* 1975; **25**:1026–8.

Brodeur C, Monplaisir J, Godbout R *et al*. Treatment of restless legs syndrome and periodic movements during sleep with l-dopa: a double-blind, controlled study. *Neurology* 1988; **38**:1845–8.

Broughton RJ, Fleming JAE, George CFP *et al*. Randomized, double-blind, placebo-controlled crossover trial of modafinil in the treatment of excessive daytime sleepiness in narcolepsy. *Neurology* 1997; **49**:444–51.

Brownell LG, West P, Sweatman P *et al*. Protriptyline in obstructive sleep apnea: a double-blind trial. *N Engl J Med* 1982; **307**:1037–42.

Burstein A, Burstein A, Freehold NJ. Treatment of night terrors with imipramine. *J Clin Psychiatry* 1983; **44**:82.

Burwell CS, Robin ED, Whaley RD *et al*. Extreme obesity associated with alveolar hypoventilation: a Pickwickian syndrome. *Am J Med* 1956; **21**:811–18.

Carpenter S, Yassa R, Ochs R. A pathologic basis for Kleine–Levin syndrome. *Arch Neurol* 1982; **39**:25–8.

Cartwright RD, Lloyd S, Lilie J *et al*. Sleep position training as treatment for sleep apnea syndrome: a preliminary study. *Sleep* 1985; **8**:87–94.

Cartwright RD, Ristanovic R, Diaz F *et al*. A comparative study of treatments for positional sleep apnea. *Sleep* 1991; **14**:546–52.

Cavallo A, Ris MD, Succop P *et al*. Melatonin treatment of pediatric residents for adaptation to night shift work. *Ambul Pediatr* 2005; **5**:172–7.

Charney DS, Kales A, Soldatos CR *et al*. Somnambulistic-like episodes secondary to combined lithium-neuroleptic treatment. *Br J Psychiatry* 1979; **135**:418–24.

Chiang ST, Lee PY, Liu SY. Pulmonary function in a typical case of Pickwickian syndrome. *Respiration* 1980; **39**:105–13.

Chiles JA, Wilkus RJ. Behavioral manifestations of the Kleine–Levin syndrome. *Dis Nerv Syst* 1976; **37**:646–8.

Chisolm T, Morehouse RL. Adult headbanging: sleep studies and treatment. *Sleep* 1996; **19**:343–6.

Clavelou P, Tournilhac M, Vidal C *et al*. Narcolepsy associated with arteriovenous malformation of the diencephalon. *Sleep* 1995; **18**:202–5.

Coleman RM, Pollack CP, Weitzman ED. Periodic movements in sleep (nocturnal myoclonus): relationship to sleep disorders. *Ann Neurol* 1980; **8**:416–21.

Connor JR, Boyer PJ, Menzies SL *et al*. Neuropathological examination suggests impaired brain iron acquisition in restless legs syndrome. *Neurology* 2003; **61**:304–9.

Connor JR, Wang XS, Patton SM *et al*. Decreased transferrin receptor expression by neuromelanin cells in restless legs syndrome. *Neurology* 2004; **62**:1563–7.

Cooper AJ. Treatment of co-existent night-terrors and somnambulism in adults with imipramine and diazepam. *J Clin Psychiatry* 1987; **48**:209–10.

Critchley M. Periodic hypersomnia and megaphagia in adolescent males. *Brain* 1962; **85**:627–56.

Critchley M, Hoffman HL. The syndrome of periodic somnolence and morbid hunger (Kleine–Levin syndrome). *BMJ* 1942; **1**:137–9.

Crocker A, Espana RA, Papadopoulou M *et al*. Concomitant loss of dynorphin NARP and orexin in narcolepsy. *Neurology* 2005; **65**:1184–8.

Crowley SJ, Lee C, Tseng CY *et al*. Combinations of bright light, scheduled dark, sunglasses, and melatonin to facilitate circadian entrainment to night shift work. *J Biol Rhythms* 2003; **18**:513–23.

Culebras A, Moore JT. Magnetic resonance findings in REM sleep behavior disorder. *Neurology* 1989; **39**:1519–23.

Czeisler CA, Richardson GS, Coleman RM *et al*. Chronotherapy: resetting the circadian clocks of patients with delayed sleep phase insomnia. *Sleep* 1981; **4**:1–21.

Czeisler CA, Johnson MP, Duffy JF *et al*. Exposure to bright light and darkness to treat physiologic maladaptation to night work. *N Engl J Med* 1990; **322**:1253–9.

Czeisler CA, Walsh JK, Roth T *et al*. Modafinil for excessive daytime sleepiness associated with shift-work sleep disorder. *N Engl J Med* 2005; **353**:476–86.

Dauvilliers Y. Follow-up of four narcolepsy patients treated with intravenous immunoglobulins. *Ann Neurol* 2006; **60**:153.

Dauvilliers Y, Mayer G, Lecendreux M et al. Kleine–Levin syndrome. An autoimmune hypothesis based on clinical and genetic analyses. Neurology 2002; 59:1739–45.

Dehoorne JL, Raes AM, van Laecke E et al. Desmopressin toxicity due to prolonged half-life in 18 patients with nocturnal enuresis. J Urol 2006; 176:754–7.

Dement WC, Rechtschaffen AR, Gulevich GD. A polygraphic study of the narcoleptic sleep attacks. Electroencephalogr Clin Neurophysiol 1964; 17:608–9.

Dement WC, Rechtschaffen AR, Gulevick GD. The nature of the narcoleptic sleep attack. Neurology 1966; 16:18–33.

Dempsey OJ, McGeoch P, de Silva RN et al. Acquired narcolepsy in an acromegalic patient who underwent pituitary irradiation. Neurology 2003; 61:537–40.

Di Gennaro G, Autret A, Mascia A et al. Night terrors associated with thalamic lesion. Clin Neurophysiol 2004; 115:2489–92.

DiMario FJ, Emery ES. The natural history of night terrors. Clin Pediatr 1987; 26:505–11.

Drachman DB, Gumnit R. Periodic alteration of consciousness in the 'Pickwickian syndrome'. Arch Neurol 1962; 6:471–7.

Drake ME. Jactatio nocturna after head injury. Neurology 1986; 36:867–8.

Dressler D, Thompson PD, Marsden CD. The syndrome of painful legs and moving toes. Mov Disord 1994; 9:13–21.

Driver HS, Shapiro CM. Parasomnias. BMJ 1993; 306:921–4.

Dyken ME, Lin-Dyken DC, Seaba P et al. Violent sleep-related behavior leading to subdural hematoma. Arch Neurol 1995; 52:318–21.

Dyken ME, Yamada T, Glenn CL et al. Obstructive sleep apnea associated with cerebral hypoxemia and death. Neurology 2004; 62:491–3.

Earley CJ, Connor JR, Beard JL et al. Abnormalities in CSF concentrations of ferritin and transferrin in restless legs syndrome. Neurology 2000; 54:1698–700.

Ebrahim IO, Sharieff MK, de Laly S et al. Hypocretin (orexin) deficiency in narcolepsy and primary hypersomnia. J Neurol Neurosurg Psychiatry 2003; 74:127–30.

Edinger JD, Wohlgemuth WK, Radtke RA et al. Cognitive behavioral therapy for treatment of chronic primary insomnia: a randomized controlled trial. JAMA 2001; 285:1856–64.

Eisensehr I, Noachter S, von Schlippenbach C et al. Hypersomnia associated with bilateral posterior hypothalamic lesions. A polysomniographic case study. Eur Neurol 2003; 49:169–72.

Ekbom KA. Restless legs syndrome. Neurology 1960; 10:868–73.

Erman M, Seiden D, Zammit G et al. An efficacy, safety, and dose-response study of ramelteon in patients with chronic primary insomnia. Sleep Med 2006; 7:17–24.

Fantini ML, Michaud M, Gosselin N et al. Periodic leg movements in REM sleep behavior disorder and related autonomic and EEG activation. Neurology 2002; 59:1889–94.

Fantini ML, Gagnon J-F, Filipini D et al. The effects of pramipexole in REM sleep behavior disorder. Neurology 2003; 61:1418–20.

Fantini ML, Cona A, Clerici S et al. Aggressive dream content without daytime aggressiveness in REM sleep behavior disorder. Neurology 2005; 65:1010–15.

Fenzi F, Simonati A, Crosato F et al. Clinical features of Kleine–Levin syndrome with localized encephalitis. Neuropediatrics 1993; 24:292–5.

Fernandez J-M, Lara I, Gila L et al. Disturbed hypothalamic pituitary axis in idiopathic recurring hypersomnia syndrome. Acta Neurol Scand 1990; 82:361–3.

Ferreira JJ, Galitzky M, Montrastruc JL et al. Sleep attacks and Parkinson's disease treatment. Lancet 2000; 355:1333–4.

Fisher C, Kahn E, Edwards A et al. A psychophysiological study of nightmares and night terrors. I. Physiological aspects of the stage 4 night terror. J Nerv Ment Dis 1973a; 157:75–98.

Fisher C, Kahn E, Edwards A et al. A psychophysiological study of nightmares and night terrors: the suppression of stage 4 night terrors with diazepam. Arch Gen Psychiatry 1973b; 28:252–9.

Forsythe WI, Butler RJ. Fifty years of enuretic alarms. Arch Dis Child 1989; 64:879–85.

Forsythe WI, Redmond A. Enuresis and spontaneous cure rate of 1129 enuretics. Arch Dis Child 1974; 49:259–63.

Fournier JCM, Helguera RAL. Postencephalitic narcolepsy and cataplexy: muscle and motor nerves electrical inexcitability during the attack of cataplexy. J Nerv Ment Dis 1934; 80:159–62.

Frey J, Darbonne C. Fluoxetine suppresses human cataplexy: a pilot study. Neurology 1994; 44:707–9.

Fritz GK, Rockney RM, Yeung AS. Plasma levels and efficacy of imipramine treatment for enuresis. J Am Acad Child Adolesc Psychiatry 1994; 33:60–4.

Frucht S, Rogers JD, Greene PE et al. Falling asleep at the wheel: motor vehicle mishaps in persons taking pramipexole and ropinirole. Neurology 1999; 52:1908–10.

Gadoth N, Kesler A, Vainstein G et al. Clinical and polysomnographic characteristics of 34 patients with Kleine–Levin syndrome. J Sleep Res 2001; 10:337–41.

Gallinek A. Syndrome of episodes of hypersomnia, bulimia and abnormal mental states. JAMA 1954; 154:1081–3.

Gallinek A. The Kleine–Levin syndrome: hypersomnia, bulimia, and abnormal mental states. World Neurology 1962; 3:235–43.

Ganji SS, Ferriss GS, Rao J et al. Hypersomnia associated with a focal pontine lesion. Clin Electroencephalogr 1996; 27:52–6.

Gann H, Feige B, Fesihi S et al. Periodic limb movements during sleep in alcohol dependent patients. Eur Arch Psychiatry Clin Neurosci 2002; 252:124–9.

Garcia-Borreguero D, Larrosa O, de la Llave Y et al. Treatment of restless legs syndrome with gabapentin. A double-blind cross-over study. Neurology 2002; 59:1573–9.

Garland H, Sumner D, Fourman P. The Kleine–Levin syndrome: some further observations. Neurology 1965; 15:1161–7.

Gemignani F, Brindani F, Negrotti A et al. Restless legs syndrome and polyneuropathy. Mov Disord 2006; 21:1254–7.

George CF, Nickerson PW, Janley PJ et al. Sleep apnoea patients have more automobile accidents. Lancet 1987; 2:447.

Gilbert GJ. Periodic hypersomnia and bulimia: the Kleine–Levin syndrome. Neurology 1964; 14:844–50.

Goldberg MA. The treatment of Kleine–Levin syndrome with lithium. Can J Psychiatry 1983; 28:491–3.

Goncalves MA, Guilleminault C, Ramos E et al. Erectile dysfunction, obstructive sleep apnea syndrome and nasal CPAP treatment. Sleep Med 2005; 6:333-9.

von Gontard A, Scaumberg H, Hollmann E et al. The genetics of enuresis: a review. J Urol 2001; 166:2438-43.

Grewal M, Hawa R, Shapiro C. Treatment of periodic limb movements in sleep with selegiline HCl. Mov Disord 2002; 17:398-401.

Guilleminault C, Mignot E, Grumet FC. Familial patterns of narcolepsy. Lancet 1989; 2:1376-9.

Guilleminault C, Aftab FA, Daradeniz D et al. problems associated with switch to modafinil – a novel alerting agent in narcolepsy. Eur J Neurol 2000; 7:381-4.

Hajak G, Rodenbeck A, Voderholzer U et al. Doxepin in the treatment of primary insomnia: a placebo-controlled, double-blind, polysomnographic study. J Clin Psychiatry 2001; 62:453-63.

Hanley PJ, Zuberi-Khokhar N. Periodic limb movements during sleep in patients with congestive heart failure. Chest 1996; 109:1497-502.

Harazin J, Berigan TR. Zolpidem tartrate and somnambulism. Mil Med 1999; 164:669-70.

Harsch HH. Cyproheptadine for recurrent nightmares. Am J Psychiatry 1986; 143:1491-2.

Hartmann M, Pfister R, Pfadenhauer K. Restless legs syndrome associated with spinal cord lesions. J Neurol Neurosurg Psychiatry 1999; 66:688-9.

Hashizume V, Yoshijima H, Uchimura N et al. Case of head banging continuing into adolescence. Psychiatry Clin Neurosci 2002; 56:255-6.

Hauri P, Fisher J. Persistent psychophysiologic (learned) insomnia. Sleep 1986; 9:38-53.

Hauser RA, Gauger L, McDowell Anderson W et al. Pramipexole-induced somnolence and episodes of daytime sleep. Mov Disord 2000; 15:658-63.

Hayakawa T, Kamei Y, Urata J et al. Trials of bright light exposure and melatonin administration in a patient with non-24 hour sleep-wake syndrome. Psychiatry Clin Neurosci 1998; 52:261-2.

Hishikawa Y, Kaneko Z. Electroencephalographic study on narcolepsy. Electroencephalogr Clin Neurophysiol 1965; 18:249-59.

Hishikawa Y, Nanno H, Tachibana M et al. The nature of sleep attack and other symptoms of narcolepsy. Electroencephalogr Clin Neurophysiol 1968; 24:1-10.

Hogl B, Frauscher B, Seppi K et al. Transient restless legs syndrome after spinal anesthesia. A prospective study. Neurology 2002; 59:1705-7.

Hohagen R, Monteero RF, Weiss E et al. Treatment of primary insomnia with trimipramine: an alternative to benzodiazepine hypnotics? Eur Arch Psychiatry Clin Neurosci 1994; 244:65-72.

Hohjoh H, Takasu M, Shishikura K et al. Significant association of the arylalkylamine N-acetyltransferase (AA-NAT) gene with delayed sleep phase syndrome. Neurogenetics 2003; 4:151-3.

Huang YS, Guilleminault C, Kao PF et al. SPECT findings in the Kleine–Levin syndrome. Sleep 2005; 28:955-60.

Hublin C, Partinen M, Heinonen EH et al. Selegiline in the treatment of narcolepsy. Neurology 1994; 44:2095-101.

Hublin C, Kaprio J, Partinen M et al. Prevalence and genetics of sleepwalking: a population-based twin study. Neurology 1997; 48:177-81.

Hublin C, Kaprio J, Partinen M et al. Nightmares: familial aggregation and association with psychiatric disorders in a nationwide twin cohort. Am J Med Genet 1999; 88:329-36.

Ikeda K, Deguchi K, Touge T et al. Painful legs and moving toes syndrome associated with herpes zoster myelitis. J Neurol Sci 2004; 219:147-50.

Iranzo A, Santamaria J. Severe obstructive sleep apnea/hypopnea mimicking REM sleep behavior disorder. Sleep 2005; 28:203-6.

Iranzo A, Munoz E, Santamaria J et al. REM sleep behavior disorder and vocal cord paralysis in Machado-Joseph disease. Mov Disord 2003; 18:1179-83.

Iranz A, Graus F, Clover L et al. Rapid eye movement sleep behavior disorder and potassium channel antibody-associated limbic encephalitis. Ann Neurol 2006; 59:178-82.

Joncas S, Zadra A, Paquet J et al. The value of sleep deprivation as a diagnostic tool in adult sleepwalkers. Neurology 2002; 58:936-40.

Kales A, Kales JD. Sleep disorders: recent findings in the diagnosis and treatment of disturbed sleep. N Engl J Med 1974; 290:487-99.

Kales A, Jacobson A, Paulson MJ et al. Somnambulism: psychophysiological correlates. Arch Gen Psychiatry 1966; 14:586-94.

Kales A, Soldatos CR, Caldwell AB et al. Somnambulism: clinical characteristics and personality patterns. Arch Gen Psychiatry 1980a; 37:1406-10.

Kales A, Soldatos CR, Bixler EO et al. Hereditary factors in sleepwalking and nightmares. Br J Psychiatry 1980b; 137:111-18.

Kales A, Soldatos CR, Caldwell AB et al. Nightmares: clinical characteristics and personality patterns. Am J Psychiatry 1980c; 137:1197-201.

Kales A, Cadieux RJ, Soldatos CR et al. Narcolepsy-cataplexy. I. Clinical and electroencephalographic characteristics. Arch Neurol 1982; 39:164-8.

Kales A, Soldatos CR, Kales JD. Sleep disorders: insomnia, sleepwalking, night terrors, nightmares and enuresis. Ann Int Med 1987; 106:582-92.

Kang SY, Sohn YH, Lee IK et al. Unilateral periodic limb movements in sleep after supratentorial cerebral infarction. Parkinsonism Relat Disord 2004; 10:429-31.

Kaplan PW, Allen RP, Buchholz DW et al. A double-blind, placebo-controlled study of the treatment of periodic limb movements in sleep using carbidopa/levodopa and propoxyphene. Sleep 1993; 16:7171-23.

Kavey NB, Whyte J, Resor SR et al. Somnambulism in adults. Neurology 1990; 40:749-52.

Kawashima T, Yamada S. Paroxetine-induced somnambulism. J Clin Psychiatry 2003; 64:483.

Kawauchi A, Inoue Y, Hashimotot T et al. Restless legs syndrome in hemodialysis patients: health-related quality of life and laboratory data analysis. Clin Nephrol 2006; 66:440-6.

Kayumov L, Brown G, Jindal R et al. A randomized, double-blind, placebo-controlled crossover study of the effect of exogenous melatonin on delayed sleep phase syndrome. *Psychosom Med* 2001; **63**:40–8.

Kellner R, Neidhardt J, Krakow B et al. Changes in chronic nightmares after one session of desensitization or rehearsal instructions. *Am J Psychiatry* 1992; **149**:659–63.

Kessler R, Chaouat A, Shinkewitch P et al. The obesity-hypoventilation syndrome revisited: a prospective study of 34 consecutive cases. *Chest* 2001; **120**:369–76.

Khazaal Y, Krenz S, Zullino DF. Bupropion-induced somnambulism. *Addict Biol* 2003; **8**:359–62.

Kim JS, Lee SB, Park SK et al. Periodic limb movement during sleep developed after pontine lesion. *Mov Disord* 2003; **18**:1403–5.

Kimura K, Tachbana N, Kohyama J et al. A discrete pontine ischemic lesion could cause REM sleep behavior disorder. *Neurology* 2000; **55**:894–5.

Kingshott RN, Vennelle M, Coleman EL et al. Randomized, double-blind, placebo-controlled crossover trial of modafinil in the treatment of residual excessive daytime sleepiness in the sleep apnea-hypopnea syndrome. *Am J Respir Crit Care Med* 2001; **163**:918–23.

Kleine W. Periodische schlafsucht. *Monatsschriff fur Psychiatrie und Neurologie* 1925; **57**:285–320.

Koerber RK, Torkelson R, Haven G et al. Increased cerebrospinal fluid 5-hydroxytryptamine and 5-hydroxyindoleacetic acid in Kleine–Levin syndrome. *Neurology* 1984; **34**:1597–600.

Kolivakis TT, Margolese HC, Beauclair L et al. Olanzapine induced somnambulism. *Am J Psychiatry* 2001; **158**:1158.

Kraiczi H, Hedner J, Dahlof et al. Effect of serotonin reuptake inhibition on breathing during sleep and daytime symptoms in obstructive sleep apnea. *Sleep* 1999; **22**:61–7.

Kramer NR, Bonitati AE, Millman RP. Enuresis and obstructive sleep apnea. *Chest* 1998; **114**:634–7.

Kravitz H, Rosenthall V, Teplitz Z et al. A study of head-banging in infants and children. *Dis Nerv Syst* 1960; **21**:203–8.

Krishnan PR, Bhatia M, Behari M. Restless legs syndrome in Parkinson's disease: a case-controlled study. *Mov Disord* 2003; **18**:181–5.

Lankford DA, Wellman J, O'Hara C. Posttraumatic narcolepsy in mild to moderate closed head injury. *Sleep* 1994; **17**(suppl. 8):S25–8.

Lee JW. Recurrent delirium associated with obstructive sleep apnea. *Gen Hosp Psychiatry* 1998; **20**:120–2.

Lee MS, Choi YC, Lee SH et al. Sleep-related periodic leg movements associated with spinal cord lesions. *Mov Disord* 1996; **11**:719–22.

Levchenko A, Provost S, Montplaisir J-Y et al. A novel autosomal dominant restless legs syndrome locus maps to chromosome 20p13. *Neurology* 2006; **67**:900–1.

Levin M. Periodic somnolence and morbid hunger: a new syndrome. *Brain* 1936; **59**:494–504.

Louden MB, Morehead MA, Schmidt HS. Activation by selegiline (Eldepryl) of REM sleep behavior disorder in parkinsonism. *W V Med J* 1995; **91**:101.

McArthur AJ, Levy AJ, Sack RL. Non-24 hour sleep-wake syndrome in a sighted man: circadian rhythm studies and efficacy of melatonin treatment. *Sleep* 1996; **19**:544–53.

Malow BA, Levy K, Maturen K et al. Obstructive sleep apnea is common in medically refractory epilepsy patients. *Neurology* 2000; **55**:1002–7.

Manconi M, Govoni V, De Vito A et al. Restless legs syndrome and pregnancy. *Neurology* 2004; **63**:1065–9.

Manconi M, Fabbrini M, Bonanni E et al. High prevalence of restless legs syndrome in multiple sclerosis. *Eur J Neurol* 2007; **14**:534–9.

Manni R, Terzaghi M, Zambrelli E et al. Interictal, potentially misleading, epileptiform EEG abnormalities in REM sleep behavior disorder. *Sleep* 2006; **29**:934–7.

Mayer G, Ewert Meier K, Hephata K. Selegiline hydrochloride treatment in narcolepsy: a double-blind, placebo-controlled study. *Clin Neuropharmacol* 1995; **18**:306–19.

Mellman TA, Uhde TW. Sleep panic attacks: new clinical findings and theoretical implications. *Am J Psychiatry* 1989a; **146**:1204–7.

Mellman TA, Uhde TW. Electroencephalographic sleep in panic disorder: a focus on sleep-related panic attacks. *Arch Gen Psychiatry* 1989b; **46**:178–89.

Mellman TA, Uhde TW. Patients with frequent sleep panic: clinical findings and response to medication treatment. *J Clin Psychiatry* 1990; **51**:513–16.

Mendelson WB. Are periodic leg movements associated with clinical sleep disturbance? *Sleep* 1996; **19**:219–23.

Mendelson WB. A review of the evidence for the efficacy and safety of trazodone in insomnia. *J Clin Psychiatry* 2005; **66**:469–76.

Mendelson WB, Garnett D, Gillin JC. Single case study: flurazepam-induced sleep apnea syndrome in a patient with insomnia and mild sleep-related respiratory changes. *J Nerv Ment Dis* 1981; **169**:261–4.

Mignot E, Lammers GJ, Ripley B et al. The role of cerebrospinal fluid hypocretin measurement in the diagnosis of narcolepsy and other hypersomnias. *Arch Neurol* 2002; **59**; 1553–62.

Mikkelsen EJ, Rapoport JL, Nee L et al. Childhood enuresis. I. Sleep patterns and psychopathology. *Arch Gen Psychiatry* 1980; **37**:1139–44.

Millman RP, Fogel BS, McNamara ME et al. Depression as a manifestation of obstructive sleep apnea: reversal with nasal continuous positive airway pressure. *J Clin Psychiatry* 1989; **50**:348–51.

Mitler MM, Shafor R, Hajdukovich R et al. Treatment of narcolepsy: objective studies on methylphenidate, pemoline, and protriptyline. *Sleep* 1986a; **9**:260–4.

Mitler MM, Browman CP, Menn SJ et al. Nocturnal myoclonus: treatment efficacy of clonazepam and temazepam. *Sleep* 1986b; **9**:385–92.

Montagna P, Cirignotta F, Sacquegna T et al. 'Painful legs and moving toes' associated with polyneuropathy. *J Neurol Neurosurg Psychiatry* 1983; **46**:399–403.

Montplaisir J, Boucher S, Poirier G et al. Clinical, polysomnographic and genetic characteristics of restless legs syndrome: a study of 133 patients diagnosed with new standard criteria. *Mov Disord* 1997; **12**:61–5.

Montplaisir J, Nicolas A, Denesle R et al. Restless legs syndrome improved by pramipexole: a double-blind randomized trial. *Neurology* 1999; **52**:938–43.

Morgenthaler TI, Silber MH. Amnestic sleep-related eating disorder associated with zolpidem. *Sleep Med* 2002; **3**:323–7.

Munoz X, Marti S, Sumalla J *et al.* Acute delirium as a manifestation of obstructive sleep apnea syndrome. *Am J Respir Crit Care Med* 1998; **158**:1306–7.

Muratori R, Bertini N, Masi G. Efficacy of lithium treatment in Kleine–Levin syndrome. *Eur Psychiatry* 2002; **17**; 232–3.

Nakamura K, Hashimoto S, Honma S *et al.* Daily melatonin intake resets circadian rhythms of a sighted man with non-24 hour sleep-wake syndrome who lacks the nocturnal melatonin rise. *Psychiatry Clin Neurosci* 1997; **51**:121–7.

Nathan PW. Painful legs and moving toes: evidence on the site of the lesion. *J Neurol Neurosurg Psychiatry* 1978; **41**:934–9.

Neveus T, Stenberg A, Lackgren G *et al.* Sleep of children with enuresis: a polysomnographic study. *Pediatrics* 1999; **103**:1193–7.

Neidhardt EJ, Krakow B, Kellner R. The beneficial effects of one treatment session and recording of nightmares on chronic nightmare sufferers. *Sleep* 1992; **15**:470–3.

Nofzinger EA, Fasiczka A, Berman S *et al.* Buropion SR reduces periodic limb movements associated with arousals from sleep in depressed patients with periodic limb movement disorder. *J Clin Psychiatry* 2000; **61**:858–62.

Nowbar S, Burkart KM, Gonzales R *et al.* Obesity-associated hypoventilation in hospitalized patients: prevalence, effects, and outcome. *Am J Med* 2004; **116**:58–9.

Odeh M, Oliven A. Coma and seizures due to severe hyponatremia and water intoxication in an adult with intranasal desmopressin therapy for nocturnal enuresis. *J Clin Pharmacol* 2001; **41**:582–4.

Ogura C, Okuma T, Nakazawa A. Treatment of periodic somnolence with lithium carbonate. *Arch Neurol* 1976; **33**:143.

Ohanna N, Peled R, Rubin AH *et al.* Periodic leg movements in sleep: effect of clonazepam treatment. *Neurology* 1985; **35**:408–11.

Olson EJ, Boeve BF, Silber MH. Rapid eye movement sleep behavior disorder: demographic, clinical and laboratory findings in 93 cases. *Brain* 2000; **123**:331–9.

Ondo W, Jankovic J. Restless legs syndrome: clinicopathologic correlates. *Neurology* 1996; **47**:1435–41.

Ondo W, Romanyshyn J, Vuong KD *et al.* Long-term treatment of restless legs syndrome with dopamine agonists. *Arch Neurol* 2004; **61**:1393–7.

Onofrj M, Luciano AL, Thomas A *et al.* Mirtazapine induces REM sleep behavior disorder (RBD) in parkinsonism. *Neurology* 2003; **60**:113–15.

Oswald I. Sudden bodily jerks on falling asleep. *Brain* 1959; **82**:92–103.

Palm L, Blennow G, Wetterberg L. Correction of non-24 hour sleep/wake cycle by melatonin in a blind retarded boy. *Ann Neurol* 1991; **29**:336–9.

Parkes JD. The parasomnias. *Lancet* 1986; **2**:1021–5.

Parkes JD, Baraitser M, Marsden CD *et al.* Natural history of symptoms and treatment of the narcoleptic syndrome. *Acta Neurol Scand* 1975; **52**:337–53.

Pedley TA, Guilleminault C. Episodic nocturnal wanderings responsive to anticonvulsant drug therapy. *Ann Neurol* 1977; **2**:30–5.

Peled R, Lavie P. Double-blind evaluation of clonazepam on periodic leg movements in sleep. *J Neurol Neurosurg Psychiatry* 1987; **50**:1679–81.

Pereira DS, Tufik S, Louzada FM *et al.* Association of the length polymorphism in the human Per3 gene with the delayed sleep phase syndrome: does latitude have an influence upon it? *Sleep* 2005; **28**:29–32.

Perlis ML, McCall WV, Krystal AD *et al.* Long-term, non-nightly administration of zolpidem in the treatment of patients with primary insomnia. *J Clin Psychiatry* 2004; **65**:1128–37.

Perroud N, Lazignac C, Baleydier B *et al.* Restless legs syndrome induced by citalopram: a psychiatric emergency? *Gen Hosp Psychiatry* 2007; **29**:72–4.

Peyron C, Faraco J, Rogers W *et al.* A mutation in a case of early onset narcolepsy and a generalized absence of hypocretin peptides in human narcoleptic brains. *Nat Med* 2000; **6**:991–7.

Pierce CM, Whitman RM, Gay ML. Enuresis and dreaming: experimental studies. *Arch Gen Psychiatry* 1961; **4**:166–70.

Pike M, Stores G. Kleine–Levin syndrome: a cause of diagnostic confusion. *Arch Dis Child* 1994; **71**:355–7.

Pillar G, Etzioni A, Shahar E *et al.* Melatonin treatment in an institutionalized child with psychomotor retardation and an irregular sleep-wake pattern. *Arch Dis Child* 1998; **79**:63–4.

Pittock SJ, Parrett T, Adler CH *et al.* Neuropathology of primary restless legs syndrome: absence of specific tau- and alpha-synucelin pathology. *Mov Disord* 2004; **19**:695–9.

Pla MER, Dillingham TR, Spellman LT *et al.* Painful legs and moving toes associated with tarsal tunnel syndrome and accessory soleus muscle. *Mov Disord* 1996; **11**:82–6.

Plazzi G, Montagna P. Remitting REM sleep behavior disorder as the initial sign of multiple sclerosis. *Sleep Med* 2002; **3**:437–9.

Plazzi G, Corsini R, Provini F *et al.* REM sleep behavior disorders in multiple system atrophy. *Neurology* 1997; **48**:1094–7.

Polydefkis M, Allen RP, Hauer P *et al.* Subclinical sensory neuropathy in late-onset restless legs syndrome. *Neurology* 2000; **55**:1115–21.

Poppe M, Freibel D, Reuner U *et al.* The Kleine–Levin syndrome – effects of treatment with lithium. *Neuropediatrics* 2003; **34**:113–19.

Poryazova R, Siccoli M, Werth E *et al.* Unusually prolonged rebound cataplexy after withdrawal of fluoxetine. *Neurology* 2005; **65**:967–8.

Quinto C, Gellido C, Chokroverty S *et al.* Posttraumatic delayed sleep phase syndrome. *Neurology* 2000; **54**:250–2.

Rangarajan S, D'Souza GA. Restless legs syndrome in Indian patients having iron deficiency anemia in a tertiary care hospital. *Sleep Med* 2007; **8**:247–51.

Rechtschaffen A, Wolpert EA, Dement WC *et al.* Nocturnal sleep of narcoleptics. *Electroencephalogr Clin Neurophysiol* 1963; **15**:599–609.

Reid KJ, Chang AM, Dubocovich ML *et al.* Familial advanced sleep phase syndrome. *Arch Neurol* 2001; **58**:1089–94.

Reid WH, Haffke EA, Chu CC. Diazepam in intractable sleepwalking: a pilot study. *Hillside J Clin Psychiatry* 1984; **6**:49–55.

Reynolds CF, Black RS, Coble P *et al.* Similarities in EEG sleep findings for Kleine–Levin syndrome and unipolar depression. *Am J Psychiatry* 1980; **137**:116–18.

Reynolds CF, Kupfer DJ, Christiansen CL *et al.* Multiple sleep latency test findings in Kleine–Levin syndrome. *J Nerv Ment Dis* 1984; **172**:41–4.

Riemann D, Klein T, Todenbeck A *et al.* Nocturnal cortisol and melatonin secretion in primary insomnia. *Psychiatry Res* 2002a; **113**:17–27.

Riemann D, Voderholzer U, Cohrs S *et al.* Trimipramine in primary insomnia: results of a polysomnographic double-blind study. *Pharmacopsychiatry* 2002b; **35**:165–74.

Rijsman RM, de Weerd AW, Stam CJ *et al.* Periodic limb movement disorder and restless legs syndrome in dialysis patients. *Nephrology* 2004; **9**:353–61.

Ringman JM, Simmons JH. Treatment of REM sleep behavior disorder with donepezil; a report of three cases. *Neurology* 2000; **55**:870–1.

Roehrs TA, Zorick FJ, Wittig RM *et al.* Alerting effects of naps in patients with narcolepsy. *Sleep* 1986; **9**:194–9.

Rogers AE, Aldrich MS, Liu X. A comparison of three different sleep schedules for reducing daytime sleepiness in narcolepsy. *Sleep* 2001; **24**:385–91.

Roizenblatt S, Guilleminault C, Poyares D *et al.* A double-blind, placebo-controlled, crossover study of sildenafil in obstructive sleep apnea. *Arch Int Med* 2006; **166**:1763–7.

Rosenfeld MR, Elchen JG, Wade DF *et al.* Molecular and clinical diversity in paraneoplastic immunity to Ma proteins. *Ann Neurol* 2001; **50**:339–48.

Sachs S, Persson HE, Hagenfeldt K. Menstruation-related periodic hypersomnia: a case study with successful treatment. *Neurology* 1982; **32**:1376–9.

Sagar RS, Khandelwal SK, Gupta S. Interepisodic morbidity in Kleine–Levin syndrome. *Br J Psychiatry* 1990; **157**:139–41.

Saletu M, Anderer P, Saletu-Zyhlarz G *et al.* Restless legs syndrome (RLS) and periodic limb movement disorder (PLMD): acute placebo-controlled sleep laboratory studies with clonazepam. *Eur Neuropsychopharmacol* 2001; **11**:153–61.

Sandberg O, Franklin KA, Bucht G *et al.* Sleep apnea, delirium, depressed mood, cognition and ADL ability after stroke. *J Am Geriatr Soc* 2001; **49**:391–7.

Sanz-Fuentenebro FJ, Huidobro A, Tejadas-Rivas A *et al.* Restless legs syndrome and paroxetine. *Acta Psychiatr Scand* 1996; **94**:482–4.

Sattar SP, Ramaswamy S, Bhatia SC, Petty F. Somnambulism due to a probable interaction of valproic acid and zolpidem. *Ann Pharmacother* 2003; **37**:1429–33.

Scammell TE, Nishino S, Mignot E *et al.* Narcolepsy and low CSF orexin (hypocretin) concentration after a diencephalic stroke. *Neurology* 2001; **56**:1751–3.

Schacter M, Parkes JD. Fluvoxamine and clomipramine in the treatment of cataplexy. *J Neurol Neurosurg Psychiatry* 1980; **43**:171–4.

Scheltens P, Visscher F, Van Keimpema ARJ *et al.* Sleep apnea syndrome presenting with cognitive impairment. *Neurology* 1991; **41**:155.

Schenck CH, Mahowald MW. Polysomnographic, neurologic, psychiatric, and clinical outcome report on 70 consecutive cases with REM sleep behavior disorder (RBD): sustained clonazepam efficacy in 89.5 percent of 57 treated patients. *Cleve Clin J Med* 1990; **57**(suppl.):S9–23.

Schenck CH, Mahowald MW. Motor dyscontrol in narcolepsy: rapid-eye-movement (REM) sleep without atonia and REM sleep behavior disorder. *Ann Neurol* 1992; **32**:3–10.

Schenck CH, Bundlie SR, Ettinger MG *et al.* Chronic behavioral disorders of human REM sleep: a new category of parasomnia. *Sleep* 1986; **9**:293–308.

Schenck CH, Bundlie SR, Patterson AL *et al.* Rapid eye movement sleep behavior disorder. A treatable parasomnia affecting older adults. *JAMA* 1987; **257**:1786–9.

Schenck CH, Milner DM, Hurwitz TD *et al.* A polysomnographic and clinical report on sleep-related injury in 100 adult patients. *Am J Psychiatry* 1989; **146**:1166–73.

Schenck CH, Bundlie SR, Mahowald MW. Delayed emergence of a parkinsonian disorder in 38% of 29 older men initially diagnosed with idiopathic rapid eye movement sleep behavior disorder. *Neurology* 1996a; **46**:388–93.

Schenck CH, Garcia-Rill E, Skinner RD *et al.* A case of REM sleep behavior disorder with autopsy-confirmed Alzheimer's disease: postmortem brain stem histochemical analyses. *Biol Psychiatry* 1996b; **40**:422–5.

Schmidauer C, Sojer M, Seppi K *et al.* Transcranial ultrasound shows migral hypoechogenicity in restless legs syndrome. *Ann Neurol* 2005; **58**:630–4.

Schmidt MH, Koshal VB, Schmidt HS. Use of pramipexole in REM sleep behavior disorder: results from a case series. *Sleep Med* 2006; **7**:418–23.

Schott GD. 'Painful legs and moving toes': the role of trauma. *J Neurol Neurosurg Psychiatry* 1981; **44**:344–6.

Schulman SI, Stokes A, Salzman PM. The efficacy and safety of oral desmopressin in children with primary nocturnal enuresis. *J Urol* 2001; **166**:2427–31.

Schwartz JRL, Feldman NT, Bogan RK. Dose effects of modafinil in sustaining wakefulness in narcolepsy patients with residual evening sleepiness. *J Neuropsychiatry Clin Neurosci* 2005a; **17**:405–12.

Schwartz DJ, Kohler WC, Katarinos G. Symptoms of depression in individuals with obstructive sleep apnea may be amenable to treatment with continuous positive airway pressure. *Chest* 2005b; **128**:1304–9.

Scrima L, Broudy M, Nay KN *et al.* Increased severity of obstructive sleep apnea after bedtime alcohol ingestion: diagnostic potential and proposed mechanism of action. *Sleep* 1982; **5**:318–28.

Sieker HO, Estes EH, Kelser GA *et al.* Cardiopulmonary syndrome with extreme obesity. *J Clin Invest* 1955; **34**:916.

Smith PL, Gold AR, Meyers DA *et al.* Weight loss in mildly to moderately obese patients with obstructive sleep apnea. *Ann Intern Med* 1985; **103**:850–5.

Smith RC. Relationship of periodic movements in sleep (nocturnal myoclonus) and the Babinski sign. *Sleep* 1985; **8**:239–43.

Smits MG, Nagtegaal EE, van der Heijden J et al. Melatonin for chronic sleep onset insomnia in children: a randomized placebo-controlled trial. J Child Neurol 2001; **16**:86–92.

Sonka K, Kemlink D, Pretl M. Cataplexy treated with escitalopram – clinical experience. Neurol Endocrinol Lett 2006; **27**:174–6.

Sours JA, Frumkin P, Indermill RR. Somnambulism: its clinical significance and dynamic meaning in late adolescence and adulthood. Arch Gen Psychiatry 1963; **9**:400–13.

Spillane JD, Nathan PW, Kelly RE et al. Painful legs and moving toes. Brain 1971; **94**:541–56.

Staedt J, Stoppe G, Kogler A et al. Nocturnal myoclonus syndrome (periodic movements in sleep) related to central dopamine D2-receptor alteration Eur Arch Psychiatry Clin Neurosci 1995; **245**:8–10.

Stahl SM, Layzer RB, Aminoff MJ et al. Continuous cataplexy in a patient with a midbrain tumor: the limp man syndrome. Neurology 1980; **30**:1115–18.

Staner L, Ertle S, Boeijinga P et al. Next-day residual effects of hypnotics in DSM-IV primary insomnia: a driving simulator study with simultaneous electroencephalographic monitoring. Psychopharmacology 2005; **181**:790–8.

Steiner MC, Ward MJ, Ali NJ. Dementia and snoring. Lancet 1999; **353**:204.

Strollo PJ, Rogers RM. Obstructive sleep apnea. N Engl J Med 1996; **334**:99–104.

Suhner A, Schlagenhauf P, Hofer I et al. Effectiveness and tolerability of melatonin and zolpidem for the alleviation of jet lag. Aviat Space Environ Med 2001; **72**:638–46.

Sutton FD, Zwillich CW, Creagh CE et al. Progesterone for outpatient treatment of Pickwickian syndrome. Ann Intern Med 1975; **83**:476–9.

Takano A, Uchiyama M, Kajimura N et al. A missense variation in human casein kinase I epsilon gene that induces functional alteration and shows an inverse association with circadian rhythm sleep disorders. Neuropsychopharmacology 2004; **29**:1901–9.

Tan A, Selgado M, Fahn S. Rapid eye movement sleep behavior disorder preceding Parkinson's disease with therapeutic response to levodopa. Mov Disord 1996; **11**:214–16.

Thirumalai SS, Shubin RA. The use of citalopram in resistant cataplexy. Sleep Med 2000; **1**:313–16.

Tinuper P, Cerullo A, Cirignotta F et al. Nocturnal paroxysmal dystonia: three cases with evidence for an epileptic frontal lobe origin of seizures. Epilepsia 1990; **31**:549–56.

Tippmann-Peikert M, Boeve BF, Keegam BM. REM sleep behavior disorder initiated by acute brainstem multiple sclerosis. Neurology 2006; **66**:1277–9.

Tippmann-Peikert M, Park G, Boeve BF et al. Pathologic gambling in patients with restless legs syndrome treated with dopaminergic agonists. Neurology 2007; **68**:301–3.

Tobin JD. Treatment of somnambulism with anticipatory awakening. J Pediatr 1993; **122**:426–7.

Trenkwalder C, Seidel VC, Gasser T et al. Clinical symptoms and possible anticipation in a large kindred of familial restless legs syndrome. Mov Disord 1996; **11**:389–94.

Trenkwalder C, Garcia-Borreguero D, Montagna P et al. Ropinirole in the treatment of restless legs syndrome: results from the TREAT RLS 1 study, a 12 week, randomized, placebo controlled study in 10 European countries. J Neurol Neurosurg Psychiatry 2004; **75**:92–7.

Turner RS, D'Amato CJ, Chervin RD et al. The pathology of REM sleep behavior disorder with comorbid Lewy body dementia. Neurology 2000; **55**:1730–2.

Uchiyama M, Isse K, Tanaka K et al. Incidental Lewy body disease in a patient with REM sleep behavior disorder. Neurology 1995; **45**:709–12.

US Modafinil in Narcolepsy Multicenter Study Group. Randomized trial of modafinil for the treatment of pathological somnolence in narcolepsy. Ann Neurol 1998; **43**:88–97.

US Modafinil in Narcolepsy Multicenter Study Group. Randomized trial of modafinil as a treatment for the excessive daytime sleepiness of narcolepsy. Neurology 2000; **54**:1166–75.

Wagner ML, Walters AS, Coleman RG et al. Randomized, double-blind, placebo-controlled study of clonidine in restless legs syndrome. Sleep 1996; **19**:52–8.

Walters AS, Hening W, Rubinstein M et al. A clinical and polysomnographic comparison of neuroleptic-induced akathisia and the idiopathic restless legs syndrome. Sleep 1991; **14**:339–45.

Walters AS, Wagner ML, Hening WA et al. Successful treatment of idiopathic restless legs syndrome in a randomized double-blind trial of oxycodone versus placebo. Sleep 1993; **16**:327–32.

Ward WA, Kelsey WM. The Pickwickian syndrome: a review of the literature and report of a case. J Pediatr 1962; **61**:745–50.

Ware JC, Brown FU, Moorad PJ et al. Nocturnal myoclonus and tricyclic antidepressants. Sleep Res 1984; **13**:72.

Watanabe T, Kajimura N, Kato M et al. Effects of phototherapy in patients with delayed sleep phase syndrome. Psychiatry Clin Neurosci 1999; **53**:231–3.

de Weerd AW, Rijsman RM, Brinkley A. Activity patterns of leg muscles in periodic limb movement disorder. J Neurol Neurosurg Psychiatry 2004; **75**:317–19.

Weitzman ED, Cseisler CA, Coleman RM et al. Delayed sleep phase syndrome. A chronobiological disorder with sleep-onset insomnia. Arch Gen Psychiatry 1981; **38**:737–46.

White DP, Zwillich CW, Pickett CK et al. Central sleep apnea. Improvement with acetazolamide therapy. Arch Int Med 1982; **142**:1816–19.

Whitney JF, Gannon DE. Obstructive sleep apnea presenting as acute delirium. Am J Emerg Med 1996; **14**:270–1.

Whyte KF, Allen MB, Jeffrey AA et al. Clinical features of the sleep apnoea/hypopnoea syndrome. Q J Med 1989; **72**:659–66.

Whyte J, Kavey NB, Gidro-Frank S. A self-destructive variant of jactatio capitis nocturna. J Nerv Ment Dis 1991; **179**:49–50.

Will RG, Young JPR, Thomas DJ. Kleine-Levin syndrome: report of two cases with onset of symptoms precipitated by head trauma. Br J Psychiatry 1988; **152**:410–12.

Wilson SAK. The narcolepsies. Brain 1928; **51**:63–109.

Wilson SJ, Lillywhite AR, Potokar JP et al. Adult night terrors and paroxetine. Lancet 1997; **350**:185.

Winkelmann JW, Chertow GM, Lazarus JM. Restless legs syndrome in end-stage renal disease. Am J Kidney Dis 1996; **28**:372–8.

Winkelmann J, Wetter TC, Collado-Seidel V *et al.* Clinical characteristics of the hereditary restless legs syndrome in a population of 300 patients. *Sleep* 2000; **23**:597–602.

Winkelmann J, Muller-Myhsok B, Wittchen H-U *et al.* Complex segregation analysis of restless legs syndrome provides evidence of an autosomal dominant mode of inheritance in early age at onset families. *Ann Neurol* 2002; **52**:297–302.

Winkelmann JW, Sethi KD, Kushida CA *et al.* Efficacy and safety of pramipexole in restless legs syndrome. *Neurology* 2006; **67**:1034–9.

Wyatt JK. Delayed sleep phase syndrome: pathophysiology and treatment options. *Sleep* 2004; **27**:1195–203.

Xu Y, Padiath QS, Shapiro RE *et al.* Functional consequences of a CKIdelta mutation causing familial advanced sleep phase syndrome. *Nature* 2005; **434**:640–4.

Yaggi HK, Concato J, Kernan WM *et al.* Obstructive sleep apnea as a risk factor for stroke and death. *N Engl J Med* 2005; **353**:2034–45.

Yang W, Dollear M, Muthukrishnan SR. One rare side effect of zolpidem – sleepwalking: a case report. *Arch Phys Med Rehabil* 2005; **86**:1265–6.

Zambelis T, Paparrigopoulos T, Soldatos CR. REM sleep behavior disorder associated with a neurinoma of the left pontocerebellar angle. *J Neurol Neurosurg Psychiatry* 2002; **72**:821–2.

Zammit GK, McNabb LJ, Caron J *et al.* Efficacy and safety of eszopiclone across 6 weeks of treatment for primary insomnia. *Curr Med Res Opin* 2004; **20**:1979–91.

Zhdanova IV, Wurtman RJ, Regan MM *et al.* Melatonin treatment for age-related insomnia. *J Clin Endocrincol Metabol* 2001; **86**:4727–30.

19

Brain tumors and hydrocephalus

19.1 BRAIN TUMORS

Neoplastic brain tumors may be broadly divided into two types, namely those neoplasms that are primary to the brain, such as gliomas or meningiomas, and those that represent metastases from systemic cancers, such as lung or breast cancer.

Clinical features

Although brain tumors may occur at any age, most patients are middle-aged or older. The onset itself ranges from acute to insidious, depending in large part on the aggressiveness of the tumor involved. Certain gliomas, such as glioblastoma multiforme, may evolve rapidly over several weeks or months, whereas some meningiomas may attain a large size without ever causing symptoms (Olivero *et al.* 1995) and may indeed be found incidentally on imaging for other reasons or at autopsy.

The symptomatology of brain tumors varies according to their location, size, the extent of peri-tumoral vasogenic edema, and the appearance of increased intracranial pressure; there is generally little room for expansion within the intracranial vault and, with growth of a tumor and, especially, expansion of vasogenic edema, there is an inevitable rise in overall intracranial pressure, which may eventually produce symptoms in its own right.

The overall symptomatology seen with brain tumors may be divided into the following domains: *headache*; *non-focal symptoms*; *focal signs and specific syndromes*, such as dementia or personality change; and *seizures*. Each of these is considered in turn below.

Headache (Forsyth and Posner 1993) may be generalized or have a unilateral predominance, in which case it may have some lateralizing value. The headache itself tends to be dull and may be severe. Classically, it is worst in the morning upon awakening and is worsened by recumbancy.

In most cases the headache reflects stretching of pain-sensitive structures; should increased intracranial pressure occur, the headache may worsen and be joined, classically, by projectile vomiting.

Non-focal symptoms often reflect increased intracranial pressure and may include dizziness, 'fuzziness' of thought, and somnolence (Davison and Demuth 1945, 1946; McKendree and Feinier 1927).

Focal signs and specific syndromes typically reflect compression of brain tissue by the tumor mass or peri-tumoral edema. Traditional focal signs, such as hemiplegia, aphasia, apraxia, and hemianopia, may occur and may serve to both lateralize and localize the tumor; compression or stretching of cranial nerves may result in appropriate cranial nerve palsies. Specific syndromes seen with tumors include, most commonly, dementia and personality change; other specific syndromes, seen in a small minority, include delirium, amnesia, mania, depression, and psychosis.

Dementia is classically seen with tumors of the frontal lobe (Sachs 1950) or corpus callosum (Alpers and Grant 1931; Moersch 1925), and in such cases it is often accompanied by apathy, dullness, and somnolence (Williamson 1896) or by a frontal lobe syndrome (Frazier 1936). Tumors of the thalamus and hypothalamus (Alpers 1937; Liss 1958; Strauss and Globus 1931) may also cause dementia, and with hypothalamic tumors one often sees additional symptoms (Beal *et al.* 1981), such as hypersomnolence, weight gain or diabetes insipidus.

Personality change may be seen with tumors of the frontal lobe (Direkze *et al.* 1971; Strauss and Keschner 1935) or temporal lobe and, rarely, with tumors of the thalamus or hypothalamus. Although this personality change may be non-specific, in cases of frontal lobe tumors one classically sees an accompanying frontal lobe syndrome (Avery 1971).

Delirium may occur with tumors of the temporal lobe (Keschner *et al.* 1936) or the hypothalamus (Alpers 1940).

Amnesia, with isolated short-term memory loss, may be seen with tumors that impinge on any part of the circuit of

Papez, for example the fornix (e.g., by a subsplenial tumor), the mamillary bodies (e.g., by a craniopharyngioma), and the thalamus.

Mania may uncommonly occur with tumors of the mesencephalon, hypothalamus, thalamus, cingulate gyrus, or frontal lobe.

Depression may rarely constitute the presentation of a tumor, as has been noted with a tumor of the anterior portion of the corpus callosum (Ironside and Guttmacher 1929).

Psychosis may occur with tumors, most commonly of the temporal lobe (Gal 1958; Keschner et al. 1936; Malamud 1967; Strobos 1953; Tucker et al. 1986); other locations include the frontal lobe (Strauss and Keschner 1935) and the corpus callosum (Murthy et al. 1997).

Finally, a few words are in order regarding tumors located in the hypothalamus. As noted earlier, these may present with dementia, personality change, delirium, amnesia, or mania. Other symptoms may also be seen, including diabetes insipidus, anorexia with profound weight loss (Heron and Johnston 1976; White et al. 1977), and hyperphagia with extreme weight gain (Fulton and Bailey 1929; Liss 1958), which may, in rare instances, be accompanied by episodic rage (Haugh and Markesbery 1983; Reeves and Plum 1969).

Seizures are eventually seen in approximately one-third of all brain tumor cases, and may be simple partial, complex partial, or grand mal in type. In some cases of small, slowly growing tumors, such as oligodendrogliomas or low-grade astrocytomas, seizures may constitute the sole symptomatology of the underlying tumor for long periods of time.

With growth of the tumor and enlargement of the area of peri-tumoral edema, the clinical picture evolves, with worsening of initial symptoms and addition of new ones. In some cases, hydrocephalus may occur, with symptoms as discussed in Section 19.2. In other cases, there may be acute clinical exacerbations due to either intratumoral hemorrhage or infarction secondary to arterial compression.

Magnetic resonance (MR) scanning should, if possible, be obtained in all cases, and this should generally be with gadolinium enhancement. Computed tomography (CT) scanning, again with enhancement, is an alternative, but far less sensitive technique.

Lumbar puncture, although not routine, may be appropriate when certain tumors are suspected, such as primary central nervous system lymphoma or leptomeningeal carcinomatosis.

Although in most cases of metastatic disease the systemic cancer is already known, in a minority of cases, perhaps up to one-quarter, the metastasis represents the presentation of the systemic cancer, and, consequently, in evaluating patients with a brain tumor who do not apparently have systemic cancer, this possibility must always be kept in mind. One clue to the metastatic nature of the disease is the number of tumors: whereas primary tumors, with the exception of primary central nervous system lymphoma, are generally singular, metastatic disease generally manifests with two or more lesions. In such cases, a diligent search must be made for a primary tumor and this may include CT of the chest, abdomen, and pelvis, and, in limiting cases, total body positron emission tomography (PET) scanning.

Course

The natural course varies widely, depending on the malignancy of the tumor itself, ranging from as little as months in the case of glioblastoma multiforme up to a decade or more with low-grade gliomas.

Etiology

As noted earlier, brain tumors may be either primary to the central nervous system or metastatic; of these two broad types, metastatic tumors are more common.

PRIMARY TUMORS

Of the primary brain tumors, *gliomas* and *meningiomas* constitute the vast majority of cases. *Primary central nervous system lymphoma*, once rare, has become increasingly common, both in immunocompromised and immunocompetent patients. Other primary brain tumors, seen in a small minority, include *neuromas*, *medulloblastoma*, *gangliocytoma*, *pituitary adenoma*, *craniopharyngioma*, *pineal tumors*, *hemangioblastoma*, and *colloid cyst of the third ventricle*. Each of these is considered further below.

Gliomas include astrocytomas, oligodendrogliomas, and ependymomas. Astrocytomas are by far the most common type and may be divided into four grades according to their malignancy, namely grades I, II, III, and IV. Grades I and II astrocytoma, or 'low-grade' astrocytomas, are slow growing, whereas grades III and IV, or 'malignant' or 'high-grade' astrocytomas, tend to be rather aggressive. Grade IV astrocytoma is also known as glioblastoma multiforme; this is the most common of the gliomas and is extremely aggressive. Astrocytomas tend to occur in the white matter of the frontal, temporal, or parietal lobes, but may also be found in the cerebellum or brainstem. On MR scanning, low-grade astrocytomas have decreased signal intensity on T1-weighted imaging and display homogenous increased signal intensity on T2-weighted imaging; there may or may not be enhancement. High-grade astrocytomas may appear heterogenous on T1- and T2-weighted imaging, and typically undergo enhancement, which, especially in the case of glioblastoma multiforme, may be ring-shaped. Over long periods of time, low-grade astrocytomas may undergo malignant transformation. A variant form of glioma is known as gliomatosis cerebri. This is a very aggressive growth characterized not by a discrete mass but by a widespread infiltration of one or both hemispheres of the cerebrum, primarily of the white matter; patients typically present with delirium, headache, and seizures, and MR scanning may reveal

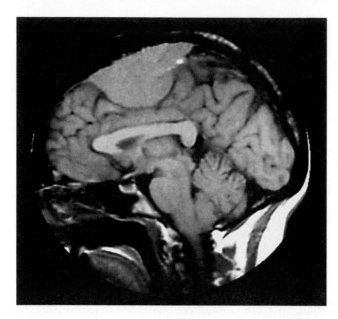

Figure 19.1 *A sagittal T1-weighted magnetic resonance scan demonstrates the clear demarcation between a meningioma and the surrounding tissue. (Reproduced from Gillespie and Jackson 2000.)*

diffusely increased signal intensity in the white matter, which may undergo enhancement.

Oligodendrogliomas arise from oligodendrocytes and are indolent growths (Wilkinson *et al.* 1987) found typically in the white matter of the frontal or temporal lobes, which often present with seizures; on MR scanning they present as non-enhancing masses with increased signal intensity on T2-weighted images, and on CT scans one may appreciate calcification.

Ependymomas, although most commonly seen in children, may present in early adult years. These tumors arise from ependymal cells of the fourth, third, or lateral ventricles, and may cause symptoms either by causing obstructive hydrocephalus or by extending into the adjacent brain parenchyma; they may undergo calcification and may show enhancement.

Meningiomas are very slow growing tumors that arise from arachnoidal cells and which have an attachment to the dura. These are well-demarcated, extra-axial tumors that produce symptoms by compression of the subjacent brain parenchyma, from which they are clearly separated, as illustrated in Figure 19.1. Although they may or may not be readily discernible on T2-weighted scans, they do undergo homogenous enhancement. There are several favored locations. Meningiomas of the falx cerebri, by compression of the medial aspects of the frontal or parietal cortices, may cause dementia or paraparesis. Lateral convexity meningiomas may cause various focal signs, such as hemiplegia or aphasia. Olfactory groove meningiomas may cause anosmia, blindness, and, by upward extension against the frontal lobe, dementia; should they attain a size capable of causing increased intracranial pressure,

a Foster Kennedy syndrome may occur, with ipsilateral anosmia, ipsilateral optic atrophy, and contralateral papilledema. Suprasellar meningiomas may cause a bitemporal hemianopia and pituitary failure, and meningiomas of the sphenoid ridge may present with extraocular nerve palsies and proptosis. All meningiomas may also be associated with seizures. Rarely, rather than presenting as a circumscribed mass, meningiomas may present 'en plaque' as a sheath-like structure.

Primary central nervous system lymphoma, once rare, has recently shown an increasing incidence, and this appears to be the case not only in immunocompromised patients, such as transplant patients (Schneck and Penn 1970) and those with AIDS (Feiden *et al.* 1993; Lang *et al.* 1989), but also in immunocompetent elderly patients. These tumors may be single or multiple and typically show bright, homogenous enhancement (Lai *et al.* 2002). Although most are found in the cerebrum, often in a periventricular location, they may also occur in the cerebellum or brainstem. They often seed into the cerebrospinal fluid (CSF), and a suspicion of primary central nervous system lymphoma is one situation where a lumbar puncture should be seriously considered.

Neuromas, although capable of arising from cranial nerves V, VII, IX, or X, are by far most commonly associated with cranial nerve VIII, in which case they are referred to as acoustic neuromas. These acoustic neuromas constitute the most common cause of a cerebellopontine angle tumor and typically present with hearing loss, accompanied in most cases by dysequilibrium and tinnitus; with growth of the tumor and compression of cranial nerves V and VII, there may be facial numbness and a peripheral facial palsy; rarely, a trigeminal neuralgia may occur (Harner and Laws 1983). In cases in which the cerebellum is compressed, there may be nystagmus and ataxia.

Medulloblastomas, although generally seen only in children, may occasionally occur in adults. These are typically found in the midline cerebellum and often protrude into the fourth ventricle, causing hydrocephalus.

Gangliocytomas (Kernohan *et al.* 1932) are composed of neural elements, and gangliogliomas (Morris *et al.* 1993) of both neural and glial elements. These are rare, indolent tumors, generally found in the temporal, frontal, or parietal cortices, which typically present with seizures.

Pituitary adenomas may be subclassified according to either their size or their endocrinologic status. Macroadenomas are larger than 1 cm, whereas microadenomas, which are more common, are smaller. Endocrinologically, more than 80 percent of adenomas are secretory, with the remainder being non-productive. Pituitary adenomas may cause symptoms by either compression of adjacent tissue or secondary to the secretion of various hormones. With compression of adjacent pituitary tissue there may be pituitary failure, with, for example, hypothyroidism or adrenocortical insufficiency. Lateral extension of a macroadenoma into the adjacent cavernous sinus may cause an oculomotor palsy or facial numbness in the areas of the first or second divisions of the trigeminal nerve.

In turn, upward extension of a macroadenoma may impinge on the optic chiasm, with a bitemporal hemianopia; on the hypothalamus, with diabetes insipidus; or, in extreme cases, on the frontal lobe, with cognitive changes and seizures. Endocrinologic changes seen with secretory tumors most commonly involve hyperprolactinemia, with amenorrhea in females and gynecomastia and erectile dysfunction in males. Excess growth hormone and adrenocorticotropic hormone (ACTH) secretion are the next most common changes and may cause acromegaly or Cushing's disease respectively. Gonadotropin and thyroid-stimulating hormone (TSH) excess are rare. Importantly, in about 10 percent of secreting adenomas, two or more hormones may be excessively produced. In addition, in some cases of macroadenomas there may be 'kinking' of the pituitary stalk, and in such cases dopamine delivery to the posterior pituitary may be impaired with a resultant secondary hyperprolactinemia. Magnetic resonance scanning is typically positive with macroadenomas; however, microadenomas of less than 3 mm in diameter may escape detection. In rare instances, pituitary adenomas may undergo hemorrhage or infarction, producing the syndrome of 'pituitary apoplexy' with severe headache, diplopia, blindness, and, critically, an acute case of adrenocortical insufficiency, which may be fatal.

Craniopharyngiomas are lobulated, calcified tumors that, although most commonly occurring in children, may occur in patients of any age. They typically arise from the junction of the infundibulum and pituitary gland, and may produce a variety of symptoms, depending on which direction they grow in. With upward extension and impingement of the hypothalamus, there may be diabetes insipidus and obesity, and with compression of the third ventricle, hydrocephalus may occur. Compression of the optic chiasm may cause a bitemporal hemianopia, and with downward extension various forms of pituitary failure may appear.

Pineal tumors include not only pinealomas but also germ cell tumors, gliomas, and teratomas. These tumors cause symptoms primarily by compression of the adjacent quadrigeminal plate and the underlying aqueduct of Sylvius, with a Parinaud syndrome (limitation of upgaze and an Argyll Robertson pupil) and obstructive hydrocephalus respectively.

Hemangioblastomas (Boughey *et al.* 1990) are cystic masses found in the cerebellum, which typically contain an enhancing nodule on MR scanning. They are found in children or young adults, usually present with cerebellar symptoms, and may occur as part of von Hippel–Lindau disease.

Colloid cysts of the third ventricle are rare cystic masses that may cause dementia (Kelly 1951), either by compression of the surrounding thalamus (Faris and Terrence 1989; Lobosky *et al.* 1984) or as a result of obstructive hydrocephalus, as illustrated in Figure 19.2. Interestingly, by virtue of a 'ball-valve' effect, in which the foramen of Monro is intermittently occluded, these tumors may also cause intermittent elevations of intraventricular pressure. Thus, patients may experience intermittent headache, unsteadiness, and confusion, and report that these symptoms are posture-dependent.

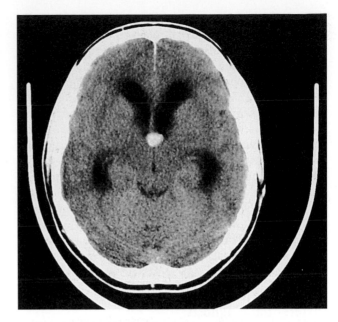

Figure 19.2 *This unenhanced computed tomography scan demonstrates a colloid cyst, which, by obstructing the foramen of Monro, has caused obstructive hydrocephalus with dilation of the lateral ventricles. (Reproduced from Gillespie and Jackson 2000.)*

METASTATIC TUMORS

Metastases may arise from various different primary tumors and almost always reach the brain via hematogenous spread. By far the most common source is lung cancer, primarily the non-small-cell type, followed by breast cancer and melanoma and then by various other tumors, including those of the colon and rectum, kidney, gallbladder, liver, thyroid, testicle, prostate, uterus or ovary, and pancreas; both systemic lymphoma (primarily of the non-Hodgkin's type) and leukemia may also metastasize to the brain. Of all these primaries, melanoma and testicular cancer, although not common, exhibit the greatest propensity for metastasis to the brain.

Two-thirds of metastases eventually settle in the brain parenchyma, whereas the remainder lodge either in the leptomeninges (where they create a condition known as leptomeningeal carcinomatosis) or in the dura. Parenchymal metastases may be found throughout the cerebrum (Delattre *et al.* 1988a); they are found in the hemispheres in about three-quarters of cases, in the cerebellum in about one-eighth, and in the brainstem or thalamus in the remainder; of those lodging in the hemispheres, all lobes may be involved, including, in descending order, the frontal, parietal, occipital, and temporal lobes.

Metastases to the parenchyma generally appear as homogenously enhancing masses, often with considerable peri-tumoral edema; in high-grade malignancies, however, central necrosis may lead to a ring-enhancing pattern. Although solitary lesions may occur, multiple tumors, as noted earlier, are more common, and indeed at autopsy one may find widespread, microscopic foci.

Leptomeningeal carcinomatosis occurs when tumor cells that are widely distributed throughout the subarachnoid space spread into subjacent tissue, leading to delirium and cranial nerve palsies; obstruction of CSF outflow may also lead to hydrocephalus. Magnetic resonance scanning typically reveals meningeal enhancement, and tumor cells may be found with lumbar puncture; this may have to be repeated multiple times, however, to avoid a false negative result. Although spread to the leptomeninges may occur with almost every type of primary tumor, it is, as noted earlier, a relatively uncommon occurrence. The exception occurs with systemic lymphoma or leukemia, which, unique among the primaries, tend to preferentially seed into the leptomeninges.

Dural metastases may occur via direct spread to the dura or by virtue of an inward extension of a calvarial metastasis. Symptoms are produced by virtue of compression of subjacent tissues and may include focal signs and seizures.

Differential diagnosis

In evaluating a mass lesion, consideration must be given not only to primary or metastatic neoplasms but also to sarcoid granulomas, syphilitic gummas, tuberculomas, and bacterial abscesses. Furthermore, in patients immuno-compromised by acquired immune deficiency syndrome (AIDS) or chemotherapy, opportunistic infections enter the differential, including toxoplasmosis and fungal infections. Patients who have undergone focal radiation treatment may subsequently develop a new mass lesion as part of a late-delayed radiation encephalopathy, and the distinction between this and tumor recurrence is discussed in Section 11.5.

In evaluating patients with metastatic lesions who develop delirium, care must be taken not to immediately attribute this to the tumor, because in most cases such a change occurs on a metabolic basis (Clouston et al. 1992). Another consideration here is the development of a para-neoplastic limbic encephalitis.

Treatment

Treatment may involve any one or a combination of surgery, radiation treatment, chemotherapy, and use of dexamethasone and anti-epileptic drugs; neurosurgical and neuro-oncologic consultation is appropriate in all cases.

Surgery may be curative in cases of single, well-demarcated, accessible lesions, such as meningiomas or low-grade gliomas. With large, highly infiltrative tumors, such as glioblastoma multiforme, cure is not expected, but debulking of the tumor may improve the patient's overall functioning. In other cases, surgery may be required to obtain tissue for diagnostic purposes.

Radiation treatment may be focal or whole brain. Focal irradiation may be considered in patients who are not good surgical candidates or in whom the tumor mass or masses are inaccessible. Whole-brain radiation may be considered when there are multiple lesions, and may also be used preventively, for example in metastatic disease in which there is a strong presumption that miliary metastases have already occurred.

With few exceptions, chemotherapy has traditionally played only a limited role; recent advances, however, may be changing this picture.

Dexamethasone is indicated in cases characterized by considerable peri-tumoral edema, and is generally given in a dose of 4 mg q.i.d.; the results are often prompt, within a day, and are at times dramatic.

Anti-epileptic drugs should generally be held in reserve until patients have seizures, as there is little evidence for a prophylactic effect. Enzyme-inducing drugs, such as phenytoin, carbamazepine, and phenobarbital, should be avoided if chemotherapy is utilized or contemplated, as they may reduce levels of chemotherapeutic agents; furthermore, the use of phenytoin in patients undergoing radiation treatment has been associated with a high incidence of severe rash (Delattre et al. 1988b). In general, other agents, such as levetiracetam, gabapentin, or divalproex, should be considered first.

In cases characterized by pituitary involvement, hormone replacement therapy is often required after surgery or radiotherapy. Prolactinomas, unique among the pituitary adenomas, may be treated medically, with bromocriptine.

The general treatment of dementia, personality change, delirium, amnesia, mania, depression, and psychosis is discussed in the respective sections.

It must be borne in mind that not all tumors require treatment. Indolent, asymptomatic tumors, such as small meningiomas or low-grade gliomas, may merely be monitored clinically and with serial MRI scans.

19.2 HYDROCEPHALUS

The overall volume of CSF is about 140 mL: about 20 mL is contained within the lateral ventricles, 5 mL within the third and fourth ventricles, with the remainder found in the subarachnoid space surrounding the brain and cord. Cerebrospinal fluid is produced at a rate of about 20 mL/hour, and about three-quarters of the total CSF production occurs in the choroid plexus, with the rest originating via transependymal flow. Cerebrospinal fluid produced within the lateral ventricles normally flows through the foramina of Monro into the third ventricle and then via the aqueduct of Sylvius into the fourth ventricle, from where it exits via the foramina of Magendie and Luschka into the subarachnoid space surrounding the brainstem. From here, the CSF circulates around the cord and brain, and finally arrives at the cerebral convexity, where it exits the subarachnoid space via the villi of the arachnoid granulations into the dural sinuses.

Hydrocephalus is characterized by an enlargement of one or more of the ventricles as a result of an increase in

CSF pressure. It may be usefully divided into two types: non-communicating and communicating. In non-communicating hydrocephalus, the overall 'communication' between the ventricular system and the brainstem subarachnoid space is partially or totally blocked at some point, thus hindering or totally preventing the egress of CSF from the ventricles into the subarachnoid space. By contrast, in communicating hydrocephalus, this 'communication' is unimpeded and CSF flows freely from the ventricular system into the brainstem subarachnoid space.

Non-communicating hydrocephalus may occur with obstruction of CSF flow at various locations. With obstruction of one of the foramen of Monro, only one of the lateral ventricles enlarges, whereas with obstruction of both foramen, both lateral ventricles become enlarged. Obstruction at the aqueduct of Sylvius is followed by enlargement of the third and both lateral ventricles, and obstruction at the exit foramina of Magendie and Luschka entails expansion of all four ventricles.

Communicating hydrocephalus typically occurs as a result of an obstruction at the level of the arachnoid villi, and is associated with enlargement of all of the ventricles. Rarely, communicating hydrocephalus may occur not because of an obstruction at any point but rather because of a grossly excessive production of CSF, which overwhelms the drainage system.

Although hydrocephalus may occur at any age, from infancy to senescence, in this text only adult or later-onset cases are considered.

Clinical features

From a clinical point of view it is very useful to divide hydrocephalus into two forms, namely acute and chronic, depending on their mode of onset.

Acute hydrocephalus is a form of non-communicating hydrocephalus in which there is a complete, or near-complete, obstruction of CSF flow. This form of hydrocephalus is characterized clinically by a rapid onset of symptoms, over days, hours, or even quicker. Patients present with headache, stupor, and vomiting, and, without treatment, coma and death may rapidly ensue.

Chronic hydrocephalus may represent either a communicating or a non-communicating condition; when it occurs as a result of non-communicating hydrocephalus, one finds only a partial obstruction. Clinically (Gustafson and Hagberg 1978; Harrison *et al.* 1974), chronic hydrocephalus typically presents gradually, or even insidiously, and is characterized by a dementia marked by forgetfulness, apathy, and a generalized slowing of thought and behavior; rarely, akinetic mutism may occur (Messert *et al.* 1966). A gait disturbance also occurs, and this may either precede or follow the onset of the dementia. The gait may be shuffling, apraxic, or 'magnetic' in type; in this last type of gait, it appears as if the patient's feet are 'stuck' to the floor, as if held there by magnets. Urinary urgency or frequency or urinary incontinence may also occur. On examination there may be generalized hyper-reflexia and bilaterally positive Babinski signs.

Although ventriculomegaly is evident on both CT and MR scanning (as illustrated in Figure 19.3), MR scanning is preferred as it is more likely to reveal the underlying cause of any obstructive hydrocephalus. In addition, on T2-weighted or fluid-attenuated inversion recovery (FLAIR) images one typically sees evidence of transependymal flow of CSF from the ventricles into the immediately subjacent white matter, producing a hazy rim of increased signal intensity in a periventricular distribution.

Lumbar puncture may or may not be necessary; in cases of non-communicating hydrocephalus, the opening pressure is normal; in cases of communicating hydrocephalus it is generally increased, except in the condition known as normal pressure hydrocephalus (see Section 19.3).

Course

Acute hydrocephalus is a catastrophic event, with a rapid evolution of symptoms. Chronic hydrocephalus, by contrast, is marked by a very slow progression of symptoms as the pressure of the CSF very slowly increases. In most cases, however, a new 'equilibrium' is eventually reached between CSF production and outflow, and in this situation, although the ventricles remain under increased pressure, they do not undergo any further expansion. When this development occurs, the previously 'active' hydrocephalus

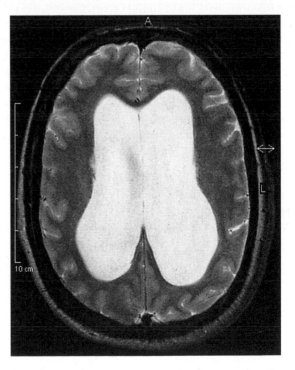

Figure 19.3 *Massive enlargement of the lateral ventricles in a case of communicating hydrocephalus, as demonstrated on a T2-weighted magnetic resonance scan. (Reproduced from Gillespie and Jackson 2000.)*

is said to have undergone 'arrest', and such 'arrested' cases of hydrocephalus clinically manifest a plateau of symptoms, with a subsequently stable clinical course.

Etiology

In non-communicating hydrocephalus the obstruction may occur at various sites and may be caused by various different lesions. Thus, the foramen of Monro may be obstructed by a tumor, such as an astrocytoma, or by a colloid cyst of the third ventricle, and the third ventricle may be occluded by a tumor (Riddoch 1936). The aqueduct of Sylvius may be stenotic (Nag and Falconer 1966; Wilkinson et al. 1966) or may suffer post-infectious scarring; it may also be compressed by adjacent tumors, such as pineal tumors. The fourth ventricle may be compressed by cerebellar lesions, such as tumors, hemorrhages, or infarctions. The exit foramina of Magendie and Luschka may be occluded by scarring, as may occur after an episode of viral or bacterial meningitis, or in the course of an indolent basilar meningitis, as may be seen in meningovascular syphilis, tuberculosis, or fungal infections; scarring and obstruction may also occur after a subarachnoid hemorrhage, either spontaneous or as may be seen with traumatic brain injury.

Communicating hydrocephalus is most commonly seen with obstruction of outflow at the arachnoid granulations. Although such obstruction most commonly occurs after subarachnoid hemorrhage (Ellington and Margolis 1969; Theander and Granholm 1967), it may also occur in a condition known as leptomeningeal carcinomatosis, discussed in Section 19.1; rarely, egress of CSF through the arachnoid villi may be slowed in cases of extremely elevated total protein values, as may be seen in some cases of spinal tumor or polyneuritis. As noted earlier, another rare mechanism underlying communicating hydrocephalus is actual overproduction of CSF, as has been seen with papilloma of the choroid plexus (Eisenberg et al. 1974). Finally, the condition known as normal pressure hydrocephalus is a very important cause of communicating hydrocephalus; this is discussed in detail in Section 19.3.

Differential diagnosis

The first task in making the differential diagnosis is to distinguish 'true' hydrocephalus from a condition known as 'hydrocephalus ex vacuo'. In true hydrocephalus, ventricular enlargement occurs as the result of an increase in pressure within the ventricles. By contrast, in hydrocephalus ex vacuo, ventricular enlargement occurs not because of any pressure increase but merely secondary to shrinkage of the surrounding brain parenchyma, as may be seen in normal ageing or in various neurodegenerative conditions such as Alzheimer's disease. There are two imaging clues that allow one to differentiate between these two forms of ventricular enlargement. First, and most importantly, one should look at the size of the cortical sulci and determine whether or not these are enlarged. In true hydrocephalus, although there may be some enlargement of the sulci, the ventricular enlargement is proportionately much greater, often markedly so. By contrast, in hydrocephalus ex vacuo, there is always sulcal enlargement, and the degree of sulcal enlargement is proportionate to the degree of ventricular enlargement. A second clue is the presence or absence of evidence of transependymal flow on MR scanning: this is present in true hydrocephalus but not in hydrocephalus ex vacuo, given that the ventricular contents are not under any increased pressure.

From a clinical point of view, the dementia seen in hydrocephalus may mimic that caused by Alzheimer's disease or Binswanger's disease; however, imaging will immediately indicate the correct diagnosis.

Treatment

Neurosurgical consultation should be considered in all cases as patients may be candidates for either ventriculoperitoneal shunting or, in cases of non-communicating hydrocephalus in which the obstruction is distal to the third ventricle, endoscopic third ventriculostomy (Farin et al. 2006). Importantly, shunting may be effective even in cases of arrested hydrocephalus (Larsson et al. 1999). The general treatment of dementia is discussed in Section 5.1.

19.3 NORMAL PRESSURE HYDROCEPHALUS

As described in the preceding section, hydrocephalus may be subdivided into communicating or non-communicating and chronic or acute types. Normal pressure hydrocephalus is a form of chronic communicating hydrocephalus that occurs on an idiopathic basis. Classically, it presents with the triad of gait disturbance, dementia, and urinary incontinence or urgency (Adams et al. 1965; Gallassi et al. 1991; Hill et al. 1967).

Clinical features

The onset of symptoms is typically gradual and generally occurs in late middle age or later.

Of the classic triad of symptoms, the gait disturbance typically constitutes the first evidence of this disorder. Patients may walk with short steps on a somewhat widened base, and sometimes there is a degree of shuffling, but the distinctive feature is what is often referred to as a 'magnetic' gait. Here, patients have difficulty initiating steps, as if their feet are held in place on the floor by a large magnet; some may complain that it feels as if their feet are 'glued to the floor'.

The dementia of normal pressure hydrocephalus is characterized by forgetfulness, slowness of thought and action, apathy, and indifference. Rarely the clinical picture may be dominated by a personality change (Rice and Gendelman 1973) or depression (Pujol *et al.* 1989), and even more rarely by aggressiveness (Crowell *et al.* 1973; Sandyk 1984) or mania (Kwentus and Hart 1987).

Urinary incontinence is considered the third symptom of the triad; however, this may be only intermittent and patients may not complain of it. At times, rather than incontinence there may only be urinary urgency.

On examination there may be generalized hyper-reflexia and the Babinski sign may be positive bilaterally; snout and grasp reflexes may also be present.

Computed tomography or MR scanning reveals enlargement of the lateral ventricles out of proportion to any sulcal enlargement that may be present. If lumbar puncture is performed, the opening pressure is typically normal.

Course

In most cases there is a gradual progression of symptoms and some patients may eventually develop akinetic mutism and an inability to stand. Often, however, the hydrocephalus may become arrested, and symptoms may 'plateau out'.

Etiology

Although, as just noted, the opening pressure on lumbar puncture is generally normal, it appears that in these patients there are indeed elevations in CSF pressure but that these elevations occur only intermittently, typically at night (Packard 1982). In this condition the hydrocephalus is of the communicating type and it appears that the intermittently increased pressure occurs secondary to an impaired outflow of CSF through the arachnoid villi (Borgesen and Gjerris 1987). The mechanism underlying this impaired outflow, however, is not known. Given this uncertainty as to the underlying cause, some authors prefer to refer to this condition not as 'normal pressure hydrocephalus' but rather as 'idiopathic chronic communicating hydrocephalus'.

The mechanism whereby symptoms appear probably relates to stretching of the long periventricular axonal fibers.

Differential diagnosis

From a clinical point of view, consideration must be given to other disorders such as Alzheimer's disease and Binswanger's disease, and certain parkinsonian disorders (e.g., diffuse Lewy body disease), and the diagnosis of normal pressure hydrocephalus may only become apparent after neuroimaging. It must be borne in mind, of course, that normal pressure hydrocephalus may co-exist with any of these other disorders, thus producing a mixed diagnostic picture.

Normal pressure hydrocephalus must also be distinguished from other causes of chronic communicating hydrocephalus, such as subarachnoid hemorrhage, as described in the preceding section.

Treatment

Ventriculoperitoneal shunting should be considered in all cases. Among patients who do respond, the gait disturbance generally improves first, followed by the dementia and urinary symptoms; at times the overall response may be dramatic (Graff-Radford *et al.* 1989; Raftapoulos *et al.* 1994).

Selecting patients for shunting is at times difficult. Certainly, in cases in which the classic triad is definitely present and imaging reveals unequivocal hydrocephalus, one should strongly consider surgery. However, these features may not all be present and in such cases one may consider a number of ancillary tests, including the 'tap test', prolonged external lumbar drainage, and the 'infusion' test (Kathlon *et al.* 2002; Sand *et al.* 1994; Walchenbach *et al.* 2002).

In both the tap test and external lumbar drainage the patient's gait is videotaped on at least two occasions and a detailed mental status examination performed. In the tap test, 30–45 mL of fluid are withdrawn within 2 hours of the test and the patient's gait re-videotaped along with a repeat performance of the mental status examination. In the external lumbar drainage procedure, an external lumbar catheter is placed and about 50 mL of fluid is withdrawn daily for 3–5 days, with repeated videotaping of gait and mental status examinations. In both of these tests one looks for an improvement in gait or cognition as evidence that chronic drainage via a ventriculoperitoneal shunt will confer long-term benefit.

In the infusion test normal saline is infused into the lumbar cistern and outflow resistance measured: increased resistance indicates the presence of impaired egress of CSF through the arachnoid villi and thus confirms the diagnostic suspicion of normal pressure hydrocephalus.

The decision as to which of these three ancillary tests to use is not straightforward and practices differ in this regard. The tap test is simplest to perform but may have false negatives; external lumbar drainage and the infusion test are more difficult to perform but are more sensitive. Overall, it may be appropriate to do a tap test first and, if this is negative, proceed to either external lumbar drainage or an infusion test. It must be borne in mind, however, that none of these tests is completely accurate in predicting the response to shunting, and they may yield false negatives in this regard. Consequently, even when these tests are all negative, one may still consider shunting in clinically appropriate cases.

REFERENCES

Adams RD, Fisher CM, Hakim S et al. Symptomatic occult hydrocephalus with 'normal' cerebrospinal fluid pressure. N Engl J Med 1965; 273:117–26.

Alpers BJ. Relation of the hypothalamus to disorders of personality: report of a case. Arch Neurol Psychiatry 1937; 38:291–303.

Alpers BJ. Personality and emotional disorders associated with hypothalamic lesions. In: Fulton JF, Ranson SW, Frantz AM eds. Research publications. Association for Research in Nervous and Mental Disease. Vol. XX. The hypothalamus and central levels of autonomic function. Baltimore: William & Wilkins, 1940.

Alpers BJ, Grant FC. The clinical syndrome of the corpus callosum. Arch Neurol Psychiatry 1931; 25:67–86.

Avery TL. Seven cases of frontal tumor with psychiatric presentation. Br J Psychiatry 1971; 119:19–23.

Beal MF, Kleinman GM, Ojemann RG et al. Gangliocytoma of third ventricle: hyperphagia, somnolence, and dementia. Neurology 1981; 31:1224–8.

Borgesen SE, Gjerris F. Relationships between intracranial pressure, ventricular size, and resistance to CSF outflow. J Neurosurg 1987; 67:535–9.

Boughey AM, Fletcher NA, Harding AE. Central nervous system haemangioblastoma: a clinical and genetic study of 52 cases. J Neurol Neurosurg Psychiatry 1990; 53:644–8.

Clouston PD, DeAngelis LM, Posner JB. The spectrum of neurological disease in patients with systemic cancer. Ann Neurol 1992; 31:268–73.

Crowell RM, Tew JM, Mark VH. Aggressive dementia associated with normal pressure hydrocephalus. Neurology 1973; 23:461–4.

Davison C, Demuth EL. Disturbances in sleep mechanism: a clinicopathologic study. I. Lesions at the cortical level. Arch Neurol Psychiatry 1945; 53:399–406.

Davison C, Demuth EL. Disturbances in sleep mechanism: a clinicopathologic study. III. Lesions at the diencephalic level (hypothalamus). Arch Neurol Psychiatry1946; 55:111–25.

Delattre JY, Krol G, Thaler HT et al. Distribution of brain metastases. Arch Neurol 1988a; 45:741–4.

Delattre JY, Safai B, Posner JB. Erythema multiforme and Stevens–Johnson syndrome in patients receiving cranial irradiation and phenytoin. Neurology 1988b; 38:194–8.

Direkze M, Bayliss SG, Cutting JC. Primary tumors of the frontal lobe. Br J Clin Pract 1971; 25:207–13.

Eisenberg HM, McComb JG, Lorenzo AV. Cerebrospinal fluid overproduction and hydrocephalus associated with choroid plexus papilloma. J Neurosurg 1974; 40:381–5.

Ellington E, Margolis G. Block of arachnoid villus by subarachnoid hemorrhage. J Neurosurg 1969; 30:651–7.

Farin A, Aryan HE, Ozgur BM et al. Endoscopic third ventriculostomy. J Clin Neurosci 2006; 13:663–70.

Faris AA, Terrence CF. Limbic system symptomatology associated with colloid cyst of the third ventricle. J Neurol 1989; 236:60–1.

Feiden W, Bise K, Steude U et al. The stereotactic biopsy diagnosis of focal intracerebral lesions in AIDS patients. Acta Neurol Scand 1993; 87:228–33.

Forsyth PA, Posner JB. Headaches in patients with brain tumors: a study of 111 patients. Neurology 1993; 43:1678–83.

Frazier CH. Tumor involving the frontal lobe alone: a symptomatic survey of one hundred and five verified cases. Arch Neurol Psychiatry 1936; 35:525–71.

Fulton JF, Bailey P. Tumors in the region of the third ventricle: their diagnosis and relation to pathological sleep. J Nerv Ment Dis 1929; 69:1–25.

Gal P. Mental symptoms in cases of tumor of the temporal lobe. Am J Psychiatry 1958; 115:157–60.

Gallassi R, Morreale A, Montagna P et al. Binswanger's disease and normal-pressure hydrocephalus: clinical and neuro-radiological comparison. Arch Neurol 1991; 48:1156–9.

Gillespie J, Jackson A. MRI and CT of the brain. London: Arnold, 2000.

Graff-Radford NR, Godersky JC, Jones MP. Variable predicting surgical outcome in symptomatic hydrocephalus in the elderly. Neurology 1989; 39:1601–4.

Gustafson L, Hagberg B. Recovery in hydrocephalic dementia after shunt operation. J Neurol Neurosurg Psychiatry 1978; 41:940–7.

Harner SG, Laws ER. Clinical findings in patients with acoustic neurinoma. Mayo Clin Proc 1983; 58:721–8.

Harrison MJG, Robert CM, Uttley D. Benign aqueductal stenosis in adults. J Neurol Neurosurg Psychiatry 1974; 37:1322–8.

Haugh RM, Markesbery WR. Hypothalamic astrocytoma: syndrome of hyperphagia, obesity and disturbances of behavior and endocrine and autonomic function. Arch Neurol 1983; 40:560–3.

Heron GB, Johnston DA. Hypothalamic tumor presenting as anorexia nervosa. Am J Psychiatry 1976; 133:580–2.

Hill ME, Lougheed WM, Barnett HJM. A treatable form of dementia due to normal-pressure, communicating hydrocephalus. Can Med Assoc J 1967; 97:1309–11.

Ironside R, Guttmacher M. The corpus callosum and its tumors. Brain 1929; 52:442–83.

Kathlon B, Sundbarg G, Rehncrona S. Comparison between the lumbar infusion and CSF tap tests to predict outcome after shunt surgery in suspected normal pressure hydrocephalus. J Neurol Neurosurg Psychiatry 2002; 73:721–6.

Kelly R. Colloid cysts of the third ventricle: analysis of twenty-nine cases. Brain 1951; 74:23–65.

Kernohan JW, Learmonth JR, Doyle JB. Neuroblastomas and gangliocytoma of the central nervous system. Brain 1932; 55:287–310.

Keschner M, Bender MB, Strauss I. Mental symptoms in cases of tumor of the temporal lobe. Arch Neurol Psychiatry 1936; 35:572–96.

Kwentus JA, Hart RP, Normal pressure hydrocephalus presenting as mania. J Nerv Ment Dis 1987; 175:500–2.

Lai R, Rosenblum MK, DeAngelis LM. Primary CNS lymphoma: a whole-brain disease? Neurology 2002; 59:1557–62.

Lang W, Miklossy J, Deruaz JP et al. Neuropathology of the acquired immune deficiency syndrome (AIDS): a report of 135 consecutive autopsy cases from Switzerland. Acta Neuropathol 1989; 77:379–90.

Larsson A, Stephenson H, Wikkelso C. Adult patients with 'asymptomatic' and 'compensated' hydrocephalus benefit from surgery. Acta Neurol Scand 1999; 99:81–90.

Liss L. Pituicytoma, a tumor of the hypothalamus. *Arch Neurol Psychiatry* 1958; **80**:567–76.

Lobosky JM, Vangilder JC, Damasio AR. Behavioral manifestations of third ventricular colloid cysts. *J Neurol Neurosurg Psychiatry* 1984; **47**:1075–80.

Malamud N. Psychiatric disorder with intracranial tumors of limbic system. *Arch Neurol* 1967; **17**:113–23.

McKendree CA, Feinier L. Somnolence: its occurrence and significance in cerebral neoplasms. *Arch Neurol Psychiatry* 1927; **17**:44–56.

Messert B, Henke TK, Langheim W. Syndrome of akinetic mutism associated with obstructive hydrocephalus. *Neurology* 1966; **16**:635–49.

Moersch FP. Psychic manifestations in cases of brain tumors. *Am J Psychiatry* 1925; **81**:707–24.

Morris HH, Estes ML, Gilmore R et al. Chronic intractable epilepsy as the only symptom of primary brain tumor. *Epilepsia* 1993; **34**:1038–43.

Murthy P, Jayakumar PN, Sampat S. Of insects and eggs: a case report. *J Neurol Neurosurg Psychiatry* 1997; **63**:522–3.

Nag TK, Falconer MA. Non-tumoral stenosis of the aqueduct in adults. *BMJ* 1966; **2**:1168–70.

Olivero WC, Lister JR, Elwood PW. The natural history and growth rate of asymptomatic meningiomas. *J Neurosurg* 1995; **83**:222–4.

Packard JD. Adult communicating hydrocephalus. *Br J Hosp Med* 1982; **27**:35–44.

Pujol J, Leal S, Fluvia X et al. Psychiatric aspects of normal pressure hydrocephalus. *Br J Psychiatry* 1989; **154**(suppl. 4):77–00.

Raftapoulos C, Deleval J, Chaskis C et al. Cognitive recovery in idiopathic normal pressure hydrocephalus: a prospective study. *Neurosurgery* 1994; **35**:397–405.

Reeves AG, Plum F. Hyperphagia, rage and dementia accompanying a ventromedial hypothalamic neoplasm. *Arch Neurol* 1969; **20**:616–24.

Rice E, Gendelman S. Psychiatric aspects of normal pressure hydrocephalus. *JAMA* 1973; **223**:409–12.

Riddoch G. Progressive dementia, without headache or changes in the optic discs, due to tumors of the third ventricle. *Brain* 1936; **59**:225–33.

Sachs E. Meningiomas with dementia as the first and presenting feature. *J Ment Sci* 1950; **96**:998–1007.

Sand T, Bovin G, Grimse R et al. Idiopathic normal pressure hydrocephalus: the CSF tap-test may predict the clinical response to shunting. *Acta Neurol Scand* 1994; **89**:311–16.

Sandyk R. Aggressive dementia in normal-pressure hydrocephalus. *S Afr Med J* 1984; **65**:114.

Schneck SA, Penn I. Cerebral neoplasms associated with renal transplantation. *Arch Neurol* 1970; **22**:226–33.

Strauss I, Globus JH. Tumor of the brain with disturbance in temperature regulation. *Arch Neurol Psychiatry* 1931; **25**:506–22.

Strauss I, Keschner M. Mental symptoms in cases of tumor of the frontal lobe. *Arch Neurol Psychiatry* 1935; **33**:986–1007.

Strobos RRJ. Tumors of the temporal lobe. *Neurology* 1953; **3**:752–60.

Theander S, Granholm L. Sequelae after spontaneous subarachnoid hemorrhage, with special reference to hydrocephalus and Korsakoff's syndrome. *Acta Neurol Scand* 1967; **43**:479–88.

Tucker GJ, Price TRP, Johnson VB et al. Phenomenology of temporal lobe dysfunction: a link to atypical psychosis: a series of cases. *J Nerv Ment Dis* 1986; **174**:348–56.

Walchenbach R, Geiger E, Thomeer RTWM et al. The value of temporary external lumbar CSF drainage in predicting the outcome of shunting on normal pressure hydrocephalus. *J Neurol Neurosurg Psychiatry* 2002; **72**:503–6.

White JH, Kelly P, Dorman K. Clinical picture of atypical anorexia nervosa associated with a hypothalamic tumor. *Am J Psychiatry* 1977; **134**:323–5.

Wilkinson HA, Lemay M, Drew JH. Adult aqueductal stenosis. *Arch Neurol* 1966; **15**:643–8.

Wilkinson IM, Anderson JR, Holmes AE. Oligodendroglioma: an analysis of 42 cases. *J Neurol Neurosurg Psychiatry* 1987; **50**:304–12.

Williamson RT. On the symptomatology of gross lesions (tumors and abscesses) involving the pre-frontal regions of the brain. *Brain* 1896; **19**:346–65.

Idiopathic psychotic, mood, and anxiety disorders

20.1 SCHIZOPHRENIA

Schizophrenia is a chronic, more or less debilitating psychosis that occurs in about 1 percent of the general population and which is equally common in males and females. This illness was first noted by Morel in 1860 (Anonymous 1954), who referred to it as démence précoce. A full description of the disease, however, had to await the efforts of Emil Kraepelin. Kraepelin, who latinized the name to dementia praecox, was a German psychiatrist of the late nineteenth and early twentieth centuries, whose work remains a guiding force for modern psychiatry. The current name for the disease, schizophrenia, was coined by Eugen Bleuler, a Swiss psychiatrist who amplified Kraepelin's original descriptions. Another guiding light in the elucidation of the disease was the German psychiatrist Kurt Schneider, who isolated certain symptoms, now known as Schneiderian first rank symptoms, which, although not pathognomonic of the disease, are very, very suggestive.

Clinical features

The age of onset of schizophrenia, although generally falling in the late teens or early twenties, may range from late childhood to the seventh decade (Brodaty *et al.* 1999; Grahame 1984). A prodrome may or may not be present; in some cases the premorbid personality may have been completely normal, whereas in others, peculiarities may have been present for years or even decades (Walker and Lewine 1990). In cases in which the prodrome begins in childhood, history may reveal introversion and peculiar interests. In cases in which the prodrome appears in teenage years or later, well after the patient's personality has formed, family members may recall a stretch of time when the patient 'changed' and was no longer 'himself'; prior interests and hobbies may have been abandoned and replaced by a certain irritable seclusiveness or perhaps suspiciousness.

The mode of onset ranges from acute to gradual. Acute onsets occur over weeks or months and may be initially marked by perplexity or depressive symptoms; patients may recognize that something is going wrong, and some may make desperate attempts to bring order and structure into a life that is rapidly fragmenting. By contrast, gradual onsets, which may span months or a year or more, may not be particularly disturbing to the patient; there may be fleeting, whispering auditory hallucinations, vague intimations, or strange occurrences.

Although the symptomatology of schizophrenia may be quite varied, in most cases one sees *hallucinations*, *delusions*, *disorganized speech*, and *catatonic* or *bizarre behavior*. *Negative symptoms* (e.g., flattening of affect) are also often seen and, as with all typologies, there is also a category of miscellaneous symptoms, the most important of which is transient disturbances of mood. Generally, based on the overall constellation of symptoms, one may classify any given case of schizophrenia into one of several *subtypes*, namely paranoid, catatonic, disorganized (also known as hebephrenic), or simple schizophrenia; in a large minority, however, there appears to be a mixture of these subtypes, and in such cases one speaks of 'undifferentiated' schizophrenia. Each of these symptoms and subtypes is now considered in some detail.

HALLUCINATIONS

Hallucinations may occur in the auditory, visual, gustatory, olfactory, and tactile realms (Mueser *et al.* 1990).

Auditory hallucinations are most common in schizophrenia and, as noted by Kraepelin (1919), it is 'the hearing of voices' (italics in original) that is by far most 'peculiarly characteristic' of schizophrenia. Voices may come from inside the body or perhaps the air; sometimes they are sent by electronic devices or emerge from the walls or furniture. They often speak in short phrases and may at times manifest as commands, which patients may or may not be able to resist. Certain auditory hallucinations, included among the Schneiderian first rank symptoms although not specific for schizophrenia, are highly suggestive: these include voices that repeat the patient's thoughts, voices that comment on what the patient is doing, and voices that argue with each other. For most patients the voices sound as real as the voice of another person, and they may talk back to them or argue with them. At times when the voices are loud or unpleasant, patients may try and drown them out by listening to music or watching television. In addition to voices, patients may also hear sounds, such as the ringing of bells, footsteps, or tapping on the walls or windows.

Visual hallucinations, although common, play a much less prominent role in the overall symptomatology than auditory hallucinations. Often they are poorly formed and indistinct and perhaps seen only fleetingly, 'out of the corner of the eye'. In some cases, however, they may be detailed, vivid, and compelling: strange people walk the halls; the devil appears in violent red straight ahead; heads may float through the air; and reptilian creatures may crawl the floors.

Gustatory and olfactory hallucinations are uncommon but may at times be quite compelling. Patients may smell poison gas and inspect the air ducts to find the source. Tastes, often foul and bitter, may appear on the tongue, and patients may become convinced that their drinks have been fouled by poisons.

Tactile hallucinations may also occur and may be quite varied. Patients may feel electric currents course over their bodies; they may complain that fluids are poured on them at night or that they are pricked by needles from behind; in some cases they may experience movements deep inside, such as crampings and twistings.

DELUSIONS

Delusions are almost universal in schizophrenia and, although their content is extremely varied, certain themes stand out, including delusions of persecution, delusions of grandeur, delusions of reference, and a number of Schneiderian first rank symptoms. These false beliefs may either grow slowly in the patient or occur suddenly, as if in an enlightenment. Although some patients may entertain some lingering doubts as to the veracity of these beliefs, for most they are as self-evidently true as any other belief. Occasionally patients may argue with others about these beliefs, and even attempt to convince others of their truth, but more often they do not press their case on the unbeliever. Most patients hold multiple delusions; these are often not well elaborated and are often poorly coordinated with each other, and they may even be contradictory. An exception to this rule is seen in the paranoid subtype of schizophrenia, in which one may find a certain degree of systematization of the patients delusions into a more or less coherent corpus of beliefs.

Delusions of persecution are particularly common. Patients may believe that there is a conspiracy against them, for example that the police have coordinated their efforts with co-workers or neighbors or that perhaps the mafia is involved or certain underground organizations. Patients may believe that they are being followed, that their telephone conversations are being listened to, and that their mail is being cleverly opened. Some patients may endure these persecutions stoically, whereas others may engage in what to them appears to be a justifiable self-defense and fight back. Some may flee the area, seeking safety in another town or state. In some cases, if the delusion of persecution is a bizarre one, the response may be proportionately bizarre: one patient, believing that 'rays' were being sent through the ceiling to kill him, proceeded to cover the ceiling in aluminum foil in order to protect himself.

Delusions of grandeur are also common and may coexist with delusions of persecution. Patients may believe that they have developed great inventions and that others persecute them out of envy. Some believe that they have been elected by God, that millions of dollars are held privately for them, that heads of state secretly await their advice on foreign affairs. Although some patients may harbour these beliefs quietly, others may feel compelled to make an announcement. One patient took out a full-page advertisement in the newspaper in which he described his plans for 'world peace' through alliances with 'extraterrestrial beings' that had chosen him as their emissary.

Delusions of reference are intimately related to delusions of persecution and to delusions of reference, and serve, as it were, to reinforce them. Here, patients believe that chance events, rather than being innocuous and unrelated to them, in fact bear special meaning and pertain specifically to them. Newspaper headlines seem to be a kind of code, which only the patient can decipher, informing him or her that the time is near; street lights which blink on are a sign to those pursuing the patient that the time has come to 'move in'. The patient with grandiose delusions may hear church bells on Sunday morning and know that they serve as an announcement of his or her glory. For patients with delusions of reference, at times all things seem pregnant with meaning: there are no more chance occurrences, no accidents, and no coincidences.

Schneiderian first rank symptoms may comprise delusions, including thought broadcasting, thought withdrawal, thought insertion, and delusions of influence, control, or passivity. In thought broadcasting, patients believe that thoughts can leave the head without being spoken or written, and that others may 'pick up' these thoughts directly; some patients say that it works 'like a radio' and they may feel no need to speak their thoughts as they assume that others, perhaps including the doctors, have already picked up the 'broadcast'. Thought withdrawal is characterized by the experience of having one's thoughts directly withdrawn from the mind. In such cases, patients suddenly become bereft of thoughts and are left with blank minds; some may elaborate on the experience and speak of electrical or magnetic devices that remove the thoughts. Patients who experience thought withdrawal while speaking may exhibit the sign known as 'thought blocking'. Here, in the middle of speaking, patients abruptly cease talking and become silent; this happens because they just as abruptly find themselves with no thoughts to speak. Thought insertion represents the converse of thought withdrawal, and in this experience patients believe that thoughts that are not their own have been 'inserted' directly into their minds; these 'alien' thoughts exist as a kind of cognitive 'foreign body', and patients may elaborate on the experience and believe that strange devices, perhaps using magnets, are responsible for their appearance. Delusions of influence, control or passivity are characterized by the belief on the patient's part that their thoughts, feelings, or actions are somehow directly influenced or controlled by some outside force or agency, and that they have somehow become like robots or passive automatons, without any independence of will. Some again may elaborate on these beliefs and speak of being under the influence of a spell or perhaps of an electrical or magnetic machine, or perhaps a distant computer.

Other delusions may also occur. Indeed, any imaginable belief may be held, no matter how fantastic: angels live in the patient's nose; a small person is seated at a chair in the external auditory canal and whispers to the patient; parents have risen from the grave, etc.

DISORGANIZED SPEECH

In considering the sign of disorganized speech we are concerned not with the content of speech, which may be composed of delusions, but rather with the form of speech. This 'formal thought disorder' is most often referred to as 'loosening of associations', but may sometimes be termed 'derailment'. Thought and speech become illogical and incoherent; thoughts are juxtaposed that have no conceivable connection and family members may complain that the patient 'doesn't make sense'; there is a lack of 'goal-directedness', and thoughts, lacking such an organizing goal, become disparate and unconnected. At its most extreme, loosening of associations produces a 'word salad' in which successive spoken words have no more inherent connection with each other than do the tossed leaves of a salad. In one case, a patient, after being asked about the previous day's activities, replied, 'The sun bestrides the mouse doctor. In the morning, if you wish. Twenty-five dollars is a lot of money! Large faces and eyes. Terrible smells. Rats in the socket. Can there be darkness? Oh, if you only knew!' Here, any inner connection between the various ideas and concepts is lost; it is as if they come at random. Typically, patients are unconcerned with their incoherence; if asked to explain what they mean, they make little, if any, effort at clarification.

In some cases, rather than loosening of associations one may see mere tangentiality or circumstantiality. In tangentiality, in response to a question, thoughts proceed off on a tangent and patients never get around to giving an answer; in circumstantiality, the responses are circuitous and patients take a long 'round about' path before they finally 'get to the point'.

Neologisms may also occur, in which, in the course of speaking, the patient may use a word that seems to have no meaning. For example, one patient, when asked if he wanted anything, replied, 'Yes, please, some bufkuf.' When asked the meaning of 'bufkuf', the patient responded, 'Oh, you know,' and made no further attempt to define or explain it.

CATATONIC OR BIZARRE BEHAVIOR

Catatonia may occur in one of two forms, namely stuporous catatonia and excited catatonia. Both forms may be seen in schizophrenia and, indeed, it is not uncommon to see individual patients with the catatonic subtype of schizophrenia exhibit both forms at different times (Morrison 1973). In stuporous catatonia one sees immobility, catalepsy, and mutism, which may be joined by posturing, echolalia or echopraxia, negativism, or automatic obedience, whereas in excited catatonia one sees bizarre, frenzied, purposeless behavior. All of these symptoms are discussed in detail in Section 3.11.

In addition to catatonic symptoms there may be other bizarre aspects to schizophrenia, including mannerisms, bizarre affect, and an overall disorganization and disintegration of behavior.

Mannerisms, as discussed in Section 4.27, represent bizarre or odd caricatures of gestures, speech, or behavior. In a manneristic gesture, the patient may offer a hand to shake with the fingers splayed out, or the fingers may intermittently writhe in a peculiar, contorted way. In manneristic speech, cadence, modulation or volume may be erratic and dysmodulated. One patient spoke in a 'sing-song' voice and, in another, random syllables were accented in a pompous way. Overall behavior may undergo manneristic transformation; one patient walked in a stiff-legged fashion, rigidly swinging only one arm with each step.

Bizarre affect may manifest in a variety of ways. In some cases facial expression appears theatrical, wooden, or under a peculiar constraint, for example patients may report feeling joy but the rapturous facial expression may appear brittle, tenuous, and disconnected. In other cases there may be inappropriate affect. Here, as described in Section 4.26, one finds a disconnection between what the patient feels and what 'shows' on his face, as, for example, in the case of a patient who, although feeling sadness at the death of a parent, was seen to involuntarily snicker.

There may also be a bizarre disintegration of the patient's overall behavior and demeanor, and it is this sign that often makes these patients 'stand out' in public. Patients become untidy and may neglect to clean their clothes or to bathe. Dress and grooming may become bizarre: several layers of clothing may be worn, even when it is hot outside, and bits of string or cloth may festoon jackets or shirts. Patients may cut off their eyebrows or make deep gashes in their arms or legs. Some seem almost analgesic: one patient bit out part of his biceps muscle; another eviscerated himself, 'just to see' what was inside. In some cases the bizarre behavior may be in response to delusions, as, for example, when a patient wrapped his legs in aluminum foil to 'keep the bugs off'.

NEGATIVE SYMPTOMS

'Negative', or 'defect', symptoms (Andreasen 1982; Andreasen and Olson 1982; Andreasen et al. 1990a) include flattening of affect, poverty of thought or speech, and avolition.

Flattening of affect, also known as mere 'blunting' of affect when less severe, is, as discussed further in Section 4.25, characterized by a lifeless and wooden facial expression accompanied by a corresponding dearth or diminution of all feelings.

Poverty of speech and poverty of thought are often referred to collectively as 'alogia'. Poverty of speech is said to be present when patients, although speaking a normal amount, seem to 'say' very little; there is a dearth of meaningful content and speech is often composed of stock phrases. In poverty of thought, by contrast, patients speak little, essentially because there is a wide-ranging and far-reaching impoverishment of their entire thinking; patients may complain that their heads are 'empty' and that, simply, nothing comes to mind; there are no stirrings.

Avolition, referred to by Kraepelin as 'annihilation of the will', is allied to poverty of thought in that avolitional patients simply do not experience any impulses, desires, stirrings or inclinations; if left undisturbed they may spend hours or days in quietude, doing nothing.

MISCELLANEOUS SYMPTOMS

Of the miscellaneous symptoms seen in schizophrenia, perhaps the most important are transient disturbances of mood, which may tend toward depression, mania, or anxiety. Patients may complain of depressive symptoms, such as feeling depressed, being tired or having trouble sleeping; some may demonstrate some euphoria and increased energy and talkativeness, whereas others may complain of feeling anxious and tremulous. Indeed, at first glance these symptoms may seem to dominate the clinical picture; however, on a closer and wider look one finds that they are transient, lasting only hours or days, are mild overall, and, relative to other symptoms, such as hallucinations and delusions, play only a very minor role in the overall clinical picture. Agitation may also be seen, and this may occur either as a non-specific part of an exacerbation of the disease or as a reaction to delusions of persecution or threatening voices.

SUBTYPES

Classifying patients as to subtype is useful not only because the various subtypes pursue different courses with different prognoses, as noted further below, but also because knowledge of a patient's subtype diagnosis may allow the clinician to predict how the patient will act in any given situation.

After discussing the paranoid, catatonic, disorganized, simple, and undifferentiated subtypes of schizophrenia, some comments will also be offered on an alternative mode of subdividing schizophrenia, namely into 'reactive' and 'process' types.

Paranoid schizophrenia tends to have a somewhat later onset, sometimes as late as in middle years, and is characterized primarily by hallucinations and delusions; disorganized speech, catatonic or bizarre behavior, and negative symptoms are either absent or relatively minor. Hallucinations are generally auditory and delusions are generally of persecution and reference. In paranoid schizophrenia, more so than in any other subtype, the delusions tend to be systematized and, on first glance, even plausible. Voices may warn patients that their supervisors are plotting against them. Patients may begin to suspect that people are talking about them, perhaps laughing at them behind their backs. Newspaper headlines pertain to them; the CIA may be involved or perhaps the FBI. At times patients may appeal to the authorities for help, but often they suffer their persecutions in rigid silence; occasionally they may try to escape, perhaps by moving to another area, or they may turn on their supposed attackers, sometimes violently. Often, allied with delusions of persecution, there may also be delusions of grandeur. Patients believe that they are being persecuted not for some trivial reason; they suspect that others know that they have developed great inventions. Rarely, grandiose delusions may be more prominent than persecutory ones, and they may even dominate the clinical picture. One patient believed himself to be the anointed of God; he heard trumpets proclaiming his advent and was prepared to announce himself to the world.

Catatonic schizophrenia, as the name obviously indicates, is dominated by catatonic symptoms. As described in Section 3.11, catatonia occurs in both stuporous and excited forms and, although some patients with catatonic schizophrenia may demonstrate only one form throughout the course of the illness, in most cases, as noted earlier, these two forms are seen to alternate in the same patient. The duration of these forms is quite variable, ranging from hours on one extreme to months or years on the other. The transition from one form to another may be quite unpredictable and, at times, quite sudden; in one case a chronically stuporous patient, without any warning, suddenly jumped from his bed, screamed incoherently, and paced agitatedly from one wall to another, only to lapse into immobility and muteness an hour later.

Disorganized schizophrenia, also known classically as hebephrenic schizophrenia, tends to have an earlier onset than the other subtypes and to develop very slowly. Although hallucinations and delusions are present, they generally play a minor role and the clinical picture is dominated by disorganized speech and bizarre behavior. Overall, the behavior of these patients seems at times to represent a caricature of childish silliness. Senselessly, they may busy themselves, first with this and then with that, generally to no purpose and often with silly, shallow giggling. At times they may be withdrawn and inaccessible. When delusions are at all prominent, they tend to be hypochondriacal in nature and very unsystematized. In some cases there may also be disorganized speech, with marked loosening of associations to the point of a fatuous, drivelling incoherence.

Simple schizophrenia (Black and Boffeli 1989; Kendler *et al.* 1994a), also known as 'simple deteriorative disorder', has the earliest age of onset, often appearing in childhood, with a very slow and insidious onset, stretching over years. Hallucinations, delusions, and disorganized speech are sparse, and indeed are for the most part absent, and the clinical picture is dominated by negative symptoms. Over the years, these patients fall away from any acquaintances that they may have had and often become distant and emotionally dead. They may appear shiftless and some may accuse them of being 'lazy'. Few thoughts, desires or inclinations disturb them and they may appear quite content to lie in bed or sit in a darkened room all day. For the most part they do little to attract the attention of others and may pass their lives in homeless shelters.

Undifferentiated schizophrenia is said to be present when the clinical picture of any given case does not fit well into any one of the foregoing subtypes. This is not uncommonly the case, and it also appears that, over long periods of time, the clinical picture, which initially did fit a particular subtype, may gradually change and become less distinctive. This transition from a recognized specific subtype to an undifferentiated presentation appears to be most common with the catatonic and disorganized subtypes; by contrast, the paranoid and simple subtypes tend to 'run true'.

As noted earlier, in addition to these classic subtypes there is an alternative proposal for classifying schizophrenia, which divides the illness into two types: 'reactive' schizophrenia, also known as 'good prognosis' or 'type I' schizophrenia, and 'process' schizophrenia, also known as 'poor prognosis' or 'type II' schizophrenia. In reactive schizophrenia, the premorbid personality tends to be normal and the onset, which is marked by depression and perplexity, is acute and occurs generally in adult years, often following some obvious social or personal stress; hallucinations and delusions, with some speech disorganization, dominate the clinical picture. In process schizophrenia, by contrast, the premorbid personality is often abnormal and the onset is insidious, often in childhood or adolescence, and without any recognizable precipitants; negative symptoms tend to dominate the clinical picture. As might be expected, the overall prognosis is favorable for 'reactive' cases and quite poor for 'process' ones.

Although this reactive–process dichotomy is useful, many patients do not fit neatly into one type or the other but rather demonstrate a mix of features. Furthermore, it is not clear whether this scheme represents an advance over the classic subtyping; indeed, one might say that the 'reactive' types represent paranoid schizophrenia whereas the 'process' types include disorganized and simple schizophrenia.

Course

Schizophrenia is a chronic, lifelong disease and most patients suffer considerable disability throughout their lives (McGlashan 1984; Tsuang *et al.* 1979). In most cases, the disease exhibits one of two courses: an overall waxing and waning course or a chronic, slow progression.

The waxing and waning course is characterized by exacerbations and partial remissions. The pattern of these changes is often quite irregular, as are the durations of the exacerbations and partial remissions, which may range from weeks to months or even years. In some cases, after a partial remission patients may develop a depressive episode, commonly referred to as 'post-psychotic depression' (Mandel *et al.* 1982); this is an important development as the risk of suicide is higher during this time. Importantly, this sustained depressive episode must not be confused with the frequently observed, transient, minor depressive symptoms that may occasionally accompany an exacerbation of psychotic symptoms. Overall, this waxing and waning course may persist throughout the life of the patient or, in many cases, it may give way, after anywhere from 5 to 20 years, to a stable chronicity.

The chronic progressive course may be evident from the onset of the disease, as for example in the simple subtype, or may become evident only after the initial onslaught has settled some. Over long periods of time, there is a very gradual progression, after which many patients eventually 'burn out' with no further changes.

As noted earlier, the subtype diagnosis may enable some predictions to be made as to course (Fenton and McGlashan 1991; Kendler *et al.* 1994b). Thus, the paranoid and catatonic subtypes tend to pursue a waxing and waning course and, of these two, the overall prognosis appears to be better for the paranoid subtype. The disorganized and simple subtypes, by contrast, tend to demonstrate a slowly progressive course.

Schizophrenia may have a fatal outcome. Patients with catatonic schizophrenia of the stuporous type may die of aspiration pneumonia or extensive decubiti. Suicide occurs in about 10 percent of patients (Tsuang 1978); overall, about one-third will make a suicide attempt (Allebeck *et al.* 1987).

Before leaving this discussion of the course of schizophrenia it is appropriate to consider whether or not, in the natural course of events and in the absence of treatment, schizophrenia ever undergoes a full, complete, and spontaneous remission. Certainly, in cases that exhibit a waxing and waning course, the partial remissions may be far-reaching and, to casual inspection, it may appear that the patient has recovered. Closer inspection, however, almost always reveals lingering residual symptoms in these 'recovered' patients, such as fleeting hallucinations, odd beliefs, mannerisms, or a certain poverty of thought. Consequently, in perusing the literature on the course of schizophrenia, one must pay careful attention to the definition used by the authors for 'recovery' or 'remission', for often it is a broad one that looks more to social functioning than to a true absence of all symptoms.

In this regard one may recall Bleuler's opinion (Bleuler 1950) that a full cure, a *restitutio ad integrum*, never occurs; although he saw 'far reaching improvements' to the point of 'social restitution', he was always able, upon careful examination, to 'see distinct signs of the disease'.

Etiology

Both computed tomographic (CT) and magnetic resonance imaging (MRI) studies have amply demonstrated the presence of ventricular dilation and cortical atrophy, most prominently in the temporal cortex (Andreasen *et al.* 1990b; Chua and McKenna 1995; Jaskiw *et al.* 1994; Nopoulos *et al.* 1995; Suddah *et al.* 1989; Turner *et al.* 1986). Furthermore, several studies have also demonstrated a correlation between the degree of atrophy seen in the left temporal cortex and the severity of such psychotic symptoms as loosening of associations and auditory hallucinations (Barta *et al.* 1990; Hirayasu *et al.* 2000; Menon *et al.* 1995; Shenton *et al.* 1992). Autopsy studies support the results of neuroimaging, demonstrating a reduced volume in the medial temporal lobe structures (Bogerts *et al.* 1985, 1990) and a prominence of ventricular enlargement in the temporal horn (Crow *et al.* 1989).

Microscopic studies have demonstrated the presence of an excessive number of interstitial neurons within the white matter (Akbarian *et al.* 1993a,b, 1996; Rioux *et al.* 2003) and neuronal disarray within the temporal lobe, specifically the hippocampus (Conrad *et al.* 1991). Furthermore, although not without controversy, some subcortical structures may suffer neuronal loss (Byne *et al.* 2002; Kreczmanski *et al.* 2007). Strikingly, and importantly, gliosis is absent (Bogerts *et al.* 1985; Bruton *et al.* 1990; Roberts *et al.* 1987).

Although the mechanism underlying these anatomic changes is not known with certainty, it is strongly suspected that they represent a disorder of neuronal migration. In the normal course of development, neurons migrate along radial glial fibers from the ventricular area through the embryonic white matter to the overlying cortical subplate, where they come to rest in an orderly fashion to create the laminated cortex. Furthermore, and again normally, a small number of these neurons fail to migrate through the white matter and remain there as interstitial neurons. The findings noted above of an increased number of interstitial neurons and neuronal disarray in the cortex are consistent with the hypothesis of a failure of normal migration in schizophrenia.

The mechanism underlying such a failure of normal migration, although not clear, may involve one or more environmental insults acting on a genetically determined vulnerability. As noted earlier, schizophrenia occurs in about 1 percent of the general population; however, among first-degree relatives the prevalence rises to about 5 percent, whereas among dizygotic twins it is about 20 percent and among monozygotic twins the concordance rate rises to about 50 percent. Furthermore, adoption studies have made clear that the increased prevalence in first-degree relatives reflects genetic and not environmental factors (Kendler and Gruenberg 1984; Kety 1987; Tienari *et al.* 2003). Of course, genetics cannot explain the entire picture or one would expect a much higher concordance rate in monozygotic twins, and consequently one must look to environmental factors. Several have been proposed, including obstetrical complications (Kendell *et al.* 1996), maternal malnutrition (Susser and Lin 1992), and *in utero* exposure to certain viral illnesses (Murray 1994), for example influenza and rubella (Brown *et al.* 2001). All of these factors can cause disorders of neuronal migration, and it may be that what is inherited in schizophrenia is not the disease *per se* but rather a defect that renders the fetal brain particularly vulnerable to certain of these factors.

If indeed the neuropathology of schizophrenia represents a non-progressive disorder of neuronal migration, one must also explain why the onset of the disease is delayed until the late teenage or early adult years. One hypothesis is that the phenotypic expression of the disease is dependent upon an interaction between the fixed neuronal migration defect and the normally evolving neuroanatomic changes seen during adolescence. During normal childhood and adolescence there is a progressive and selective 'pruning' of dendrites, and, according to this hypothesis, the ability of the fixed neuronal migration defect to express itself clinically may have to wait until a specific degree and type of 'pruning' has 'cleared the way'.

Although this neurodevelopmental theory of the etiology of schizophrenia has much to recommend it, the case is not proven and readers are encouraged to watch the literature.

Differential diagnosis

Although a host of disorders enters the differential diagnosis, only certain of them play a large part, thus making the differential task a little less daunting. These include mood disorders (i.e., bipolar disorder and major depressive disorder), schizoaffective disorder, delusional disorder, alcoholic psychoses, several personality disorders, and two putative disorders known as schizophreniform disorder and brief psychotic disorder.

Bipolar disorder, discussed in Section 20.5, is characterized by episodes of mania and depression, whereas major depressive disorder, as noted in Section 20.6, is marked by depressive episodes alone. Both manic episodes, as seen in bipolar disorder, and depressive episodes, as seen in either bipolar disorder or major depressive disorder, may be characterized by psychotic symptoms.

Manic episodes, discussed in Section 6.3, often show a progression in which typical manic symptoms are joined by hallucinations and delusions and, in some, disorganized speech, and if one sees the patient at this stage of mania and if there is no history, consideration might be given to a diagnosis of hebephrenic, catatonic or paranoid schizophrenia.

If, however, one has a reliable history, the differential diagnosis is fairly straightforward. In mania, mood symptoms, namely heightened mood, increased energy, and decreased need for sleep, occur first and are present in a sustained and prominent fashion before the onset of hallucinations, delusions, or disorganized speech. By contrast, in schizophrenia one finds that the course is marked by the presence of hallucinations before the onset of any mood symptoms; furthermore, as noted earlier, any manic symptoms seen in schizophrenia are transient and relatively mild. Certain other features may also help in the differential diagnosis between mania and schizophrenia. In mania, euphoria is typically 'infectious' and deeply felt, and this contrasts with the euphoria seen, for example, in hebephrenic schizophrenia, which is shallow and silly and which, rather than being infectious, typically leaves the interviewer unmoved. Furthermore, the hyperactivity of mania is typically outgoing and extroverted, and this is in marked contrast to the behavior of the excited catatonic patient, who typically avoids contact. Finally, in cases in which the heightened mood is one of irritability rather than euphoria, the manic patient is typically 'on the attack', which contrasts with the irritable paranoid schizophrenic, who is more 'on guard'; although both irritable manics and irritable paranoid schizophrenics are dangerous, the manic patient is recklessly so, in contrast to the paranoid schizophrenic, who may become violent only if approached in what appears, to the patient at least, to be a potentially hostile manner.

Depression, as discussed in Section 6.1, may likewise, at its depth, be characterized by hallucinations and delusions, and this may be seen in depressive episodes of either bipolar disorder or major depressive disorder. As with manic symptoms, however, the differential is fairly straightforward providing that one has a reliable history: in depression characterized by hallucinations and delusions, these symptoms only occur well after the typical depressive symptoms have become well-established and severe; by contrast, in schizophrenia, delusions and hallucinations precede the advent of depressive symptoms. Furthermore, the depressive symptoms seen in schizophrenia are generally transient and are typically not severe. The nature of the delusions seen in depression may also be helpful. In depression, the delusions are 'mood-congruent' in that they 'make sense' in light of the prevailing mood. Thus, patients with depression may come to believe that they have committed unpardonable sins or that their insides are drying up and dying, as is only fitting for such miserable sinners. By contrast, in schizophrenic patients who experience some depressive symptoms, the delusions are often 'mood-incongruent' and indeed often bear no conceivable relationship to depression, as, for example, in the case of a schizophrenic who complained of feeling depressed and then went on to talk about the 'telepathy' that made his toe tingle. Finally, consideration may be given to differentiating a severe depressive episode from a catatonic stupor. In both conditions one may see immobility and mutism; however, with prolonged observation one may chance to see a sudden 'lysis' of catatonic stupor, either into relatively normal mobility or into a brief period of excitation; such a lysis, occurring over seconds or minutes, simply is not seen in depression.

Schizoaffective disorder, as described further in Section 20.2, is an illness characterized by the chronic presence of psychotic symptoms, such as hallucinations, delusions, or disorganized speech, and by intermittent episodes of either mania or depression, during which the pre-existing psychotic symptoms undergo an exacerbation. The differential point that allows a distinction from schizophrenia is that the mood disturbances, whether manic or depressed, are full, severe, and sustained, generally lasting at least weeks, in marked contrast to the mood changes that may be seen in schizophrenia, which are fragmentary, mild, and transient.

Delusional disorder, as noted in Section 20.3, is characterized by delusions and thus may be confused with paranoid schizophrenia. The differential here rests on the degree of plausibility and systematization of the delusions and on the absence of other symptoms. Delusional disorder is marked by delusions that are often quite plausible and typically very well systematized, and by the absence of other symptoms, in particular hallucinations, disorganized speech, and bizarre behavior. By contrast, although there may be some plausibility and systematization to the delusions seen in paranoid schizophrenia, close inspection typically reveals some fragmentation and inconsistencies and almost always at least some hints of auditory hallucinations, speech disorganization, and bizarreness.

Alcoholic psychoses, namely alcoholic hallucinosis and alcoholic paranoia, discussed in Sections 22.9 and 22.10, respectively, may be characterized by delusions and hallucinations, and thus mimic paranoid schizophrenia. The differential here rests on the history: if the psychosis in question occurred only after many years of alcoholism with repeated episodes of delirium tremens, then a case may be made for an alcoholic psychosis; in cases, however, in which delusions or hallucinations occurred early on, perhaps in adolescence or early adult years, and only after a relatively brief drinking career, then one would be hard pressed to explain them on the basis of alcoholism.

Several personality disorders, namely those of the paranoid, borderline, and schizotypal types, may occasionally offer some diagnostic difficulties. Patients with paranoid personality disorder are chronically distrustful and on guard, quick to take offense and to read malevolence into what others do, and prone to harbor deep, long-standing resentments; under great stress they may develop delusions of persecution and thus may resemble patients with paranoid schizophrenia. In patients with paranoid schizophrenia, however, close inspection will reveal other symptoms, such as delusions of other types (e.g., delusions of grander) or hallucinations, which are not seen in the personality disorder; furthermore, in paranoid schizophrenia one often also sees some lack of full systematization of the delusions, in contrast to the personality disorder in which logic is preserved. Borderline personality disorder is characterized by a chronic instability in all aspects of the patient's life, accompanied by intense loneliness and dramatic and stormy emotions; when under great stress, these patients may at times also develop delusions, either of persecution or reference, and may also experience auditory hallucinations. The distinction from schizophrenia rests on the stormy instability that characterizes these patients' lives and on the fact that the psychotic symptoms appear only at times of great stress; this is in contrast to schizophrenia, in which they are present throughout the course, even during stress-free periods. Schizotypal personality disorder is characterized by chronic aloofness and by peculiar thoughts and behavior, and thus may mimic simple schizophrenia. The differential here rests on the overall course: in the personality disorder there is no deterioration, whereas in simple schizophrenia one sees a very slow progression.

Schizophreniform disorder and brief psychotic disorder (also known as brief reactive psychosis) are both characterized by symptoms that are similar to those seen in schizophrenia; however, where they differ is in their supposed course. Patients who experience a full, complete, and spontaneous remission within 1 month are said to have brief psychotic disorder, whereas those whose illness lasts longer than 1 month but less than 6 months are said to have schizophreniform disorder. However, there is a debate as to whether such disorders actually exist. Certainly, there are patients with schizophrenia who are treated with antipsychotics early in the course of the illness and who experience a complete, antipsychotic-induced remission of symptoms; however, in these cases, if treatment is discontinued, symptoms gradually recur. What is at issue here is whether there are, in fact, cases in which symptoms spontaneously and completely undergo a lasting remission without treatment. I have never seen such a case, nor am I aware of any such well-documented cases in the literature.

Other causes of psychosis are discussed in Section 7.1 and, although most of these are rare, the reader is encouraged to gain familiarity with them.

Treatment

In almost all cases, treatment involves the use of an antipsychotic drug. These agents may be broadly divided into two different categories, namely first-generation and second-generation or, as they are often also termed, typical and atypical agents.

First-generation agents are further subdivided into 'high-potency' (haloperidol, fluphenazine, perphenazine, trifluoperazine, and thiothixene), 'low-potency' (chlorpromazine and thioridazine), and 'medium-potency' (loxapine and molindone) drugs. High-potency drugs require lower milligram doses and are more likely to cause extrapyramidal side-effects (e.g., parkinsonism, dystonia, akathisia, akinesia). Low-potency drugs require higher doses and are less likely to cause extrapyramidal side-effects, but are prone to cause sedation, hypotension, and anticholinergic effects. Medium-potency drugs, as might be expected, fall in-between regarding both milligram

dosage and side-effects. Of these first-generation agents, both haloperidol and fluphenazine are available in intramuscular 'depot' formulations, which are given, on average, once every 4 or 2 weeks respectively. All other things being equal, of the first-generation agents, haloperidol is probably a reasonable first choice.

Second-generation agents include clozapine, olanzapine, risperidone, quetiapine, aripiprazole, and ziprasidone. Choosing among these agents is not straightforward. With regard to effectiveness, clozapine is clearly superior; however, its side-effect profile, especially the risk of agranulocytosis, limits its use to treatment-resistant cases. Of the other agents, although there is controversy here, it appears that olanzapine may have an edge in terms of overall effectiveness (Lieberman et al. 2005). This advantage, however, is severely tempered by the tendency of olanzapine to cause metabolic derangements, including weight gain, hyperlipidemia, and diabetes. Both risperidone and quetiapine may also cause these metabolic derangements, but are much less likely to do so; risperidone, alone among the second-generation agents, is available in a long-acting intramuscular 'depot' formulation, providing benefit for 2 weeks. Aripiprazole and ziprasidone stand out in that they are not associated with metabolic changes. Overall, and all other things being equal, if a second-generation agent is used, it may be reasonable to start with risperidone; however, again, it must be acknowledged that this is an area of great controversy.

In deciding which antipsychotic, whether first or second generation, to prescribe, the first step is to obtain an accurate treatment history, and this may require not only questioning the patient but also reviewing records and interviewing family members. If there is a history of a good response combined with good tolerability, then it makes sense to use the same drug again. In treatment-naive patients, or in cases in which prior treatments were unsatisfactory, other considerations come into play. Although not without controversy, it appears that, overall, second-generation agents are more effective and better tolerated than first-generation ones, and, consequently, it may be reasonable to select a second-generation agent. Of the second-generation agents, risperidone, as noted above, is a reasonable choice, both regarding efficacy and side-effects, and this also allows one to move to intramuscular 'depot' treatments in cases of non-compliance. It must be emphasized, however, that the choice of an agent is not simple or straightforward, and often multiple trials of different agents must be performed before a regimen is found that is reasonably effective and well-tolerated.

Regardless of which agent is chosen, it is important that one gives it an 'adequate' trial before moving on to another, not only in terms of dose but also duration. In general, assuming an adequate dose is used, one should observe the patient for at least 2 weeks to get a reasonable idea as to response. In cases characterized by significant agitation, one may, as described in Section 6.4, consider adding adjunctive lorazepam to either risperidone or haloperidol, and continuing this until the agitation has passed, after which the patient may be continued on the antipsychotic alone. If the overall initial response is only partial, but otherwise promising, one may elect to observe the patient for another 4 weeks and, if the response is good, then move to maintenance treatment, as described below. If the response to the first agent is poor, or the side-effects are unacceptable, then a trial with a different agent should be considered. Should patients fail to get a good response to adequate trials of two agents, one may be dealing with a treatment-resistant case. In such cases several options are available, including a trial of clozapine, trials of other agents, or simply 'living with' a less than optimal treatment regimen. As regards effectiveness, clozapine is clearly head and shoulders above all other antipsychotics in treatment-resistant cases, and indeed may yield some of the most gratifying treatment responses in all of medical practice; however, its side-effect profile gives pause to many patients and physicians. If clozapine is not an option, some clinicians will try trial after trial of different agents, hoping to find one that 'works'; provided that patients have the fortitude, this is not an unreasonable strategy, as in some cases patients will simply have idiosyncratic and unpredictable 'good' responses to one agent but not others. In some cases, however, patients will opt to stay with a regimen that, although perhaps providing less relief than is hoped for, is at least tolerable.

Maintenance treatment is appropriate in almost all cases. Initially, patients should be maintained on a dose that is similar to, if not identical to, that utilized during initial treatment. Once patients are stable, cautious dose adjustments may be considered every 3–4 months. As noted earlier, in many cases the course of schizophrenia is characterized by gradually occurring exacerbations and partial remissions, and in such cases it is appropriate to try to 'titrate' the dose to the underlying severity of the disease, always seeking the lowest possible dose consistent with acceptable symptomatic control. This serves not only to reduce cost and side-effect burden but also reduces the risk of tardive dyskinesia (this dreaded complication of long-term treatment with antipsychotics, primarily first-generation agents, is discussed further in Section 22.2). In a minority of cases, the underlying course is so favorable, and the partial spontaneous remissions so profound, that it may be possible to taper the dose to almost nothing, at which point some patients and physicians may consider stopping treatment. This is a difficult decision. Schizophrenia is a chronic disease and, although far-reaching spontaneous partial remissions do occur, exacerbations may be expected at some point in the future. Consequently, it is necessary to continue seeing patients in regular follow-up visits and to discuss with them, and with family, the importance of calling immediately should symptoms recur.

In both initial and maintenance treatment phases there are two side-effects that must always be kept in mind, namely akinesia and akathisia. Akinesia, as noted in Section 3.9, may leave patients psychomotorically retarded and, in the unwary clinician, may prompt a misdiagnosis of depression (King et al. 1995; Van Putten and May 1978). Akathisia, described in Section 3.10, classically renders patients restless but at times may manifest only with an exacerbation of psychotic symptoms (Van Putten 1975; Van Putten et al. 1974); unless this is properly diagnosed, a 'vicious cycle' may occur, in which the exacerbation is mistakenly attributed to the underlying schizophrenia, prompting an increased dose of the antipsychotic with a consequent worsening of the psychosis. Although these side-effects are classically seen with first-generation agents, they may also, albeit rarely, occur with second-generation ones.

Post-psychotic depression may occur after psychotic symptoms have partially remitted, either spontaneously or by virtue of antipsychotic treatment. These sustained depressions must be treated as they carry a significant risk of suicide. Treatment may be accomplished with an antidepressant (Siris et al. 1987), such as a selective serotonin reuptake inhibitor (SSRI), or, in severe cases, with electroconvulsive therapy (ECT). Of interest, ECT may also be effective in the acute treatment of catatonic schizophrenia.

In addition to treatment with antipsychotics and routine supportive care, many patients will also require extensive assistance in gaining housing and sheltered employment; social skills training and cognitive–behavioral treatment may also be beneficial. Insight-oriented or psychodynamically oriented psychotherapy is generally contraindicated, as it may make patients worse.

Hospitalization is required for most patients at some point in their illness and, in many cases, repeated admissions occur. In some cases involuntary hospitalization is required and may be life-saving. Partial hospitalization or 'day hospitals' may enable some severely ill patients to be maintained in the community.

20.2 SCHIZOAFFECTIVE DISORDER

The term 'schizoaffective' has had many definitions since it was first coined by Kasanin in 1933. As conceived of here, schizoaffective disorder is characterized by chronic, unremitting psychotic symptoms, similar to those seen in schizophrenia, upon which are superimposed full episodes of either depression or mania, during which the pre-existing psychotic symptoms undergo an exacerbation. Although the prevalence of schizoaffective disorder is not known with certainty, it is probably far less common than schizophrenia.

Clinical features

The onset is typically in the late teens or early twenties, and, viewed over time, this disorder, as suggested above, appears to represent a superimposition of a mood disorder, such as major depressive disorder or bipolar disorder, upon schizophrenia. Thus, these patients typically present with a psychosis similar to that described in the preceding section for schizophrenia, and the symptoms (e.g., hallucinations, delusions, disorganized speech, etc.) persist in a chronic, generally lifelong fashion. Periodically, however, these chronic symptoms are joined by either a depressive episode or a manic episode (with symptoms as described in Sections 6.1 and 6.3 respectively). Characteristically, whenever a depressive or manic episode does occur, the chronically persistent psychotic symptoms become more severe, only to eventually return to their previous level of severity once the mood episode has run its course.

Course

Although it is clear that the psychotic symptoms remain chronic, the frequency with which episodes of depression or mania occur has not been well studied. In some cases it appears that only depressive episodes occur, and here one speaks of schizoaffective disorder, depressed type; in others one sees both depressive and manic episodes or manic episodes alone, and in these cases one speaks of schizoaffective disorder, bipolar type. The overall outcome of this disorder, although not as favorable as that of the mood disorders, is better than that seen in schizophrenia (Jager et al. 2004).

Etiology

Family studies suggest that schizoaffective disorder may either 'run true' or result from a 'double loading' of genetic susceptibilities for both schizophrenia and either major depressive disorder or bipolar disorder (Angst et al. 1979; Cohen et al. 1972; Kendler et al. 1995; Lauren et al. 2005; Pope et al. 1980).

Differential diagnosis

Schizoaffective disorder must be distinguished both from schizophrenia and from mood disorders.

In schizophrenia, as noted in the preceding section, one may see mood disturbances, but these differ fundamentally from the episodes of depression or mania seen in schizoaffective disorder. The mood changes seen in schizophrenia are transient, fragmentary, and generally mild, whereas those seen in a depressive or manic episode are sustained, pervasive and severe, typically enduring at least for weeks. Post-psychotic depression (McGlashan and Carpenter 1976), as seen in some cases of schizophrenia, is distinguished by the fact that there is no exacerbation of psychotic symptoms during the depression.

In major depressive disorder or bipolar disorder, episodes of mood disturbance may, when severe, be accompanied by delusions and hallucinations; however, the differential may be easily made if one simply attends to the overall course of the illness. In mood episodes of major depressive disorder or bipolar disorder, psychotic symptoms occur only within the context of the mood episode, generally at their height, and are not present in the intervals between mood episodes. By singular contrast, in schizoaffective disorder, psychotic symptoms are always present: they are present during the mood episodes and also in the intervals between these episodes.

Treatment

As might be expected, the treatment of schizoaffective disorder borrows heavily from the treatments for schizophrenia and for either major depressive disorder or bipolar disorder. In general, most patients are treated with an antipsychotic, following the scheme described for schizophrenia in the preceding section. This will generally control psychotic symptoms and may also decrease the severity of mood symptoms in some cases. In cases in which either depressive or manic episodes continue to occur to a problematic degree of severity despite antipsychotic treatment, one may consider use of an antidepressant or a mood stabilizer (e.g., lithium, carbamazepine, or divalproex). In patients with schizoaffective disorder, depressed type, an antidepressant alone may be adequate to bring the depressive episode under control, and once this has been accomplished one may consider using an antidepressant on a preventive basis. In patients with schizoaffective disorder, bipolar type, a mood stabilizer may be used. This may not only control depressive or manic episodes but may also prevent their occurrence. In cases in which depressive symptoms seen in the bipolar type are not controlled by a mood stabilizer alone, one may add an antidepressant, but it is critical to make sure that the patient is 'covered' with a mood stabilizer first to guard against the emergence of an antidepressant-induced manic episode.

Other modalities of treatment are as discussed in the sections on schizophrenia (Section 20.1), major depressive disorder (Section 20.6), and bipolar disorder (Section 20.5).

20.3 DELUSIONAL DISORDER

Delusional disorder is a chronic disorder characterized by the gradual appearance of one or more delusions that eventually elaborate into a coherent system (Kendler 1980, 1988; Kraepelin 1921). In contrast to the delusions seen in schizophrenia, the delusions of delusional disorder have a certain plausibility, and the eventual delusional system is within itself quite logical.

The traditional name for this disorder, as originally bestowed by Kraepelin, was paranoia, and although this term is still seen in the literature, delusional disorder is probably a better name, for two reasons. First, it emphasizes the cardinal aspect of this disorder, namely the presence and prominence of delusions. Second, it avoids the unfortunate association of paranoia with persecution, and reminds us that delusions of persecution are but one of many types of delusions seen in this disorder.

This is an uncommon disorder, with a lifetime prevalence falling between 0.01 and 0.05 percent.

Clinical features

The onset is generally in early adult years, although some may not fall ill until the age of 50 years (Winokur 1977). Generally, these patients experience a lengthy prodrome, with evanescent delusions or perhaps intimations that things are not 'right'. Eventually, persistent and clear-cut delusions occur, and the illness begins to assume its definitive form. This transition to active illness may at times be sudden, and patients may experience a sort of 'epiphany' in which lurking suspicions and concerns suddenly crystallize into beliefs; often, however, the transition from prodrome to active illness is gradual, almost furtive.

Although the most common type of delusion seen in delusional disorder is that of persecution, other themes may be prominent: jealousy, grandiosity, erotic longing, litigiousness, and bodily concerns may all occur. Regardless of which delusion is most prominent, however, one typically also sees delusions of reference. Furthermore, as noted earlier, the delusions experienced by these patients often fit together quite logically, and the entire corpus of beliefs is well systematized. Often, one finds that all of the delusions appear to stem from one delusional 'premise' and that this premise often has a certain plausibility to it.

Traditionally, delusional disorder has been divided into several subtypes, depending on the type of delusion present (Winokur 1977); thus, there are persecutory, grandiose, erotomanic, jealous, and somatic subtypes, and these are described further below. However, this division is somewhat artificial given that, although one type of delusion will dominate the picture, two or more may be present, thus creating a 'mixed' picture.

In the persecutory subtype the dominant delusion is one of being persecuted or conspired against. Patients feel singled out; they are watched and followed. Delusions of reference typically appear, and patients may believe that people on the street talk about them. Patients may move to another city to avoid their persecutors, and may feel safe for a while, but eventually their persecutors catch up with them. These patients may at times be dangerous and may attack others in what, to them, appears to be justified self-defense (Kennedy et al. 1992).

The litigious subtype may be the most difficult to diagnose as the initial delusion may appear very plausible and the ensuing delusions may have an almost unassailable logic to them. During the onset of the illness, patients are typically involved in legal proceedings that go badly for them. A suit may be lost or, if won, the award may appear to the patient to be too low. Patients become convinced that someone is at fault: their attornies are incompetent; the judges were biased; the juries were prejudiced. Patients may pore over trial manuscripts until, finally, some irregularity, no matter how minor, is found. New attornies are then hired and appeals are filed, and a series of legal proceedings is embarked upon. With each failed legal manuever, patients may become more convinced that the legal system as a whole is conspiring in the denial of justice. Eventually,

the disparity between the magnitude of the patients' sense of being unjustly harmed and the trivial, insignificant nature of the original inciting insult to their sense of justice brings to light the pathologic nature of their behavior.

In the grandiose subtype, the dominant theme of grandiosity may come to light in a variety of ways. Patients may believe themselves to be secret 'captains of industry' whose advice is sought by leaders in the financial community. Others may entertain delusions of high descent. One man believed that his mother was an heiress who, out of shame for her out-of-wedlock pregnancy, gave him up for adoption to a poor family; the patient, believing that an inheritance would soon be his, quit his job as he felt no need for his income anymore. Others may believe themselves to be great, although unrecognized, inventors, and toil on in their homes, littering their walls with fantastic diagrams and sketches of their magnificent creations.

In the erotomanic subtype (also known as de Clerambault's syndrome), patients come to believe that they are loved by someone else, generally someone of much higher social station. The clinical picture is dominated by the patient's belief that the imagined lover, for some reason or other, cannot openly express the love. For example, one woman believed that the mayor was in love with her and was unable to tell her this openly as he was married. She saw him at a political rally and he turned his gaze from her, a move she interpreted as evidence that he could not bear the unrequited longing he surely must have felt had he looked at her. The newspaper hinted at a strain in his marriage, and the patient believed that, had it not been for the mayor's high moral character, he would immediately have divorced his wife. This attitude of hopeful expectation lasted for years, throughout which the patient occasionally sent 'secret' letters to the mayor at this office. Eventually, unable to wait longer she began stalking the mayor's wife, and called him to say that she would soon 'dispose' of his wife, thus freeing him.

In the jealous subtype, the patient becomes convinced that his or her spouse or lover is being unfaithful. The patient not only 'sees' evidence for the infidelity but may seek it out. The spouse is a few minutes late getting home from work and the patient believes that only passionate lovemaking could have caused the delay. Sheets and underclothing are inspected for telltale stains; telephone conversations are listened in on; a private detective may be hired. The patient may insist that the spouse stay at home, and at times spouses may become virtual prisoners in their own homes.

In the somatic subtype patients believe, despite reassurances to the contrary from their physicians, that they have a serious disease. Although the 'symptoms' may be mild, perhaps a minor headache, patients are convinced that the underlying disease is severe, perhaps a brain tumor. Two atypical variations on this subtype deserve mention, namely the olfactory reference syndrome (Videbech 1966) and parasittosis (Andrews et al. 1986; Mitchell 1989). In the olfactory reference syndrome patients are convinced that they are emanating a foul odor from the mouth or some other orifice, and may anxiously ask others if they smell it also.

In parasitosis patients believe that the skin is infested: they may complain that they feel bugs crawling and may dig under the skin to find them.

In addition to delusions, some patients with delusional disorder may also have hallucinations, but these generally play only a minor role in the clinical picture and are consistent with the delusions. For example, a persecuted patient may hear a voice warning him that his life is in danger or an erotomanic patient may hear voices whispering caressing words. Mood and affect may be unremarkable or may show changes, again consistent with the delusions: the persecuted patient may become quite irritable and the grandiose patient may experience a shallow, contented euphoria.

Overall, regardless of subtype, the behavior of these patients may be quite normal in areas of their lives that are not touched by their delusions. For example, a patient with the persecutory subtype who believed that co-workers at the factory were conspiring against him, but who was free of delusional concerns regarding all others, led an unremarkable life at home and sang in the choir at church, took his children to baseball games, and was considered a 'good neighbor'.

Course

Although partial remissions may occur, for the most part delusional disorder appears to pursue a chronic waxing and waning course (Opjordsmoen and Rettersol 1991).

Etiology

Although the etiology is not known, delusional disorder appears to be familial; importantly, there is no evidence of any genetic relationship with schizophrenia (Kendler *et al.* 1982, 1985; Watt 1985; Winokur 1985).

Differential diagnosis

Schizophrenia is distinguished on two counts, namely the lack of systematization and the presence of other symptoms. As noted, in delusional disorder the various delusions are logically connected into a well-systematized corpus of beliefs. By contrast, in schizophrenia there is always some lack of connectedness among the various delusions, which at times may be flatly contradictory. Furthermore, in schizophrenia one sees other symptoms, such as bizarre delusions, prominent hallucinations, speech disorganization, etc. In some cases, however, it may be difficult to differentiate paranoid schizophrenia from the persecutory subtype of delusional disorder. In paranoid schizophrenia, the patient's guardedness and suspiciousness may be such that only the fact of the 'conspiracy' is leaked to the physician, with all else held in secret. Thus the patient may not reveal certain bizarre beliefs, for example that a listening device has been placed in his abdomen or that he constantly

hears voices telling him that a 'super computer' is monitoring his thoughts. However, this very refusal to confide in the physician is a valuable clue. In paranoid schizophrenia, suspicions are mercurial and focus on others in seconds; thus the physician may be suspected moments after the interview begins. In delusional disorder, by contrast, patients take time to size others up, and indeed are often quite willing to confide in the physician.

Of the multiple other causes of psychosis considered in Section 7.1, special consideration should be given to alcoholic paranoia. This is one of the alcoholic psychoses and, as noted in Section 22.10, is characterized by delusions of persecution or jealousy; however, in this condition one always finds a history of chronic alcoholism that precedes the onset of the delusions by years or decades.

Hypochondriasis may enter the differential for the somatic subtype of delusional disorder. As noted in Section 7.7, however, in hypochondriasis the patient's concerns about having a serious illness do not amount to delusions; patients with hypochondriasis do respond, albeit perhaps only temporarily, to reassurance from the physician, whereas patients with the somatic subtype of delusional disorder do not.

Treatment

Treatment generally involves the use of an antipsychotic; however, in most cases, gaining the patient's agreement to take medication may be quite difficult. These patients see nothing wrong with themselves or their beliefs, and if told they have 'delusions' may be quite offended. Consequently, great tact and diplomacy are required, and the subject of medication may often have to be approached obliquely; whereas the persecuted patient might never accept a prescription for 'psychosis', he might well agree to 'try' a medicine to help him maintain his composure in the face of all the tribulations he is facing. An antipsychotic may be chosen using the scheme discussed in the section on schizophrenia; importantly, one should choose a medication with a low propensity for side-effects and start at a low dose, as patients with delusional disorder are typically prone to seize on the occurrence of a side-effect, no matter how trivial, as a reason to never take medication of any sort again. The somatic subtype may constitute an exception to the foregoing as there are case reports of this subtype responding to antidepressants such as clomipramine (Wada *et al.* 1999) or paroxetine (Hayashi *et al.* 2004).

Occasionally, hospitalization may be required to protect others, for example in the persecutory or erotomanic subtypes.

20.4 POST-PARTUM PSYCHOSIS

Post-partum psychosis, also known as puerperal psychosis, is a rare disorder, occurring in less than 2 per 1000 deliveries; it is more common in primaparous than multiparous women.

Clinical features

Symptoms generally have an abrupt onset, anywhere from days to a few weeks after delivery (Brockington *et al.* 1981; Munoz 1985). Clinically (Bagedahl-Strindlund 1986; Brockington *et al.* 1981; Hadley 1941; Kumar *et al.* 1983; Munoz 1985), mood changes are prominent and, although depressive features may occur, manic symptoms are much more common. Delusions may appear and often center on the baby, who may variously be considered evil or the Messiah; auditory hallucinations may also occur and may be command in type, instructing the patient to do things to the baby. Confusion and variable disorientation may also be seen. Infanticide may occur in up to 4 percent of cases, and suicide may also occur.

Course

In the natural course of events, symptoms undergo a gradual, spontaneous, and full remission after a matter of weeks or months. Close to one-third of patients will have another episode should they have another child (Davidson and Robertson 1985; Kendell *et al.* 1987).

Etiology

Although the etiology is not known, it is strongly suspected that the psychosis occurs secondary to the effects of profoundly changing hormonal levels on the central nervous system (Ahokas *et al.* 2000a,b).

Differential diagnosis

Both schizophrenia and schizoaffective disorder may undergo symptomatic exacerbation in the post-partum period; however, here, given that these are chronic illnesses, one also sees symptoms before delivery, indeed typically long before the patient became pregnant.

In bipolar disorder there is an increased risk of mania in the post-partum period (Bratfos and Haug 1966), thus presenting a picture similar to that of post-partum psychosis. In most cases, however, one will find a history of prior episodes of mania (or depression) occurring outside the post-partum time span.

Eclampsia may present with delirium immediately post-partum; however, here one finds associated symptoms, such as hypertension and proteinuria. There are also rare case reports of psychosis occurring secondary to treatment with bromocriptine (Canterbury *et al.* 1987), which may be used to suppress lactation.

Treatment

Hospitalization is generally indicated. When manic symptoms are prominent, case reports suggest the usefulness of lithium, and divalproex may also be considered; they may be used as described in Section 20.5. In other cases one may use an antipsychotic, and the choice among these may be made utilizing the guidelines offered in Section 20.1. Consideration may also be given to sublingual estradiol: in one non-blind study, 1 mg four to five times daily yielded impressive results (Ahokas *et al.* 2000b). Regardless of which pharmacologic strategy is employed, it should always be possible, given the natural course of this disorder, to eventually taper and discontinue treatment.

As patients begin to improve, attempts should be made to gradually guide them into appropriate interactions with their babies; however, these visits should always be closely monitored until patients have recovered.

Subsequent to recovery, patients should be counselled regarding the risk of recurrence after future pregnancies. If patients do become pregnant again, close monitoring is required post-partum, and a case may also be made for prophylactic use of lithium (Austin 1992; Stewart 1988) or whichever other agent was effective during the earlier episode, with treatment beginning either immediately post-delivery or, in some highly selected cases, shortly before anticipated delivery.

20.5 BIPOLAR DISORDER

Bipolar disorder is characterized by the occurrence of at least one manic or mixed-manic episode during the patient's lifetime; most patients will also have one or more depressive episodes at other times. In the intervals between these episodes, most patients return to their normal state of well-being. Thus, bipolar disorder is properly considered an 'episodic', 'periodic', or 'cyclic' illness, with patients 'cycling' up into a manic or mixed-manic episode, then returning to normal and cycling 'down' into a depressive episode, from which they likewise eventually more or less fully recover.

Bipolar disorder has a lifetime prevalence of roughly 1.5 percent and is equally common in males and females.

A synonym for bipolar disorder is 'manic-depressive illness, circular type'; however, this terminology is gradually fading from use. In the past it was believed that patients with what is now termed bipolar disorder and patients with major depressive disorder actually suffered from the same illness, namely manic-depressive illness, which merely manifested in different forms. Those who had both manic episodes and depressive episodes during their lifetimes were considered to have the 'circular' form, whereas those who had only depressive episodes during their lifetimes were considered to have the 'depressive' form. Given that it is now clear that bipolar disorder and major depressive disorder are different diseases, it may be appropriate to leave the term 'manic-depressive illness' to history.

Clinical features

The onset of bipolar disorder is heralded by the appearance of a first episode of illness, which may be manic, depressive, or mixed-manic. In general, most patients have their first episode in their late teens or early twenties, and by the age of 50 years, over 90 percent of patients will have had their first episode. The range of age of onset is, however, wide, from as young as 11 years (McHarg 1954) up to the eighth decade (Charron *et al.* 1991), even as late as the age of 79 years (Summers 1983). Each type of episode is described in turn.

MANIC EPISODE

Manic episodes are often preceded by a prodrome, lasting from a few days to a few months, of mild and often indistinct manic symptoms. At times, however, there may be little or no prodrome and the episode may appear quite abruptly; when this occurs, patients often unaccountably wake up in the middle of the night full of energy and vigor, thus manifesting the so-called 'manic alert'.

The overall symptomatology of mania has been well described (Abrams and Taylor 1981; Black and Nasrallah 1989; Bowman and Raymond 1931; Brockington *et al.* 1980; Carlson and Goodwin 1973; Kraepelin 1921; Lipkin *et al.* 1970; Rosenthal *et al.* 1979, 1980; Stevens 1904; Winokur 1984). As discussed in Section 6.3, mania may be divided into three stages: hypomania or stage I mania; acute mania or stage II mania; and delirious mania or stage III mania. All patients who enter a manic episode experience hypomania and most progress to acute mania; however, only a minority eventually reach delirious mania. By convention, patients whose manic episodes never pass beyond hypomania are said to have 'bipolar II disorder', whereas those who, during at least one episode of mania, pass beyond hypomania are said to have 'bipolar I disorder'.

The rapidity with which patients pass from hypomania through acute mania and on to delirious mania varies from a week to a few days to, rarely, hours; indeed, in hyperacute onsets, patients may already have passed through hypomania before being brought to medical attention. The duration of an entire manic episode varies from the extremes of only a few days up to many years, or even a decade (Wertham 1929). On average, however, most first episodes of mania last from several weeks to several months. In general, once the peak of the episode is reached, symptoms gradually subside and, after remission finally occurs, many patients, looking back over what they did, often feel guilt and remorse.

Hypomania, or stage I mania, is characterized by the cardinal manic symptoms of heightened mood, increased energy and decreased need for sleep, pressure of speech and flight of ideas, and pressure of activity (Abrams and Taylor 1976a; Beigel and Murphy 1971a; Clayton *et al.* 1965; Loudon *et al.* 1977; Taylor and Abrams 1973; Winokur and Tsuang 1975; Winokur *et al.* 1969). The heightened mood may be one of either euphoria or irritability, or a mixture of the two, and is often quite labile. Euphoric patients are in great good cheer and wish to share their immense enjoyment with others; they are often full of jokes, puns, and wisecracks, and their humor is often irresistibly infectious to those around them. Indeed, it is the rare physician who can resist at least inwardly smiling when in the presence of a euphoric manic. Irritable manics, by contrast, are irascible, fault-finding, and accusatory, and when their intemperate demands are not immediately met, they may erupt into a tirade of curses and threats, and indeed may become violently assaultive. Increased energy leaves these patients strangers to fatigue and in little need of sleep. Pressured speech is rapid and voluble. Patients have much to say, their thoughts come rapidly and race pell-mell, and in extreme cases they cannot speak fast enough to express them. Although patients may, with great urging, be able momentarily to dam up their words, such respites, when an interviewer may be able to get a few words in, are but transient events before the dam bursts and the interviewer is again inundated with a torrent of words. Such pressured speech is also typically characterized by flight of ideas, in which patients' interests change abruptly from one subject to another, successive subjects having little in common with each other. Pressure of activity impels patients to be ever on the go and perpetually involved in schemes, plans, projects, and activities, activities in which they also often seek to involve others. Patients may also demonstrate distractibility, in which their attention changes mercurially from one subject to another. As might be expected, hypomanic patients often become involved in impetuous and ill-considered ventures: there may be spending sprees, intense, injudicious, and often sexual, relationships, and ruinous business ventures. Attempts to reason with such patients, and to bring them back to some good judgment, are typically in vain. Hypomanic patients rarely see anything wrong with themselves; indeed, they often opine that if only others saw as they did, and partook of their confidence, all would be well.

Acute, or stage II, mania is characterized by an intensification of all of the symptoms seen in hypomania and by the appearance of delusions. The mood becomes extraordinarily heightened and labile, and irritability may be quite pronounced, with unpredictable assaults and tirades. Energy seems boundless, and the pressure of activity and speech may begin to fragment the overall behavior; patients may shout, then cry, hop on the floor or race to the nurses' station, making one demand, then an opposite one, and be completely incapable of channelling themselves towards any one overall purpose. Delusions are typically either of grandeur or of persecution, according to the mood of the patient. Euphoric patients may announce their divinity or lavish listeners with promises to share their great wealth; irritable patients may accuse others of irrationally thwarting and persecuting them. Patients may also hear voices.

Delirious, or stage III, mania represents the height of mania and is characterized by a sometimes startling metamorphosis. The cardinal symptoms of mania may fade, and speech and behavior may become profoundly fragmented (Bond 1980). Loosening of associations may occur, and patients are often confused; some may become mute. Hallucinations and delusions abound and, in addition to delusions of grandeur or persecution, one may also see bizarre delusions, including Schneiderian first rank symptoms (Jampala *et al.* 1989). Catatonic stupor may appear, with immobility, waxy flexibility, and bizarre posturing (Abrams and Taylor 1976b; Taylor and Abrams 1977).

DEPRESSIVE EPISODE

As discussed in Section 6.1, depression manifests with depressed or irritable mood, low self-esteem or guilt, pessimism, difficulty with concentration and forgetfulness, anhedonia, anergia, sleep and appetite disturbances, and psychomotor change. In depression seen in bipolar disorder there tends to be an increased need for sleep and increased appetite and psychomotor retardation, which may be profound (Beigel and Murphy 1971b; Hartmann 1968; Johnson 1984; Mitchell *et al.* 2001). Delusions and hallucinations may occur (Guze *et al.* 1975) and are 'mood-congruent', in that they seem fitting when viewed in the context of the patient's overall mood. Patients may believe themselves to be the worst of sinners and that they are to be taken into imprisonment or to execution. Voices may accuse and condemn them, urging them on to suicide. Depressive episodes of bipolar disorder tend to come on subacutely, over several weeks (Casper *et al.* 1985; Winokur *et al.* 1993), and last 6 months or so; the range here, however, is wide, from as little as weeks up to years.

MIXED MANIC EPISODE

Mixed mania (Himmelhoch *et al.* 1976; Kotin and Goodwin 1972; McElroy *et al.* 1992) is a variant of mania in which there is a strong admixture of depressive symptoms. In some cases, manic and depressive symptoms may rapidly alternate, and in others they may exist simultaneously. Euphoric patients, singing and proclaiming their glory and beneficence, may suddenly be thrust into the profoundest of despair, weeping, bereft of all hope and energy, and intensely suicidal. Mixtures of manic and depressive symptoms may present a startling clinical picture: one patient strode through the ward, shouting unstoppably that he was the greatest of sinners and would die of unspeakable tortures; another, weeping uncontrollably with a look of utter despair, proclaimed to feel wonderful, at peace and transcendently happy.

Mixed manic episodes are relatively uncommon and tend to last longer than straight manic ones.

Course

As noted earlier, bipolar disorder is an episodic disorder and its course is characterized in most patients by the intermittent appearance, over the lifespan, of episodes of illness, in-between which most patients experience 'euthymic' intervals during which they more or less return to their normal state of health. Both the duration of the euthymic intervals and the sequencing of episodes varies widely among patients.

The duration of the euthymic interval varies from as little as a few hours or days (Bunney *et al.* 1972; Sitaram *et al.* 1978) up to years, or even decades. In contrast to this inter-patient variability, however, one may often find a remarkable intrapatient regularity, and indeed in some patients the euthymic intervals are so regular that it is possible to predict, even to the month, when the next episode will occur. Occasionally, one may also see a seasonal pattern, with manic episodes more likely in the spring or early summer, and depressive ones in the fall or winter. Manic episodes in patients with bipolar disorder may also become 'entrained' to certain biologic events, such as the puerperium (Bratfos and Haug 1966; Viguera *et al.* 2000) or the premenstruum (D'Mello *et al.* 1993).

The total number of episodes experienced by a patient depends, of course, not only on the duration of the euthymic interval but also on the duration of the episodes themselves. On one extreme, the euthymic interval may be so long that patients have only a couple of episodes in their lifetimes; indeed, in the natural course of events, some patients may die before they were 'scheduled' for another episode, and thus they end up having only one episode in their entire life. On the other extreme, patients with very brief episodes and brief intervals may have literally hundreds of episodes per year (Bunney and Hartmann 1965; Jenner *et al.* 1967); such an extremely high frequency of episodes, however, is very rare. Patients with more than four episodes per year are termed 'rapid cyclers' (Bauer *et al.* 1994; Dunner *et al.* 1977). Interestingly, it appears that, in some instances, rapid cycling is associated with subclinical hypothyroidism (Bauer *et al.* 1990; Cowdry *et al.* 1983) (as may be induced by treatment with lithium [Terao 1993]).

The sequence of episodes is also quite variable. It is rare to find patients whose courses are characterized by regularly alternating manic and depressive episodes. Most patients experience either a preponderance of manic or a preponderance of depressive episodes throughout their lives. Thus, to look at two extremes, whereas one patient may have six episodes of depression and only one of mania throughout his life, another might have a dozen episodes of mania but only one of depression. Indeed, albeit very rarely, one may encounter 'unipolar' manic patients who have only manic episodes throughout their lives, never experiencing a depressive one (Pfohl *et al.* 1982; Shulman and Tohen 1994).

Bipolar disorder may present with either a depressive episode or a manic one. Importantly, in cases in which the first episode is depressive, it appears that, in over 90 percent of cases, a manic episode will ensue within either 10 years or a total of five episodes of depression, whichever comes first (Dunner *et al.* 1976).

As noted earlier, during the intervals between episodes, most patients are euthymic and free of mood symptoms. In about one-quarter of cases, however, the intervals may be 'colored' by very mild mood symptoms, and the 'direction' or 'polarity' of this coloring correlates with the preponderance of episodes. Thus, a patient who tends to have very mild, 'sub-hypomanic' symptoms during the interval is more likely to have manic than depressive episodes, whereas a patient whose intervals are clouded by minor depressive symptoms is more likely to have depressive than manic episodes.

Occasionally, one may find cases in which certain events, pharmacologic or otherwise, may more or less reliably precipitate a manic episode. These include serotoninergic agents, such as tryptophan or 5-hydroxytryptophan; noradrenergic or dopaminergic agents, such as cocaine, amphetamine, methylphenidate, various sympathomimetics, levodopa, or direct-acting dopaminergics such as bromocriptine; alcohol or sedative–hypnotic withdrawal, or sudden discontinuation of clonidine; and treatment with steroids, such as prednisone. Most notably, antidepressants may also precipitate mania; although this is more likely with tricyclic antidepressants, it has also been noted with newer antidepressants such as SSRIs, venlafaxine, and bupropion. Other agents capable of inducing mania include herbal preparations, such as St. John's wort (Moses and Mallinger 2000), and phototherapy.

Suicide occurs in 10–20 percent of patients with bipolar disorder, and although most suicides tend to occur during a depressive episode, patients in the uncommon mixedmanic episodes are actually at highest risk.

Etiology

Bipolar disorder has a definite genetic component. The incidence of bipolar disorder is higher among the first-degree relatives of probands than among the general population (Gershon et al. 1982; Tsuang et al. 1985), and the monozygotic concordance rate is higher than the dizygotic one (Bertelsen et al. 1977; Kieseppa et al. 2004). Furthermore, adoption studies have demonstrated that the prevalence of bipolar disorder is several-fold higher among the biologic parents of patients with bipolar disorder than among their adoptive parents (Mendlewicz and Rainer 1977). Although genetic studies have offered tantalizing clues, replication of positive findings has been difficult. In all likelihood, multiple genes on multiple different chromosomes are involved, each conferring a susceptibility to the disease.

Neuropathologic findings are sparse but suggest hypothalamic and brainstem involvement. Within the hypothalamus, overall neuronal loss has been noted in the paraventricular nucleus (Manaye et al. 2005), with, however, an increased number of corticotrophin-releasing hormone (CRH)-containing cells (Bao et al. 2005); within the brainstem, disturbances have been noted in the locus ceruleus and the dorsal raphe nucleus (Baumann and Bogerts 2001).

Endocrinologic changes strongly suggest hypothalamic disturbances: the dexamethasone suppression test (DST) is generally positive (Rush et al. 1997; Watson et al. 2004), and the thyroid-stimulating hormone (TSH) response to thyrotropin-releasing hormone (TRH) stimulation is blunted (Extein et al. 1980). It also appears that there may be a disturbance of cholinergic transmission in bipolar disorder: the infusion of physostigmine reliably precipitates depression in patients who are currently manic (Janowsky et al. 1973), and the latency to rapid eye movement (REM) sleep upon infusion of arecoline is shortened in bipolar patients compared with control subjects.

Although speculative, taken together these findings are consistent with the notion that bipolar disorder represents an inherited disturbance of the structure or function of hypothalamic and brainstem nuclei.

Differential diagnosis

In considering a diagnosis of bipolar disorder, the first step is to ensure that the patient either has had a manic episode or is in the midst of one. As noted in Section 6.3, hypomania is a distinctive syndrome and is difficult to confuse with anything else. Difficulties arise, however, when one either lacks this history or happens to see the patient when the stage of hypomania has already been passed and the patient is now in acute mania or delirious mania. Acute mania may be confused with the syndrome of psychosis, given the presence of delusions and hallucinations; however, in acute mania the cardinal manic symptoms (e.g., heightened mood, increased energy, etc.) are still prominent and offer a clue. In delirious mania, however, these cardinal symptoms, as noted above, may fade from the picture and, at this point, in addition to a syndromal diagnosis of psychosis, one may also entertain syndromal diagnoses of catatonia or delirium. It must be emphasized that the easiest and best way to make a correct syndromal diagnosis of mania is to obtain an accurate history. This may be laborious at times as patients in acute mania or delirious mania are generally unable to provide a reliable history, and consequently one may have to contact friends, family members, or co-workers; the best diagnostic strategy is to establish a typical clinical evolution of symptoms, from normalcy to hypomania and then on to acute and perhaps delirious mania.

Once the syndromal diagnosis of mania is established, the next step is to determine the cause of the mania. Although bipolar disorder is by far the most common cause of mania, multiple other etiologies, as discussed in Section 6.3, are possible. Of the disorders discussed there, the idiopathic ones, namely cyclothymia, schizoaffective disorder, and post-partum psychosis, figure most prominently on the differential. Cyclothymia is in all likelihood merely a forme fruste of bipolar disorder (Akiskal et al. 1977), and patients experience recurrent episodes of very mild hypomania and correspondingly very mild depression. Schizoaffective disorder is immediately distinguished by the course. In schizoaffective disorder the intervals between episodes of mania or depression are marked by psychotic symptoms, such as delusions, hallucinations, and loosening of associations, and this is in stark contrast to the intervals of bipolar disorder, in which such psychotic symptoms are never seen. Post-partum psychosis is characterized by a psychosis, often with prominent manic symptoms, occurring in the post-partum period, and is distinguished from bipolar disorder by its course. In post-partum psychosis, symptoms occur only in the post-partum period, whereas in bipolar disorder, although episodes of mania may occur post-partum, they are also seen at other times in the patient's life. Other disorders noted in Section 6.3, although less common, must also be considered, and the reader is encouraged to review that section.

Treatment

The treatment of bipolar disorder involves acute, continuation, and preventive treatments for manic and mixed-manic episodes and for depressive episodes. This almost always involves the use of one of the mood-stabilizer agents, including lithium, carbamazepine, divalproex, and lamotrigine.

MANIC AND MIXED–MANIC EPISODES

Acute treatment of a manic or mixed-manic episode almost always involves the administration of one of the mood stabilizers (lithium, divalproex, or carbamazepine; lamotrigine has not been shown to be effective in the acute treatment of mania) or an antipsychotic (either a second-generation agent [olanzapine, risperidone, quetiapine, aripiprazole, or ziprasidone] or a first-generation agent [e.g., chlorpromazine or haloperidol]) or, most commonly, a combination of a mood stabilizer plus one of the antipsychotics. Although there are no hard and fast guidelines for choosing which agent or agents to use, some general guidelines may be offered. Certainly, if the patient has a history of an excellent response to a particular agent or combination of agents, then this should be seriously considered. Lacking such a history, and assuming that there are no significant contraindications, then one should consider either lithium or divalproex; although lithium has by far the longest track record, divalproex is extraordinarily easy to use and may have an edge over lithium in mixed episodes. Another definite advantage of divalproex is the rapidity of response when a 'loading' strategy is used, with patients often showing a response within a matter of days, in contrast to the week or two 'lag period' seen with lithium. Carbamazepine is not as well tolerated as either divalproex or lithium, and may be a little less effective than lithium. Among the antipsychotics, the first choice is probably olanzapine, as it has the longest track record in this regard. However, if for some reason chronic treatment with an antipsychotic is anticipated, concerns about the metabolic effects of olanzapine might prompt one to consider a different antipsychotic, such as quetiapine or risperidone.

When symptoms are relatively mild, as may be seen in hypomania, utilization of a mood stabilizer alone may be sufficient. However, when acute or delirious mania has occurred, one typically has to use a combination of a mood stabilizer plus an antipsychotic. In very severe cases that fail to respond to combination treatment, one may also consider ECT.

Most manic patients require admission to a locked unit. Stimulation, including visitors, phone calls, and mail, should be kept to an absolute minimum, as they routinely exacerbate symptoms. In some cases seclusion is required, and certain patients, still possessed of some insight, may demand seclusion as they know that the reduced stimulation of the seclusion room will allow for some reduction in their symptoms.

Continuation treatment is designed to prevent the recurrence of symptoms once they have been brought under control during the acute phase of treatment. Generally, this is accomplished by continuing the regimen that was effective during the acute phase, and doing so for the anticipated duration of the manic episode. In many cases, if a combination of a mood stabilizer plus an antipsychotic were required, it may be possible to discontinue the antipsychotic and maintain the patient on the mood stabilizer alone; should symptoms recur, the antipsychotic may be restarted. As noted earlier, most manic episodes last on average from weeks to months; however, given the wide variability here, the best guide is the individual patient's past history.

If a decision is made not to enter into a preventive phase of treatment, then continuation treatment may be discontinued after the current episode has gone into a spontaneous remission. This is sometimes difficult, especially if one does not have a reliable history regarding the length of earlier episodes. Certainly, if the patient is having *any* manic symptoms, no matter how mild, treatment should be continued, and in general it is best to hold off on discontinuing treatment until the patient's personal life is fairly stable.

Before moving on to a consideration of the preventive phase of treatment, some further words are in order regarding lithium. If lithium was used during the acute phase it may be necessary to reduce the dose once symptoms have been brought under control; in many patients, even though the dose of lithium is held constant, the blood level will rise as symptoms come under control, and patients may develop significant, and unexpected, side-effects. Furthermore, if lithium was used during continuation treatment and the decision is to forego preventive treatment, then the dose of lithium should be tapered gradually over a few weeks, as it appears that abrupt discontinuation of lithium may predispose to a recurrence of mania (Baldessarini *et al.* 1996, 1997). Although this effect has not been demonstrated for divalproex or carbamazepine, prudence dictates following a similar strategy.

Preventive treatment should be seriously considered in all cases, and the decision as to whether or not to embark on preventive treatment should be made with reference to several factors, including the frequency of episodes, the rapidity with which they develop, and the anticipated side-effect burden. Frequent episodes, perhaps occurring more than once every 2 years, usually constitute an indication for preventive treatment; a frequency of once every 5 years or more, however, may be such that the risk of another episode is outweighed by the need to take the medicine chronically and having to suffer any attendant side-effects. Severe episodes, however, even if infrequent, may warrant prevention. In cases in which episodes develop very slowly, patients may be able to 'catch' themselves in time, and treatment may be instituted on an outpatient basis; in cases in which episodes come on acutely, however, patients may be defenseless and thus in need of preventive treatment.

If preventive treatment is elected, the patient may be maintained on the agent or combination of agents that proved effective during continuation treatment. Of the mood stabilizers, lithium has the longest track record and, all other things being equal, is the treatment of first choice; however, carbamazepine and divalproex also constitute reasonable alternatives. If lithium is utilized, the blood level should be kept between 0.6 and 1 mEq/L. The optimum preventive doses for divalproex and carbamazepine have not been determined; prudence suggests continuing the same dose as was effective in the continuation phase of treatment. Should 'breakthrough' symptoms of mania occur it is critical to determine thyroid status, as even 'chemical' hypothyroidism, with a normal free thyroxine (T_4) but an elevated TSH, may blunt the effectiveness of a mood stabilizer. Should breakthrough mania occur despite normal thyroid status and good compliance, consideration may be given to switching to monotherapy with another mood stabilizer or to using a combination of mood stabilizers (e.g., lithium plus divalproex or lithium plus carbamazepine).

Some clinicians may opt for using an antipsychotic such as olanzapine for preventive treatment; however, although this is becoming increasingly popular, caution may be necessary for two reasons. First, although olanzapine has been shown to be effective in this regard, its track record is not as long as that of lithium, for example. Second, this may be a problematic option if the potential long-term side-effects of olanzapine occur, such as weight gain, diabetes, and hyperlipidemia.

DEPRESSIVE EPISODES

Treatment of a depressive episode of bipolar disorder may involve the use of a mood stabilizer alone; traditionally, if this is ineffective an antidepressant is added. If patients are not already taking a mood stabilizer, one should be started; in this regard, although lamotrigine has not been shown to be effective in the acute treatment of mania, it is effective in the acute treatment of depression. If the patient is taking lithium or divalproex and a depression occurs, it may be appropriate to switch to either carbamazepine or lamotrigine, as these may be more effective against depression. In evaluating the effectiveness of this strategy, one must keep in mind that two or more weeks may be required before depression lifts.

In cases in which depression persists, or is so severe that one does not wish to risk a failure of a mood stabilizer, it is appropriate to consider adding an antidepressant. Importantly, however, given that all antidepressants may precipitate a manic episode, antidepressants should not be used alone but must always be used in combination with a mood stabilizer. In this regard, given the relative ineffectiveness of lamotrigine as an anti-manic agent, if one is adding an antidepressant it is prudent to have one of the other mood stabilizers (i.e., lithium, divalproex, or carbamazepine) in place. The choice of an antidepressant is discussed in Section 20.6. If possible, some clinicians prefer avoiding the use of antidepressants, not only because they may precipitate manic episodes but also because there is some evidence that they may alter the course of the illness, making future episodes of mania more likely (Altschuler et al. 1995).

Recently demonstrated additional options for the acute treatment of depression include the combination of olanzapine plus fluoxetine and, interestingly, monotherapy with quetiapine.

Once depressive symptoms have been relieved, treatment should be continued to prevent a reappearance of symptoms. If the depression has responded to a mood stabilizer alone, one may then simply continue this. If, however, in addition to a mood stabilizer an antidepressant has been required, the ongoing risk of an antidepressant-precipitated mania will dictate an attempt at some point to discontinue the antidepressant and see if the patient can be maintained on the mood stabilizer alone. Deciding when to discontinue an antidepressant is not straightforward. Certainly, if a reliable history indicates that the patient's depressive episodes routinely last for a more or less definite and predictable length of time, one could discontinue the antidepressant if that time has elapsed. Lacking this guidance, however, one may wish to wait until the patient has been euthymic for a significant period of time, at least weeks, before attempting a discontinuation; should symptoms recur, then one may simply restart the antidepressant.

Once the current depressive episode has run its course, patients may be considered for preventive treatment with a mood stabilizer: carbamazepine, lithium, or lamotrigine are effective, with lamotrigine being more effective than lithium in the prevention of depressive episodes.

SUMMARY

In planning the treatment of a chronic disorder such as bipolar disorder, the most important decision to make is which drug to use over the long haul. Although not without controversy, it is probably appropriate to consider one of the mood stabilizers for long-term treatment. Among the mood stabilizers, lithium remains the 'one to beat' as it is effective in all phases of treatment; carbamazepine is also effective in all phases but its side-effect burden is typically significantly greater. Divalproex is a reasonable choice for mania predominant cases of bipolar disorder; however, the lack of demonstrated effectiveness in the acute or preventive treatment of depression may give the clinician pause in recommending this agent. Lamotrigine, until it is shown to be effective for mania, should probably be reserved for cases that are heavily depression predominant.

These summary recommendations, however, must be taken as only the broadest possible of guidelines, and treatment must be individualized, with due regard to the peculiarities of each case.

20.6 MAJOR DEPRESSIVE DISORDER

Major depressive disorder, often referred to simply as major depression, is characterized by the occurrence of one or more depressive episodes during the patient's lifetime. Synonyms for this disorder include unipolar affective disorder, melancholia, and manic-depressive illness, depressed type. 'Unipolar' highlights the critical difference between major depressive disorder and bipolar disorder, namely the fact that the patient with major depressive disorder has episodes that go only toward one 'pole', namely the depressive one, whereas the patient with bipolar disorder, in addition to depressive episodes, will also have episodes that go to the other, or manic, pole. Melancholia is the most ancient term for this disorder; it comes from the Greek word meaning 'black bile', reflecting the Greek's humoral theory of this disorder. Manic-depressive illness, depressed type, the final synonym for this disorder, is problematic for two reasons. First, as originally conceived by Kraepelin, manic-depressive illness was a disorder that subsumed what today are recognized as two disorders, namely major depressive disorder and bipolar disorder. Kraepelin felt that these two disorders were merely variants or subtypes of one overarching disorder, but recognizing the clinical differences of these variants he spoke of a 'depressive' type and a 'circular' type. Given the separateness of major depressive disorder and bipolar disorder, however, it may no longer be appropriate to use the overarching term. The second reason has to do with common usage. In the United States, when clinicians use the term 'manic-depressive illness', most are referring to bipolar disorder, and hence to use it to refer to major depressive disorder may lead to confusion.

Major depressive disorder is a common disorder, occurring in at least 5 percent of the general population; amongst adults it is twice as common in women as in men.

Clinical features

Major depression is characterized by the occurrence of episodes of depression, in between which patients return to more or less normal functioning. Although the first episode of depression generally appears in the mid-twenties, the range in age of onset is wide, from childhood to the ninth decade.

Depressive episodes tend to appear gradually, even insidiously. Typically, there is a long prodrome, often lasting months, characterized by fleeting and often indefinite symptoms such as moodiness, anxiety or fatigue. Furthermore, when the depressive episode finally does settle in, the various symptoms often appear haltingly and with differing severities, and it is consequently rare that a patient can date the onset idiopath with any sort of precision. This is not to say, however, that acute and obvious onsets are not seen. They do occur,

and some patients may describe a rapid fall from emotional well-being into a full depressive episode in as little as a week or two. Such acute onsets, however, are the exception rather than the rule. In about 50 percent of cases the duration of a depressive episode of major depressive disorder ranges from 6 to 12 months; longer durations, up to 2 years, may be seen in about 10 percent of cases. Eventually, symptoms gradually undergo a more or less full remission.

At times depressive episodes may appear to be precipitated by a stressful life event, typically a serious loss, such as the death of a loved one, divorce, or the loss of a job. At times, however, close enquiry will reveal that the stressful life event, rather than actually precipitating the depressive episode, was itself caused by the depressive episode. For example, a married person, in the midst of a long prodrome, may be sufficiently irritable to cause the spouse to leave. In such cases, although the patient may blame the depression on the separation, in fact it was the depressive prodrome that caused the separation. This is not to say, of course, that independent precipitating events do not at times trigger depressive episodes, for they do. However, it appears that in this group of patients with precipitated depressive episodes, subsequent episodes tend to become independent and to occur autonomously without any precipitating events (Brown *et al.* 1994; Frank *et al.* 1994).

As discussed in Section 6.1, depressive episodes are characterized by a number of symptoms, including depressed or irritable mood; low self-esteem, guilt or pessimism; suicidal ideation; difficulty with concentration or forgetfulness; anhedonia; anergia; sleep disturbance; appetite disturbance; and psychomotor change. Patients may also describe an overall diurnal variation in the severity of their depression, with symptoms being more intense in the morning. Delusions and hallucinations may also occur, as may certain other symptoms, such as anxiety attacks.

Mood is typically depressed but may be primarily irritable; some patients may also complain of anxiety. In some cases, however, although possessed of a depressed affect, patients may deny feeling depressed but may rather speak of a sense of discouragement, lassitude, or a feeling of being weighed down. Occasionally one may see patients who 'put on' a 'happy face', and feign a normal affect despite experiencing a depressed mood. Such a 'smiling depression' may mislead the diagnostician who fails to specifically enquire after the patient's mood.

Self-esteem typically sinks and the workings of conscience become prominent. Patients may consider themselves worthless and as having never done anything of value; in looking over their past, they see their sins multiplied. Indeed, in reviewing the past, patients seem 'blind' to any accomplishments and fix only on their misdeeds and shortcomings, which, as they recall them, may become magnified to heinous proportions. Some patients may give way to rumination, in which their failings and defects repeat themselves again and again in a litany of hopelessness. Pessimism is common and patients see no hope for the future; to them there are no prospects and all appears bleak.

Suicidal ideation is almost always present. At times this may be merely passive and patients may wish aloud that they might die of some disease or accident. Conversely, it may be active, and patients may consider hanging or shooting themselves, jumping from bridges, or overdosing on their medications. Often, and seemingly paradoxically, the risk of suicide is greatest as patients begin to recover. Still seeing themselves as worthless and hopeless sinners, these patients, now with some relief from fatigue, may find themselves with enough energy to carry out their suicidal plans. The overall suicide rate in major depressive disorder is about 4 percent; among those with depressive episodes severe enough to prompt hospitalization, however, the rate rises to about 9 percent.

Difficulty with concentration (Roy-Byrne et al. 1986) may be particularly troubling. Patients may complain of a dull heavy-headedness, as if they are 'in a fog'; attempts to read may be especially painful as patients read and re-read the same paragraph but never find themselves understanding what they read. Short-term memory may become difficult, and patients may be unable to recall where they put their keys or what was said just minutes before. Making decisions, even simple ones, may become an almost insuperable task; everything appears too complicated, with too many possibilities and choices. In some cases of severe depression in the elderly, cognitive decrements may be severe enough to constitute a dementia (Rabins et al. 1984), which may be particularly severe. One 76-year-old became disoriented to time, was unable to recall any items after 3 minutes, and presented cachectic and curled up in a fetal position (McAllister and Price 1982); a 66-year-old was disoriented to time and place, confused, and incontinent (Kramer 1982); both recovered with adequate antidepressant treatment.

Anhedonia manifests with a lack of interest in formerly pleasurable activities; sports and hobbies, etc. no longer arouse patients and, if they force themselves to partake, they take no pleasure in such activities and merely go through the motions. Libido is routinely lost and there is no pleasure in sexual activity.

Anergia manifests with a dearth of energy, and patients may complain of feeling tired, fatigued, lifeless, or drained. Occasionally, patients may complain of having too much energy; however, on closer questioning one finds rather that patients have a 'nervous energy', more akin to agitation; such 'increased energy' is useless to the patient and is always overshadowed by a sense of imminent and impending exhaustion.

Sleep disturbance tends toward insomnia, which may be a torment to the patient. Although many complain of what is technically known as 'initial' insomnia, or trouble falling asleep, the most characteristic kind of insomnia in depression comes later in the night as either 'middle' or 'terminal' insomnia. In middle insomnia the patient awakens in the middle of the night for no particular reason and then has great difficulty falling back to sleep, often lying awake for an hour or more before sleep finally comes. Terminal insomnia, also known as 'early morning awakening', comes later in the night, and, here, once awake, the patient cannot fall back to sleep at all. As they lie awake, many patients experience ruminations or restless, unproductive thoughts. When the morning finally does come, patients find themselves unrefreshed and exhausted, as if they had not slept at all. Rarely, rather than experiencing insomnia, patients with major depressive disorder may complain of hypersomnia, wherein they sleep excessively, sometimes for up to 18 hours.

Appetite is routinely lost and many patients lose weight, sometimes in substantial amounts (Stunkard et al. 1990). Food may lose its taste or become unpalatable, and some patients may complain that food tastes like cardboard or leaves them nauseated. Uncommonly, patients may experience an increased appetite and may gain weight.

Psychomotor change tends toward agitation. When slight, this agitation may be experienced as a mere inner restlessness. When more severe, however, there may be hand-wringing and incessant pacing: patients may complain that they cannot keep still; they may lament their fate out loud and give way to wailing and repetitive pleas for help. The tension of these patients may be extreme, almost palpable, and yet, despite their piteous pleas for help, they cannot be comforted, no matter what is done for them. Psychomotor retardation, although uncommon, may also occur. In this, thoughts come slowly and sluggishly, if at all, and speech, when it occurs, is slow and halting. Some patients may sit immobile for hours, and if asked to do something may complain that they can't, that it is too difficult. In severe cases patients may not move for any reason; they may go without bathing or changing their clothes, and some may defecate or urinate in the chair or on the bed.

Delusions and hallucinations may occur in about 15 per cent of the depressive episodes of major depressive disorder, most commonly in cases in which the depressive symptoms are quite severe (Lykouras et al. 1986; Maj et al. 1990). Delusions are mood-congruent in that, in some extreme, fantastic way, they are appropriate to the patients' moods and views of themselves. Guilt may be extreme and patients may confess to unspeakable sins: they have poisoned their children; family or friends are imprisoned for crimes that they, the patients, have committed. They may believe that they are condemned to Hell, that they have only hours to live. Delusions of persecution are common and have a peculiar twist to them. In contrast to patients with schizophrenia, who have delusions of persecution and protest that they are innocent victims, depressive patients with delusions of persecution typically feel that they deserve their persecutions for their miserable sins and shortcomings. Delusions of poverty and nihilistic delusions may also occur and are entirely consistent with these patients' views of themselves as worthless and hopeless. They may believe that they are without any funds and are completely bankrupt and unable to pay any bills, and that their families will go destitute. Those with nihilistic delusions may believe that they are near death: their insides have turned to dust or concrete; their brains have shrivelled up; the heart has dried up for lack of blood. In extreme cases patients may believe that they are dead, and some may believe that all are dead, that death has finally achieved complete dominion over the world. Auditory hallucinations may also occur and generally reflect the patients' delusions. Voices may accuse them of crimes or sins, or announce that their well-deserved punishment is at hand. Visual hallucinations occasionally occur, and patients may see corpses or accusatory spirits. In some cases patients may develop stuporous catatonia (Starkstein *et al.* 1996).

Other symptoms seen during a minority of depressive episodes include anxiety attacks (Van Valkenburg *et al.* 1984) and what have been called 'anger attacks', in which generally hostile and irritable patients occasionally experience episodes of violence and autonomic arousal (Fava *et al.* 1993). Obsessions and compulsions may also appear: a particularly common obsession is the 'horrific temptation' to use a knife or gun to kill a loved one, and a consequent overwhelming necessity to rid the house of all potential weapons and to avoid any contact with them outside the house.

Course

Major depressive disorder is a relapsing and remitting illness (Thase 1990), characterized in most patients by the recurrence of depressive episodes throughout their lives, in between which they return to a more or less normal mood.

As noted earlier, in about 50 percent of cases, depressive episodes will undergo a spontaneous remission within 6–12 months. The duration of the interval between successive episodes ranges widely, from as little as 1 year up to decades, with an overall average of about 5 years. In general, however, with repeated episodes the interval between episodes tends to shorten, and the episodes themselves tend to lengthen, such that, over a very long period of time, successive episodes may eventually 'merge' to create a chronic, non-remitting condition.

Recently, much attention has been focused on patients whose depressive episodes seem entrained to the changing seasons. In patients with this seasonal pattern of illness, depressive episodes appear to occur far more commonly in the fall or winter than in the spring or summer.

Etiology

Hereditary factors appear to play a role: the prevalence of major depression is higher in the relatives of patients than of control subjects, and the monozygotic concordance rate is significantly higher than the dizygotic one (McGuffin *et al.* 1996). To date, however, genetic studies have not identified genes or loci that may be confidently associated with this illness, indicating in all likelihood that, from a genetic point of view, this is a complex disorder, involving multiple genes and multiple modes of inheritance.

Hereditary factors, although clearly important, do not appear to provide a complete account, and environmental factors also seem to play a role. Among the various environmental events proposed, it appears that early childhood loss may be the most important. Events may also serve as precipitants for episodes in adult life; however, as noted earlier, the importance of precipitants fades with successive episodes to the point where, over long periods of time, episodes become, as it were, autonomous.

There is abundant evidence for endocrinologic disturbances in depression, all of which point to disturbances in the hypothalamus. Within the hypothalamus, for example, the level of messenger RNA for CRH in the paraventricular nucleus is elevated (Raadsheer *et al.* 1995), as is the cerebrospinal fluid (CSF) level of CRH (Nemeroff *et al.* 1984); consistent with this, the low-dose DST test is generally positive (Carroll *et al.* 1968, 1976). The thyroid axis also shows disturbances: the CSF level of TRH is elevated (Banki *et al.* 1988), and, consistent with this, the response of TSH to exogenous TRH is blunted (Prange *et al.* 1972).

Abnormalities in brainstem structures responsible for REM sleep are suggested by the fact that REM sleep latency is reduced in depression (Hauri *et al.* 1974; Rush *et al.* 1986), and by the response to cholinergic agents. Normally, REM sleep may be induced by cholinergic stimulation; however, in patients with major depressive disorder the latency to REM sleep with such cholinergic agents as arecoline (Gillin *et al.* 1991) and donepezil (Perlis *et al.* 2002) is shorter than in control subjects.

The undoubted success of antidepressant medications has focused attention on biogenic amines. Given that all antidepressants have effects on either noradrenergic or serotoninergic functioning, it appears reasonable to assume that there is a complementary disturbance in these amines in patients with major depressive disorder. Despite enormous research efforts, however, it has been difficult to isolate definite abnormalities here. One notable exception involves the effects of tryptophan depletion. Tryptophan is the dietary precursor of serotonin and, in patients with an antidepressant-induced remission of depression, tryptophan depletion is promptly followed by a relapse of depressive symptoms (Aberg-Wistedt *et al.* 1998; Delgado *et al.* 1990; Smith *et al.* 1997).

Relatively speaking, neuropathologic studies are in their infancy in this disorder. Some studies have suggested changes in the dorsolateral prefrontal cortex; however, in my opinion the endocrinologic and sleep abnormalities point rather to the diencephalon or brainstem as the most likely sites for any changes. In this regard, several, albeit preliminary, findings have been reported, including the following; an increased number of neurons in the mediodorsal nucleus of the thalamus (Young *et al.* 2004); an overall decreased number of neurons in the paraventricular nucleus of the hypothalamus (Manaye *et al.* 2005) with a relative increase in the number of CRH-containing neurons in the same nucleus (Bao *et al.* 2005).

Integrating all of the foregoing findings into a coherent theory is problematic and involves some speculation. With this caveat in mind, however, it may be reasonable to propose that major depressive disorder represents an interaction between certain environmental events and an inherited abnormality of noradrenergic, serotoninergic or cholinergic functioning, of variable degree, associated with subtle neuroanatomic changes in the thalamus, hypothalamus or mesencephalon.

Differential diagnosis

The first step in differential diagnosis is to ensure that the patient either has, or has had, a depressive episode, for without this, of course, a diagnosis of major depressive disorder cannot be made. As discussed in Section 6.1, not all patients who complain of depression or who appear depressed have a true depressive episode; almost all persons, at some point in their lives, will have some depressive symptoms as a normal reaction to adverse life circumstances, and these must be distinguished, using the guidelines outlined in that section, from a depressive episode.

Once it has been determined that a true depressive episode has occurred, the next step is to determine whether this has been caused by a major depressive disorder or one of the many other causes of depression discussed in Section 6.1, a section that the reader is strongly advised to review.

Treatment

The overall pharmacologic treatment of major depressive disorder is conveniently divided into three phases: acute treatment designed to initially relieve symptoms during a depressive episode; continuation treatment to prevent the re-emergence of symptoms; and maintenance or prophylactic treatment aimed at preventing the occurrence of subsequent episodes. Although this text focuses on pharmacologic treatment, consideration may also be given, in mild to moderate cases, to psychotherapy (e.g., cognitive-behavioral therapy).

ACUTE TREATMENT

Before beginning treatment a decision must be made as to whether or not to admit the patient. Indications for hospitalization include the following: significant suicide risk; depressive symptoms of such severity as to preclude independent functioning at home and work; significant concurrent illness that requires inpatient monitoring; and a need for acute treatment with ECT.

Acute treatment generally begins with the selection of an antidepressant medication from one of the following groups: tricyclics (e.g., nortriptyline), SSRIs (e.g., escitalopram), monoamine oxidase inhibitors (MAOIs; e.g., selegiline), and a large miscellaneous group (including duloxetine, venlafaxine, mirtazapine, bupropion, and trazodone). Several considerations come into play when making this selection, including overall effectiveness, a personal or family history of response to a particular agent, anticipated side-effects, potential drug–drug interactions, and, finally, lethality in overdose.

Overall, although the various antidepressants are of approximately equal effectiveness, there is some evidence that tricyclics and venlafaxine may have an edge over the others, and that trazodone may be somewhat less effective. These differences, however, are modest at best.

A personal history of a good response to a particular agent is a good predictor of future response, and a family history of a good response may also predict a good response, but this relationship may not be as robust.

Side-effects sometimes loom large in the patient's overall reaction to an antidepressant. Where weight gain is a concern, SSRIs, duloxetine, and bupropion are good choices, and certainly preferable, in this regard, to tricyclics and mirtazapine. Sexual side-effects (e.g., erectile dysfunction, decreased vaginal lubrication, decreased libido) are common with most antidepressants, with the notable exceptions of mirtazapine and bupropion. Orthostatic hypotension, of particular concern in the elderly, is unlikely with SSRIs, venlafaxine, mirtazapine, and bupropion, but common with tricyclics and trazodone. Cardiac arrhythmias may be induced by tricyclics, but SSRIs are particularly benign in this regard. The seizure threshold may be reduced by tricyclics, venlafaxine, and bupropion; in this regard, particular attention must be given to any history of bulimia nervosa, as such patients appear to be particularly at risk for seizures if treated with bupropion. Sedation may be problematic with tricyclics (with the exception of nortriptyline, desipramine, and protriptyline), mirtazapine, and trazodone, but is generally negligible with the other agents.

Drug–drug interactions are a constant concern, and in this regard the SSRIs (especially citalopram and escitalopram) are the 'cleanest' of agents. Conversely, there are so many drug–drug interactions with MAOIs that these agents generally constitute a last choice.

Lethality in overdose is always a concern in prescribing for depressed patients, and in this regard the SSRIs are by far the safest agents, followed by duloxetine, venlafaxine, mirtazapine, and bupropion; the tricyclics and MAOIs are by far the most dangerous of the antidepressants.

All other things being equal, and lacking clear guidance from a personal or strong family history, a first choice may reasonably be made from the following: an SSRI, duloxetine, venlafaxine, mirtazapine, or bupropion. Regardless of which agent is chosen it must be given an 'adequate' trial, which involves not only an 'adequate' dose but also an 'adequate' duration. Even with an average or above-average dose, one should not expect to see any improvement for the first week or two; by the fourth week, however, if there has been no improvement at all it is unlikely that the patient will get a response, at least at the dose used (Quitkin *et al.* 1996). If there is improvement by the fourth week, then the patient should be advised that it may take up to 3 months to see a full response.

In cases in which there has been little or no response by 4 weeks, one should, if not already done, check the free T_4 and TSH levels. Hypothyroidism, even if only 'chemical' (with a normal free T_4 but an elevated TSH), blunts the response to antidepressants and must be corrected. If the patient is euthyroid, and the side-effect burden is readily tolerable, one may at this point consider simply increasing the dose; with the sole exception of nortriptyline (which has a true 'therapeutic window') it appears that for most other antidepressants the dose–response curve is linear, and thus it is a reasonable strategy to gradually push the dose to the maximum recommended, waiting weeks each time to see if there is an initial response.

If the patient does not respond to an increased dose, or if side-effects preclude this approach, then one may consider either switching to a different antidepressant or trying a combination of agents. Switching antidepressants is a viable option but in doing so one should probably switch to an antidepressant of a different pharmacologic class; changing from one SSRI to another, or from one tricyclic to another, makes little sense. In making a switch one must be wary of drug–drug interactions. For example, given the long half-life of some SSRIs and their ability to inhibit the metabolism of tricyclics, in switching from an SSRI to a tricyclic one must either allow time for the SSRI to wash out or alternatively start with a low dose of the tricyclic. Combination treatment is also viable but only a few combinations have been found to be effective, including lithium plus a tricyclic or an SSRI; triiodothyronine (50 μg) plus a tricyclic or an SSRI; olanzapine plus fluoxetine; aripiprazole plus an SSRI or venlafaxine; and, finally, an MAOI plus a tricyclic. This last option is potentially dangerous and should probably only be undertaken by a specialist. Regardless of whether one switches or uses a combination strategy, one must again allow for an 'adequate trial', ensuring that doses are adequate and that at least 4 weeks are allowed to assess the response.

Should depression prove resistant to a switch or to a combination, one might consider different single agents or different combinations. How far one goes with this approach depends largely on the severity of the depression. If the symptoms are tolerable and the risk of suicide is low, then further trials may be reasonable; if however, symptoms are severe or there is a significant risk of death, one should strongly consider ECT.

Although the foregoing schema for the acute treatment of depression is in general applicable to most cases, exceptions do occur. First, in severe cases requiring hospitalization, many physicians will routinely check thyroid status and begin either with high-dose monotherapy or with a combination. Second, for the highly suicidal patient, or in other life-threatening cases (e.g., in severely debilitated elderly patients), moving immediately to ECT may be appropriate, as ECT is clearly not only the most effective treatment for depression but also, with proper technique, remains quite safe. Third, there is some controversy regarding the treatment of 'psychotic depression', that is depression that is accompanied by delusions or hallucinations. Traditionally, patients with psychotic depression have been treated with the combination of an antipsychotic plus an antidepressant, or with ECT. However, it appears that in many of these cases, prolonged treatment with high-dosage monotherapy may be just as effective.

Before leaving this discussion of the acute treatment of depression, some words are in order regarding certain other treatments, including herbal remedies (i.e., St. John's wort), omega-3 fatty acids, phototherapy, alprazolam, buspirone, vagal nerve stimulation, and transcranial magnetic stimulation. St. Johns wort and omega-3 fatty acids may be beneficial in mild depressions, but cannot be counted on in anything more severe. Phototherapy is generally reserved for mild depressions occurring in patients whose illnesses demonstrate a seasonal pattern, as described earlier. Alprazolam may be effective in mild to moderate depressions, but the 3–6 mg dose required carries such a significant risk of neuroadaptation that most clinicians shy away from using it. Buspirone, in doses of 60 mg or more daily, may be effective in mild to moderate depression, but is not commonly employed. Vagal nerve stimulation has not been shown to be effective in double-blind studies and cannot be recommended. Although the place of transcranial magnetic stimulation is still not clear, it is my belief that this will emerge as a viable option.

CONTINUATION TREATMENT

Once acute treatment has effected a remission of depressive symptoms, continuation treatment is required. It must be kept in mind that antidepressants, rather than 'curing' depression, merely suppress symptoms, and consequently if treatment is discontinued before the depressive episode has run its course, symptoms will gradually recur. In general, continuation treatment involves a continuation of the regimen that was effective for acute treatment. In a minority of cases it may be possible to scale back treatment without any loss of effectiveness (e.g., in monotherapy cases, allowing a dose reduction, or in combination therapy, discontinuing one of the agents); however, this must be carried out carefully given the risk of relapse. If ECT was required, one should consider either 'continuation ECT' or antidepressant treatment, for example either with an SSRI (e.g., paroxetine) or with a combination of nortriptyline and lithium.

Continuation treatment should persist for the duration of the depressive episode. In cases in which the patient has a history of depressive episodes of fairly uniform and discrete duration, this may be used as a guide for determining the length of continuation treatment. In most cases, however, such guidance is not available, either because the current episode is the first or because prior episodes were of such indistinct onset and offset that a reliable estimation of their duration is not possible. In these cases, continuation treatment should probably be performed until the patient has been symptom free for 6 consecutive months (Altamura and Percudani 1993; Kupfer et al. 1992; Prien and Kupfer 1986; Reimherr et al. 1998). This guideline is based on the assumption that no treatment is perfect and that, given the waxing and waning nature of symptoms, one will find that, when symptoms rise to a 'peak', they 'break through' the antidepressant 'barrier' to the point where they cause distress. Furthermore, the longer a patient goes without such a breakthrough, the more likely it becomes that the underlying episode has finally gone into a spontaneous remission, and it appears that 6 months represents a reasonable duration for this to occur. When the time does come to consider discontinuation of treatment, given that a small risk of relapse still exists, one may wish to schedule the discontinuation for a time in the patient's life when a relapse would not have disastrous consequences.

MAINTENANCE TREATMENT

Given that the majority of patients will eventually have another episode, it is reasonable to discuss maintenance or preventive treatment. Prevention should be strongly considered in cases in which past history suggests that, in the natural course of events, the euthymic interval between episodes is less than 2 years, or in cases in which, regardless of the frequency of episodes, the episodes themselves have been so severe that one would not wish to risk a relapse, no matter how far in the future that might occur. If patients do elect for maintenance therapy one may simply continue the antidepressant regimen used in continuation therapy. In cases in which ECT was required for continuation therapy it is not clear whether ongoing ECT is required, and one may opt for an antidepressant regimen.

20.7 PREMENSTRUAL DYSPHORIC DISORDER

Premenstrual dysphoric disorder, also known as the premenstrual syndrome or late luteal phase dysphoric disorder, is characterized by recurrent, relatively brief, depressive episodes that are tightly entrained to the events of the menstrual cycle. This is a common disorder, occurring in about 5 percent of all menstruating females.

Clinical features

The onset of this disorder is generally between menarche and the late twenties, and its most remarkable aspect is the timing of the depressive episodes, which have a fairly abrupt onset, anywhere from 3 to 10 days before menstruation begins, and then just as rapidly remit, 2–3 days after menstrual flow commences.

During the depressive episode, the mood (Bloch *et al.* 1997) is variously depressed, sad, anxious, or, classically, irritable; often there is considerable lability with inexplicable crying spells or unwonted anger, and many patients complain of feeling 'out of control'. Patients may have difficulty with concentration or paying attention to things, and may lose interest in work, hobbies, or sexual activity. There may be prominent fatigue, and some may become lethargic. Sleep disturbance is common and may be toward either insomnia or hypersomnia. Appetite may also change and is often increased with associated cravings for sweets or chocolates. Other symptoms may also occur, including

headache, mastalgia, bloating (particularly with swelling of the hands and feet), clumsiness, nausea, and constipation.

Some patients, concerned over their irritability, may voluntarily isolate themselves, and family members may soon learn to 'leave well enough alone' during this part of the menstrual cycle.

Course

Over long periods of time the depressive episodes may become more severe and may appear progressively earlier in the menstrual cycle, to the point where, in some cases, the episode may begin 3 weeks before menstrual flow. Eventually, with menopause, the episodes cease to occur.

Etiology

Premenstrual dysphoric disorder is familial and may bear a relationship to major depressive disorder, given that the prevalence of major depressive disorder is higher in the relatives of probands than in the general population.

There is ample evidence for a disturbance in serotoninergic functioning in patients with premenstrual dysphoric disorder. Fenfluramine, a serotoninergic agent, normally stimulates prolactin secretion, and the prolactin response to this agent in premenstrual dysphoric disorder is blunted (Fitzgerald *et al.* 1997). Furthermore, symptoms may be exacerbated either by administration of a serotonin-blocking agent (Roca *et al.* 2002) or by tryptophan depletion (Menkes *et al.* 1994). Finally, whereas serotoninergic agents (e.g., SSRIs) are effective in this disorder, non-serotoninergic antidepressants (e.g., desipramine [Freeman *et al.* 1999] and bupropion [Pearlstein *et al.* 1997]) are not.

Overall, although speculative, it may be reasonable to hypothesize that in premenstrual dysphoric disorder there is an inherited disturbance of serotoninergic functioning, probably in mesencephalic or hypothalamic structures, that is episodically triggered by the dramatic hormonal changes seen during the transition from the follicular to the luteal phase of the normal menstrual cycle.

Differential diagnosis

The key to making this diagnosis is to monitor the patient over at least several menstrual cycles to establish the classic onset and duration of the episodes and, very importantly, to demonstrate that during the follicular phase patients are symptom free. Essentially, there is no other disorder that mimics this remarkable pattern.

Of the multiple other causes of depression discussed in Section 6.1, major depressive disorder, bipolar disorder, and post-partum depression may also be kept in mind. In these disorders, depressive episodes may be quite prolonged and may undergo an exacerbation during the luteal phase. If this exacerbation is sufficiently severe, patients may mistakenly report that they feel 'better' during the follicular phase, thus lulling the diagnostician into a mistaken conclusion. Close examination in these cases, however, reveals that, although patients do indeed feel better during the follicular phase, this is only relatively so, and in fact the depressive symptoms are present throughout all phases of the menstrual cycle, in stark contrast to the pattern seen in premenstrual dysphoric disorder.

Dysmenorrhea, characterized by cramps, headaches, and bloating, is easily distinguished by its course, beginning not before but after the commencement of menstrual flow.

Treatment

SSRIs, including fluoxetine (20 mg) (Cohen *et al.* 2002; Pearlstein and Stone 1994; Pearlstein *et al.* 1997; Steiner *et al.* 1995), paroxetine (20 mg) (Landen *et al.* 2007), and sertraline (50–150 mg) (Freeman *et al.* 1999, 2004; Yonkers *et al.* 1997; Young *et al.* 1998), constitute the mainstay of treatment, and these may be taken either chronically on a daily basis or on a timed basis relative to the timing of the episode itself, such that they are started just before the anticipated onset of symptoms and then stopped several days into menstrual flow. Venlafaxine (50–200 mg) (Freeman *et al.* 2001), taken chronically, is another option, as is alprazolam (1–4 mg) (Freeman *et al.* 1995), taken during the luteal phase. Recently, effectiveness has also been demonstrated for an herbal preparation, *Vitex agnus-castus* (Atmaca *et al.* 2003; Schellenberg 2001). In my opinion, treatment should begin with one of the SSRIs; venlafaxine may also be considered, but alprazolam, given the risks of neuroadaptation, should probably be held in reserve. The place of *Vitex agnus-castus* is not as yet clear.

20.8 POST-PARTUM DEPRESSION

In the strict sense used here, post-partum depression is characterized by the occurrence of depressive episodes only in the post-partum period (Cooper and Murray 1995); as such it must be distinguished from cases of major depressive disorder, for example, in which depressive episodes, although at times occurring in the post-partum period, also occur at other times in the patient's life. This is probably a common disorder.

Clinical features

The onset of the depressive episode is anywhere from several weeks to several months post-partum. Mood is depressed and often accompanied by a considerable amount of anxiety (Hendrick *et al.* 2000). Self-esteem falls, particularly in regard to the patient's estimate of her abilities as a mother. There may be poor concentration, anhedonia, fatigue, initial insomnia, and anorexia. Obsessions may occur and typically involve 'horrific temptations' to do harm to the baby (Wisner *et al.* 1999). Rarely, infanticide may occur, and, as with any depression, suicide remains a risk.

Course

Although most patients experience a spontaneous remission within months or years, the depression may be chronic in a minority. Those who do recover are at increased risk for another episode after a subsequent pregnancy.

Etiology

Post-partum depression may occur secondary to an unusual sensitivity of mood-regulating central nervous system structures to the profound endocrinologic changes that occur post-partum. One particularly interesting study (Bloch *et al.* 2000) looked at two groups of women: both groups had a history of depressive episodes, but in one they were confined to the post-partum period, whereas in the other, depressive episodes occurred at times outside this period. All patients were euthymic at the time of the study, and all were given supraphysiologic doses of estradiol and progesterone for 8 weeks, after which these hormones were abruptly discontinued. In the group of women with a history of post-partum depression, the hormone withdrawal was followed by a depressive episode in the majority, whereas in the group with a history of depression outside the post-partum period, there were no depressions.

Differential diagnosis

Of the many causes of depression discussed in Section 6.1, several figure prominently in the differential diagnosis of post-partum depression, including major depressive disorder, bipolar disorder, post-partum blues, and hypothyroidism. Patients with major depressive disorder or bipolar disorder may have depressive episodes in the post-partum period; however, as stressed earlier, these patients also have episodes at other times. In cases in which a depressive episode occurring in the post-partum period represents the first ever episode in the patient's life, long-term follow-up will be required to determine whether any future episodes occur and, if so, whether they are unrelated to pregnancy or are confined to the post-partum period. The post-partum blues are distinguished by their early onset, within days, and rapid resolution, within 2 weeks; there are also symptomatic differences here, with the post-partum blues being marked by prominent lability. Hypothyroidism, especially that due to Hashimoto's thyroiditis, is not uncommon post-partum, and determining a free T_4 level and a TSH level should be part of the work-up.

Sheehan's syndrome is suggested by a failure of lactation, persistent amenorrhea, and, often, by loss of pubic and axillary hair.

Treatment

Various treatment modalities are available. Double-blind studies support the effectiveness of antidepressants, such as fluoxetine (Appleby et al. 1997), sertraline, and nortripty-line (Wisner et al. 2006). One double-blind study also found transdermal estrogen to be effective (Gregoire et al. 1996), and an open study suggested effectiveness for sublingual estradiol (Ahokas et al. 2001). Both cognitive–behavioral and interpersonal therapy also appear to be effective.

Given the risk of recurrence with subsequent pregnancies, attempts have been made to develop preventive treatments. In this regard, one double-blind study found that sertraline was effective (Wisner et al. 2004), whereas another surprisingly found no preventive effect with nortriptyline (Wisner et al. 2001).

20.9 POST–PARTUM BLUES

The post-partum blues, also known as maternity blues or baby blues, is a common disturbance, seen in about half of all women. Although such a high incidence may suggest that this is a 'normal' phenomenon, the fact that the symptomatology is often strikingly out of character for the patient argues rather that the 'blues' represent a specific disorder.

Clinical features

Clinically (Pitt 1973; Rohde et al. 1997; Yalom et al. 1968), the onset is acute, usually within the first few days post-partum. Mood may be depressed, irritable or fearfully anxious. Crying spells are frequent, and there may be a striking lability of affect; crying spells may come and go with remarkable rapidity, and at times the patient may actually be laughing and claim to feel happy with her delivery, yet be absolutely unable to stop the tears cascading down past her smile. There may also be minor degrees of difficulty with concentration, fatigue, and insomnia. Symptoms tend to peak within a couple of days and then gradually undergo a full remission by the end of the second post-partum week.

Course

Although the post-partum blues may recur after subsequent pregnancies, they tend to be less severe.

Etiology

Although the post-partum blues is almost certainly related to the profound hormonal and neurophysiologic changes present in the immediate post-partum period, as yet it has not been possible to develop a unified theory. One study found a relationship with lower post-partum progesterone levels (Harris et al. 1994), whereas another did not (Kuevi et al. 1983); one study noted a relationship with lower allopregnanolone levels (Nappi et al. 2001). Disturbances in tryptophan metabolism have also been suggested: one study found lower levels in relation to post-partum blues (Kohl et al. 2005), whereas another, although finding normal levels, demonstrated a reduced ratio of tryptophan to other large neutral amino acids (Bailara et al. 2006); notably, however, treatment with tryptophan is not effective (Harris 1980). Finally, two studies have noted an association between an increased number of platelet alpha-2 autoreceptors and the occurrence of the blues (Best et al. 1988; Metz et al. 1983).

Differential diagnosis

Post-partum depression is distinguished by its later onset (usually at least several weeks post-partum), longer duration (at least months), and by the absence of lability. It must be borne in mind, however, that, like any other post-partum women, patients with the post-partum blues may go on to develop a post-partum depression and hence any persistence of symptoms beyond a couple of weeks should prompt a diagnostic re-evaluation.

Treatment

Given the brevity of the syndrome, treatment with antidepressants is not indicated, as a spontaneous remission may be anticipated before an antidepressant could be expected to take effect. Support, reassurance, and assistance are generally sufficient; in some cases a brief course of treatment with a benzodiazepine, such as lorazepam, may be considered, but it must be kept in mind that these drugs do appear in the breast milk.

20.10 PANIC DISORDER

Panic disorder is characterized by the repeated occurrence of discrete anxiety attacks, which, in the context of this disorder, are referred to as 'panic attacks'. This is a common disorder, with a lifetime prevalence of 1–2 percent, and is several times more common in females than males.

Clinical features

The first panic attack generally occurs in late adolescence or early adult years; later onsets, in the fourth decade, are not uncommon and, albeit rarely, onsets have been noted in childhood or the fifth decade.

The panic attack itself usually comes on acutely, often within a minute, and symptoms crescendo rapidly. Anxiety is typically severe, and patients may report the classic 'sense of impending doom', as if some catastrophic event were looming; some fear that they are having a heart attack, others that they are about to 'go crazy'. Uncommonly, however, one may see attacks in which the feeling of anxiety is mild relative to other symptoms, and rarely patients may deny any significant anxiety at all; although the existence of these 'panic attacks without panic' was initially controversial, there is no doubt that they do in fact occur (Russell *et al.* 1991). Other symptoms include tremor, tachycardia, palpitations, chest pain, dyspnea, dizziness, nausea, diaphoresis, and acral parasthesiae; rarely, one may see hemianesthesia, macropsia, or microspia (Coyle and Sterman 1986). Chest pain may be most alarming to patients, and, as this pain may at times radiate to the left shoulder or left side of the neck, it may likewise cause some alarm in emergency room physicians. The attack itself generally lasts about 5–15 minutes, but may persist for up to an hour; symptoms then remit over a few minutes, after which patients may feel 'shaken', drained, and apprehensive for up to a few hours. Although most attacks occur during waking hours, some patients may have nocturnal attacks (Mellman and Uhde 1989a), and, in a small minority, attacks may only occur nocturnally (Mellman and Uhde 1990). Nocturnal attacks arise from non-rapid eye movement (NREM) sleep (Mellman and Uhde 1989b) and often awaken the patient, who typically has trouble falling back asleep and is able to recall the panic the next morning (Hauri *et al.* 1989).

In most cases, panic attacks occur spontaneously, without any precipitating factors; patients may complain that they 'come out of the blue' and strike without warning.

Course

The frequency with which panic attacks occur varies widely among patients, from the extremes of multiple attacks daily to only one attack every few months. The overall course of the disorder appears to follow one of two patterns. In one, the frequency of attacks may vary over years or decades, with the patient never experiencing any prolonged attack-free interval. In the other, one does see prolonged attack-free intervals, and in patients with this pattern one may speak of panic disorder with an episodic course; the 'episodes', characterized by recurrent attacks, are separated from each other by prolonged intervals in which no spontaneous attacks occur.

Over time, and with repeated attacks, most patients begin to develop a chronic, anxious apprehension that another attack may be just around the corner. This 'anticipatory anxiety' may induce patients to avoid situations in which, should they have an attack, they might not be able to find immediate help; thus patients may avoid travelling by plane or boat, or even on limited access highways. Should this anticipatory anxiety become very severe, patients may develop the syndrome of agoraphobia, described in the next section.

Abuse of alcohol or benzodiazepines is a serious risk. Some patients may use these to quell their anticipatory anxiety, whereas others will consume them during the attack itself, in the mistaken belief that oral administration of these agents will result in pharmacologic blood levels before the attack runs its course. In cases in which chronic use of these agents leads to neuroadaptation, any attempt to stop them may lead to a withdrawal state that, in turn, may precipitate further attacks, thus setting up a vicious cycle.

Etiology

Panic disorder is probably hereditary: as the degree of consanguinity rises from unrelated persons to first-degree relatives, then to dizygotic and finally monozygotic twins, so too does the risk of having panic disorder (Crowe *et al.* 1983; Noyes *et al.* 1986; Torgerson 1990). Genetic studies, however, have not as yet yielded robust findings, and neither the mode of inheritance nor candidate loci have been clearly demonstrated.

The discovery of 'panicogens' has been one of the major fruits of the research efforts into panic disorder. Panicogens are substances that, although innocuous in normal control subjects, reliably produce panic attacks in patients with panic disorder. Importantly, these panicogen-induced attacks are identical to spontaneously occurring attacks and, furthermore, may be prevented by the same medicines that are effective in the treatment of panic disorder. Panicogens include inhalation of 5 percent or 35 percent carbon dioxide (Gorman *et al.* 1988), intravenous sodium lactate (Cowley and Arana 1990; Liebowitz *et al.* 1984), caffeine (Charney *et al.* 1985), yohimbine (Charney *et al.* 1992), isoproterenol (Pohl *et al.* 1988), intravenous meta-chlorophenylpiperazine (Kahn and Wetzler 1991), flumazenil (Nutt *et al.* 1990) (although not all studies concur with this [Strohle *et al.* 1998]), and cholecystokinin tetrapeptide (Bradwejn *et al.* 1991).

Various neurotransmitters have also been implicated, including norepinephrine, serotonin, and GABA. Norepinephrine is implicated by the panicogenic effects of caffeine, yohimbine, and isoproterenol, and also by studies reporting a blunted response of growth hormone to clonidine administration. Serotonin involvement is suggested by the response to the panicogen meta-chlorophenylpiperazine and by studies involving manipulation of serotonin levels. For example, depletion of the serotonin precursor tryptophan increases the effectiveness of panicogens such as flumazenil (Bell *et al.* 2002), whereas the administration of L-5-hydroxytrptophan, a serotonin precursor, will blunt the panicogenic effect of carbon dioxide inhalation (Schruers *et al.* 2002). GABAergic involvement is suggested by the panicogenic effect of flumazenil and also by studies that have demonstrated reduced levels of GABA within the occipital cortex (Goddard *et al.* 2001).

Although there are no neuropathologic findings, imaging studies have yielded interesting results. Gray matter density appears lower in the left parahippocampal gyrus (Massana *et al.* 2003a), and positron emission tomography (PET) studies have revealed altered metabolism in the left parahippocampal gyrus (Bisaga *et al.* 1998; Nordahl *et al.*

1990); furthermore, a recent study demonstrated atrophy of both amygdalae (Massana *et al.* 2003b). Finally, a single photon emission computed tomography (SPECT) study revealed a decrease in presynaptic serotonin reuptake transporters within the midbrain, thalamus, and temporal lobes (Maron *et al.* 2004).

Integrating all of these findings into a coherent theory regarding the pathophysiology of panic disorder is problematic and does require some speculation. With this caveat in mind it appears plausible to say that panic disorder results from an inherited disturbance in the metabolism of norepinephrine, serotonin, and/or GABA in one or more of the central nervous system structures that subserve the experience of anxiety. Candidate structures include the locus ceruleus, the dorsal raphe nucleus, the parahippocampal gyrus, hippocampus, and amygdala. The locus ceruleus is noradrenergic and the dorsal raphe nucleus is serotoninergic, and both send fibres to a large number of structures, including the parahippocampus, hippocampus, and amygdala, structures that are rich in GABA receptors. Stimulation of the parahippocampus, hippocampus, and, especially, the amygdala is well-known to produce anxiety. If one considers the amygdala as being the 'final common pathway' in the development of anxiety, then dysfunction of any one of these upstream structures, or of the amygdala itself, could produce an attack. It has been proposed that one possible 'trigger' for the activation of this circuitry is an abnormal sensitivity of brainstem structures to disturbances in the acid–base balance (Klein 1993). Such a sensitivity, in turn, could explain the panicogenic effects of lactate infusion and carbon dioxide inhalation.

Before leaving this section on etiology, some words are in order regarding mitral valve prolapse. Although there is a clear association between this disorder and panic disorder (Katerndahl 1993), it is probably not etiologic in a direct sense. In all likelihood the association is probably secondary to some, as yet unidentified, common factor that underlies both disorders.

Differential diagnosis

As noted earlier, the term 'panic attack' refers to an anxiety attack that happens to occur secondary to panic disorder, and, consequently, in pursuing the differential diagnosis of panic disorder one must consider the various other causes of anxiety attacks, as discussed in Section 6.5.

Occasionally, an otherwise normal individual will have an anxiety attack, and, after thorough investigation, no clear cause may be found. In such cases one is tempted to make a diagnosis of panic disorder; however, by convention, this diagnosis should probably be withheld until subsequent attacks have occurred and one is able to demonstrate that, at least at some point in the course, a frequency of once monthly or more has been observed.

Anxiety attacks may also be seen as part of the depressive episodes of either major depressive disorder or bipolar disorder; if their occurrence is confined solely within the limits of the depressive episode, an additional diagnosis of panic disorder is not warranted. However, if one can demonstrate that the anxiety attacks preceded the onset of the depressive episode, or persisted beyond the resolution of the episode, then the additional diagnosis is appropriate.

Of the other causes of anxiety attacks noted in Section 6.5, some of the most common are simple phobia, social phobia, post-traumatic stress disorder, and obsessive–compulsive disorder. In all of these disorders, however, the anxiety attacks are precipitated. For example, if the simple phobic has to approach a snake, the social phobic public speaking, the post-traumatic patient a situation reminiscent of the original trauma, or the obsessive–compulsive a contaminated object, a severe anxiety attack may indeed occur. If however, these precipitating situations may be avoided, these patients remain free of attacks.

Of the less common causes of anxiety attacks noted in Section 6.5, special consideration should be given to myocardial infarction or angina, paroxysmal atrial tachycardia, hypoglycemia, hyperventilation, and simple partial seizures. As noted earlier, panic attacks may be accompanied by chest pain, which may radiate to the neck or shoulder, hence suggesting a diagnosis of cardiac disease, and in these cases the general medical setting is very helpful. Clearly, if the patient is elderly and has known risk factors and no history of panic attacks, then one would lean toward a diagnosis of coronary artery disease; by contrast, if the patient is young and lacks risk factors, one might be inclined to lean toward a diagnosis of panic disorder. An episode of paroxysmal atrial tachycardia may occasionally prompt considerable anxiety in the sufferer. However, here one finds a hyperacute onset of the tachycardia, over a second or so, in contrast to the build-up of a panic attack, which occurs over a minute or so; furthermore, in paroxysmal atrial tachycardia a valsalva manuever may terminate the attack, whereas such a manuever has no effect on a panic attack. Hypoglycemia should be suspected in the case of a diabetic who has missed a meal, and in whom the attack is associated with hunger; prompt relief with glucose confirms the suspicion. Hyperventilation is suggested by the prominent dyspnea and by relief with re-breathing through a paper bag. Simple partial seizures are suggested by an exquisitely paroxysmal onset, over seconds, and by a history in most cases of other, more obvious seizure types, such as complex partial seizures or grand mal seizures.

Treatment

Pharmacologic treatment of panic disorder has as its goal the prevention of future panic attacks, and the first step is to choose one of the various medications that are effective in this regard, including antidepressants (SSRIs, tricyclics, or MAOIs), benzodiazepines, and inositol. Cognitive–behavioral therapy (Beck *et al.* 1992) also appears to be effective; if this is tried first and is less than fully effective, then one may simply proceed to pharmacologic treatment.

Among the antidepressants, the following SSRIs, with their average effective doses, may be used: fluoxetine (20 mg) (Michelson *et al.* 2001), paroxetine (40 mg) (Ballenger *et al.* 1998; Oehrberg *et al.* 1995), sertraline (50–150 mg) (Dohl *et al.* 1998; Londborg *et al.* 1998), citalopram (20 mg) (Wade *et al.* 1997), escitalopram (10 mg) (Stahl *et al.* 2003), and fluvoxamine (150 mg) (Hoehn-Saric *et al.* 1993). Of the tricyclics, one may use imipramine (150–200 mg) (Mavissakalian and Perel 1989) or clomipramine (50–150 mg) (Modigh *et al.* 1992). Of the MAOIs, one may use phenelzine (30–90 mg). As all of these are of approximately equal effectiveness, the choice among them is generally based on side-effect profile and ease of use, and with these criteria as guides, an SSRI is probably the first choice (with the exception of fluvoxamine, whose side-effects and many problematic drug–drug interactions make this a second choice). A tricyclic, such as imipramine, constitutes a reasonable alternative; however, the MAOI phenelzine, given the difficulty with its use, should be held in distant reserve. Regardless of which antidepressant is chosen, it is important to start with a low dose, as initiation of treatment at a full dose may cause a 'flurry' of panic attacks. Thus, one should start with anywhere from one-tenth to one-third of the full dose (breaking up tablets, if need be), followed by upward titration in similar increments every week or so. Importantly, however, although most patients require, and eventually tolerate, a full dose, there is a small minority of patients who do not tolerate anything more than a minimal dose, which they do benefit from; consequently, if patients do not tolerate a dose escalation, one option is to continue with a low dose and see if they respond. Once an optimum dose has been reached, it may take up to 3 months to see a good prophylactic effect.

Among the benzodiazepines, choices include clonazepam (Rosenbaum *et al.* 1997; Tesar *et al.* 1991), alprazolam (Ballenger *et al.* 1988), lorazepam (Schweizer *et al.* 1990), and diazepam (Noyes *et al.* 1996). Each should be started at a low dose, with the understanding that dose increases may be required to prevent attacks. Total daily starting doses and potential final doses are as follows: clonazepam, starting at 0.5–1.5 mg, increasing to 1–4 mg; aprazolam, starting at 0.75–1.5 mg, increasing to 1.5–6 mg; lorazepam, starting at 1–2 mg, increasing to 2–6 mg; and diazepam, starting at 4–10 mg and increasing to 10–60 mg. In general, the total daily dose should be divided into a twice- or thrice-daily schedule. Clearly, given the wide ranges of starting and potential final doses here, considerable clinical judgment is required. Importantly, however, and unlike the antidepressants, these benzodiazepines are immediately effective once the 'right' dose has been reached; consequently, if patients continue to have attacks, this is an indication that their current dose will not be effective and that the dose should promptly be increased.

Many clinicians, concerned about the possibility of neuroadaptation with benzodiazepines, and the risk of precipitating a flurry of attacks if the patient runs out of medication or tapers the dose too rapidly (Pecknold *et al.* 1988; Rickels

et al. 1993a), lean toward trying an antidepressant first. However, in some cases, especially those characterized by very frequent attacks and considerable anticipatory anxiety, some clinicians will 'split the difference' and start the patient on a combination of a benzodiazepine and an antidepressant (e.g., clonazepam and an SSRI), with plans to gradually taper the benzodiazepine once enough time has passed for the antidepressant to take effect.

Inositol is a naturally occurring isomer of glucose that is normally converted to inositol 1,4,5-triphosphate, which in turn functions as an intracellular second messenger, and doses of 6000–9000 mg b.i.d. have been found to be superior to placebo and comparable to fluvoxamine in preventing panic attacks (Palatnik *et al.* 2001). Although experience with inositol is relatively limited, it would certainly be a reasonable option in cases of intolerance to other agents or for patients who prefer 'natural' remedies.

20.11 AGORAPHOBIA

Agoraphobia is derived from the Greek meaning literally a fear of the marketplace or, more generally, a fear of open spaces. However, on close questioning, what becomes apparent is that patients suffering from agoraphobia do not in fact fear a particular place or situation, but rather the possibility of becoming ill or incapacitated in some fashion or other and either not being able to escape or not being able to get immediate help.

As discussed further below, there are probably two kinds of agoraphobia (Horwarth *et al.* 1993; Lelliott *et al.* 1989). In one type, seen in the vast majority of cases, agoraphobia represents a complication of panic disorder, and what patients fear is being incapacitated by a panic attack while away from home and safety; in the other type, there is no history of panic disorder, and patients seem unable to clearly delineate what they fear might happen.

The lifetime prevalence of agoraphobia ranges from 1 to 5 percent; it is probably two to four times more common in females than males.

Clinical features

The onset is generally in the twenties or thirties; in those cases in which agoraphobia represents a complication of panic disorder, anywhere from as little as a few days to up to a year or more may elapse between the occurrence of the first panic attack and the onset of the agoraphobia.

A large number of places and situations may be feared and avoided (Page 1994), including travelling on airplanes or trains, travelling across bridges or through tunnels, and, in extreme cases, simply waiting in long lines, and the prospect of being caught in such a situation may fill patients with a catastrophic, yet difficult to describe, sense of dread (Goisman *et al.* 1995). Some patients become completely housebound and literally may never set foot outside the house for years.

Interestingly, in many cases patients are able to temporarily overcome their agoraphobia if they take their 'safety' with them by travelling with a good and trusted friend.

Course

Agoraphobia is a chronic disorder and tends to gradually worsen over long periods of time.

Etiology

In cases occurring secondary to panic disorder, the normal anticipatory anxiety about having another panic attack becomes so severe and pervasive that patients cannot bear venturing into 'unsafe' situations. In those cases that occur in the absence of panic disorder, patients, although describing well the dread they feel over being in agoraphobic situations, cannot clearly explain, either to themselves or others, what it is they fear might happen, and the etiology in these cases is simply not known.

Differential diagnosis

In social phobia of the generalized subtype (also known as social anxiety disorder), patients may fear and avoid many different situations. The difference here is that social phobics fear that they will do something that embarrasses or humiliates them, whereas agoraphobics fear that something will happen to them, such as a panic attack.

In illnesses characterized by delusions of persecution, patients may avoid going out for fear that people will talk about them, spy on them, assault them, etc. This may be seen in schizophrenia, schizoaffective disorder, the persecutory subtype of delusional disorder, and depressive episodes of either major depressive disorder or bipolar disorder.

Treatment

Agoraphobia may be treated either with cognitive–behavioral therapy or a behavioral program of graded exposure, in which the patient gradually and sequentially takes progressively greater 'steps' toward and into the feared situation. Critically, however, in those cases occurring secondary to panic disorder, one must first treat the panic disorder and render the patient free of panic attacks. The occurrence of even one panic attack can, and often does, destroy any gains made by cognitive–behavioral or exposure therapy.

20.12 SPECIFIC (SIMPLE) PHOBIA

The patient with a specific phobia, or, as it was formerly known, a simple phobia, experiences extreme anxiety upon approaching something that for others arouses little or no apprehension. Although adult patients acknowledge the irrationality of their fear, they go out of their way to avoid the feared object. First described by Hippocrates, this condition is quite common, occurring in at least 10 percent of the general population; it is about twice as frequent in females as in males.

In the past it was fashionable to subdivide specific phobia according to the feared object or situation, and thus one reads of arachnophobia, acrophobia, claustrophobia, etc. For the most part, however, this subdividing added little to our understanding of the disorder, with one probable exception, namely blood-injury phobia, which, as noted below, may be a unique specific phobia.

Clinical features

The age of onset of specific phobia ranges from childhood to early adult years: animal phobias and blood-injury phobia tend to first appear in childhood, whereas the other phobias may first appear at any point from childhood to adult years (Marks and Gelder 1966).

A wide range of objects or situations may come to be feared, including snakes, spiders, heights, being in closed spaces, darkness, storms, and the sight of blood. Although most patients with specific phobia have only one phobia, in a minority two or more may be present.

On approaching the feared object or situation, or even upon simply imagining doing so, patients experience the acute onset of an anxiety attack, characterized by anxiety, tremor, tachycardia, diaphoresis, and piloerection; in some cases, these symptoms may be accompanied by depersonalization. Some patients may be able to steel themselves and stay nearby, but for the most part the fear and anxiety is so great that they must escape, no matter how humiliating or embarrassing such behavior might be for them. Importantly, as soon as patients can get away, the anxiety ceases and patients, although perhaps a little 'shaken' by the experience, promptly return to normal.

Blood-injury phobia, as indicated earlier, may be unique. A common example is found in patients who are phobic about having a venipuncture (Chapman et al. 1993). If these patients can force themselves to hold still for the phlebotomist, they typically experience a biphasic symptomatology. Initially, there is anxiety and tachycardia, similar to that seen in the anxiety attack just described; soon after, however, these sympathetic symptoms give way to a parasympathetic response, with hypotension and either pre-syncope or actual fainting (Curtis and Thyer 1983). It is this second phase that gives blood-injury phobia its unique status.

Course

Phobias with an onset in childhood tend to remit within months or a year or so. In cases of childhood-onset phobias that persist, and in cases characterized by later onsets in adolescence or early adult years, the course tends to be chronic.

Etiology

Specific phobias run in families (Fyer *et al.* 1990), although it is not clear whether this reflects environmental or genetic factors, or both. Some authors believe that children become phobic by virtue of modeling their parents' behavior; however, this theory begs the question as to the source of the parents' phobias. Other authors suggest that phobias represent a vestigial remnant from our ancient evolutionary history, when an instinctual avoidance of certain objects, such as snakes, could have conferred considerable survival value. In support of this evolutionary view is the fact that certain monkeys who have never had any contact with a snake nevertheless react with extreme fear upon seeing one.

In the case of blood-injury phobia, it appears that there is an underlying chronic dysfunction of the autonomic nervous system, which predisposes these patients to the development of vaso-vagal syncope (Accurso *et al.* 2001; Donadio *et al.* 2007).

Differential diagnosis

Specific phobia must be distinguished from social phobia of the circumscribed type, certain cases of obsessive–compulsive disorder, and post-traumatic stress disorder. Social phobia of the circumscribed type may be distinguished from specific phobia by the fact that, in social phobia, what is feared is humiliation or embarrassment in certain situations, rather than the situation *per se*. For example, the patient with a circumscribed social phobia of public speaking, although terrified at the prospect of speaking when others are present, may, when rehearsing the speech in private, have little or no anxiety: here, it is the apprehension of embarrassing oneself when speaking, rather than speaking itself, which the patient fears. This is in contrast to the patient with a specific phobia, for example of snakes, who reacts with anxiety upon seeing the snake regardless of whether this occurs in public or in private. Certain cases of obsessive–compulsive disorder may also cause diagnostic concern, for example when patients have a fear of contamination and avoid various objects or situations, such as shaking hands or using a public restroom. In these cases, however, the reaction to the feared object or situation persists long after contact ceases, for example when the patient with obsessive–compulsive disorder washes his or her hands repeatedly; this is in contrast to specific phobia, in which patients return to normal promptly upon disengaging from the phobic object or situation. Post-traumatic stress disorder may be confused with specific phobia when post-traumatic patients report avoiding certain situations. Here, however, one finds that the avoided situations have a specific meaning for patients in that they are reminiscent of an earlier traumatic event; this is in contrast to social phobia, in which patients admit that the fear is 'irrational' and not based on any earlier event.

Treatment

Both desensitization and cognitive–behavioral therapy are effective. The place of pharmacologic therapy of specific phobias is not entirely clear. Many patients are prescribed benzodiazepines on a chronic basis; however, there is no research support for this and it runs the risk of neuro-adaptation. Brief, 'one time' use of benzodiazepines may, however, have a place, as for example in the pre-treatment of a claustrophobic patient before an MRI study in a 'closed' system. There is also one study that found paroxetine to be superior to placebo (Benjamin *et al.* 2000).

20.13 SOCIAL PHOBIA

In social phobia, patients fear that if they attempt to do certain things in public they will appear inept, foolish, or inadequate, and thus suffer shame, humiliation, or embarrassment. Feeling this way, patients, although admitting that their fears are perhaps groundless, nevertheless become intensely anxious on approaching these situations and may go to great lengths to avoid them.

Importantly, there are two subtypes of social phobia, namely the generalized type (also known as social anxiety disorder) and the circumscribed type (Heimberg *et al.* 1990; Mannuzza *et al.* 1995). The generalized subtype is characterized by fears that span multiple situations, whereas in the circumscribed subtype only one or two specific situations are feared.

This is a common disorder, occurring in anywhere from 3 to 13 percent of the adult population; it is more frequent in females than males.

Clinical features

The onset of social phobia ranges from late childhood to the early adult years, with most patients falling ill in their mid-teens (Marks and Gelder 1966). Pre-morbidly, in some cases there is a history of shyness and easy blushing. The actual onset itself is heralded by the first wave of irrational anxiety over doing something in public.

In the generalized subtype, patients fear multiple situations, including, for example, answering questions in class, asking others out for dates, or attending meetings; in some cases patients may have a global fear of interacting socially in any situation.

In the circumscribed subtype there may be a fear of public speaking, or fears that one will tremble when writing in public, misplay notes when giving a musical performance, choke when eating in public, or, in males, be unable to urinate in a public restroom. Regardless of the specific circumscribed fear involved, it is important to note that it is not the activity itself that is feared but rather the performance of that activity in public. Thus, the patient with a fear of public speaking who is paralyzed into muteness upon approaching the podium with an audience present may nevertheless be able to make the speech flawlessly on rehearsal in an empty hall.

If patients do approach the phobic situation (or at times, merely imagine doing so), they experience an anxiety attack of variable severity, with anxiety, tremor, tachycardia, diaphoresis, and dyspnea. In some cases patients may be able to endure the anxiety and proceed with the performance; however, in many cases the anxiety is simply 'too much' and patients may refuse to go on. One variation on this reaction is known as erythrophobia. Here, what patients are concerned about is excessive blushing in public. In some cases there may actually be an obvious, scarlet blush; however, in others the blush is actually not noted by others but is simply experienced by the patient as a sense of flushing or uncomfortable warmth.

Course

Social phobia appears to be a chronic disorder.

Etiology

The etiology of the two types of social phobia may not be the same, and hence they are considered separately.

Generalized social phobia, which has been subjected to the most study, appears to be familial (Fyer *et al.* 1993) and to be associated with disturbances in various neurotransmitter systems, including serotonin, endogenous benzodiazepines, and dopamine. With regard to serotonin, several abnormalities have been noted, including an aggravation of symptoms with depletion of the serotonin precursor tryptophan (Argyropoulos *et al.* 2004), a decrease in the serotonin-1A binding potential both on platelets and neurons in the amygdala and cingulate cortex (Lanzenberger *et al.* 2007), and an augmented cortisol response to the serotoninergic agent fenfluramine (Tancer *et al.* 1994). In looking at endogenous benzodiazepine function, there appears to be a reduced number of platelet benzodiazepine receptors (Johnson *et al.* 1998). Finally, both a reduced density of dopamine receptors in the striatum (Schneier *et al.* 2000) and a decrease in striatal dopamine reuptake sites (Tiihonen *et al.* 1997a) have also been noted.

Regarding the circumscribed type of social phobia, little can be said except that it is suspected to reflect a disturbance in noradrenergic functioning.

Differential diagnosis

Agoraphobia may be distinguished from the generalized type of social phobia by the source of the patients' fear about going out in public. In the agoraphobic, what is feared is having a panic attack, whether anyone is around or not; this is in contrast to social phobics who fear that they will do something humiliating or embarrassing.

Specific phobia may be readily distinguished from social phobia of the circumscribed type by asking patients whether they can engage in the fearful behavior when in private; the patient with a specific phobia, for example of snakes, is no more able to approach the snake in private than in public, whereas the patient with a circumscribed social phobia, for example of speaking in public, may, as noted earlier, go through a rehearsal of the speech without anxiety, provided that there is no audience.

Similarly to the generalized type of social phobia, body dysmorphic disorder is characterized by a fear of humiliation or embarrassment in public; however, in body dysmorphic disorder the fear arises from the patients' beliefs that they are in some way misshapen or deformed, rather than from a concern that they might suffer embarrassment because of something they do.

Certain conditions, by their very symptoms, may occasion some embarrassment, and in such cases a separate diagnosis of social phobia is not made. Examples include the tremor of essential tremor or Parkinson's disease, and developmental stuttering.

One must also distinguish between normal fears and social phobia. Most individuals experience some apprehension or 'stage fright' when first approaching certain situations; however, in contrast to social phobia, the fear is not overwhelming and, importantly, diminishes after a few 'dress rehearsals'.

Treatment

A large number of medications are effective in the generalized type of social phobia, including various antidepressants, clonazepam, and two anti-epileptic drugs, gabapentin and pregabalin. Effective antidepressants include sertraline 50–200 mg/day (Katzelnick *et al.* 1995), paroxetine 20–40 mg/day (Allgulander 1999; Baldwin *et al.* 1999; Stein *et al.* 1998), escitalopram 10–20 mg/day (Kasper *et al.* 2005), fluvoxamine 150 mg/day (Stein *et al.* 1999; van Vliet *et al.* 1994), venlafaxine 75–225 mg/day (Liebowitz *et al.* 2005), and phenelzine 60–90 mg/day (Heimberg *et al.* 1998; Liebowitz *et al.* 1992; Versiani *et al.* 1992). The benzodiazepine clonazepam 0.5–3.0 mg/day (Davidson *et al.* 1993) is also effective, as are the anti-epileptics gabapentin 900–3600 mg/day (Pande *et al.* 1999) and pregabalin 600 mg/day (Pande *et al.* 2004). All other things being equal, one of the antidepressants (with the exception of phenelzine, which, given the difficulty in its use, should be held in reserve) is a reasonable first choice. Although experience with gabapentin and pregabalin is limited in social phobia, they might be a reasonable second choice; of the two, gabapentin is probably preferable. Although clonazepam is often used, the potential for neuroadaptation may give one pause. Cognitive–behavioral therapy may be considered but appears to be slightly less effective than medication.

Circumscribed social phobia, especially fears of speaking, writing, or giving a musical performance, may be treated with a beta-blocker such as propranolol, given on an 'as needed' (p.r.n.) basis in anticipation of the public performance (Brantigan *et al.* 1982; Hartley *et al.* 1983; James *et al.* 1977; Liden and Gottfries 1974). The dose of propranolol ranges from 20 to 60 mg, and the drug appears to work not so much by reducing anxiety *per se* as by reducing autonomic symptoms, such that patients no longer 'shake like a leaf'. Behavioral desensitization may also be helpful.

20.14 OBSESSIVE–COMPULSIVE DISORDER

Obsessive–compulsive disorder is characterized by obsessions and compulsions (Rasmussen and Tsuang 1986). It is a common disorder, with a lifetime prevalence of 2–5 percent.

Clinical features

Most patients fall ill in adolescence or early adult years; although onset in childhood is not rare, onset past the age of 40 years is quite rare.

The majority of patients experience both obsessions and compulsions (Foa *et al.* 1995). Somewhat less than 25 percent will have only obsessions and about 5 percent will have only compulsions; very rarely one finds patients with a subtype known as primary obsessive slowness.

Obsessions are unwanted, intrusive, and troubling ideas, impulses or images, often related to sexual or violent themes. A minister recurrently found himself thinking of bestiality; a neurologist found himself repeatedly experiencing an urge to question his patients about their bowel movements; and a young mother, to her distress, continually had thoughts of her toddler being run over by a truck. Most patients are, at the very least, distressed by these obsessions, and many are horrified. All, at least initially, will try their best to somehow stop the obsessions from occurring.

Compulsions arise in response to irrational fears or concerns, and in some way or other they serve to allay these fears. These strong urges give patients no peace, typically waxing ever stronger as patients try to resist carrying them out. Compulsions are often categorized according to what patients feel compelled to do: thus, for example, there are checkers, washers, touchers, counters, and arrangers. A 'checker', after going upstairs to bed, had doubts that he had turned off the electric light downstairs and felt compelled to go back downstairs to check on it; despite finding the light off, however, the fear again arose once he had returned upstairs, forcing him to go back once again, the process being repeated many times before the patient could finally get to bed (Tuke 1894). 'Washers' are convinced that they have been contaminated in some way, perhaps by dirt, 'germs', or fecal material, and feel compelled to wash their hands, no matter how clean they may be or how many times they have already been washed; some may wash to the point of rawness, yet still feel unclean. 'Counters' feel compelled to count to a certain number and do it repeatedly, whereas 'arrangers', under the compulsion to arrange things 'just so', may spend much time arranging and then rearranging things on the desk or in the closet, always finding afterwards on inspection, however, that some critical point of symmetry has been missed. These counters and arrangers are sometimes at a loss to explain what they fear might happen should they fail to act; it is as if a there is a nameless dread motivating them. Although most compulsive behaviors are visible and evident to others, some patients may at times engage in 'silent' or private compulsions, for example repeating the Lord's Prayer to themselves a certain number of times. Almost all patients, at least initially, recognize the 'senselessness' or irrationality of their compulsions and will attempt to resist them (Stern and Cobb 1978); over the years, however, many will give in, carrying out the compulsions without even a token show of resistance. In a small minority of cases, patients may lose insight into the irrationality of their compulsive behavior and become convinced, to a delusional degree, that their behavior is in fact reasonable and appropriate (Eisen and Rasmussen 1993; Insel and Akiskal 1986). Such patients with psychotic obsessive–compulsive disorder, now finding their compulsions reasonable, pursue them with purpose rather than resisting them. One patient (Gordon 1950), after 25 years of resisting the urge to repeat his prayers for fear that he had left a word out, eventually came to believe that he was in fact a sinner and that God had given him the compulsion to specifically ensure that he said the prayers with the perfection that salvation and eternal life demanded; subsequently, he freely gave himself to the repeating of his prayers whenever he had the slightest doubt that he had left anything out.

Primary obsessive slowness is characterized by the transformation of routine daily activities into lengthy, meticulous rituals. Dressing or preparing a meal may take literally hours; the sequence and form of each step in the process is carefully and scrupulously observed, and any deviation leads to an accretion of severe anxiety. Only when completely satisfied that the job has been perfectly done can the patient move on to the next task of the day. Patients with primary obsessive slowness typically have had, or continue to have, other compulsions, such as checking or washing.

Course

Although obsessive–compulsive disorder generally pursues a chronic course, exceptions do occur: in a small minority, perhaps 5 percent, symptoms undergo a complete, or near-complete, spontaneous remission; in such cases, however, relapses generally occur in the following years. Although in most chronic cases symptoms tend to wax and wane in severity and frequency over long periods of time, in 10–15 percent the course is progressively downhill until patients' lives are literally consumed by their obsessions and compulsions.

Etiology

Obsessive–compulsive disorder is familial (Grabe *et al.* 2006; Pauls *et al.* 1995), and genetic research, although inconclusive, is promising (Shugart *et al.* 2006); in some cases it appears that obsessive–compulsive disorder may represent a phenotypic variant of the same genes responsible for Tourette's syndrome (Apter *et al.* 1993; Frankel *et al.* 1986). Although neuropathologic studies are lacking, PET studies (Baxter *et al.* 1987, 1992; Benkelfat *et al.* 1990; Perani *et al.* 1995; Saxena *et al.* 2002) have demonstrated increased metabolic activity in the orbitofrontal cortex, caudate, and thalamus. Furthermore, several lines of evidence suggest a disturbance in serotoninergic functioning: all of the medicines effective in this disorder are serotoninergic; meta-chlorophenylpiperazine, a mixed agonist/antagonist at post-synaptic serotonin receptors, generally increases the severity of symptoms (Broocks *et al.* 1998; Hollander *et al.* 1992); and SPECT studies suggest disturbances in serotonin binding within the midbrain (Hasselbach *et al.* 2007) and caudate (Adams *et al.* 2005), and serotonin reuptake mechanisms within the thalamus and brainstem (Hesse *et al.* 2005).

In a minority of childhood-onset cases it appears that obsessive–compulsive disorder occurs on an autoimmune basis, via a mechanism similar to that seen in Sydenham's chorea, and such patients are said to have one of the 'PANDAS' or '*pediatric autoimmune neuropsychiatric disorders associated with streptococcal infections*' (Swedo *et al.* 1998). In these cases, as in Sydenham's chorea, a preceding beta-hemolytic streptococcal pharyngitis initiates an autoimmune attack on the basal ganglia, resulting in obsessions and compulsions. Whether this group of patients should be considered to have obsessive–compulsive disorder or a phenotype is a nosologic question that has not as yet been answered. In any case, PANDAS should be suspected in cases in which either the onset of the disorder or exacerbations are related to streptococcal pharyngitides, and the work-up should proceed as outlined for Sydenham's chorea in Section 17.10.

Importantly, there is no relationship between obsessive–compulsive disorder and obsessive–compulsive personality disorder. Although in the past, the personality disorder was felt to provide the 'fertile' soil for the development of obsessive–compulsive disorder, there is no evidence for this, and patients with obsessive–compulsive disorder are no more likely to have a pre-existing obsessive–compulsive personality disorder than any other personality disorder (Baer *et al.* 1990; Black *et al.* 1993; Joffe *et al.* 1988).

Differential diagnosis

The differential diagnosis of obsessions and compulsions is discussed in detail in Section 4.17, and the reader is encouraged to review that section.

Treatment

Effective therapy involves the use of a serotoninergic medication or either the behavioral techniques of exposure and response prevention (Foa *et al.* 1984; Steketee *et al.* 1982) or cognitive–behavioral therapy; most patients do best with a combination of medication and one of these two techniques (Foa *et al.* 2005).

Serotoninergic drugs effective in obsessive–compulsive disorder include clomipramine, venlafaxine, and the SSRIs. Clomipramine is effective in the dose range 200–250 mg/day (Clomipramine Collaborative Study Group 1991), venlafaxine in a dose of 300 mg (Denys *et al.* 2003), fluoxetine (Bergeron *et al.* 2002; Pigott *et al.* 1990) in doses of 20–60 mg/day (Tollefson *et al.* 1994), fluvoxamine (Freeman *et al.* 1994; Hollander *et al.* 2003a; Koran *et al.* 1996) in doses of 100–300 mg/day, sertraline in doses of 50–200 mg/day (Bergeron *et al.* 2002; Greist *et al.* 1995; Krong *et al.* 1999), paroxetine (Hollander *et al.* 2003b; Zohar and Judge 1996) in doses of 40–60 mg/day, and escitalopram in a dose of 20 mg/day (Stein *et al.* 2007). Most clinicians will start with an SSRI, given their favorable side-effect profile relative to clomipramine (Zohar and Judge 1996); venlafaxine represents a new addition to this armamentarium, and its place is not as yet clear. Importantly, regardless of which medication is used, 6 weeks must be allowed to see an initial response, and a full response may not be seen for 3 months.

When an initial trial of medication fails, several strategies are available. First, one may consider an increased dose, for example increasing the dose of sertraline up to 400 mg (Ninan *et al.* 2006). If dosage increase is either not tolerated or ineffective, then one may consider switching from one agent to another, for example from an SSRI to clomipramine or venlafaxine. Another option is to add an antipsychotic, such as risperidone (1–3 mg) (Li *et al.* 2005; McDougle *et al.* 2000), haloperidol (2–5 mg) (Li *et al.* 2005; McDougle *et al.* 1994, 2000), quetiapine (300–400 mg) (Denys *et al.* 2004), or olanzapine (5–20 mg) (Bystritsky *et al.* 2004). Of these antipsychotics, risperidone is probably the treatment of first choice, as it is better tolerated than haloperidol (Li *et al.* 2005); experience with quetiapine is limited; and the long-term metabolic effects of olanzapine give one pause. Importantly, these antipsychotics are effective only as augmenting agents and are not useful in monotherapy. In severe and treatment-resistant cases, consideration may be given to cingulotomy (Baer *et al.* 1995; Dougherty *et al.* 2002; Hay *et al.* 1993), anterior capsulotomy, or deep brain stimulation of the anterior capsules (Greenberg *et al.* 2006).

In acute cases of obsessive–compulsive disorder occurring as part of PANDAS, it is tempting to consider utilizing the same sort of acute treatment as is recommended for Sydenham's chorea; although prednisone has not been studied in this regard, one study did report benefit from plasma exchange (Perlmutter *et al.* 1999). In chronic cases one might also consider preventive treatment with benzathine penicillin.

20.15 POST-TRAUMATIC STRESS DISORDER

Post-traumatic stress disorder (PTSD) may occur in practically anyone who has been exposed to an overwhelmingly traumatic event, for example combat (Lee *et al.* 1995), torture (Basoglu *et al.* 1994; Ramsey *et al.* 1993), concentration camps (Kinzie *et al.* 1984), mass shootings (North *et al.* 1994), earthquakes (Goenjian *et al.* 1994), or fire, as in the famous Coconut Grove disaster in Boston in 1943 (Adler 1943). Subsequent to the trauma, patients, in various fashions, re-experience the event over and over again; there is also a general withdrawal from present life, and patients tend to be anxious and easily startled. This is probably a common disorder, occurring in anywhere from 1 to 9 percent of the general population; it is probably more frequent in females than males.

Clinical features

As trauma may occur at any age, so too may PTSD; however, given that the most common precipitants for PTSD, such as combat, occur in early adult years, most cases have an onset in the twenties. Symptoms may appear either acutely, within days or weeks after the trauma, or in a delayed fashion, after a latency of months to many years (Watson *et al.* 1988); indeed, in one case of PTSD secondary to combat in World War II, the syndrome was delayed for three decades (Van Dyke *et al.* 1985). In cases of delayed onset, the latency period is generally, but not always, marked by dysphoria and a tendency to avoid situations reminiscent of the original trauma. Although delayed onsets typically occur subacutely, occasionally the latent interval will end abruptly if the patient experiences a new trauma similar to the original one. Although it is not possible to predict with any degree of certainty who, after a trauma, will go on to develop PTSD, it appears that a history of dissociation during the trauma portends a greater risk (Birmes *et al.* 2003; Koopman *et al.* 1994; Shalev *et al.* 1996).

Clinically (Gersons and Carlier 1992), in one fashion or another, patients become numb to the world around them. Events that used to arouse interest now leave them unaffected and unmoved; they may complain of feeling 'dead inside' or of having no feelings at all, and some may appear listless and detached.

The experience of the trauma lives on in these patients, and they typically have intense, intrusive, and vivid memories of it. Nightmares are common and, unlike most nightmares, these have little of the fantastic in them; rather they tend to stick to the persistently disturbing facts. At times the waking recollections of the trauma may be more compelling and vivid than the patients' actual surroundings, and they may experience 'flashbacks' in which they act as if the original trauma were actually occurring; in extreme cases, these flashbacks may be characterized by visual and auditory hallucinations that recreate the original trauma.

Situations that remind patients of the trauma tend to be avoided. Veterans may refuse to view war movies, and World War II concentration camp survivors may avoid anything German. If unavoidably trapped in such a situation, patients become intensely anxious and some may have an anxiety attack.

Patients tend to be anxious, tense, and easily startled. Although often fatigued, they try to remain alert, as if on guard against some fresh onslaught. There may be difficulty with concentration, insomnia, and lability of mood; irritability is common, and patients may become enraged with little or no provocation.

Over time, a full depressive episode may occur, and alcohol abuse or alcoholism may also occur, in which case one typically sees a florid exacerbation of the symptoms of PTSD.

Course

In about 50 percent of cases, symptoms undergo a gradual and spontaneous remission within months of the onset, and this appears to be more common in cases with an acute onset shortly after the original trauma. A chronic course may also occur, and this appears likely when either symptoms have persisted beyond 6 months or the onset was delayed. When the course is chronic, symptoms tend to wax and wane over years or decades.

Etiology

By far the best predictor of PTSD is the type and severity of the trauma itself. Products of human cruelty, such as torture or incarceration in a concentration camp, commonly produce this disorder. Furthermore, events that catch persons by surprise and then leave them without social support afterward, such as a typhoon that devastates a community, likewise provide fertile ground for the development of this disorder. Conversely, certain traumatic events, such as mild motor vehicle accidents, are less likely to precipitate PTSD.

However, the fact that not all persons exposed to severe trauma develop the disorder, coupled with the finding that some individuals may develop PTSD after relatively mild trauma (Feinstein and Dolan 1991; McFarlane 1989), indicates that other factors are involved. Twin studies have suggested a genetic susceptibility; however, it is not clear whether the inherited factor is a susceptibility to the development of PTSD *per se* or rather a tendency to become involved in high-risk activities.

Endocrinologic and biochemical studies have yielded interesting results. The autonomic symptomatology seen in this disorder, such as a heightened startle response (Butler *et al.* 1990; Shalev *et al.* 1992) and sensitivity to stimuli reminiscent of the original trauma (Pitman *et al.* 1987), immediately suggests disturbances of catecholamines, and indeed both CSF (Geracioti *et al.* 2001) and 24-hour urine levels (Young and Breslau 2004) of norepinephrine are increased; furthermore, intravenous administration of yohimbine, a noradrenergic agonist, will increase the severity of symptoms (Southwick *et al.* 1993). Of the endocrinologic studies carried out on PTSD, the hypothalamic–pituitary–adrenal axis has been most extensively studied and shows unique abnormalities. Cerebrospinal fluid levels of CRH are increased (Baker *et al.* 1999, 2005), and this is similar to what is seen in major depressive disorder. However, the cortisol response to dexamethasone, rather than being blunted as is seen in depression, is enhanced in PTSD (Goenjian *et al.* 1996; Yehuda *et al.* 1993, 2004).

Hippocampal atrophy has been demonstrated by some (Bremner *et al.* 1995, 2003; Lindauer *et al.* 2006; Villarreal *et al.* 2002), but not all (Bonne *et al.* 2001; Jatzko *et al.* 2006; Woodward *et al.* 2006), studies. The significance of this finding is not clear. There are, at present, no prospective MRI studies of patients before and after trauma, and hence it is not clear if hippocampal atrophy precedes the trauma and perhaps represents an underlying anatomic vulnerability, or merely represents an epiphenomenon, perhaps related to the physiologic effects of stress.

There is, apparently, only one neuropathologic study of PTSD (Bracha *et al.* 2005). This study demonstrated a reduction in neuronal cell number in the locus ceruleus in PTSD patients compared with control subjects.

Overall, it appears reasonable to invoke a 'stress–diathesis' model for the etiology of PTSD. However, although the 'stress' is clear, the nature of the diathesis is not. It may be, however, that there are changes in certain structures that subserve emotional reactivity and remembrance, such as the locus ceruleus and the hippocampus, which may in turn be related to disturbances in catecholamine activity and the function of the hypothalamic–pituitary–adrenal axis.

Differential diagnosis

After a significant trauma, rather than developing PTSD, individuals may develop a major depressive disorder, and the resulting depressive episode may at times be difficult to distinguish from the symptoms seen in PTSD. Certain features, however, may enable a differential diagnosis to be made. Patients with depression have a depressed mood rather than a sense of numbness or detachment; furthermore, patients with depression may experience ruminations, which are heavy, leaden recollections of misfortune, thus standing in contrast to the starkly vivid and mercurial recollections and flashbacks seen in PTSD. As noted earlier, patients with PTSD may develop a depressive episode, but in these cases one sees clear-cut PTSD preceding the onset of the depression.

In cases in which the original trauma was a head injury, one must distinguish the features of a traumatic brain injury or a post-concussion syndrome from PTSD, and this may be difficult. Certainly, one cannot entertain the diagnosis of PTSD in such cases unless patients display evidence of involuntarily re-experiencing the original event, such as vivid memories, nightmares or flashbacks. In post-head trauma patients who do display such symptoms, other symptoms, such as poor concentration, fatigue, insomnia, lability, and irritability, may individually occur secondary to a combined effect of the traumatic brain injury (or post-concussion syndrome) and PTSD.

Malingerers and those with factitious illness, as discussed in Section 7.8, may feign PTSD. In those feigning combat-related PTSD, a review of military records may reveal the lie; in cases, however, in which an actual trauma did occur, for example a motor vehicle accident, the diagnosis may have to wait upon resolution of pending litigation, after which the 'PTSD' magically resolves.

Treatment

Cognitive–behavioral therapy appears to be effective. Certain antidepressants are also effective, including phenelzine (Frank *et al.* 1988), imipramine (Davidson *et al.* 1990), venlafaxine (Davidson *et al.* 2006), mirtazapine (Davidson *et al.* 2003), and the SSRIs fluoxetine (Connor *et al.* 1999; Martenyi *et al.* 2002; van der Kolk *et al.* 1994), paroxetine (Marshall *et al.* 2001; Tucker *et al.* 2001), and sertraline (Brady *et al.* 2000; Davidson *et al.* 2001), (although not all studies are in agreement regarding the effectiveness of fluoxetine [Martenyi *et al.* 2007] or sertraline [Freidman *et al.* 2007]). Of the antidepressants, the SSRIs have the longest track record, and one of these is generally used first; consideration, however, may also be given to mirtazapine or venlafaxine; imipramine is generally not as well tolerated, and phenelzine is difficult to use. Regardless of which antidepressant is chosen, a high dose may be required, and at least 6 weeks should be allowed to pass before assessing any effects. In cases in which the antidepressant is either poorly tolerated or ineffective, consideration may be given to switching to a different antidepressant or, in patients on an SSRI, to augmentation with either risperidone (1–2 mg) (Bartzokis *et al.* 2005; Reich *et al.* 2004) or olanzapine (10 mg) (Stein *et al.* 2002); of these two antipsychotics, risperidone is generally better tolerated over the long haul and should probably be tried first. Another medication to consider is prazosin. This alpha-1 antagonist has been shown in double-blind work to reduce the nightmares seen in PTSD (Raskind *et al.* 2003, 2007), and may be started at 1 mg in the evening, with the dose increased in similar increments every few days until patients obtain relief or limiting side-effects occur; most patients respond to a dose of about 13 mg. There is also suggestive work indicating that daytime prazosin may provide further relief (Taylor *et al.* 2006). A non-blind study also suggests that cyproheptadine, in a night-time dose of 4–12 mg, may reduce nightmares (Gupta *et al.* 1998).

As noted earlier, alcohol abuse or alcoholism not uncommonly accompany PTSD, and when this is the case it is critical to treat these, either first or concomitantly with the PTSD.

20.16 GENERALIZED ANXIETY DISORDER

Generalized anxiety disorder is characterized by a persistent, 'free-floating' anxiety, which is accompanied by autonomic symptoms such as tremor. Although the lifetime prevalence of this disorder has been estimated to be as high as 5 percent, there has been some doubt expressed regarding this; as noted below, it may be difficult to distinguish generalized anxiety disorder from a chronic agitated depression, and such misdiagnoses may have inflated the prevalence figures.

Clinical features

The onset is gradual and may occur in either teenage or early adult years.

Clinically (Anderson et al. 1984; Hoehn-Saric et al. 1989; Marten et al. 1993; Nisita et al. 1990; Starcevic et al. 1994), patients experience a chronic, pervasive sense of anxious apprehension and tension. They frequently worry about the future and are easily startled. Some complain of a sense of shakiness, and there may be a mild degree of a fine postural tremor of the hands. There is occasionally tachycardia, and the skin is often cold and clammy. Insomnia may occur, and many complain of nausea and headache. Some patients can offer no explanation for their symptoms, whereas others will offer 'reasons' and blame their state on some life event or other. Observation over time, however, reveals that the anxiety is in fact autonomous and 'free-floating'.

Course

This appears to be a chronic disorder, with symptoms waxing and waning in intensity over the years or decades. In some cases there appear to be spontaneous remissions; however, it is not clear in what percentage of these cases relapses eventually occur.

Etiology

Both family (Newman and Bland 2006; Noyes et al. 1987) and twin studies (Hettema et al. 2001; Kendler et al. 1992) suggest a genetic role in generalized anxiety disorder, and although it is not entirely clear what is inherited, several findings suggest abnormalities in GABAergic and noradrenergic functioning. GAGAergic dysfunction is indicated by the effectiveness of benzodiazepines in this disorder and by the finding of reduced benzodiazepine receptor sites, not only on peripheral blood lymphocytes (Rocca et al. 1998) but also in the left temporal pole (Tiihonen et al. 1997b). Noradrenergic dysfunction is suggested both by the resemblance of the symptoms seen in generalized anxiety disorder and those produced by noradrenergic agents and also by the presence of a reduced number of alpha-2 adrenergic receptors on platelets (Cameron et al. 1990).

Differential diagnosis

The most important disorder on the differential is a chronic depressive episode of a major depressive disorder.

In some patients, depressive episodes may be marked by psychomotor change with agitation, and such patients may experience restlessness, hand-wringing, and considerable tension, thus mimicking the picture seen in generalized anxiety disorder. Closer inquiry, however, will reveal additional symptoms in the depressed patient that are not seen in generalized anxiety disorder, such as crying spells, anhedonia, and anergia.

Other causes of persistent anxiety are discussed in Section 6.5. Of these, particular attention should be given to chronic use of caffeine or sympathomimetics, and to alcohol or sedative–hypnotic withdrawal.

Treatment

Both cognitive–behavioral therapy and numerous medications appear to be effective. Various antidepressants are effective, including imipramine (Hoehn-Saric et al. 1988; Kahn et al. 1986; Rickels et al. 1993b), trazodone (Rickels et al. 1993b), venlafaxine (Davidson et al. 1999; Gelenberg et al. 2000; Rickels et al. 2000), duloxetine (Endicott et al. 2007), and the SSRIs paroxetine (Ball et al. 2005; Bielski et al. 2005; Pollack et al. 2001; Rickels et al. 2003), sertraline (Allgulander et al. 2004; Ball et al. 2005; Brawman-Mintzer et al. 2006; Dahl et al. 2005), and escitalopram (Bielski et al. 2005). Alprazolam (Elie and Lamontagne 1984; Enkelmann 1991; Hoehn-Saric et al. 1988), lorazepam (Laakmann et al. 1998), and diazepam (Elie and Lamontagne 1984; Rickels et al. 1993b) are likewise effective, and consideration may also be given to hydroxyzine (Lader and Scotto 1998; Llorca et al. 2002), buspirone (Enkelmann 1991; Laakmann et al. 1998; Lader and Scotto 1998; Rickels et al. 1988; Sramek et al. 1996), and pregabalin (Montgomery et al. 2006; Rickels et al. 2005). The antidepressants should be given in doses comparable to those used in depression; total daily doses for the other agents are 2–6 mg for alprazolam, 3 mg for lorazepam, 15–25 mg for diazepam, 50 mg for hydroxyzine, 15 mg for buspirone, and 300–600 mg for pregabalin. Although choosing among the various medications is not straightforward, all other things being equal it is probably reasonable to start with an antidepressant: venlafaxine, duloxetine, or one of the SSRIs constitute reasonable first choices. Antidepressants take weeks to become effective, however, and many clinicians lean toward using one of the benzodiazepines, given their prompt onset of effect; however, this advantage must be weighed against the high probability of neuroadaptation and the rebound anxiety that accompanies any missed doses or attempts at tapering. Hydroxyzine is also rapidly effective; however, although it does not cause neuroadaptation, it does carry a considerable anticholinergic side-effect burden. Buspirone remains a reasonable alternative but has never become particularly popular. Pregabalin is the newest agent available for use in this disorder, and its place in the armamentarium is not as yet clear.

REFERENCES

Aberg-Wistedt A, Hasselmark L, Stain-Malmgren R et al. Serotoninergic 'vulnerability' in affective disorder: a study of the tryptophan depletion test and relationships between peripheral and central serotonin indexes in citalopram responders. Acta Psychiatr Scand 1998; 97:374–8.

Abrams R, Taylor MA. Manic and schizoaffective disorder, manic type: a comparison. Am J Psychiatry 1976a; 133:1445–7.

Abrams R, Taylor MA. Catatonia: a prospective clinical study. Arch Gen Psychiatry 1976b; 33:579–81.

Abrams R, Taylor MA. Importance of schizophrenic symptoms in the diagnosis of mania. Am J Psychiatry 1981; 138:658–61.

Accurso V, Winnicki M, Shamsuzzaman AS et al. Predisposition to vasovagal syncope in subjects with blood/injury phobia. Circulation 2001; 104:903–7.

Adams KH, Hansen ES, Pinborg LH et al. Patients with obsessive–compulsive disorder have increased 5-HT2A receptor binding in the caudate nuclei. Int J Neuropsychopharmacol 2005; 8:391–401.

Adler A. Neuropsychiatric complications in victims of Boston's Coconut Grove disaster. JAMA 1943; 123:1098–101.

Ahokas A, Aito M, Turianinen S. Association between oestradiol and puerperal psychosis. Acta Psychiatr 2000a; 101:167–9.

Ahokas A, Aito M, Rimon R. Positive treatment effect of estradiol in postpartum psychosis: A pilot study. J Clin Psychiatry 2000b; 61:166–9.

Ahokas A, Kaukrnta J, Wahlbek K et al. Estrogen deficiency in severe postpartum depression: successful treatment with sublingual physiologic 17 beta-estradiol: a preliminary study. J Clin Psychiatry 2001; 62:332–6.

Akbarian S, Bunney WE, Potkin SG et al. Altered distribution of nicotinamide-adenine dinucleotide phosphate-diaphorase cells in frontal lobe of schizophrenics implies disturbances of cortical development. Arch Gen Psychiatry 1993a; 50:169–77.

Akbarian S, Vinuela A, Kim JJ et al. Distorted distribution of nicotinamide-adenine dinucleotide phosphate-diaphorase neurons in temporal lobe of schizophrenics implies anomalous cortical development. Arch Gen Psychiatry 1993b; 50:178–87.

Akbarian S, Kim JJ, Potkin SG et al. Maldistribution of interstitial neurons in prefrontal white matter of the brains of schizophrenic patients. Arch Gen Psychiatry 1996; 53:425–36.

Akiskal HS, Djenderedjian AM, Rosenthal RH et al. Cyclothymic disorder: validating criteria for inclusion in the bipolar affective group. Am J Psychiatry 1977; 134:1227–33.

Allebeck P, Varla A, Kristjansson E et al. Risk factor for suicide among patients with schizophrenia. Acta Psychiatr Scand 1987; 76:414–19.

Allgulander C. Paroxetine in social anxiety disorder: a randomized placebo-controlled study. Acta Psychiatr Scand 1999; 100:193–8.

Allgulander C, Dahl AA, Austin C et al. Efficacy of sertraline in a 12-week trial for generalized anxiety disorder. Am J Psychiatry 2004; 161:1642–9.

Altamura AC, Percudani M. The use of antidepressants for long-term treatment of recurrent depression: rationale, current methodologies, and future directions. J Clin Psychiatry 1993; 54(suppl. 8):29–37.

Altschuler LL, Post RM, Leverich GS. Antidepressant-induced mania and cycle acceleration: a controversy revisited. Am J Psychiatry 1995; 152:1130–8.

Anderson JD, Noyes R, Crowe RR. A comparison of panic disorder and generalized anxiety disorder. Am J Psychiatry 1984; 141:572–5.

Andreasen NC. Negative symptoms in schizophrenia: definition and reliability. Arch Gen Psychiatry 1982; 39:784–8.

Andreasen NC, Olson S. Negative versus positive schizophrenia: definition and validation. Arch Gen Psychiatry 1982; 39:789–94.

Andreasen NC, Flaum M, Swayze VW et al. Positive and negative symptoms in schizophrenia: a critical reappraisal. Arch Gen Psychiatry 1990a; 47:615–21.

Andreasen NC, Swayze VW, Flaum M et al. Ventricular enlargement in schizophrenia: evaluation with computed tomographic scanning. Arch Gen Psychiatry 1990b; 47:1008–15.

Andrews E, Ballard J, Walter-Ryan WG. Monosymptomatic hypochondriacal psychosis manifesting as delusions of infestation: case studies of treatment with haloperidol. J Clin Psychiatry 1986; 47:188–90.

Angst J, Felder W, Lohmeyer B. Schizoaffective disorders. I. Results of a genetic investigation. J Affect Disord 1979; 1:139–53.

Anonymous. Historical notes: earliest use of the term dementia praecox. Am J Psychiatry 1954; 111:470.

Appleby L, Warner R, Whitton A et al. A controlled study of fluoxetine and cognitive behavioral counselling in the treatment of postnatal depression. BMJ 1997; 314:932–6.

Apter A, Pauls DL, Bleich A et al. An epidemiologic study of Gilles de la Tourette's syndrome in Israel. Arch Gen Psychiatry 1993; 50:734–8.

Argyropoulos SV, Hood SD, Adrover M et al. Tryptophan depletion reverses the therapeutic effect of selective serotonin reuptake inhibitors in social anxiety disorder. Biol Psychiatry 2004; 56:503–9.

Atmaca M, Kumru S, Tezcan E. Fluoxetine versus agnus castus extract in the treatment of premenstrual dysphoric disorder. Hum Psychopharmacol 2003; 1:191–5.

Austin MP. Puerperal affective psychosis: is there a case for lithium prophylaxis? Br J Psychiatry 1992; 161:692–4.

Baer L, Jenike MA, Ricciardi JN et al. Standardized assessment of personality disorders in obsessive-compulsive disorder. Arch Gen Psychiatry 1990; 47:826–30.

Baer L, Rauch SL, Ballantine HT et al. Cingulotomy for intractable obsessive-compulsive disorder: prospective long-term follow-up of 18 patients. Arch Gen Psychiatry 1995; 52:384–92.

Bagedahl-Strindlund M. Postpartum mental illness: timing of illness onset and its relation to symptoms and sociodemographic characteristics. Acta Psychiatr Scand 1986; 74:490–6.

Bailara KM, Henry C, Lestage J et al. Decreased brain tryptophan availability as a partial determinant of post-partum blues. Psychoneuroendocrinology 2006; 31:407–13.

Baker DG, West SA, Nicholson WE et al. Serial CSF corticotropin-releasing hormone levels and adrenocortical activity in combat veterans with posttraumatic stress disorder. Am J Psychiatry 1999; 156:585–8.

Baker DG, Ekhator NN, Kasckow JW *et al.* Higher levels of basal serial CSF cortisol in combat veterans with posttraumatic stress disorder. *Am J Psychiatry* 2005; **162**:992–4.

Baldessarini RJ, Tondo L, Faeda GL *et al.* Effects of the rate of discontinuing lithium maintenance treatment in bipolar disorder. *J Clin Psychiatry* 1996; **57**:441–8.

Baldessarini RJ, Tondo L, Floris G *et al.* Reduced morbidity after gradual discontinuation of lithium treatment for bipolar I and II disorders: a replication study. *Am J Psychiatry* 1997; **154**:551–3.

Baldwin D, Bobes J, Stein DJ *et al.* Paroxetine in social phobia/social anxiety disorder: randomized, double-blind, placebo-controlled study. *Br J Psychiatry* 1999; **175**:120–6.

Ball SG, Kuhn A, Wall D *et al.* Selective serotonin reuptake inhibitor treatment for generalized anxiety disorder: a double-blind, prospective comparison between paroxetine and sertraline. *J Clin Psychiatry* 2005; **66**:94–9.

Ballenger JC, Burows CD, DuPont RL *et al.* Alprazolam in panic disorder and agoraphobia: results from a multicenter trial. I. Efficacy in short-term treatment. *Arch Gen Psychiatry* 1988; **45**:413–22.

Ballenger JC, Wheadon DE, Steiner M *et al.* Double-blind, fixed-dose, placebo-controlled study of paroxetine in the treatment of panic disorder. *Am J Psychiatry* 1998; **155**:36–42.

Banki CM, Bissette G, Arato M *et al.* Elevation of immunoreactive CSF TRH in depressed patients. *Am J Psychiatry* 1988; **145**:1525–31.

Bao A-M, Hestiantoro A, Van Someren EJW *et al.* Colocalization of corticotropin-releasing hormone and oestrogen receptor-alpha in the paraventricular nucleus of the hypothalamus in mood disorders. *Brain* 2005; **128**:1301–13.

Barta PE, Pearlson GD, Powers RE *et al.* Auditory hallucinations and smaller superior temporal gyral volume in schizophrenia. *Am J Psychiatry* 1990; **146**:1457–62.

Bartzokis G, Lu PH, Turner J *et al.* Adjunctive risperidone in the treatment of chronic combat-related posttraumatic stress disorder. *Biol Psychiatry* 2005; **57**:474–9.

Basoglu M, Paker M, Paker O *et al.* Psychological effects of torture: a comparison of tortured with nontortured political activists in Turkey. *Am J Psychiatry* 1994; **151**:76–81.

Bauer MS, Whybrow PC, Winokur A. Rapid cycling bipolar affective disorder. I. Association with grade I hypothyroidism. *Arch Gen Psychiatry* 1990; **47**:427–32.

Bauer MS, Calabrese J, Dunner DL *et al.* Multisite data reanalysis of the validity of rapid cycling as a course modifier for bipolar disorder in DSM-IV. *Am J Psychiatry* 1994; **151**:506–15.

Baumann B, Bogerts B. Neuroanatomical studies on bipolar disorder. *Br J Psychiatry* 2001; **41**(suppl.):142–7.

Baxter LR, Phelps ME, Mazziotta JC *et al.* Local cerebral glucose metabolic rates in obsessive-compulsive disorder: a comparison with rates in unipolar depression and in normal controls. *Arch Gen Psychiatry* 1987; **44**:211–18.

Baxter LR, Schwartz JM, Bergman KS *et al.* Caudate glucose metabolic rate changes with both drug and behavior therapy for obsessive-compulsive disorder. *Arch Gen Psychiatry* 1992; **49**:681–9.

Beck AT, Sokol L, Clark DA *et al.* A crossover study of focused cognitive therapy for panic disorder. *Am J Psychiatry* 1992; **149**:778–83.

Beigel A, Murphy DL. Assessing clinical characteristics of the manic state. *Am J Psychiatry* 1971a; **128**:688–94.

Beigel A, Murphy DL. Unipolar and bipolar affective illness: differences in clinical characteristics accompanying depression. *Arch Gen Psychiatry* 1971b; **24**:215–20.

Bell C, Forshall S, Andover M *et al.* Does 5-HT restrain panic? A tryptophan depletion study in panic disorder patients recovered on paroxetine. *Psychopharmacol* 2002; **16**:5–14.

Benjamin J, BenZion IZ, Karbofsky E *et al.* Double-blind placebo-controlled pilot study of paroxetine for specific phobia. *Psychopharmacology* 2000; **149**:194–6.

Benkelfat C, Nordahl TE, Semple WE *et al.* Local cerebral glucose metabolic rates in obsessive-compulsive disorder: patients treated with clomipramine. *Arch Gen Psychiatry* 1990; **47**:840–8.

Bergeron R, Ravindram AV, Chaput Y *et al.* Sertraline and fluoxetine treatment of obsessive-compulsive disorder: results of a double-blind, 6-month treatment study. *J Clin Psychopharmacol* 2002; **22**:148–54.

Bertelsen A, Harvald B, Hauge M. A Danish twin study of manic-depressive disorders. *Br J Psychiatry* 1977; **130**:330–51.

Best NR, Wiley M, Stump K *et al.* Binding of tritiated yohimbine to platelets in women with maternity blues. *Psychol Med* 1988; **18**:837–42.

Bielski RJ, Bose A, Chang CC. A double-blind comparison of excitalopram and aroxetine in the long-term treatment of generalized anxiety disorder. *Ann Clin Psychiatry* 2005; **17**:65–9.

Birmes P, Brunet A, Carreras D *et al.* The predictive power of peritraumatic dissociation and acute stress symptoms for posttraumatic stress symptoms: a three-month prospective study. *Am J Psychiatry* 2003; **160**:1337–9.

Bisaga A, Katz JL, Antonini A *et al.* Cerebral glucose metabolism in women with panic disorder. *Am J Psychiatry* 1998; **155**:1178–83.

Black DW, Boffeli TJ. Simple schizophrenia: past, present and future. *Am J Psychiatry* 1989; **146**:1267–73.

Black DW, Nasrallah H. Hallucinations and delusions in 1,715 patients with unipolar and bipolar affective disorders. *Psychopathology* 1989; **22**:28–34.

Black DW, Noyes R, Pfohl B *et al.* Personality disorder in obsessive-compulsive volunteers, well comparison subjects, and their first-degree relatives. *Am J Psychiatry* 1993; **150**:1226–32.

Bleuler E. *Dementia praecox or the group of schizophrenias.* New York: International Universities Press, 1950.

Bloch M, Schmidt PJ, Rubinow DR. Premenstrual syndrome: evidence of symptom stability across cycles. *Am J Psychiatry* 1997; **154**:1741–6.

Bloch M, Schmidt PJ, Danaceau M *et al.* Effects of gonadal steroids in women with a history of postpartum depression. *Am J Psychiatry* 2000; **157**:924–30.

Bogerts B, Meertz E, Schonfeldt-Bausch R. Basal ganglia and limbic system pathology in schizophrenia: a morphometric study of brain volume and shrinkage. *Arch Gen Psychiatry* 1985; **42**:784–91.

Bogerts B, Falkai P, Haupts M *et al.* Post-mortem volume measurements of limbic system and basal ganglia structures in chronic schizophrenics. Initial results from a new brain collection. *Schizophren Res* 1990; **3**:295–301.

Bond TC. Recognition of acute delirious mania. *Arch Gen Psychiatry* 1980; **37**:553–4.

Bonne O, Brandes D, Gilboa A *et al.* Longitudinal MRI study of hippocampal volume in trauma survivors with PTSD. *Am J Psychiatry* 2001; **158**:1248–51.

Bowman KM, Raymond AF. A statistical study of hallucinations in the manic-depressive psychoses. *Am J Psychiatry* 1931; **88**: 299–309.

Bracha HS, Garcia-Rill E, Mrak RE *et al.* Postmortem locus coeruleus neuron count in three American veterans with probable or possible war-related PTSD. *J Neuropsychiatry Clin Neurosci* 2005; **17**:503–9.

Bradwejn J, Koszycki D, Shriqui C. Enhanced sensitivity to cholecystokinin tetrapeptide in panic disorder. Clinical and behavioral findings. *Arch Gen Psychiatry* 1991; **48**:603–10.

Brady K, Pearlstein T, Asnis GM *et al.* Efficacy and safety of sertraline treatment of posttraumatic stress disorder: a randomized controlled trial. *JAMA* 2000; **283**:1837–44.

Brantigan CO, Brantigan TA, Joseph N. Effect of beta blockade and beta stimulation on stage fright. *Am J Med* 1982; **72**:88–94.

Bratfos O, Haug JO. Puerperal mental disorders in manic-depressive females. *Acta Psychiatr Scand* 1966; **42**:285–94.

Brawman-Mintzer O, Knapp RG, Rynn M *et al.* Sertraline treatment for generalized anxiety disorder: a randomized, double-blind, placebo-controlled study. *J Clin Psychiatry* 2006; **67**:874–81.

Bremner JD, Randall P, Scott TM *et al.* MRI-based measurement of hippocampal volume in patients with combat-related posttraumatic stress disorder. *Am J Psychiatry* 1995; **152**:973–81.

Bremner JD, Vythilingam M, Vermetten E *et al.* MRI and PET study of deficits in hippocampal structure and function in women with childhood sexual abuse and posttraumatic stress disorder. *Am J Psychiatry* 2003; **160**:924–32.

Brockington IF, Wainwright S, Kendell RE. Manic patients with schizophrenic or paranoid symptoms. *Psychol Med* 1980; **10**:73–83.

Brockington IF, Cernik KF, Schofield EM *et al.* Puerperal psychosis: phenomena and diagnosis. *Arch Gen Psychiatry* 1981; **38**:829–33.

Brodaty H, Sachdev P, Rose N *et al.* Schizophrenia with onset after age 50 years. I. Phenomenology and risk factors. *Br J Psychiatry* 1999; **175**:410–15.

Broocks A, Pigott TA, Hill JL *et al.* Acute intravenous administration of ondansetron and m-CPP, alone and in combination, in patients with obsessive-compulsive disorder (OCD): behavioral and biological results. *Psychiatry Res* 1998; **79**:11–20.

Brown AS, Cohen P, Harkavy-Friedman J *et al.* Prenatal rubella, premorbid abnormalities, and adult schizophrenia. *Biol Psychiatry* 2001; **49**:473–86.

Brown GW, Harris TO, Hepworth C *et al.* Life events and endogenous depression: a puzzle re-examined. *Arch Gen Psychiatry* 1994; **51**:525–34.

Bruton CJ, Crow TJ, Frith CD *et al.* Schizophrenia and the brain: a prospective clinico-pathological study. *Psychol Med* 1990; **20**:285–304.

Bunney WE, Hartmann EL. Study of a patient with a 48-hour manic-depressive cycle. *Arch Gen Psychiatry* 1965; **12**:611–18.

Bunney WE, Murphy DL, Goodwin FK *et al.* The 'switch process' in manic-depressive illness. *Arch Gen Psychiatry* 1972; **27**:295–302.

Butler RW, Braff DL, Rausch J *et al.* Physiological evidence of exaggerated startle response in a subgroup of Vietnam veterans with combat-related posttraumatic stress disorder. *Am J Psychiatry* 1990; **147**:1308–12.

Byne W, Buschbaum MS, Mattiace LA *et al.* Postmortem assessment of thalamic nuclear volumes in subjects with schizophrenia. *Am J Psychiatry* 2002; **159**:59–65.

Bystritsky A, Ackerman DL, Rosen RM *et al.* Augmentation of sertraline reuptake inhibition in refractory obsessive-compulsive disorder using adjunctive olanzapine: a placebo-controlled trial. *J Clin Psychiatry* 2004; **65**:565–8.

Cameron OG, Smith CB, Lee MA *et al.* Adrenergic status in anxiety disorders: platelet alpha-2-adrenergic receptor binding, blood pressure, pulse and plasma catecholamines in panic and generalized anxiety disorder patients and in normal subjects. *Biol Psychiatry* 1990; **28**:2–20.

Canterbury RJ, Haskins B, Kahn N *et al.* Postpartum psychosis induced by bromocriptine. *South Med J* 1987; **80**:1463–4.

Carlson GA, Goodwin FK. The stages of mania: a longitudinal analysis of the manic episode. *Arch Gen Psychiatry* 1973; **28**:221–8.

Carroll BJ, Martin FI, Davis B. Pituitary-adrenal function in depression. *Lancet* 1968; **2**:1373–4.

Carroll BJ, Curtis GC, Mendels J. Neuroendocrine regulation in depression. *Arch Gen Psychiatry* 1976; **33**:1039–44.

Casper RC, Redmond E, Katz MM *et al.* Somatic symptoms in primary affective disorder: presence and relationship to the classification of depression. *Arch Gen Psychiatry* 1985; **42**:1098–104.

Chapman TF, Fyer AJ, Mannuzza S *et al.* A comparison of treated and untreated simple phobia. *Am J Psychiatry* 1993; **150**:816–18.

Charney DS, Henninger GR, Jatlow PI. Increased anxiogenic effects of caffeine in panic disorders. *Arch Gen Psychiatry* 1985; **42**:233–43.

Charney DS, Woods SW, Krystal JH *et al.* Noradrenergic neuronal dysregulation in panic disorder: the effects of intravenous yohimbine and clonidine in panic disorder patients. *Acta Psychiatr Scand* 1992; **86**:273–82.

Charron M, Fortin L, Paquette I. De novo mania among elderly people. *Acta Psychiatr Scand* 1991; **84**:503–7.

Chua SE, McKenna PJ. Schizophrenia – a brain disease? A critical review of structural and functional cerebral abnormality in the disorder. *Br J Psychiatry* 1995; **166**:563–82.

Clayton P, Pitts FN, Winokur G. Affective disorders. IV. Mania. *Compr Psychiatry* 1965; **3**:313–22.

Clomipramine Collaborative Study Group. Clomipramine in the treatment of patients with obsessive-compulsive disorder. *Arch Gen Psychiatry* 1991; **48**:730–8.

Cohen LS, Mier C, Brown EW *et al.* Premenstrual daily fluoxetine for premenstrual dysphoric disorder: a placebo-controlled, clinical trial using computerized diaries. *Obstet Gynecol* 2002; **100**:435–44.

Cohen SM, Allen MG, Pollin W et al. Relationship of schizoaffective psychosis to manic-depressive psychosis and schizophrenia: findings in 15,909 veteran pairs. Arch Gen Psychiatry 1972; 26:539–46.

Connor KM, Sutherland SM, Tupler LA et al. Fluoxetine in post-traumatic stress disorder. Br J Psychiatry 1999; 175:17–22.

Conrad AJ, Abebe T, Austin R et al. Hippocampal pyramidal cell disarray in schizophrenia as a bilateral phenomenon. Arch Gen Psychiatry 1991; 48:413–17.

Cooper PJ, Murray L. Course and recurrence of postnatal depression. Evidence for the specificity of the diagnostic concept. Br J Psychiatry 1995; 166:191–5.

Cowdry RW, Wehr TA, Zis AP et al. Thyroid abnormalities associated with rapid-cycling bipolar illness. Arch Gen Psychiatry 1983; 40:414–20.

Cowley DS, Arana GW. The diagnostic utility of lactate sensitivity in panic disorder. Arch Gen Psychiatry 1990; 47:277–84.

Coyle PK, Sterman AB. Focal neurologic symptoms in panic attacks. Am J Psychiatry 1986; 143:648–9.

Crow TJ, Ball J, Bloom SR et al. Schizophrenia as an anomaly of development of cerebral asymmetry: a post-mortem study and a proposal concerning the genetic basis of the disease. Arch Gen Psychiatry 1989; 46:1145–50.

Crowe RR, Noyes R, Pauls DL et al. A family study of panic disorder. Arch Gen Psychiatry 1983; 40:1065–9.

Curtis GC, Thyer B. Fainting on exposure to phobic stimuli. Am J Psychiatry 1983; 140:771–4.

Dahl AA, Ravindran A, Allgulander C et al. Sertraline in generalized anxiety disorder: efficacy in treating the psychic and somatic anxiety factors. Act Pschiatr Scand 2005; 111:429–35.

Davidson J, Robertson E. A follow-up study of postpartum illness, 1946–1978. Acta Psychiatr Scand 1985; 71:451–7.

Davidson JRT, Kudler HS, Smith R et al. Treatment of posttraumatic stress disorder with amitriptyline and placebo. Arch Gen Psychiatry 1990; 47:259–66.

Davidson J, Potts N, Richichi E et al. Treatment of social phobia with clonazepam and placebo. J Clin Psychopharmacol 1993; 13:423–8.

Davidson JRT, DuPont RL, Hedges D et al. Efficacy, safety, and tolerability of venlafaxine extended release and buspirone in outpatients with generalized anxiety disorder. J Clin Psychiatry 1999; 60:528–35.

Davidson JRT, Rothbaum BO, van der Kolk BA et al. Multicenter, double-blind comparison of sertraline and placebo in the treatment of posttraumatic stress disorder. Arch Gen Psychiatry 2001; 58:485–92.

Davidson JR, Weisler RH, Butterfield MI et al. Mirtazapine vs placebo in posttraumatic stress disorder: a pilot trial. Biol Psychiatry 2003; 53:188–91.

Davidson J, Baldwin D, Stein DJ et al. Treatment of posttraumatic stress disorder with venlafaxine extended release: a 6-month randomized controlled trial. Arch Gen Psychiatry 2006; 63:1158–65.

Delgado PL, Charney DS, Price LH et al. Serotonin function and the mechanism of antidepressant action: reversal of antidepressant-induced remission by rapid depletion of plasma tryptophan. Arch Gen Psychiatry 1990; 47:411–18.

Denys D, van der Wee N, van Megen HJGM et al. A double blind comparison of venlafaxine and paroxetine in obsessive-compulsive disorder. J Clin Psychopharmacol 2003; 23:568–75.

Denys D, de Geus F, van Megen HJGM et al. A double-blind, randomized, placebo-controlled trial of quetiapine addition in patients with obsessive-compulsive disorder refractory to serotonin reuptake inhibitors. J Clin Psychiatry 2004; 65:1040–8.

D'Mello DA, Pinheiro AL, Lalinet-Michaud M. Premenstrual mania: two case reports. J Nerv Ment Dis 1993; 181:330–1.

Dohl RB, Wolkow RM, Clary CM. Sertraline in the treatment of panic disorder: a double-blind multicenter trial. Am J Psychiatry 1998; 155:1189–95.

Donadio V, Liguori R, Elam M et al. Arousal elicits exaggerated inhibition of sympathetic nerve activity in phobic syncope patients. Brain 2007; 130:1653–7.

Dougherty DD, Baer L, Cosgrove GR et al. Prospective long-term follow-up of 44 patients who received cingulotomy for treatment-refractory obsessive-compulsive disorder. Am J Psychiatry 2002; 159:269–75.

Dunner DL, Fleiss JL, Fieve RR. The course of development of mania in patients with recurrent depression. Am J Psychiatry 1976; 133:905–8.

Dunner DL, Patrick V, Fieve RR. Rapid cycling manic depressive patients. Compr Psychiatry 1977; 18:561–6.

Eisen JL, Rasmussen SA. Obsessive-compulsive disorder with psychotic features. J Clin Psychiatry 1993; 54:373–9.

Elie R, Lamontagne Y. Alprazolam and diazepam in the treatment of generalized anxiety. J Clin Psychopharmacol 1984; 4:125–9.

Endicott J, Russell JM, Raskin J et al. Duoxetine treatment for role functioning in generalized anxiety disorder: three independent studies. J Clin Psychiatry 2007; 68:518–24.

Enkelmann R. Alprazolam versus buspirone in the treatment of outpatients with generalized anxiety disorder. Psychopharmacology 1991; 105:428–32.

Extein I, Pottash AL, Gold MS et al. Differentiating mania from schizophrenia by the TRH test. Am J Psychiatry 1980; 137:981–2.

Fava M, Rosenbaum JF, Pava JA et al. Anger attacks in unipolar depression. I. Clinical correlates and response to fluoxetine treatment. Am J Psychiatry 1993; 150:1158–63.

Feinstein A, Dolan R. Predictors of post-traumatic stress disorder following physical trauma: an examination of the stressor criterion. Psychol Med 1991; 21:85–91.

Fenton WS, McGlashan TH. Natural history of schizophrenia subtypes. I. Longitudinal study of paranoid, hebephrenic and undifferentiated schizophrenia. Arch Gen Psychiatry 1991; 48:969–77.

Fitzgerald M, Malone KM, Li S et al. Blunted serotonin response to fenfluramine challenge in premenstrual dysphoric disorder. Am J Psychiatry 1997; 154:556–8.

Foa EB, Steketee G, Grayson JB et al. Deliberate exposure and blocking of obsessive compulsive rituals: immediate and long-term effect. Behav Ther 1984; 15:450–72.

Foa EB, Kozak MJ, Goodman WK et al. DSM-IV field trial: obsessive-compulsive disorder. Am J Psychiatry 1995; 152:90–6.

Foa EB, Liebowitz MR, Kozak MJ et al. Randomized, placebo-controlled trial of exposure and ritual prevention, clomipramine, and their combination in the treatment of obsessive-compulsive disorder. *Am J Psychiatry* 2005; **162**:151–61.

Frank E, Anderson B, Reynolds CF *et al.* Life events and the research diagnostic criteria endogenous subtype: a confirmation of the distinction using the Bedford College methods. *Arch Gen Psychiatry* 1994; **51**:519–24.

Frank JB, Kosten TR, Giller EL *et al.* A randomized clinical trial of phenelzine and imipramine for posttraumatic stress disorder. *Am J Psychiatry* 1988; **145**:1289–91.

Frankel M, Cummings JL, Robertson MM *et al.* Obsessions and compulsions in Gilles de la Tourette's syndrome. *Neurology* 1986; **36**:378–82.

Freeman CP, Trimble MR, Deakin JF *et al.* Fluvoxamine versus clomipramine in the treatment of obsessive-compulsive disorder: a multi-center, randomized, double-blinded, parallel group comparison. *J Clin Psychiatry* 1994; **55**:301–5.

Freeman EW, Rickels K, Sondheimer SJ *et al.* A double-blind trial of oral progesterone, alprazolam and placebo in the treatment of severe premenstrual syndrome. *JAMA* 1995; **27**:51–4.

Freeman EW, Rickels K, Sondheimer SJ *et al.* Differential response to antidepressants in women with premenstrual syndrome/premenstrual dysphoric disorder: a randomized controlled trial. *Arch Gen Psychiatry* 1999; **56**:932–9.

Freeman EW, Rickels K, Yonkers KA *et al.* Venlafaxine in the treatment of premenstrual dysphoric disorder. *Obstet Gynecol* 2001; **98**:737–44.

Freeman EW, Rickels K, Sondheimer SJ *et al.* Continuous or intermittent dosing with sertraline for patients with severe premenstrual syndrome or premenstrual dysphoric disorder. *Am J Psychiatry* 2004; **161**:343–51.

Freidman MJ, Marmar CR, Baker DG *et al.* Randomized, double-blind comparison of sertraline and placebo for posttraumatic stress disorder in a Department of Veterans Affairs setting. *J Clin Psychiatry* 2007; **68**:711–20.

Fyer AJ, Mannuzza S, Gallops MS *et al.* Familial transmission of simple phobias and fears: a preliminary report. *Arch Gen Psychiatry* 1990; **47**:252–6.

Fyer AJ, Mannuzza S, Chapman TF *et al.* A direct interview family study of social phobia. *Arch Gen Psychiatry* 1993; **50**:286–93.

Gelenberg AJ, Lydiard RB, Rudolph RL *et al.* Efficacy of venlafaxine extended-release capsules in nondepressed outpatients with generalized anxiety disorder. *JAMA* 2000; **283**:3082–8.

Geracioti TD, Baker DG, Ekhatur NN *et al.* CSF norepinephrine concentrations in posttraumatic stress disorder. *Am J Psychiatry* 2001; **158**:1227–30.

Gershon ES, Hamovit J, Guroff JJ *et al.* A family study of schizoaffective, bipolar I, bipolar II, unipolar and normal control probands. *Arch Gen Psychiatry* 1982; **39**:1157–67.

Gersons BPR, Carlier IVE. Post-traumatic stress disorder: the history of a recent concept. *Br J Psychiatry* 1992; **161**:742–8.

Gillin JC, Sutton L, Ruiz C *et al.* The cholinergic rapid eye movement induction test with arecoline in depression. *Arch Gen Psychiatry* 1991; **48**:264–70.

Goddard AW, Mason GF, Almai A *et al.* Reductions in occipital cortex GABA levels in panic disorder detected with 1h-magnetic resonance spectography. *Arch Gen Psychiatry* 2001; **58**:556–61.

Goenjian AK, Najarian LM, Pynoos RS *et al.* Posttraumatic stress disorder in elderly and younger adults after the 1988 earthquake in Armenia. *Am J Psychiatry* 1994; **151**:895–901.

Goenjian AK, Yehuda R, Pynoos RS *et al.* Basal cortisol dexamethasone suppression of cortisol and MHPG in adolescents after the 1988 earthquake in Armenia. *Am J Psychiatry* 1996; **153**:929–34.

Goisman RM, Warshaw MG, Steketee GS *et al.* DSM-IV and the disappearance of agoraphobia without a history of panic disorder: new data on a controversial diagnosis. *Am J Psychiatry* 1995; **152**:1438–43.

Gordon A. Transition of obsessions into delusions. *Am J Psychiatry* 1950; **107**:455–8.

Gorman JM, Fyer MR, Goetz R *et al.* Ventilatory physiology of patients with panic disorder. *Arch Gen Psychiatry* 1988; **45**:31–9.

Grabe HJ, Ruhrmann S, Ettelt S *et al.* Familiarity of obsessive-compulsive disorder in nonclinical and clinical subjects. *Am J Psychiatry* 2006; **163**:1986–92.

Grahame PS. Schizophrenia in old age (late paraphrenia). *Br J Psychiatry* 1984; **145**:493–5.

Greenberg BD, Malone DA, Friehs GM *et al.* Three-year outcomes in deep brain stimulation for highly resistant obsessive-compulsive disorder. *Neuropsychopharmacology* 2006; **31**:2384–93.

Gregoire AJ, Kumar L, Everitt B *et al.* Transdermal oestrogen for treatment of severe postnatal depression. *Lancet* 1996; **347**:930–3.

Greist J, Chouinard G, DuBoff E *et al.* Double-blind parallel comparison of three dosages of sertraline and placebo in outpatients with obsessive-compulsive disorder. *Arch Gen Psychiatry* 1995; **52**:289–95.

Gupta S, Popli A, Bathurst E *et al.* Efficacy of cyproheptadine for nightmares associated with posttraumatic stress disorder. *Compr Psychiatry* 1998; **39**:160–4.

Guze SB, Woodruff RA, Clayton PJ. The significance of psychotic affective disorders. *Arch Gen Psychiatry* 1975; **32**:1147–50.

Hadley HG. A case of puerperal psychosis recovering from four attacks. *J Nerv Ment Dis* 1941; **94**:540–1.

Harris B. Prospective trial of L-tryptophan in maternity blues. *Br J Psychiatry* 1980; **137**:233–5.

Harris B, Lovett L, Newcombe RG *et al.* Maternity blues and major endocrine changes: Cardiff puerperal mood and hormone study II. *BMJ* 1994; **308**:949–53.

Hartley LR, Ungapen S, Davie I *et al.* The effect of beta adrenergic blocking drugs on speakers' performance and memory. *Br J Psychiatry* 1983; **142**:512–17.

Hartmann E. Longitudinal studies of sleep and dream patterns in manic-depressive patients. *Arch Gen Psychiatry* 1968; **19**:312–29.

Hasselbach SG, Hansen ES, Jakosen TB *et al.* Reduced midbrain-pons serotonin receptor binding in patients with obsessive-compulsive disorder. *Acta Psychiatr Scand* 2007; **115**:388–94.

Hauri PJ, Chernik D, Hawkins D *et al.* Sleep of depressed patients in remission. *Arch Gen Psychiatry* 1974; **31**:386–91.

Hauri PJ, Friedman M, Ravaruis CL. Sleep in patients with spontaneous panic attacks. *Sleep* 1989; **12**:323–37.

Hay P, Sachdev P, Cummings S et al. Treatment of obsessive-compulsive disorder by psychosurgery. Acta Psychiatr Scand 1993; 87:197–207.

Hayashi H, Oshino S, Ishikawa J et al. Paroxetine treatment of delusional disorder, somatic subtype. Hum Psychopharmacol 2004; 19:351–2.

Heimberg RG, Hope DA, Dodge CS et al. DSM-III-R subtypes of social phobia: comparison of generalized social phobics and public speaking phobics. J Nerv Ment Dis 1990; 178:172–9.

Heimberg RG, Liebowitz MR, Hope DA et al. Cognitive behavioral group therapy vs. phenelzine therapy for social phobia. Arch Gen Psychiatry 1998; 55:1133–41.

Hendrick V, Altshuler L, Strouse T et al. Postpartum and non postpartum depression: differences in presentation and response to pharmacologic treatment. Depress Anxiety 2000; 11:66–72.

Hesse S, Muller U, Lincke T et al. Serotonin and dopamine transporter imaging in patients with obsessive-compulsive disorder. Psychiatry Res 2005; 140:63–72.

Hettema JM, Prescott CA, Kendler KS. A population-based twin study of generalized anxiety disorder in men and women. J Nerv Ment Dis 2001; 189:413–20.

Himmelhoch JM, Mulla D, Neil JF et al. Incidence and significance of mixed affective states in a bipolar population. Arch Gen Psychiatry 1976; 33:1062–6.

Hirayasu Y, McCarley RW, Salisbury DF et al. Planum temporale and Heschl gyrus volume reduction in schizophrenia: a magnetic resonance imaging study of first-episode patients. Arch Gen Psychiatry 2000; 57:692–9.

Hoehn-Saric R, McLeod DR, Zimmerli WD. Differential effects of alprazolam and imipramine in generalized anxiety disorder: somatic versus psychic symptoms. J Clin Psychiatry 1988; 49:293–301.

Hoehn-Saric R, McLeod DR, Zimmerli WD. Somatic manifestations in women with generalized anxiety disorder. Arch Gen Psychiatry 1989; 46:1113–19.

Hoehn-Saric R, McLeod DR, Hipsley PA. Effect of fluvoxamine on panic disorder. J Clin Psychopharmacol 1993; 13:321–6.

Hollander E, DeCaria CM, Nitescu A et al. Serotoninergic function in obsessive-compulsive disorder: behavioral and neuroendocrine responses to m-chlorophenylpiperazine and fenfluramine in patients and healthy volunteers. Arch Gen Psychiatry 1992; 49:21–8.

Hollander E, Koran LM, Goodman WK et al. A double-blind, placebo-controlled study of the efficacy and safety of controlled-release fluvoxamine in patients with obsessive-compulsive disorder. J Clin Psychiatry 2003a; 64:640–7.

Hollander E, Allen A, Steiner M et al. Acute and long-term treatment and prevention of relapse of obsessive-compulsive disorder with paroxetine. J Clin Psychiatry 2003b; 64:1113–21.

Horwarth E, Lish JD, Johnson J et al. Agoraphobia without panic: clinical reappraisal of an epidemiologic finding. Am J Psychiatry 1993; 150:1496–501.

Insel TR, Akiskal HS. Obsessive-compulsive disorder with psychotic features: a phenomenologic analysis. Am J Psychiatry 1986; 143:1527–33.

Jager M, Bottlender R, Strauss A et al. Fifteen-year follow-up of ICD-10 schizoaffective disorders compared with schizophrenia and affective disorders. Acta Psychiatr Scand 2004; 109:30–7.

James IM, Griffith DNW, Pearson RM et al. Effect of oxyprenolol on stage-fright in musicians. Lancet 1977; 2:952–4.

Jampala VC, Taylor MA, Abrams R. The diagnostic implication of formal thought disorder in mania and schizophrenia: a reassessment. Am J Psychiatry 1989; 146:459–63.

Janowsky DS, El-Yousof MK, David JM et al. Parasympathetic suppression of manic symptoms by physostigmine. Arch Gen Psychiatry 1973; 28:542–7.

Jaskiw GE, Juliano DM, Goldberg TE et al. Cerebral ventricular enlargement in schizophreniform disorder does not progress. A seven year follow-up study. Schizophren Res 1994; 14:23–8.

Jatzko A, Rothenhofer S, Schmitt A et al. Hippocampal volume in chronic posttraumatic stress disorder (PTSD): MRI study using two different evaluation methods. J Affect Disord 2006; 94:121–6.

Jenner FA, Gjessing LR, Cox JR et al. A manic depressive psychotic with a persistent forty-eight hour cycle. Br J Psychiatry 1967; 113:895–910.

Joffe RT, Swinson RP, Regan JJ. Personality features of obsessive-compulsive disorder. Am J Psychiatry 1988; 145:1127–9.

Johnson J. Stupor: review of 25 cases. Acta Psychiatr Scand 1984; 70:370–7.

Johnson MR, Marazziti D, Brawman-Mintzer O et al. Abnormal peripheral benzodiazepine receptor density associated with generalized social phobia. Biol Psychiatry 1998; 43:306–9.

Kahn RJ, McNair DM, Lipman RS et al. Imipramine and chlordiazepoxide in depressive and anxiety disorders. II. Efficacy in anxious outpatients. Arch Gen Psychiatry 1986; 43:79–85.

Kahn RS, Wetzler S. m-Chlorophenylpiperazine as a probe of serotonin function. Biol Psychiatry 1991; 30:1139–66.

Kasper S, Stein DJ, Loft H et al. Escitalopram in the treatment of social anxiety disorder: randomized, placebo-controlled, flexible-dosage study. Br J Psychiatry 2005; 186:222–6.

Katerndahl DA. Panic and prolapse: meta-analysis. J Nerv Ment Dis 1993; 181:539–44.

Katzelnick DJ, Kobak KA, Greist JH et al. Sertraline for social phobia: a double-blind, placebo-controlled crossover study. Am J Psychiatry 1995; 152:1368–71.

Kendell RE, Chalmers JC, Platz C. Epidemiology of puerperal psychoses. Br J Psychiatry 1987; 150:662–73.

Kendell RE, Juszczak E, Cole SK. Obstetric complications and schizophrenia: a case control study based on standardized obstetric records. Br J Psychiatry 1996; 168:556–61.

Kendler KS. The nosological validity of paranoia (simple delusional disorder): a review. Arch Gen Psychiatry 1980; 37:699–706.

Kendler KS. Kraepelin and the diagnostic concept of paranoia. Compr Psychiatry 1988; 29:4–11.

Kendler KS, Gruenberg AM. An independent analysis of the Danish Adoption Study of Schizophrenia. IV. The relationship between psychiatric disorders as defined by DSM-III in the relatives and adoptees. Arch Gen Psychiatry 1984; 41:555–64.

Kendler KS, Gruenberg AM, Strauss JS. An independent analysis of the Copenhagen sample of the Danish Adoption Study of Schizophrenia. III. The relationship between paranoid psychosis (delusional disorder) and the schizophrenia spectrum disorders. *Arch Gen Psychiatry* 1982; **38**:985–7.

Kendler KS, Masterson CC, Davis KL. Psychiatric illness in first-degree relatives of patients with paranoid psychosis, schizophrenia and medical illness. *Br J Psychiatry* 1985; **147**:524–31.

Kendler KS, Neale MC, Kessler RC *et al*. Generalized anxiety disorder in women: a population-based twin study. *Arch Gen Psychiatry* 1992; **49**:267–72.

Kendler KS, McGuire M, Gruenberg AM *et al*. An epidemiologic, clinical and family study of simple schizophrenia in County Roscommon, Ireland. *Am J Psychiatry* 1994a; **151**:27–34.

Kendler KS, McGuire M, Gruenberg AM *et al*. Outcome and family study of the subtypes of schizophrenia in the West of Ireland. *Am J Psychiatry* 1994b; **151**:849–56.

Kendler KS, McGuire M, Gruenberg AM *et al*. Examining the validity of DSM-III-R schizoaffective disorder and its putative subtypes in the Roscommon family study. *Am J Psychiatry* 1995; **152**:755–64.

Kennedy HG, Kemp LI, Dyer DE. Fear and anger in delusional (paranoid) disorder: the association with violence. *Br J Psychiatry* 1992; **160**:488–92.

Kety SS. The significance of genetic factors in the etiology of schizophrenia: results from the national study of adoptees in Denmark. *J Psychiatr Res* 1987; **21**:423–9.

Kieseppa T, Partonen I, Haukka J *et al*. High concordance of bipolar I disorder in a nationwide sample of twins. *Am J Psychiatry* 2004; **161**:1814–21.

King DJ, Burke M, Lucas RA. Antipsychotic drug-induced dysphoria. *Br J Psychiatry* 1995; **167**:480–2.

Kinzie JD, Fredrickson RH, Ben R *et al*. Posttraumatic stress disorder among survivors of Cambodian concentration camps. *Am J Psychiatry* 1984; **141**:645–50.

Klein DF. False suffocation alarms, spontaneous panics, and related conditions: an integrative hypothesis. *Arch Gen Psychiatry* 1993; **50**:306–17.

Kohl C, Walch T, Huber R *et al*. Measurement of tryptophan, kynurenine and neopterin in women with and without postpartum blues. *J Affect Disord* 2005; **86**:135–42.

van der Kolk BA, Dreyfuss D, Michaels M *et al*. Fluoxetine in posttraumatic stress disorder. *J Clin Psychiatry* 1994; **55**:517–22.

Koopman C, Classen C, Spiegel D. Predictors of posttraumatic stress symptoms among survivors of the Oakland/Berkeley, Calif., firestorm. *Am J Psychiatry* 1994; **151**:888–94.

Koran LM, McElroy SL, Davidson JR *et al*. Fluvoxamine versus clomipramine for obsessive-compulsive disorder: a double-blind comparison. *J Clin Psychopharmacol* 1996; **16**:121–9.

Kotin J, Goodwin FK. Depression during mania: clinical observations and theoretical implications. *Am J Psychiatry* 1972; **129**:679–86.

Kraepelin E. *Dementia praecox and paraphrenia*, 1919. Huntington, New York: Robert E. Krieger, 1971.

Kraepelin E. *Manic-depressive insanity and paranoia*, 1921. New York: Arno Press, 1976.

Kramer BA. Depressive pseudodementia. *Compr Psychiatry* 1982; **23**:538–44.

Kreczmanski P, Heinsen H, Mantua V *et al*. Volume, neuron density and total neuron number in five subcortical regions in schizophrenia. *Brain* 2007; **130**:678–92.

Krong MH, Apter J, Asnis G *et al*. Placebo-controlled multicenter study of sertraline treatment for obsessive-compulsive disorder. *J Clin Psychopharmacol* 1999; **19**:172–6.

Kuevi V, Causon R, Dixson AF *et al*. Plasma amine and hormone changes in 'post-partum blues'. *Clin Endocrinol* 1983; **19**:39–46.

Kumar R, Issacs S, Meltzer E. Recurrent post-partum psychosis: a model for prospective clinical investigation. *Br J Psychiatry* 1983; **142**:618–20.

Kupfer DJ, Frank E, Perel JM *et al*. Five-year outcome for maintenance therapies in recurrent depression. *Arch Gen Psychiatry* 1992; **49**:769–73.

Laakmann G, Schule C, Lorkowski G *et al*. Buspirone and lorazepam in the treatment of generalized anxiety disorder in outpatients. *Psychopharmacology* 1998; **136**:357–66.

Lader M, Scotto JC. A multicentre double-blind comparison of hydroxyzine, buspirone and placebo in patients with generalized anxiety disorder. *Psychopharmacology* 1998; **139**:402–6.

Landen M, Nissbrandt H, Allgulander C *et al*. Placebo-controlled trial comparing intermittent and continuous paroxetine in premenstrual dysphoric disorder. *Neuropsychopharmacology* 2007; **32**:153–61.

Lanzenberger RR, Mitterhauser M, Spindelegger C *et al*. Reduced serotonin-1A receptor binding in social anxiety disorder. *Biol Psychiatry* 2007; **61**:1081–9.

Lauren TM, Labouriau R, Licht RW *et al*. Family history of psychiatric illness as a risk factor for schizoaffective disorder: A Danish register-based cohort study. *Arch Gen Psychiatry* 2005; **62**:841–8.

Lee KA, Vaillant GE, Torrey WC *et al*. A 50-year prospective study of the psychological sequelae of World War II combat. *Am J Psychiatry* 1995; **152**:516–22.

Lelliott P, Marks I, McNamee G *et al*. Onset of panic disorder with agoraphobia. *Arch Gen Psychiatry* 1989; **46**:1000–8.

Li X, May RS, Tolbert LC *et al*. Risperidone and haloperidol augmentation of serotonin reuptake inhibitors in refractory obsessive-compulsive disorder: a crossover study. *J Clin Psychiatry* 2005; **66**:736–43.

Liden S, Gottfries CG. Beta-blocking agents in the treatment of catecholamine-induced symptoms in musicians. *Lancet* 1974; **2**:529.

Lieberman JA, Stroup TS, McEvoy JP *et al*. Effectiveness of antipsychotic drugs in patients with chronic schizophrenia. *N Engl J Med* 2005; **353**:1209–23.

Liebowitz MR, Fyer AJ, Gorman IM *et al*. Lactate provocation of panic attacks. I. Clinical and behavioral findings. *Arch Gen Psychiatry* 1984; **41**:764–70.

Liebowitz MR, Schneier F, Campeas R *et al*. Phenelzine versus atenolol in social phobia: a placebo-controlled comparison. *Arch Gen Psychiatry* 1992; **39**:290–300.

Liebowitz MR, Gelenberg AJ, Munjack D. Venlafaxine extended release vs placebo and paroxetine in social anxiety disorder. *Arch Gen Psychiatry* 2005; **62**:190–8.

Lindauer RJ, Olff M, van Meijel EP *et al.* Cortisol, learning, memory and attention in relation to smaller hippocampal volume in police officers with posttraumatic stress disorder. *Biol Psychiatry* 2006; **59**:171–7.

Lipkin KM, Dyrud J, Meyer GD. The many faces of mania; therapeutic trial of lithium carbonate. *Arch Gen Psychiatry* 1970; **22**:262–7.

Llorca P-M, Spadone C, Sol L *et al.* Efficacy and safety of hydroxyzine in the treatment of generalized anxiety disorder: a 3-month double-blind study. *J Clin Psychiatry* 2002; **63**:1020–7.

Londborg PD, Wolkow R, Smith WT *et al.* Sertraline in the treatment of panic disorder. *Br J Psychiatry* 1998; **173**:54–60.

Loudon JB, Blackburn IM, Ashworth CM. A study of the symptomatology and course of manic illness using a new scale. *Psychol Med* 1977; **7**:723–9.

Lykouras E, Malliargas D, Christdoulou GN *et al.* Delusional depression: phenomenology and response to treatment. *Acta Psychiatr Scand* 1986; **73**:324–9.

McAllister TW, Price TRP. Severe depressive pseudodementia with and without dementia. *Am J Psychiatry* 1982; **139**:626–9.

McDougle CJ, Goodman WK, Leckman JF *et al.* Haloperidol addition to fluvoxamine-refractory obsessive-compulsive disorder: a double-blind, placebo-controlled study in patients with and without tics. *Arch Gen Psychiatry* 1994; **51**: 302–8.

McDougle CJ, Epperson CN, Pelton GH *et al.* A double-blind, placebo-controlled study of risperidone addition in serotonin reuptake inhibitor-refractory obsessive-compulsive disorder. *Arch Gen Psychiatry* 2000; **57**:794–801.

McElroy SL, Keck PE, Pope HG *et al.* Clinical and research implications of the diagnosis of dysphoric or mixed mania. *Am J Psychiatry* 1992; **149**:1633–44.

McFarlane AC. The aetiology of post-traumatic morbidity: predisposing, precipitating and perpetuating factors. *Br J Psychiatry* 1989; **154**:221–8.

McGlashan TH. The Chestnut Lodge Follow-Up Study. II. Long-term outcome of schizophrenia and the affective disorders. *Arch Gen Psychiatry* 1984; **41**:586–601.

McGlashan TH, Carpenter WT. Postpsychotic depression in schizophrenia. *Arch Gen Psychiatry* 1976; **33**:231–9.

McGuffin P, Katz R, Watkins S *et al.* A hospital-based twin register of the heritability of DSM-IV unipolar depression. *Arch Gen Psychiatry* 1996; **53**:129–36.

McHarg JF. Mania in childhood: report of a case. *Arch Neurol Psychiatry* 1954; **72**:531–9.

Maj M, Pirozzi R, DiCaprio EL. Major depression with mood-congruent psychotic features: a distinct diagnostic entity or a more severe subtype of depression? *Acta Psychiatr Scand* 1990; **82**:439–44.

Manaye KF, Lei DL, Tizabi Y *et al.* Selective neuron loss in the paraventricular nucleus of hypothalamus in patients suffering from major depression and bipolar disorder. *J Neuropathol Exp Neurol* 2005; **64**:224–9.

Mandel MR, Severe JB, Schooler NR *et al.* Development and prediction of postpsychotic depression in neuroleptic-treated schizophrenia. *Arch Gen Psychiatry* 1982; **39**:197–203.

Mannuzza S, Schneier FR, Chapman TF *et al.* Generalized social phobia: reliability and validity. *Arch Gen Psychiatry* 1995; **52**:230–7.

Marks IM, Gelder MG. Different ages of onset in varieties of phobia. *Am J Psychiatry* 1966; **123**:218–21.

Maron E, Kuikka JT, Shlik J *et al.* Reduced brain serotonin transporter binding in patients with panic disorder. *Psychiatry Res* 2004; **132**:173–81.

Marshall RD, Beebe KL, Oldham M *et al.* Efficacy and safety of paroxetine treatment for chronic PTSD: a fixed-dose, placebo-controlled study. *Am J Psychiatry* 2001; **158**:1982–8.

Marten PA, Brown TA, Barlow DH *et al.* Evaluation of the ratings comprising the associated symptom criteria of DSM-III-R generalized anxiety disorder. *J Nerv Ment Dis* 1993; **181**:676–82.

Martenyi F, Brown EB, Zhang H *et al.* Fluoxetine versus placebo in posttraumatic stress disorder. *J Clin Psychiatry* 2002; **63**:199–206.

Martenyi F, Brown EB, Caldwell CD. Failed efficacy of fluoxetine in the treatment of posttraumatic stress disorder: results of a fixed-dose. placebo-controlled study. *J Clin Psychopharmacol* 2007; **27**:166–70.

Massana G, Serra-Grabulosa JM, Salgado-Pineda P *et al.* Parahippocampal gray matter density in panic disorder: a voxel-based morphometric study. *Am J Psychiatry* 2003a; **160**:566–8.

Massana G, Serra-Grabulosa JM, Salgado-Pineda P *et al.* Amygdalar atrophy in panic disorder patients detected by volumetric magnetic resonance imaging. *Neuroimage* 2003b; **19**:80–90.

Mavissakalian MR, Perel JM. Imipramine dose-response relationship in panic disorder with agoraphobia: preliminary findings. *Arch Gen Psychiatry* 1989; **46**:127–31.

Mellman TA, Uhde TW. Sleep panic attacks: new clinical findings and theoretical implications. *Am J Psychiatry* 1989a; **146**:1204–7.

Mellman TA, Uhde TW. Electroencephalographic sleep in panic disorder: focus on sleep-related panic attacks. *Arch Gen Psychiatry* 1989b; **46**:178–89.

Mellman TA, Uhde TW. Patients with frequent sleep panic: clinical findings and response to medication treatment. *J Clin Psychiatry* 1990; **51**:513–16.

Mendlewicz J, Rainer JD. Adoption study supporting genetic transmission in manic-depressive illness. *Nature* 1977; **268**:327–9.

Menkes DB, Coates DC, Fawcett JP. Acute tryptophan depletion aggravates premenstrual syndrome. *J Affect Disord* 1994; **32**:37–44.

Menon RR, Barta PE, Aylward EH *et al.* Posterior superior temporal gyrus in schizophrenia: grey matter changes and clinical correlates. *Schizophren Res* 1995; **16**:127–35.

Metz A, Stump K, Cowen PJ *et al.* Changes in platelet alpha 2-autoreceptor binding post partum: possible relation to maternity blues. *Lancet* 1983; **1**:495–8.

Michelson D, Allgulander C, Dantendorfer K *et al.* Efficacy of usual antidepressant dosing regimens of fluoxetine in panic disorder: randomized, placebo-controlled trial. *Br J Psychiatry* 2001; **179**:514–18.

Mitchell C. Successful treatment of chronic delusional parasittosis. *Br J Psychiatry* 1989; **155**:556–7.

Mitchell PB, Wilhelm K, Parker G *et al*. The clinical features of bipolar depression: a comparison with matched major depressive patients. *J Clin Psychiatry* 2001; **62**:212–16.

Modigh K, Westberg P, Eriksson E. Superiority of clomipramine over imipramine in the treatment of panic disorder: a placebo-controlled trial. *J Clin Psychopharmacol* 1992; **12**:251–61.

Montgomery SA, Tobias K, Zornberg GL *et al*. Efficacy and safety of pregabalin in the treatment of generalized anxiety disorder: a 6-week multicenter, randomized, double-blind, placebo-controlled comparison of pregabalin and venlafaxine. *J Clin Psychiatry* 2006; **67**:771–82.

Morrison JR. Catatonia: retarded and excited types. *Arch Gen Psychiatry* 1973; **28**:39–41.

Moses EL, Mallinger AG. St. John's wort: three cases of possible mania induction. *J Clin Psychopharmacol* 2000; **20**:115–17.

Mueser KT, Bellack AS, Brady EU. Hallucinations in schizophrenia. *Acta Psychiatr Scand* 1990; **82**:26–9.

Munoz RA. Postpartum psychosis as a discrete entity. *J Clin Psychiatry* 1985; **46**:182–4.

Murray RM. Neurodevelopmental schizophrenia: the rediscovery of dementia praecox. *Br J Psychiatry* 1994; **165**(suppl. 25):6–12.

Nappi RE, Petraglia F, Luisi S *et al*. Serum allopregnanolone in women with postpartum 'blues'. *Obstet Gynecol* 2001; **97**:77–80.

Nemeroff CB, Widerlow E, Bissete G *et al*. Elevated concentrations of CSF corticotropin-releasing factor-like immunoreactivity in depressed patients. *Science* 1984; **226**:1342–4.

Newman SC, Bland RC. A population-based family study of DSM-III generalized anxiety disorder. *Psychol Med* 2006; **36**:1275–81.

Ninan PT, Koran LM, Kiev A *et al*. High-dose sertraline strategy for nonresponders to acute treatment of obsessive-compulsive disorder; a multicenter double-blind trial. *J Clin Psychiatry* 2006; **67**:15–22.

Nisita C, Petracca A, Akiskal HS *et al*. Delimitation of generalized anxiety disorder: clinical comparisons with panic and major depressive disorder. *Compr Psychiatry* 1990; **31**:409–15.

Nopoulos P, Torres I, Flaun M *et al*. Brain morphology in first-episode schizophrenia. *Am J Psychiatry* 1995; **152**:1721–3.

Nordahl TE, Semple WE, Gross M *et al*. Cerebral glucose metabolic differences in patients with panic disorder. *Neuropsychopharmacology* 1990; **3**:261–72.

North CS, Smith EM, Spitznagel EL. Posttraumatic stress disorder in survivors of a mass shooting. *Am J Psychiatry* 1994; **151**:82–8.

Noyes R, Crowe RR, Harris EL *et al*. Relationship between panic disorder and agoraphobia. A family study. *Arch Gen Psychiatry* 1986; **43**:227–32.

Noyes R, Clarkson C, Crow RR *et al*. A family study of generalized anxiety disorder. *Am J Psychiatry* 1987; **144**:1019–24.

Noyes R, Burows GD, Reich JH *et al*. Diazepam versus alprazolam for the treatment of panic disorder. *J Clin Psychiatry* 1996; **57**:349–55.

Nutt DJ, Glue P, Lawson C *et al*. Flumazenil provocation of panic attacks: evidence for altered benzodiazepine receptor sensitivity in panic disorder. *Arch Gen Psychiatry* 1990; **47**:917–25.

Oehrberg S, Christiansen PE, Behnke K *et al*. Paroxetine in the treatment of panic disorder: a randomized, double-blind, placebo-controlled study. *Br J Psychiatry* 1995; **167**:374–9.

Opjordsmoen R, Rettersol N. Delusional disorder: the predictive validity of the concept. *Acta Psychiatr Scand* 1991; **84**:250–4.

Page AC. Distinguishing panic disorder and agoraphobia from social phobia. *J Nerv Ment Dis* 1994; **182**:611–17.

Palatnik A, Frolov K, Fux M *et al*. Double-blind, controlled, crossover trial of inositol versus fluvoxamine for the treatment of panic disorder. *J Clin Psychopharmacol* 2001; **21**:335–9.

Pande AC, Davidson JRT, Jefferson JW *et al*. Treatment of social phobia with gabapentin: a placebo-controlled study. *J Clin Psychopharmacol* 1999; **19**:341–8.

Pande AC, Feltner DE, Jefferson JW *et al*. Efficacy of the novel anxiolytic pregabalin in social anxiety disorder: a placebo-controlled, multicenter study. *J Clin Psychopharmacol* 2004; **24**:141–9.

Pauls DL, Alsobrook JP, Goodman W *et al*. A family study of obsessive-compulsive disorder. *Am J Psychiatry* 1995; **152**:76–84.

Pearlstein TB, Stone AB. Long-term fluoxetine treatment of late luteal phase dysphoric disorder. *J Clin Psychiatry* 1994; **55**:332–5.

Pearlstein TB, Stone AB, Lund SA *et al*. Comparison of fluoxetine, bupropion, and placebo in the treatment of premenstrual dysphoric disorder. *J Clin Psychopharmacol* 1997; **17**:261–6.

Pecknold JC, Swinson RP, Krich K *et al*. Alprazolam in panic disorder and agoraphobia: results from a multicenter trial. III. Discontinuation effects. *Arch Gen Psychiatry* 1988; **45**:429–36.

Perani D, Colombo C, Bressi S *et al*. [18F]FDG PET study in obsessive-compulsive disorder: a clinical/metabolic correlation study after treatment. *Br J Psychiatry* 1995; **166**:244–50.

Perlis ML, Smith MT, Orff HJ *et al*. The effects of orally administered cholinergic agonists on REM sleep in major depression. *Biol Psychiatry* 2002; **51**:457–62.

Perlmutter SJ, Leitman SF, Garvey MA *et al*. Therapeutic plasma exchange and intravenous immunoglobulin for obsessive-compulsive disorder and tic disorders in childhood. *Lancet* 1999; **354**:1153–8.

Pfohl B, Vaquez N, Nasrallah H. Unipolar vs. bipolar mania: a review of 247 patients. *Br J Psychiatry* 1982; **141**:453–8.

Pigott TA, Pato MT, Bernstein SE *et al*. Controlled comparisons of clomipramine and fluoxetine in the treatment of obsessive-compulsive disorder: behavioral and biological results. *Arch Gen Psychiatry* 1990; **47**:926–32.

Pitman RK, Orr SP, Forgue DF *et al*. Psychophysiologic assessment of post-traumatic stress disorder imagery in Vietnam combat veterans. *Arch Gen Psychiatry* 1987; **44**:970–5.

Pitt B. Maternity blues. *Br J Psychiatry* 1973; **122**:431–3.

Pohl R, Yeragani VK, Balon R *et al*. Isoproterenol-induced panic attacks. *Biol Psychiatry* 1988; **24**:891–902.

Pollack MH, Zaninelli R, Goddard A *et al*. Paroxetine in the treatment of generalized anxiety disorder: results of a placebo-controlled, flexible-dosage trial. *J Clin Psychiatry* 2001; **62**:350–7.

Pope HG, Lipinski JF, Cohen BM *et al*. 'Schizoaffective disorder', an invalid diagnosis? A comparison of schizoaffective disorder, schizophrenia and affective disorder. *Am J Psychiatry* 1980; **137**:921-7.

Prange AJ, Lara PP, Wilson IC *et al.* Effect of thyrotropin-releasing hormone in depression. *Lancet* 1972; **2**:999-1002.

Prien RF, Kupfer DJ. Continuation drug therapy for major depression episodes: how long should it be maintained? *Am J Psychiatry* 1986; **143**:18-23.

Quitkin FM, McGrath PJ, Stewart JW *et al.* Chronological milestones to guide drug change. When should clinicians switch antidepressants? *Arch Gen Psychiatry* 1996; **53**:785-92.

Raadsheer FC, van Heerikhuize JJ, Lucassen PJ *et al.* Corticotropin-releasing hormone mRNA in the paraventricular nucleus of patients with Alzheimer's disease and depression. *Am J Psychiatry* 1995; **152**:1372-6.

Rabins PV, Merchant A, Nestadt G. Criteria for diagnosing reversible dementia caused by depression: validation by 2-year follow-up. *Br J Psychiatry* 1984; **144**:488-92.

Ramsey R, Gorst-Unsworth C, Turner S. Psychiatric morbidity in survivors of state violence including torture. *Br J Psychiatry* 1993; **162**:55-9.

Raskind MA, Peskind ER, Kanter ED *et al.* Reduction of nightmares and other PTSD symptoms in adult veterans by prazosin: a placebo-controlled study. *Am J Psychiatry* 2003; **160**:371-3.

Raskind MA, Peskind EF, Hoff DJ *et al.* A parallel group placebo controlled study of prazosin for trauma nightmares and sleep disturbances in combat veterans with post-traumatic stress disorder. *Biol Psychiatry* 2007; **61**:928-34.

Rasmussen SA, Tsuang MT. Clinical characteristics and family history in DSM-III obsessive-compulsive disorder. *Am J Psychiatry* 1986; **143**:317-22.

Reich DB, Winternitz S, Hennen J *et al.* A preliminary study of risperidone in the treatment of posttraumatic stress disorder related to childhood abuse in women. *J Clin Psychiatry* 2004; **65**:1601-6.

Reimherr FW, Amsterdam JD, Quitkin FM *et al.* Optimal length of continuation therapy in depression: a prospective assessment during long-term fluoxetine treatment. *Am J Psychiatry* 1998; **155**:1247-53.

Rickels K, Schweizer E, Csanalosi I *et al.* Long-term treatment of anxiety and risk of withdrawal: prospective comparison of clorazepate and buspirone. *Arch Gen Psychiatry* 1988; **45**:444-50.

Rickels K, Schweizer E, Weiss S *et al.* Maintenance drug treatment for panic disorder. II. Short- and long-term outcome after drug taper. *Arch Gen Psychiatry* 1993a; **50**:61-8.

Rickels K, Downing R, Schweizer E *et al.* Antidepressants for the treatment of generalized anxiety disorder: a placebo-controlled comparison of imipramine, trazodone and diazepam. *Arch Gen Psychiatry* 1993b; **50**:884-95.

Rickels K, Pollack MH, Sheehan DV *et al.* Efficacy of extended-release venlafaxine in nondepressed outpatients with generalized anxiety disorder. *Am J Psychiatry* 2000; **157**:968-74.

Rickels K, Zaninelli R, McCafferty J *et al.* Paroxetine treatment of generalized anxiety disorder: a double-blind, placebo-controlled study. *Am J Psychiatry* 2003; **160**:745-56.

Rickels K, Pollack MH, Feltner DE *et al.* Pregabalin for treatment of generalized anxiety disorder. A 4-week, multicenter, double-blind, placebo-controlled trial of pregabalin and alprazolam. *Arch Gen Psychiatry* 2005; **62**:1022-33.

Rioux L, Nissanov J, Lauber K *et al.* Distribution of microtubule-associated protein MAP2-immunoreactive interstitial neurons in the parahippocampal white matter in subjects with schizophrenia. *Am J Psychiatry* 2003; **160**:149-55.

Roberts GW, Colter N, Lofthouse RM *et al.* Is there gliosis in schizophrenia? Investigation of the temporal lobe. *Biol Psychiatry* 1987; **22**:1459-68.

Roca CA, Schmidt PJ, Smith MJ *et al.* Effects of metergoline on symptoms in women with premenstrual dysphoric disorder. *Am J Psychiatry* 2002; **159**:1876-81.

Rocca P, Beoni AM, Eva C *et al.* Peripheral benzodiazepine receptor messenger RNA is decreased in lymphocytes of generalized anxiety disorder patients. *Biol Psychiatry* 1998; **43**:767-73.

Rohde LA, Busnello E, Wolf A *et al.* Maternity blues in Brazilian women. *Acta Psychiatr Scand* 1997; **95**:231-5.

Rosenbaum JF, Moroz G, Bowden CL *et al.* Clonazepam in the treatment of panic disorder with or without agoraphobia: a dose-response study of efficacy, safety and discontinuance. *J Clin Psychopharmacol* 1997; **17**:390-6.

Rosenthal NE, Rosenthal LN, Stallone F *et al.* Psychosis as a predictor of response to lithium maintenance treatment in bipolar affective disorder. *J Affect Disord* 1979; **1**:237-45.

Rosenthal NE, Rosenthal LN, Stallone F *et al.* Toward the validation of RDC schizoaffective disorder. *Arch Gen Psychiatry* 1980; **37**:804-10.

Roy-Byrne PR, Weingartner H, Bierer LM *et al.* Effortful and automatic cognitive processes in depression. *Arch Gen Psychiatry* 1986; **43**:265-7.

Rush AJ, Erman MK, Giles DE *et al.* Polysomnographic findings in recently drug free and clinically remitted depressed patients. *Arch Gen Psychiatry* 1986; **43**:878-84.

Rush AJ, Giles DE, Schlesser MA *et al.* Dexamethasone response, thyrotropin-releasing hormone stimulation, rapid eye movement latency and subtypes of depression. *Biol Psychiatry* 1997; **41**:915-28.

Russell JL, Kushner MG, Beitman BD *et al.* Nonfearful panic disorder in neurology patients validated by lactate challenge. *Am J Psychiatry* 1991; **148**:361-4.

Saxena S, Brody AL, Ho ML *et al.* Differential cerebral metabolic changes with paroxetine treatment of obsessive-compulsive disorder vs major depression. *Arch Gen Psychiatry* 2002; **59**:250-61.

Schellenberg R. Treatment for the premenstrual syndrome with agnus castus fruit extract: prospective, randomized, placebo controlled study. *BMJ* 2001; **322**:134-7.

Schneier FR, Liebowitz MR, Abi-Dargham A *et al.* Low dopamine D(2) receptor binding potential in social phobia. *Am J Psychiatry* 2000; **157**:457-9.

Schruers K, van Diest R, Overbeek T *et al.* Acute L-5-hydroxytryptophan administration inhibits carbon-dioxide-induced panic in panic disorder patients. *Psychiatry Res* 2002; **113**:237-43.

Schweizer E, Pohl R, Balon R *et al.* Lorazepam vs. alprazolam in the treatment of panic disorder. *Pharmacopsychiatry* 1990; **23**:90-3.

Shalev AY, Orr SP, Peri T *et al*. Physiologic responses to loud tones in Israeli patients with posttraumatic stress disorder. *Arch Gen Psychiatry* 1992; **49**:870–5.

Shalev AY, Peri T, Cangetti L *et al*. Predictors of PTSD in injured trauma survivors: a prospective study. *Am J Psychiatry* 1996; **153**:219–25.

Shenton ME, Kikinis R, Jolesz FA *et al*. Abnormalities of the left temporal lobe and thought disorder in schizophrenia: a quantitative magnetic resonance imaging study. *N Engl J Med* 1992; **327**:604–12.

Shugart YY, Samuels J, Willour VL *et al*. Genomewide linkage scan for obsessive-compulsive disorder: evidence for susceptibility loci on chromosomes 3q, 7p, 15q, and 6q. *Mol Psychiatry* 2006; **11**:736–70.

Shulman KI, Tohen M. Unipolar mania revisited: evidence from an elderly cohort. *Br J Psychiatry* 1994; **164**:547–9.

Siris SG, Morgan V, Fagerstrom R *et al*. Adjunctive imipramine in the treatment of postpsychotic depression: a controlled trial. *Arch Gen Psychiatry* 1987; **44**:533–9.

Sitaram N, Gillen JC, Bunney WE. The switch process in manic-depressive illness: circadian variation in time of switch and sleep and manic ratings before and after switch. *Acta Psychiatr Scand* 1978; **58**:267–78.

Smith KA, Fairburn CG, Cowen PJ. Relapse of depression after rapid depletion of tryptophan. *Lancet* 1997; **349**: 915–19.

Southwick SM, Krystal JH, Morgan CA *et al*. Abnormal noradrenergic function in post-traumatic stress disorder. *Arch Gen Psychiatry* 1993; **50**:31–7.

Sramek JJ, Tansman M, Suri A *et al*. Efficacy of buspirone in generalized anxiety disorder with coexisting mild depressive symptoms. *J Clin Psychiatry* 1996; **57**:287–91.

Stahl SM, Gergel I, Li D. Escitalopram in the treatment of panic disorder; a randomized, double-blind, placebo-controlled trial. *J Clin Psychiatry* 2003; **64**:1322–7.

Starcevic V, Fallon S, Uhlenhuth EH. The frequency and severity of generalized anxiety disorder symptoms: toward a less cumbersome conceptualization. *J Nerv Ment Dis* 1994; **182**:80–4.

Starkstein SE, Petraca G, Teson A *et al*. Catatonia in depression: prevalence, clinical correlates, and validation of a scale. *J Neurol Neurosurg Psychiatry* 1996; **60**:326–32.

Stein DJ, Anderson EW, Tonnoir B *et al*. Escitalopram in obsessive-compulsive disorder: a randomized, placebo-controlled, paroxetine-referenced, fixed-dose, 24-week study. *Curr Med Res Opin* 2007; **23**:701–11.

Stein MB, Liebowitz MD, Lydiard RB *et al*. Paroxetine treatment of generalized social phobia (social anxiety disorder). *JAMA* 1998; **280**:708–13.

Stein MB, Fyer AJ, Davidson JRT *et al*. Fluvoxamine treatment of social phobia (social anxiety disorder): a double-blind, placebo-controlled study. *Am J Psychiatry* 1999; **156**:756–60.

Stein MB, Kline NA, Matloff JL. Adjunctive olanzapine for SSRI-resistant combat-related PTSD: a double-blind, placebo-controlled study. *Am J Psychiatry* 2002; **159**:1777–9.

Steiner M, Steinberg S, Stewart D *et al*. Fluoxetine in the treatment of premenstrual dysphoria. *N Engl J Med* 1995; **332**:1529–34.

Steketee F, Foa EB, Grayson JB. Recent advances in the behavioral treatment of obsessive-compulsives. *Arch Gen Psychiatry* 1982; **39**:1365–71.

Stern RS, Cobb JP. Phenomenology of obsessive-compulsive neurosis. *Br J Psychiatry* 1978; **132**:233–9.

Stevens JW. Manic-depressive insanity, with the report of a typical case. *J Nerv Ment Dis* 1904; **31**:513–25.

Stewart DE. Prophylactic lithium in postpartum affective psychosis. *J Nerv Ment Dis* 1988; **176**:485–9.

Strohle A, Kellner M, Yassouridis A *et al*. Effect of flumazenil in lactate-sensitive patients with panic disorder. *Am J Psychiatry* 1998; **155**:610–12.

Stunkard AJ, Fernstrom MH, Price A *et al*. Direction of weight gain in recurrent depression: consistency across episodes. *Arch Gen Psychiatry* 1990; **47**:857–60.

Suddah RL, Casanova MF, Goldberg TE *et al*. Temporal lobe pathology in schizophrenia: a quantitative magnetic resonance imaging study. *Am J Psychiatry* 1989; **146**:464–72.

Summers WK. Mania with onset in the eighth decade: two cases and a review. *J Clin Psychiatry* 1983; **44**:141–3.

Susser ES, Lin SP. Schizophrenia after prenatal exposure to the Dutch Hunger Winter of 1944–1945. *Arch Gen Psychiatry* 1992; **49**:983–8.

Swedo SE, Leonard HL, Garvey M *et al*. Pediatric autoimmune neuropsychiatric disorders associated with streptococcal infections: clinical description of the first 50 cases. *Am J Psychiatry* 1998; **155**:264–71.

Tancer ME, Mailman RB, Stein MB *et al*. Neuroendocrine responsivity to monoaminergic system probe in generalized social phobia. *Anxiety* 1994; **1**:216–23.

Taylor FB, Lowe K, Thompson C *et al*. Daytime prazosin reduces psychological distress to trauma specific cues in civilian trauma posttraumatic stress disorder. *Biol Psychiatry* 2006; **59**:577–81.

Taylor MA, Abrams R. The phenomenology of mania: a new look at some old patients. *Arch Gen Psychiatry* 1973; **29**:520–2.

Taylor MA, Abrams R. Catatonia: prevalence and importance in the manic phase of manic-depressive illness. *Arch Gen Psychiatry* 1977; **34**:1223–5.

Terao T. Subclinical hypothyroidism in recurrent mania. *Biol Psychiatry* 1993; **38**:853–4.

Tesar GE, Rosenbaum JF, Pollack MH *et al*. Double-blind, placebo-controlled comparison of clonazepam and alprazolam for panic disorder. *J Clin Psychiatry* 1991; **52**:69–76.

Thase ME. Relapse and recurrence in unipolar major depression: short-term and long-term approaches. *Compr Psychiatry* 1990; **51**(suppl. 26):51–7.

Tienari P, Wynne LC, Laksy K *et al*. Genetic boundaries of the schizophrenic spectrum: evidence from the Finnish adoptive family study. *Am J Psychiatry* 2003; **160**:1587–94.

Tiihonen J, Kuikka J, Bergstrom K *et al*. Dopamine reuptake site densities in patients with social phobia. *Am J Psychiatry* 1997a; **154**:239–42.

Tiihonen J, Kuikka J, Rasanen P et al. Cerebral benzodiazepine receptor binding and distribution in generalized anxiety disorder: a fractal analysis. Mol Psychiatry 1997b; 2:463–71.

Tollefson GD, Rampey AH, Potvin JH et al. A multicenter investigation of fixed-dose fluoxetine in the treatment of obsessive-compulsive disorder. Arch Gen Psychiatry 1994; 51:559–67.

Torgerson S. Comorbidity of major depression and anxiety disorders in twin pairs. Am J Psychiatry 1990; 147:1199–202.

Tsuang MT. Suicide in schizophrenics, manics, depressives, and surgical controls: a comparison with general population suicide mortality. Arch Gen Psychiatry 1978; 35:153–5.

Tsuang MT, Woolson RF, Fleming JA. Long-term outcome of major psychoses. I. Schizophrenia and affective disorders compared with psychiatrically symptom-free surgical controls. Arch Gen Psychiatry 1979; 36:1295–304.

Tsuang MT, Faraone SV, Fleming JA. Familial transmission of major affective disorders: is there evidence supporting the distinction between unipolar and bipolar disorders? Br J Psychiatry 1985; 146:268–71.

Tucker P, Zaninelli R, Yehuda R et al. Paroxetine in the treatment of chronic posttraumatic stress disorder: results of a placebo-controlled, flexibile dosage trial. J Clin Psychiatry 2001; 62:860–8.

Tuke DH. Imperative ideas. Brain 1894; 17:179–97.

Turner SW, Toone BK, Brett-Jones JR. Computerized tomographic scan changes in early schizophrenia – preliminary findings. Psychol Med 1986; 16:219–25.

Van Dyke C, Zilberg NJ, McKinnon JA. Posttraumatic stress disorder: a thirty-year delay in a World War II veteran. Am J Psychiatry 1985; 142:1070–3.

Van Putten T. The many faces of akathisia. Compr Psychiatry 1975; 16:43–7.

Van Putten T, May PRA. 'Akinetic depression' in schizophrenia. Arch Gen Psychiatry 1978; 35:1101–7.

Van Putten T, Multalipassi LR, Malkin MD. Phenothiazine-induced decompensation. Arch Gen Psychiatry 1974; 30:102–5.

Van Valkenburg C, Winokur G, Behar D et al. Depressed women with panic attacks. J Clin Psychiatry 1984; 45:367–9.

Versiani M, Nardi AE, Mundim FD et al. Pharmacotherapy of social phobia: a controlled study with moclobemide and phenelzine. Br J Psychiatry 1992; 161:353–60.

Videbech T. Chronic olfactory paranoid syndromes. Acta Psychiatr Scand 1966; 42:183–213.

Viguera AC, Nonacs R, Cohen LS et al. Risk of recurrence of bipolar disorder in pregnant and nonpregnant women after discontinuing lithium maintenance. Am J Psychiatry 2000; 157:179–84.

Villarreal G, Hamilton DA, Petropoulos H et al. Reduced hippocampal volume and total white matter volume in posttraumatic stress disorder. Biol Psychiatry 2002; 52:119–25.

van Vliet IM, den Boer JA, Westenberg HG. Psychopharmacological treatment of social phobia: a double blind placebo controlled study with fluvoxamine. Psychopharmacology 1994; 115:128–34.

Wada T, Kawakatsu S, Nadaoka T et al. Clomipramine treatment of delusional disorder, somatic type. Int Clin Psychopharmacol 1999; 14:181–3.

Wade AG, Lepola U, Koponen HJ et al. The effect of citalopram in panic disorders. Br J Psychiatry 1997; 170:549–53.

Walker E, Lewine RJ. Prediction of adult-onset schizophrenia from childhood home movies of the patients. Am J Psychiatry 1990; 147:1052–6.

Watson CG, Kucala T, Manifold V et al. Differences between post traumatic stress disorder patients with delayed and undelayed onset. J Nerv Ment Dis 1988; 176:568–72.

Watson S, Gallagher P, Ritchie JC et al. Hypothalamic-pituitary-adrenal axis function in patients with bipolar disorder. Br J Psychiatry 2004; 184:496–502.

Watt JAG. The relationship of paranoid states to schizophrenia. Am J Psychiatry 1985; 142:1456–8.

Wertham FI. A group of benign psychoses: prolonged manic excitements. Am J Psychiatry 1929; 86:17–78.

Winokur G. Delusional disorder (paranoia). Compr Psychiatry 1977; 18:511–21.

Winokur G. Psychosis in bipolar and unipolar affective illness with special reference to schizo-affective disorder. Br J Psychiatry 1984; 145:236–42.

Winokur G. Familial psychopathology in delusional disorder. Compr Psychiatry 1985; 26:241–8.

Winokur G, Tsuang MT. Elation versus irritability in mania. Compr Psychiatry 1975; 16:435–6.

Winokur G, Clayton PJ, Reich T. Manic depressive illness. St. Louis, MO: Mosby, 1969.

Winokur G, Coryell W, Endicott J et al. Further distinction between manic-depressive illness (bipolar disorder) and primary depressive disorder (unipolar depression). Am J Psychiatry 1993; 150:1176–81.

Wisner KL, Peindel KS, Gigliotti T et al. Obsessions and compulsions in women with postpartum depression. J Clin Psychiatry 1999; 60:17–80.

Wisner KL, Perel JM, Peindel KS et al. Prevention of postpartum depression: a randomized clinical trial. J Clin Psychiatry 2001; 62:82–6.

Wisner KL, Perel JM, Peindel KS et al. Prevention of postpartum depression: a pilot randomized clinical trial. Am J Psychiatry 2004; 161:1290–2.

Wisner KL, Hanusa BH, Perel JM et al. Postpartum depression: a randomized trial of sertraline versus nortriptyline. J Clin Psychopharmacol 2006; 26:353–60.

Woodward SH, Kaloupek DG, Streeter CC et al. Hippocampal volume, PTSD, and alcoholism in combat veterans. Am J Psychiatry 2006; 163:674–81.

Yalom ID, Lunde DT, Moos RH et al. 'Postpartum blues' syndrome: a description and related variables. Arch Gen Psychiatry 1968; 18:16–27.

Yehuda R, Southwick SM, Krystal JH et al. Enhanced suppression of cortisol following dexamethasone administration in posttraumatic stress disorder. Am J Psychiatry 1993; 150:83–6.

Yehuda R, Golier JA, Hallian SL et al. The ACTH response to dexamethasone in PTSD. Am J Psychiatry 2004; 161:1397–403.

Yonkers KA, Halbreich U, Freeman E et al. Symptomatic improvement of premenstrual dysphoric disorder with sertraline treatment: a randomized controlled trial. *JAMA* 1997; **278**:983–8.

Young EA, Breslau N. Cortisol and catecholamines in posttraumatic stress disorder: an epidemiologic community study. *Arch Gen Psychiatry* 2004; **61**:394–401.

Young KA, Holcomb LA, Yazdani U *et al.* Elevated neuron number in the limbic thalamus in major depression. *Am J Psychiatry* 2004; **161**:1270–7.

Young SA, Hurt PH, Benedek DM *et al.* Treatment of premenstrual dysphoric disorder with sertraline during the luteal phase: a randomized, double-blind, placebo-controlled crossover trial. *J Clin Psychiatry* 1998; **59**:76–80.

Zohar J, Judge R. Paroxetine versus clomipramine in the treatment of obsessive-compulsive disorder. *Br J Psychiatry* 1996; **169**:468–74.

21

Substance use disorders

21.1 STIMULANTS

Of the many stimulants that are used for intoxication, amphetamine, dextroamphetamine, and methamphetamine are most commonly utilized; some patients may also abuse methylphenidate. These drugs may be taken orally or, after being crushed and dissolved, intravenously. Occasionally they may be 'snorted' intranasally, and purified methamphetamine ('ice') may also be smoked.

Clinical features

Mild intoxication (Hollister and Gillespie 1970) is characterized by increased energy, varying degrees of elation, increased self-confidence, and talkativeness; the pupils are dilated, the blood pressure, both systolic and diastolic, is increased, the heart rate may be increased or reflexively decreased, and the deep tendon reflexes are diffusely brisk. With more severe intoxication there may be agitation and some bizarre behavior: often patients take a particular interest in things mechanical, and hours may be spent first taking apart, and then trying to put back together, various items, such as clocks, radios, televisions, etc. Fleeting delusions of persecution and auditory hallucinations may occur. In severe intoxication a delirium may ensue, with confusion, incoherence, and disorientation. Abnormal movements, such as bruxism, chorea (Lundh and Tunving 1981), and, in some cases, generalized dystonia, may occur; intracerebral hemorrhage has also been reported (Harrington et al. 1983; Yen et al. 1994) and grand mal seizures may also occur. The temperature rises, there may be extreme diaphoresis, and patients may experience nausea, vomiting, abdominal cramping, and diarrhea. Arrhythmias may appear, and with severe elevations of blood pressure

there may be a hypertensive encephalopathy. Regardless of the degree of intoxication, most patients recover within hours to a day or so.

In some cases, delusions and hallucinations, rather than being fleeting, may dominate the clinical picture of the intoxication, and in some of these cases, such symptoms may persist beyond the resolution of the intoxication, thus yielding a stimulant-induced psychosis. Although this is typically seen only with intravenous stimulant use, it has been reported after high-dosage oral use. In this psychosis (Angrist and Gershon 1970; Bell 1973; Derlet et al. 1989; Ellinwood 1967; Griffith et al. 1972; Iwanami et al. 1994) patients experience delusions of persecution and reference, and, in some cases, hallucinations, which may in turn be either auditory or visual. In some cases there may be bizarre delusions, including Schneiderian first rank symptoms (Janowsky and Risch 1979). Rarely, patients with delusions of persecution have resorted to murder to 'protect' themselves (Ellinwood 1971). This amphetamine-induced psychosis generally clears within a matter of days or weeks, but it may occasionally last many months. Those who resume daily use of stimulants may display 'sensitization', in which the psychosis recurs at progressively lower and lower doses.

With chronic use of stimulants, both tolerance and withdrawal may occur. With the development of tolerance, patients require ever larger doses to achieve euphoria, in some cases up to several grams daily. A withdrawal syndrome (Kramer et al. 1967; Watson et al. 1972) may appear with abstinence after long-term use, and is characterized by irritability, fatigue, suicidal ideation, and sleep disturbance, either hypersomnia or less commonly insomnia. This 'crash', as the withdrawal syndrome is often referred to, typically undergoes considerable clearing within days or a week or more; however, mild symptomatology may linger for weeks or months.

Course

Recreational use of stimulants is not uncommon, and such occasional use generally causes few, if any, consequences. Some patients may develop an abusive pattern of use, however, and continue to seek intoxication despite suffering social or legal consequences. Addiction is said to occur when a craving develops for the stimulant, accompanied by the phenomena of tolerance and withdrawal; such patients may use stimulants on a daily basis, in relatively modest doses, or display a 'binge' pattern (Kramer *et al.* 1967), in which they use ever-escalating doses until, after a matter of days or more, they either run out of money or become so debilitated that they have to stop, after which they suffer through a withdrawal syndrome before going on yet another binge.

Etiology

It appears that the euphoria seen with stimulants occurs secondary to dopamine release within the ventral striatum (Drevets *et al.* 2001), whereas the autonomic symptomatology is mediated by enhanced noradrenergic tone (Nurnberger *et al.* 1984).

Differential diagnosis

Intoxication with cocaine may be clinically indistinguishable from stimulant intoxication, and the differential may rest on history or drug screening.

Lacking a history (as is often the case, given the deceit and denial seen in many cases), the elation and talkativeness of the intoxication may suggest mania, and the irritability, fatigue, and sleep disturbance of withdrawal may suggest depression. Drug screening is helpful here; however, observation in a controlled environment will also tell the tale, as the symptoms resolve over the expected time period.

The stimulant-induced psychosis represents one of the toxic psychoses, discussed in Section 7.1, and is suggested by its emergence during an intoxication and its resolution during enforced abstinence.

Treatment

Intoxication, if mild, may be managed with simple observation. In severe cases one may utilize an antipsychotic such as haloperidol, in a dose of approximately 5 mg, either as the concentrate or parenterally, with repeat doses every hour or so until the patient is calm, limiting side-effects occur or a maximum dose of approximate 20 mg is reached.

Stimulant psychosis may be treated with an antipsychotic, such as haloperidol (5–10 mg) or risperidone (2–4 mg), with the understanding that the medication may, given the natural course of the disorder, be eventually discontinued.

Withdrawal symptomatology, if severe and accompanied by suicidal ideation, may require hospitalization. Pharmacologic treatment is generally not indicated.

The overall treatment of stimulant addiction has as its goal abstinence. Hospitalization is often required to break the pattern of use, and long-term involvement with groups such as Cocaine Anonymous or Narcotics Anonymous may be helpful.

21.2 COCAINE

Several different preparations of cocaine are available illegally. Cocaine hydrochloride is a white powder that may be insufflated ('snorted') into the nasal passages where it is absorbed through the nasal mucosa; it is also water soluble and thus may be dissolved and injected intravenously. Cocaine hydrochloride is destroyed by heat and is thus not suitable for smoking; it may, however, be treated with sodium bicarbonate and then either extracted with ether to yield a 'free base' preparation or warmed to create a 'rock' of 'crack' cocaine. Both the free base and crack preparations evaporate with heating and thus may be smoked.

Clinical features

The onset of intoxication varies according to the preparation used; after snorting, peak levels are reached within 30–60 minutes, whereas after intravenous injection or smoking, peak levels occur within seconds, creating a much more intense intoxication. During intoxication (Kleber and Gawin 1984), patients become euphoric, hyperalert, talkative, and grandiose. Hyperactivity is common, and with higher doses agitation may occur (Fischman *et al.* 1976). Some patients may experience visual hallucinations, and these are typically of insects, which are often referred to as 'cocaine bugs'; these hallucinations may be accompanied by tactile hallucinations of bugs crawling beneath the skin, and some patients may excoriate themselves in an attempt to 'get' them. With mild intoxication libido increases, and in males there may be delayed ejaculation; with more severe intoxication, however, there may be erectile dysfunction. In severe intoxication, especially after intravenous use or smoking, a delirium may occur, with confusion, incoherence, lability, and delusions and hallucinations. Other symptoms and signs include mydriasis, hypertension, headache, nausea and vomiting, tachycardia, and arrhythmias or cardiac arrest (Hsue *et al.* 2007). Uncommonly, there may be chorea ('crack dancing') (Daras *et al.* 1994), tics (Pascual-Leone and Dhuna 1990), myocardial infarction (Virmani *et al.* 1988), rhabdomyolysis (Roth *et al.* 1988), stroke (due to infarction, intracerebral hemorrhage or subarachnoid hemorrhage [Klonoff *et al.* 1989; Lichtenfeld *et al.* 1986; Nolte *et al.* 1996]), and, with chronic, repeated use, a cerebral vasculitis (Fredericks *et al.* 1991; Krendel *et al.* 1990).

Intoxication after snorting cocaine lasts from 30 to 60 minutes, whereas after intravenous administration or smoking it lasts only 5–20 minutes.

Cocaine is rapidly metabolized by plasma and hepatic esterases to such inactive metabolites as benzoylecgonine, and this metabolite may be found in the urine for up to a week; of note, in some cases the level of this metabolite may fluctuate, such that a 'negative' urine test may occasionally be followed by a 'positive' one (Burke *et al.* 1990).

Shortly after resolution of the intoxication, most patients will experience a 'crash', lasting from hours to a day, characterized by fatigue, depressed mood, irritability, and anxiety. Given that this 'crash' may occur with first-time use of cocaine as well as after widely spaced repeat intoxications, it may not be appropriate to consider it a withdrawal syndrome. Clear-cut withdrawal, however, does occur with chronic use and indeed may appear after only a few days of heavy use. The withdrawal symptoms (Weddington *et al.* 1990) include not only those seen in the 'crash' but also anhedonia, hyperphagia, insomnia, and, often, suicidal ideation; furthermore, during withdrawal there is typically a tense craving for more cocaine. This withdrawal reaches a maximum of severity within a few days and then gradually remits over days or weeks. Rarely, dystonia may appear during withdrawal (Choy-Kwong and Lipton 1989).

Tolerance may develop rapidly with repeated use; indeed, with a 'run' of intravenous use, tolerance may appear within a day. Unfortunately, this tolerance applies only to the euphoriant effects of cocaine and not to its potentially lethal cardiovascular effects.

After approximately two or more years of frequent cocaine use, intoxications may become characterized by delusions of persecution and of reference, and by auditory hallucinations (Brady *et al.* 1991; Rosse *et al.* 1994; Satel *et al.* 1991; Sherer *et al.* 1988). Although initially these symptoms tend to resolve shortly after the intoxication resolves (Brady *et al.* 1991), over time, and with repeated episodes, they appear with lower doses and also tend to last much longer (Bartlett *et al.* 1997), in some cases creating a psychosis that may persist for weeks (Manschreck *et al.* 1987), despite abstinence.

Course

Recreational use of cocaine, that is occasional intoxications without consequences, is generally seen only with 'snorting'. Abusive use, with legal, social, and medical consequences, may also occur with snorting but is more common when cocaine is taken intravenously or smoked. Cocaine is one of the most, perhaps the most, addictive substances in the world, and craving may develop rapidly, leading to chronic, frequent use and the development of tolerance and withdrawal. When addiction does set in, the pattern of cocaine use may be either continuous or episodic. Continuous use is characterized by daily intoxication, either via snorting, injection, or smoking. Episodic use is characterized by 'binges', lasting anywhere from hours to a week, during which cocaine may be injected or smoked very frequently, sometimes every 10 or 15 minutes; with such frequent use, however, the euphoria of the intoxication becomes progressively briefer and the crashes progressively more severe, until finally either exhaustion or a lack of funds ends the binge. The intervals between binges vary widely, from only a few days to up to weeks or months.

Etiology

Within the central nervous system cocaine both inhibits the reuptake and facilitates the release of monoamines by pre-synaptic neurons. Although both serotonin and norepinephrine are involved, it appears that the euphoriant effects of cocaine are related to the increased concentration of dopamine at the terminals of the mesolimbic and mesocortical dopaminergic pathways.

Differential diagnosis

A clinical differentiation of cocaine intoxication from stimulant intoxication may not be possible, and the differential often rests on history or a drug screen.

Withdrawal may suggest depression and, when the history of cocaine use is unavailable, the differential may rest on observation in a controlled environment, which will reveal the fairly rapid resolution of symptoms.

The diagnosis of a persistent cocaine psychosis is generally straightforward as it is difficult to hide the history of chronic cocaine addiction. If, however, this history is not available, then the differential for psychosis, as discussed in Section 7.1, must be pursued.

Treatment

For most cases of intoxication and post-intoxication 'crashes', simple observation is sufficient. Even in cases of severe intoxication with delirium, observation, given the brevity of the intoxication, is again generally all that is required; if, however, agitation is severe, one may give a dose of parenteral haloperidol in a dose of 5–10 mg. Patients with severe withdrawal and suicidal ideation may require hospitalization to protect themselves; hospitalization may also be required in cases of cocaine abuse or addiction to effect a period of abstinence, during which other measures may be initiated.

The overall goal of treatment of cocaine abuse or addiction is abstinence from cocaine and other substances, such as alcohol, benzodiazepines, and opioids. Patients may be referred to organizations such as Cocaine Anonymous or Narcotics Anonymous, and some may undergo cognitive behavioral therapy. The efficacy of pharmacologic treatment for cocaine addiction is uncertain. Earlier claims for the effectiveness of dopaminergic agents, such as amantadine, levodopa or direct-acting dopaminergic agents (e.g., bromocriptine) have not survived attempts at replication. More recent work has focused on other agents, such as modafinil (Dackis *et al.* 2005), baclofen (Shoptaw *et al.* 2003), disulfiram (Carroll *et al.* 2004), tiagabine (Gonzalez *et al.* 2007), topiramate (Kampman *et al.* 2004), and ondansetron (Johnson *et al.* 2006), but, in my opinion, experience with these more recent pharmacologic approaches is as yet too limited to warrant their widespread use.

21.3 HALLUCINOGENS

The hallucinogens (also known as psychotomimetics) can be roughly divided into two groups, namely the indolealkylamines and the phenylalkylamines. Of the indolealkylamines, the prototype is lysergic acid diethylamide (LSD); other members include psilocybin, dimethyltryptamine (DMT), and 5 methoxy-*N,N*-diisopropyltryptamine ('Foxy'). Among the phenylalkylamines, mescaline is the prototype, and this is joined by numerous other compounds including dimethoxymethylamphetamine (DOM), dimethoxyamphetamine (DMA), methylenedioxyamphetamine (MDA), 3,4-methylenedioxy-N-cthylamphctamine (MDEA or 'Evc'), and the very popular 3,4-methylenedioxymethamphetamine (MDMA or 'Ecstasy'). With the exception of DMT, which must be insufflated, smoked, or injected (Strassman *et al.* 1994a,b), all of the hallucinogens are active orally and are usually taken in this fashion.

Clinical features

Intoxication begins within 20 60 minutes after oral ingestion and is characterized by a profound, 'cosmic' sense, without any drowsiness or sedation (Bercel *et al.* 1956; Freedman 1968; Hollister *et al.* 1960; Isbell *et al.* 1956; Ungerleider *et al.* 1966). Patients may experience vivid memories, and commonplace events may appear exceedingly meaningful. Visual illusions and hallucinations are common, and a minority may experience synesthesiae or simple auditory hallucinations; importantly, patients maintain insight during intoxication and recognize the hallucinations as being unreal. Mild degrees of tachycardia, elevated blood pressure, mydriasis, fine tremor, hyperreflexia, and poor coordination may be seen, and the temperature may be elevated. In a minority of cases the intoxication may turn into a 'bad trip', with the development of severe anxiety, which may be accompanied by delusions of persecution and of reference (Kuramochi and Takahashi 1964). Most intoxications last in the order of 6–24 hours; exceptions include psilocybin and DMT, which produce shorter intoxications lasting 2–6 hours.

Intoxication with MDMA ('Ecstasy') deserves special mention for several reasons. First, unlike the other hallucinogens, intoxication is characterized by an initial, often quite intense 'rush', which is then followed by a heightened sense of empathy and connectedness with others. Second, it has become immensely popular, especially among young adults who may use it during all-night parties known as 'raves'. Third, in addition to the possibility of a 'bad trip' (Kosten and Price 1992; Liester *et al.* 1992; Whitaker-Azmita and Aronson 1989; Winstock 1991), MDMA may cause significant complications, including arrhythmias, cardiac arrest, severe hyponatremia, hyperpyrexia, rhabdomyolysis with renal failure, and hepatitis (Fahal *et al.* 1992; Greene *et al.* 2003; Hartung *et al.* 2002; Shearman *et al.* 1992). In addition to these immediately obvious sequelae, there is also evidence that MDMA may cause long-lasting, and perhaps permanent, short-term memory loss (Bolla *et al.* 1998; Gouzoulis-Mayfrank *et al.* 2000; Zakzanis *et al.* 2001).

Tolerance develops rapidly to the intoxicating effects of all of the hallucinogens (with the sole exception of DMT), and most patients must wait a few days before they can again achieve intoxication (Isbell *et al.* 1956). Interestingly, despite the occurrence of tolerance, withdrawal phenomena do not occur.

A small minority of patients may develop certain sequelae after intoxication, including flashbacks, mood changes, or a psychosis.

Flashbacks (Abraham 1983; Frosch *et al.* 1965; Horowitz 1969) may occur in up to one-quarter of patients, during which, although not intoxicated, patients re-experience one or more of the symptoms that occurred during a prior intoxication; classically, patients experience visual hallucinations, which may be complex or quite simple, or may consist of 'trailing', a kind of palinopsia in which afterimages follow along after patients divert their gaze away from an object. As with the hallucinations occurring during intoxication, patients retain insight and recognize the flashbacks as unreal. Flashbacks may occur spontaneously or may be precipitated by moving into a darkened area or by the use of alcohol, cannabis, or an antipsychotic drug. Flashbacks may be infrequent or occur multiple times daily, and they may remit spontaneously after a few weeks or months or persist indefinitely. When flashbacks occur frequently, chronically, and cause distress, by convention one speaks of 'hallucinogen persisting perception disorder'.

Mood changes may appear shortly after intoxication resolves, generally within a few days, and may consist of depression or, less commonly, mania. These mood changes are typically quite brief, lasting in the order of days, and only rarely weeks, after which patients return to their baseline.

Psychosis (McGuire *et al.* 1994) may emerge with resolution of the intoxication; it is generally characterized by one or more of the hallucinations or delusions seen during the intoxication, with the critical difference that insight is lost and patients now experience them as real and react to them accordingly. Although this 'hallucinogen-induced psychotic disorder' generally remits spontaneously after a few days, in a small minority it may persist for weeks, months, or longer.

Course

Recreational use of hallucinogens is very common among adolescents and young adults; it is typically confined to occasional use without consequences at parties or social gatherings. Hallucinogen abuse, that is repeated use despite significant consequences, is relatively rare. Neither craving nor, as pointed out earlier, withdrawal occur, and addiction is not seen.

Etiology

All of the hallucinogens exhibit complex agonist and antagonist effects at either pre- or post-synaptic serotonin receptors, and in the case of MDMA there may be destruction of serotoninergic neurons (McCann et al. 1998; Ricaurte et al. 1988).

Differential diagnosis

Mild intoxication with phencyclidine may be quite similar to that seen with hallucinogens, but is suggested by nystagmus, dysarthria, and ataxia.

Hallucinogen-induced flashbacks, mood changes, and psychosis are all indicated by the preceding intoxication. When this history is lacking, disorders noted in the differential diagnosis for hallucinations, depression, mania, and psychosis may be considered.

Treatment

'Bad trips' may be managed by supportive observation; in some cases lorazepam may be helpful. Post-intoxication mood changes, if severe, may require hospitalization for supportive care until they run their course. Post-intoxication psychosis may likewise require hospitalization and, if prolonged, may be treated with an antipsychotic such as olanzapine. Flashbacks generally do not require treatment but, if frequent and troubling, consideration may be given to the use of clonazepam in a dose of 2 mg daily (Lerner et al. 2003).

21.4 PHENCYCLIDINE AND KETAMINE

Phencyclidine and its closely related derivative ketamine are both arylcyclohexylamines that were developed as 'dissociative' anesthetics. The frequent occurrence of post-operative psychosis with phencyclidine has led to its abandonment in medical practice; however, ketamine is still used, both as an anesthetic and as an analgesic. Both drugs are used as intoxicants, and the use of ketamine in this regard appears to be on the rise. Phencyclidine is also known as PCP, 'angel dust', 'hog', and 'peace pill', and ketamine may be referred to as 'K', 'special K', 'vitamin K', 'cat valium', 'kat' or 'kit-kat'.

Clinical features

Intoxication with phencyclidine may be roughly characterized as mild, moderate, or severe; ketamine is less potent than phencyclidine and only rarely produces the severe and potentially life-threatening intoxication not uncommonly seen with phencyclidine. Both of these drugs may be ingested, 'snorted' intranasally, smoked, or injected.

Mild intoxication (Javitt and Zukin 1991; Luby et al. 1959; McCarron et al. 1981; Meyer et al. 1959; Pearlson 1981; Weiner et al. 2000) is characterized by euphoria and a peculiar sense of detachment or dissociation. Patients may feel as if they are floating, and their bodies may, to them, appear misshapened. Lability, agitation, or lethargy may appear, and behavior may become bizarre and unpredictable, with violence in some cases. Patients may complain of nausea, vomiting, or vertigo, and examination may disclose dysarthria, ataxia, nystagmus (which may be rotatory, horizontal, or vertical), myoclonus, tremor, increased deep tendon reflexes, decreased pin-prick sensation in the extremities, and autonomic signs, such as an elevated temperature, tachycardia, an elevated respiratory rate, elevated blood pressure, diaphoresis, and flushing; rather than mydriasis, however, one typically sees miosis.

Moderate intoxication is characterized by a delirium, which may be accompanied by delusions and visual hallucinations (Allen and Young 1978). Abnormal movements may appear, including facial grimacing, posturing, stereotypies, dystonia, and opisthotonus; grand mal seizures may also occur (Alldredge et al. 1989). Agitation may be extreme, and in some cases rhabdomyolysis occurs, with renal failure.

Severe intoxication is characterized by stupor or coma (McCarron et al. 1981). In stupor, patients may be quite still or may evidence random, purposeless movements; myoclonus is frequent and the deep tendon reflexes are greatly increased. With even higher doses coma supervenes; this is a kind of 'coma vigil' in which the eyes are open and the patient appears vigilant, but shows no response to pain or to anything else. The temperature rises further, as does the blood pressure, and in some cases a hypertensive encephalopathy occurs. The electroencephalogram (EEG) in these cases shows profound generalized slowing.

The duration of intoxication with ketamine, which has a half-life of about 3 hours, is approximately 4–6 hours. Phencyclidine intoxication is longer for two reasons. First, the half-life of phencyclidine is longer, anywhere from 7 to 20 hours. Second, phencyclidine is a weak base and hence is 'trapped' in the stomach; phencyclidine is also lipophilic and is therefore taken up into adipocytes. Thus protected from hepatic metabolism, phencyclidine may linger for prolonged periods, and indeed may be detectable in the blood for weeks or longer after a single dose. Overall, intoxication with phencyclidine tends to last from half a day up to many days and, during the overall resolution of phencyclidine intoxication, the clinical picture may fluctuate fairly widely.

Tolerance does not appear to occur and it is unclear if a withdrawal syndrome exists. Some patients, shortly after resolution of the intoxication, may complain of a 'letdown' lasting a day or so, with dysphoria, irritability, and insomnia; however, as this can occur after the first dose of either drug, and does not worsen with prolonged use, it is probably not appropriate to consider it a withdrawal syndrome.

A minority of patients may experience persistent sequelae after intoxication, including mood changes, psychosis, delirium, or dementia. Although these are described below as discrete entities, it must be borne in mind that individual patients may at times have a mixture of these sequelae.

Mood changes tend toward mania, and manic symptoms may persist for days to a week or more. Depression may also occur but tends to be seen only in long-term, heavy users; such depressions may be relatively long-lasting, persisting sometimes for many weeks.

Psychosis is characterized by a persistence of the delusions and hallucinations that are seen in moderate degrees of intoxication; although this syndrome tends to resolve spontaneously within days to a week or so, there are rare reports of a chronic psychosis occurring after heavy use of phencyclidine.

Delirium, as noted earlier, may be seen during moderate intoxication, and this may persist beyond the resolution of other signs and symptoms, lasting from days up to a week.

Dementia constitutes a rare sequela of prolonged and very heavy use of phencyclidine, and this may persist for months and up to a year or more, despite abstinence. Patients may develop decreased short-term memory, concreteness, an expressive aphasia, and a personality change with dysphoria, irritability, and impulsivity.

Course

Occasional recreational use of either phencyclidine or ketamine, without consequences, is not uncommon in late adolescence or early adult years. Prolonged and repeated use, despite medical or social consequences, appears uncommon, and such abuse of these drugs tends to resolve while patients are still in their twenties. Craving does not appear to occur and addiction is not seen.

Etiology

Both phencyclidine and ketamine act as non-competitive antagonists at cation channels within the N-methyl-D-aspartic acid (NMDA) receptor complex, and, although numerous other receptors are also affected, it is this action at the NMDA receptor that appears to be responsible for the intoxicating effect of these drugs.

Differential diagnosis

Hallucinogen intoxication resembles mild intoxication with phencyclidine or ketamine, although it lacks some of the characteristic signs seen in arylcyclohexylamine intoxication, including dysarthria, ataxia, and nystagmus; furthermore, in hallucinogen intoxication one sees mydriasis rather than the miosis of arylcyclohexylamine intoxication.

In the absence of a history of ingestion, the delirium of moderate intoxication and the stupor or coma of severe intoxication may present a diagnostic puzzle in the emergency room, with the differential being pursued as outlined in Section 5.3.

The various post-intoxication sequelae are suggested by the history of intoxication; lacking this, the differential expands, as discussed in the sections on the respective syndromes.

Treatment

Intoxicated patients should be observed in a supervised setting. Patients should be separated from unnecessary stimulation, and isolation in a quiet, dimly lit, well-protected room with constant monitoring is often best; unlike hallucinogen-intoxicated patients, arylcyclohexylamine-intoxicated patients do not respond well to verbal support, and cannot be 'talked down'. Restraints may be required but should be used sparingly given that patients who struggle against them may undergo worse rhabdomyolysis (Lahmeyer and Stock 1983). Agitation, delusions, and hallucinations, if problematic, may be treated with an antipsychotic such as haloperidol (Giannini et al. 1984). Dystonia, if severe, and opisthotonus may be treated with intravenous lorazepam, and seizures may be treated with intravenous lorazepam and, if repetitive, fosphenytoin. Vigorous general medical care may be required for hyperthermia, hypertension, and rhabdomyolysis.

In the case of phencyclidine, which is 'trapped' in the gastric fluid, consideration may be given to treatment with activated charcoal followed by continuous nasogastric suctioning.

The treatment of the various post-intoxication sequelae is discussed in the respective sections on these syndromes.

Once intoxication and any post-intoxication sequelae have resolved, efforts should be undertaken to ensure abstinence, which may include involvement in Narcotics Anonymous.

21.5 ALCOHOL

This section deals with the various disorders and phenomena associated with alcohol use, including alcohol intoxication, blackouts, pathological intoxication, tolerance to alcohol, alcohol withdrawal, alcohol withdrawal seizures, delirium tremens, and various other disorders often seen in association with alcohol use, such as head trauma. The full panoply of these is often seen in alcoholism, and this disorder is also discussed.

Clinical features

Alcohol intoxication of mild degree is characterized by euphoria, talkativeness, and a degree of disinhibition; in some patients there may be some irritability or dysphoria rather than euphoria. In moderate intoxication, the behavior becomes coarse and the thinking is slow and unclear. There is facial flushing, conjunctival injection, dysarthria, nystagmus, and ataxia. With severe intoxication there is drowsiness, stupor, and disabling ataxia; coma may ensue, with respiratory depression and death.

The blood alcohol level (BAL) is customarily reported in milligrams/deciliter or, as it is often worded, milligrams percent (mg%). In an alcohol-naive subject, mild intoxication is seen at 100 mg%, moderate intoxication at 200 mg%, and severe intoxication at 300 mg%; in the alcohol-naive patient, levels of 400 mg% generally cause coma, and levels of approximately 500 mg%, respiratory depression.

In general, in a 70-kg subject, the rapid consumption of 15 mL of pure, 100% ethanol will elevate the BAL by about 15–20 mg%, and this amount of pure ethanol is generally found in one mixed drink, one can of beer, or one glass of wine. In those with normal hepatic function, ethanol is metabolized at a rate of 5–10 mL/hour. Of interest, females tend to become intoxicated with a smaller amount of ingested alcohol than males, and this may be because of a reduction in gastric alcohol dehydrogenase activity, thus allowing a greater percentage of the ingested alcohol to escape this initial metabolic step (Frezza *et al.* 1990).

After the intoxication has passed, patients may experience a 'hangover', which may last from hours up to a day. This is characterized by headache, malaise, dysphoria, nausea, mild tremulousness, and diaphoresis.

Blackouts may occur during moderate or severe alcohol intoxication and consist of transient episodes of anterograde amnesia, lasting anywhere from minutes to days, depending on how long the BAL remains high (Goodwin 1971; Goodwin *et al.* 1969a). During a blackout, patients' behavior may, to casual inspection, not appear to be changed: patients may recall what they were doing at the start of the blackout and may also be able to keep track of ongoing events sufficiently well that they are able to keep up a conversation, play cards, etc. If, however, short-term memory is tested during the blackout, one finds that patients are unable to recall anything that happened much more than 5 minutes earlier. Furthermore, once the blackout ends, the time period covered by the blackout remains an 'island of amnesia' to patients, who can recall little or nothing of the events that transpired during the blackout.

Should blacked-out patients fall asleep during the blackout, they may, upon awakening the next day, anxiously ask acquaintances what they did the night before. Those who are still awake when the blackout abruptly ends may be quite startled at their situation; one patient (Goodwin *et al.* 1969b) 'found himself dancing with no recollection of what he had been doing during the previous six hours'. A variant of blackouts, known as 'brownouts', may occur in which

the amnesia is not complete and patients can recall some of what happened (Tamerin *et al.* 1971).

Pathological intoxication (Perr 1986), although long written of (Banay 1944; May and Ebaugh 1953), is a controversial diagnosis (Coid 1979). Putatively, patients, after only a small amount of alcohol, undergo a dramatic change, becoming uncharacteristically irritable and often violent. One study was able to reproduce these symptoms in patients thought to have suffered pathologic intoxication (Maletzky 1976), whereas another was not (Bachy-Rita *et al.* 1971); if indeed pathologic intoxication does exist, it is probably rare.

Tolerance to alcohol typically develops gradually with chronic, repeated intoxications, and greater and greater amounts must be drunk to achieve the desired intoxication. Thus, whereas in the alcohol-naive patient levels of 100 mg% typically cause intoxication, those with tolerance may need to reach a level of 300 mg% before they begin to 'feel' the alcohol; indeed, in some cases alcohol-tolerant patients may sustain levels of 500 mg% without loss of consciousness (Adachi *et al.* 1991; Minion *et al.* 1989). Interestingly, late in the course of alcoholism, some patients may fairly rapidly 'lose' their tolerance. In such cases, patients who had previously been able to consume a liter of liquor and still be standing may now find themselves hopelessly and severely intoxicated after only a few drinks.

Alcohol withdrawal (Isbell *et al.* 1955), colloquially known as the 'shakes', although generally seen only in alcoholics, may be seen in anyone who engages in heavy, prolonged drinking. The symptoms appear gradually, anywhere from 4 to 12 hours after the BAL has fallen below the patient's 'threshold' for intoxication. Importantly, this implies that for some patients, such as alcoholics who have developed tolerance, withdrawal symptoms may appear while the patient is still drinking, provided that the alcohol consumption has 'slowed down' sufficiently.

Symptoms include tremulousness, anxiety, easy startability, poor memory and concentration, fleeting and poorly formed visual or auditory hallucinations, insomnia (Johnson *et al.* 1970), elevated temperature, pulse and systolic blood pressure, mydriasis, generalized hyper-reflexia, diaphoresis, nausea and vomiting, and diarrhea. The most prominent symptom of alcohol withdrawal, however, is tremor, and it is from this that the syndrome derives its colloquial name. The tremor is postural, rapid, and ranges in amplitude from fine to coarse; it may be confined to the outstretched hands or be more widespread, even generalized, involving the eyelids and tongue in severe cases. Rarely one may see transient myoclonus or chorea.

Most patients recognize that a drink will 'solve' their problem, and many will take some 'hair of the dog that bit you'. This does offer temporary relief of the shakes but of course threatens to set off a vicious cycle.

Alcohol withdrawal generally peaks within a couple of days and then gradually settles over the next 2 or 3 days. Among recreational or abusive drinkers, the symptoms may gradually resolve fully within a week, but among alcoholics, residual symptoms may persist for up to 6 months.

Alcohol withdrawal seizures, also known as 'rum fits', are a rare accompaniment of the alcohol withdrawal syndrome, seen only in a few percent of alcoholics (Schuckit *et al.* 1993); typically they occur only after many years of heavy drinking and repeated episodes of alcohol withdrawal. They may occur within hours to 2 days after either a cessation of alcohol use or a substantial reduction in the amount consumed and typically consist of grand mal seizures, which may, in about one-quarter of cases, have focal features. Most patients have only one seizure; occasionally patients may experience two or three, or even a half-dozen, and very rarely status epilepticus may occur.

Delirium tremens (Lundquist 1961; Nielsen 1965; Rosenbaum *et al.* 1941), also known as alcohol withdrawal delirium or simply the 'DTs', is generally seen only in alcoholics who have been drinking heavily for many years and who have had repeated episodes of alcohol withdrawal; the presence of a concurrent illness, such as pneumonia, hepatic failure, or gastrointestinal bleeding, increases the risk. Clinically, patients first develop a typical alcohol withdrawal syndrome, and in about 10 percent of cases there may be an alcohol withdrawal seizure. After anywhere from hours to a week or more, but generally within 2–3 days, there is a dramatic exacerbation of the typical alcohol withdrawal symptoms accompanied by the appearance of delirium. In addition to confusion, disorientation, and short-term memory loss, patients typically also experience hallucinations and delusions. Visual hallucinations are most common, and they tend to be extremely vivid and complex, typically involving animals or insects: dogs may circle the bed; rats eat at the toes; bugs crawl on the arms and face and the patient may try and swat them away. Tactile hallucinations may accompany the visual ones, and the patient may feel animals tearing at the flesh or bugs biting into the skin. Auditory hallucinations may occur. Patients may hear bells, whistles, or alarms, and at times voices; when voices do occur they tend to be critical and persecutory. Delusions are common and tend to be persecutory and referential. Patients may believe that staff are conspiring against them to have them killed and may believe that chance conversations refer especially to them.

Delirium tremens is fatal in 5–20 percent of cases, with patients succumbing to concurrent illnesses such as pneumonia, hepatic failure, cardiac arrhythmias, or hypovolemic shock. Those who survive generally experience a gradual remission of symptoms within a day to 2 or 3 weeks, with most recovering within several days.

Rarely, one may see a variant of delirium tremens known as delirium tremens sine tremore (trembling delirium without tremor). Here, the tremor and other autonomic symptoms classically associated with delirium tremens are either minimal or absent, and patients present with a 'quiet' delirium, seemingly undisturbed while all the time experiencing confusion, hallucinations, and delusions.

Other disorders often accompany alcohol intoxication, especially in patients with alcoholism. Falls and motor vehicle accidents are common, and traumatic brain injury (Section 7.5), especially with subdural hematoma (Section 11.1), is not uncommon. Vitamin deficiencies may occur: thiamine deficiency may cause a Wernicke's encephalopathy (Section 13.4), and the much less commonly seen niacin deficiency may cause the acute, encephalopathic form of pellagra (Section 13.3). Among alcoholics, recurrent attacks of alcoholic hepatitis may lead to hepatic cirrhosis and, in some, to a hepatic encephalopathy (Section 13.19). Alcoholics are also prone to infection and aspiration pneumonia is not uncommon; bacterial meningitis may also occur but this is relatively rare. Hypoglycemia may occur, not only due to malnourishment but also to the direct inhibitory effect alcohol has on hepatic gluconeogenesis; hypomagnesemia may also be seen. Gastritis, bleeding esophageal varices, and pancreatitis may likewise occur. Chronic hyponatremia may be seen in some cases, and its overly rapid correction may cause central pontine myelinolysis (Section 13.17).

Patients who have survived a Wernicke's encephalopathy may be left with the chronic amnesia of Korsakoff's syndrome (Section 13.4). Long-term, chronic alcoholism may also be associated with the gradual development of various other disorders, including alcoholic dementia (Section 22.8), alcohol hallucinosis (Section 22.9), alcoholic paranoia (Section 22.10), Marchiafava–Bignami disease (Section 22.11), alcoholic cerebellar degeneration, and alcoholic polyneuropathy.

Course

Recreational or 'social' use of alcohol is almost ubiquitous in most parts of the world, but the intoxications here are generally mild and, although a significant minority of recreational drinkers may experience blackouts and some may suffer head trauma, the other consequences of alcohol use described above do not occur. Alcohol abuse is characterized by recurrent intoxication despite significant medical, social, and legal consequences, and these patients, in addition to episodes of intoxication of moderate or severe degree, commonly experience blackouts and may develop a degree of tolerance and experience minor episodes of the alcohol withdrawal syndrome; these patients, however, do not have a craving for alcohol and, albeit with some effort, are able to either moderate their drinking or stop altogether. Alcoholism emerges from alcohol abuse and is signalled by the development of craving, with an inability to 'leave it alone', and by clear-cut tolerance and frequent episodes of moderate or severe alcohol withdrawal; alcoholics are also prone to alcohol withdrawal seizures, delirium tremens, and all of the other disorders described earlier, such as head trauma and Wernicke's encephalopathy.

Alcoholism is a common disorder, seen in about 10 percent of the adult population in the United States, and is much more frequent in males than females. In most cases of alcoholism, excessive alcohol use begins in the late teens or early twenties, and progressively and gradually worsens until the full clinical picture is reached after a decade or so; exceptions to this pattern do occur, however, and in some cases the onset may be delayed until middle years or the progression may be unusually rapid. Among alcoholics, drinking becomes the primary need in life, and patients continue to drink despite disastrous consequences. Denial is ubiquitous, and almost all alcoholics will strenuously deny that they have a problem with drinking or they will attempt to rationalize it in one way or another. Most alcoholics, at least initially, will try at times to control their drinking, perhaps after a hospital stay, incarceration for driving while intoxicated, or the angry departure of a spouse, and some may experience some success at this, only to soon find themselves again hopelessly intoxicated. The overall course of alcoholism may be episodic or chronic. The episodic course is characterized by more or less lengthy episodes, or 'binges', during which there are frequent, closely spaced intoxications; these binges may last anywhere from weeks to months, and in between them patients generally remain abstinent. The chronic course may be apparent from the onset of the alcoholism or may supervene upon a prior episodic course; in this chronic course there are repeated, more or less closely spaced intoxications without any intervening periods of sobriety of any significant length. Regardless of whether the course is episodic or chronic, spontaneous, full remissions are rare and most alcoholics continue to drink despite losing jobs, friends, families, and their health, and indeed they continue to do so until they are either institutionalized or dead.

Etiology

Alcohol intoxication may reflect not only increases in membrane fluidity, with consequent changes in ion channel function, but also alcohol-mediated sensitization of gamma-aminobutyric acid (GABA) receptors and inhibition of NMDA glutamate receptors. With repeated, frequent intoxications, it is suspected that there is a chronic down-regulation of GABA receptors and an up-regulation of NMDA receptors, and that it is these changes that predispose to the development of the alcohol withdrawal syndrome and delirium tremens. The mechanisms underlying blackouts, pathologic intoxication, and alcohol withdrawal seizures are not clear. Although the etiology of alcoholism itself is not known, it is clear that hereditary factors play a major role, accounting for approximately 60 percent of cases.

Differential diagnosis

Alcohol intoxication may be mimicked by intoxication with various other substances, but certain signs allow for a differential. In the case of intoxication with benzodiazepines

(or other sedative–hypnotics) and ethylene glycol, there is no odor of alcohol on the breath, and in the case of ethylene glycol one will also see an increased anion gap. Both isopropyl alcohol and methanol intoxication may be accompanied by an odor of alcohol; however, in these intoxications there is prominent nausea and vomiting and, furthermore, in methanol intoxication one finds bilateral dimming or loss of vision. Consideration must also be given to some of the other disorders that may accompany intoxication, especially in cases in which intoxicated patients fail to sober up within the expected time frame, including especially head trauma, infection, hypoglycemia, and hypomagnesemia.

Blackouts must be distinguished from certain other causes of episodic anterograde amnesia, as discussed in Section 5.4. Transient global amnesia and pure epileptic amnesia are distinguished by the absence of other signs of intoxication, such as dysarthria. Concussion may occur during intoxication, but the evidence of head injury is generally obvious.

Alcohol withdrawal may be clinically indistinguishable from withdrawal from benzodiazepines or other sedative–hypnotics, and the diagnosis therefore rests on the history of substance use, keeping in mind that many patients will also use these other agents in addition to alcohol. Hypoglycemia, not uncommonly seen in intoxicated alcoholics, may produce a similar picture (Fredericks and Lazor 1963; de Moura *et al.* 1967) and, as noted below, a blood glucose determination should be standard.

Alcohol withdrawal seizures, in a sense, should be considered a 'rule-out' diagnosis, given the large number of other conditions that may produce grand mal seizures in alcoholics. To begin with, patients with epilepsy of any cause are more likely to have seizures during alcohol withdrawal. Seizures may also occur secondary to some of the other disorders noted above, including head trauma, Wernicke's encephalopathy, hepatic encephalopathy, hypoglycemia, hypomagnesemia, and the rare cases of bacterial meningitis or Marchiafava–Bignami disease.

Delirium tremens may be clinically indistinguishable from benzodiazepine or sedative–hypnotic withdrawal delirium, and the differential here rests on the history of substance use. Other disorders capable of causing a 'trembling delirium' with marked autonomic signs include the serotonin syndrome, the neuroleptic malignant syndrome, thyroid storm, and hypoglycemia. In some cases, alcohol withdrawal may be accompanied by a delirium secondary to one of the other disorders seen in alcoholics, thus producing a clinical picture that may be easily passed off as delirium tremens rather than an etiologically multifactorial delirium; consideration should therefore be given to the presence of Wernicke's encephalopathy, hepatic encephalopathy, traumatic brain injury, hypomagnesemia, encephalopathic pellagra, Marchiafava–Bignami disease, meningitis, pneumonia with sepsis, and, in patients who have undergone correction of hyponatremia, central pontine myelinolysis.

Treatment

Alcohol intoxication is generally managed by observation and routine general medical supportive care. An estimate should be made as to the time of the last drink and a BAL should be obtained, after which one may calculate the time required for the alcohol to wash out. With very high blood levels respiratory failure may occur, necessitating intubation, and in some cases hemodialysis may be appropriate.

In older, debilitated, or alcoholic patients, or those who demonstrate withdrawal or seizures, routine laboratory tests should be obtained, including a complete blood count (CBC), electrolytes, glucose, magnesium, ammonia, bilirubin, liver enzymes, stool for occult blood, and an electrocardiogram (ECG); if there is any suspicion of pneumonia or head trauma, a chest radiograph or computed tomography (CT) scan, respectively, should also be obtained. Patients should also receive 100 mg of thiamine parenterally, followed by 100 mg daily of parenteral or oral thiamine; glucose and food should, if possible, be withheld until 2 hours have passed from the administration of the initial dose of parenteral thiamine.

Blackouts are managed by simple observation until serial mental status examinations have demonstrated a recovery of short-term memory function.

Pathological intoxication is likewise managed by observation; however, here, seclusion and, at times, restraints may be required until the intoxication has passed.

Alcohol withdrawal may or may not require pharmacologic treatment. For some alcoholics and alcohol abusers, the 'shakes' may constitute a valuable lesson that strengthens the motivation for sobriety, and provided that their general medical condition is such that the overall autonomic symptomatology does not constitute a risk, it may be appropriate to simply let such patients 'shake it out'. However, when autonomic symptoms are intolerable, serve no instructive purpose, or pose a threat to the patient (e.g., as may occur in those with epilepsy or cardiac disease), then pharmacologic treatment is indicated. Traditionally, a benzodiazepine has been used; however, either carbamazepine or dialproex constitute reasonable alternatives, and, as discussed further below, a combination of a benzodiazepine plus one of these anti-epilepsy drugs (AEDs) may also be used. Some clinicians advocate the use of alcohol itself, generally via an intravenous drip; however, the hepatotoxicity of alcohol may give one pause here.

Of the benzodiazepines, lorazepam, given its short half-life and lack of metabolites, is recommended. Oral administration is preferred; however, if this is not practicable, roughly the same dose may be given parenterally. Initially 2 mg is given (or less in the elderly or debilitated), followed by 2 mg every 2 hours until the tremor is controlled and the patient is calm. The next day the patient is placed on a regular total daily dose that is roughly equivalent to the total amount that was required on the first day, with this total dose divided into three or four doses; provision is also made for ongoing as-needed doses of 1 or 2 mg every 2

hours for breakthrough tremor, and on succeeding days the total daily dose is increased until eventually the regular dose is sufficient to control tremor without the need for any further as-needed doses. At this point, as-needed doses are discontinued and the patient is then placed on a tapering dose whereby the total daily dose is decreased every succeeding day by an amount that is approximately equal to 20 percent of the total required for control; in this fashion the dose may be tapered and then discontinued over about 4 or 5 days. Other benzodiazepines may also be considered, such as chlordiazepoxide (25–50 mg) or diazepam (5–10 mg); however, these agents have long half-lives and active metabolites making them more difficult to use. Regardless of which benzodiazepine is used, such a program generally requires admission. Most outpatients are simply unable to discipline themselves to follow the program and will either abort it, take enough of the benzodiazepine to cause intoxication, or resume drinking.

Both carbamazepine (Malcolm *et al.* 1989; Seifert *et al.* 2004; Stuppacek *et al.* 1992) and divalproex (Reoux *et al.* 2001) are generally equally as effective as a benzodiazepine in suppressing the tremor and other autonomic symptomatology of alcohol withdrawal. In otherwise healthy patients with normal hepatic function, one may begin with carbamazepine in a dose of 200 mg three or four times daily or with divalproex in a total daily loading dose of 20 mg/kg, divided into two or three doses; subsequent dose adjustments may then be made based on the clinical response, side-effects, and blood levels. As both of these agents may take a day or two to quell the symptoms of alcohol withdrawal, many clinicians will combine their use with as-needed doses of lorazepam, as described above; generally, after 3 days at the most, no further lorazepam will be required, and the patient may then be continued on the AED alone for about a week, that is to say, long enough for the alcohol withdrawal to run its natural course, after which it may be rapidly tapered and discontinued. Some clinicians, however, may elect to continue divalproex for a matter of months. As noted earlier, among alcoholics the withdrawal syndrome may persist in a smoldering fashion for up to 6 months, and in such cases, after discharge, the temptation to drink or take sedatives to quell these symptoms, particularly the insomnia, may be very strong. Continuing divalproex has been shown to be useful in this regard, and may therefore actually increase the chances of long-term sobriety. One of the great advantages of using an AED is that it ends the struggle that may occur between the patient who demands ever more lorazepam and the clinician who suspects that the patient's demands reflect not the pain of withdrawal but rather a desire for intoxication.

There is debate as to whether a course of benzodiazepines or a course of an AED is preferable. Given that lorazepam, as noted below, is effective both in preventing recurrent withdrawal seizures and in treating delirium tremens, whereas the AEDs have not been shown to be effective in these regards, many clinicians feel safer using lorazepam. Others, noting that the combination strategy provides coverage with lorazepam during the first few days of withdrawal, when the risk of seizures and delirium tremens is highest, and the advantage of getting away from potentially intoxicating substances as soon as possible, find the combination strategy acceptable. Clinical judgment is clearly required here. Certainly, if there is a history of withdrawal seizures or delirium tremens, then one should strongly consider a full course of lorazepam, or, if a combination strategy is otherwise very attractive, a longer initial course of lorazepam should be considered before phasing into treatment with an AED alone.

Alcohol withdrawal seizures generally present in the context of an alcohol withdrawal syndrome, and it has been shown that after a first seizure the intravenous administration of 2 mg of lorazepam will reduce the risk of a second seizure over the next 6 hours (D'Onofrio *et al.* 1999). It is therefore probably reasonable to treat these patients with lorazepam, as described for alcohol withdrawal, either throughout the course of the withdrawal or, if a combination strategy is used, for the first few days, after which carbamazepine or divalproex may be used alone. Should status epilepticus occur, most clinicians will give fosphenytoin.

Delirium tremens represents a medical emergency. Patients should be treated with intravenous lorazepam in doses of 2 mg every 1–2 hours until they are lightly sedated, and massive doses may be required to accomplish this. Once patients are comfortable and the autonomic signs are well controlled, the dose of lorazepam may then be gingerly tapered, generally in daily decrements approximately equivalent to 10 percent of the total daily dose required for initial control. In many cases, lorazepam, although capable of calming patients and quelling tremor and other autonomic symptoms, does not control hallucinations and delusions, and in these cases an antipsychotic should be considered, such as haloperidol or risperidone. Haloperidol may be given in a dose of 1–5 mg, and risperidone in doses of 0.25–1 mg every hour, until symptoms are acceptably controlled, limiting side-effects occur, or a maximum dose of approximately 20 mg of haloperidol or 5 mg of risperidone is achieved. Once symptoms are controlled, the antipsychotic should be continued in approximately the same total daily dose (divided into two or three doses) until the symptoms have been well controlled for at least a few consecutive days, after which the drug may generally be tapered and discontinued over the following few days. Further suggestions for the overall treatment of delirium are discussed in Section 5.3.

In addition to the routine laboratory tests described earlier, a careful search should be made for other illnesses, such as pneumonia, pancreatitis, gastrointestinal bleeding, hepatic failure, etc., as one or more of these is usually present. Diaphoresis, vomiting, and diarrhea may cause dehydration, and massive fluid replacement may be required.

In those rare cases of delirium tremens sine tremore, antipsychotics alone, coupled with other measures discussed in Section 5.3, may be all that is required.

Overall, the goal of treatment of alcoholism is abstinence. Although attempts have been made to enable alcoholics to continue drinking in a 'controlled' fashion, these are not reliable and cannot be recommended: the goal of abstinence must be stated to alcoholics clearly, starkly, and unmistakably. Whether the same applies to alcohol abusers is not clear; however, given the risk that alcohol abuse may evolve into alcoholism or that, if it doesn't, further drinking may get out of control with disastrous consequences, it is prudent to advance the same goal to alcohol abusers.

Although some alcoholics are able to stop drinking by an extraordinary act of will, this is rare and the vast majority will continue to drink unless they receive help. In such cases, various psychosocial methods are helpful and may be offered. Pharmacologic treatment of alcoholism, utilizing acamprosate, naltrexone, topiramate, disulfiram, or divalproex, although at times helpful, is adjunctive only and cannot replace psychosocial treatments.

Various psychotherapies, such as cognitive behavioral therapy, have been utilized, and in some cases are successful. A referral to Alcoholics Anonymous (AA), however, should be considered, regardless of whether patients are referred to psychotherapy. Many patients are also hospitalized in residential treatment facilities, and this may be necessary to effect a period of sobriety of sufficient length to allow patients to begin to think clearly again; during such stays patients are often engaged in various psychotherapies and, importantly, are often taken to AA meetings.

Alcoholics Anonymous is the oldest treatment approach to alcoholism and, if participated in fully, has an excellent success rate. The key word here is 'fully': no treatment works unless patients are compliant, and AA is no exception. Patients must be told that much will be expected of them but that, if they persist, they will become sober. Alcoholics Anonymous meetings are available around the world, and in the United States contact may be made by simply calling directory assistance in virtually any city. Patients should be instructed to attend meetings as frequently as possible, ideally attending 'ninety meetings in ninety days', and to get an AA 'sponsor'. Should patients protest that they don't have the time to go to a meeting every day, they may be gently, but clearly, reminded that they have a debilitating and potentially fatal disease, and that the time spent at meetings will pay off not only in keeping them alive but also in salvaging what is left of their careers and relationships.

Of the medications to be considered, naltrexone, acamprosate, and possibly topiramate may each partially reduce either the urge to drink or the intoxication that occurs with drinking; disulfiram, by contrast, induces a toxic 'Antabuse reaction' if patients do drink, thus adding another motivation to remain sober, and divalproex, as noted earlier, may ease some of the lingering residual withdrawal symptoms, especially insomnia, thus removing these as motivations to drink or use sedatives.

Naltrexone, given only to patients with normal hepatic function, is used orally in a dose of 50 mg daily, and acamprosate, in patients with normal renal function, is given in a dose of 666 mg three times daily; it appears that naltrexone is more effective than acamprosate (Morley *et al.* 2006), although the combination of naltrexone plus acamprosate appears to be more effective than naltrexone alone (Kiefer *et al.* 2003). Topiramate is used in total daily doses of approximately 100–200 mg (Johnson *et al.* 2003). Each one of these three agents has been shown to reduce the number of drinking days in patients who do 'slip' and drink, although the overall results are modest at best. Disulfiram is begun in a dose of 500 mg daily, with the dose reduced to 250 mg daily after 1 or 2 weeks; patients should be given a graphic description of the toxic reaction that they may expect should they ingest even a miniscule amount of alcohol, and, given the potential toxicity of disulfiram, treatment is generally maintained for only a matter of months. Divalproex neither reduces the urge to drink nor the intoxication that occurs with drinking, but may, in doses similar to those used for alcohol withdrawal, reduce lingering withdrawal symptomatology. Choosing among these medications is not straightforward. Out of naltrexone, acamprosate, and topiramate, all other things being equal, it is probably reasonable to begin with naltrexone. Given its toxicity, disulfiram should be reserved for highly motivated patients. The place of divalproex is not as yet clear; however, if it has been used during treatment of alcohol withdrawal, and one can predict a lingering withdrawal, it is reasonable to continue it.

Although these medications may be helpful, patients must not be allowed to think that their use can substitute for involvement in psychosocial treatments. Many patients fondly hope for a 'magic bullet' that will resolve their alcoholism, and such hopes must be firmly dashed. The overall role of the physician in the treatment of alcoholism *per se* is generally limited to treatment of some of the complications of alcoholism (e.g., hepatic failure) and to treatment of any concurrent disorders, such as depression, panic disorder, or schizophrenia. As a general rule, in prescribing medications for these or any other conditions, potentially intoxicating drugs, such as benzodiazepines or opioids, should be avoided as they may trigger off a desire to drink; exceptions to this rule are few.

Alcoholism is a chronic disease and hence relapses are to be expected; these occur most frequently in the first 6 months of treatment. Relapses, or 'slips', therefore, although certainly undesirable, should not be taken as an indication of failure but rather as an indication for patients to redouble their efforts.

21.6 SEDATIVES, HYPNOTICS, AND ANXIOLYTICS

The sedatives, hypnotics, and anxiolytics, including the benzodiazepines and related drugs, comprise a large group of agents, often collectively referred to as the 'sedative–hypnotics', each of which has an effect similar to that of alcohol. Although most commonly used in conjunction with alcohol or other substances, such as opioids, stimulants or cocaine, they may at times be used in isolation. Table 21.1 lists these various agents, grouped according to their half-lives, as short acting (generally less than 6 hours), intermediate acting (6–18 hours) or long acting (generally over 24 hours). This classification is useful as it allows one to make a rough prediction as to when withdrawal, withdrawal seizures, or withdrawal delirium is likely to occur.

The popularity of these various agents has changed over time. The barbiturates, meprobamate, and chloral hydrate, once commonly abused, have been supplanted by the benzodiazepines, among which alprazolam, lorazepam, and diazepam are most popular.

Clinical features

As indicated, the clinical features of sedative–hypnotic use are similar to those of alcohol, and thus one may see sedative–hypnotic intoxication, blackouts, tolerance, withdrawal, withdrawal seizures, and withdrawal delirium. Each of these is discussed below in turn.

When mild, sedative–hypnotic intoxication with barbiturates (Curran 1938, 1944; Isbell *et al.* 1950), meprobamate (Roache and Griffiths 1987), or benzodiazepines is characterized by euphoria, a degree of affective lability, and disinhibition. With moderate intoxication, reaction time is slowed, lethargy and drowsiness appear, and patients often develop nystagmus, dysarthria, and ataxia; falls may occur, with possible head injury. With severe intoxication stupor or coma may occur, with respiratory depression and death.

Sedative–hypnotic blackouts are quite similar to those seen with alcohol; although possible with long-acting

Table 21.1 Sedative–hypnotics grouped by duration of effect

Short-acting (less than 6 hours)	Triazolam
	Alprazolam
	Zolpidem
	Zaleplon
Intermediate-acting (6–18 hours)	Oxazepam
	Temazepam
	Lorazepam
	Chlordiazepoxide
	Meprobamate
	Chloral hydrate
Long-acting (greater than 24 hours)	Quazepam
	Prazepam
	Halazepam
	Flurazepam
	Clonazepam
	Diazepam
	Amobarbital
	Secobarbital
	Pentobarbital
	Phenobarbital
	Butalbital

benzodiazepines such as diazepam (Wolkowitz *et al.* 1987), they are more common with short-acting, high-potency benzodiazepines (Scharf *et al.* 1987) such as triazolam (Ewing *et al.* 1988; Greenblatt *et al.* 1991; Morris and Estes 1987).

Tolerance may appear with long-term use and at times may be quite remarkable: some patients may end up taking hundreds of milligrams of diazepam daily, with little or no evidence of sedation.

Sedative–hypnotic withdrawal, as seen with benzodiazepines (Busto *et al.* 1986; Covi *et al.* 1973; Hollister *et al.* 1961; Juergens and Morse 1988; Murphy *et al.* 1984, 1989; Rickels *et al.* 1990; Shader *et al.* 1993; Tyrer *et al.* 1983) and barbiturates (Fraser *et al.* 1958; Isbell *et al.* 1950), is characterized by anxiety, irritability, insomnia, tremor, tachycardia, diaphoresis, nausea and vomiting, and postural hypotension. The onset of the withdrawal syndrome varies according to the half-life of the agent: roughly speaking, for short-acting agents withdrawal starts in less than a day; for intermediate-acting agents, 2–3 days; and for long-acting agents, 2–6 days. For certain very-long-acting agents, such as diazepam or phenobarbital, the blood level may fall so slowly that there is, in effect, a 'self-tapering', with, in many cases, a substantially less severe withdrawal syndrome. The duration of withdrawal likewise varies with the half-life of the agent. Roughly speaking, for short- and intermediate-acting agents, symptoms peak within 1–3 days and persist for 1–2 weeks, whereas for long-acting agents the peak arrives in 5–7 days and the syndrome may persist for up to 2 or 3 weeks. As with alcohol withdrawal, some patients may experience lingering, low-level withdrawal symptoms for weeks or months after withdrawing from benzodiazepines (Ashton 1984; Shader *et al.* 1993). In addition to this typical picture of withdrawal, a recent report described the occurrence of stuporous catatonia as a withdrawal phenomenon of benzodiazepines (Rosebush and Mazurek 1996).

Sedative–hypnotic withdrawal seizures typically occur within the context of withdrawal symptomatology and, although these may occur with benzodiazepines (e.g., aprazolam [Breier *et al.* 1984; Noyes *et al.* 1986]), they are much more common with barbiturates, in which case there is a significant risk of multiple seizures and status epilepticus.

Sedative–hypnotic withdrawal delirium, noted with benzodiazepines (such as alprazolam [Levy 1984; Zipursky *et al.* 1985] and flunitrazepam, lorazepam, and triazolam [Heritch *et al.* 1987; Martinez-Cano *et al.* 1995]) and barbiturates (Fraser *et al.* 1958; Isbell *et al.* 1950), typically emerges out of a withdrawal syndrome and is characterized by an intensification of those symptoms, accompanied by confusion, disorientation, agitation, hallucinations, and persecutory delusions. In the natural course of events, the delirium tends to clear in anywhere from days to a couple of weeks.

Course

Recreational use of these agents, particularly the benzodiazepines, is common among adolescents and young adults.

Sedative–hypnotic abuse is said to occur when patients continue to seek intoxication despite experiencing blackouts and social or legal consequences, and the onset of addiction is heralded by the development of craving, tolerance, and withdrawal phenomena, such as a withdrawal syndrome, seizures, or delirium. As noted earlier, concurrent use of other substances, especially alcohol, is common, and 'pure-culture' sedative–hypnotic abuse or addiction is relatively rare.

Etiology

Both the benzodiazepines and the barbiturates, by somewhat different mechanisms, enhance chloride flux via GABA receptors upon stimulation by endogenous GABA, and it is by virtue of this that intoxication occurs. Presumably, with prolonged use, down-regulation of these receptors occurs, with the consequent development of tolerance and withdrawal phenomena.

Differential diagnosis

Sedative–hypnotic intoxication is clinically indistinguishable from alcohol, isopropyl alcohol, and methanol intoxication except for the fact that sedative–hypnotic-intoxicated patients do not have an odor of alcohol on their breath. Ethylene glycol intoxication, which also lacks an odor of alcohol, is distinguished by an increased anion gap. In cases in which patients fail to recover from an intoxication within the expected time frame, other disorders, for example traumatic brain injury, should be considered.

Sedative–hypnotic blackouts must be distinguished from other causes of episodic anterograde amnesia, as discussed in Section 5.4.

Sedative–hypnotic withdrawal is basically indistinguishable from alcohol withdrawal, and the diagnosis must rest on an accurate history of substance use, keeping in mind that many patients may have a 'mixed' picture of both sedative–hypnotic and alcohol withdrawal.

Sedative–hypnotic seizures, as with alcohol-withdrawal seizures, constitute a 'rule-out diagnosis', and consideration must be given to pre-existing epilepsy and head trauma.

Sedative–hypnotic withdrawal delirium may be indistinguishable from delirium tremens and the diagnosis may rest on an accurate history, keeping in mind that, as for withdrawal, a 'mixed' picture may be present. Consideration may also be given to other causes of delirium with tremor, including the serotonin syndrome, the neuroleptic malignant syndrome, thyroid storm, and hypoglycemia.

Treatment

Sedative–hypnotic intoxication typically requires only observation and general medical support. In cases of benzodiazepine intoxication in which respiratory depression threatens, flumazenil may be given (Brogden and Goa 1991); however, caution is needed here in cases in which tolerance has developed, as flumazenil may precipitate a withdrawal syndrome with seizures.

Sedative–hypnotic blackouts require only observation until serial mental status examinations have revealed a restoration of short-term memory, and the intoxication itself has resolved.

Sedative–hypnotic withdrawal should probably be treated with the same agent that the patient is addicted to. This is particularly the case for barbiturate withdrawal, which is not controlled by benzodiazepines, and alprazolam withdrawal, which may not respond to other benzodiazepines such as diazepam (Zipursky *et al.* 1985). For benzodiazepine withdrawal, a strategy similar to that described for the treatment of alcohol withdrawal in the preceding section may be utilized, with equivalent doses (e.g., lorazepam 2 mg, alprazolam 1 mg, diazepam 10 mg, chlordiazepoxide 25 mg). In the case of barbiturate withdrawal it is traditional to utilize phenobarbital, with doses of 90–120 mg every 1–2 hours until symptoms are controlled, after which the dose may, as with the benzodiazepines, be gradually tapered.

An alternative to consider in the case of benzodiazepine withdrawal is carbamazepine (Schweizer *et al.* 1991). Once symptoms have been adequately controlled with the benzodiazepine, one may add carbamazepine in a dose of 200 mg three or four times daily, after which the benzodiazepine may be rapidly tapered over a day or two. Importantly, carbamazepine is not effective for barbiturate withdrawal and may also be ineffective in the case of alprazolam.

Sedative–hypnotic withdrawal seizures should be treated by rapidly reinstituting the sedative–hypnotic in question, with the goal of completely controlling any concurrent withdrawal symptomatology.

Sedative–hypnotic withdrawal delirium demands vigorous treatment of the withdrawal syndrome, with the goal of producing a light degree of sedation. Should hallucinations and delusions persist in a troubling fashion, an antipsychotic, as described in Section 5.3, may be required. Once symptoms have been brought under control, the sedative–hypnotic may be gradually tapered in daily decrements approximately equivalent to 10 percent of the total daily dose initially required to effect control.

Overall, the goal of treatment in the case of abuse or addiction is abstinence. Those addicted to sedative–hypnotics alone, or to a combination of a sedative–hypnotic and alcohol, may do well in AA.

21.7 INHALENTS (SOLVENTS)

The volatile ingredients of many readily available products are often inhaled for intoxication. These include airplane or model glue, paint thinner, kerosene, gasoline, fingernail polish remover, the propellants in aerosol sprays and spray paints, and typewriter correction fluid. Each of these products contains various mixtures of aliphatic and aromatic hydrocarbons, some of which may be halogenated; of all of these intoxicating hydrocarbons, toluene appears to be the most significant.

Clinical features

Intoxication is obtained either by soaking a rag in the volatile substance and holding it to the face or by placing the substance in a plastic or paper bag and then inhaling; when a bag is used it may leave a telltale circular rash on the face. The intoxication (Evans and Raistrick 1987) occurs within minutes and is characterized by a dreamy euphoria, drowsiness, dizziness, dysarthria, diplopia, nystagmus, and ataxia. Some may also experience confusion and hallucinations, which may be either visual or, less commonly, auditory, and others may become irritable and impulsive. Cardiac arrhythmias may occur and may be fatal (GS King *et al.* 1985; Steffee *et al.* 1996). Convulsions, coma, and respiratory depression may also be seen (King *et al.* 1981), as may acute hepatitis and renal failure (Gupta *et al.* 1991; Taverner *et al.* 1988). If leaded gasoline is sniffed, intoxication may be accompanied by chorea and myoclonus (Goldings and Stewart 1982).

Tolerance may develop and, when this occurs, withdrawal may also appear. Withdrawal (Evans and Raistrick 1987; Watson 1979) occurs within 1–2 days of abstinence and is characterized by irritability, sweating, tremulousness, and insomnia, all of which generally remit within a matter of days.

With long-term use a dementia may occur (discussed in Section 22.12), as may a severe motor peripheral polyneuropathy (Altenkirch *et al.* 1977; PJ King *et al.* 1985).

Course

Occasional, recreational use of inhalants is not uncommon among adolescents; abuse and addiction appear to be far less common. In many cases other substances are also used, especially alcohol and opioids.

Etiology

Although the intoxicating hydrocarbons clearly have an effect on lipid neuronal cell membranes, the precise mechanism whereby intoxication occurs is not known.

Differential diagnosis

Intoxication with alcohol or sedative–hypnotics may yield a somewhat similar clinical picture. The odor of solvents on clothing or skin may be a clue, as may a rash on the face; if toluene has been used it may be detected in the blood for days (King *et al.* 1981).

Treatment

Simple observation is generally sufficient. Patients who also abuse or are dependent on alcohol or opioids may be referred to Alcoholics Anonymous or Narcotics Anonymous; the optimal treatment of those who are solely involved with inhalants is not clear.

21.8 CANNABIS

The name 'cannabis' comes from the Greek word for hemp and refers specifically to the flowering tops of the hemp plant, *Cannabis sativa*. In the United States, the two most common preparations of cannabis are marijuana and hashish. Marijuana (also known as 'grass', 'pot', 'reefer', 'weed' or 'Mary Jane') is simply a dried collection of the flowers and nearby leaves and sprouts of the hemp plant and, although at times ingested, it is usually rolled into a cigarette and smoked. Hashish is a more potent preparation, composed of the resin scraped from the leaves and flowers of the plant, and is usually smoked.

Clinical features

Intoxication with cannabis (Allentuck and Bowman 1942; Bromberg 1934; Clark and Nakashima 1968; Clark *et al.* 1970; Klonoff *et al.* 1973; Melges 1976) is characterized by a dreamy sense of well-being, an unusual heightening of the senses, and a feeling that time is slowing down or disintegrating (Melges *et al.* 1970). Thinking becomes slowed and patients often develop a heightened sense of the ridiculous, laughing and giggling at otherwise prosaic things; in some cases depersonalization or derealization may occur. Typically, intoxication is accompanied by conjunctival injection, dry mouth, increased appetite, mild ataxia, mild tachycardia, and a combination of increased supine blood pressure and orthostatic hypotension. In general, symptoms undergo substantial resolution after 3 or 4 hours. Tetrahydrocannabinol (THC) or its metabolites, however, may be detected in the urine for 2–6 days in infrequent users, and in chronic heavy users the urine may remain positive for several weeks.

In a minority of cases of intoxication, complications may occur, including anxiety, psychosis, and delirium.

Anxiety may occur during otherwise unremarkable intoxications and may at times crescendo to constitute an anxiety attack (Bromberg 1934), with tremor, tachycardia, and palpitations; typically the anxiety resolves as does the intoxication.

Psychosis (Kroll 1975; Mathers and Ghodse 1992; Talbott and Teague 1969; Weil 1970) may also occur during an intoxication and patients may develop delusions of persecution, which may be accompanied by auditory or visual hallucinations. Patients may become quite agitated in the midst of this, and some will flee the scene or seek safety in some other way. This 'cannabis-induced psychotic disorder' generally outlasts the intoxication itself and indeed may persist for days. Before leaving this discussion of psychosis, mention should also be made of the possible occurrence of a chronic psychosis secondary to cannabis use. This is a controversial notion. Although there is no doubt that, in the midst of chronic cannabis use, some patients will develop a psychosis with delusions of persecution and auditory hallucinations which may persist for years into abstinence, what is in doubt is whether this psychosis was caused by cannabis or merely represents the occurrence of paranoid schizophrenia in a patient who also happens to have a history of chronic cannabis use.

Delirium (Chopra and Smith 1974; Palsson *et al.* 1982) may also occur during an intoxication, but generally only when very high doses have been taken. Patients become confused, agitated, and at times incoherent; delusions and hallucinations may also occur. This delirium may either clear as the intoxication does, or may persist for up to a few days.

Tolerance to cannabis can develop and is manifest by a decreased euphoric response and a diminution of the tachycardia and elevated supine blood pressure normally seen during intoxication.

Withdrawal (Duffy *et al.* 1996; Haney *et al.* 1999; Mendelson *et al.* 1984) may occur in tolerant patients, and typically appears anywhere from 3 to 12 hours after the resolution of intoxication. Symptoms are typically mild and consist of anxiety, irritability, restlessness, a fine tremor, diaphoresis, and insomnia. Withdrawal symptoms reach a peak intensity within 1–2 days and then resolve after a total of 4–5 days.

Course

Recreational use of cannabis is extremely common among adolescents and young adults, and most of these individuals either stop entirely or greatly reduce their use as they begin to assume adult responsibilities. Cannabis abuse is marked by frequent intoxication despite social and legal consequences, and dependence is heralded by the onset of tolerance and withdrawal. Overall, abuse and dependence are far less common than recreational use, occurring in no more than 5 percent of adolescents and young adults.

Etiology

The principal intoxicant in cannabis is the delta-9 isomer of THC (Isbell *et al.* 1967). Marijuana contains anywhere from 1 to 15 percent THC, whereas the more potent hashish contains anywhere from 10 to 60 percent. THC is highly lipid soluble and readily crosses the blood–brain barrier. Two endogenous cannabinoid receptors have been identified within the central nervous system, namely CB1 and CB2; CB1 receptors appear to be responsible for the euphoria and are concentrated in the cerebral cortex, hippocampus, basal ganglia, and cerebellar cortex, and recent data suggest that different polymorphisms in the gene for CB1 may confer different risks for the development of cannabis addiction (Hopfer *et al.* 2006).

Differential diagnosis

Uncomplicated intoxication with cannabis may be mimicked by intoxication with alcohol, sedative–hypnotics, inhalants, and opioids, and cannabis intoxication complicated by psychosis or delirium may be confused with hallucinogen or phencyclidine intoxication; furthermore, many patients may present with a mixed intoxication, having utilized both cannabis and one or more of these other substances. History and urine drug screens may be required to make the differential diagnosis.

Treatment

Uncomplicated intoxication generally requires only observation until the intoxication has passed. Anxiety, if troubling, may be relieved by diazepam, in a dose of 10 mg. Psychosis, if problematic, may be treated with a dose of an antipsychotic, such as 5 mg of haloperidol or 1–2 mg of risperidone, with repeat doses as needed. Delirious patients should be closely monitored until the delirium has passed, and may be treated as outlined in Section 5.3. Cannabis withdrawal generally does not require treatment.

The overall goal of treatment in abusers and addicts is abstinence, and various forms of psychotherapy have been attempted. Unfortunately, many adolescents and young adults simply see nothing wrong with their use, and often drop out of treatment.

21.9 OPIOIDS

An opiate is any intoxicant normally found in opium. The term 'opioid' is more general and refers to any substance, either natural or synthetic, that has effects similar to opium.

Opium is obtained from the juice of the poppy plant, and two opiates are found within opium, namely morphine and codeine. Synthetic and semi-synthetic derivatives include heroin, oxycodone, hydromorphone, meperidine, pentazocine, methadone, and buprenorphine: these last two derivatives, although often used in the treatment of opioid withdrawal and addiction, may also be used for intoxication (Torrens *et al.* 1993). Of all of the opioids, oxycodone and heroin are the most commonly used for intoxication.

Although these drugs may be taken orally for intoxication, most users prefer a parenteral route as the effect is more immediate and intense; tablets may be crushed, dissolved, and filtered (often utilizing cigarette filters) to yield a more or less adulterated and contaminated liquid, which is then injected. Most addicts progress from 'skin popping', or subcutaneous injection, to 'mainlining' the drug intravenously. Occasionally heroin may be snorted or smoked, or, in the process known as 'chasing the dragon', heated, with subsequent inhalation of the heroin vapor.

Clinical features

Intoxication with opioids is intensely seductive. Within moments of intravenous injection, the user may be rewarded by an intense 'rush'. The body is suffused with warmth, and orgasmic sensations may be experienced. In less than a minute the rush tends to pass, to be replaced by a drowsy, vaguely euphoric feeling that may last for hours and which is accompanied by difficulty with concentration and dysarthria. The pupils are generally constricted, peristalsis is slowed, and constipation ensues; urinary hesitancy or retention may also occur.

Meperidine and pentazocine intoxication have distinctive features. Meperidine is metabolized to normeperidine, and this metabolite may cause agitation, tremor, mydriasis, increased deep tendon reflexes, and, occasionally, myoclonus or seizures (Kaiko *et al.* 1983). Pentazocine intoxication, when high doses are utilized, may be accompanied by dysphoria, anxiety, hallucinations, and bizarre thoughts, along with dizziness and diaphoresis (Challoner *et al.* 1990).

Overdoses of opioids are not uncommon. The purity of 'street' heroin varies widely, and the unwary user may unintentionally take a lethal amount; furthermore, some addicts, after a period of abstinence during which tolerance is lost, may resume use with a dose that, although prior to the loss of tolerance produced only intoxication, is now sufficient to cause overdose. Overdose itself is characterized by stupor or coma, accompanied by hypotension and respiratory depression. Pupils are initially pinpoint; however, with the advent of cerebral anoxia, mydriasis appears. Pulmonary edema and seizures may occur, and death is usually due to respiratory arrest. Those who survive may be left with an anoxic dementia or sequelae of watershed infarctions.

Tolerance may develop to almost all of the effects of opioids (with the exception of miosis and constipation) and addicts may progressively increase their doses to obtain intoxication, sometimes to stunning levels of a gram or more of morphine.

Withdrawal is characterized initially by a sense of uneasiness and a craving for the drug; soon after, yawning, lacrimation, and rhinorrhea appear, accompanied in some cases by diaphoresis. After several hours, patients may fall into a restless sleep known as 'yen' sleep. Upon awakening, all of the earlier symptoms intensify and patients become irritable, dysphoric, restless, and demanding. Patients begin to experience waves of goose flesh that may be so severe that they resemble the skin of a plucked turkey, an appearance that prompted the phrase 'going cold turkey'. Intense bone and muscle pain, especially in the back, arms, and legs, also occurs, and patients may engage in seemingly involuntary kicking movements, a phenomenon that gave rise to another synonym for opioid withdrawal, namely 'kicking the habit'. Insomnia may be severe. The pupils are dilated and the temperature, pulse, and blood pressure are all increased. Nausea, vomiting, intestinal cramping, and diarrhea occur, and the resulting fluid loss may be so severe that it causes circulatory collapse.

Withdrawal usually begins within the first day of abstinence, peaks in a matter of days, and then generally subsides over a week or so; in heavy users, however, a protracted withdrawal syndrome may persist for weeks up to 6 months, and is characterized by dysphoria, irritability, anhedonia, insomnia, and drug craving (Martin and Jasinski 1969).

Other disorders may accompany opioid abuse or addiction. Intravenous use brings the risk of bacteremia with pulmonary abscess, endocarditis, cerebral abscess, cerebral mycotic aneurysm, meningitis, osteomyelitis, and tetanus. Parenteral users often share needles and are thus at risk for acquired immune deficiency syndrome (AIDS), syphilis, and hepatitis. Furthermore, the presence of particulates in the injected fluid (as may occur when cigarette filters are used) may lead to pulmonary fibrosis, pulmonary hypertension, and cor pulmonale. Particulates may also collect in regional lymph nodes causing a chronic lymphadenopathy with edema, especially of the hands.

'Skin popping' may be followed by cellulitis or ulceration, and those who inject heroin intramuscularly may develop a myositis, with, in some cases, ossification.

Patients who 'chase the dragon' and inhale heroin vapor may develop a leukoencephalopathy with dementia accompanied by other signs such as ataxia, mutism, or quadriparesis. (Kriegstein et al. 1999).

Illegally manufactured 'street' meperidine may be contaminated with a by-product, methyl-phenyl-tetrahydropyridine (MPTP), which in turn may cause a chronic parkinsonian condition.

Course

Recreational use of opioids is uncommon and most patients pass fairly rapidly to abuse and addiction. Although some addicts, notably physicians who may have ready access to opioids, are able to maintain their social positions, most addicts quickly lose whatever gainful employ they may have had and turn to crime to support their addiction. Those who become deeply involved in the drug 'subculture' are liable to have a violent death at the hands of others; suicide attempts are also not uncommon, and those who do survive often end up losing all in their pursuit of the drug.

Etiology

The intoxicant effects of opioids are mediated by their binding to mu and, to a lesser extent, kappa receptors within the central nervous system. Genetic factors appear to increase the risk of addiction, as does the childhood environment of most patients who become addicted, whose parents are often themselves afflicted with opioid addiction, alcoholism, or other substance use disorders.

Differential diagnosis

Opioid intoxication may be partially mimicked by intoxication with alcohol, sedative–hypnotics or inhalants; however, these intoxications generally lack the intense miosis characteristic of most opioid intoxications; in doubtful cases drug screening will resolve the issue. It must be borne in mind, however, that many patients will use other substances in addition to opioids: cocaine may be used to reduce sedation, and alcohol or sedative–hypnotics may be employed to ease the pain of withdrawal.

Treatment

Intoxication, if mild, may require only simple observation. In severe intoxication, however, consideration should be given to treatment with naloxone; however, care must be taken to avoid 'overshooting' in addicts and producing a hyperacute withdrawal syndrome.

Withdrawal should generally only be attempted on a secure inpatient unit, and, given the intense drug craving seen during withdrawal, patients should be confined to the ward until the withdrawal has run its course; visitation, if allowed at all, must be closely and continuously supervised.

Currently, there are three traditional approaches that remain standard for withdrawal: 'cold turkey', withdrawal with opioids, or treatment with clonidine. Recent work also suggests effectiveness for buspirone.

Very few patients opt to go 'cold turkey'; however, as withdrawal is not life threatening, this may be appropriate for some. Prochlorperazine may be given for nausea and vomiting, diphenoxylate for diarrhea, and amitriptyline (in a dose of approximately 50 mg at bedtime) for insomnia (Srisurapanont and Jarusuraisin 1998), and these may also be made available for those who undergo treatment with either opioids or clonidine.

Withdrawal utilizing an opioid may be accomplished with methadone, buprenorphine, or, if the patient had been using another illicit substance (e.g., oxycodone), with that agent. Treatment is generally commenced as withdrawal symptoms appear. Methadone may be started in a dose of 10–20 mg, with repeat doses every 4 hours as needed to suppress symptoms. Most patients are stabilized on a dose ranging from 20 to 40 mg daily, after which the total daily dose may be reduced in decrements of 5–10 mg daily. Buprenorphine may be given sublingually in an initial dose of 4–6 mg, with repeat doses as needed every 2 hours until symptoms are suppressed, a process that generally requires anywhere from 8 to 32 mg; once the patient is stabilized, the dose may be gradually tapered in daily decrements of 2–4 mg.

Clonidine (Charney *et al.* 1981; Gold *et al.* 1978; Jasinski *et al.* 1985) is not nearly as effective at suppressing withdrawal symptoms as opioids. Overall, it is most effective against nausea and diarrhea, and insomnia may also be partially relieved; however, clonidine has little effect on drug craving, restlessness, and 'kicking'. Once withdrawal begins, clonidine is given in a dose ranging from 0.1 to 0.3 mg, with repeat doses every 2–3 hours until maximum effect is obtained. The initial total dose is then given on a daily basis in four divided doses, with provision for further as-needed doses, after which the total daily dose is titrated up based on how much is given in as-needed doses until no further as-needed doses are required; most patients are stabilized by a total daily dose ranging from 0.6 to 2.4 mg. The patient is then generally 'covered' by this final dose for about a week to a week and a half, that is to say for the expected duration of the withdrawal, after which the dose may be tapered over 3 or 4 days and then discontinued.

Buspirone, in a remarkable double-blind study (Buydens-Branchey *et al.* 2005), was as effective in opioid withdrawal as methadone. Patients were treated with a total dose of 30 or 45 mg of buspirone, and this was maintained throughout a 12-day withdrawal period.

Choosing among these treatment options for withdrawal is not straightforward, with one exception: pregnant females should be withdrawn with opioids as any of the other options risks fetal death. Presuming that the patient is not pregnant, however, any one of these options is viable. Going 'cold turkey', as noted, is rarely chosen by patients given the intense suffering associated with withdrawal; however, some may prefer this. In those who do want pharmacologic treatment, most prefer withdrawal with opioids. However, a case may be made for treatment with clonidine or, perhaps, a combination of clonidine and buspirone; in this scenario, patients may be started on buspirone immediately and 'covered' with clonidine for any breakthrough symptoms, with the buspirone continued for the anticipated duration of the withdrawal.

Before leaving this discussion of the treatment of withdrawal, some words are in order regarding what is known as 'rapid' or 'ultra-rapid' detoxification. Although details differ among various programs, in most cases patients are first 'covered' with clonidine and an anti-emetic and then either sedated or anesthetized. In this state they are then given naloxone and naltrexone and a hyperacute withdrawal is produced. Consciousness is then allowed to return and patients are continued on the naltrexone and, temporarily, on the clonidine and anti-emetic. Although these programs are heavily advertised, it has not been established whether they increase the odds of abstinence or whether any purported successes outweigh the risks of anesthesia.

Overall, in some cases the goal is abstinence from all opioids, whereas in others the goal is to reduce the frequency of intoxication by providing maintenance treatment with either methadone or buprenorphine.

Abstinence, although very difficult to achieve, is clearly preferable, and patients desiring this option may be seen in psychotherapy or referred to Narcotics Anonymous; many also require a lengthy inpatient stay, not only to get over withdrawal but also to begin their rehabilitation efforts. Consideration may also be given to treatment with 50 mg of naltrexone daily, which blocks opioid-induced euphoria and thus effectively blocks the overwhelmingly reinforcing 'rush' that patients get if they 'slip'.

In the United States, methadone maintenance is available only in specially licensed facilities. In some cases indefinite maintenance is anticipated, and such patients are generally treated with doses of 80–120 mg of methadone daily. In other cases consideration is given to eventual abstinence, and here patients are initially maintained on doses ranging from 20 to 60 mg; once patients have consistently tested drug free for a year or so, attempts are then made to reduce the dose of methadone in decrements of 5–10 percent of the total daily dose every week until the drug can be discontinued.

Buprenorphine maintenance, given the less stringent controls imposed on its use, is becoming popular, and is conducted by individual physicians on an outpatient basis. Treatment is conducted with a combination product of sublingual buprenorphine and naloxone: naloxone itself is not absorbed, but its presence serves as a deterrent to anyone who would consider crushing the tablet and taking it intravenously, as the intravenously active naloxone will block the intoxication. Most patients are managed with doses ranging from 16 to 32 mg three times weekly. As with methadone, some patients are continued indefinitely on the drug, whereas in other cases attempts may be made to eventually taper it.

Maintenance with either methadone or buprenorphine clearly 'works' in that such maintained patients are less likely to become intoxicated with illicitly obtained opioids or to engage in the criminal behavior that often accompanies addiction. Both methadone and buprenorphine, however, as noted earlier, may produce intoxication, and supplies obtained through maintenance programs have been used for this purpose.

21.10 NICOTINE

Although nicotine is the substance in question here, this section might just as well be entitled 'tobacco', for tobacco is the only 'vehicle' by which abuse or addiction to nicotine occurs. Of the various ways that tobacco is used, cigarette smoking is by far the most clinically important; although both chewing tobacco and smoking cigars or pipes can cause addiction, their numbers pale in comparison to cigarettes. With each cigarette smoked, anywhere from 1 to 3 mg of nicotine is delivered (Benowitz and Henningfield 1994).

Clinical features

Intoxication with nicotine is mild: especially with the first cigarette of the day, there is a sense of satisfaction and a reduction in any irritability. With this intoxication there may be a mild tachycardia, elevation of blood pressure, and an increase in peristaltic activity, and in some cases there may be palpitations; tobacco-naive patients may also experience nausea and vomiting. Overall, appetite decreases and frequent smokers may lose some weight.

Tolerance occurs rapidly and, by the end of a day spent smoking, there is little effect from a cigarette. Such tolerance, however, rapidly decreases, such that by the next day intoxication may again be achieved. Despite these daily fluctuations, however, a chronic tolerance does develop. Whereas a tobacco-naive patient may, as noted above, experience toxic nausea and vomiting with one cigarette, the nicotine addict may be able to smoke dozens of cigarettes a day without any immediate adverse effects.

Withdrawal symptoms (Hughes and Hatsukami 1986; Hughes et al. 1991a) may appear within anywhere from hours to a day of abstinence. There is a restless craving for a cigarette, and patients become tense and irritable. Headache, difficulty concentrating, and insomnia may occur, as may increased appetite with, in some, substantial weight gain. Withdrawal generally peaks within days and then gradually subsides over a matter of weeks; in some, however, mild withdrawal symptoms may persist for months, and in many cases the craving for a cigarette may recur intermittently for years, often at times of stress.

Other disorders may appear in association with tobacco use, and these occur not as a result of the effects of nicotine itself but rather of the by-products of tobacco. Smoked tobacco produces over 4000 different compounds, in both gaseous and particulate form. Gaseous components include carbon monoxide and hydrogen cyanide, whereas particulates contain a substance known as 'tar', which for the most part contains polycyclic aromated hydrocarbons. With chronic smoking, patients are at risk for cancer of the mouth, larynx, and lung, chronic obstructive pulmonary disease (COPD), coronary artery disease, cerebrovascular disease, peripheral vascular disease, Raynaud's phenomenon, gingivitis, gastroesophageal reflux, cancer of the esophagus, and peptic ulcer disease. Smoking during pregnancy may cause spontaneous abortion, abruptio placentae, and low birth weight.

Course

Recreational use of nicotine is very rare; those who start smoking usually either stop in short order or go on to fairly rapidly develop nicotine addiction (with craving, tolerance, and withdrawal) and persistent use, despite the development of one or more of the other disorders associated with tobacco use.

Etiology

Although the mechanisms that determine which patients will stop and which will go on to develop addiction are not clearly understood, genetic factors appear to play a significant role (Kendler et al. 2000).

Differential diagnosis

There is generally no diagnostic difficulty; in those who deny smoking, but who appear to be doing so, one may obtain a urine screen for cotinine, one of the metabolites of nicotine, which has a half-life of about 20 hours.

Treatment

Patients should choose a 'quit date', which ideally should fall during a relatively stress-free time in the not-too-distant future. Patients should be instructed to stop smoking on that day and to avoid, if possible, situations or gatherings where smoking is likely to occur. Individual or group therapy with a cognitive–behavioral approach is helpful and should be offered to patients. Various pharmacologic approaches are also available, including varenicline, bupropion, nortriptyline, and various preparations of nicotine. Importantly, both bupropion and nortriptyline are effective regardless of whether patients are depressed or not.

Varenicline is a partial agonist at alpha4beta2 nicotinic acetylcholine receptors, and reduces both nicotine intoxication and craving. Treatment is begun 1 week before the quit date with 0.5 mg/day for 3 days, then 0.5 mg twice daily for 3 days, and finally 1 mg twice daily thereafter, with treatment continued for 3–12 months.

Bupropion is started 1 week before the quit date at 150 mg daily and increased 3 days later to 150 mg twice daily, and then continued for 3–12 months.

Nortriptyline is started 1 week before the quit date at 25 mg daily, increased to 50 mg daily after 3 days, and then to 75 mg 3 days later, after which it is continued for 3–12 months. Although studies measuring blood levels have not been performed, it would not be unreasonable to check a blood level after a week or so of the full dose and to make appropriate adjustments based on the results.

Nicotine is available in a 24-hour patch delivering various strengths of nicotine (commonly 7, 14, and 21 mg) and, for as-needed dosage, in lozenges and gum tablets (both available in 2-mg sizes) and a nasal spray (delivering 0.5 mg). If a nicotine preparation is used, it should be started on the quit date. If the patch is used, the 21-mg size should be used for a 'pack a day' smoker, with lower doses used for those who smoke less; the initial strength is then continued until the patient has been abstinent for at least a couple of weeks, after which one steps down to the next lowest size, which is then continued until the patient has been abstinent for at least another 2 continuous weeks, until finally the patch is discontinued. The as-needed preparations are utilized with the goal of gradually reducing the number of doses until they too can be discontinued.

Overall, it appears that varenicline is superior to bupropion (Gonzales et al. 2006), which in turn appears superior

Greden JF. Anxiety or caffeinism: a diagnostic dilemma. *Am J Psychiatry* 1974; **131**:1089–92.

Greenblatt DJ, Harmatz JS, Shapiro L *et al.* Sensitivity to triazolam in the elderly. *N Engl J Med* 1991; **324**:1691–8.

Greene SL, Dargan PI, O'Connor N *et al.* Multiple toxicity from 3,4-methlenedioxymethamphetamine ('Ecstasy'). *Am J Emerg Med* 2003; **21**:121–4.

Griffith JD, Cavanaugh J, Held J *et al.* Dextroamphetamine: evaluation of psychotomimetic properties in man. *Arch Gen Psychiatry* 1972; **26**:97–100.

Griffiths RR, Evans SM, Heishman SJ *et al.* Low-dose caffeine physical dependence in humans. *J Pharmacol Exp Ther* 1990; **255**:1123–32.

Guggenheim MA, Couch JR, Weinberg W. Motor dysfunction as a permanent complication of methanol intoxication: presentation of a case with a beneficial response to levodopa treatment. *Arch Neurol* 1971; **24**:550–4.

Gupta RK, van der Meulen J, Johny KV. Oliguric acute renal failure due to glue-sniffing. Case report. *Scand J Urol Nephrol* 1991; **25**:247–50.

Haney M, Ward AS, Comer SD *et al.* Abstinence symptoms following oral THC administration to humans. *Psychopharmacology* 1999; **141**:385–94.

Harrington H, Heller HA, Dawson D *et al.* Intracerebral hemorrhage and oral amphetamine. *Arch Neurol* 1983; **40**:503–7.

Hartung TK, Schofield E, Short AI *et al.* Hyponatremic states following 3,4-methylenedioxymethamphetamine (MDMA, 'ecstasy') ingestion. *Q J Med* 2002; **95**:431–7.

Heritch AI, Capwell R, Roy-Byrne PR. A case of psychosis and delirium following withdrawal from triazolam. *J Clin Psychiatry* 1987; **48**:168–9.

Hollister LE, Gillespie HK. Marijuana, ethanol, and dextroamphetamine: mood and mental function alterations. *Arch Gen Psychiatry* 1970; **23**:199–203.

Hollister LE, Prusmack JJ, Paulsen JAS *et al.* Comparison of three psychotropic drugs (psilocybin, JB-329, IT-290) in volunteer subjects. *J Nerv Ment Dis* 1960; **131**:428–34.

Hollister LE, Motzenbecker FP, Degan RO. Withdrawal reactions from chlordiazepoxide (Librium). *Psychopharmacology* 1961; **2**:63–8.

Hopfer CJ, Young SE, Purcell S *et al.* Cannabis receptor haplotype associated with fewer cannabis dependence symptoms in adolescents. *Am J Genet B Neuropsychiatr Genet* 2006; **141**:895–901.

Horowitz MJ. Flashbacks: recurrent intrusive images after the use of LSD. *Am J Psychiatry* 1969; **126**:565–9.

Hovda KE, Hunderi OH, Tajjord AB *et al.* Methanol outbreak in Norway: epidemiology, clinical features and prognostic signs. *J Intern Med* 2005; **258**:181–90.

Hsue PY McManus D, Selby V *et al.* Cardiac arrest in patients who smoke crack cocaine. *Am J Cardiol* 2007; **99**:822–4.

Hughes JR, Hatsukami D. Signs and symptoms of tobacco withdrawal. *Arch Gen Psychiatry* 1986; **43**:289–94.

Hughes JR, Gust SW, Skoog K *et al.* Symptoms of tobacco withdrawal: a replication and extension. *Arch Gen Psychiatry* 1991a; **48**:52–9.

Hughes JR, Higgins ST, Bickel WK *et al.* Caffeine self-administration, withdrawal, and adverse effects among coffee drinkers. *Arch Gen Psychiatry* 1991b; **48**:611–17.

Isbell H, Altschul S, Kornetsky CH *et al.* Chronic barbiturate intoxication. *Arch Neurol Psychiatry* 1950; **64**:1–28.

Isbell H, Fraser HF, Wickler A *et al.* An experimental study of etiology of 'rum fits' and delirium tremens. *Q J Stud Alcohol* 1955; **16**:1–33.

Isbell H, Belleville RE, Fraser HF *et al.* Studies on lysergic acid diethylamide (LSD-25). I. Effects in former morphine addicts and development of tolerance during chronic intoxication. *Arch Neurol Psychiatry* 1956; **76**:468–78.

Isbell H, Gorodetzky CW, Jasinski D *et al.* Effects of (–) 9-trans-tetrahydrocannabinol in man. *Psychopharmacologia* 1967; **11**:184–8.

Iwanami A, Sugiyama A, Kuroki N *et al.* Patients with methamphetamine psychosis admitted to a psychiatric hospital in Japan. *Acta Psychiatr Scand* 1994; **89**:428–32.

Janowsky DS, Risch C. Amphetamine psychosis and psychotic symptoms. *Psychopharmacology* 1979; **65**:73–7.

Jasinski DR, Johnson RE, Kocher TR. Clonidine in morphine withdrawal: differential effects on signs and symptoms. *Arch Gen Psychiatry* 1985; **42**:1063–6.

Javitt DC, Zukin SR. Recent advances in the phencyclidine model of schizophrenia. *Am J Psychiatry* 1991; **148**:1301–8.

Johnson BA, Ait-Daoud N, Bowden CL *et al.* Oral topiramate for treatment of alcohol dependence: a randomized controlled trial. *Lancet* 2003; **361**:1677–85.

Johnson BA, Roache JD, Ait-Daoud N *et al.* A preliminary randomized double-blind, placebo-controlled study of the safety and efficacy of ondansetron in the treatment of cocaine dependence. *Drug Alcohol Depend* 2006; **84**:256–63.

Johnson LC, Burdick JA, Smith J. Sleep during alcohol intake and withdrawal in the chronic alcoholic. *Arch Gen Psychiatry* 1970; **22**:406–18.

Jorenby DE, Leischow SJ, Nides MA *et al.* A controlled trial of sustained release bupropion, a nicotine patch, or both for smoking cessation. *N Engl J Med* 1999; **340**:685–91.

Juergens SM, Morse RM. Alprazolam dependence in seven patients. *Am J Psychiatry* 1988; **145**:625–7.

Kaiko RF, Foley KM, Grabinski PY *et al.* Central nervous system excitatory effects of meperidine in cancer patients. *Ann Neurol* 1983; **13**:180–5.

Kampman KM, Pettinati H, Lynch KG *et al.* A pilot trial of topiramate for the treatment of cocaine dependence. *Drug Alcohol Depend* 2004; **75**:233–40.

Kaplan K. Methyl alcohol poisoning. *Am J Med Sci* 1962; **244**:170–4.

Kendler KS, Thornton LM, Pedersen NL. Tobacco consumption in Swedish twins reared apart and reared together. *Arch Gen Psychiatry* 2000; **57**:886–92.

Kiefer F, Jahn H, Tarnaske T *et al.* Comparing and combining naltrexone and acamprosate in relapse prevention of alcoholism: a double-blind, placebo-controlled study. *Arch Gen Psychiatry* 2003; **60**:92–9.

King GS, Smialek JE, Trouthman WG. Sudden deaths in adolescents resulting from inhalation of typewriter correction fluid. *JAMA* 1985; **253**:1604–9.

King MD, Day RE, Oliver JS et al. Solvent encephalopathy. BMJ 1981; 283:663–5.

King PJ, Morris JG, Pollard JD. Glue sniffing neuropathy. Aust N Z J Med 1985; 15:293–9.

Kleber HD, Gawin FH. The spectrum of cocaine abuse and its treatment. J Clin Psychiatry 1984; 45(suppl. 2):18–23.

Klonoff DC, Andrews BT, Obana WG. Stroke associated with cocaine use. Arch Neurol 1989; 46:989–93.

Klonoff H, Low M, Marcus A. Neuropsychological effects of marijuana. Can Med Assoc J 1973; 108:150–7.

Kosten TR, Price LH. Phenomenology and sequelae of 3,4-methylenedioxymethamphetamine use. J Nerv Ment Dis 1992; 180:353–4.

Kramer JC, Fischman VS, Littlefield DC. Amphetamine abuse patterns and effects of high doses taken intravenously. JAMA 1967; 201:305–9.

Krendel DA, Ditter SM, Frankel MR. Biopsy-proven cerebral vasculitis associated with cocaine abuse. Neurology 1990; 40:1092–4.

Kriegstein AR, Shungu DC, Millar WS et al. Leukoencephalopathy and raised brain lactate from heroin vapor inhalation ('chasing the dragon'). Neurology 1999; 53:1765–73.

Kroll P. Psychoses associated with marijuana abuse in Thailand. J Nerv Ment Dis 1975; 161:149–56.

Kuramochi H, Takahashi R. Psychopathology of LSD intoxication: study of experimental psychosis induced by LSD-25: description of LSD symptoms in normal oriental subjects. Arch Gen Psychiatry 1964; 11:151–61.

Lacouture PG, Watson S, Abrams A et al. Acute isopropyl alcohol intoxication: diagnosis and management. Am J Med 1983; 75:680–4.

Lahmeyer HW, Stock PG. Phencyclidine intoxication, physical restraint and acute renal failure. J Clin Psychiatry 1983; 44:184–5.

Lerner AG, Gelkopf M, Skladman I et al. Clonazepam treatment of lysergic acid diethylamide-induced hallucinogen persisting perception disorder with anxiety features. Int Clin Psychopharmacol 2003; 18:101–5.

Levy AB. Delirium and seizures due to abrupt alprazolam withdrawal: case report. J Clin Psychiatry 1984; 45:38–9.

Lichtenfeld J, Rubin DB, Feldman RS. Subarachnoid hemorrhage precipitated by cocaine snorting. Arch Neurol 1986; 41:223–4.

Liester MB, Grob CS, Bravo GL et al. Phenomenology and sequelae of 3,4-methylenedioxymethamphetamine use. J Nerv Ment Dis 1992; 180:345–52.

Luby ED, Cohen BD, Rosenbaum G et al. Study of a new schizophrenomimetic drug – Sernyl. Arch Neurol Psychiatry 1959; 81:363–9.

Lundh H, Tunving K. An extrapyramidal choreiform syndrome caused by amphetamine addiction. J Neurol Neurosurg Psychiatry 1981; 44:728–30.

Lundquist G. Delirium tremens: a comparative study of pathogenesis, course and prognosis. Acta Psychiatr Neurol Scand 1961; 36:443–66.

McCann UD, Szabo Z, Scheffel U et al. Positron emission tomographic evidence of toxic effect of MDMA ('Ecstasy') on brain serotonin neurons in human beings. Lancet 1998; 352:1433–7.

McCarron MM, Schulze BW, Thompson GA et al. Acute phencyclidine intoxication: clinical patterns, complications, and treatment. Ann Emerg Med 1981; 10:290–7.

McGuire PK, Cope H, Fahy TA. Diversity of psychopathology associated with use of 3–4,methylenedioxyamphetamine ('Ecstasy'). Br J Psychiatry 1994; 165:391–5.

McLean DR, Jacobs H, Mielke BW. Methanol poisoning: a clinical and pathological study. Ann Neurol 1980; 8:161–7.

Malcolm R, Ballenger JC, Sturgis ET et al. Double-blind controlled trial comparing carbamazepine to oxazepam treatment of alcohol withdrawal. Am J Psychiatry 1989; 146:617–21.

Maletzky BM. The diagnosis of pathological intoxication. Q J Stud Alcohol 1976; 37:1215–28.

Manschreck TC, Allen DF, Neville M. Freebase psychosis: cases from a Bahamian epidemic of cocaine abuse. Compr Psychiatry 1987; 28:555–64.

Martin WA, Jasinski DR. Physiological parameters of morphine dependence in man – tolerance, early abstinence and protracted abstinence. J Psychiatr Res 1969; 7:7–9.

Martinez-Cano H, Vela-Bueon A, de Iceta M et al. Benzodiazepine withdrawal syndrome seizures. Pharmacopsychiatry 1995; 28:257–62.

Mathers DC, Ghodse AH. Cannabis and psychotic illness. Br J Psychiatry 1992; 161:648–53.

May PRA, Ebaugh FG. Pathological intoxication, alcoholic hallucinosis, and other reactions to alcohol: a clinical study. Q J Stud Alcohol 1953; 14:200–27.

Melges FT. Tracking difficulties and paranoid ideation during hashish and alcohol intoxication. Am J Psychiatry 1976; 133:1024–8.

Melges FT, Tinklenberg JR, Hollister LE et al. Temporal disintegration and depersonalization during marijuana intoxication. Arch Gen Psychiatry 1970; 23:204–10.

Mendelson JH, Mello NK, Lex BW et al. Marijuana withdrawal syndrome in a woman. Am J Psychiatry 1984; 141:1289–90.

Meyer JS, Greifenstein F, Devault M. A new drug causing symptoms of sensory deprivation. J Nerv Ment Dis 1959; 129:54–61.

Minion GE, Slovid CM, Boutiette L. Severe alcohol intoxication: a study of 204 consecutive patients. Clin Toxicol 1989; 27:375–84.

Morley KC, Teesson M, Reid SC et al. Naltrexone versus acamprosate in the treatment of alcohol dependence: a multi-centre, randomized, double-blind, placebo-controlled trial. Addiction 2006; 101:1451–62.

Morris HH, Estes ML. Traveler's amnesia: transient global amnesia due to triazolam. JAMA 1987; 258:945–6.

Murphy SM, Owen RT, Tyrer PJ. Withdrawal symptoms after six weeks' treatment with diazepam. Lancet 1984; 2:1389.

Murphy SM, Owen RT, Tyrer PJ. Comparative assessment of efficacy and withdrawal symptoms after 6 and 12 weeks' treatment with diazepam or buspirone. Br J Psychiatry 1989; 154:529–34.

Nielsen J. Delirium tremens in Copenhagen. Acta Psychiatr Scand 1965; 41(suppl. 187):1–92.

Nolte KB, Brass LM, Fletterick CF. Intracranial hemorrhage associated with cocaine abuse: a prospective autopsy study. Neurology 1996; 46:1291–6.

Noyes R, Perry PJ, Crowe RR *et al.* Seizures following withdrawal of alprazolam. *J Nerv Ment Dis* 1986; **174**:50–2.

Nurnberger JL, Simmons-Aling S, Kessler L *et al.* Separate mechanisms for behavioral, cardiovascular, and hormonal responses to dextroamphetamine in man. *Psychopharmacology* 1984; **84**:200–4.

Paasma R, Hovda KE, Tikkerberi A *et al.* Methanol mass poisoning in Estonia: outbreak in 154 patients. *Clin Toxicol* 2007; **45**:152–7.

Palsson A, Thulin SO, Tunving K. Cannabis psychosis in south Sweden. *Acta Psychiatr Scand* 1982; **66**:311–21.

Pascual-Leone A, Dhuna A. Cocaine-associated multifocal tics. *Neurology* 1990; **40**:999–1000.

Pearlson GD. Psychiatric and medical syndromes associated with phencyclidine (PCP) abuse. *Johns Hopkins Med J* 1981; **148**:25–33.

Perr IN. Pathological intoxication and alcohol idiosyncratic intoxication. I. Diagnostic and clinical aspects. *J Forensic Sci* 1986; **31**:806–11.

Rapoport JL, Jensvold M, Elkins R *et al.* Behavioral and cognitive effects of caffeine in boys and adult males. *J Nerv Ment Dis* 1981; **169**:726–32.

Reoux JP, Saxon AJ, Malte CA *et al.* Divalproex sodium in alcohol withdrawal: a randomized double-blind placebo-controlled trial. *Alcohol Clin Exp Res* 2001; **25**:1324–9.

Ricaurte GA, Forno LS, Wilson MA *et al.* ($\pm$)3,4-methylenedioxymethamphetamine selectively damages central serotoninergic neurons in nonhuman primates. *JAMA* 1988; **260**:51–5.

Rich J, Scheife RT, Katz N *et al.* Isopropyl alcohol intoxication. *Arch Neurol* 1990; **47**:322–4.

Rickels K, Schweizer E, Case G *et al.* Long-term therapeutic use of benzodiazepines. I. Effects of abrupt discontinuation. *Arch Gen Psychiatry* 1990; **47**:899–907.

Roache J, Griffiths RR. Lorazepam and meprobamate dose effects in humans: behavioral effects and abuse liability. *J Pharmacol Exp Ther* 1987; **243**:978–88.

Rosebush PI, Mazurek MF. Catatonia after benzodiazepine withdrawal. *J Clin Psychopharmacol* 1996; **16**:315–19.

Rosenbaum M, Lewis M, Piker P *et al.* Convulsive seizures in delirium tremens. *Arch Neurol Psychiatry* 1941; **45**:486–93.

Rosse RB, Collins JP, Fay-McCarthy M *et al.* Phenomenologic comparison of the idiopathic psychosis of schizophrenia and drug-induced cocaine and phencyclidine psychoses: a retrospective study. *Clin Neuropharmacol* 1994; **17**:349–69.

Roth D, Alarcon FJ, Fernandez JA. Acute rhabdomyolysis associated with cocaine intoxication. *N Engl J Med* 1988; **319**:673–7.

Satel SL, Southwick SM, Gawin FH. Clinical features of cocaine-induced paranoia. *Am J Psychiatry* 1991; **148**:495–8.

Scharf MB, Saskin P, Fletcher K. Benzodiazepine-induced amnesia: clinical laboratory findings. *J Clin Psychiatry* 1987; Monograph 5:14–17.

Schuckit MA, Smith TL, Anthenelli R *et al.* Clinical course of alcoholism in 636 male inpatients. *Am J Psychiatry* 1993; **150**:786–92.

Schweizer E, Rickels KV, Case WG *et al.* Carbamazepine treatment in patients discontinuing long-term benzodiazepine therapy: effects on withdrawal severity and outcome. *Arch Gen Psychiatry* 1991; **48**:448–52.

Seifert J, Peters E, Jahn K *et al.* Treatment of alcohol withdrawal: clomethiazole vs. carbamazepine and the effect on memory performance – a pilot study. *Addict Biol* 2004; **9**:43–51.

Shader RI, Greenblatt DJ. Use of benzodiazepines in anxiety disorders. *N Engl J Med* 1993; **328**:1398–405.

Sharpe JA, Hostovsky M, Bilbao JM *et al.* Methanol optic neuropathy: a histopathological study. *Neurology* 1982; **32**:1093–100.

Shearman JD, Chapman RWG, Satsangi J *et al.* Misuse of ecstasy. *BMJ* 1992; **305**:309.

Sherer MA, Kumor KM, Cone EJ *et al.* Suspiciousness induced by four-hour intravenous infusion of cocaine. Preliminary findings. *Arch Gen Psychiatry* 1988; **45**:673–7.

Shoptaw S, Yang X, Rotheram-Fuller EJ *et al.* Randomized placebo-controlled trial of baclofen for cocaine dependence: preliminary effects for individuals with chronic patterns of cocaine use. *J Clin Psychiatry* 2003; **64**:1440–8.

Silverman K, Evans SM, Strain EC *et al.* Withdrawal syndrome after the double-blind cessation of caffeine consumption. *N Engl J Med* 1992; **327**:1109–14.

Srisurapanont M, Jarusuraisin N. Amitriptyline vs. lorazepam in the treatment of opiate-withdrawal insomnia: a randomized double-blind study. *Acta Psychiatr Scand* 1998; **97**:233–5.

Steffee CH, Davis GJ, Nicol KK. A whiff of death: fatal volatile solvent inhalation abuse. *South Med J* 1996; **89**:879–84.

Strain EG, Mumford GK, Silverman K *et al.* Caffeine dependence syndrome: evidence from case histories and experimental evaluations. *JAMA* 1994; **272**:1043–8.

Strassman RJ, Qualls CR. Dose–response study of N,N-dimethyltryptamine in humans. I. Neuroendocrine, autonomic, and cardiovascular effects. *Arch Gen Psychiatry* 1994a; **51**:85–97.

Strassman, RJ, Qualls CR, Uhlenhuth EH *et al.* Dose-response of N,N-dimethyltryptamine in humans. II. Subjective effects and preliminary results of a new rating scale. *Arch Gen Psychiatry* 1994b; **51**:98–108.

Stuppacek CH, Pycha R, Miller C *et al.* Carbamazepine versus oxazepam in the treatment of alcohol withdrawal: a double-blind study. *Alcohol Alcoholism* 1992; **27**:153–8.

Talbott JA, Teague JW. Marijuana psychosis. *JAMA* 1969; **210**:299–302.

Tamerin JS, Weiner S, Poppen R *et al.* Alcohol and memory: amnesia and short-term memory function during experimentally induced intoxication. *Am J Psychiatry* 1971; **128**:1659–64.

Taverner D, Harrison DJ, Bell GM. Acute renal failure due to interstitial nephritis induced by 'glue sniffing' with subsequent recovery. *Scott Med J* 1988; **33**:246–7.

Torrens M, San L, Cami J. Buprenorphine versus heroin dependence: comparison of toxicologic and psychopathologic characteristics. *Am J Psychiatry* 1993; **150**:822–4.

Tyrer HR, Owen R, Dawling S. Gradual withdrawal of diazepam after long-term therapy. *Lancet* 1983; **1**:1402–6.

Ungerleider JT, Fisher DD, Fuller M. The dangers of LSD. *JAMA* 1966; **197**:389–92.

Virmani R, Robinowitz M, Smialek JE *et al.* Cardiovascular effects of cocaine: an autopsy study of 40 patients. *Am Heart J* 1988; **115**:1068–76.

Wagena EJ, Knipschild PG, Huibers MJ *et al.* Efficacy of bupropion and nortriptyline for smoking cessation among people at risk of or with chronic obstructive pulmonary disease. *Arch Int Med* 2005; **165**:2286–92.

Watson JM. Glue sniffing: two case reports. *Practitioner* 1979; **222**:845–7.

Watson R, Hartmann E, Schildkraut JJ. Amphetamine withdrawal: affective state, sleep patterns, and MHPG excretion. *Am J Psychiatry* 1972; **129**:263–9.

Weddington WW, Brown BS, Haertzen CA *et al.* Changes in mood, craving, and sleep during short-term abstinence reported by male cocaine addicts. *Arch Gen Psychiatry* 1990; **47**:861–8.

Weil AJ. Adverse reactions to marijuana. *N Engl J Med* 1970; **282**:997–1000.

Weiner AL, Vieira L. McKay CA *et al.* Ketamine abusers presenting to the emergency department: a case series. *J Emerg Med* 2000; **18**:447–51.

Whitaker-Azmita PM, Aronson TA. 'Ecstasy' (MDMA)-induced panic. *Am J Psychiatry* 1989; **146**:119.

Winstock AR. Chronic paranoid psychosis after misuse of MDMA. *BMJ* 1991; **302**:1150–1.

Wolkowitz OM, Weingartner H, Thompson K *et al.* Diazepam-induced amnesia: a neuropharmacological model of an 'organic amnesic syndrome'. *Am J Psychiatry* 1987; **144**:25–9.

Wood CA, Buller F. Poisoning by wood alcohol. Cases of death and blindness from Columbian spirits and other methylated preparations. *JAMA* 1904; **43**:972–7, 1058–62, 1117–23, 1213–21.

Yen DJ, Wang SJ, Ju TH *et al.* Stroke associated with methamphetamine inhalation. *Eur Neurol* 1994; **34**:16–22.

Zakzanis KK, Young DA. Memory impairment in abstinent MDMA ('Ecstasy') users: a longitudinal investigation. *Neurology* 2001; **56**:966–9.

Zipursky RB, Baker RW, Zimmer B. Alprazolam withdrawal delirium unresponsive to diazepam: case report. *J Clin Psychiatry* 1985; **46**:344–5.

Medication and substance-induced disorders

22.1 NEUROLEPTIC MALIGNANT SYNDROME

The neuroleptic malignant syndrome is a rare and potentially fatal disorder characterized by delirium, fever, rigidity, and autonomic instability, which occurs secondary to an abrupt diminution of dopaminergic tone, either due to the use of a dopamine-blocking agent, such as an antipsychotic, or, much less commonly, to discontinuation of a dopaminergic agent, such as levodopa.

Before proceeding further, some words are in order regarding the name of this syndrome. This syndrome was first described in association with the use of antipsychotics; at the time, the original name for an antipsychotic, namely 'neuroleptic', was in use, and consequently this malignant syndrome was referred to as the neuroleptic malignant syndrome. With the discovery that a reduction in dopaminergic tone secondary to discontinuation of a dopaminergic agent could also cause the syndrome, it might have been appropriate to change the name, perhaps to something like 'hypodopaminergic malignant syndrome'; however, this didn't occur. Another name change might also have been appropriate when 'neuroleptic' fell out of favor and the term 'antipsychotic' gained currency, such as to 'antipsychotic malignant syndrome'; however, this too failed to occur. Hence we are left with 'neuroleptic malignant syndrome', a term that, apparently, is going to persist.

Clinical features

The onset is usually within a day or two of the diminution in dopaminergic tone; exceptionally, the syndrome may appear within an hour or, at the other extreme, be delayed for weeks (Keck *et al.* 1987).

The full syndrome, as noted, is characterized by delirium, fever, rigidity, and autonomic instability, and, although it typically presents with rigidity, any one of these elements may be the presenting feature (Addonizio *et al.* 1987; Caroff 1980; Kellam 1987; Pope *et al.* 1986; Rosebush and Stewart 1989; Velamoor *et al.* 1994). Delirium may be profound, and patients may also develop stuporous catatonia (Koch *et al.* 2000). Fever is generally over 38.9°C (102°F) and, although most patients have at least some temperature elevation, there are rare reports of the syndrome occurring without fever (Peiris *et al.* 2000). Rigidity may be of either the lead pipe or cogwheel type, is typically generalized, and may be profound, to the point of compromising chest wall movement. Rigidity may be accompanied by a generalized, coarse tremor and, in some cases, dystonia or chorea may occur. Autonomic instability manifests with pallor, diaphoresis, tachycardia, and elevated blood pressure, which may be quite labile.

Rhabdomyolysis may occur (Jones and Dawson 1989), with myoglobinuria and, in some cases, acute renal failure. The white blood cell count is typically elevated to around 15 000 cells/mm^3, and the creatine phosphokinase level is likewise increased, often to around 15 000 units/L. Lactate dehydrogenase, serum glutamic oxaloacetic transaminase, and alkaline phosphatase levels are also often elevated. Aspiration or pulmonary emboli may occur and, in some cases, respiratory failure may occur secondary to extreme rigidity of the chest wall. A minority of patients develop disseminated intravascular coagulation.

Course

The mortality rate is between 10 and 20 percent. Those who survive generally recover without sequelae within a week or two, although an exception to this rule occurs in the case of the neuroleptic malignant syndrome occurring secondary to treatment with long-acting depot preparations of the antipsychotics fluphenazine, haloperidol or risperidone, in which the syndrome generally extends for a month or more.

Rarely, rigidity or catatonia may persist for months, even in cases in which a depot antipsychotic has not been used (Caroff *et al.* 2000).

Etiology

As noted earlier, the syndrome occurs secondary to an abrupt diminution of dopaminergic tone, and most commonly this occurs secondary to either initiation of treatment with an antipsychotic or a substantial dose increase (Kellam 1990). Although most cases have occurred secondary to treatment with first-generation agents, such as haloperidol, the neuroleptic malignant syndrome has also been seen with second-generation agents, such as risperidone (Levin *et al.* 1996; Meterissian 1996), olanzapine (Levenson 1999; Suh *et al.* 2003), quetiapine (Sing *et al.* 2002), aripiprazole (Brunelle *et al.* 2007), ziprasidone (Ozen *et al.* 2007), and clozapine (Anderson and Powers 1991; Das Gupta and Young 1991; Miller *et al.* 1991; Sachdev *et al.* 1995). Other dopamine blockers may also cause the syndrome, such as metoclopramide (Friedman *et al.* 1987) and promethazine (Mendhekar and Andrade 2005). The syndrome has also occurred secondary to treatment with the antidepressant amoxapine (Taylor and Schwartz 1988); however, in all likelihood the cause here is not amoxapine but one of its metabolites, loxapine, which is also a first-generation antipsychotic. There are also reports of the syndrome occurring after an antidepressant was added to a stable dose of an antipsychotic, for example with the addition of venlafaxine to trifluoperazine (Nimmagadda *et al.* 2000) or paroxetine to olanzapine (Kontaxakis *et al.* 2003).

The neuroleptic malignant syndrome has also been seen upon the cessation of treatment with not only levodopa (Friedman *et al.* 1984; Gibb and Griffith 1986; Keyser and Rodnitzky 1991; Sechi *et al.* 1984; Toru *et al.* 1981) but also amantadine (Cunningham *et al.* 1991; Harsch 1987) and a combination of levodopa and bromocriptine (Figa-Talamanca *et al.* 1985). In addition, the neuroleptic malignant syndrome has been reported secondary to the use of the dopamine-depleting drug tetrabenazine (Ossemann *et al.* 1996).

Although the mechanism by which this abrupt diminution of dopaminergic tone produces the syndrome is not known with certainty, it is suspected that there is a corresponding profound disturbance of hypothalamic functioning, and indeed in one autopsied case necrotic changes were present in the anterior and lateral hypothalamic nuclei (Horn *et al.* 1988).

Differential diagnosis

Malignant hyperthermia is distinguished by its association with the use of inhalational anesthetic agents or succinylcholine.

Heat stroke is suggested by the appearance of symptoms during a 'heat wave' or secondary to strenuous exercise in hot weather; furthermore, in heat stroke the skin is hot and dry and there is no rigidity, in contest to the diaphoresis and rigidity seen in the neuroleptic malignant syndrome.

Recently, a very similar syndrome has been described secondary to abrupt discontinuation of long-term treatment with either oral (Turner and Gainsborough 2001) or intrathecal (Coffey *et al.* 2002) baclofen. Whether this represents a distinct syndrome or merely a subtype of the neuroleptic malignant syndrome is not clear; in any case, symptoms subside with reinstitution of treatment.

Patients with parkinsonism, for example patients with Parkinson's disease, who become febrile, for example secondary to an infection, may resemble patients with the neuroleptic malignant syndrome. Here, however, history may reveal that the doses of the patient's dopaminergic agents have not been reduced; furthermore, the tremor seen in parkinsonism is typically pill-rolling, in contrast to the coarse tremor of the neuroleptic malignant syndrome.

Moderate or severe intoxication with phencyclidine is distinguished by the absence of rigidity and by the presence of nystagmus or myoclonus. Severe intoxication with stimulants or with cocaine (Daras *et al.* 1995) may produce delirium with diaphoresis, elevated temperature and pulse, and, in some cases, rigidity; hence, whenever there is doubt, a drug screen should be ordered.

Stauder's lethal catatonia, discussed in Section 3.11, may arise out of excited catatonia and is characterized by severe agitation with fever, tachycardia, and a leukocytosis; with progression, stupor may supervene. As almost all cases of excited catatonia occur in schizophrenia, and as most patients with schizophrenia are treated with an antipsychotic, the overall clinical picture may appear similar to the neuroleptic malignant syndrome. Helpful diagnostic points include the history of preceding excited catatonia and the fact that lethal catatonia first presents with an increase in agitation, in contrast to the neuroleptic malignant syndrome, which typically presents with rigidity and delirium (Castillo *et al.* 1989).

Treatment

The neuroleptic malignant syndrome constitutes a medical emergency. Intensive supportive care is required, with particular attention to fluid and electrolyte balance; adequate hydration must be assured to reduce the risk of renal failure. Cooling blankets may be required, as may ventilatory support. In addition to these measures it is critical to restore dopaminergic tone as quickly as possible. Thus, if a neuroleptic agent is at fault it should be discontinued, and if a dopaminergic agent has been stopped it should be restarted. Another strategy includes the use of bromocriptine and/or dantrolene (Granato *et al.* 1983; Guze and Baxter 1985; May *et al.* 1983; Mueller *et al.* 1983). Although these agents have not been assessed in controlled trials, anecdotal reports support their use. Bromocriptine is given orally, by nasogastric tube if necessary, in doses ranging from 2.5 to 20 mg t.i.d., and dantrolene is given intravenously in a dose of 1–2 mg/kg, which is repeated as necessary to a maximum of 10 mg/kg/24 hours. Recent double-blind work in cases secondary to withdrawal of dopaminergic agents in patients with Parkinson's disease demonstrated that the addition of intravenous methylprednisolone (1000 mg daily) to combined treatment with bromocriptine (7.5 mg daily) and dantrolene (75 mg daily) for a 3-day course not only further reduced the severity of the syndrome but also shortened its overall course (Sato *et al.* 2003). Finally, there are case reports (Lattanzi *et al.* 2006; Wang and Hsieh 2001) of the successful use of subcutaneous apomorphine, which may be given in a dose of 2 mg every 3 hours for 2 days, then every 6 hours for an additional 2 days (Lattanzi *et al.* 2006).

Another very important treatment option is electroconvulsive therapy (ECT) (Caroff *et al.* 2000; Davis *et al.* 1991; Hermesh *et al.* 1987; Troller and Sachdev 1999), which appears to be safe and effective in the treatment of antipsychotic-induced neuroleptic malignant syndrome.

In many cases of the neuroleptic malignant syndrome occurring secondary to an antipsychotic, patients require ongoing treatment. In such cases it has been found possible to reinstitute treatment with an antipsychotic (Rosebush *et al.* 1989) provided that one waits for at least 2 weeks after the neuroleptic malignant syndrome has entirely cleared and then reintroduces the antipsychotic cautiously, starting with a low dose and increasing very gradually. Although there are case reports of the successful reinstitution of treatment with the same agent that caused the syndrome, prudence dictates using a different antipsychotic. Thus, if a high-potency first-generation agent was used, one should probably choose either a low-potency first-generation agent or a second-generation one. If the syndrome has occurred secondary to a second-generation agent, then one might consider an alternate second-generation agent with a statistically lower chance of producing extrapyramidal side-effects

22.2 TARDIVE DYSKINESIA

Tardive dyskinesia is a movement disorder occurring as a side-effect of chronic treatment with antipsychotic drugs. In contrast to the more common typical 'extrapyramidal' side-effects seen with these agents, however, tardive dyskinesia does not remit promptly when the offending medication is discontinued, but rather persists for prolonged periods and may be permanent.

The most typical, and by far the most common, form of tardive dyskinesia is a choreiform one, often with bucco-lingual-masticatory movements. Less commonly, one encounters dystonic and akathetic forms, and rarely one may see tics or pain. Although some authors treat these less common forms as separate entities, this distinction appears unwarranted. Another nosologic dispute centers on the question of whether there is any fundamental difference between those cases that are permanent and those in which the abnormal movements remit spontaneously within a few months of the discontinuation of the antipsychotic. Some have referred to the latter form as 'withdrawal dyskinesia', but this distinction too may be unwarranted; in all likelihood, tardive dyskinesia, like many disorders, varies in severity, with some cases demonstrating permanent symptomatology and others displaying a spontaneous remission.

The overall prevalence of tardive dyskinesia in those treated chronically with first-generation antipsychotics is in the order of 20 percent (Woerner *et al.* 1991); the prevalence in those treated with second-generation agents is far less (Beasley *et al.* 1999; Tenback *et al.* 2005).

Clinical features

Although some cases of tardive dyskinesia have been reported after only a month of treatment with an antipsychotic, this is quite rare; in general, at least 6 months are required, and often 1 or more years pass before the abnormal movements appear. An exception to this rule is seen in the elderly, in whom the latency between initiation of treatment and the appearance of abnormal movements may be much shorter (Kane and Smith 1982; Saltz *et al.* 1991).

The mode of onset may be either acute or gradual. An acute onset may occur when the antipsychotic is discontinued or the dose rapidly decreased, in which case an abrupt 'unmasking' occurs with an equally abrupt appearance of abnormal movements. Conversely, if the dose is maintained, or decreased only slightly, the abnormal movements may make their appearance gradually or insidiously.

As noted earlier, tardive dyskinesia may manifest with chorea, dystonia, akathisia, tics, or pain, and each of these presentations is considered in turn.

Choreiform movements in tardive dyskinesia are most commonly found in the lower part of the face (Burke *et al.* 1982; Kang *et al.* 1986), less so in the extremities, and only rarely in the trunk, and range in severity from mild to disabling (Kennedy 1969). Classically, one sees buccolinguomasticatory movements in the face, with pursing or puckering of the lips, chewing motions, and repetitive tongue protrusions. Facial grimacing may also be seen, but this, importantly, spares the forehead. Extremity involvement may present with shoulder-shrugging or a restless piano-playing movement of the fingers and hands; in the lower extremities there may be foot-tapping. Truncal involvement may manifest with axial to-and-fro rocking or with pelvic thrusting. Uncommonly, respiratory dyskinesias may occur, with irregular, grunting respirations (Chiang *et al.* 1985; Ivanovitch *et al.* 1993; Rich and Radwany 1994; Yassa and Lal 1986a). Critically, the choreiform movements of tardive dyskinesia tend to be repetitive and stereotyped (Stacy *et al.* 1993); furthermore, they tend to wax and wane in severity throughout the day, and they disappear in sleep. Some patients are able to suppress them voluntarily, but such suppression is at best temporary and they inevitably reappear.

Dystonic movements (Burke *et al.* 1982; Kang *et al.* 1986; Kiriakakis *et al.* 1998; Sachdev 1993a; Wojcik *et al.* 1991; Yassa *et al.* 1986) typically appear focally and most commonly involve the face or neck, followed by the upper extremity, the trunk, and the lower extremity. Over a long period of time, segmental spread to adjacent body parts may occur, and, rarely, the dystonia may become generalized (Burke *et al.* 1982; Wojcik *et al.* 1991). Facial involvement may manifest with blepharospasm (Ananth *et al.* 1988; Glazer *et al.* 1983; Weiner *et al.* 1981), oromandibular dystonia (Tan and Jankovic 2000), or oculogyric crises (FitzGerald and Jankovic 1989; Sachdev 1993b). As with chorea, the severity of tardive dystonia ranges from mild to disabling (Yadalam *et al.* 1990). Importantly, many patients with tardive dystonia will also have choreiform movements (Sachdev 1993a; Wojcik *et al.* 1991).

Akathisia occurring on a tardive basis is symptomatically very similar to that occurring as an acute extrapyramidal side-effect of an antipsychotic, with restlessness, marching in place, and 'restless' thoughts (Burke *et al.* 1989; Dufresne and Wagner 1988; Lang 1994; Sachdev and Loneragan 1991).

Tics may be either focal or multifocal, and at times are so extensive as to mimic the picture seen in Tourette's syndrome (Bharucha and Sethi 1995; Stahl 1980), thus prompting the term 'tardive tourettism'.

Pain represents the rarest expression of tardive dyskinesia, and patients may complain of burning pain in the mouth or genital area; this typically occurs in the setting of choreiform movements or akathisia (Ford *et al.* 1994).

Course

The course of tardive dyskinesia has been most thoroughly studied with reference to the choreiform type. In situations in which the antipsychotic is continued at a constant dose, there is a gradual worsening of symptoms; although in most cases the severity eventually reaches and stays at a plateau, in a minority one sees a relentless progression (Gardos *et al.* 1988, 1994; Glazer *et al.* 1984; Yagi and Itoh 1987). Should the dose of the antipsychotic be substantially increased, there is a 'masking' of symptoms; however, this is temporary and they eventually reappear. Conversely, if the dose is decreased, symptoms worsen. If the antipsychotic is discontinued there is typically a pronounced worsening of symptoms, which is followed, however, over the succeeding weeks or months, by at least some diminution of symptoms, after which one of two eventualities may ensue (Glazer *et al.* 1990). In some cases, perhaps one-third, abnormal

movements continue to lessen and, after many months or a year or more, they go into a spontaneous remission. In the remainder, however, only a partial remission occurs, after which the abnormal movements persist indefinitely. This chronic course is more likely in the elderly and in those who have been treated with very high doses.

Interestingly, choreiform movements in tardive dyskinesia are worsened by anticholinergics (Greil *et al.* 1984), such as benztropine (Reunanen *et al.* 1982), and also may vary with mood. Patients who develop a depressive syndrome typically experience a worsening of symptoms (Sachdev 1989), whereas during mania there may be a partial remission (de Potter *et al.* 1983; Yazici *et al.* 1991); symptom improvement has also been noted during catatonic stupor (Assmann and van Woerkom 1987).

Etiology

Although the vast majority of cases of tardive dyskinesia occur secondary to treatment with antipsychotics, cases have also been reported with other dopamine blockers, such as metoclopramide (Sewell and Jeste 1992; Sewell *et al.* 1994), and secondary to chronic treatment with the antidepressant amoxapine (Huang 1986; Thornton and Stahl 1984); in this latter case, however, it is probably not amoxapine that is at fault but rather one of its metabolites, loxapine, which is an antipsychotic.

Given that all of the drugs capable of causing tardive dyskinesia have one thing in common, namely a blockade of post-synaptic dopamine receptors, and given that the risk of tardive dyskinesia increases with higher doses (Morganstern and Glazer 1993) and a longer duration of treatment (Glazer *et al.* 1993; Kane *et al.* 1988), it seems reasonable to suppose that it is some effect of the chronic dopamine blockade that is etiologic in this disorder, and, indeed, this is the basis for the dopamine up-regulation hypothesis. According to this hypothesis, with chronic dopamine blockade there is a gradually worsening compensatory up-regulation of the post-synaptic receptors to the point at which, if the dose of the dopamine blocker is reduced, the 'unmasking' of these up-regulated receptors leads to a hyperdopaminergic state and the production of the abnormal movements. Further support for a disturbance in dopamine transmission is provided by the response to anticholinergics in tardive dyskinesia. Dopaminergic and cholinergic systems exist in a balance in the basal ganglia, such that an increase in dopaminergic tone may be mimicked by a reduction in cholinergic tone and vice versa. Given this one would predict that, in patients with tardive dyskinesia, a reduction in cholinergic tone, as might occur with the administration of an anticholinergic medication, would increase the abnormal movements, and this is generally what happens (Klawans and Rubovits 1974).

As attractive as this dopamine theory is, it does not account for several important findings. First, the fact that acute antipsychotic-induced parkinsonism can co-exist with tardive dyskinesia (Richardson and Craig 1982) argues against any generalized hyperdopaminergic state, as theoretically this should bring a relief of the parkinsonism. Second, some cases of the dystonic subtype of tardive dyskinesia may, as noted below, be relieved by, rather than worsened by, anticholinergic agents. Finally, if it were simply a matter of the compensatory up-regulation of the postsynaptic dopamine receptors, then providing that the dose of a neuroleptic were held constant, with no dose decrease, one should not see any abnormal movements as there would be no 'unmasking' and thus no hyperdopaminergic state. Unfortunately for the theory, however, tardive dyskinesia does in fact emerge while patients continue at the same dose, a fact strongly suggesting that some other process, in addition perhaps to a progressive up-regulation, is at work.

The nature of this other process is not clear. Theories include disturbances in GABAergic transmission, glutamate toxicity, and progressive neuronal destruction by free radicals produced in the course of neuroleptic treatment. This last theory is of some interest given the evidence, noted below, for the treatment efficacy of vitamin E, an antioxidant.

Differential diagnosis

In evaluating a patient with abnormal movements the diagnosis of tardive dyskinesia cannot be considered unless the patient has undergone chronic treatment with an antipsychotic. The overall differential diagnoses of chorea, dystonia, akathisia, and tics are discussed in Sections 3.4, 3.7, 3.10, and 3.3 respectively; of the disorders discussed in these sections, several deserve special consideration.

Choreiform movements may occur in both Huntington's disease and schizophrenia, and both of these disorders are typically treated with antipsychotics. With regard to Huntington's disease, genetic testing is of course diagnostic; however, certain clinical features may also allow a differentiation to be made, including the presence of forehead chorea and a 'dancing and prancing' gait, both of which may be seen in Huntington's disease but not in tardive dyskinesia. The nature of the chorea itself provides another differential point: in Huntington's disease it is extremely transient, flickering from one part of the body to another in an almost random pattern, whereas in tardive dyskinesia the chorea tends to be stereotyped, repetitive, and persistently recurring in the same area. Schizophrenia may at times be characterized by choreiform movements, as pointed out by Kraepelin in the early part of the twentieth century (Kraepelin 1971) and confirmed by subsequent investigators (Farran-Ridge 1926; Mettler and Crandall 1959; Owens et al. 1982; Yarden and Discipio 1971); these choreiform movements, however, are mild, generally involve the face, and are present before any treatment with antipsychotics.

Both dystonia and akathisia may occur as *acute* extrapyramidal side-effects of antipsychotics but are readily distinguished from tardive dystonia or tardive akathisia by their course: acute side-effects occur shortly after the initiation or dose increase of an antipsychotic and subside with a dose decrease or discontinuation; by contrast, tardive dystonia and akathisia come on only after a long period of treatment and worsen when the dose is decreased or the antipsychotic is discontinued.

Tourette's syndrome typically has an onset in childhood, and the presence of tics before treatment with antipsychotics makes the diagnosis straightforward. As noted in Section 8.25, however, after a full or partial remission in late adolescence, there may be a relapse decades later, and if this relapse should occur in a patient being treated with an antipsychotic for another reason, diagnostic confusion may ensue; in such cases it is critical to obtain a childhood history, with special reference to the symptomatology of the prior tics to allow a comparison with the current ones.

Treatment

The best 'treatment' is prevention, and chronic antipsychotic treatment should not be undertaken for those disorders for which other medications with better side-effect profiles would be as effective.

When tardive dyskinesia does first appear, a decision must be made as to whether ongoing treatment with a neuroleptic is required, carefully weighing the risk of worsening dyskinesia against the risk of relapse. In the case of schizophrenia, the balance often tips towards continuing neuroleptic treatment. If treatment is continued, efforts, if not already in place, should be made to keep the dose as low as possible, consistent with adequate symptomatic control. In the past it was felt that intermittent 'drug holidays' for patients with schizophrenia might reduce the risk of tardive dyskinesia, but subsequent studies have suggested that drug holidays may actually *increase* the risk (Goldman and Luchins 1984; van Harten et al. 1998; Jeste et al. 1979). In cases due to treatment with a first-generation antipsychotic, consideration should be given to switching to a second-generation agent; with such a switch, adequate symptom control is maintained or improved and the risk of worsening tardive dyskinesia with further treatment is lessened.

In cases in which treatment cannot be discontinued, or in cases in which discontinuation is possible but symptoms fail to go into remission, various medical treatments may be considered, including vitamin E, vitamin B6, melatonin, branched chain amino acids, piracetam, and dopamine depletors, such as tetrabenazine, alpha-methyldopa or reserpine. In selected cases botulinum toxin may be considered, and in severe, treatment-resistant cases both ECT and deep brain stimulation constitute options.

Vitamin E, in doses ranging from 1200 to 1600 IU daily (divided into three doses), has been shown to be effective in most (Adler et al. 1993, 1998; Akhtar et al. 1993; Dabiri et al. 1994; Egan et al. 1992; Elkashef et al. 1990; Lohr and Caligiuri 1996; Lohr et al. 1988; Zhang et al. 2004), but not all (Adler *et al.* 1999; Shriqui *et al.* 1992), studies; weeks or months may be required to see a treatment response. Vitamin B6 may be given in a dose of 300 mg (Lerner *et al.* 2001), and melatonin in a dose of 10 mg (Shamir *et al.* 2001). From a pharmacologic viewpoint branched chain amino acids constitute an interesting option (Richardson *et al.* 2003). Administration of a combination of valine, isoleucine, and leucine (given in a ratio of 3:3:4 at a dose of 222 mg/kg three times daily) is followed by a fall in the plasma levels of the aromatic amino acids tyrosine and tryptophan, with presumably a fall in central nervous system levels of dopamine and serotonin, and it is this change that presumably accounts for the improvement in the tardive dyskinesia. Piracetam (not available in the United States), in a dose of 4800 mg/day, was recently found to be effective (Libov *et al.* 2007). The dopamine depleters tetrabenazine (Ondo *et al.* 1999) (not available in the United States), alpha-methyldopa, and reserpine (Huang *et al.* 1981) are likewise effective, presumably because of the reduction in dopaminergic tone.

Of these options, the vitamins and melatonin are the most benign, and one of these should probably be tried first; vitamin E has by far the most support and is a reasonable starting point. In some cases combination treatment with two or more of these agents may be appropriate. Branched chain amino acid treatment is also generally benign, but should not be used in diabetics. The dopamine depleters, given their unfavorable side-effect profile, should generally be held in reserve.

Botulinum toxin may be considered in cases in which the abnormal movement is well-localized, as may be seen with certain choreiform movements or, more especially, dystonia.

Anecdotally, ECT is effective for tardive dyskinesia (Adityanjee 1990), especially in cases in which the patient is depressed (Hay *et al.* 1990). Deep brain stimulation of the globus pallidus is effective (Damier *et al.* 2007) but for obvious reasons constitutes a last option.

Other options exist for tardive dystonia and for tardive akathisia. In the case of tardive dystonia, anecdotal reports support treatment with high-dose anticholinergic agents (Burke *et al.* 1982), such as 20 mg trihexyphenidyl (Fahn 1983); however, in cases in which the dystonia is accompanied by choreiform movements, these may worsen. Anecdotally, tardive akathisia may respond to propranolol (Yassa *et al.* 1988); however, high doses may be required.

22.3 SUPERSENSITIVITY PSYCHOSIS

Supersensitivity psychosis represents a very rare side-effect of chronic treatment with antipsychotic drugs. As such, it bears a strong etiologic relationship to tardive dyskinesia, and indeed this syndrome is also referred to as 'tardive psychosis'. This is, for some, a controversial diagnosis. As noted below (see Differential diagnosis) it may be difficult to distinguish supersensitivity psychosis from an exacerbation

of schizophrenia, and indeed some observers have held that all reported cases of supersensitivity psychosis represent merely such exacerbations. However, the occurrence of this supersensitivity psychosis in patients treated with antipsychotics who have never had symptoms of schizophrenia, or any other psychosis, clearly indicates that the syndrome, although rare, does exist (Moore 1986).

Clinical features

After a year or more of treatment with an antipsychotic, the syndrome emerges. This emergence may be fairly abrupt if the antipsychotic is discontinued or there is a rapid dose reduction; in other cases a more gradual onset may occur, for example when the dose of the antipsychotic is held constant or only gradually and modestly decreased.

Clinically (Chouinard and Jones 1980; Kirkpatrick *et al.* 1992; Moncrieff 2006; Steiner *et al.* 1990), patients develop a psychosis characterized by delusions and hallucinations. Tardive dyskinesia may or may not accompany this development.

Course

Although the course has not been well-studied, it appears that, in cases in which the antipsychotic is discontinued, symptoms very gradually lessen; the percentage of cases that go on to full remission or a stable chronicity is not known.

Etiology

Although the etiology is not known, it is speculated that with chronic treatment with antipsychotics there is an up-regulation of post-synaptic dopamine receptors within the limbic system leading to a chronic hyperdopaminergic state. Of note, cases have also been described secondary to chronic treatment with the dopamine-blocker metoclopramide (Lu *et al.* 2002).

Differential diagnosis

The diagnosis should only be entertained in patients who have been treated chronically with an antipsychotic or other dopamine blocker.

As most patients treated chronically with antipsychotics have schizophrenia, the main differential for supersensitivity psychosis is an exacerbation of the schizophrenia. For example, consider the case of a patient with schizophrenia who had been doing well and whose antipsychotic dose had been substantially reduced, after which there was a reappearance of hallucinations or delusions. The question here is whether this appearance of hallucinations and delusions represents merely the schizophrenia or whether the patient now has two disorders, namely schizophrenia and supersensitivity psychosis. One helpful differential point here lies in the course of the development of the hallucinations and delusions: exacerbations of schizophrenia are generally leisurely affairs, spanning weeks or months; by contrast, supersensitivity psychosis appears fairly promptly, often within days.

Patients with major depression or with bipolar disorder may also be treated chronically with antipsychotics, and the emergence of delusions and hallucinations in such patients may or may not represent a supersensitivity psychosis. The guiding differential point here is whether the delusions and hallucinations emerge in the context of a severe depression or mania. If they do then they may well be simply part of the expression of the underlying mood disorder; if, however, the patient was euthymic during the emergence of the psychosis, then the diagnosis of supersensitivity psychosis is more likely.

Treatment

The best treatment is prevention, and antipsychotics should not be used chronically in conditions that may respond to other agents.

In cases in which it is possible to discontinue the antipsychotic, this should be carried out, in the hope of achieving a gradual spontaneous remission. In cases in which ongoing treatment is required, or when discontinuation is not followed by a spontaneous remission, consideration may be given to increasing the dose of the antipsychotic to suppress symptoms; in such instances, if a first-generation agent has been at fault it is probably appropriate to switch to a second-generation one. Whether or not some of the treatments effective for tardive dyskinesia, such as vitamin E, are effective here is not certain; however, given the benign nature of these treatments a trial would be appropriate.

22.4 RABBIT SYNDROME

The rabbit syndrome is an uncommon movement disorder that generally occurs secondary to chronic treatment with an antipsychotic (Chiu et al. 1993; Yassa and Lal 1986b); although first-generation agents are the most common causes, cases have been reported with second-generation agents.

Clinical features

The onset is gradual, usually after a year or more of antipsychotic treatment. Clinically (Decina et al. 1990; Deshmukh et al. 1990; Todd et al. 1983), the syndrome is characterized by a rhythmic rest tremor of the jaw, with a frequency and amplitude such that the appearance is that of a rabbit chewing. Importantly, there is no involvement of the tongue or tremor elsewhere, nor is there any associated rigidity or bradykinesia.

Course

With continued antipsychotic treatment the tremor becomes more pronounced; with discontinuation of the antipsychotic the tremor gradually decreases in amplitude over weeks or months and, in most, but not all, cases, eventually remits.

Etiology

Apart from the fact that this disorder generally occurs secondary to antipsychotic treatment, the etiology is not known. Whether it represents a kind of acute, antipsychotic-induced parkinsonism, or rather a form of tardive dyskinesia, is simply not clear. To complicate matters further there are rare reports of the rabbit syndrome occurring secondary to treatment with antidepressants, such as imipramine (Fornazzari et al. 1991) and citalopram (Parvin and Swartz 2005).

Differential diagnosis

Essential tremor can produce a tremor of the jaw and chin; however, the tremor here is generally more rapid than the 'rabbit chewing' movement seen in the rabbit syndrome; furthermore in essential tremor one also finds a tremor in the hands, something that is absent in the rabbit syndrome.

Parkinsonism may also cause a jaw tremor; however, in parkinsonism this is accompanied by tremor of the hands and, at some point, rigidity and bradykinesia, findings absent in the rabbit syndrome.

Tardive dyskinesia may be considered, but the bucco-lingual-masticatory movement with repetitive tongue protrusion is fundamentally different from the chewing motion of the rabbit syndrome, in which the tongue is spared. Furthermore, anticholinergics worsen tardive dyskinesia, whereas, as noted below, they are of benefit in the rabbit syndrome.

Treatment

If possible, the antipsychotic should be discontinued to allow for a spontaneous resolution of the syndrome. If this is not possible, or if symptoms fail to fully remit, treatment with an anticholinergic agent, such as benztropine (Todd et al. 1983), is effective.

22.5 SEROTONIN SYNDROME

The serotonin syndrome, characterized classically by delirium and myoclonus, is a potentially fatal complication arising from any pharmacologic maneuver that abruptly increases serotoninergic tone within the central nervous system.

Clinical features

The onset occurs within hours or days of one of the pharmacologic maneuvers noted below (see Etiology).

Clinically (Bodner *et al.* 1995; Boyer and Shannon 2005; Feighner *et al.* 1990; Mason *et al.* 2000; Sternbach 1991), patients present with varying admixtures of delirium, myoclonus, dysarthria or ataxia, and hyper-reflexia (especially in the lower extremities). Other signs and symptoms may include extensor plantar responses, coarse tremor, shivering, and diaphoresis. In severe cases one may see hyperthermia, seizures, rhabdomyolysis, renal failure, cardiac arrhythmias, and disseminated intravascular coagulation.

Course

Although potentially fatal, most patients recover, and if nothing else is done besides discontinuing the offending medications, the syndrome gradually remits within anywhere from a day to a week.

Etiology

This syndrome occurs secondary to any of a large number of pharmacologic maneuvers, all of which have in common the effect of abruptly increasing serontoninergic tone within the central nervous system. Although, as noted below, the syndrome has been reported after monotherapy with serotoninergic agents, this is very rare (except in the case of overdose) and the vast majority of cases occur secondary to combinations of agents. Of these combinations, the one with by far the highest risk is an monamine oxidase inhibitor (MAOI) and a selective serotonin reuptake inhibitor (SSRI), and this combination should not be used.

Other combinations of some concern include the following: an MAOI with a tricyclic or with venlafaxine; and an SSRI with a tricyclic. With regard to the tricyclics, special attention should be paid to the use of clomipramine, as it has strong serotoninergic effects. Although these combinations can cause the syndrome, this is quite uncommon, and indeed the combination of an MAOI and a tricyclic is one of the recommended treatments for resistant depression.

Various other combinations have also been reported to cause the syndrome, but in general these combinations are quite safe. They include an MAOI with duloxetine, cyclobenzaprine or meperidine; an SSRI in combination with any one of the following: a triptan (e.g., sumatriptan), a second-generation antipsychotic (e.g., risperidone, olanzapine or quetiapine), an opioid (e.g., tramadol, fentanyl, hydromorphone, meperidine or pentazocine), carbamazepine, trazodone, mirtazapine, bupropion, buspirone, and, finally, levodopa; and lithium with a tricyclic, venlafaxine or a triptan. Unusual combinations include trazodone with venlafaxine, buspirone or bupropion; buspirone and bupropion; and cyclobenzaprine and duloxetine.

Monotherapy with serotoninergic agents at therapeutic doses can cause the syndrome, but this is quite rare; it has been reported for SSRIs, tricyclics, venlafaxine, mirtazapine, and trazodone. With overdoses of SSRIs, however, the syndrome is not uncommon.

Before leaving this discussion, mention should be made of tryptophan and of a relatively new antibiotic, linezolid. Tryptophan, a serotonin precursor, has been banned in the United States but may be found in various 'supplements', some of which may not be labelled as such, and the syndrome has occurred with the combination of tryptophan and an MAOI, an SSRI or a tricyclic. Linezolid, in addition to being an antibiotic, also inhibits MAO, and there has been some concern that it could have the same ability to cause the serotonin syndrome as do the other MAOIs. As it turns out, however, these fears are generally unfounded; although cases have been reported with the combination of linezolid and an SSRI, they appear to be rare.

Differential diagnosis

The occurrence of delirium in the setting of any of the pharmacologic maneuvers noted above, under Etiology, should suggest the serotonin syndrome. In some cases, however, the medication history may not be available, and here consideration must be given to other causes of the combination of delirium and myoclonus, including uremic encephalopathy, hepatic encephalopathy, hyperosmolar non-ketotic hyperglycemia, Hashimoto's encephalopathy, baclofen withdrawal, complex partial status epilepticus, and encephalopathic pellagra.

Treatment

The offending medications must be discontinued and vigorous supportive care should be provided; in cases of severe hyperthermia, consideration should be given to paralysis with a non-depolarizing agent. Agitation may be treated with lorazepam; however, specific treatment with cyproheptadine, a serotonin antagonist, should be undertaken. Cyproheptadine may be given in a dose of 4–8 mg every 2 hours, or in a loading dose of 12 mg followed by 2 mg every 2 hours, until symptoms are controlled or a maximum dose of 32 mg is reached. Most patients respond within a day; additional doses may or may not be required, depending, in part, on the half-lives of the medications at fault.

22.6 ANTICHOLINERGIC DELIRIUM

In sufficient dosage, any drug with anticholinergic properties that crosses the blood–brain barrier may cause a delirium. Old age and medical frailty increase the risk, and anticholinergic toxicity is a prominent cause of delirium in hospitalized patients (Han *et al.* 2001), especially in post-operative cases (Tune *et al.* 1981).

Of some literary interest is the possibility that the Reverend Dimmesdale, of Nathaniel Hawthorne's *The Scarlet Letter*, may himself have succumbed to an herbal preparation with anticholinergic properties, administered by the good Doctor Chillingworth (Khan 1984).

Clinical features

Clinically (Itil and Fink 1966), there is delirium and restlessness or agitation, often accompanied by visual hallucinations. On examination, the temperature and pulse are elevated, the skin is typically dry and flushed (at times to a scarlet hue), the pupils are dilated, and the deep tendon reflexes are brisk. Urinary retention may occur and, in severe cases, there may be seizures, coma, respiratory depression, and death.

Course

In the natural course of events, provided that the offending medication is discontinued, there is a gradual remission of symptoms, consistent with the half-life of the anticholinergic in question.

Etiology

Any of a large number of drugs with anticholinergic properties may, if given in sufficient dose, cause a delirium (Tune *et al.* 1981); although in most cases relatively high doses are required, individual sensitivity varies widely, and in some patients, especially the elderly, seemingly innocuous doses can have devastating results. Anticholinergically active drugs to consider include the following: atropine, scopolamine (Vonderahe 1929; Ziskind 1988), and homatropine ophthalmic drops (Tune *et al.* 1992); anticholinergic antiparkinsonian agents (De Smet *et al.* 1982) such as benztropine, biperidin, and trihexyphenidyl (Porteous and Ross 1956); tricyclic antidepressants (Goodwin 1983; Preskorn and Simpson 1982); antihistamines such as diphenhydramine (Tejera *et al.* 1994) and hydroxyzine; low-potency first-generation antipsychotics; cyclobenzaprine (Engel and Chapron 1993); and oxybutynin and tolteridone (Tsao and Heilman 2003). Delirium has also been noted with 'recreational' intoxication with Angel's trumpet (*Datura stramonium*) (Hall *et al.* 1977; Oberndorfer *et al.* 2002). Of all of these agents, diphenhydramine stands out (Agostino *et al.* 2001), not so much because of its inherent toxicity but because of the frequency with which it is used in hospitalized patients.

Differential diagnosis

Heat stroke is clinically similar to anticholinergic delirium; however, in heat stroke the temperature is often at 41.1°C (106°F), whereas in simple anticholinergic delirium it rarely rises above 40°C (104°F). Certainly, the diagnosis of heat stroke should not be considered unless the ambient temperature is quite high; however, in some cases of high ambient temperature when patients are taking anticholinergics, one may be confronted with an etiologically mixed picture in which the anticholinergic, by reducing sweating, sets the stage for the dramatic temperature increases seen in heat stroke.

Treatment

The anticholinergic should be stopped and, if ingestion is recent, consideration may be given to gastric lavage or activated charcoal. General supportive measures include intravenous fluids and, if the temperature is significantly elevated, cooling blankets. Seizures may be treated with lorazepam.

In emergent situations, treatment with physostigmine (Beaver and Gavin 1998; Burns *et al.* 2000; Duvoisin and Katz 1968; Stern 1983) may be considered; however, as noted below, this carries some risk. Physostigmine may be given intravenously in a dose of 0.5–2 mg, at a rate no faster than 1 mg/min, with repeat doses every 5–10 minutes until the patient is out of danger. Given the half-life of most anticholinergics, repeat doses of physostigmine are often required, initially every 30–60 minutes. A failure to respond to physostigmine essentially rules out a diagnosis of anticholinergic delirium. Physostigmine is not a benign treatment and patients may develop bradycardia, asystole or seizures; furthermore, in cases of tricyclic overdose, physostigmine has no effect on the development of arrhythmia, which is the main concern in this situation. Consequently, many clinicians will opt for conservative treatment and simply let the offending agent 'wash out', allowing the delirium to resolve on its own. In severe cases, however, with significant temperature elevations, seizures, coma or respiratory depression, treatment is justified.

22.7 CHOLINERGIC REBOUND

The abrupt discontinuation of medications with significant anticholinergic properties may, in about one-third of cases, be followed by a syndrome known as cholinergic rebound, or cholinergic overdrive.

Clinical features

The onset of cholinergic rebound is in large part determined by the half-life of the drug that has just undergone abrupt discontinuation; thus, in the case of most tricyclic antidepressants, the onset may be anticipated within 36–48 hours.

Clinically (Dilsaver 1989; Dilsaver *et al.* 1983a; Petti and Law 1981), patients present with depressed mood, anxiety, malaise, and insomnia; typically, there is also nausea and abdominal cramping, with, at times, vomiting and diarrhea.

Course

In the natural course of events, symptoms subside over 1–3 days.

Etiology

With chronic treatment with any drug possessing anti-cholinergic properties there is a compensatory up-regulation of post-synaptic acetylcholine receptors; if the drug is abruptly discontinued and there is insufficient time for a gradual 'down-regulation', the increased number of receptors is 'unmasked', resulting in an increase in cholinergic transmission and the symptoms seen in this disorder (Dilsaver et al. 1983b; Luchins et al. 1980). This has been noted with tricyclic antidepressants (Dilsaver et al. 1983a; Wolfe 1997), low-potency first-generation antipsychotics, the second-generation antipsychotic clozapine (Delassus-Guenault et al. 1999), and anti-parkinsonian anticholiner-gics, such as benztropine, atropine, and scopolamine.

Differential diagnosis

The appearance of depressed mood and insomnia shortly after stopping a tricyclic antidepressant may suggest a relapse of depression; however, the abruptness of the onset of symptoms is inconsistent with a relapse of depression, which would not be expected for at least a matter of weeks after stopping an antidepressant.

Treatment

The best treatment is prevention, and medications with strong anticholinergic effects should be tapered over 3 or 4 days. In cases in which rebound does occur, some patients may elect to simply wait it out. When symptoms are severe, however, one may restart the original medication, or, if this is not feasible, use another anticholinergic medication (e.g., benztropine in a dose of 1–2 mg), and adjust the dose to suppress symptoms, after which a gradual tapering may be undertaken (Wolfe 1997).

22.8 ALCOHOLIC DEMENTIA

Alcoholic dementia is one of the most common causes of dementia and indeed may account for approximately one-fifth of all cases among the institutionalized elderly (Carlen et al. 1994). Among chronic alcoholics, approximately 10 percent will develop this dreaded complication.

Clinical features

Alcoholic dementia presents insidiously, generally after decades of alcoholism. Clinically (Lee et al. 1979; Lishman 1981), patients typically present with a personality change, with frontal lobe features: there is a general coarsening of personality and a heedless disregard for social conventions; judgment becomes poor and some patients may become apathetic. Over time cognitive deficits gradually accrue, including short-term memory loss and concreteness; some patients may also develop minor 'cortical' signs such as apraxia, agnosia, and a minor degree of aphasia, but these signs are often almost subclinical and never play a major role in the overall clinical picture.

Computed tomography (CT) (Carlen et al. 1981; Gurling et al. 1984; Harper et al. 1985) and magnetic resonance (MR) (Jernigan et al. 1991; Schroth et al. 1988) scanning reveal both cortical atrophy and ventricular dilation, and there is a correlation between the extent of atrophy and the severity of the dementia (Carlen et al. 1981; Carlsson et al. 1979).

Course

With continued drinking the dementia progresses and may become profound; with abstinence a variable degree of recovery may be expected over about a 6-month period (Grant et al. 1984; Hambidge 1990), after which any remaining deficits tend to persist indefinitely.

Etiology

Alcohol, in all likelihood, is directly toxic to the white matter and perhaps also to cortical neurons. Autopsy studies have demonstrated a reduction in brain weight (Harper and Blumbergs 1982; Torvik et al. 1982) with overall cerebral atrophy (Harper and Krill 1985; Lynch 1960; Neuberger 1957), due primarily to loss of white matter (Harper et al. 1985; Jensen and Pakkenberg 1993); there is also some evidence for neuronal loss, particularly in the superior frontal cortex (Krill et al. 1997). Of note, it appears that some of these changes may be reversible: with sobriety, MR scanning has revealed re-expansion of the brain (Pfefferbaum et al. 1995; Schroth et al. 1988; Zipursky et al. 1989), primarily as a result of enlargement of the white matter (Agartz et al. 2003).

Differential diagnosis

Given the denial seen in alcoholism, at times this critical historical fact will be obscured, and in such cases the differential, as discussed in Section 5.1, is fairly wide, encompassing various dementias of gradual or subacute onset, often lacking in distinctive features, such as

Alzheimer's disease, Pick's disease, frontotemporal dementia, Binswanger's disease, etc.; given the propensity of alcoholics for falling, chronic subdural hematoma should also be considered. In cases in which the history of alcoholism is clear, one should also bear in mind that cognitive deficits associated with withdrawal may persist for some time; hence, the diagnosis of alcoholic dementia should probably be only tentative until a month or more of sobriety has been maintained.

Alcoholic dementia must also be distinguished from Korsakoff's syndrome; however, this should not be difficult. As discussed in Section 13.5, Korsakoff's syndrome is one of the amnestic syndromes, characterized by short-term memory loss and lacking the personality change and concreteness seen in alcoholic dementia.

Treatment

Adequate nutrition, including thiamine and niacin, and, above all, abstinence are essential. The overall treatment of alcoholism is discussed in Section 21.5. In cases in which patients are unable to participate successfully in rehabilitative efforts, institutionalization may be required.

22.9 ALCOHOL HALLUCINOSIS

Alcohol hallucinosis, also known as alcohol-induced psychotic disorder with hallucinations, is seen only in chronic alcoholics, typically after one or more decades of severe, heavy drinking. This psychosis is an uncommon disorder and may be more common in men than women.

Clinical features

The onset is typically abrupt, over a matter of days, and generally occurs in the context of either alcohol withdrawal or delirium tremens. Clinically (Victor and Hope 1958; Soyka 1990), the principal symptom of alcohol hallucinosis is auditory hallucinations. These are often extremely vivid and clear, and the patient has no doubt as to their reality. For the most part they are critical, deprecatory, and often persecutory. Generally, more than one voice is heard, and, curiously, the voices often talk among themselves. Visual hallucinations may also occur, but these are far less prominent than auditory hallucinations. Delusions of persecution and reference often accompany the auditory hallucinations, and are generally congruent with them. Patients may believe that others are plotting against them, or that the police are following them. Occasionally there may be Schneiderian first rank delusions, such as thought-broadcasting or delusions of influence (Soyka 1990). Patients are often constrained and very watchful, and tend to be irritable and querulous.

Course

With continued drinking, symptoms persist and may worsen. With abstinence, a gradual remission of symptoms of variable extent may occur over the following weeks or months. Should patients commence drinking again, symptoms typically recur, and, with another period of abstinence, the remission is generally not as substantial. Eventually, with repeated relapses, there may be a chronic persistence of symptoms, even with long-sustained sobriety.

Etiology

Although the etiology of alcohol hallucinosis is not clear, it does appear that the risk for developing this disorder rises in direct proportion to the severity of the alcoholism and, more importantly, to the frequency with which alcohol withdrawal and delirium tremens occurs. With this in mind, some investigators have proposed that alcohol hallucinosis is the end result of repeated 'kindling' within the temporal lobes. Importantly, alcohol hallucinosis is not etiologically related to paranoid schizophrenia (Schuckit and Winokur 1971).

Differential diagnosis

Delirium tremens may cause auditory hallucinations, and the fact that alcohol hallucinosis often has an onset in the course of delirium tremens sets the stage for some diagnostic difficulty. The question, however, may be resolved by observing the patient during enforced abstinence: in cases in which delirium tremens alone are present, all symptoms, including auditory hallucinations, gradually resolve; in cases, however, in which alcohol hallucinosis has appeared, the auditory hallucinations will persist despite resolution of other symptoms of delirium tremens, such as confusion, disorientation, tremor, etc.

Alcoholic paranoia, discussed in the next section, is distinguished by the prominence of delusions of persecution in the relative absence of any hallucinations.

Of the other causes of psychosis discussed in Section 7.1, the one that occasions the most diagnostic difficulty is paranoid schizophrenia. Patients with schizophrenia may also develop alcoholism; however, in these cases the psychosis generally occurs either before the onset of the alcoholism or relatively early on, in contrast to alcohol hallucinosis, which occurs only after a decade or more of heavy drinking. Certain symptoms may also enable a differential diagnosis to be made: loosening of associations, bizarre delusions, and bizarre behavior, although common in paranoid schizophrenia, are not seen in alcohol hallucinosis.

Treatment

Abstinence is essential, and the overall treatment of alcoholism is discussed in Section 21.5. Unfortunately, the very symptoms that are characteristic of alcohol hallucinosis often make it impossible for patients to participate in rehabilitative efforts, and hence treatment with antipsychotics is generally required. The choice of which of these agents to use may be made following the same principles given in Section 20.1 for the treatment of schizophrenia. Given the natural course of alcohol hallucinosis, an attempt should be made to gradually taper the dose of the antipsychotic after the patient has been sober and free of symptoms for a matter of months.

22.10 ALCOHOLIC PARANOIA

Alcoholic paranoia, also known as alcohol-induced psychotic disorder with delusions, like alcohol hallucinosis, is seen only in chronic alcoholics, after many years of severe, heavy drinking. Although the prevalence of this disorder has not been clearly determined, I have found it to be relatively common amongst chronic alcoholics.

Clinical features

The onset is gradual, and symptoms appear without any direct connection with either alcohol withdrawal or delirium tremens. Clinically (Albert *et al.* 1995), patients gradually develop either delusions of persecution or of jealousy. Those with delusions of persecution may believe that the police are following them or that intruders are hiding in the house; patients may peek out of windows to try and catch a glimpse of the police they are sure are 'staking out' the house, or they may feel compelled to go from room to room, perhaps with a weapon, looking for intruders. Those with delusions of jealousy typically suspect their spouse or lover of infidelity, and they may follow them or look for clues of the suspected romantic encounters. Occasionally there may be some hallucinations but these never dominate the clinical picture; indeed, if they do occur they typically play a very minor role, for example the persecuted patient may hear footsteps outside or the jealous patient may smell an unaccustomed cologne or perfume.

Course

In general, with continued drinking there is a gradual worsening of symptoms until eventually a 'plateau' of severity is reached, after which symptoms remain stable, despite ongoing drinking. With abstinence, symptoms gradually lessen over months to up to 2 years, and then either go into remission or settle into a stable, low-level chronicity.

Etiology

The mechanism by which this disorder occurs is not clear.

Differential diagnosis

Alcohol hallucinosis, discussed in the preceding section, is distinguished by its abrupt onset during alcohol withdrawal or delirium tremens, and by the prominence of hallucinations.

Of the other causes of psychosis discussed in Section 7.1, delusional disorder most closely resembles alcoholic paranoia. In delusional disorder, however, the history of chronic alcoholism is lacking.

Treatment

Abstinence is essential, and the overall treatment of alcoholism is discussed in Section 21.5. Treatment with antipsychotics should be considered, especially in cases in which delusions of persecution hinder the patient's efforts to engage in rehabilitation. The choice of antipsychotic is based on the same principles as outlined for schizophrenia in Section 20.1; given the natural history of alcoholic paranoia, attempts should eventually be made to taper the dose after the patient has been symptom free and sober for at least a few months.

22.11 MARCHIAFAVA–BIGNAMI DISEASE

Marchiafava–Bignami disease is a very rare disorder that was first described by Drs Marchiafava and Bignami (1903) in Italian alcoholics. It may present in one of two fashions, either acutely, with a delirium, or chronically, with a dementia.

Clinical features

Acute onsets are marked by delirium, stupor, or coma, often accompanied by seizures, either focal or generalized, long-tract signs, aphasia, or ataxia (Bohrod 1942; Ironside *et al.* 1961; Kamaki *et al.* 1993; Koeppen and Barron 1978; Rosa *et al.* 1991).

Chronic cases present gradually with a dementia that may be accompanied by a frontal lobe syndrome and, classically, signs of callosal disconnection, such as left-sided apraxia or agnosia (Lechevalier *et al.* 1977; Lhermitte *et al.* 1977; Mayer *et al.* 1987).

Magnetic resonance scanning (Johkura *et al.* 2005; Kamaki *et al.* 1993; Kawamura *et al.* 1985; Menegon *et al.* 2005) reveals distinctive changes. In acute cases, increased signal intensity on T2-weighted, fluid-attenuated inversion recovery (FLAIR), and diffusion-weighted imaging is seen in the corpus callosum and, in some cases, the adjacent white matter of the cerebral hemispheres; in severe cases, similar changes have also been noted in the frontal and parietal cortices. In chronic cases, atrophy and cystic changes may be noted in the same areas. One remarkable MRI study captured the entire evolution of these MRI changes (Chang *et al.* 1992).

Course

Those with acute onsets generally progress to coma and death within days to weeks; recovery, although uncommon, has been reported (Helenius *et al.* 2001). In chronic cases, should alcohol use persist, there is a steady progression to death within 3–8 years; with abstinence there may be a variable, but not complete, degree of recovery.

Etiology

Pathologically (Bohrod 1942; Ironside *et al.* 1961; Poser 1973), demyelinization with relative axonal sparing is found in the central portion of the corpus callosum, sparing the dorsal and ventral areas, and this may extend laterally in a symmetric fashion to involve adjacent areas of the centrum semiovale. Demyelinization may also be seen in the anterior and posterior commisures and the middle cerebellar peduncles. In severe cases, cystic changes may occur.

The cause of this demyelinization is not clear. Originally it was believed that there was an association with the consumption of cheap red wine by Italian men, as most of the original cases fit this description; however, it has become quite clear that this disease may occur in alcoholics who consume whiskey, beer, or white wine, and also in non-Italians (Ironside *et al.* 1961). Indeed, there are also rare reports of the disease occurring in association with severe malnutrition in non-alcoholics (Leong 1979). Presumably, the demyelinization occurs secondary to a vitamin deficiency; however, the nature of this deficiency is not clear, nor is it clear if a genetic susceptibility is involved.

Differential diagnosis

Marchiafava–Bignami disease must be distinguished from other disorders typically seen in chronic alcoholism. Acute cases may be mimicked clinically by delirium tremens, Wernicke's encephalopathy, hepatic encephalopathy, and encephalopathic pellagra, whereas chronic cases may be mistaken for alcoholic dementia. In practice, the diagnosis is generally only suspected when MR scanning reveals the distinctive findings noted above.

Treatment

Abstinence and adequate nutrition are critical, and it is appropriate to give thiamine, niacin, and folic acid.

22.12 INHALENT-INDUCED DEMENTIA

Inhalent intoxication (discussed in Section 21.7), if chronic and repeated, may cause a dementia.

Clinical features

The onset of dementia is gradual in the setting of ongoing, chronic inhalent use. Clinically (Fornazzari *et al.* 1983; Grabski 1961; Hormes *et al.* 1986; Knox and Nelson 1966; Lazar *et al.* 1983; Lewis *et al.* 1981; Rosenberg *et al.* 1988), patients become apathetic and concrete, and have difficulty with memory; in general, 'cortical' signs, such as aphasia, are lacking. In concert with the dementia, cerebellar signs are very common, including ataxia, dysarthria, titubation, intention tremor, and ocular abnormalities such as nystagmus or opsoclonus; a minority of patient may also have spasticity. In some cases there may also be a peripheral neuropathy (Korobkin *et al.* 1975).

Computed tomography scanning reveals cerebral and cerebellar cortical atrophy (Fornazzari *et al.* 1983; Hormes *et al.* 1986; Lazar *et al.* 1983); in addition to the atrophy, T2-weighted MR imaging also reveals diffuse, increased signal intensity in the cerebral and cerebellar white matter, with, in some cases, decreased signal intensity in the thalami or basal ganglia (Aydin *et al.* 2002; Filley *et al.* 1990; Rosenberg *et al.* 1988).

Course

With continued use a progression occurs; with abstinence there may be a gradual, but generally only partial, remission.

Etiology

Autopsy studies have revealed both cerebral and cerebellar atrophy, with widespread demyelinization (Escobar and Aruffo 1980; Kornfeld *et al.* 1994; Rosenberg *et al.* 1988).

Differential diagnosis

Consideration may be given to other disorders capable of causing dementia in combination with ataxia, as discussed in Section 5.1; however, the history of chronic inhalent use is hard to miss.

Treatment

Abstinence is essential and may require institutionalization. There is no specific treatment.

REFERENCES

Addonizio G, Susman VL, Roth SD. Neuroleptic malignant syndrome: review and analysis of 115 cases. *Biol Psychiatry* 1987; **22**:1004–20.

Adityanjee, Jayaswal SK, Chan TM *et al.* Temporary remission of tardive dystonia following electroconvulsive therapy. *Br J Psychiatry* 1990; **156**:433–5.

Adler LA, Peselow E, Rotrosen J *et al.* Vitamin E in the treatment of tardive dyskinesia. *Am J Psychiatry* 1993; **150**:1405–7.

Adler LA, Edson R, Lavori P *et al.* Long-term treatment effects of vitamin E for tardive dyskinesia. *Biol Psychiatry* 1998; **43**:868–72.

Adler LA, Rotrosen J, Edson R *et al.* Vitamin E treatment for tardive dyskinesia. *Arch Gen Psychiatry* 1999; **56**:863–41.

Agartz I, Brag S, Franck J *et al.* MR volumetry during acute alcohol withdrawal and abstinence: a descriptive study. *Alcohol Alcohol* 2003; **38**:71–8.

Agostino JV, Leo-Summers LS, Inouye SK. Cognitive and other adverse effects of diphenhydramine use in hospitalized older patients. *Arch Int Med* 2001; **161**:2091–7.

Akhtar S, Jajor TR, Kumar S. Vitamin E in the treatment of tardive dyskinesia. *J Postgrad Med* 1993; **39**:124–6.

Albert A, Mirza S, Mirza KAH *et al.* Morbid jealousy in alcoholics. *Br J Psychiatry* 1995; **167**:668–72.

Ananth J, Edelmuth E, Dargan B. Meige's syndrome associated with neuroleptic treatment. *Am J Psychiatry* 1988; **145**:513–15.

Anderson ES, Powers PS. Neuroleptic malignant syndrome associated with clozapine use. *J Clin Psychiatry* 1991; **52**:102–4.

Assmann VCCA, van Woerkom TCAM. Disappearance of tardive dyskinesia during catatonic stupor. *Acta Psychiatr Scand* 1987; **76**:217–18.

Aydin K, Sencer S, Demir T *et al.* Cranial MR findings in chronic toluene abuse by inhalation. *AJNR* 2002; **23**:1173–9.

Beasley CM, Dellva MA, Tamura RN *et al.* Randomized double-blind comparison of the incidence of tardive dyskinesia in patients with schizophrenia during long-term treatment with olanzapine or haloperidol. *Br J Psychiatry* 1999; **174**:23–30.

Beaver KM, Gavin TJ. Treatment of acute anticholinergic poisoning with physostigmine. *Am J Emerg Med* 1998; **16**:505–7.

Bharucha KJ, Sethi KD. Tardive Tourettism after exposure to neuroleptic therapy. *Mov Disord* 1995; **10**:791–3.

Bodner RA, Lynch T, Lewis L *et al.* Serotonin syndrome. *Neurology* 1995; **45**:219–23.

Bohrod MG. Primary degeneration of the corpus callosum (Marchiafava's disease): report of the second American case. *Arch Neurol Psychiatry* 1942; **47**:465–73.

Boyer EW, Shannon M. The serotonin syndrome. *N Engl J Med* 2005; **352**:1112–20.

Brunelle J, Guigueno S, Gouin P *et al.* Aripiprazole and neuroleptic malignant syndrome. *J Clin Psychopharmacol* 2007; **27**:212–14.

Burke RE, Fahn S, Jankovic J *et al.* Tardive dyskinesia: late-onset and persistent dystonia caused by antipsychotic drugs. *Neurology* 1982; **32**:1335–46.

Burke RE, Kang UK, Jankovic J *et al.* Tardive akathisia: an analysis of clinical features and response to open therapeutic trials. *Mov Disord* 1989; **4**:157–75.

Burns MJ, Linden CH, Graudins A *et al.* A comparison of physostigmine and benzodiazepines for the treatment of anticholinergic poisoning. *Ann Emerg Med* 2000; **35**:374–81.

Carlen PL, Wilkinson DA, Wotzman G *et al.* Cerebral atrophy and functional deficits in alcoholics without clinically apparent liver disease. *Neurology* 1981; **31**:377–85.

Carlen PL, McAndrews MP, Weiss RT *et al.* Alcohol-related dementia in the institutionalized elderly. *Alcohol Clin Exp Res* 1994; **18**:1330–4.

Carlsson C, Claeson L-E, Karlsson K-I *et al.* Clinical, psychometric and radiological signs of brain damage in chronic alcoholism. *Acta Neurol Scand* 1979; **60**:85–92.

Caroff SN. The neuroleptic malignant syndrome. *J Clin Psychiatry* 1980; **41**:79–83.

Caroff SN, Massa SC, Keck PE *et al.* Residual catatonic state following neuroleptic malignant syndrome. *J Clin Psychopharmacol* 2000; **2**:257–9.

Castillo E, Rubin RT, Holsboer-Trachsler E. Clinical differentiation between lethal catatonia and neuroleptic malignant syndrome. *Am J Psychiatry* 1989; **146**:324–8.

Chang KH, Cha SH, Han MH *et al.* Marchiafava–Bignami disease: serial changes in corpus callosum on MRI. *Neuroradiology* 1992; **34**:480–2.

Chiang E, Pitts WM, Rodriguez-Garcia M. Respiratory dyskinesia: review and case reports. *J Clin Psychiatry* 1985; **46**:232–4.

Chiu HFK, Lan LCW, Chung DWS. Prevalence of the rabbit syndrome in Hong Kong. *J Nerv Ment Dis* 1993; **181**:264–5.

Chouinard G, Jones BD. Neuroleptic-induced supersensitivity psychosis: clinical and pharmacologic characteristics. *Am J Psychiatry* 1980; **137**:16–21.

Coffey RJ, Edgar TS, Francsco GE *et al.* Abrupt withdrawal from intrathecal baclofen: recognition and management of a potentially life-threatening syndrome. *Arch Phys Med Rehabil* 2002; **83**:1479.

Cunningham MA, Darby DG, Donnan GA. Controlled-release delivery of L-dopa associated with nonfatal hyperthermia, rigidity and autonomic dysfunction. *Neurology* 1991; **41**:942–3.

Dabiri LM, Pasta D, Darby JK *et al.* Effectiveness of vitamin E for the treatment of long-term tardive dyskinesia. *Am J Psychiatry* 1994; **151**:925–6.

Damier P, Thobois S, Witjas T *et al.* Bilateral deep brain stimulation of the globus pallidus to treat tardive dyskinesia. *Arch Gen Psychiatry* 2007; **64**:170–6.

Daras M, Kakkouras L, Tuchman AJ *et al.* Rhabdomyolysis and hyperthermia after cocaine abuse: a variant of the neuroleptic malignant syndrome? *Acta Neurol Scand* 1995; **92**:161–5.

Das Gupta K, Young A. Clozapine-induced neuroleptic malignant syndrome. *J Clin Psychiatry* 1991; **52**:105–7.

Davis JM, Janicak PG, Sakkas P *et al.* Electroconvulsive therapy in the treatment of the neuroleptic malignant syndrome. *Convulsive Ther* 1991; **7**:111–20.

Decina P, Caracci G, Spichio PL. The rabbit syndrome. *Mov Disord* 1990; **5**:263–6.

Delassus-Guenault N, Jegouzo A, Odou P *et al.* Clozapine-olanzapine: a potentially dangerous switch. A report of two cases. *J Clin Pharmacol Ther* 1999; **24**:191–5.

Deshmukh DK, Joshi VS, Agarwal MR. Rabbit syndrome – a rare complication of long-term neuroleptic medication. Br J Psychiatry 1990; 157:293.

De Smet Y, Ruberg M, Serdaru M et al. Confusion, dementia and anticholinergics in Parkinson's disease. J Neurol Neurosurg Psychiatry 1982; 45:1161–4.

Dilsaver SC. Antidepressant withdrawal syndromes: phenomenonology and pathophysiology. Acta Psychiatr Scand 1989; 79:113.

Dilsaver SC, Feinberg M, Greden JF. Antidepressant withdrawal symptoms treated with anticholinergic agents. Am J Psychiatry 1983a; 140:249–51.

Dilsaver SC, Kronfol Z, Sackellares JC et al. Antidepressant withdrawal syndrome: evidence supporting the cholinergic overdrive hypothesis. J Clin Psychopharmacol 1983b; 3:157–64.

Dufresne RL, Wagner RL. Antipsychotic-withdrawal akathisia versus antipsychotic-induced akathisia: further evidence for the existence of tardive akathisia. J Clin Psychiatry 1988; 49:435–8.

Duvoisin RC, Katz R. Reversal of central anticholinergic syndrome in man by physostigmine. JAMA 1968; 206:1963–5.

Egan MF, Hyde TM, Albers GW et al. Treatment of tardive dyskinesia with vitamin E. Am J Psychiatry 1992; 149:773–7.

Elkashef AM, Ruskin PE, Bacher N et al. Vitamin E in the treatment of tardive dyskinesia. Am J Psychiatry 1990; 147:505–6.

Engel PA, Chapron D. Cyclobenzaprine-induced delirium in two octogenarians. J Clin Psychiatry 1993; 54:39.

Escobar A, Aruffo C. Chronic thinner intoxication: clinico-pathologic report of a human case. J Neurol Neurosurg Psychiatry 1980; 43:986–94.

Fahn S. High dosage anticholinergic therapy in dystonia. Neurology 1983; 33:1255–61.

Farran-Ridge C. Some syndromes referable to the basal ganglia occurring in dementia praecox and epidemic encephalitis. J Ment Sci 1926; 72:513–23.

Feighner JP, Boyer WF, Tyler DL et al. Adverse consequences of fluoxetine–MAOI combination therapy. J Clin Psychiatry 1990; 51:222–5.

Figa-Talamanca L, Gualandi C, Di Meo L et al. Hyperthermia after discontinuance of levodopa and bromocriptine therapy: impaired dopamine receptors a possible cause. Neurology 1985; 35:258–61.

Filley CM, Heaton RK, Rosenberg NL. White matter dementia in chronic toluene abuse. Neurology 1990; 40:532–4.

FitzGerald PM, Jankovic J. Tardive oculogyric crises. Neurology 1989; 39:1434–7.

Ford B, Greene P, Fahn S. Oral and genital tardive pain syndromes. Neurology 1994; 44:2115–19.

Fornazzari L, Wilkinson DA, Kapur BM et al. Cerebellar, cortical and functional impairment in toluene abusers. Acta Neurol Scand 1983; 67:319–29.

Fornazzari L, Ichise M, Remington G et al. Rabbit syndrome, antidepressant use, and cerebral perfusion SPECT scan findings. J Psychiatry Neurosci 1991; 16:227–9.

Friedman J, Feinberg SS, Feldman RG. A neuroleptic malignant-like syndrome due to L-dopa withdrawal. Ann Neurol 1984; 16:126–7.

Freidman LS, Weinrauch LA, D'Elia JA. Metoclopramide-induced neuroleptic malignant syndrome. Arch Int Med 1987; 147:1495–7.

Gardos G, Cole JO, Haskell D et al. The natural history of tardive dyskinesia. J Clin Psychopharmacol 1988; 8(suppl. 4):31–3.

Gardos G, Casey D, Cole JO et al. Ten year outcome of tardive dyskinesia. Am J Psychiatry 1994; 151:836–41.

Gibb W, Griffith D. Levodopa withdrawal syndrome identical to neuroleptic malignant syndrome. Postgrad Med J 1986; 62:59–60.

Glazer WM, Moore DC, Hansen TC et al. Meige syndrome and tardive dyskinesia. Am J Psychiatry 1983; 140:798–9.

Glazer WM, Moore DC, Schooler NR et al. Tardive dyskinesia: a discontinuation study. Arch Gen Psychiatry 1984; 41:623–7.

Glazer WM, Morgenstern H, Schooler N et al. Predictors of improvement in tardive dyskinesia following discontinuation of neuroleptic medication. Br J Psychiatry 1990; 157:585–92.

Glazer WM, Morgenstern H, Doucette JT. Predicting the long-term risk of tardive dyskinesia in outpatients maintained on neuroleptic medication. J Clin Psychiatry 1993; 54:133–9.

Goldman MB, Luchins DJ. Intermittent neuroleptic therapy and tardive dyskinesia: a literature review. Hosp Comm Psychiatry 1984; 35:1215–19.

Goodwin CD. Case report of tricyclic-induced delirium at a therapeutic drug concentration. Am J Psychiatry 1983; 140:1517–18.

Grabski DA. Toluene sniffing producing cerebellar degeneration. Am J Psychiatry 1961; 118:461–2.

Granato JE, Stern BJ, Ringel J et al. Neuroleptic malignant syndrome: successful treatment with dantrolene and bromocriptine. Ann Neurol 1983; 14:89–90.

Grant I, Adams KM, Reed R. Aging, abstinence, and medical risk factors in the prediction of neuropsychologic deficit among long-term alcoholics. Arch Gen Psychiatry 1984; 41:710–18.

Greil W, Haag H, Rossnagl G et al. Effect of anticholinergics on tardive dyskinesia: a controlled discontinuation study. Br J Psychiatry 1984; 145:304–10.

Gurling HMD, Reveley MA, Murray RM. Increased cerebral ventricular volume in monozygotic twins discordant for alcoholism. Lancet 1984; 1:986–8.

Guze BH, Baxter LR. Current concepts: neuroleptic malignant syndrome. N Engl J Med 1985; 313:163–6.

Hall RCW, Popkin MK, McHenry LE. Angel's trumpet psychosis: a central nervous system anticholinergic syndrome. Am J Psychiatry 1977; 134:312–14.

Hambidge DM. Intellectual impairment in male alcoholics. Alcohol Alcoholism 1990; 25:555–9.

Han L, McCusker J, Cole M et al. Use of medications with anticholinergic effect predicts clinical severity of delirium symptoms in older medical inpatients. Arch Int Med 2001; 161:1099–105.

Harper CG, Blumbergs PC. Brain weights in alcoholics. J Neurol Neurosurg Psychiatry 1982; 45:838–40.

Harper CG, Krill JJ. Brain atrophy in chronic alcoholic patients – a quantitative pathological study. J Neurol Neurosurg Psychiatry 1985; 48:211–17.

Harper CG, Krill JJ, Holloway RL. Brain shrinkage in chronic alcoholics: a pathological study. BMJ 1985; 290:501–4.

Harsch HH. Neuroleptic malignant syndrome: physiological and laboratory findings in a series of nine cases. J Clin Psychiatry 1987; 48:328–33.

van Harten PN, Hoek HW, Matroos GE et al. Intermittent neuroleptic treatment and risk of tardive dyskinesia: Curacao extrapyramidal syndromes study III. Am J Psychiatry 1998; 155:565–7.

Hay DP, Hay L, Blackwell B et al. ECT and tardive dyskinesia. J Geriatr Psychiatr Neurol 1990; 3:106–9.

Helenius J, Tatlisumak T, Soinne L et al. Marchiafava–Bignami disease: two cases with favorable outcome. Eur J Neurol 2001; 8:269–72.

Hermesh H, Aizenburg D, Weizman A. A successful electroconvulsive treatment of neuroleptic malignant syndrome. Acta Psychiatr Scand 1987; 75:237–9.

Hormes JT, Filley CM, Rosenberg NL. Neurologic sequelae of chronic solvent vapor abuse. Neurology 1986; 36:698–702.

Horn E, Lach B, Lapierre Y et al. Hypothalamic pathology in the neuroleptic malignant syndrome. Am J Psychiatry 1988; 145:617–20.

Huang CC. Persistent tardive dyskinesia associated with amoxapine therapy. Am J Psychiatry 1986; 143:1069–70.

Huang CC, Wang RI, Haegawa A et al. Reserpine and alpha-methyldopa in the treatment of tardive dyskinesia. Psychopharmacology 1981; 73:359–62.

Ironside R, Bosanquet FD, McMenemy WH. Central demyelination of the corpus callosum (Marchiafava–Bignami disease): with report of a second case in Great Britain. Brain 1961; 84:212–30.

Itil T, Fink M. Anticholinergic drug-induced delirium: experimental modification, quantitative EEG, and behavioral correlations. J Nerv Ment Dis 1966; 143:492–507.

Ivanovitch M, Glantz R, Bone RC et al. Respiratory dyskinesia presenting as acute respiratory distress. Chest 1993; 103:314–16.

Jensen GB, Pakkenberg B. Do alcoholics drink their neurons away? Lancet 1993; 342:1201–4.

Jernigan TL, Butters N, Ditraglia G et al. Reduced cerebral grey matter in alcoholics using MRI. Alcoholism Clin Exp Res 1991; 15:418–27.

Jeste DV, Potkin SG, Sinha S et al. Tardive dyskinesia – reversible and persistent. Arch Gen Psychiatry 1979; 36:585–90.

Johkura K, Naito M, Naka T. Cortical involvement in Marchiafava–Bignami disease. AJNR 2005; 26:670–3.

Jones EM, Dawson A. Neuroleptic malignant syndrome: a case report with post-mortem brain and muscle pathology. J Neurol Neurosurg Psychiatry 1989; 52:1006–9.

Kamaki M, Kawamura M, Moriya H et al. 'Crossed homonymous hemianopia' and a 'crossed left hemispatial neglect' in a case of Marchiafava–Bignami disease. J Neurol Neurosurg Psychiatry 1993; 56:1027–32.

Kane JM, Smith JM. Tardive dyskinesia: prevalence and risk factors, 1959–1979. Arch Gen Psychiatry 1982; 39:473–81.

Kane JM, Woerner M, Lieberman J. Tardive dyskinesia: prevalence, incidence and risk factors. J Clin Psychopharmacol 1988; 8:52S–56S.

Kang UJ, Burke RE, Fahn S. Natural history and treatment of tardive dystonia. Mov Disord 1986; 1:193–208.

Kawamura M, Shiota J, Yagishita T et al. Marchiafava–Bignami disease: computed tomographic scan and magnetic resonance imaging. Ann Neurol 1985; 18:103–4.

Keck PE, Pope HG, McElroy SL. Frequency and presentation of neuroleptic malignant syndrome: a prospective study. Am J Psychiatry 1987; 144:1344–6.

Kellam AMP. Neuroleptic malignant syndrome, so-called. A survey of the world literature. Br J Psychiatry 1987; 150:752–9.

Kellam AMP. The (frequently) neuroleptic malignant syndrome. Br J Psychiatry 1990; 157:169–73.

Kennedy PF. Chorea and phenothiazines. Br J Psychiatry 1969; 115:103–4.

Keyser DL, Rodnitzky RL. Neuroleptic malignant syndrome in Parkinson's disease after withdrawal or alteration of dopaminergic therapy. Arch Int Med 1991; 151:794–6.

Khan JA. Occasional notes: atropine poisoning in Hawthorne's The Scarlet Letter. N Engl J Med 1984; 311:414–17.

Kiriakakis V, Bhatia K, Quinn NP et al. The natural history of tardive dystonia: a long-term follow-up study of 107 cases. Brain 1998; 121:2053–66.

Kirkpatrick B, Alphs L, Buchanen RW. The concept of supersensitivity psychosis. J Nerv Ment Dis 1992; 180:265.

Klawans HL, Rubovits R. Effect of cholinergic and anticholinergic agents on tardive dyskinesia. J Neurol Neurosurg Psychiatry 1974; 37:941–7.

Knox JW, Nelson JR. Permanent encephalopathy from toluene inhalation. N Engl J Med 1966; 275:1494–6.

Koch M, Chandragiri S, Rizvi S et al. Catatonic signs in neuroleptic malignant syndrome. Compr Psychiatry 2000; 41:73–5.

Koeppen AH, Barron KD. Marchiafava–Bignami disease. Neurology 1978; 28:290–4.

Kontaxakis VP, Havaki-Kontaxaki BJ, Pappa DA et al. Neuroleptic malignant syndrome after addition of paroxetine to olanzapine. J Clin Psychopharmacol 2003; 23:671–2.

Kornfeld M, Moser AB, Moser HW et al. Solvent vapor abuse leukoencephalopathy. Comparison to adrenoleukodystrophy. J Neuropathol Exp Neurol 1994; 53:389–98.

Korobkin R, Asbury AK, Sumner AJ et al. Glue-sniffing neuropathy. Arch Neurol 1975; 32:158–62.

Kraepelin E. Dementia praecox and paraphrenia. Huntington, NY: Robert E. Krieger, 1971.

Krill JJ, Halliday GM, Svoboda MD et al. The cerebral cortex is damaged in chronic alcoholics. Neuroscience 1997; 79:983–98.

Lang AE. Withdrawal akathisia: case reports and a proposed classification of chronic akathisia. Mov Disord 1994; 9:188–92.

Lattanzi L, Mungai F, Romano A et al. Subcutaneous apomorphine for neuroleptic malignant syndrome. Am J Psychiatry 2006; 163:1450–1.

Lazar RB, Ho SU, Melen O *et al.* Multifocal central nervous system damage caused by toluene abuse. *Neurology* 1983; **33**:1337–40.

Lechevalier B, Anderson JC, Morin P. Hemispheric disconnection syndrome with a 'crossed avoiding' reaction in a case of Marchiafava–Bignami disease. *J Neurol Neurosurg Psychiatry* 1977; **40**:483–97.

Lee K, Moller L, Hardt F *et al.* Alcohol induced brain damage and liver damage in young males. *Lancet* 1979; **2**:759–61.

Leong ASV. Marchiafava–Bignami disease in a non-alcoholic Indian male. *Pathology* 1979; **11**:241–9.

Lerner V, Miodownik C, Kapstan A *et al.* Vitamin B6 in the treatment of tardive dyskinesia: a double-blind, placebo-controlled, crossover study. *Am J Psychiatry* 2001; **158**:1511–14.

Levenson JL. Neuroleptic malignant syndrome after the initiation of olanzapine. *J Clin Psychopharmacol* 1999; **19**:477–8.

Levin GM, Lazowick AL, Powell HS. Neuroleptic malignant syndrome with risperidone. *J Clin Psychopharmacol* 1996; **16**:192–3.

Lewis JD, Moritz D, Mellis LP. Long-term toluene abuse. *Am J Psychiatry* 1981; **138**:368–70.

Lhermitte F, Marteau R, Serdaru M *et al.* Signs of interhemispheric disconnection in Marchiafava–Bignami disease. *Arch Neurol* 1977; **34**:254–7.

Libov I, Miodowni C, Bersudsky Y *et al.* Efficacy of piracetam in the treatment of tardive dyskinesia in schizophrenic patients: a randomized, double-blind, placebo-controlled crossover study. *J Clin Psychiatry* 2007; **68**:1031–7.

Lishman WA. Cerebral disorder in alcoholism: syndromes of impairment. *Brain* 1981; **104**:373–410.

Lohr JB, Caligiuri MP. A double-blind placebo-controlled study of vitamin E in the treatment of tardive dyskinesia. *J Clin Psychiatry* 1996; **57**:167–73.

Lohr JB, Cadet JL, Lohr MA *et al.* Vitamin E in the treatment of tardive dyskinesia: the possible involvement of free radical mechanisms. *Schizophr Bull* 1988; **14**:291–6.

Lu ML, Pan JJ, Teng HW *et al.* Metoclopramide-induced supersensitivity psychosis. *Ann Pharmacother* 2002; **36**:1387–90.

Luchins DJ, Freed WJ, Wyatt RJ. The role of cholinergic supersensitivity in the medical symptoms associated with withdrawal of antipsychotic drugs. *Am J Psychiatry* 1980; **137**:1395–8.

Lynch MJG. Brain lesions in chronic alcoholism. *Arch Pathol* 1960; **69**:342–53.

Marchiafava E, Bignami A. Sopra un alterazione del corpo callsos osservata in sogetti alcoolisti. *Riv Patol Nerv Mentale* 1903; **8**:544–9.

Mason PI, Morris VA, Balcezak TJ. Serotonin syndrome. Presentation of 2 cases and review of the literature. *Medicine* 2000; **79**:201–9.

May EDC, Morris SW, Stewart RM *et al.* Neuroleptic malignant syndrome: response to dantrolene sodium. *Ann Intern Med* 1983; **98**:183–4.

Mayer JM, De Liege P, Netter JM *et al.* Computerized tomography and nuclear magnetic resonance imaging in Marchiafava–Bignami disease. *J Neuroradiol* 1987; **14**:152–8.

Mendhekar DN, Andrade CR. Neuroleptic malignant syndrome with promethazine. *Aust N Z J Psychiatry* 2005; **39**:310.

Menegon P, Sibon I, Pachia C *et al.* Marchiafava–Bignami disease: diffusion-weighted MRI in corpus callosum and cortical lesions. *Neurology* 2005; **65**:475–7.

Meterissian GB. Risperidone-induced neuroleptic malignant syndrome: a case report and review. *Can J Psychiatry* 1996; **41**:52–4.

Mettler FA, Crandall A. Neurologic disorders in psychiatric institutions. *J Nerv Ment Dis* 1959; **128**:148–59.

Miller DD, Sharafuddin MJA, Kathol RG. A case of clozapine-induced neuroleptic malignant syndrome. *J Clin Psychiatry* 1991; **52**:99–101.

Moncrieff J. Does antipsychotic withdrawal provoke psychosis? Review of the literature on rapid onset psychosis (supersensitivity psychosis) and withdrawal-related relapse. *Acta Psychiatr Scand* 2006; **114**:3–13.

Moore DP. Tardive psychosis. *J Ky Med Assoc* 1986; **84**:351–3.

Morganstern H, Glazer WM. Identifying risk factors for tardive dyskinesia among the long-term outpatients maintained with neuroleptic medications. *Arch Gen Psychiatry* 1993; **50**:723–33.

Mueller PS, Vester JW, Fermaglich J. Neuroleptic malignant syndrome – successful treatment with bromocriptine. *JAMA* 1983; **249**:386–8.

Neuberger KT. The changing neuropathological picture of chronic alcoholism. *Arch Pathol* 1957; **63**:1–6.

Nimmagadda SR, Ryan DH, Atkin SL. Neuroleptic malignant syndrome after venlafaxine. *Lancet* 2000; **354**:289–90.

Oberndorfer S, Grisold W, Hinterholzer G *et al.* Coma with focal neurological signs caused by *Datura stramonium* intoxication in a young man. *J Neurol Neurosurg Psychiatry* 2002; **73**:458–9.

Ondo WG, Hanna PA, Jankovi J. Tetrabenazine treatment for tardive dyskinesia: assessment by randomized videotape protocol. *Am J Psychiatry* 1999; **156**:1279–81.

Ossemann M, Sindic CJM, Laterre C. Tetrabenazine as a cause of neuroleptic malignant syndrome. *Mov Disord* 1996; **11**:95.

Owens DGC, Johnstone EC, Frith CD. Spontaneous involuntary disorders of movement: their prevalence, severity and distribution in chronic schizophrenics with and without treatment with neuroleptics. *Arch Gen Psychiatry* 1982; **39**:452–61.

Ozen ME, Yumru M, Savas HA *et al.* Neuroleptic malignant syndrome induced by ziprasidone on the second day of treatment: a case report. *World J Biol Psychiatry* 2007; **8**:133–4.

Parvin MM, Swartz CM. Dystonic rabbit syndrome from citalopram. *Clin Neuropharmacol* 2005; **28**:289–91.

Peiris DTS, Kuruppuarachchi KALA, Weeasena LP *et al.* Neuroleptic malignant syndrome without fever: a report of three cases. *J Neurol Neurosurg Psychiatry* 2000; **69**:277–8.

Petti TA, Law W. Abrupt cessation of high-dose imipramine treatment in children. *JAMA* 1981; **246**:768–9.

Pfefferbaum A, Sullivan EV, Mathalon DH *et al.* Longitudinal changes in magnetic resonance imaging brain volumes in abstinent and relapsed alcoholics. *Alcohol Clin Exp Res* 1995; **19**:1177–91.

Pope HG, Keck PE, McElroy SL. Frequency and presentation of neuroleptic malignant syndrome in a large psychiatric hospital. *Am J Psychiatry* 1986; **143**:1227–33.

Porteous HB, Ross DN. Mental symptoms in parkinsonism following benzhexol hydrochloride therapy. *BMJ* 1956; **2**:138–40.

Poser CM. Demyelinization in the central nervous system in chronic alcoholism, central pontine myelinolysis, and Marchiafava–Bignami's disease. *Ann NY Acad Sci* 1973; **215**:373–81.

de Potter RW, Linkowski P, Mendelwicz J. State-dependent tardive dyskinesia in manic-depressive illness. *J Neurol Neurosurg Psychiatry* 1983; **46**:666–8.

Preskorn SH, Simpson S. Tricyclic-antidepressant-induced delirium and plasma drug concentrations. *Am J Psychiatry* 1982; **139**:822–3.

Reunanen M, Kaarnen P, Vaisanen E. The influence of anticholinergic treatment on tardive dyskinesia caused by neuroleptic drugs. *Acta Psychiatr Scand* 1982; **65**(suppl. 90):278–9.

Rich MW, Radwany SM. Respiratory dyskinesia: an underrecognized phenomenon. *Chest* 1994; **105**:1826–32.

Richardson MA, Craig TJ. The coexistence of Parkinsonism-like symptoms and tardive dyskinesia. *Am J Psychiatry* 1982; **139**:341–3.

Richardson MA, Vevans ML, Read LL *et al.* Efficacy of branched-chain amino acids in the treatment of tardive dyskinesia. *Am J Psychiatry* 2003; **160**:1117–24.

Rosa A, Demiati M, Cartz L *et al.* Marchiafava–Bignami disease, syndrome of interhemispheric disconnection, and right-handed agraphia in a left-hander. *Arch Neurol* 1991; **48**:986–8.

Rosebush P, Stewart T. A prospective analysis of 24 episodes of neuroleptic malignant syndrome. *Am J Psychiatry* 1989; **146**:717–25.

Rosebush PI, Stewart TED, Gelelberg AJ. Twenty neuroleptic rechallenges after neuroleptic malignant syndrome in 15 patients. *J Clin Psychiatry* 1989; **50**:295–8.

Rosenberg NL, Kleineschmidt-DeMasters BK, Davis KA *et al.* Toluene abuse causes diffuse central nervous system white matter changes. *Ann Neurol* 1988; **23**:611–14.

Sachdev PS. Depression-dependent exacerbation of tardive dyskinesia. *Br J Psychiatry* 1989; **155**:253–5.

Sachdev P. Clinical characteristics of 15 patients with tardive dystonia. *Am J Psychiatry* 1993a; **150**:498–500.

Sachdev P. Tardive and chronically recurrent oculogyric crises. *Mov Disord* 1993b; **8**:93–7.

Sachdev P, Loneragan C. The present status of akathisia. *J Nerv Ment Dis* 1991; **179**:381–91.

Sachdev P, Kruk J, Kneebone M *et al.* Clozapine-induced neuroleptic malignant syndrome: review and report of new case. *J Clin Psychopharmacol* 1995; **15**:365–71.

Saltz BL, Woerner MG, Kane JM *et al.* Prospective study of tardive dyskinesia incidence in the elderly. *JAMA* 1991; **266**:2402–6.

Sato Y, Asoh T, Metoki N *et al.* Efficacy of methylprednisolone pulse therapy on neuroleptic malignant syndrome in

Parkinson's disease. *J Neurol Neurosurg Psychiatry* 2003; **74**:574–6.

Schroth G, Naegele T, Klose U *et al.* Reversible brain shrinkage in abstinent alcoholics, measured by MRI. *Neuroradiology* 1988; **30**:385–9.

Schuckitt MA, Winokur G. Alcohol hallucinosis and schizophrenia: a negative study. *Br J Psychiatry* 1971; **119**:549–53.

Sechi GP, Tanda F, Mutani R. Fatal hyperpyrexia after withdrawal of levodopa. *Neurology* 1984; **34**:249–51.

Sewell DD, Jeste DV. Metoclopramide-associated tardive dyskinesia: an analysis of 67 cases. *Arch Fam Med* 1992; **1**:271–8.

Sewell DD, Kodsi AB, Caligiuri MP *et al.* Metoclopramide and tardive dyskinesia. *Biol Psychiatry* 1994; **36**:630–2.

Shamir E, Varak Y, Shalman I *et al.* Melatonin treatment for tardive dyskinesia. A double-blind, placebo-controlled, crossover study. *Arch Gen Psychiatry* 2001; **58**:1049–52.

Shriqui CL, Bradwejn J, Annable L *et al.* Vitamin E in the treatment of tardive dyskinesia: a double-blind placebo-controlled study. *Am J Psychiatry* 1992; **149**:391–3.

Sing KJ, Ramaekers GMGI, van Harten PN. Neuroleptic malignant syndrome and quetiapine. *Am J Psychiatry* 2002; **159**:149–50.

Soyka M. Psychopathological characteristics in alcohol hallucinosis and paranoid schizophrenia. *Acta Psychiatr Scand* 1990; **81**:255–9.

Stacy M, Cardoso F, Jankovic J. Tardive stereotypy and other movement disorders in tardive dyskinesias. *Neurology* 1993; **43**:937–41.

Stahl SM. Tardive Tourette syndrome in an autistic patient after long-term neuroleptic administration. *Am J Psychiatry* 1980; **137**:1267–9.

Steiner W, Laporta M, Chouinard G. Neuroleptic-induced supersensitivity psychosis in patients with bipolar affective disorder. *Acta Psychiatr Scand* 1990; **81**:437–40.

Stern TA. Continuous infusion of physostigmine in anticholinergic delirium: case report. *J Clin Psychiatry* 1983; **44**:463–4.

Sternbach H. The serotonin syndrome. *Am J Psychiatry* 1991; **148**:705–13.

Suh H, Bronson B, Martin R. Neuroleptic malignant syndrome and low-dose olanzapine. *Am J Psychiatry* 2003; **160**:796.

Tan E-K, Jankovic J. Tardive and idiopathic oromandibular dystonia: a clinical comparison. *J Neurol Neurosurg Psychiatry* 2000; **68**:186–90.

Taylor NE, Schwartz HI. Neuroleptic malignant syndrome following amoxapine overdose. *J Nerv Ment Dis* 1988; **176**:249–51.

Tejera CA, Saravay SM, Goldman E *et al.* Diphenhydramine-induced delirium in elderly hospitalized patients with mild dementia. *Psychosomatics* 1994; **35**:399–402.

Tenback DE, van Harten PN, Slooff CJ *et al.* Effects of antipsychotic treatment on tardive dyskinesia: a 6-month evaluation of patients from the European Schizophrenia Outpaient Health Outcomes (SOHO) Study. *J Clin Psychiatry* 2005; **66**:1130–3.

Thornton NE, Stahl SM. Case report of tardive dyskinesia and parkinsonism associated with amoxapine therapy. *Am J Psychiatry* 1984; **141**:704–5.

Todd R, Lippmann S, Manshadi M et al. Recognition and treatment of rabbit syndrome, an uncommon complication of neuroleptic therapies. Am J Psychiatry 1983; 140:1519–20.

Toru M, Matsuda O, Makiguchi K et al. Single case study: neuroleptic malignant syndrome-like state following withdrawal of antiparkinsonian drugs. J Nerv Ment Dis 1981; 169:324–7.

Torvik A, Lindboe CF, Rogde S. Brain lesions in alcoholics. A neuropathological study with clinical correlations. J Neurol Sci 1982; 56:233–48.

Troller JN, Sachdev PS. Electroconvulsive treatment of neuroleptic malignant syndrome: a review and report of cases. Aust N Z J Psychiatry 1999; 33:650–9.

Tsao JW, Heilman KM. Transient memory impairment and hallucination associated with tolteridone use. N Engl J Med 2003; 349:2274–5.

Tune LE, Dainloth NF, Holland A et al. Association of postoperative delirium with raised serum levels of anticholinergic drugs. Lancet 1981; 2:651–3.

Tune LE, Bylsma FW, Hilt DC. Anticholinergic delirium caused by topical homatropine ophthalmic solution: confirmation by anticholinergic radioreceptor assay in two cases. J Neuropsychiatry Clin Neurosci 1992; 4:195–7.

Turner MR, Gainsborough N. Neuroleptic malignant-like syndrome after abrupt withdrawal of baclofen. J Psychopharmacol 2001; 15:61–3.

Velamoor VR, Norman RMG, Caroff SN et al. Progression of symptoms in neuroleptic malignant syndrome. J Nerv Ment Dis 1994; 182:168–73.

Victor M, Hope JM. The phenomenon of auditory hallucinations in chronic alcoholism. J Nerv Ment Dis 1958; 126:451–8.

Vonderahe AR. Lilliputian hallucinations: report of a case of hyoscine poisoning. Arch Neurol Psychiatry 1929; 22:585–8.

Wang H-C, Hsieh Y. Treatment of neuroleptic malignant syndrome with subcutaneous apomorphine therapy. Mov Disord 2001; 16:765–7.

Weiner WJ, Nausieda PA, Glantz RH. Meige syndrome (blepharospasm–oromandibular dystonia) after long-term neuroleptic therapy. Neurology 1981; 31:1555–6.

Woerner M, Kane JM, Lieberman JA et al. The prevalence of tardive dyskinesia. J Clin Psychopharmacol 1991; 11:34–42.

Wojcik JD, Falk WE, Fink JS et al. A review of 32 cases of tardive dystonia. Am J Psychiatry 1991; 148:1055–9.

Wolfe RM. Antidepressant withdrawal reactions. Am Fam Physician 1997; 56:455–62.

Yadalam KG, Korn ML, Simpson GM. Tardive dystonia: four case histories. J Clin Psychiatry 1990; 51:17–20.

Yagi G, Itoh H. Follow-up study of 11 patients with potentially reversible tardive dyskinesia. Am J Psychiatry 1987; 144:1596–8.

Yarden PE, Discipio WJ. Abnormal movements and prognosis in schizophrenia. Am J Psychiatry 1971; 128:317–23.

Yassa R, Lal S. Respiratory irregularity and tardive dyskinesia: a prevalence study. Acta Psychiatr Scand 1986a; 73:506–10.

Yassa R, Lal S. Prevalence of the rabbit syndrome. Am J Psychiatry 1986b; 143:656–7.

Yassa R, Nair V, Dimitry A. Prevalence of tardive dystonia. Acta Psychiatr Scand 1986; 73:629–33.

Yassa R, Iskander H, Nastase C. Propranolol in the treatment of tardive akathisia: a report of two cases. J Clin Psychopharmacol 1988; 8;283–5.

Yazici O, Kantemir E, Tastaban Y et al. Spontaneous improvement of tardive dystonia during mania. Br J Psychiatry 1991; 158:847–50.

Zhang XY, Zhou DF, Cao LY et al. The effect of vitamin E treatment on tardive dyskinesia and blood superoxide dismutase: a double-blind, placebo-controlled trial. J Clin Psychopharmacol 2004; 24:83–6.

Zipursky RB. Lim KC, Pfefferbaum A. MRI study of brain changes with short-term abstinence from alcohol. Alcohol Clin Exp Res 1989; 13:664–6.

Ziskind AA. Transdermal scopolamine-induced psychosis Postgrad Med 1988; 84:73–6.

Index

anterograde amnesias   183–4, 184–5,
      185–6
   in Korsakoff syndrome   471
   with retrograde component *see*
      retrograde amnesia
   seizures   256
   transient global   184, 447
antibiotics
   Lyme disease   511, 512
   streptococcal pharyngitis/rheumatic
      fever   558, 560
   syphilis   510
   tuberculosis   512–13
   Whipple's disease   513
antibodies
   in autoimmune disorders
         (autoantibodies)
      anti-phospholipid syndrome   552
      Hashimoto's encephalopathy   541,
         557, 558
      Hashimoto's thyroiditis   540, 541,
         556
      limbic encephalitis   554
      Sjögren's syndrome   551
      Sneddon's syndrome   552
      systemic lupus erythematosus   549
   detection in CSF   34
   in Sydenham's chorea   559
   see also monoclonal antibody therapy
anticholinergics
   delirium with   690–1
   in Parkinson's disease   348
   rebound following discontinuation
      691–2
anticholinesterases, Alzheimer's disease
   339
anticipation
   in myotonic dystrophy   372
   in panic attacks   632
anticonvulsants *see* anti-epileptic drugs
antidepressants
   adverse/side-effects   627
      delirium   177
      serotonin syndrome   690
   attention-deficit/hyperactivity disorder
      420
   autism   418
   in depression   214, 281–2, 627–8
      in Alzheimer's disease   339–40
      in bipolar disorder   623
      in diffuse Lewy body disease   352
      major depression   627–8
      in multiple sclerosis   548
      in Parkinson's disease   350
      in post-concussion syndrome   458
      resistance to   628
      in traumatic brain injury   292
   generalized anxiety disorder   642
   interactions with other drugs   627
   mechanism of action   626
   obsessive–compulsive disorder   639
   panic disorder   634

   post-traumatic stress disorder   641
   premenstrual syndrome   630
   social phobia   637
   Tourette's syndrome   371
antidiuretic hormone (ADH; vasopressin)
   analog (desmopressin), in nocturnal
      enuresis   575
   syndrome of inappropriate secretion, in
      subarachnoid hemorrhage   281
anti-epileptic drugs (AEDs)   272–5
   prenatal exposure causing mental
      retardation   189
   therapeutic use   272–5
      alcohol withdrawal   665–6
      brain tumors   600
      status epilepticus   274–5
      stroke patients   288
      traumatic brain injury   293
      tuberous sclerosis patients   405
antifungal drugs   516
antihypertensive drugs, hypertensive
      encephalopathy   444
anti-nuclear antibodies *see* nuclear
      components
anti-phospholipid antibodies
   in anti-phospholipid syndrome   552,
      553
   in Sneddon's syndrome   552
anti-phospholipid syndrome   552–3
   chorea gravidarum associated with
      560
   clinical features
      dementia   172
      thrombotic infarctions   283
   differential diagnosis   553
      Sneddon's syndrome   552
anti-platelet agents, ischemic stroke   287
antiprotozoals in toxoplasmosis   516
antipsychotics (neuroleptics)   613–14,
      683–9
   1st generation   613, 684
   2nd generation   613, 684
   adverse effects   614, 683–9
      akathisia   92, 614, 686, 687
      akinesia   91, 614
      dystonia   85, 686
      mannerisms   140
      rabbit syndrome   689
      seizures   262–3
      supersensitivity psychosis   240,
         688–9
      tardive dyskinesia *see* tardive
         dyskinesia (antipsychotic-induced)
      see also neuroleptic malignant
         syndrome
   therapeutic use   613–14
      agitation   173, 223–5
      Alzheimer's disease   340
      autism   418
      ballism   83
      cannnabis users   671
      chorea   81

   delirium   182–3, 224
   delusional disorder   617
   diffuse Lewy body disease   352
   mania (incl. bipolar disorder)   222,
      225, 622, 689
   obsessive–compulsive disorder   639
   post-partum psychosis   618
   post-traumatic stress disorder   641
   psychosis (in general)   244
   schizoaffective disorder   615
   schizophrenia   613–14
   stuttering   424
   Tourette's syndrome   370–1
antiretroviral agents, AIDS   495
anti-thyroid antibodies *see* thyroid gland
antituberculous agents   512–13
antiviral agents
   AIDS   495
   cytomegalovirus   496
   herpes simplex virus   499
Anton's syndrome   61
anxiety (and fear)   225–7
   acute *see* panic attacks
   anticipatory   632
   clinical features   6, 225
   differential diagnosis   227
      agitation   223
      normal fears vs social phobia   637
      simple partial seizures   270
   etiology   225–6, 538
      cannabis   670
      Cushing's syndrome   534
      drug related   225, 282, 350
      hyperthyroidism   226, 537, 538
      seizures   252, 259
      stroke   282
   observing for   6
   persistent   225, 225–6
   treatment   227, 282
   tremor and   73, 74
anxiety disorders   631–42
   generalized   641–2
anxiolytics *see* benzodiazepines;
      sedative–hypnotics
apathy   214–15
   Alzheimer's disease   340
   frontal lobe syndrome   214, 244, 245
   hyperthyroidism   538
   traumatic brain injury   292
aphasia   45–9
   atypical   47–8
   clinical features   45–8
   differential diagnosis   48–9
      apraxia   56
      aprosodia   55
      delirium   48–9, 182
      foreign accent syndrome   137
      stuttering   120
      visual agnosia   58
   etiology   48
   progressive, dementia presenting with
      163, 164, 167

to nortriptyline (Wagena *et al.* 2005). Consideration may also be given to combination treatment with bupropion plus nicotine or nortriptyline plus nicotine, and it appears that the combination of bupropion and nicotine may be modestly more effective than bupropion alone (Jorenby *et al.* 1999). The combination of varenicline and nicotine is not recommended. Nicotine alone, although superior to placebo, is the least effective of the pharmacologic approaches. Overall, it appears reasonable to start with varenicline; should that prove ineffective or not tolerated, then consideration may be given to bupropion with or without supplemental nicotine. An exception to this general rule is major depressive disorder. For reasons that are not clear, patients with major depressive disorder, even if they are not currently in the midst of a depressive episode, are at high risk for recurrence of depression in the first few months of abstinence from nicotine (Glassman *et al.* 2001), and for such patients it is appropriate to consider treatment with either bupropion or nortriptyline. Although the combination of varenicline and bupropion has not been formally evaluated, it may be considered an option in some cases.

Regardless of which approach is used, during the first year at least, relapses are the rule rather than the exception, and such 'slips' should not be seen as failures. As weight gain is common during the first year, patients should be warned about this and instructed to begin a program of diet and exercise should they start to gain weight.

21.11 CAFFEINE

Caffeine is the most commonly used substance in the Western world. A cup of coffee contains about 100 mg of caffeine, a cup of tea about 50 mg, and over-the-counter 'stimulant', analgesic, and 'cold' remedies may contain anywhere from 25 to 200 mg.

Clinical features

In caffeine-naive patients, about 100 mg of caffeine produces an increased sense of alertness and decreased fatigue. At doses ranging from 200 to 500 mg, however, intoxication (Hughes *et al.* 1991b; Rapoport *et al.* 1981) occurs, with apprehensiveness, restlessness, tremor, tachycardia, headache, and insomnia. With higher doses, up to 1000 mg, an anxiety attack may occur, and some patients may become very agitated; tremor and tachycardia are pronounced and there may be premature beats and muscle twitches. At doses of 5 g or more, severe intoxication occurs and there may be serious ventricular arrhythmias, grand mal seizures, respiratory depression, and death (Curatolo and Robertson 1983). Most intoxications clear within 6–12 hours.

Tolerance to caffeine may appear after only a couple of weeks' use of 500 mg or more daily. In cases in which tolerance has occurred, withdrawal symptoms (Griffiths *et al.* 1990; Hughes *et al.* 1991b; Silverman *et al.* 1992; Strain *et al.* 1994) may appear anywhere from 12 to 24 hours after the last dose, with headache, poor concentration, fatigue, anxiety, and depressed mood; these withdrawal symptoms tend to gradually subside within days to a week of abstinence.

Other disorders associated with chronic caffeine use include gastroesophageal reflux disease, peptic ulcer, fibrocystic disease, and hypertension; caffeine may also precipitate anxiety attacks seen in panic disorder (Boulenger *et al.* 1984; Charney *et al.* 1985).

Course

Recreational use of caffeine is extraordinarily common. Abusive use, that is continued use despite recurrent intoxication or the aggravation of some of the other disorders seen in association with caffeine use, is relatively uncommon. Craving for caffeine does not appear to occur.

Etiology

The intoxicating effects of caffeine appear to be mediated by its competitive blockade of central nervous system adenosine receptors.

Differential diagnosis

There is generally little difficulty here as the history is readily obtained. Occasionally, patients with chronic caffeine intoxication may present a picture which is similar to that seen in generalized anxiety disorder; however, the differential is straightforward provided that the patient can abstain from caffeine for a few days (Greden 1974).

Treatment

With the exception of severe intoxication (which may require intensive supportive care), specific treatment is generally not required. In those with troublesome withdrawal, patients may be gradually tapered off their regular dose in daily decrements approximately equal to 10 percent of the initial total daily dose.

21.12 METHANOL

Methanol, also known as methyl alcohol or 'wood alcohol', is found in 'canned heat' preparations such as 'Sterno', in certain solvents and paint thinners, and as a 'denaturant' added to ethanol, which is then sold tax-free as 'denatured alcohol' for use as a cleaner. Methanol is at times used by desperate alcoholics when no other source of intoxication is at hand; methanol intoxication may also occur accidentally with inhalation of fumes, absorption through the skin, or inadvertent ingestion.

Methanol is metabolized first via alcohol dehydrogenase to formaldehyde and then via aldehyde dehydrogenase to formic acid, which is the ultimate cause of the devastating sequelae of methanol intoxication; formic acid is not only directly toxic to neuronal mitochondria but also produces a severe systemic acidosis. Importantly, this is the same metabolic pathway used by ethanol, a fact of considerable importance regarding not only the evolution of methanol intoxication but also one of the traditional treatments of this intoxication.

Clinical features

Clinically (Bennet *et al.* 1953; Erlanson *et al.* 1965; Hovda *et al.* 2005; Kaplan 1962; Paasma *et al.* 2007; Wood and Buller 1904) the intoxication seen with methanol evolves in a biphasic fashion. The initial response, occurring in response to the methanol itself, is characterized by euphoria, headache, and nausea, all accompanied by an odor of alcohol on the breath. Subsequently, as formic acid begins to accumulate in the following hours, there may be delirium, restlessness, dizziness, vomiting, and bilateral blurring or dimming of vision; with more severe intoxication, seizures, respiratory depression, and coma may supervene. Methanol levels are generally above 30 mg/dL, and a metabolic acidosis is present with an increased anion gap reflecting the presence of formic acid. Untreated, methanol intoxication may be fatal in up to one-third of cases; those who survive generally recover from the intoxication in 1–3 days, but may be left with one or more sequelae, such as visual loss (Wood and Buller 1904), parkinsonism (Guggenheim *et al.* 1971), or dementia (McLean *et al.* 1980). Magnetic resonance scanning may reveal areas of increased signal intensity on fluid-attenuated inversion recovery (FLAIR) and diffusion-weighted images in the putamina and subcortical white matter.

Course

Repeated ingestion of methanol is uncommon, as most alcoholics learn their lesson.

Etiology

Secondary to the direct toxicity of formic acid, there are widespread petechial hemorrhages involving the cortex, putamen (Erlanson *et al.* 1965; McLean *et al.* 1980), retina, and optic nerve (Benton and Calhoun 1953; Sharpe *et al.* 1982).

Differential diagnosis

Ethanol and isopropanol intoxication are distinguished by the absence of features such as visual loss and delirium, and

ethylene glycol intoxication by the absence of an odor of alcohol.

A confusing diagnostic picture may emerge when both methanol and ethanol are consumed, as may occur when denatured alcohol is ingested. As noted earlier, ethanol inhibits the metabolism of methanol to formic acid, and hence the evolution of the second phase of methanol intoxication may be delayed until the ethanol is cleared, after which the remaining methanol is converted to formic acid.

Treatment

Methanol intoxication constitutes a medical emergency. If patients are seen within 2 hours of ingestion, gastric lavage may be performed. Throughout treatment one must monitor pH, bicarbonate levels, the anion gap, and methanol levels: initial methanol levels above 20 mg/dL are considered toxic, and levels above 50 mg/dL are potentially life-threatening.

The cornerstone of treatment rests on delaying the transformation of methanol to formic acid. In the past this was accomplished by giving ethanol, which binds preferentially to the enzymes responsible for the metabolism of methanol to formic acid, thus preventing an overly rapid accumulation of formic acid. A more recent, and far better, option involves the administration of fomepizole, a drug that inhibits alcohol dehydrogenase (Brent *et al.* 2001). Folic acid hastens the excretion of formic acid and may be given in doses of 50 mg intravenously every 6 hours. In cases in which the foregoing measures are ineffective, hemodialysis may be utilized to remove formic acid.

21.13 ISOPROPANOL

Isopropanol, also known as isopropyl alcohol, is found in aftershave lotions, hand lotions, hair tonics, and in 'rubbing alcohol'. Among desperate alcoholics it may be known as 'rubby dubby', with reference to the source in rubbing alcohol, or as 'blue heaven', the latter name derived from the blue coloring often added to rubbing alcohol. In part, isopropyl alcohol is metabolized via alcohol dehydrogenase to acetone.

Clinical features

Intoxication (Lacouture *et al.* 1983; Rich *et al.* 1990) is characterized by mild euphoria, an odor of alcohol on the breath, dizziness, and ataxia, and may also be accompanied by headache, nausea, vomiting, and, in some cases, hematemesis. With high doses, severe intoxication may occur, with coma and respiratory depression. Isopropanol, as noted, is converted to acetone, leading to both acetonemia and acetonuria. The intoxication generally passes within 12 hours.

Tolerance may occur; whereas 250 mL may constitute a lethal dose in a non-tolerant patient, alcoholics may be able to consume this much with little untoward effect. Although withdrawal probably occurs, this has not been documented.

Course

Isopropanol is generally taken by alcoholics for want of something better and, once alcohol is available, its use is abandoned.

Etiology

The mechanism whereby isopropanol produces intoxication is probably similar to that for ethanol.

Differential diagnosis

The prominent nausea, with, in some cases, hematemesis, helps to distinguish isopropanol from ethanol or methanol intoxication; furthermore, the absence of dimming of vision argues against methanol intoxication. Ethylene glycol intoxication is suggested by an absence of the odor of alcohol on the breath.

Treatment

If patients are seen within 2 hours of ingestion, gastric lavage may be performed. Hemodialysis (Freireich *et al.* 1967) should be considered in cases of severe intoxication or when the isopropanol level is over 400 mg/dL.

REFERENCES

Abraham HD. Visual phenomenology of the LSD flashback. *Arch Gen Psychiatry* 1983; **40**:884–9.

Adachi J, Mizoi Y, Fukunaga T *et al.* Degrees of alcohol intoxication in 117 hospitalized cases. *J Stud Alcohol* 1991; **52**:448–53.

Alldredge BK, Lowenstein DH, Simon RP. Seizures associated with recreational drug abuse. *Neurology* 1989; **39**:1037–9.

Allen RM, Young SJ. Phencyclidine induced psychosis. *Am J Psychiatry* 1978; **135**:1081–4.

Allentuck S, Bowman SM. The psychiatric aspects of marijuana intoxication. *Am J Psychiatry* 1942; **99**:248–50.

Altenkirch H, Mager J, Stoltenburg G *et al.* Toxic polyneuropathies after sniffing a glue thinner. *J Neurol* 1977; **214**:137–52.

Angrist B, Gershon S. The phenomenology of experimentally induced amphetamine psychosis. *Biol Psychiatry* 1970; **2**:95–107.

Ashton H. Benzodiazepine withdrawal: an unfinished story. *BMJ* 1984; **288**:1135–40.

Bach-y-Rita G, Lion JR, Climent CE *et al.* Episodic dyscontrol: a study of 130 violent patients. *Am J Psychiatry* 1971; **127**:1473–8.

Banay RS. Pathologic reaction to alcohol. I. Review of the literature and original case reports. *Q J Stud Alcohol* 1944; **4**:580–605.

Bartlett E, Hallin A, Chapman B *et al.* Selective sensitization to the psychosis-inducing effects of cocaine: a possible marker for addiction relapse vulnerability? *Neuropsychopharmacology* 1997; **16**:77–82.

Bell DS. The experimental reproduction of amphetamine psychosis. *Arch Gen Psychiatry* 1973; **29**:35–40.

Bennet IL, Cary FM, Mitchell GL *et al.* Acute methyl alcohol poisoning: a review based on experience in an outbreak of 323 cases. *Medicine* 1953; **32**:431–63.

Benowitz NL, Henningfield JE. Establishing a nicotine threshold for addiction. The implications for tobacco regulation. *N Engl J Med* 1994; **331**:123–5.

Benton ED, Calhoun FP. The ocular effects of methyl alcohol poisoning. Report of a catastrophe involving 320 persons. *Arch Ophthalmol* 1953; **36**:1677–85.

Bercel NA, Travis LE, Olinger LB *et al.* Model psychoses induced by LSD-25 in normals. I. Psychophysiological investigations, with special reference to the mechanism of the paranoid reaction. *Arch Neurol Psychiatry* 1956; **75**:588–611.

Bolla KI, McCann UD, Ricaurte GA. Memory impairment in abstinent MDMA ('Ecstasy') users. *Neurology* 1998; **51**:1532–7.

Boulenger JP, Uhde TW, Wolff EA *et al.* Increased sensitivity to caffeine in patients with panic disorder: preliminary evidence. *Arch Gen Psychiatry* 1984; **41**:1067–71.

Brady KT, Lydiard RB, Malcolm R *et al.* Cocaine-induced psychosis. *J Clin Psychiatry* 1991; **52**:509–12.

Breier A, Charney DS, Nelson JC. Seizures induced by abrupt discontinuation of alprazolam. *Am J Psychiatry* 1984; **141**:1606–7.

Brent J, McMartin K, Phillips S *et al.* Fomepizole for the treatment of methanol poisoning. *N Engl J Med* 2001; **344**:424–9.

Brogden RN, Goa KL. Flumazenil. A reappraisal of its pharmacological properties and therapeutic efficacy as a benzodiazepine antagonist. *Drugs* 1991; **42**:1061–89.

Bromberg W. Marijuana intoxication. *Am J Psychiatry* 1934; **91**:303–30.

Burke WM, Ravi NV, Dhopesh V *et al.* Prolonged presence of metabolite in urine after compulsive cocaine use. *J Clin Psychiatry* 1990; **51**:145–8.

Busto U, Sellers EM, Naranjo CA *et al.* Withdrawal reactions after long-term therapeutic use of benzodiazepines. *N Engl J Med* 1986; **315**:854–7.

Buydens-Branchey L, Brancey M, Reel-Brander C. Efficacy of buspirone in the treatment of opioid withdrawal. *J Clin Psychopharmacol* 2005; **25**:230–6.

Carroll KM, Fenton LR, Ball SA *et al.* Efficacy of disulfiram and cognitive behavior therapy in cocaine-dependent outpatients: a randomized placebo-controlled trial. *Arch Gen Psychiatry* 2004; **61**:264–72.

Challoner KR, McCarron MM, Newton EJ. Pentazocine (Talwin) intoxication: report of 57 cases. *J Emerg Med* 1990; **8**:67–74.

Charney DS, Sternberg DE, Kleber HD *et al.* The clinical use of clonidine in abrupt withdrawal from methadone: effects on blood pressure and specific signs and symptoms. *Arch Gen Psychiatry* 1981; **38**:1273–7.

Charney DS, Heninger GR, Jatlow PI. Increased anxiogenic effects of caffeine in panic disorders. *Arch Gen Psychiatry* 1985; **42**:233–43.

Chopra GS, Smith JW. Psychotic reactions following marijuana use in East Indians. *Arch Gen Psychiatry* 1974; **30**:24–7.

Choy-Kwong M, Lipton RB. Dystonia related to cocaine withdrawal: a case report and pathogenic hypothesis. *Neurology* 1989; **39**:996–7.

Clark LD, Nakashima EN. Experimental studies of marijuana. *Am J Psychiatry* 1968; **125**:379–84.

Clark LD, Hughes R, Nakashima EN. Behavioral effects of marijuana. *Arch Gen Psychiatry* 1970; **23**:193–8.

Coid J. Mania a potu: a critical review of pathological intoxication. *Psychol Med* 1979; **9**:709–19.

Covi L, Lipman RS, Pattison JH *et al.* Length of treatment with anxiolytic sedatives and response to their sudden withdrawal. *Acta Psychiatr Scand* 1973; **49**:51.

Curatolo PW, Robertson D. The health consequences of caffeine. *Ann Intern Med* 1983; **98**:641–53.

Curran FJ. The symptoms and treatment of barbiturate intoxication and psychosis. *Am J Psychiatry* 1938; **95**:73–85.

Curran FJ. Current views on the neuropsychiatric effects of barbiturates and bromides. *J Nerv Ment Dis* 1944; **100**:142–69.

Dackis CA, Kampman KM, Lynch KG *et al.* A double-blind, placebo-controlled trial of modafinil for cocaine dependence. *Neuropsychopharmacology* 2005; **30**:205–11.

Daras M, Koppel BS, Atos-Radzion E. Cocaine-induced choreoathetoid movements ('crack dancing'). *Neurology* 1994; **44**:751–2.

de Moura MC, Correla JP, Madeira F. Clinical alcohol hypoglycemia. *Ann Int Med* 1967; **66**:893–905.

Derlet RW, Rice P, Horowitz BZ *et al.* Amphetamine toxicity: experience with 127 cases. *J Emerg Med* 1989; **7**:157–61.

D'Onofrio G, Rathlev NK, Ulrich AS *et al.* Lorazepam for the prevention of recurrent seizures related to alcohol. *N Engl J Med* 1999; **340**:915–19.

Drevets WC, Gautier C, Price JC *et al.* Amphetamine-induced dopamine release in human ventral striatum correlates with euphoria. *Biol Psychiatry* 2001; **49**:81–96.

Duffy A, Millin R. Case study: withdrawal syndrome in adolescent chronic cannabis users. *J Am Acad Child Adol Psychiatry* 1996; **35**:1618–21.

Ellinwood EH. Amphetamine psychosis. I. Description of the individuals and the process. *J Nerv Ment Dis* 1967; **144**:273–83.

Ellinwood EH. Assault and homicide associated with amphetamine abuse. *Am J Psychiatry* 1971; **127**:1170–5.

Erlanson P, Fritz H, Hagstam KE *et al.* Severe methanol intoxication. *Arch Med Scand* 1965; **177**:393–408.

Evans AC, Raistrick D. Phenomenology of intoxication with toluene-based adhesives and butane gas. *Br J Psychiatry* 1987; **150**:769–73.

Ewing JA, Elliot WJ, Maio LD *et al.* You don't have to be a neuroscientist to forget everything with triazolam but it helps. *JAMA* 1988; **259**:350–2.

Fahal IH, Sallomi DF, Yaqoob M *et al.* Acute renal failure after ecstasy. *BMJ* 1992; **305**:29.

Fischman MW, Schuster CR, Resnekov L *et al.* Cardiovascular and subjective effects of intravenous cocaine administration in humans. *Arch Gen Psychiatry* 1976; **33**:983–9.

Fraser HF, Wiler A, Essig CF *et al.* Degree of physical dependence induced by secobarbital or pentobarbital. *JAMA* 1958; **166**:126–9.

Fredericks EJ, Lazor MZ. Recurrent hypoglycemia associated with acute alcoholism. *Ann Int Med* 1963; **59**:90–4.

Fredericks RK, Lefkowitz DS, Challa VR *et al.* Cerebral vasculitis associated with cocaine abuse. *Stroke* 1991; **22**:1437–9.

Freedman DX. On the use and abuse of LSD. *Arch Gen Psychiatry* 1968; **18**:330–47.

Freireich AW, Cinqu TJ, Xanthaky G *et al.* Hemodialysis for isopropanol poisoning. *N Engl J Med* 1967; **277**:699.

Frezza M, di Padova C, Pozzato G *et al.* High blood alcohol levels in women: the role of decreased gastric alcohol dehydrogenase activity and first-pass metabolism. *N Engl J Med* 1990; **322**:95–9.

Frosch WA, Robbins ES, Stern M. Untoward reactions to lysergic acid diethylamide (LSD) resulting in hospitalization. *N Engl J Med* 1965; **273**:1235–9.

Giannini AJ, Eighan MS, Loiselle RH *et al.* Comparison of haloperidol and chlorpromazine in the treatment of phencyclidine psychosis. *J Clin Pharmacol* 1984; **24**:202–4.

Glassman AH, Covey LS, Stetner F *et al.* Smoking cessation and the course of major depression: a follow-up study. *Lancet* 2001; **357**:1929–32.

Gold MS, Redmond DE, Kleber HD. Clonidine blocks acute opiate withdrawal symptoms. *Lancet* 1978; **2**:599.

Goldings AS, Stewart RM. Organic lead encephalopathy: behavioral change and movement disorder following gasoline inhalation. *J Clin Psychiatry* 1982; **43**:70–2.

Gonzales D, Rennard ST, Nides M *et al.* Varenicline, an alpha4beta2 nicotinic acetylcholine receptor partial agonist, vs. sustained-release bupropion and placebo for smoking cessation: a randomized controlled trial. *JAMA* 2006; **296**:47–55.

Gonzalez D, Desai R, Sofuoglu M *et al.* Clinical efficacy of gabapentin versus tiagabine for reducing cocaine use among cocaine dependent methadone-treated patients. *Drug Alcohol Depend* 2007; **87**:1–9.

Goodwin DW. Two species of alcoholic 'blackout.' *Am J Psychiatry* 1971; **127**:1665–70.

Goodwin DW, Crane JB, Guze SB. Alcoholic 'blackouts': a review and clinical study of 100 alcoholics. *Am J Psychiatry* 1969a; **126**:191–8.

Goodwin DW, Crane JB, Guze SB. Phenomenological aspects of the alcoholic 'blackout'. *Br J Psychiatry* 1969b; **115**:1033–8.

Gouzoulis-Mayfrank E, Daumann J, Tuchtenhagen F *et al.* Impaired cognitive performance in drug free users of recreational ecstasy (MDMA). *J Neurol Neurosurg Psychiatry* 2000; **68**:719–25.